W R Gassard, MD
2202 Quenby
Houston, TX 77005

FRACTURES

Volume 1

Volume 1

FRACTURES

edited by

Charles A. Rockwood, Jr., M.D.

Professor and Chairman, Division of Orthopaedics, The University of Texas Medical School at San Antonio, San Antonio, Texas

and

David P. Green, M.D.

Associate Professor of Orthopaedics, and Chief, Hand Surgery Service, The University of Texas Medical School at San Antonio, San Antonio, Texas

with 26 contributors

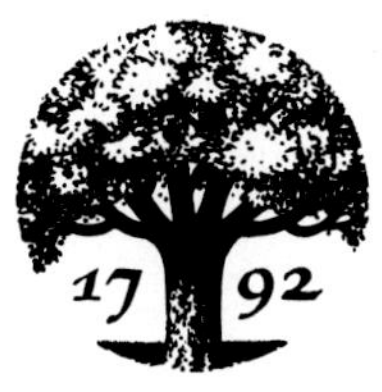

J. B. Lippincott Company

Philadelphia *Toronto*

ISBN 0-397-50339-3

Library of Congress Catalog Card Number 74-32299

Printed in the United States of America

3 5 6 4

Library of Congress Cataloging in Publication Data

Rockwood, Charles A.
Fractures.

1. Fractures. I. Green, David P., Joint author.
II. Title. [DNLM: 1. Dislocations—Fractures. WE175 R684f]
RD101.R69 617'.15 74-32299
ISBN 0-397-50339-3

To our parents and our teachers, who helped us understand

and

to our wives, Patsy and Marjorie, who understand us

Contributors

Lewis D. Anderson, M.D.
Professor of Orthopaedic Surgery and Associate Dean, University of Tennessee College of Medicine; Staff Member, Campbell Clinic, Memphis, Tennessee

Thomas D. Brower, M.D.
Professor and Chairman, Division of Orthopaedic Surgery, University of Kentucky College of Medicine, Lexington, Kentucky

D. Kay Clawson, M.D.
Professor and Chairman, Department of Orthopaedics, University of Washington School of Medicine, Seattle, Washington

Richard L. Cruess, M.D., F.R.C.S.(C)
Professor of Surgery, McGill University; Orthopaedic Surgeon-in-Charge, Royal Victoria Hospital, and Chief Surgeon, Shriners Hospital for Crippled Children, Montreal, Quebec

James H. Dobyns, M.D.
Assistant Professor of Orthopaedic Surgery, Mayo Medical School, and Consultant in Orthopaedic Surgery and Surgery of the Hand, Mayo Clinic, Rochester, Minnesota

Jacques Dumont, M.D., F.R.C.S.(C)
Assistant Professor of Orthopaedic Surgery, McGill University; Orthopaedic Surgeon, Royal Victoria Hospital, Shriners Hospital, Queen Elizabeth Hospital, Montreal, Quebec

Richard H. Eppright, M.D.
Assistant Professor of Orthopaedics, Baylor College of Medicine; Clinical Associate Professor, The University of Texas Medical School at Houston, Houston, Texas

Charles H. Epps, Jr., M.D.
Professor and Chief, Division of Orthopaedic Surgery, Howard University College of Medicine, Washington, D.C.

C. McCollister Evarts, M.D.
Professor and Chairman, Department of Orthopaedics, University of Rochester School of Medicine and Dentistry; Orthopaedic Surgeon-in-Chief, Strong Memorial Hospital, Rochester, New York

Nicholas J. Giannestras, M.D.
Associate Clinical Professor of Surgery, Division of Orthopaedics, Department of Surgery, University of Cincinnati Medical Center; Director of Orthopaedics, Good Samaritan Hospital, and Director of the Foot Clinic, University of Cincinnati Medical Center, Cincinnati, Ohio

David P. Green, M.D.
Associate Professor of Orthopaedics, and Chief, Hand Surgery Service, The University of Texas Medical School at San Antonio, San Antonio, Texas

Charles F. Gregory, M.D.
W. B. Carrell—Scottish Rite Professor and Chairman, Division of Orthopaedic Surgery, The University of Texas Health Science Center at Dallas, Southwestern Medical School, Dallas, Texas

James W. Harkess, M.B., Ch.B.
Kosair Professor of Orthopaedics, University of Louisville School of Medicine, and Chief of Orthopaedic Surgery, Louisville General Hospital, Louisville, Kentucky

Mason Hohl, M.D.
Associate Clinical Professor/Orthopaedic Surgery, University of California at Los Angeles, School of Medicine, and Attending Physician/Orthopaedic Surgery, Veterans' Administration, Sawtelle Facility, Los Angeles, California

William J. Kane, M.D., Ph.D.
Ryerson Professor and Chairman, Department of Orthopaedic Surgery, Northwestern University Medical School, Chicago, Illinois

Herbert Kaufer, M.D.
Associate Professor of Surgery, Section of Orthopaedic Surgery, The University of Michigan Medical School, Ann Arbor, Michigan

Robert L. Larson, M.D.
Senior Clinical Instructor in Orthopaedics, University of Oregon Medical School, Portland; Director of Athletic Medicine and Orthopaedic Consultant, University of Oregon Athletic Department, Eugene, Oregon

Robert E. Leach, M.D.
Professor and Chairman, Department of Orthopaedic Surgery, Boston University Medical School, Boston, Massachusetts

Ronald L. Linscheid, M.D.
Associate Professor of Orthopaedic Surgery, Mayo Medical School, and Consultant in Orthopaedic Surgery and Surgery of the Hand, Mayo Clinic, Rochester, Minnesota

Peter J. Melcher, M.D.
Associate in Orthopaedics, University of Washington School of Medicine, Seattle, Washington

Vert Mooney, M.D.
Associate Clinical Professor of Orthopaedic Surgery, University of Southern California School of Medicine, Los Angeles, and Chief, Amputation and Problem Fracture Service, Problem Back Treatment Center, Rancho Los Amigos Hospital, Downey, California

Charles S. Neer II, M.D.
Professor of Clinical Orthopaedic Surgery, Columbia University College of Physicians and Surgeons; Attending Orthopaedic Surgeon and Chief of Fracture Service, New York Orthopaedic Hospital, Columbia-Presbyterian Medical Center, New York, New York

Charles A. Rockwood, Jr., M.D.
Professor and Chairman, Division of Orthopaedics, The University of Texas Medical School at San Antonio, San Antonio, Texas

Spencer A. Rowland, M.D.
Clinical Associate Professor of Orthopaedics, and Consultant, Hand Surgery Service, The University of Texas Medical School at San Antonio; Chief, Department of Orthopaedic Surgery, Santa Rosa Medical Center; Consultant in Hand Surgery, Brooke Army Medical Center, San Antonio, Texas

G. James Sammarco, M.D.
Assistant Clinical Professor of Surgery, Division of Orthopaedics, Department of Surgery, University of Cincinnati Medical Center, Cincinnati, Ohio

E. Shannon Stauffer, M.D.
Associate Clinical Professor of Surgery (Orthopaedics), University of Southern California School of Medicine, Los Angeles, and Director, Spinal Injuries Service, Rancho Los Amigos Hospital, Downey, California

Kaye E. Wilkins, M.D.
Assistant Professor of Orthopaedics, The University of Texas Medical School at San Antonio, San Antonio, Texas

Frank C. Wilson, M.D.
Professor and Chairman, Division of Orthopaedic Surgery, University of North Carolina School of Medicine, Chapel Hill, North Carolina

FRACTURES

Volume 1

Foreword

Drs. Rockwood and Green have embarked on a much needed project. As stated in their Preface, they intend to provide an authoritative discussion on most musculoskeletal injuries. This is, indeed, a monumental task. The old classics on fracture treatment are mostly out of print and, so, unavailable to the young orthopaedist.

In the last 15 years many major treatment advances have been made in almost every field of skeletal injury. Although the literature is replete with articles on individual injuries, nowhere is there a complete up-to-date treatise on the whole subject.

Then too, the number of orthopaedists in the country has increased dramatically in the last 15 years. These young men will, by and large, concentrate their efforts on trauma, at least in the early years of their practice. A comprehensive volume such as this will be a very welcome addition to the personal library of any orthopaedist, encompassing as it does, the whole field in a single source. Indeed, we oldsters welcome it too.

A personal word about the senior editor, Charles A. Rockwood, Jr. I have followed Charles' career through medical school, very closely through 5 years of training, and since that time during his years in the Armed Forces. He accepted the professorship of orthopaedic surgery at the University of Texas at San Antonio and has done an exemplary job in building a fine training program and developing an excellent orthopaedic department in this young school. This man has made amazing progress, and with his energy, integrity, perseverance, and his indefatigable work, he has become a potent force in orthopaedics. He has become very much involved in the education of orthopaedists, and his many contributions to the literature have added a new dimension in methods of teaching. I know that he will long be an influential member of our specialty.

I have great confidence in this book. I know it will be an accurate, complete, and authoritative source to be recommended very highly to teachers, students, and practitioners of our specialty. My congratulations to these fine young men and their many collaborators for a job well done.

Don H. O'Donoghue, M.D.
Professor Emeritus of Orthopaedic Surgery
University of Oklahoma Medical School
Oklahoma City, Oklahoma

Foreword

It is my great privilege to contribute a foreword to this excellent volume on fractures. With the steady increase in the number of accident cases seen in emergency rooms each year, the management of trauma is more important now than ever before.

The editors, Drs. Rockwood and Green, and their illustrious group of co-authors, have spent 2 years on this work. The rapid rate of growth in this field, much of it due to the expanding interest in athletic injuries, biomechanics, and the development of new systems of implants, internal fixation, and fracture bracing, have made it clear that to do this work adequately was beyond the capacity of any one person. They have produced a scholarly text that stresses a clear explanation of fundamental principles of fracture care as well as a complete discussion of the various methods of treating the given injury. Each author has set forth his preferred method of treatment, which reflects his clinical experience and expertise. This is an essential feature so often missing in a collaboration of this kind.

Among the outstanding attractions of this book are the excellent line drawings, x-ray reproductions, and the extensive bibliography.

In the preface, the editors state that there is a need for a comprehensive and up-to-date textbook on bone and joint injuries. The authors and the editors have done a superb piece of work in fulfilling that requirement. Residents, medical students, and experienced fracture surgeons will all derive benefit and valuable assistance from this book.

I congratulate all on the success of their effort.

Frank E. Stinchfield, M.D.
Professor of Orthopaedic Surgery
New York Orthopaedic Hospital
Columbia Presbyterian Medical Center
New York, New York

Preface

Orthopaedists agree on the need for a comprehensive, up-to-date reference book on fractures. Texts that once filled this role are now either out of date or unavailable. Since the most recent of those books was published—a short span of some 14 years—significant advances have been made in the recognition and management of bone and joint injuries. For example, improved methods of external and internal fixation have been devised, a more sophisticated appreciation of the ligamentous anatomy of the knee has led to improved operative repair of damaged structures, and innovative thinking in regard to the management of spine injuries has revolutionized the management of patients with spinal cord injuries.

One cannot properly discuss fractures and exclude dislocations and ligamentous injuries and, indeed, our intent has been to cover the entire range of bone and joint injuries in adults.

We recognize that much controversy exists in the treatment of musculoskeletal injuries and that there may be several "correct" methods of treating any given injury. Realizing this, our goals in this book are (1) to present the historical background, diagnosis and pathological anatomy of virtually every bone and joint injury the orthopaedist is called upon to treat; (2) to offer a thorough discussion of the various alternative methods of treating each injury, discussing, when pertinent, the relative advantages and disadvantages of each; (3) to allow each author, chosen for his recognized competence in the management of the injuries about which he is writing, to present the methods he has come to prefer; and (4) to provide a comprehensive list of references at the end of each chapter, in order to give the reader as complete a compilation as possible of valuable sources for further study. It is our hope that we have succeeded.

Charles A. Rockwood, Jr., M.D.
David P. Green, M.D.

Acknowledgments

A great many individuals have contributed generously of time and talent to this undertaking. This book is a synthesis of those labors, and we wish to express our deep appreciation to each of them:

To our 26 contributing authors, whose efforts are manifestly visible in these pages. When we started this project, we honestly wondered how these extremely busy men could find the time to accumulate the necessary data and compile the comprehensive text we were planning. Now, seeing the results of their efforts, we are still wondering where they did in fact find the time to do just that. Their dedication to this task has been admirable and remarkable, their cooperation superb, and their labors prodigious. We are deeply grateful to each of them.

To Lewis Reines, Editor of Medical Books at J. B. Lippincott Company, without whom this book would not exist. Over six years ago, he saw the need for a comprehensive book on bone and joint injuries, and he embarked on a one man crusade to see that it came about. His dogged persistence resulted in our agreeing to undertake this project, and his unbounded enthusiasm and unfailing optimism have helped to sustain us over the many months from inception to publication.

To Suzanne Boyd, our copy editor, whose difficult and unrewarding job has been to try to create some semblance of continuity and consistency throughout the book without altering the diverse writing styles of the many authors.

To J. Stuart Freeman, Jr., Editor of Medical Books at J. B. Lippincott Company, whose advice and assistance with the editing has been most helpful.

To Betty Montgomery, Coordinator of Graphic Arts here at our Health Science Center, whom we consider to be one of the most talented and efficient medical illustrators in her profession. We are grateful to her for the illustrations in our own two chapters and in those of Drs. Hohl and Larson.

To Miles Johnson, Medical Photographer at the Audie Murphy VA Hospital in San Antonio, whose skills have contributed substantially to the quality of this book. He took a large number of roentgenograms whose important features were difficult to see clearly and using the LogEtronic technique, produced optimally readable prints.

To our residents, Drs. Jimmy Adams, Will Allison, George Armstrong, Robert Boone, Jesse DeLee, and John Richards, who provided us with much raw data and historical background material for several of the chapters.

To our secretaries, Jean Jordan, Beth Fecci, Rachel Gardner, Jean McCoy, Norma Tawil, and Blanche Murphy, and to all the other secretaries not mentioned by name, who labored many evening and weekend hours typing manuscripts and gathering references.

To Colleen Mann and Anna Verstegen, who provided special help in the development and preparation of the section on shoulder dislocations.

To the staff of the University of Texas Health Science Center Library, for tracking down difficult and obscure references.

To our residents, past, present, and future, who are a constant source of stimulation and inspiration. The endless stream of questions, challenges, and new insights into old problems by residents everywhere is what changes the face of orthopaedics.

And finally—and perhaps most importantly—to our teachers, who have shown us the way. As a physician or surgeon grows and his knowledge matures, he often forgets where he acquired the many facts, concepts, and principles he has assimilated into a philosophy of practice that he comes to call his own. To those by whom we have been and continue to be taught, we are grateful.

CHARLES A. ROCKWOOD, JR., M.D.
DAVID P. GREEN, M.D.

Contents

Volume 1

Volume 2

FRACTURES
Volume 1

1 Principles of Fractures and Dislocations

James W. Harkess, M.B., Ch.B.

DESCRIPTION OF FRACTURES

Fractures may be categorized in several ways: (1) by their anatomical location (proximal, middle, or distal third of the shaft; supracondylar; subtrochanteric); (2) by the direction of the fracture line (transverse, oblique, spiral); and (3) by whether the fracture is linear or comminuted (i.e., with multiple extensions, giving rise to many small fragments). Greenstick fractures so common in children are rarely, if ever, found in adults, but occasionally, an incomplete fracture or infraction may be seen. When the shaft of a long bone is driven into its cancellous extremity it is said to be impacted. This is common in fractures of the upper humerus, but I believe the so-called impacted fracture of the femoral neck is really a misnomer for an incomplete or partial fracture.

Fractures may be open, when the overlying soft tissues have been breached, exposing the fracture to the external environment, or closed, when the skin is still intact. The archaic terms compound and simple have nothing to recommend them and should be dropped.

While most fractures occur as the result of a single episode by a force powerful enough to fracture normal bone, there are two types of fracture in which this is not so.

Pathological Fracture

A pathological fracture is one in which a bone is broken, through an area weakened by preexisting disease, by a degree of stress that would have left a normal bone intact. Osteoporosis, from whatever cause, may be a source of pathological fracture and is one of the important factors implicated in the high incidence of fractures in the aged. Although fractures through any type of lesion may reasonably be called pathological, sometimes the term is used in a rather more restricted sense to denote a fracture through a malignant lesion such as osseous metastasis or a primary tumor such as myeloma. Pentecost *et al.* have suggested the term "insufficiency fracture" for those fractures occurring in bones affected with nontumorous disease.[130]

Stress Fracture

Bone reacts to repeated loading as do other materials. On occasion, it becomes fatigued, and a crack develops, which may go on to complete fracture. These fractures are seen most frequently in military installations where recruits are undergoing rigorous training. However, they are sometimes found in ballet dancers and athletes, and no age group or occupation is immune.[46,47] Recently Baker and Frankel[10] have suggested that these fractures occur only after muscle fatigue and the absence of functioning muscles allows abnormal stress concentration with subsequent failure of the bone.

BIOMECHANICS OF FRACTURES

Biomechanics, for many people, is an inherently dry subject, but an understanding of some principles is necessary in order to treat fractures rationally. What follows constitutes a rather elementary review of the subject, which I hope will serve as an introduction for the uninitiated.

Extrinsic Factors[18,19,63,165]

Whether or not a bone fractures under stress depends on both extrinsic and intrinsic factors.

The extrinsic factors important in the production of fractures are the magnitude, duration, and direction of the forces acting on the bone as well as the rate at which the bone is loaded. For the purposes of subsequent discussion, it might be well to define some terms. A force is an action or influence, such as a push or pull, which, when applied to a free body, tends to accelerate or deform it (force = mass × acceleration). Forces, having both magnitude and direction, may be represented by vectors. A load is a force sustained by a body. If no acceleration results from the application of a load, it follows that a force of equal magnitude and opposite direction opposes it (i.e., a reaction, Newton's Third Law).

Stress may be defined as the internal resistance to deformation or the internal force generated within a substance as the result of the application of an external load. Stress is calculated by the formula $\text{Stress} = \frac{\text{Load}}{\text{Area on which the load acts}}$ and cannot be measured directly. Both stress and force may be classified as tension, compression, or shear. Tension forces attempt to pull a substance or material apart; compression does the reverse. The stresses evoked by such forces resist the lengthening or squashing; since these stresses act at right angles to the plane under consideration, they are called normal stresses. A shear stress, in contradistinction, acts in a direction parallel to the plane being considered.

Stress is force per unit area and is usually expressed as pounds per square inch (p.s.i.) or kilograms per square centimeter (kg./cm.^{2}). However, purists point out that kilograms and pounds are measurements of mass and not force, so that the rather clumsy terms "pound force" and "kilogram force" have been introduced to differentiate force from mass. To further complicate matters, other units of force have been created: dynes, poundals, Newtons, kiloponds and hectobars (see Glossary, p. 90).[38]

Strain is defined as the change in linear dimensions of a body resulting from the application of a force or a load. Tensile strain and compression strain are respectively, the increase or decrease, in length per unit of the starting length and may be expressed as inches per inch, centimeters per centimeter, or merely as a percentage of the starting length. Shear strain has been defined as the relative movement of any two points perpendicular to the line joining them expressed as a fraction of the length of that line.

Intrinsic Factors

Gaynor Evans[57] lists the properties of bone that are important in determining its susceptibility to fracture as: energy-absorbing capacity, modulus of elasticity (Young's modulus), fatigue strength, and density.

Energy Absorbing Capacity. Energy is the capacity to do work, and work is the product of a force moving through a displacement (i.e., work = force × distance). Work and energy are measured in foot pounds (ft. lbs.) or kilogram centimeters (kg. cm.).

Strain energy is the energy a body is capable of absorbing by changing its shape under the application of an external load. The more rapidly a bone is loaded, the greater will be the energy absorption prior to failure. Thus the fractures associated with slow loading are generally linear, whereas high-energy fractures usually show severe comminution. At failure an explosion of the bone takes place when rapid loading infuses enormous strain energy.

According to Frankel and Burstein,[63] the energy absorbed to produce failure of a femoral neck has been found experimentally to be 60 kg. cm. However, in falls, kinetic energy far in excess of this level is produced. This energy—if it can be dissipated by muscle action, elastic and plastic strain of the soft tissues, and other mechanisms—will save the bone from fracture. In old age, these mechanisms become progressively impaired, and this is a potent factor in the production of fractures in the elderly.

Young's Modulus and Stress-Strain Curves.[19,57,63,165] When a rubber band is stretched, once the deforming force is removed, the band will revert to its resting length, i.e., there has been a stretch deformation which is recoverable, and this is known as elastic strain. However, if greater stress is applied to the material, its power to recover may be exceeded, and it remains permanently deformed. This is known as plastic strain. Eventually, if the strain increases, a point will come when the material fails. This is known as the break point. If stress and strain are plotted on a graph, a curve results (Fig. 1-1).

It can be seen that the first portion of the curve to point A is linear. The strain increases proportionately to the stress. After point A, the strain becomes relatively greater than the stress producing it. Point A is known as the yield point, or limit of proportionality. From O to A is the elastic region of the stress-strain curve, and its gradient, known as the modulus of elasticity or Young's modulus, is the ratio of unit stress to unit strain. It is, therefore, a measure of the stiffness or rigidity of a material.

Between A and B it can be seen that smaller increments of stress produce greater increments of strain until, from point B onward, strain increases without any further increase in the magnitude of the stress. Point B represents the ultimate tensile strength (UTS), which is the maximum stress a material can tolerate before fracturing.

The point C represents the break point or breaking strain of the material, and the portion of the curve from A to C represents the range of plastic deformity or the range of strain from which there is no recovery (i.e., where the material remains permanently deformed). Point B is also known as the ductility of the material, the amount of strain which the material withstands before failure. The concept of the stress-strain curve is important not only from the point of view of bone and fracture, but it is also helpful in assessing the desirability of metals for use in implants.

Fatigue Strength. When a material is subjected to repeated or cyclical stresses, the material may fail, even though the magnitude of these individual stresses is much lower than the ultimate tensile strength of the material. This is known as fatigue failure. After each repetition of the loading,

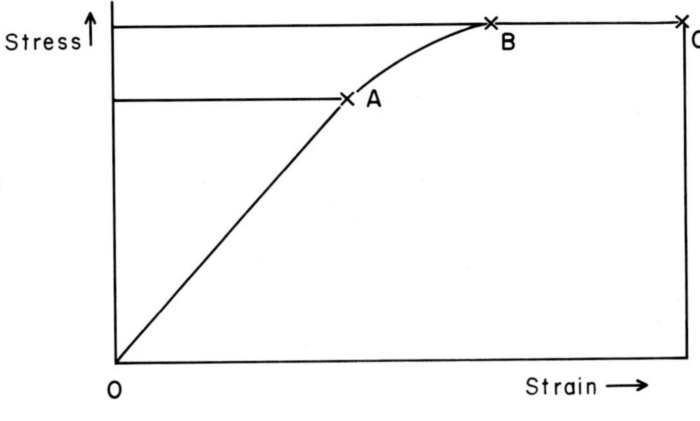

Fig. 1-1. This is an imaginary stress-strain curve. A is the yield point, or limit of proportionality; B, the ultimate tensile strength; and C, the break point.

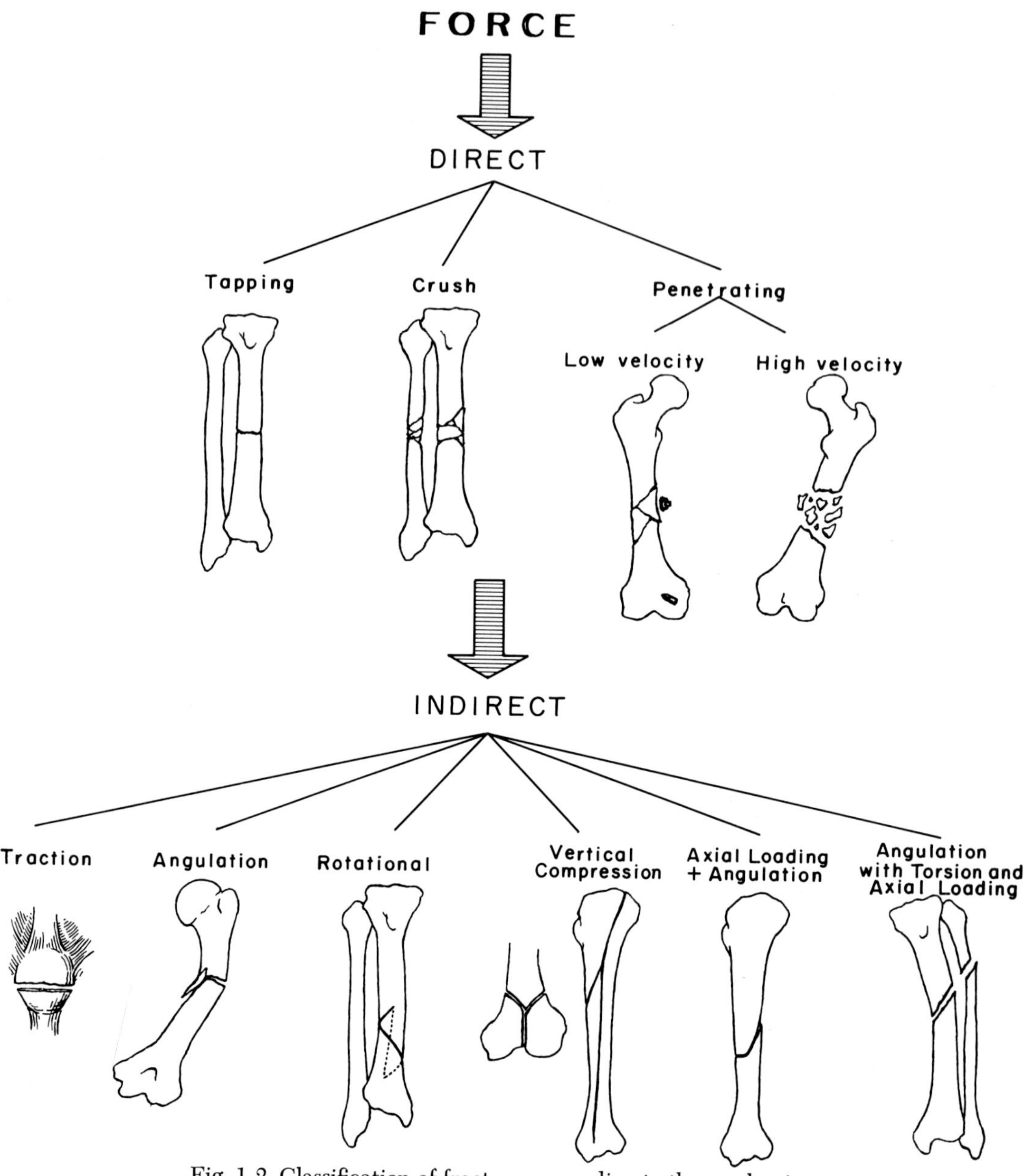

Fig. 1-2. Classification of fractures according to the mechanism.

some strain energy is retained in the material until the cumulative effect exceeds the material's capacity and failure results. The fatigue strength of a material may be illustrated by plotting the stress range against the number of cycles necessary to produce failure. From this curve the fatigue limit and endurance limits can be read. There are materials that will never undergo fatigue failure, no matter how many cycles they undergo, provided that the level of stress never rises above a critical level.

Density. The strength of a bone is directly related to its density (bone mass per unit volume). When bone density is reduced by osteoporosis or osteomalacia, the stresses necessary to produce fracture are much smaller.

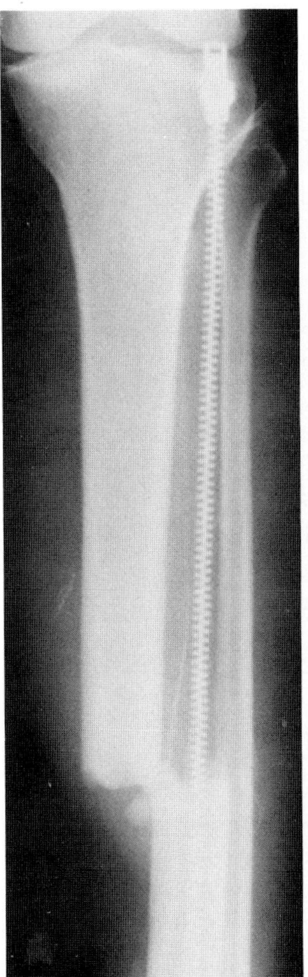

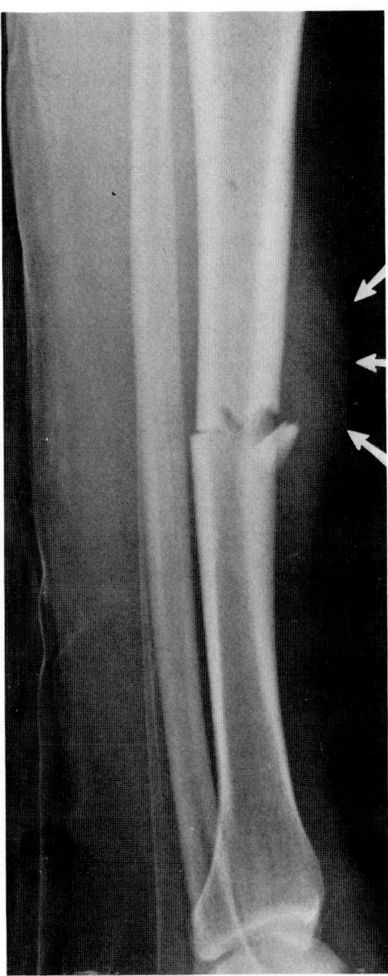

Fig. 1-3. Anteroposterior and lateral views of the left tibia, showing a typical tapping fracture. The fracture is transverse with comminution of one cortex, and the fibula is intact. Note the fracture hematoma overlying the point of impact (*arrows*).

CLASSIFICATION OF FRACTURES BY THE MECHANISM OF INJURY

Deducing the probable mechanism of injury by interpreting the clinical and radiographic features of a fracture is not merely a sterile academic exercise. Knowing how a fracture was produced has therapeutic implications. Bones fracture both from direct and indirect forces, which may be classified (Fig. 1-2).

Direct Trauma

Perkins divides fractures due to direct application of the force to the fracture site into tapping fractures, crush fractures, and penetrating fractures.[131] Essentially, they are due, respectively, to a small force acting on a small area, a large force acting on a large area, and a large force acting on a small area.

Tapping fractures occur when a force of dying momentum is applied over a linear area. The identifying features of this fracture are the transverse fracture line; and the finding that, frequently, in the arm or leg only one bone is fractured. Since most of the energy is absorbed by the bone, there is very little soft-tissue damage, although a small area of the overlying skin may be split or bruised. This fracture is frequently inflicted by kicks on the shin or blows with nightsticks or other blunt weapons (Fig. 1-3).

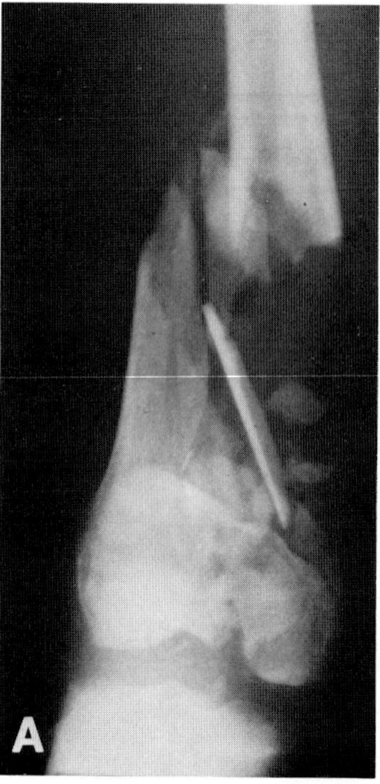

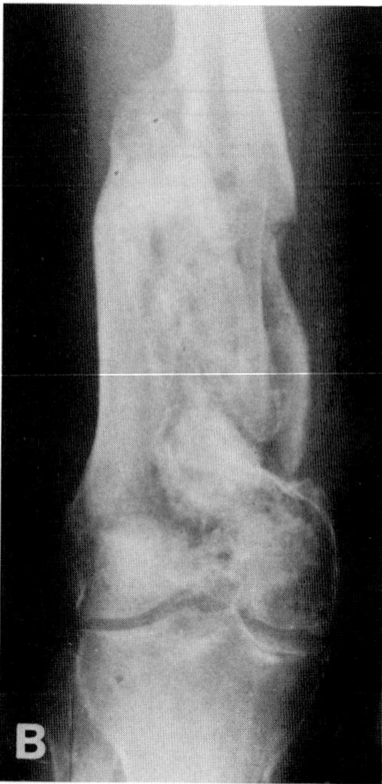

Fig. 1-4. (*A*) A crush fracture of the distal end of the right femur. This woman attempted suicide by jumping from an overpass on an interstate highway and was struck by a speeding truck. Note the gross comminution of the fracture. (*B*) The end result of this fracture after treatment by traction and active motion of the knee. After 8 months the defects in the femur have healed in by periosteal new bone.

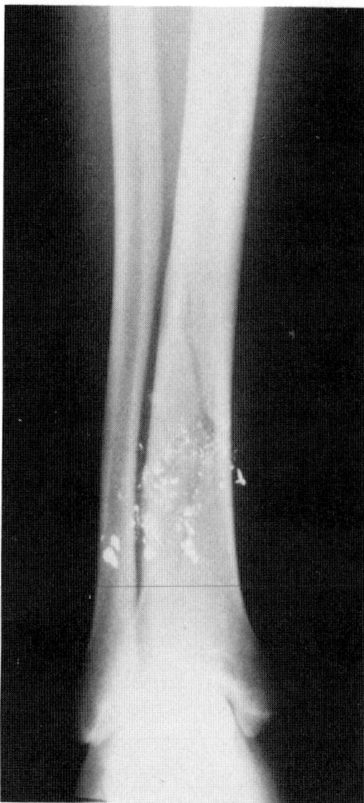

Fig. 1-5. Low-velocity gunshot wound of the left tibia. The fracture line is linear without displacement, and the bullet has disintegrated on contact with the bone.

Crush fractures may be accompanied by extensive soft-tissue damage. The bone is either extensively comminuted or broken transversely. In the forearm or leg, both bones fracture at the same level (Fig. 1-4).

Penetrating fractures are produced by projectiles, and for all intents and purposes we can call them gunshot fractures. A distinction should be made between high-velocity and low-velocity missiles. There is some contradiction in the literature as to what constitutes a high-velocity weapon. Dimond and Rich quote the *Wound Ballistics Manual* of the Office of the Surgeon General as stating that muzzle velocity greater than 2500 feet per second constitutes high velocity.[47A] DeMuth and Smith consider anything over 1800 feet per second high velocity.[45A] Regardless of the precise definition of a high-velocity missile, however, the distinction has important implications in the management of gunshot wounds, since the kinetic energy of the

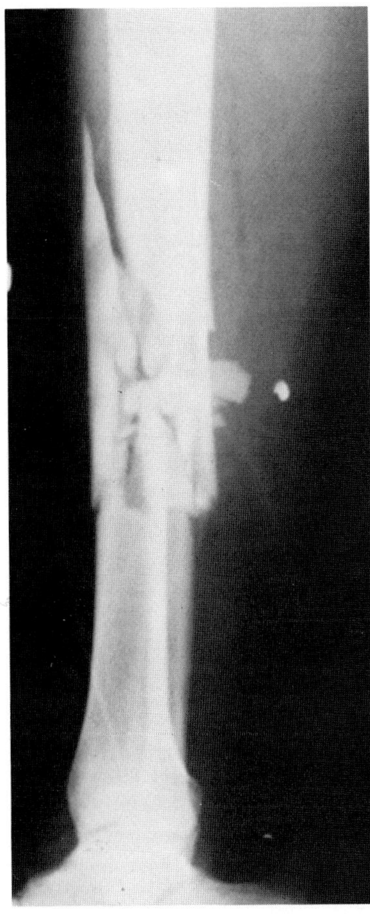

Fig. 1-6. High-velocity gunshot wound sustained during a robbery attempt. The patient was shot by police with an M-16 rifle. Note in this case the extreme comminution of the fracture fragments due to the greater energy imparted to the bone. (Compare Figs. 1-5 and 1-65.)

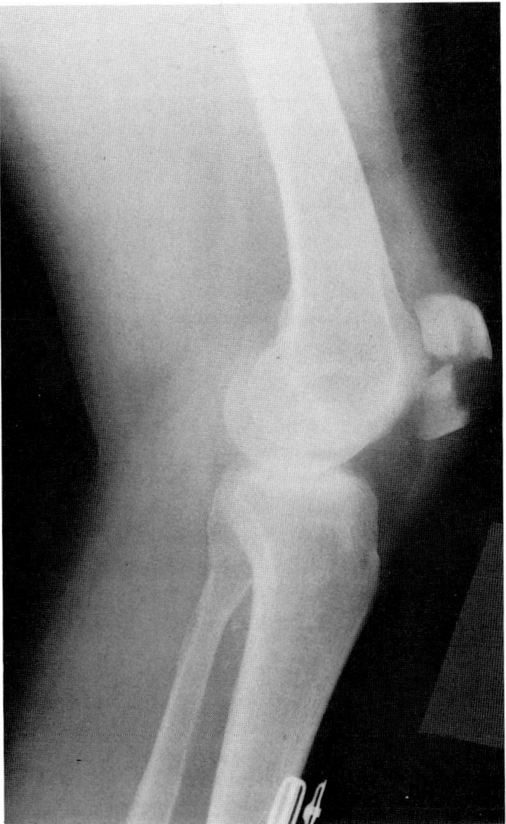

Fig. 1-7. Fractures of the patella may occur as the result of a flexion force being applied to the knee while the quadriceps is in contraction, giving rise to a separated transverse fracture.

bullet varies directly with the square of its velocity and only linearly with its mass. Low-velocity missiles produce little in the way of soft-tissue damage. They may splinter the shaft of a bone or embed themselves in cancellous ends. On the other hand, high-velocity injuries from military rifles cause extensive soft-tissue damage, and the fragments of the bone, which disintegrates on being struck, become secondary missiles (Figs. 1-5, 1-6).

Indirect Trauma

Fractures produced by a force acting at a distance from the fracture site are said to be caused by indirect trauma.

Traction or Tension Fracture. The shaft of a long bone is most unlikely to be pulled apart by a traction or tension force, but this can happen to the patella or olecranon, when the knee or elbow is forcibly flexed while the extensor muscles are contracting (Fig. 1-7). Similarly, the medial malleolus may be pulled off by the deltoid ligament in eversion and external rotation injuries of the ankle. The fracture line in tension fractures is transverse.

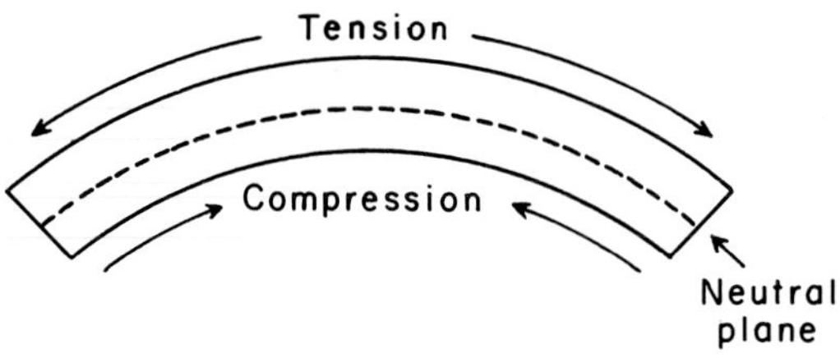

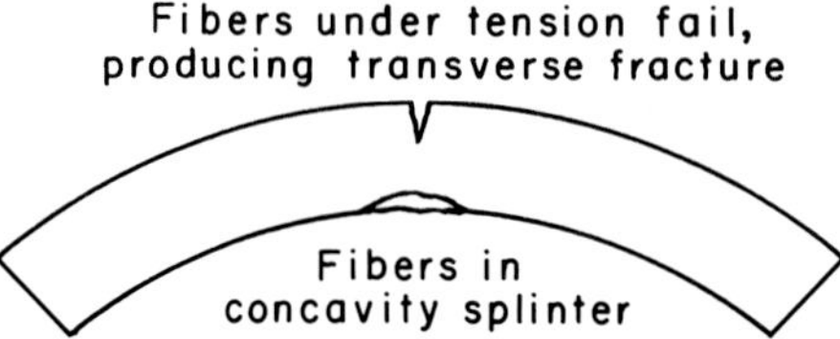

Fig. 1-8. Mechanism of an angulation fracture. If a bone is angulated, tension stresses will be present over the convexity, while compression stresses will be present in concavity. Since bone is most likely to fail in tension, the fibers over the convexity will rupture first, throwing the stress onto the fibers immediately adjacent until a transverse fracture is produced. Commonly, the bone in the concavity of the angulation will fail in compression, giving rise to some splintering of the cortex.

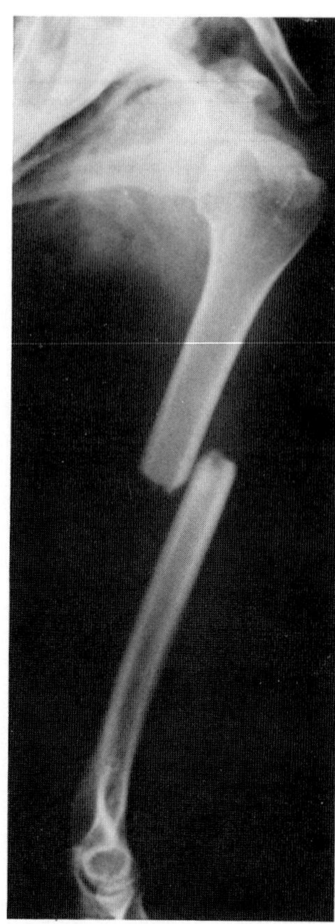

Fig. 1-9. Transverse fracture of the humerus due to an angulation force.

Angulation Fracture. If a lever is angulated (as in Fig. 1-8), the convexity is under a tension stress; the concavity is under compression; and somewhere between there is a neutral plane (under neither tension nor compression). Were this lever made of wood or bone, the fibers over the convexity would fail first, throwing more stress on the fibers immediately adjacent, which would then fail in turn. This progression gives rise to a transverse fracture, although frequently the cortex under compression splinters before the fracture is complete (Fig. 1-9).

Rotational Fracture. When a rotational stress, or torque, is applied to a stick of chalk, it fails with a spiral fracture line at 45 degrees to its long axis. The upper and lower ends of the fracture are connected by a vertical component (Figs. 1-10, 1-11, 1-16).

As Alms points out, a pure rotational stress is a very rare occurrence, and twisting forces on a bone are usually accompanied by axial loading.[3] The torque may be resolved into a normal tension stress and a tangential shear stress at 45 degrees to the long axis of the bone. Similarly, the compression stress may be resolved into a shear force in the same direction plus a normal compression stress. When the bone fractures, it fails in shear, usually at about 45 degrees to the long axis of the shaft. Theoretically, the greater the axial compression the more vertical the shear line should be, but the plane of greatest weakness is not much over 45 degrees. Alms also states that the forces of rotation are not very powerful on the lower tibia, and that rather than the shaft of the tibia failing, there is more likely to be a fracture-dislocation of the ankle. However, in old people with osteoporosis, this no longer holds true.

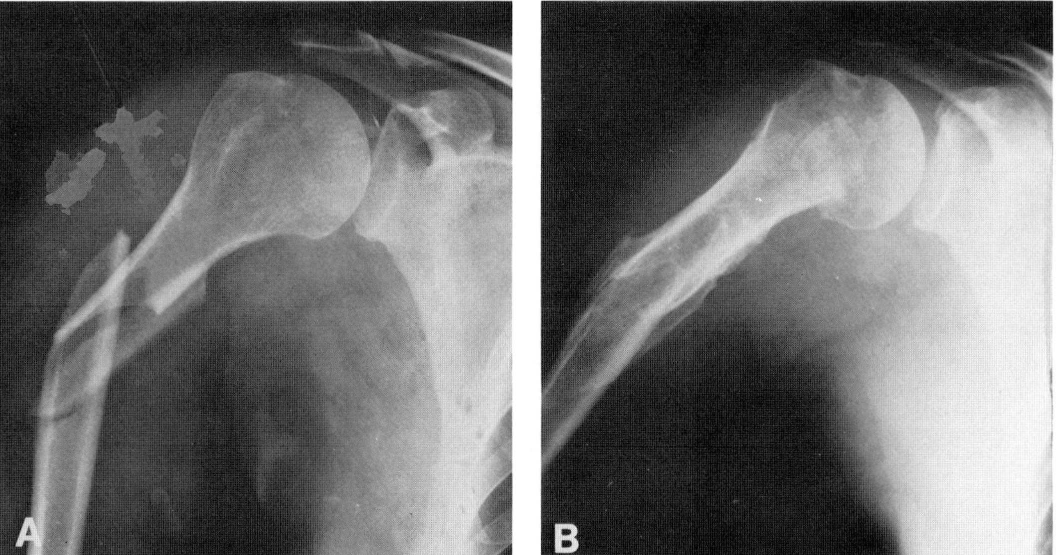

Fig. 1-10. (*A*) At the age of 67 this man sustained a spiral fracture of the left humerus with a loose butterfly fragment. (*B*) Ten years later this fracture seems to be well healed. After a fall, he sustained an impacted fracture of the humeral neck.

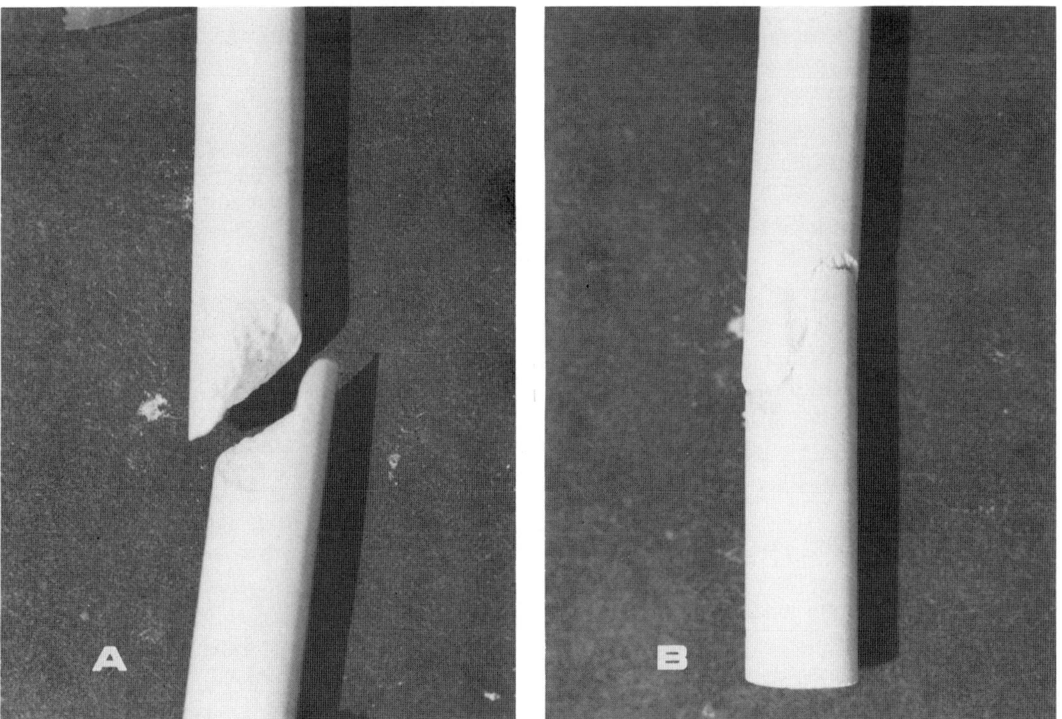

Fig. 1-11. (*A*) A model of a spiral fracture produced by torque. (*B*) The vertical fracture line joining the upper and lower extremities of the spiral fracture.

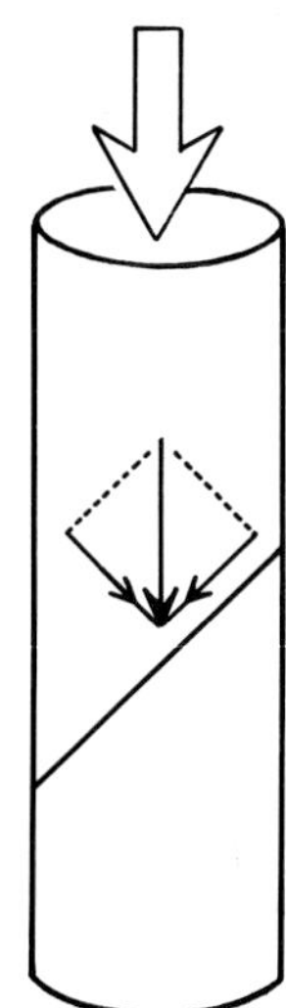

Fig. 1-12. If a column of a uniform material is vertically loaded, it will tend to fail in shear at an angle of 45 degrees to the long axis of the column. This is due to the fact that if the force is resolved into two components, as shown here, the maximum shear force will be at 45 degrees to the long axis of the column.

A spiral fracture commonly occurs in the distal third of the shaft, which is under the greatest axial compression by the calf muscles.

Brooks *et al.* disagree that spiral fractures are produced by shear forces and in their experimentally produced fractures showed that the bone failed along planes of maximum tensile stresses.[21] It is their contention that bone is weaker in tension than in shear.

Compression Fracture. If one were to take a uniform cylinder of a homogeneous material and load it axially until it failed, it would fracture along a linear plane at an angle of almost 45 degrees (Fig. 1-12). However, long bones are not uniform cylinders or columns and are only rarely fractured by a pure compression force. When this does happen, the hard shaft of the long bone is driven into the cancellous end, giving rise to the **T**- or **Y**-shaped fracture (e.g., at the lower end of the humerus or femur;[3] Fig. 1-13).

Less commonly, compression in the longitudinal axis of the tibia sometimes produces longitudinal fractures without displacement. Perkins has christened these "teacup fractures," comparing them to a cracked cup which does not break and is still usable[132] (Fig. 1-14A). These fractures do not become displaced, need no treatment, and always heal.

Fractures Due to Angulation and Axial Compression. Fractures are usually produced by a combination of forces rather than a single one. In his analysis of fracture mechanics, Alms states that when a beam is loaded axially with a force insufficient to cause failure and then angulated, this will result in the compressive force being diminished on the convex side of the beam and increased on the concave.[3] As a result, failure might start by shearing at an angle of 45 degrees where the bone is under compression; or alternatively, the failure may start at right angles to the shaft, owing to tension stress over the convexity. In either case, the resultant fracture line is curved, consisting of an oblique component due to compression and a transverse component due to angulation (Fig. 1-14B). The magnitude of each will be proportional to the size of the respective force. Frequently, the fragment of bone bearing the oblique surface is sheared off, forming a butterfly fragment.

Fractures Due to Angulation Rotation.[3] The result of combined angulation and rotation is the equivalent of an angulation about an oblique axis and gives rise to an oblique fracture. If the shaft of a long bone is also loaded axially, then the tendency to fracture is increased with a shear force at 45 degrees to the long axis (Fig. 1-15).

This type of fracture is sometimes confused with spiral fractures. Perkins makes the statement that the broken ends of a spiral fracture are "long and sharp and pointed like pen nibs" (Fig. 1-16C); whereas in oblique fractures they are "short, blunted and rounded like a garden

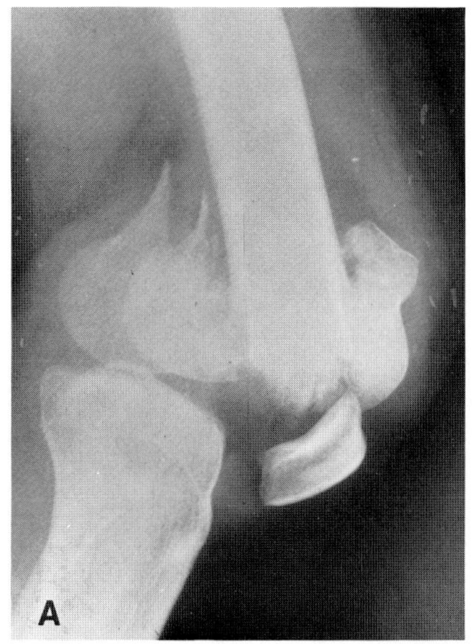

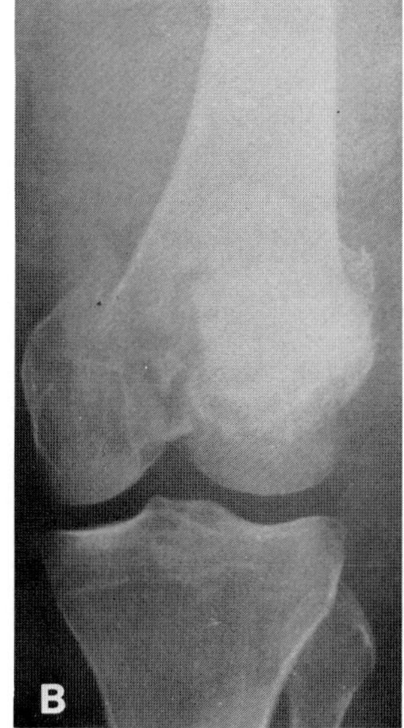

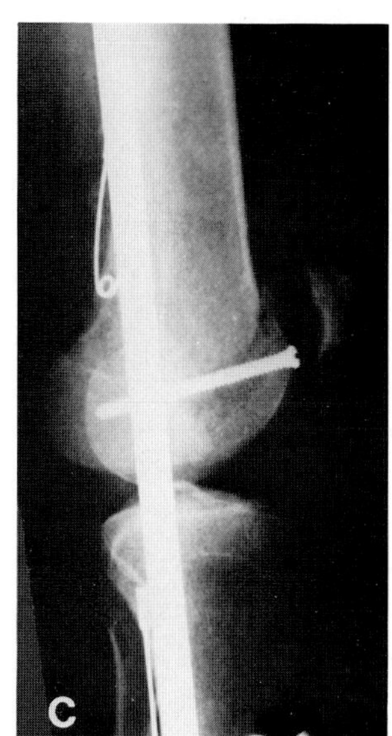

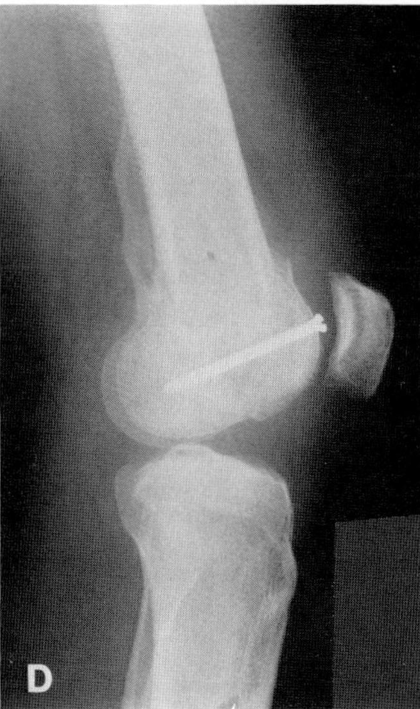

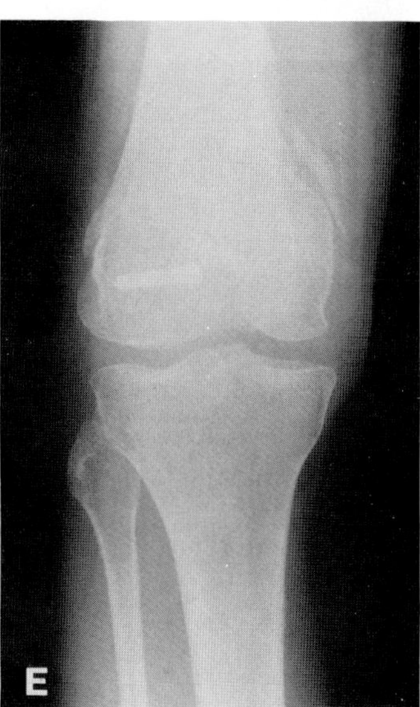

Fig. 1-13. (*A*, *B*) Compression fracture of the lower end of the femur where the femoral shaft has been driven through the condyles, giving rise to a supracondylar **T** fracture plus a vertical fracture of the lateral femoral condyle. (*C*) Open reduction was carried out with internal fixation of the lateral condyle by a screw. (*D*, *E*) Long-term follow-up showing healing of the fracture. This patient has a full range of motion of the knee in spite of a defect in the lateral femoral condyle.

trowel."[132] Charnley notes that, "if truly spiral it will be impossible for a clear gap to be seen through the fracture by any orientation of the radiograph."[33]

CLINICAL FEATURES OF FRACTURES

In the majority of fractures, the diagnosis is self-evident, but the following signs and symptoms, alone or in combination, should alert the surgeon to the possibility of a fracture.

Pain and Tenderness

All fractures give rise to pain in neurologically intact individuals, although the intensity may vary considerably. Minor compression fractures of the vertebrae, for example, often go untreated because the

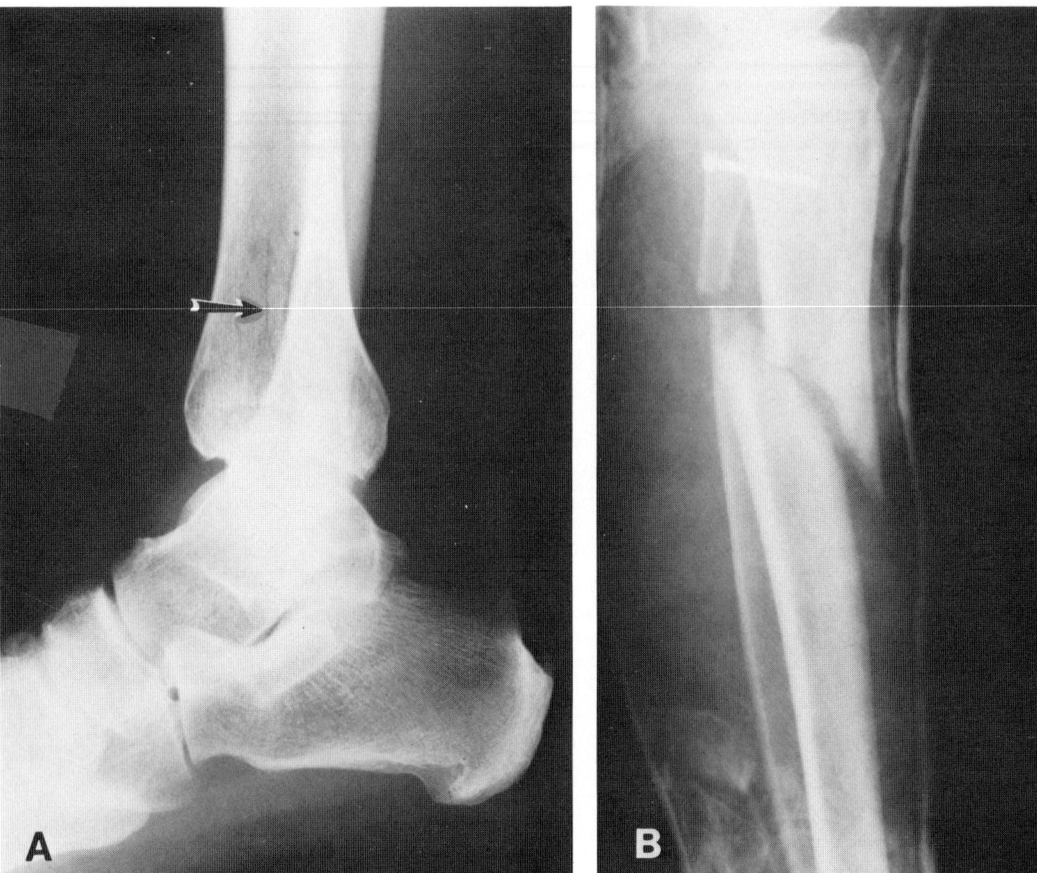

Fig. 1-14. (*A*) This 45-year-old man fell from a chair and landed heavily on his foot. Pain developed in his distal tibia and ankle. He has vertical fracture lines traversing the articular surfaces of the joint, but without displacement. This is a typical "teacup fracture," as described by Perkins. (*B*) This patient was riding a motorcycle and sustained this fracture in a collision when his foot struck the ground. The fracture has both oblique and transverse elements, due to a combination of vertical compression and angulation. The head of the fibula was also dislocated, and resection of the fibular shaft was necessary to reduce the dislocation and relieve the tension on the common peroneal nerve. The tibial fracture became very unstable and required stabilization by a plate.

pain is not severe enough for the patient to seek medical advice. On the other hand, pain and tenderness may be the only evidence of fracture (e.g., a fractured scaphoid and fatigue fractures; Fig. 1-17).

In an examination of the injured patient, gentle palpation will generally confirm the presence of tenderness, and once this has been established, there is little point in reconfirming the observation at the expense of the patient's discomfort.

Loss of Function

Function is lost due to pain and the loss of a lever arm in most fractures, but not all. In incomplete fractures of the femoral neck, it is not uncommon for the patient to continue to walk or even ride a bicycle.

Deformity

The hemorrhage resulting from fracture generally gives rise to perceptible swelling, and fractures commonly give rise to angu-

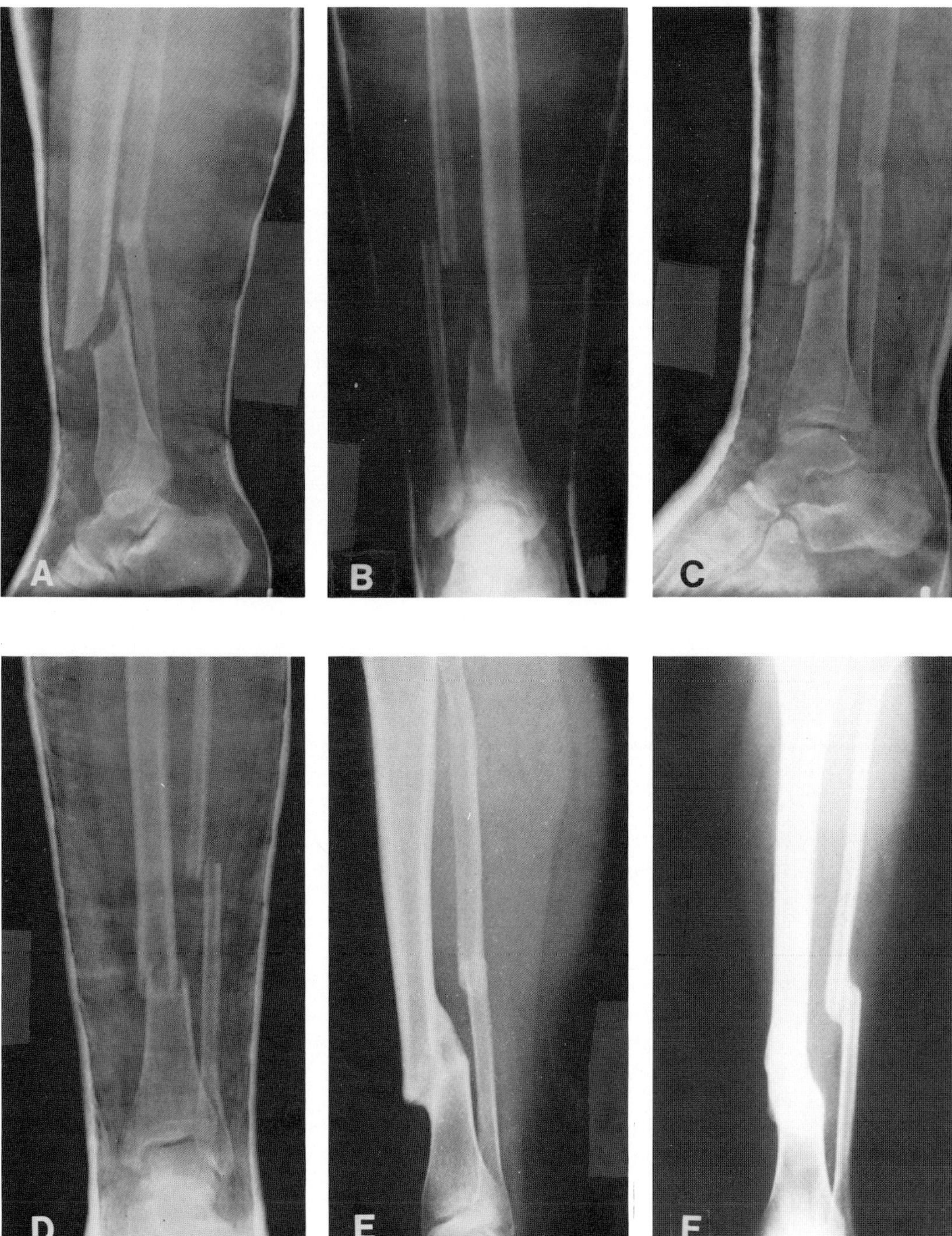

Fig. 1-15. (*A, B*) Anteroposterior and lateral views of an oblique fracture. The proximal fragment is shaped like a trowel. This reduction, obtained by a tyro, is inadequate. Note the large air space at the upper end of the tibia where the cast has lost contact with the tibia. (*C, D*) After remanipulation and the application of three-point fixation, the proximal and distal fragments are parallel in both planes, and there is little or no shortening. (*E, F*) The fracture has united by periosteal callus. In spite of the off-set, the cosmetic and functional results are excellent.

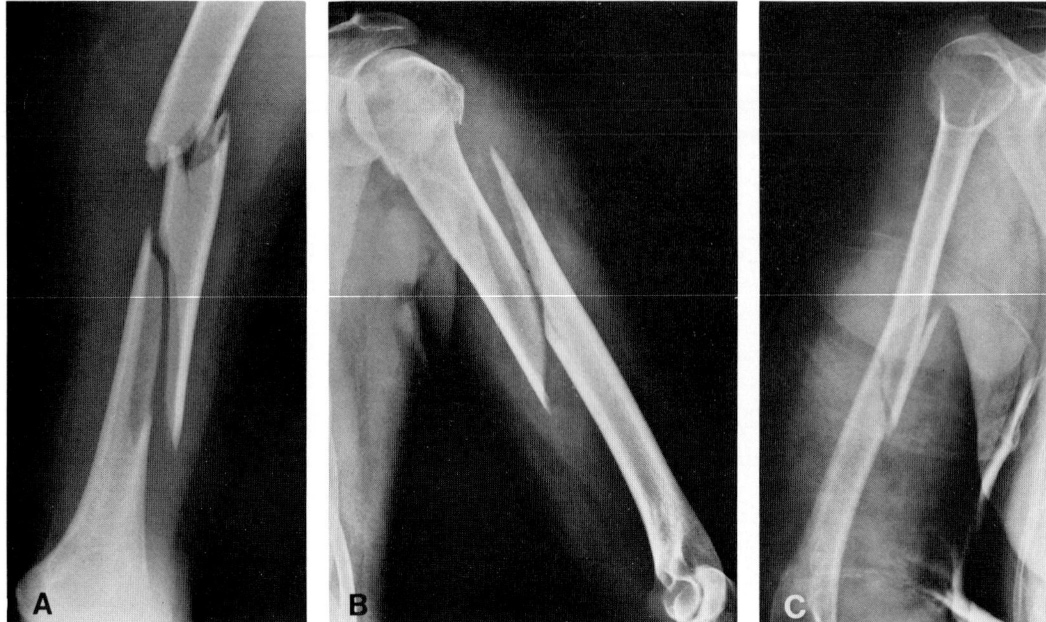

Fig. 1-16. (*A*) This girl was riding the pillion of a motorcycle that ran off the road. The segmental fracture is produced by an oblique fracture proximally and a spiral distally. (*B*) A combination of an impacted humeral neck proximally and spiral fracture distally as a result of a fall and torque to the humerus. (*C*) Spiral fracture of the humerus with butterfly fragment. Note the sharp ends of the fracture fragments "like pen-nibs" which, according to Perkins, characterize spiral fractures.

lation or rotational deformities and, especially where there is marked muscle spasm, shortening.

Attitude

The attitude of patients is sometimes diagnostic. The patient with a fractured clavicle generally supports the affected upper extremity with the opposite hand and rotates his head to the side of the fracture. When a patient sits up from the supine position holding his head with his hands, a fracture of the odontoid is very probably the cause.

Abnormal Mobility and Crepitus

When motion is possible in the middle of a long bone, there can be little doubt that it is fractured. Such motion may also provoke crepitus, the transmitted grating sensation of bone fragments rubbing on each other. Since eliciting these signs is painful to the patient and potentially dangerous, they should never be sought deliberately.

Neurovascular Injury

No examination for suspected fracture is complete without careful evaluation of peripheral nerve function and vascularity.

Roentgenographic Examination

Ultimately, the proof of the pudding is the roentgenographic demonstration of fracture. There are pitfalls to avoid in this regard.[132] Fractures will be missed if the proper views are not requested. The roentgenograms should include the joints at each end of the bone. Technically poor films should not be accepted. Fractures of the carpal bones may not show immediately or if the proper view has not been

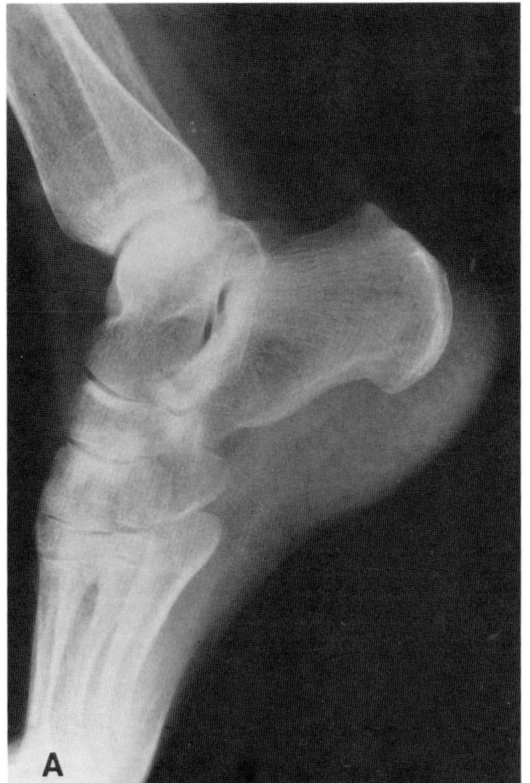

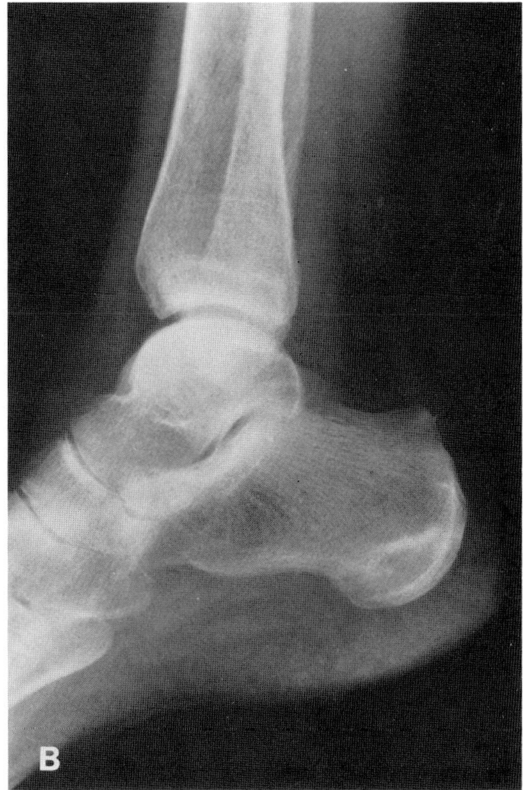

Fig. 1-17. (*A*) This lady complained of severe pain in her heel, but on the original roentgenogram there is no evidence of fracture. (*B*) Films of the foot taken 1 month later show a linear density of endosteal callus in the posterior tuberosity of the os calcis, indicating a healing fatigue fracture.

taken, and stress fractures may not be evident until some considerable time after the onset of pain (Fig. 1-17).

Fractures of the axial skeleton are the most likely to be missed, and cervical spine films should always be taken where patients have head injuries and are unconscious.

DISLOCATIONS

A dislocation is a complete disruption of a joint so that the articular surfaces are no longer in contact (Fig. 1-18). Subluxations are minor disruptions of joints where articular contact still remains. Perkins states that most subluxations are associated with fractures of the joint, and with this I agree[132] (Fig. 1-19).

Clinical Features of Dislocations

Pain. Like other injuries, dislocations are associated with pain which may be severe and may persist until the joint is relocated.

Loss of Normal Contour and Relationship of Bony Joints. In anterior dislocation of the shoulder, the flattening of the deltoid and the loss of the greater tuberosity as the most lateral point of the shoulder confirms the diagnosis. When the elbow is flexed 90 degrees, the epicondyles and olecranon form an equilateral triangle, and with the joint fully extended, a straight line. This is disrupted in dislocation.

Loss of Motion. In all dislocations both active and passive motion are grossly limited or impossible.

Attitude. The position in which the limb

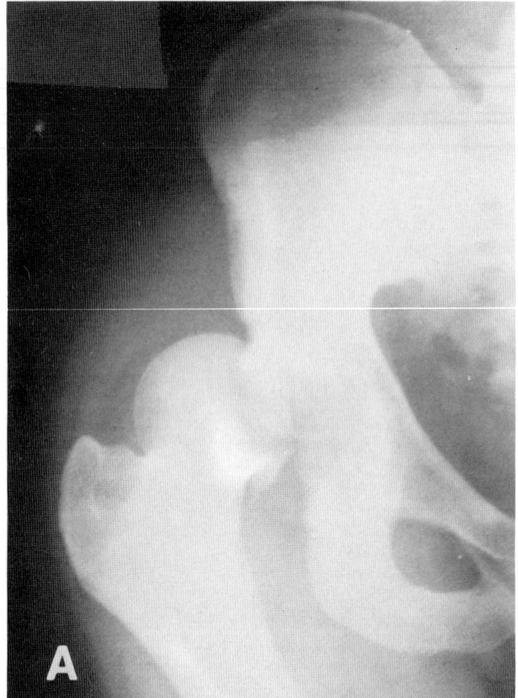

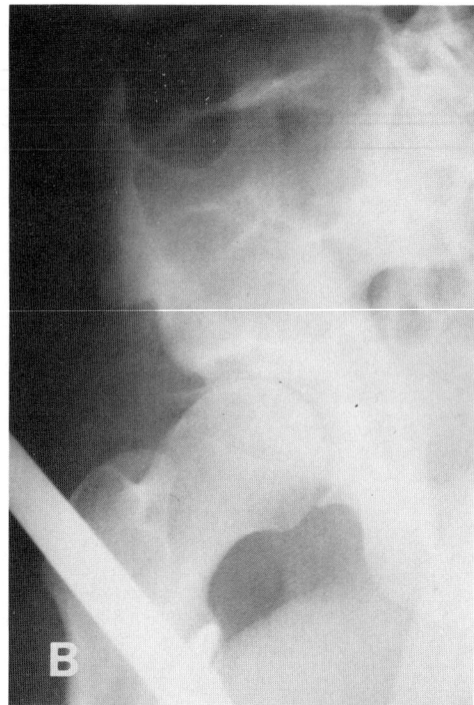

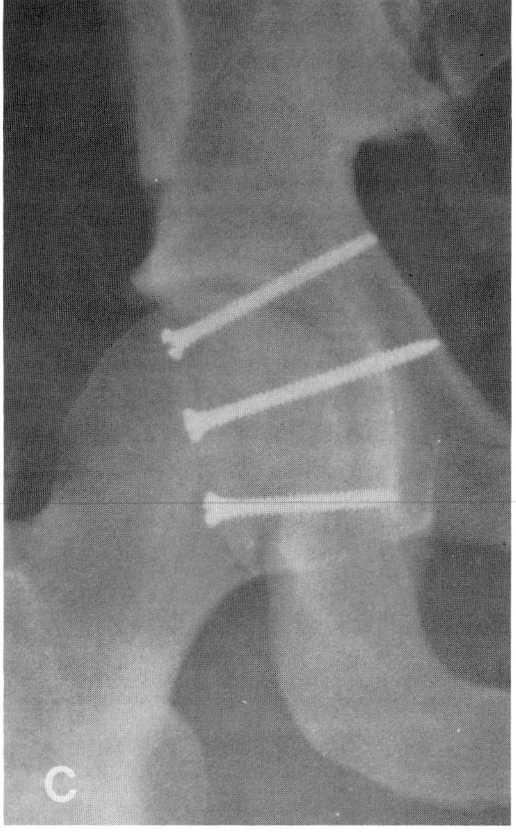

Fig. 1-18. (*A*) A classical posterior dislocation of the hip, with the hip held in the flexed, adducted, and internally rotated position. (*B*) Attempted closed reduction of the hip shows that bony fragments have been reduced into the acetabulum and this hip is unstable. (*C*) After open reduction of the hip and the internal fixation of the fragments from the posterior lip.

is held is diagnostic in dislocations of the hip. The flexed, adducted, internal rotation deformity of the posterior dislocation and the abducted, externally rotated lower extremity with apparent lengthening of an anterior dislocation are both diagnostic.

As in fractures, roentgenography is an indispensable part of the evaluation. If this is omitted, catastrophes will occur, because associated fractures will go unrecognized. Roentgenographic examination without clinical examination is equally reprehensible. A distressingly high proportion of posterior dislocations of the shoulder go unrecognized, because the limitation of motion is not elicited and the appropriate axillary or angle-up views are not taken.

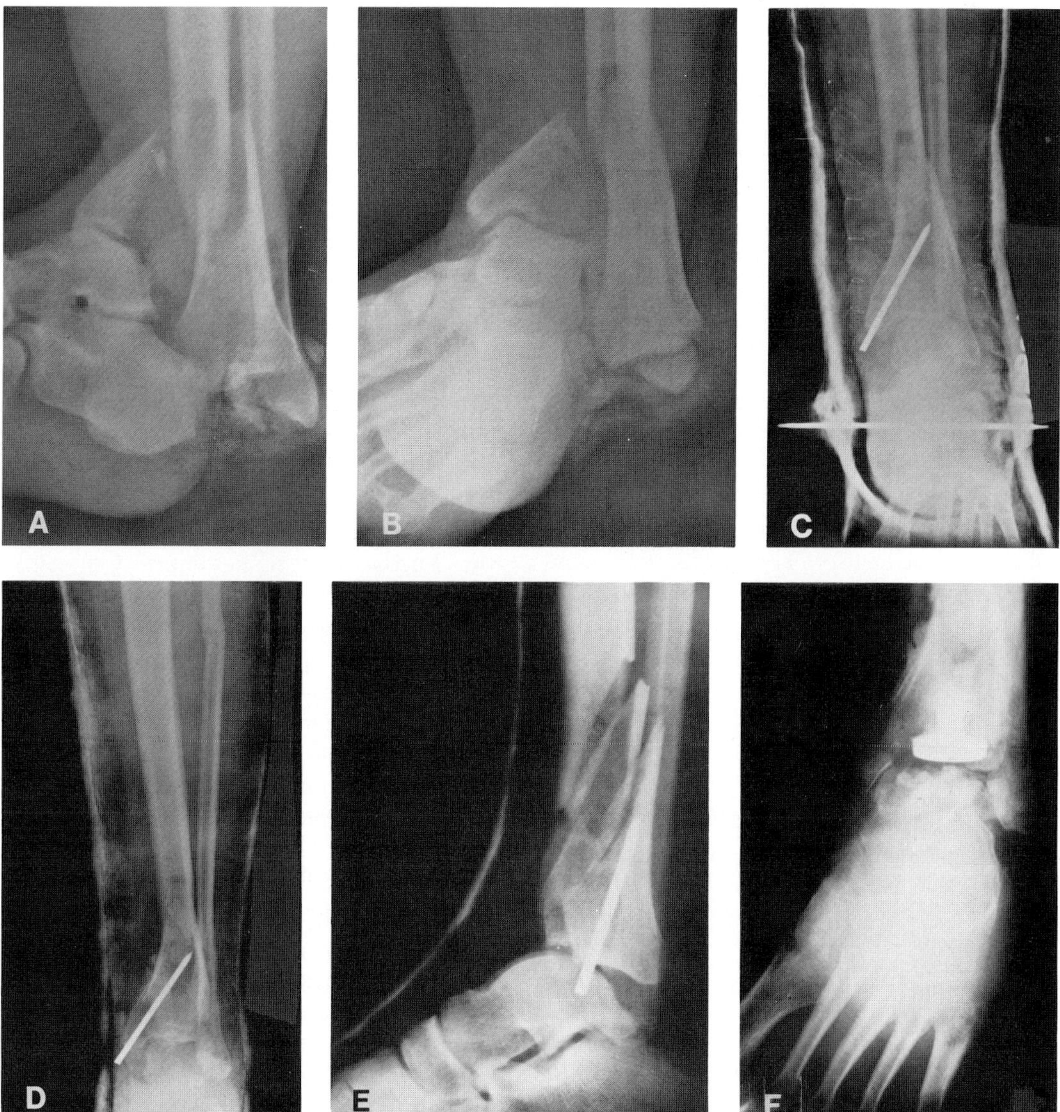

Fig. 1-19. (*A, B*) Views of the left ankle of a worker who fell 50 feet from a bosun's chair and plunged through a rooftop. He sustained a comminuted open fracture-dislocation of the ankle, and had pitch from the rooftop embedded in the distal end of his tibia and fibula. (*C*) The immediate postoperative film after debridement and reconstruction of the ankle. Due to the instability of the ankle, transfixation pins were passed through the os calcis and proximal tibia to maintain stability. (*D, E*) Four months later, while the anteroposterior view looks reasonably good, the ankle shows anterior subluxation due to the absence of the anterior lip of the tibia in spite of all efforts to keep it reduced. (*F*) Appearance of the ankle after bone grafting for nonunion and attempting to reconstruct the ankle joint by a total prosthesis.

As for fractures, a neurological examination must be done. The incidence of neurological damage is much higher with dislocations than with fractures. The sciatic nerve is often contused in posterior dislocations of the hip with the common peroneal division taking the brunt. The common peroneal nerve is also pulled asunder by varus dislocations of the knee. Shoulder dislocations are often associated with brachial plexus or axillary nerve stretching and radial head dislocations, with injury to the posterior interosseous nerve.

EMERGENCY MANAGEMENT OF FRACTURES

The treatment of fractures may be divided into three phases: emergency care, definitive treatment, and rehabilitation.

Unfortunately, physicians are rarely present to give the initial treatment at the site of the accident, and of necessity we have delegated this role to others. We cannot, however, completely abrogate our responsibility in this matter. The burden for teaching ambulance attendants, firemen, policemen, and others must rest with the medical profession.

SPLINTING

". . . Not only should the technical use (of splints) be appreciated by the men, but it should also be appreciated that all unnecessary handling of the injured part without splinting should be avoided. It cannot be too strongly emphasized that a wound which may be of moderate seriousness may become greatly increased in importance by careless or incompetent handling in the transport to or from the hospital." Joel E. Goldthwait, Lt. Col. M.C. *In* Jones, Robert (ed.): *Orthopaedic Surgery of Injuries*. London, Oxford Medical Publications. Published by the Joint Committee of Henry Frowde, Hodder, & Stoughton, 1921.

One of the most highly touted and least frequently obeyed maxims in emergency care is: Splint them where they lie. London, in his investigation of ambulance services in England states, "Little formal splintage was used; when questioned, crews often said that with a journey that was usually short they did not think that the time spent on applying splints was justifiable."[106] In the same paper, London makes the following observations: "Crews were encouraged to think in terms of comfortable support rather than splintage or immobilization . . . What was disappointing was the infrequent use of inflatable splints."

What is true in England is, I believe, equally true in the United States. Even after being seen in emergency rooms, the majority of patients are shuffled off to radiology departments sans splints. Even worse, those arriving with splints not infrequently have them removed before they are sent for roentgenographic examination. In an informal survey of five emergency rooms in Louisville, we found that less than 20 per cent of patients with fractures had been splinted prior to being seen by an orthopaedist.

Adequate splinting is desirable for the following reasons:

1. Further soft tissue injury (especially to nerves and vessels) may be averted and, most importantly, closed fractures are saved from becoming open.
2. Immobilization relieves pain.
3. Splinting may well lower the incidence of clinical fat embolism and shock.
4. Patient transportation and the taking of roentgenograms are facilitated.

Improvised Splints

The excuse should never be used that no splints were available. Almost anything rigid can be pressed into service—walking sticks, umbrellas, slats of wood—padded by almost any material that is soft. Folded newspapers or magazines make admirable splints for the arm or forearm, and when all else fails, bandaging the lower extremities together or fixing the arm to the trunk will help. For injuries of the legs and ankles a pillow pinned or bandaged around the injured limb immobilizes by its bulk.

Conventional Splints

Basswood splints, still found in first-aid kits and some hospitals, are hallowed by tradition and really fall in the category of improvised splints.

Universal arm and leg splints, rather ludicrous looking, are aluminum and prefabricated to fit the leg or upper limb.

These splints, which look like portions of discarded armor, are designed to fit everyone and so fit no one.

Cramer wire splints resemble miniature ladders with malleable metal uprights and wire rungs. They can be bent into appropriate shapes, padded, and bandaged to the extremities. They do not appreciably interfere with x-ray examinations and are most useful. This is the type of splinting advocated in *Emergency War Surgery*, the NATO handbook for the Armed Forces.[52]

Thomas splints have a long and honorable history in the emergency care of lower extremity fractures. Their introduction in World War I by Sir Robert Jones reduced the horrendous mortality from fractures of the femur from 80 to 20 per cent, and its use was continued by the British Army into World War II where, with the addition of plaster-of-paris, it became the Tobruk splint.

The Thomas splint and its modifications are still in widespread use. In most emergency services, the half ring type is used, and in fact is required ambulance equipment by National Standards. Traction is usually accomplished by a padded hitch over the shoe with a Spanish windlass, and the leg is held firmly in place with Velcro fasteners. Such special accessories for the Thomas splint are not essential. I prefer to apply the splint with triangular bandages. A narrow-fold bandage made into a clove hitch and placed over the shoe or boot without constricting the ankle, provides the traction. There are devices, such as the Millbank clip, that grasp the heel of the shoe, or spats with traction tapes which may be used. Broad-fold bandages are then tied at intervals along the splint to support the limb. The whole process takes only a few minutes.

Inflatable splints are among the most widely used emergency splints in the United States today. They consist of a double-walled polyvinyl jacket with a zip fastener which is placed around the injured limb. A valve on the outer wall then allows the jacket to be inflated, either by mouth or by a pump.

These splints have been enthusiastically endorsed as being easy to apply, comfortable, effective, and safe. They are said to control swelling and bleeding, and they are the splint of choice in fractured limbs that are burned.[153,170] I am considerably less enthusiastic than most. Frequently, I find they have been applied to the leg to splint fractures of the femur and barely reach the fracture site (see Fig. 1-55). Meanwhile the ambulance attendant or policeman feels he has splinted "the fracture," and the patient is certainly no better–and perhaps even worse–off as a result of his ministrations. Although the air splints are excellent for forearm, wrist, and ankle injuries, the feeling that they are the answer to all extremity injuries is unfounded.

Ashton has shown that these splints when inflated to a pressure of 40 mm. Hg markedly reduced blood flow in the limbs of all of 15 subjects tested, and that there was complete cessation of flow in six of them.[7] Inflation to 30 mm. Hg caused a similar but less pronounced reduction in flow which was further aggravated by elevation of the extremity, so that five out of the six subjects tested had complete cessation of flow. It would seem that when splints are inflated to pressures that are efficient, there is danger of circulatory embarrassment, and at lower pressures they are ineffective.

These splints should not be applied over clothing, since folds give high pressure points and blistering. We have also had trouble removing splints that had adhered to areas of abrasion and other exudating surfaces such as burns.

Structural Aluminum Malleable Splint (SAM).[153] If one were to enumerate the properties of the ideal first-aid splint, they might be as follows: It should be efficient, light, inexpensive, easily applied to a variety of anatomic locations, easily stored or carried, and radiolucent.

In Louisville we have been trying out a splint invented by Dr. Sam Scheinberg, which seems to have these virtues. The splint consists of a strip of soft aluminum, .02 inches thick and available in varying widths. These strips are coated with polyvinyl and can be rolled up like a bandage or stored flat in a small space, and thus are easily carried by soldiers, ski-patrols, and ambulances. When they are folded longitudinally (the "structural bend") these floppy, malleable strips change as if by magic to rigid members. The structural bend gives the splint a configuration like the slat from a venetian blind. Sugar-tong splints can be made to immobilize the forearm and humerus. A two-poster splint can be made to stabilize the cervical spine, and the femur can be splinted by an aluminum Liston splint. The excess length may either be folded on itself or easily trimmed with bandage scissors. Much to our surprise, we found that these splints could be used many times without developing fatigue fractures. They may be washed with soap and water and do not stain. Happily, they present no impediment to x-rays, and excellent roentgenograms can be obtained without removing the splint. This splint is not commercially available at the time of this writing, but it is hoped that it will be in the near future.

Open Fractures

Open fractures should be splinted exactly as closed fractures are, except that the wound should be covered as early as possible. Even if sterile dressings are unavailable, a socially clean handkerchief over the wound is better than nothing. Gratuitous interference with wounds outside the operating room is the worst kind of meddling, and external bleeding is best managed by local pressure over the wound.

DEFINITIVE TREATMENT OF FRACTURES

The definitive treatment of fractures must be delayed until the general condition of the patient has stabilized. The establishment and maintenance of an adequate airway, the treatment of chest, abdominal, and other life-threatening injuries all take precedence over the management of fractures.

The fact that large volumes of blood may be lost even in closed fractures should not be forgotten. Fractures of the femur may be associated with a blood loss of 1 to 2.5 liters; tibial fractures, with 0.5 to 1.5 liters. Fractures of the pelvis are notoriously treacherous in this regard and may result in exsanguination. Any patient who has sustained multiple fractures has lost a lot of blood and should have blood drawn immediately for cross-matching. Even if the patient appears in no great distress, it is circumspect in these cases to have a large needle or catheter in at least one vein and kept open with saline or some other physiologic solution. Open fractures, of course, are even more dangerous from this point of view; and it is good practice to estimate what the possible blood loss has been, as well as monitoring the patient's physical signs.[34,35,36,59]

The objectives of the treatment of a fracture are to have the bone heal in such a position that the function and cosmesis of the extremity is unimpaired, and to return the patient to his vocation and avocations in the shortest possible time with the least expense. Unfortunately, these objectives are sometimes incompatible, and which goals are to be stressed depends on the desires and needs of the patient.

It is customary to talk about the conservative and the operative treatment of fractures. But conservative does not mean nonoperative. The meaning of this word has become so corrupted by modern usage that this connotation should be dropped. I much prefer to talk of open and closed methods of treatment. Either may, on occasion, be radical or conservative, depending on one's point of view.

CLOSED TREATMENT

The closed treatment of fractures generally consists of some form of manipulation or "reduction" followed by the application of a device to maintain the reduction until healing has occurred.

The Reduction

The sooner the reduction of a fracture is attempted, the better, since swelling of the extremity tends to increase for 6 to 12 hours after the injury. This hemorrhage and edema in the soft tissues make them inelastic and a barrier to an adequate reduction. To wait until the swelling has subsided is often to miss the boat. On the other hand, a closed fracture is not a surgical emergency, and the life of a patient must never be jeopardized by the desire to obtain an early reduction.

Prior to embarking on the manipulative reduction, adequate radiographs must be taken to determine what the objectives of the manipulation are to be or if, indeed, a reduction is necessary. Perkins says that closed reduction is contraindicated when:

1. There is no significant displacement
2. The displacement is of little concern (e.g., humeral shaft)
3. No reduction is possible (e.g., comminuted fracture of the head and neck of humerus)
4. The reduction, if gained, cannot be held (e.g., compression fracture of the vertebral body)
5. The fracture has been produced by a traction force (e.g., displaced fracture of the patella).[132]

In order to achieve a reduction, it is usually advised (1) to apply traction in the long axis of the limb, (2) to reverse the mechanism that produced the fracture, and (3) to align the fragment that you can control with the one that you cannot.

Traction

Traction can achieve a reduction only where the fragments are connected by a soft-tissue bridge (Fig. 1-20). Indeed, no manipulative reduction can be successful without some form of soft-tissue linkage, and great care must be taken not to disrupt these soft-tissue connections by ill-advised, over-strenuous manipulations. When you pull on the limb, the distal fragment guided by the soft tissue hinge falls into place.

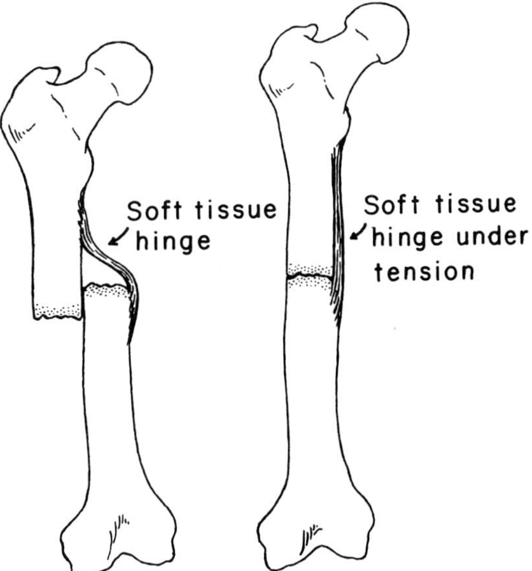

Fig. 1-20. In most fractures a soft-tissue hinge will be present between the bone ends. This hinge will lie in the concavity of the angulation in a transverse fracture, or along the vertical component of a spiral fracture. This soft-tissue hinge is the linkage that allows the fracture to be reduced, and under appropriate tension it will stabilize the fracture once it has been reduced.

Unhappily, traction by itself does not always achieve this felicitous result. Where bone fragments penetrate overlying muscles, it may be impossible to disengage the fragments, so that there is a soft-tissue obstruction to reduction. One might suspect this to be so when no sensation of crepitus is present on manipulation.

A second obstruction to reduction by traction, described by Charnley, is the presence of a large hematoma in the thigh in conjunction with a fracture of the femur. To accommodate this blood, the thigh becomes grossly swollen and tense with an increase in its transverse diameter. As a result, the elasticity of the soft tissues is

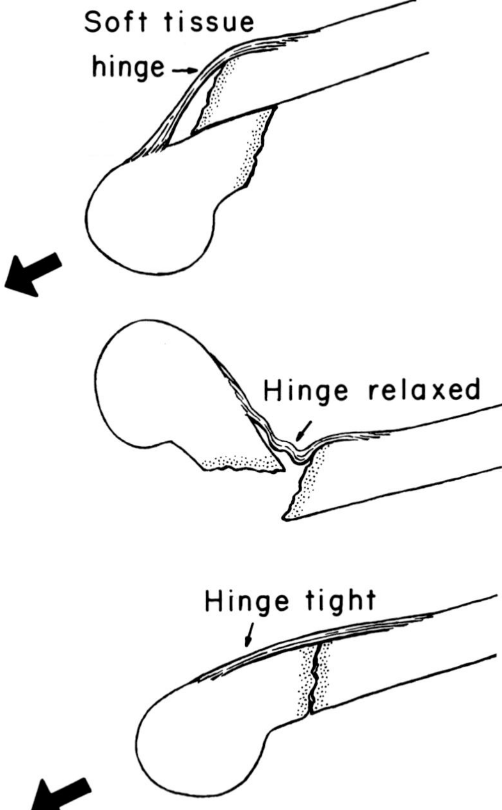

Fig. 1-21. The soft-tissue hinge may act as an obstruction to reduction by traction when the fragment ends are interlocked. Excessive traction will rupture the soft-tissue hinge, making further attempts at reduction fruitless. Under these circumstances the fracture should be angulated to relax the soft-tissue hinge, and then further traction and angulation in the opposite direction will reduce and stabilize the fracture.

grossly reduced, and the fragments cannot be pulled out to length owing to the soft tissue resistance.[33]

A third mechanism, the description of which Charnley ascribes to Beveridge Moore, is that of soft-tissue interlocking[33] (Fig. 1-21). In this circumstance, the bone ends are overlapped, and the soft-tissue hinge then acts as an obstruction to the reduction. Traction, if pursued with vigor, will rupture the hinge, making the fracture completely unstable, and will lead to overdistraction. In order to reduce such a fracture, it must be "toggled" (i.e., the angulation is increased until the bone ends disengage, after which the bone ends are latched on and the fracture is reduced by gentle traction and reversal of the angulation).

By and large, traction should be reserved for fractures that are overlapped (e.g., fractures of the femur where the pull of the quadriceps shortens the bone). It must also be remembered that unless the bone ends can be locked on and are stable, once the traction is discontinued, the shortening will recur.

Reversing the Mechanism of Injury

It seems axiomatic that if a fracture is produced by an external torque then it should be reduced by making the distal fragment retrace its steps—by twisting it internally. Similarly, angulation in one direction should be reduced by angulation in the opposite direction. An initial period of longitudinal traction may aid in fracture reduction by overcoming muscle pull and disimpacting the fracture, but the definitive reduction should be accomplished by reversing the mechanism of injury. For example, a Colles' fracture, which is produced by supination and dorsal angulation, should be reduced not by prolonged traction on the fingers but by pronating and flexing the distal fragment.

Reduction by this method depends on the presence of a soft-tissue linkage. In oblique and transverse fractures, the soft-tissue hinge is in the concavity of the angulation, and in spiral fractures, in the region of the vertical fracture line. Where there is no soft-tissue hinge, closed reduction is not feasible.

Align the Fragment That You Can Control

By and large, this advice is somewhat simplistic. Essentially, the fragment that can be controlled is the distal fragment, and one tries to line this up with the proximal fragment. The proximal fragment adopts a position dictated by the pull of the muscles attached to it. In fractures of the forearm, the key to reduction is the position of the proximal radial fragment. If the fracture is through the proximal third, the proximal fragment will be strongly supinated by the supinator and biceps; and the forearm must be manipulated accordingly. A fracture at a lower level adds the action of the pronator teres, so that the proximal fragment is now in a position midway between full supination and full pronation. Since few surgeons nowadays treat fractures of the forearm by closed reduction, this precept is only of value in children's fractures. Similarly, in the closed management of transverse subtrochanteric fractures, the proximal fragment is flexed, abducted, and externally rotated, and the distal fragment must be aligned in this manner for a successful reduction.

Immobilization

Once a satisfactory reduction has been achieved, it must then be maintained until primary union has taken place. Immobilization may be provided by a plaster-of-paris cast, continuous traction, or some form of splint.

Plaster-of-Paris Casts*

The use of splints for the maintenance of fracture reduction has been practiced from times immemorial. Albucasis immobilized fractures by bandages made stiff with egg albumin. The genius who first impregnated a dressing with dehydrated gypsum to be used in the treatment of battlefield injuries was a Flemish military surgeon named Antonius Mathysen.[113] This invention, which eventually developed into the modern plaster bandage, is second in importance only to roentgenography in the history of the treatment of fractures.

The plaster-of-paris bandage consists of a roll of muslin stiffened by dextrose or starch and impregnated with the hemihydrate of calcium sulfate. When water is added, the calcium sulfate takes up its water of crystallization ($CaSO_4 \cdot H_2O + H_2O \rightleftharpoons CaSO_4 \cdot 2H_2O$ + heat). This is an exothermic reaction, and after a few minutes, the plaster-of-paris becomes a homogenous, rock-like mass. Accelerator substances are added to the bandages to afford a spectrum of available setting rates ranging from slow to extra-fast. When greater retardation of setting time is needed, common salt may be added to the water. Setting may be accelerated by increasing the temperature of the water or by adding alum.

Methods of Applying Plaster-of-Paris Casts. Every orthopaedist has his own pet method of applying plaster-of-paris casts, but in essence, there are three schools.

The skin-tight cast was advocated by Böhler, the famous Viennese fracture surgeon. The plaster-of-paris bandage is applied directly to the skin without any intervening padding, in an effort to gain the most efficient immobilization possible. This type of cast is rarely (if ever) used now. It required a great deal of skill to apply and was fraught with the danger of pressure sores and circulatory embarrassment, and it was uncomfortable to remove because the patient's hair was incorporated into the cast.

The Bologna cast, emanating from the Rizzoli Institute, is advocated by Charnley, and in contrast to Böhler's method, generous amounts of cotton wadding are applied to the limb and compressed by the plaster bandage with "just the right amount of tension."[33] This technique is said by Charnley to be demanding, so that most people (including me) split the difference and apply a padded cast without tension. We shall call this the Third Way.

In the Third Way most people use stockinette, a tubular knitted stocking, which

* Although the correct term is plaster-of-paris cases, or casings, it does seem rather pedantic, and I shall use the incorrect but common appellation, cast.

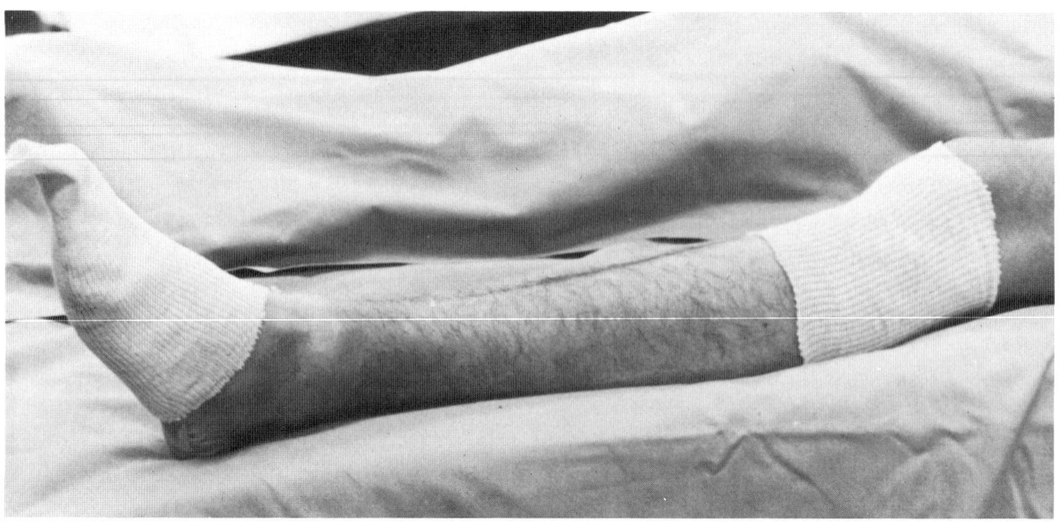

Fig. 1-22. It is necessary to use stockinette only at the upper and lower extremities of the cast. Not only is this economical, but it prevents tension of the stockinette over bony prominences which may later give rise to burning pain and even pressure sores.

stretches freely in diameter but sparingly in length. It may be applied over the entire member to be immobilized, but my preference is to cut two segments to cover the upper and lower ends of the casts (Fig. 1-22). This, I feel, is its main use. It makes the cast look tidy and pads the sharp margins. It is probably best to avoid stockinette in postoperative casts where swelling is anticipated.

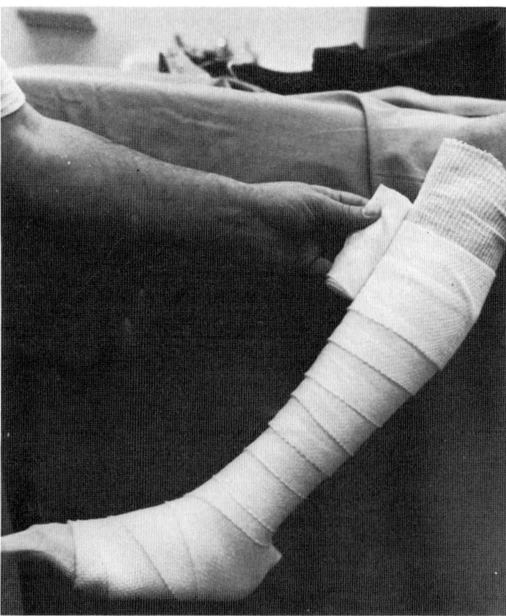

Fig. 1-23. Padding should be applied from distal to proximal, taking care to apply the padding evenly. Each turn should be overlapped by 50 per cent of the succeeding turn.

Following the stockinette, sheet wadding is applied from the distal to proximal end of the limb, as smoothly as possible. Each turn should be applied transversely, tearing the border that traverses the greater diameter of the limb so that it lies smoothly (Fig. 1-23). Various types of wadding are available; my own personal preference is for the rather soft, quilted variety that can be stretched easily. The more densely compressed forms of wadding are more likely to exert a tourniquet effect if they become wadded or displaced. The amount of wadding to be used depends on how much swelling one anticipates after the application of the cast. Too much padding reduces the efficacy of the cast, and the more padding, the more plaster is necessary. Thighs are so well padded by nature that I apply the plaster directly on the stockinette without any padding. It is circumspect to apply a little extra padding to the heel and malleoli. If felt pads are to be used, they must be applied as the most superficial layer, immediately under the plaster. Since they adhere to the plaster, they do not produce an embarrassing pressure sore by getting displaced.

The rolled plaster bandage must be thoroughly immersed in water until air bubbles stop rising. At this point the bandage is saturated with water and should be held with one end in each hand and gently and lovingly squeezed. It never should be wrung out like a wash cloth, since this tends to leave the plaster-of-paris in the pail rather than in the bandage. It is also prudent to unwrap the first 2 or 3 inches before wetting so that the tail of the bandage can be located easily. Use the largest bandage you can handle—8-inch for the thigh, 6-inch for the leg, 4-inch for the hand and forearm. When the plaster is applied with the bandage held vertically, the central core tends to drop out. This can be prevented by pushing it back at intervals with the left thumb.

The plaster bandage should be rolled onto the limb in the same direction as the wadding. At all times the bandage should be in contact with the limb; if it is rolled on by the fingertips, it can never be too tight. Each turn of the bandage should overlap the preceding turn by half and the bandage should always be moving (Fig. 1-24). It is permissible to put two turns in the same place only at the upper and lower extremities of the cast. In this way the cast is uniformly thick throughout its length. Areas of uneven thickness act as stress risers, and the cast tends to break at the juncture between thick and thin.

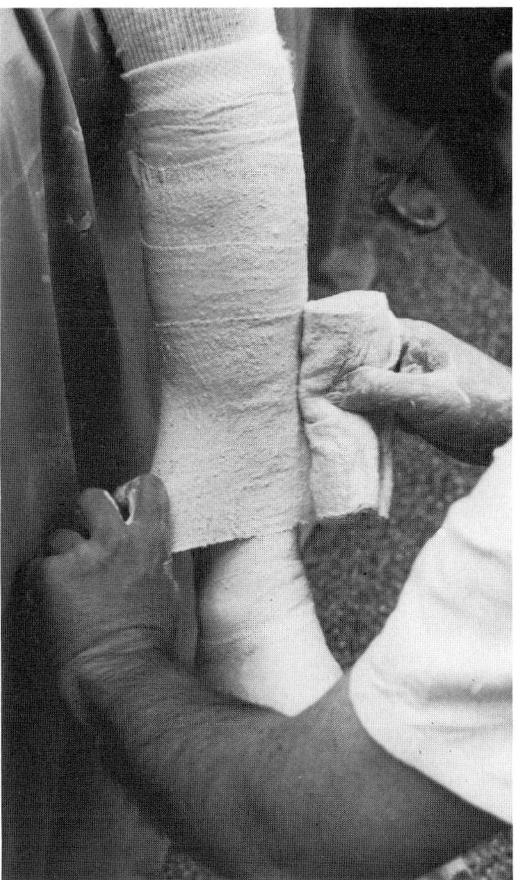

Fig. 1-24. The plaster-of-paris bandage should be applied in the same direction as the wadding. The roll should be applied with the fingertips and must never be removed from the extremity. In order to make the bandage conform to the varying circumferences of the arm or leg, tucks should be taken in it with the left hand.

The bandage should always be laid on transversely, and tucks are taken in the lower border by the left hand to accommodate for the changing circumference of the limb. Each turn is smoothed by the left thenar eminence as it is laid down, and the bandage is smoothed by the palms of both hands after it is applied, so that every layer is melded with the others into a homogenous whole. Where this is not done, the cast is lamellated and much weaker than it should be. A plaster bandage should never be reversed, as may be done when applying a gauze bandage. If one does so, the bandage runs against the grain and cannot be applied properly.

A cast should always be made too long and then be trimmed to size with a sharp knife or cast saw. I prefer a scalpel, and it should be held with the four fingers and the palm while the thumb is braced against

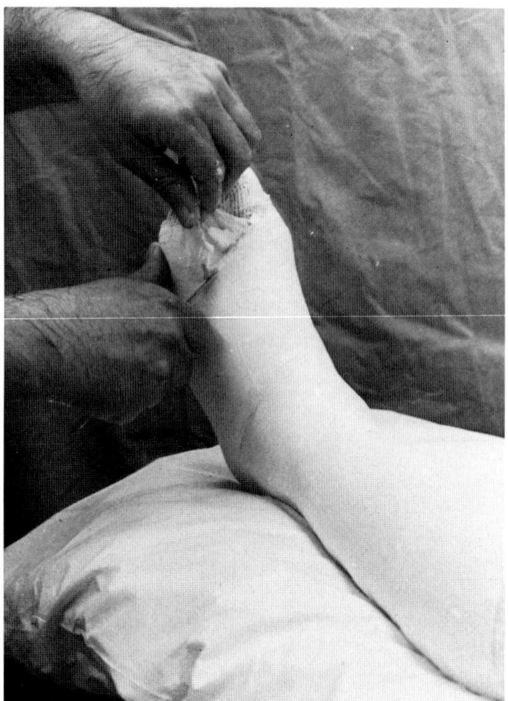

Fig. 1-25. In trimming the extremities of plaster-of-paris casts, a good method is to brace the thumb against the plaster and hold a sharp knife in the remaining four fingers. Tension is applied to the plaster to be removed by the other hand as the knife cuts.

the cast to prevent slipping. The plaster to be removed is held in the left hand and pulled against the scalpel blade (Fig. 1-25). After trimming, the stockinette is folded over the cut edge and fixed by a turn of bandage or by a plaster strip (Fig. 1-26).

In reducing fractures, it is often necessary to manipulate the fracture through the wet cast for the final adjustment. This requires the cast to be applied as quickly and as dexterously as possible. These manipulations must be done with the palms and thenar eminences (Fig. 1-27). On no account must the cast be indented by a fingertip, as this will almost certainly produce a pressure sore in the underlying skin. In molding the cast to achieve a three-point fixation, one hand must exert pressure over the fracture site on the side opposite the soft-tissue bridge, while the other hand gently massages the distal fragment in the proper direction to close the gap. As Charnley advises, it takes a curved cast to produce a straight bone (Fig. 1-28).

Upper Extremity Casts. Casts on the upper extremity may extend above the elbow or be limited to the forearm and hand. In either case, the cast should be trimmed along the line of the knuckles on the dorsum and obliquely across the proximal flexion crease of the palm on the volar side to allow unrestricted motion of the fingers. A hole should be cut out around the thumb just large enough to allow it unrestricted motion. The edges of this thumb hole must be carefully everted, so that the sharp edge does not cut the skin (Fig. 1-44). Occasionally, the thumb may be included in the cast. Some surgeons prefer to treat fractured carpal scaphoids with the thumb immobilized.

Lower Extremity Casts. Long leg casts may be applied with the knee flexed or extended; but if weight bearing is to be allowed, the knee should be neutral or in 5 degrees of flexion. The cast should be trimmed in line with the metatarsal heads on the plantar aspect and at the base of the toes dorsally. The fifth toe must be entirely free; this is a common site for a plaster sore (Fig. 1-26). Perkins feels that it is most important not to immobilize the forefoot in varus, and he leaves the metatarsal heads free to bear weight. If a toe plate is used, the MP joints must not be held in hyperextension. In fractures of the lower third of the tibia, dorsiflexion of the foot frequently causes angulation of the fracture. It is quite permissible under these circumstances to immobilize the foot in plantar flexion, although in fractures of the ankle this would be proscribed. When the foot is immobilized in plantar flexion and a walking heel is applied, the contralateral shoe should be raised to equalize leg lengths.

Böhler walking irons have apparently be-

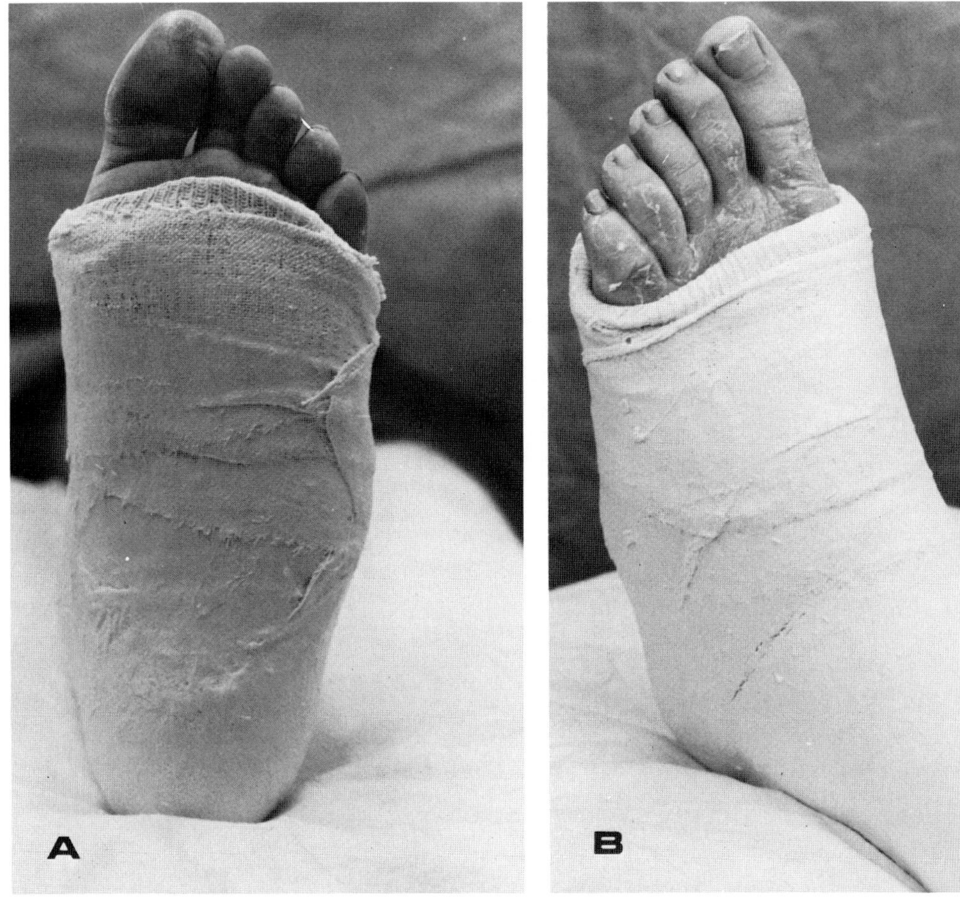

Fig. 1-26. (*A, B*) Casts should be trimmed so that the fingers and toes are free to move. The stockinette is then folded over the cut edges of the cast and anchored with a plaster-of-paris strip. Care should always be taken to make sure that the lateral border of the cast does not impinge on the fifth toe.

come passé in the United States, having been replaced by a bewildering variety of rubber walking heels. The sole of the cast should be reinforced by several layers of splints when these are applied, and care should be taken not to place them too far anteriorly since this will tend to crack the cast at the ankle (Fig. 1-29). Weight bearing should be proscribed for 48 hours.

I much prefer commercially available plaster boots to a walking heel. The patient walks with a much better gait and can take the boot off at bedtime.

Many orthopaedists reinforce their casts by applying splints to the posterior aspect of the cast. This adds weight without adding much strength. The same amount of plaster applied anteriorly as a fin strengthens the cast immeasurably, making fracture of the cast at the ankle virtually impossible (Fig. 1-30).

Patellar-Tendon-Bearing Casts[149] were devised by Sarmiento to immobilize fractures of the tibial shaft and at the same time allow the knee to bend. I have tended to use an above-knee cast, as recommended by Dehne, for the first 2 or 3 weeks following reduction, then replacing it with a

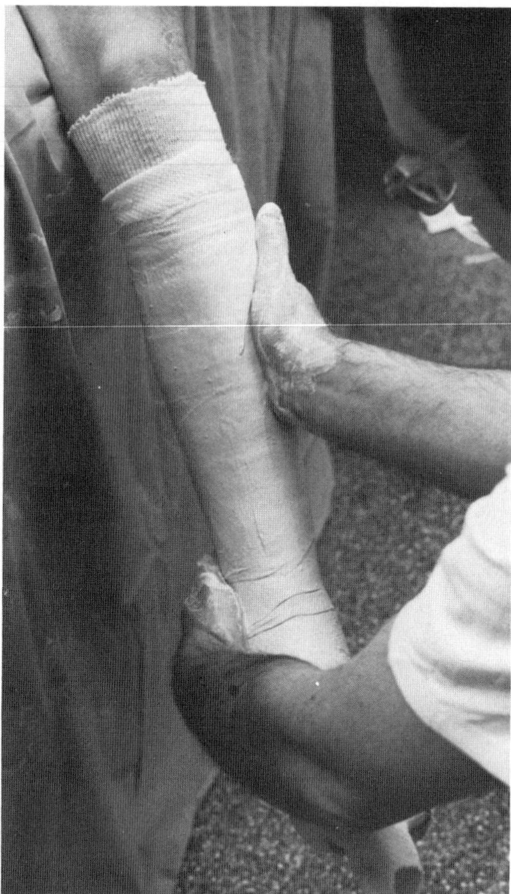

Fig. 1-27. When manipulating through a wet cast or rubbing in the turns of the bandage, always use the palms of the hands and thenar eminences and never the fingertips.

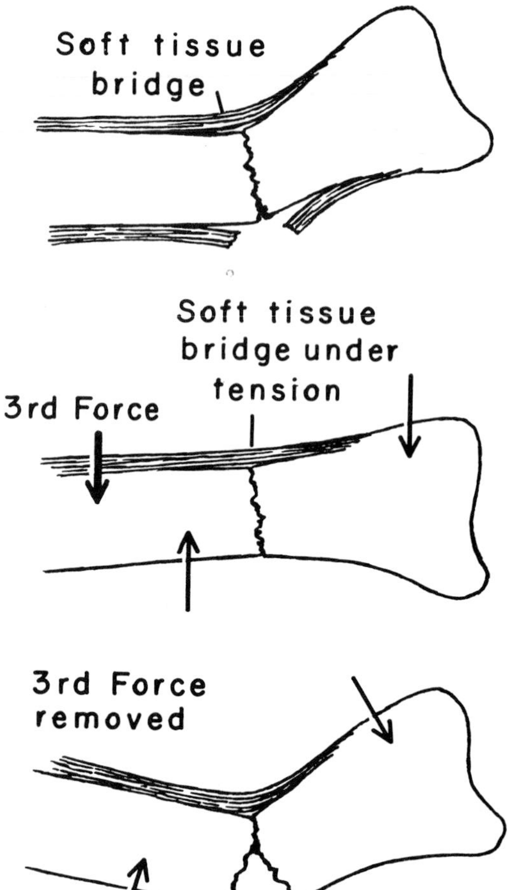

Fig. 1-28. In order to maintain the reduction of the fracture, a three-point system must be utilized. The cast should be molded so that the soft-tissue bridge is under tension. This means that the forces must be applied as in this diagram, and should one of the three forces be removed, the system becomes unstable. (After Charnley)

patellar tendon bearing cast.[43,44] This is probably irrational, and, I suspect patellar-tendon-bearing casts may be quite as effective if used immediately. This type of cast must be applied with care over minimal padding and is applied in segments. In applying the upper portion of the cast, the knee should be flexed to a right angle and the cast molded flat over the upper calf to give a triangular cross section. Meanwhile the cast is molded anteriorly around the patella, and an indentation is made over the patellar tendon (Fig. 1-31). The cast is trimmed to look like a patellar-tendon-bearing prosthesis, and it is most important to trim the cast like a wing-back chair around the femoral condyles to prevent rotation of the proximal tibia on weight bearing (Fig. 1-32).

Cast braces have been a significant contribution to the closed management of fractures of the femoral shaft, supracondylar fractures of the femur, and tibial plateau fractures.[115] After preliminary treatment by

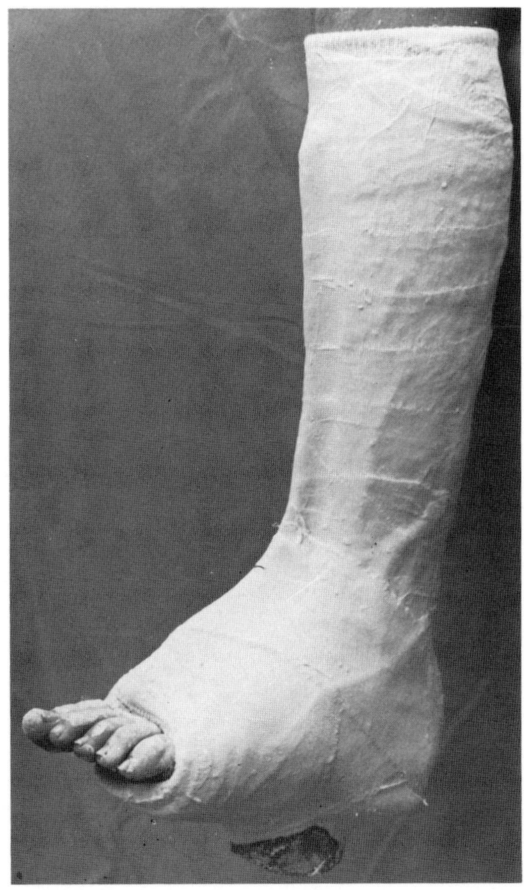

Fig. 1-29. The plantar aspect of the cast should be reinforced with splints and a walking heel applied. Care should be taken not to apply the walking heel too far anteriorly since this tends to break the cast at the ankle. The single door-stop heel should be in line with the tibial shaft.

traction, the cast brace is applied when the fracture is "stable and firm" (although this period seems to be shrinking progressively). In essence, this is a long-leg cast applied over a long Spandex stocking, with the upper end molded to the shape of a quadrilateral socket or a plastic socket incorporated in the cast. The knee is cut out and hinged (see Chap. 15).

Hip and Shoulder Spicas. I abhor the use of both these casts, since they are large, heavy, and cumbersome and are highly inefficient in the immobilization of fractures in adults. Frequently, patients are sent home in hip spicas to make space in hospitals. In their home environment, no one may care for them; and they lie, unturned, soaking in their own urine and feces manufacturing immense decubitus ulcers. I have seen a paraplegic woman with a fractured spine

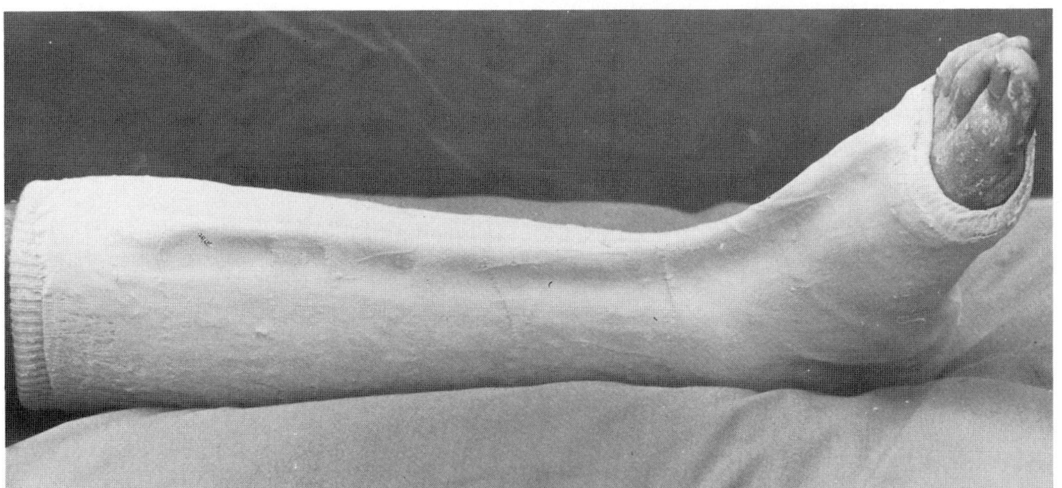

Fig. 1-30. To reinforce the cast with a splint, it is much better to apply it in the concavity of an angulation, as an I-beam or fin, than to apply it over a convexity, such as a lamina. Such a fin increases substantially the strength of the ankle, whereas the same amount of plaster applied posteriorly would have very little effect.

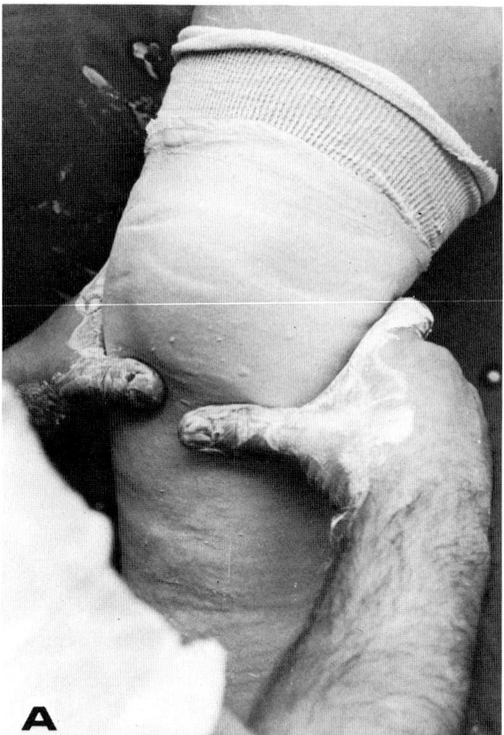

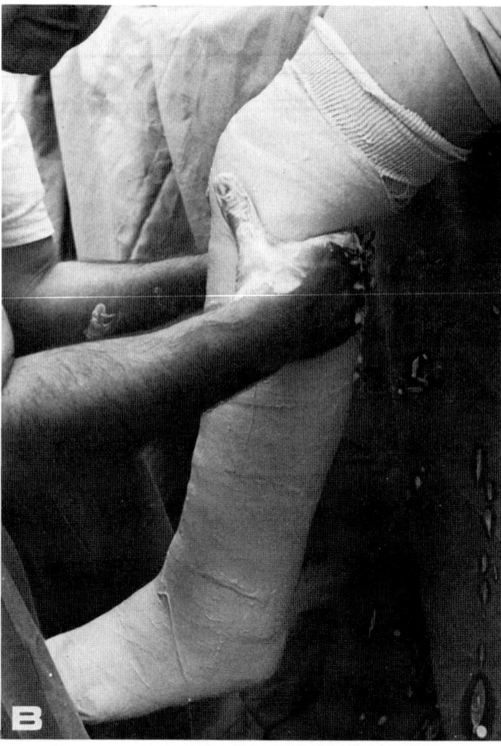

Fig. 1-31. (*A, B*) In the application of a patellar-tendon-bearing cast, indentation must be made over the patellar tendon, and the cast must be carefully molded around the patella. At the same time, the posterior calf must be molded to make a triangular cross-section at the upper end of the leg.

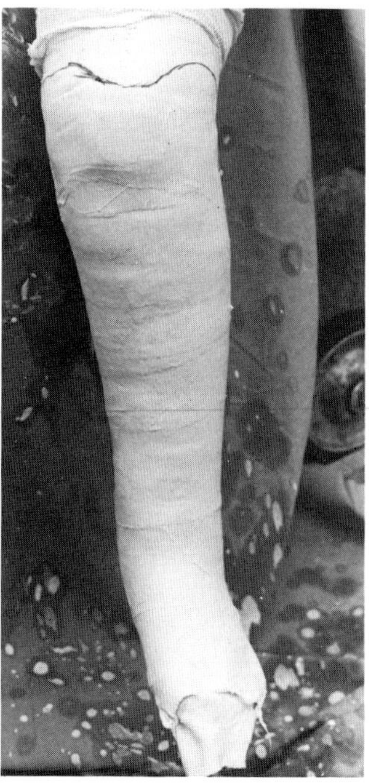

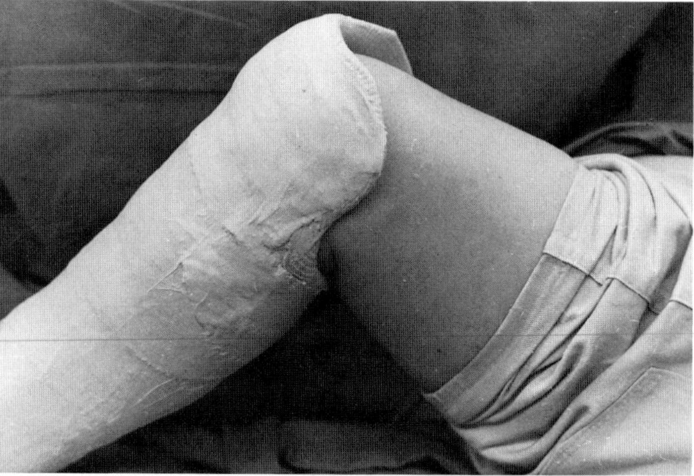

Figure 1-32. The patellar-tendon-bearing cast should be cut out to resemble a patellar-tendon-bearing prosthesis, and it is particularly important to trim the lateral portion like a wing-back chair. When the knee is flexed, pressure is taken from the patellar tendon, but in full extension, pressure is exerted on the thick skin over the tendon.

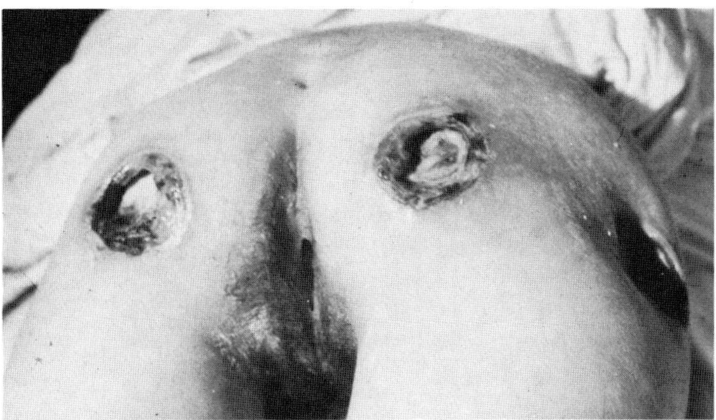

Fig. 1-33. This woman with paraplegia was transported in a double hip spica. On arrival at her new hospital she had large decubiti over both ischial tuberosities, both greater trochanters, and both anterior superior iliac spines. The application of circular casts or spicas in patients without sensation is fraught with terrible danger and should rarely, if ever, be done.

transported in a double hip spica, who on arrival had bone showing over both iliac spines, both greater trochanters, and her sacrum (Fig. 1-33). In the past I have used one-legged spicas for early weight bearing in femoral shaft fractures, although recent refinements in cast bracing have made even this passé. It is only under the most unusual circumstances that I now advocate the use of the hip spica in fractures.

In order to reduce the weight of these casts and make the patient more comfortable, a substantial window should be cut out over the belly. This portion of the cast contributes nothing to its strength, but it should always be circular or oval and never rectangular, since corners act as stress risers. This means that the window has to be cut with a knife. If one waits too long, cutting the hard plaster can be tedious. The task is made easier by outlining the window with the knife and then making a cross with the plaster saw within the circle. The free corners may then be pried up and the cutting of the circumference completed with ease (Fig. 1-34).

All of us at some time or other in our careers have been embarrassed by the disconcerting habit that spicas have of breaking at the hip. This is sometimes due to a triangular area, commonly known as the intern's angle, at the junction of the limb and trunk which does not receive its fair share of the plaster. It is also due, as St. Clair Strange has pointed out, to the juncture of the body and leg being an open section and thus very much weaker than the circular portions of the cast[146] (Fig. 1-35). In order to strengthen this weak point, fin-like reinforcements are applied anteriorly, posteriorly, and laterally, much in the same way that the walking cast might be reinforced (Fig. 1-30).

Wedging Plaster-of-Paris Casts. After an attempted closed reduction and the application of a circular cast, there may be some residual varus or valgus angulation or posterior bow. Under these circumstances, it is quite permissible to make a transverse cut two-thirds of the way around the cast (leaving a hinge opposite the convexity of the angulation) and open up the cut until the angulation is adequately corrected. The cut edges of the cast must then be everted with molders, or, if these are not available, pliers. Some surgeons place little blocks of wood or corks to hold the wedge cast open, but these are unnecessary and potentially dangerous, since they could conceivably exert pressure on the underlying skin. I generally

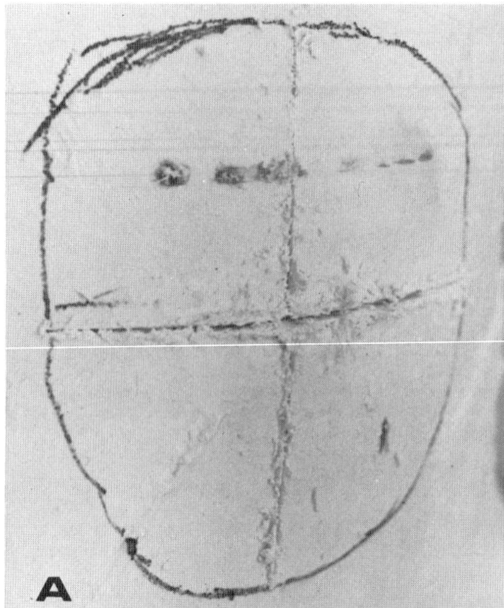

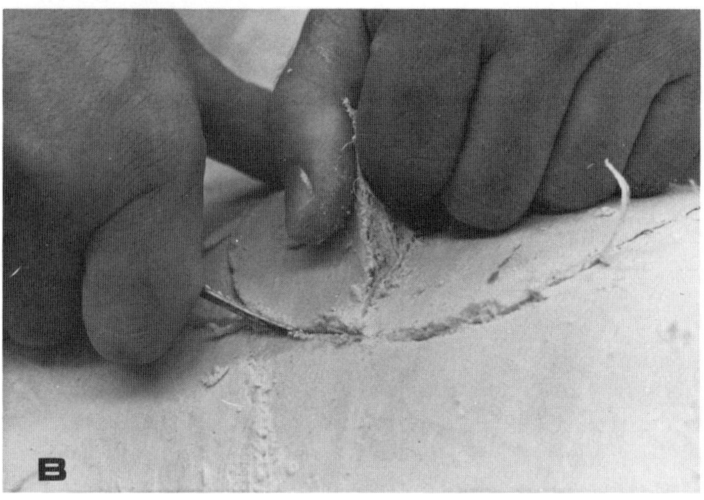

Fig. 1-34. (*A*, *B*) Cutting a belly-hole in a plaster jacket or spica can be tedious, especially when the plaster is hard. The easiest method is to outline the dimensions of the hole with a pencil and then divide the area into four quadrants with a reciprocating plaster saw. The circle is then outlined with a knife along the pencil marks and the free edges of the quadrant can be pried upwards and the periphery cut with the knife. It is always safer to brace the thumb against the cast to prevent the knife from slipping.

pack some sheet wadding in the defect and repair the cast while holding the limb in the corrected position. To gain the greatest mechanical advantage, the wedge should be made at the point where the central long axes of both fragments intersect; and this point can be ascertained by drawing the appropriate lines on the radiograph.[33] It must be stressed, however, that wedging will correct only angulation, never lateral shift or rotation. In my hands, I find the greatest use for wedging in fractures of the tibia, where the correction tends to be comparatively small. If large corrections are to be made, a combination opening wedge on the concave side with a closing wedge on the convex side is safer, since a large opening wedge will elongate the cast and apply undue pressure on the dorsum of the foot. However, if large corrections are necessary, I usually apply a new cast.

Windows in Casts. There are times when it is necessary to inspect wounds under casts, and making windows to do so seems reasonable. If at the time of the application of the cast you know that such a window will be necessary, it is a good plan to apply a large bolus of dressings over the wound, so that it sticks out. One may then take a sharp knife and cut around the periphery of this wad, leaving an oval hole. A rectangular hole cut with a saw makes the cast weak, since the corners act as stress risers. The cast might reasonably be reinforced by a dorsal fin to make up for the weakness of the open section.

These windows are hazardous if left open, especially if there is any tendency of the limb to swell. The soft tissue may herniate through the hole, becoming grossly edematous, and the skin tends to break down from the pressure produced by the margins of the defect. To avoid this complication, I generally cut a piece of felt or sponge rubber to the size of the hole and bandage this snugly in place over the dressings with an Ace bandage to provide uniform compression.

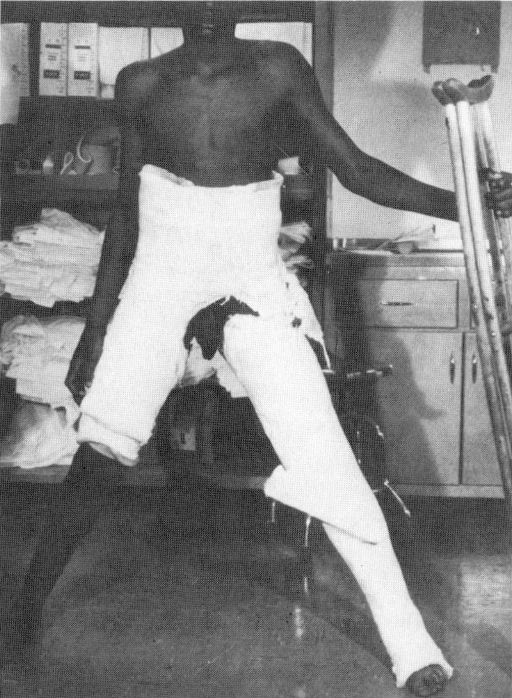

Fig. 1-35. This sporting patient walked in his spica, which failed at its weakest point, the open section of the thigh and the "intern's angle."

Plaster-of-Paris Splints

Thus far I have been describing circular casts, where the entire circumference of the anatomical part is encased. However, plaster-of-paris may be used in the form of splints, either as first-aid or, in some cases, as the definitive treatment.

The two commonest types of splint are the radial slab and the sugar tong. In adult fracture work, both of these splints are used in the treatment of Colles' fractures.

Radial Slab. The radial slab consists of eight to ten thicknesses of 6-inch plaster with a thumb hole cut in it. No padding other than stockinette is used, and the wet plaster is applied to the radial side of the forearm overlapping the dorsal and the volar surfaces of the wrist and forearm. This splint is applied with the forearm and hand strongly pronated and in as much ulnar deviation as possible. It is then bandaged on with a wet gauze bandage (2 or 3-inch) and allowed to set. Due to the tendency of the fingers to swell after Colles' fractures, I sometimes apply a hand dressing of fluffs or absorbent cotton on top of the splint with only the fingertips showing and elevate the arm. Should there be any circulatory embarrassment, the splint is easily removed with a pair of scissors.

Sugar Tongs. The radial slab has not been popular in America, but the sugar-tong splint has. After reduction of the fracture, a splint is run from the knuckles on the dorsum over the flexed elbow and over the volar aspect of the forearm to the midpalmar crease. Padding is applied either before the plaster or as a longitudinal strip along with the plaster. It is molded while setting and bandaged on with gauze or an elastic wrap. This, of course, limits the motion of the elbow and, like the radial slab, is easily removed. I have an aversion to the sugar tong for Colles' fractures, probably due to my own ineptitude, but I never feel that I can adequately control the radial shift, which is the key to mastery of this troublesome fracture. I do not have the same reservations, however, about the treatment of fractures of the humeral shaft. A sugar tong running from axilla medially to shoulder laterally, combined with a collar and cuff or a stockinette Velpeau, is an admirable way to treat these fractures.

The Efficacy of Plaster Immobilization

The object of applying a plaster-of-paris cast is to keep the bone ends in apposition and the fractures aligned until the fracture heals. It has been said that immobilization by plaster will only work where the soft-tissue hinge is intact, where there is inherent stability of the reduced fracture, and where the cast is properly applied using a three-point system. When a bone is fractured and not widely separated, the soft-tissue hinge in the concavity of the angulation or around the vertical fracture in a spiral fracture is, as we have seen, the linkage that allows us to reduce the fracture with manipulation. If no soft-tissue bridge is present, reduction by manipulation is not feasible. In the usual intracapsular femoral neck fracture of the elderly, the posterior retinacular fibers remain intact, while those subjected to tension stress are torn asunder. Reduction by traction and internal rotation is achieved solely by tightening this intact posterior retinaculum. Conversely, when young people sustain such fractures in automobile wrecks, the violence is often so great that all the retinacular fibers are torn, and no reduction is possible unless the joint capsule is opened and the fragments are manipulated under vision. A fracture will stay reduced only if the soft-tissue bridge remains under tension. This requires three-point fixation, which is achieved by molding the wet cast in a similar manner to the way the fracture was reduced initially. Two of these three points, therefore, are applied by the hands. Two forces acting alone, a couple, cannot stabilize a fracture; a third force must be present. This is the cast over the proximal portion of the limb (Fig. 1-28). With over-reduction the bridge is under the greatest tension and the reduction is even more stable—"a 'curved' plaster is necessary in order to make a straight limb."[33]

Charnley divides fractures into three categories: those with inherent stability against shortening (transverse fractures), those with potential stability against shortening (oblique fractures less than 45 degrees to the long axis of the bone), and those with no stability against shortening (oblique, spiral, and comminuted fractures). Only the first two categories, he feels, are suitable for immobilization by casts alone.[33]

However, there is another factor: the hydrodynamic effect of the cast. Since the soft tissues are semifluid, the hydrostatic pressure increases when they are compressed by a cast. This increased tension tends to keep the limb from shortening as it most certainly would do were it unsupported. I believe it is this factor that makes possible the success of the Dehne method of early ambulation in fractures of the tibia. We have treated many oblique, spiral, and indeed comminuted fractures of the tibia by this method with no more than 1.25 cm. of shortening. I would admit, however, that some such fractures do need a little help with transfixation pins for 3 or 4 weeks to prevent undue shortening. But the conviction is growing on me that the resort to pins is related more to the skill of the surgeon than to the instability of the fracture.

One would be very naive to believe that absolute immobilization can ever be achieved by any type of external splint. Patients are often quite conscious of movement of the fracture fragments in the early days, but with the production of callus and its progressive stiffening, this disappears.

Hicks applied casts to two lower limbs that had been amputated through the distal third of the femur.[78] These casts were applied "more tightly than would ever have been risked in clinical practice." When he windowed the cast over the fracture site, he was able to produce a lateral shift of 2.5 cm. in one and over 3 cm. in the other merely by pushing with his fingers. "Rotation to the extent of 20 degrees and angulation to the extent of 6 degrees were just as easily obtained."

Hicks has shown that plaster-of-paris casts applied ostensibly to immobilize fracture fragments may have the reverse effect and increase the amplitude of motion at the fracture site.[78] A slavish obedience to the rule of immobilizing the joints proximal and distal to the fracture does not necessarily insure better fixation of the fracture. In fractures of the forearm an above-elbow cast prevents the muscles spanning the elbow from exerting their action on the joint. As a result their pull is transmitted distally to the fracture sites. Sarmiento has drawn attention to the deforming action of the brachioradialis in Colles' fractures, and Hughston, to its role in the displacement of Galeazzi fractures of the distal radius.[86,148] London has shown recently that when forearm fractures in children are treated with forearm casts, late redisplacement of the fractures do not occur.[105] Although this means of treatment does not seem applicable to fractures of the forearm in adults, owing to their "inherent lack of stability," Sarmiento has recently reported on the management of 42 forearm fractures by a functional brace that allows "early freedom of motion of all joints."[151] No one who has suffered through the travail of trying to achieve union in indolent supracondylar fractures of the humerus or femur with ankylosis of the knee or elbow can doubt that the immobilization of a joint has a deleterious effect on the healing of a contiguous fracture.

Furthermore, Hicks has also demonstrated that if, in an amputated specimen with a fractured tibia, the action of the peroneal tendon is simulated, the subtalar joint is fixed by the cast and the lower fragment of the tibia is rotated externally.[78] Alternatively, simulated invertor action is accompanied by rotation of this fragment in the reverse direction. A total range of 12 degrees of rotation is produced by this means. This experimental evidence lends support to the clinical evidence of Sarmiento that free motion of the foot and ankle is not deleterious in the treatment of tibial fractures.[149,150]

It would appear, then, that for at least some fractures of the forearm and leg better immobilization is obtained by casts employing three-point fixation of the fractures and not of the joints.

Fiberglass Casts

Recently, light-curing plastics have been used in lieu of plaster-of-paris bandages. Casts made of this material are lightweight, long-wearing and radiolucent. Other advantages are that the patient may get the cast wet (particularly appreciated by children in the summertime) and that weight bearing can be commenced immediately in a short-leg walking cast, without requiring the drying time necessary for plaster casts. The fiberglass cast has very limited application in the treatment of fresh fractures, but it is quite useful as the second or subsequent cast. It is particularly indicated in the patient with an open fracture and a large soft-tissue wound that requires local care. The cast can easily be windowed and the wound treated with whirlpool, soaks or other forms of wet therapy, because the integrity of the cast is not compromised by water.

There are a few disadvantages with the fiberglass cast which have discouraged some orthopaedists from using it. While my own experience is still rather limited in its use, I have found the curing process to be a bottle-neck in a busy clinic when many patients need cast changes. Forearm and short-leg casts are easily cured, but more extensive casts present something of a problem. Application of the cast itself can be rather tedious, due to the plastic strip backing, which must be removed as the bandage unrolls, but with some practice, the time of application is not necessarily longer than with plaster casts.

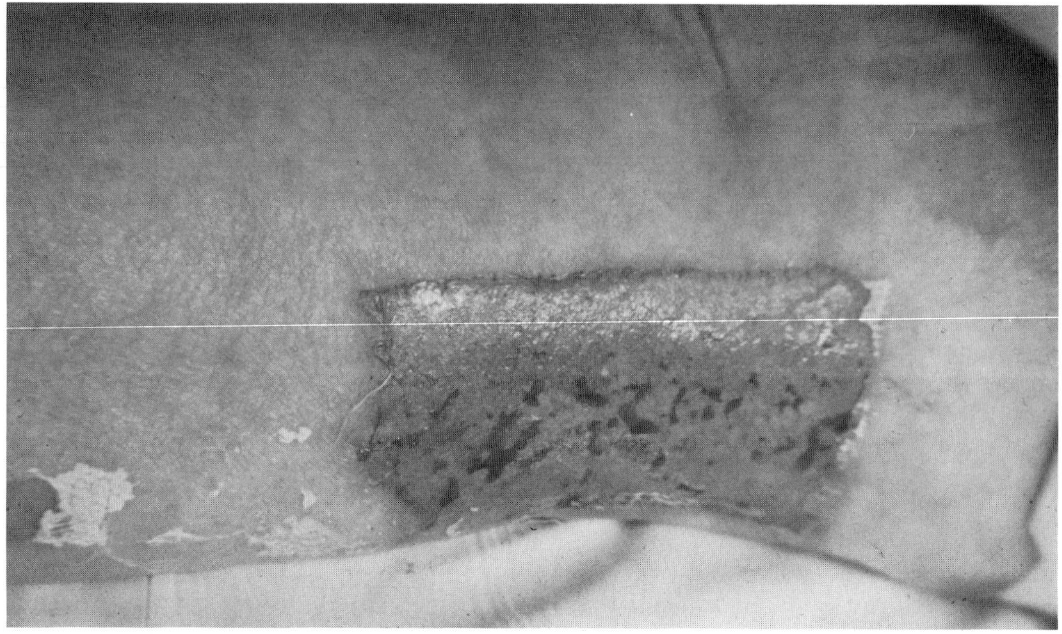

Fig. 1-36. When skin traction is applied utilizing regular adhesive tape, superficial layers of the skin may be avulsed. The result is a weeping, angry excoriation.

Achieving a snug fit with the fiberglass cast may be more difficult to accomplish than with plaster. I have been able to obtain a better fit by applying the fiberglass as longitudinal strips cut to the exact length, overlapping other splints running in the same direction. Reinforcements at the upper and lower ends and where necessary can be applied at right angles in a circular fashion.

Although at the present time the fiberglass cast is only a useful adjunct to plaster-of-paris, I believe that in all likelihood plaster-of-paris will eventually be supplanted by some such material.

Immobilization by Continuous Traction

Some fractures are so unstable that maintenance of a reduction by plaster-of-paris casts is impossible, or casts may be, for one reason or another, impractical. In these cases the bone can be reduced and held to length by means of continuous traction, provided a soft-tissue linkage still exists.

It does seem extraordinary that, although traction had been used for millenia in the reduction of fractures and dislocations and many elaborate machines and devices were invented to apply it, the use of continuous traction was not employed until the 19th century.[129]

Continuous traction may be applied through traction tapes attached to the skin by adhesives or by a direct pull through pins transfixing the skeleton.

Skin Traction. Although Gurdon Buck did not invent skin traction (nor did he claim to have done so), isotonic skin traction has come to be known by his name. It was used extensively in the Civil War and later spread to Europe and Britain, where it was called the American Method.[129] Skin, however, is designed to bear compression forces and not shear. If much more than 8 pounds is applied for any length of time, the superficial layers of the skin are pulled off, leaving an irritated, exuding surface. The force exerted by skin traction is dissipated in the soft tissues, so that this form of traction in adult fracture work is used only as a temporary measure to make the patient comfortable while awaiting more definitive therapy.

When skin traction is to be used, I prefer moleskin for the traction tape. Ordinary adhesive tape must never be used. Since it is impervious to moisture, it allows the underlying skin to become sodden with perspiration. The tape then creeps, pulling off the superficial layers of the skin, leaving a weeping, angry excoriation (Fig. 1-36). On no account should the leg be shaved. The superficial layers of the skin have a protective function, and tape on shaved skin causes irritation and discomfort. Some surgeons feel that tincture of benzoin applied to the skin prior to the application of adhesive traction protects the skin, but there is no good evidence to support this contention.

The malleoli must be protected from the traction tape by padding *proximal* to them. Pressure sores may result from padding applied directly to the malleoli. The moleskin tapes should be applied evenly without wrinkles, and if necessary, oblique cuts may be made in the borders in order to make them conform. The traction tapes are applied to a block or spreader and through this to a cord, which passes over a pulley to an attached weight. The moleskin is held in place by an elastic bandage carefully applied from the ankle to the knee, which must be checked regularly to make sure it does not exert a tourniquet effect by becoming disarranged.

Recently, a variety of prepackaged skin traction devices have been made available which are easily and quickly applied. Some of these are adherent while others exert their action by the friction of sponge rubber against the skin so that they may be removed and reapplied as often as is desired.

Skeletal Traction. Skeletal traction was first achieved by the use of tongs, but skeletal traction as we know it today, applied by a pin transfixing bone, was introduced by Fritz Steinmann. Kirschner also invented a similar device using a very fine wire which required a special traction bail to keep the wire under tension.[129] The idea of using a wire of small diameter which does minimal damage to the tissues is most attractive but, unhappily, Kirschner wires, especially after the long haul, have a propensity for cutting through the bone like wire through cheese.

My own preference is for Steinmann pin traction using a threaded pin rather than one that is smooth. Smooth pins tend to loosen rapidly, so that they slip in and out frequently giving rise to soft-tissue infection and, on occasion, to osteomyelitis of the host bone. In current American practice, the most common indication for skeletal traction is for fractures of the femur, although occasionally traction is indicated for fractures of the humerus in a patient with multiple injuries. It is also commonly used in supracondylar fractures of the humerus and tibial plateau where these difficult fractures are to be treated with early motion (Apley's traction).[4] On occasion, it is used in the treatment of tibial fractures, particularly where there are associated burns. It is said, however, that nonunion or delayed union of the tibia is encouraged by this treatment.[173]

Traction Through the Olecranon. A medium or small threaded Steinmann pin is inserted from the medial side 1½ inches distal to the tip of the olecranon. The course of the ulnar nerve is kept in mind; the flat posteromedial surface of the ulna is palpated; and the pin is drilled through. The traction may be in the side-arm position, or the humerus may be held vertically with the forearm supported by a felt sling. In the side-arm position, skin traction with a spreader may be used to support the forearm (Fig. 1-37).

Traction for the Lower Extremity. Three sites are commonly used for traction in lower extremity fractures: the supracondylar region of the femur, the proximal tibia, and the os calcis. The proximal tibia is the site of choice for traction in femoral fractures. Although one would imagine that traction through the distal femur would be

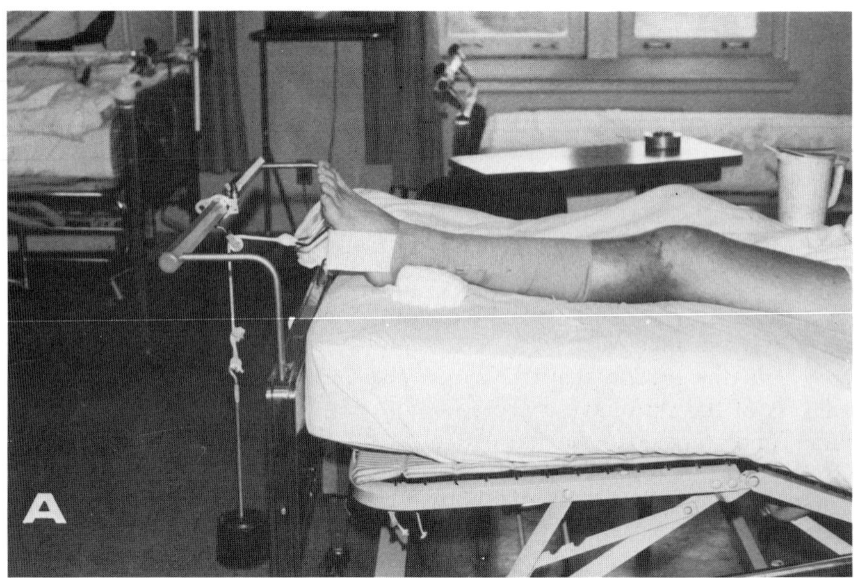

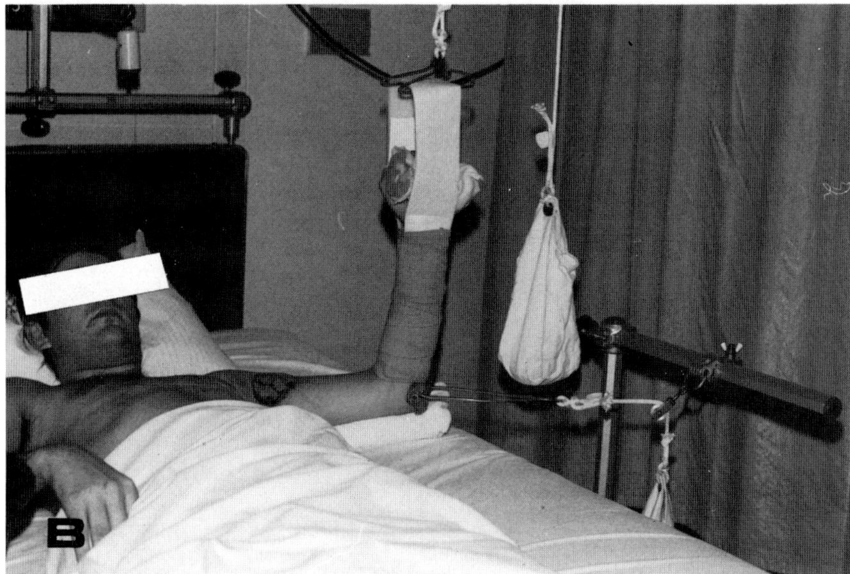

Fig. 1-37. (*A*) Skin traction should be applied only as a temporary expedient. Padding is applied *superior to* the malleoli and the traction tapes are bandaged by an elastic bandage from the ankle to the knee. (*B*) Olecranon traction is sometimes used in the treatment of fractures of the humerus, especially supracondylar fractures. The pin is inserted through the ulnar shaft immediately distal to the olecranon, taking care to avoid the ulnar nerve. The forearm and hand are supported by skin traction.

much more efficient, it has the inherent disadvantage that the pin may provoke binding down of the quadriceps, particularly when the pin tract becomes infected.[33] The main indication for the use of this site is where the ligaments of the knee have been injured on the ipsilateral side of a femoral fracture. In supracondylar fractures, where

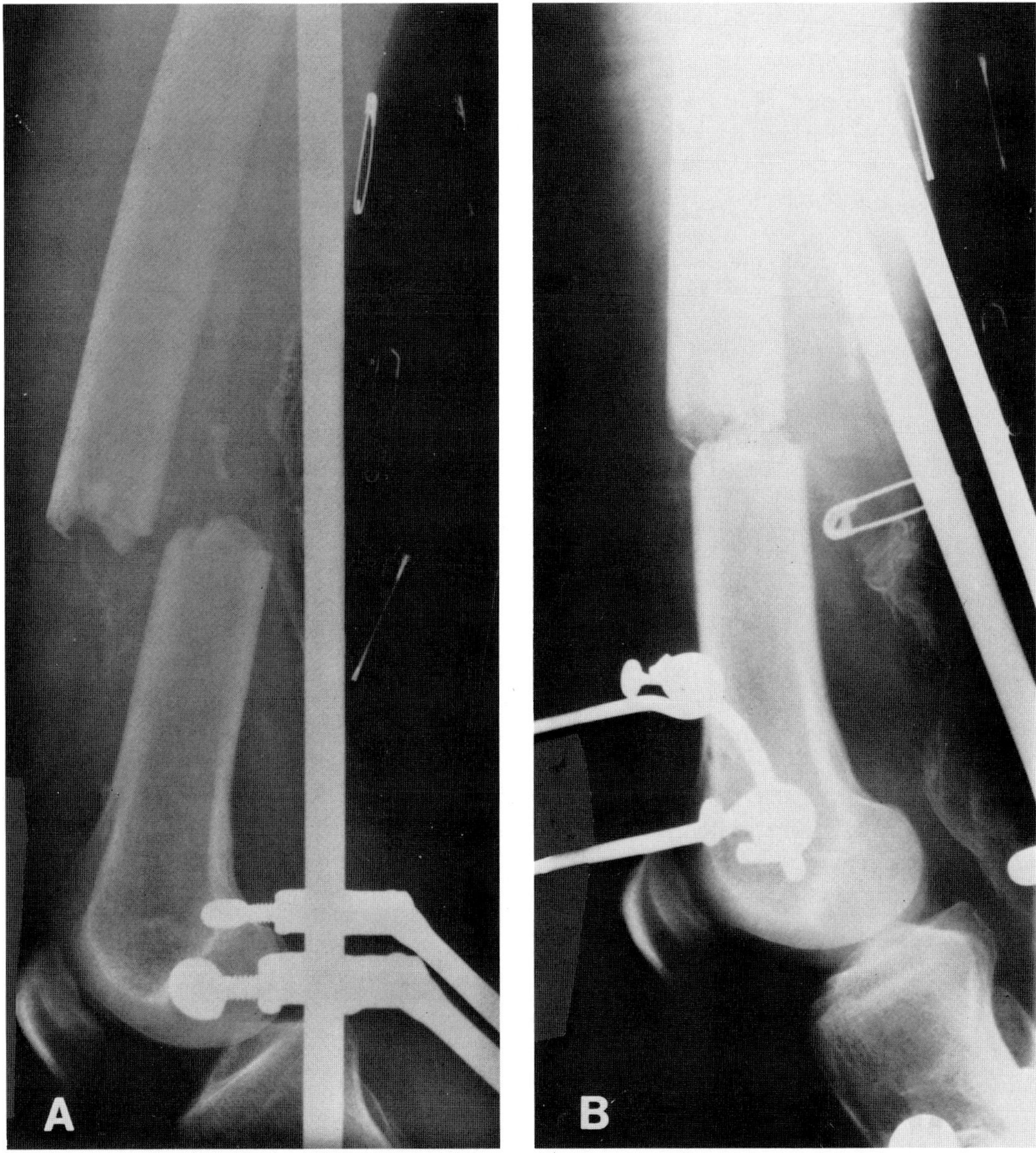

Fig. 1-38. (*A, B*) This femoral fracture could not be reduced by simple longitudinal traction alone. With the addition of a Steinmann pin through the distal fragment at the level of the upper border of the patella with anterior traction a better position was produced.

the posterior tilt of the distal fragment cannot be controlled by other means, a pin or Kirschner wire may be inserted at the level of the superior border of the patella and the recalcitrant fragment pulled anteriorly (Fig. 1-38). The Steinmann pin is best inserted from the medial to the lateral side (to avoid any risk to the femoral vessels) and immediately proximal to the condyles.

Proximal Tibial Traction. The tibial tubercle is palpated, and the pin is drilled from lateral to medial side, 2 cm. posterior to the tibial tubercle. In osteoporotic patients, it is prudent to go distally into the bone of the shaft. This purchase is less likely to fail than one in the weak bone of the metaphysis.

Os Calcis Traction. This site may be used in the treatment of tibial or femoral fractures, but I tend to avoid it whenever possible, because osteomyelitis of the calcaneus is such a chronic and disabling condition. When it must be used, great care should be exercised to avoid skewering the subtalar joint. Choose a point 2.5 cm. posterior and 2.5 cm. inferior to the lateral malleolus or, as Charnley advises, pick "a point 1 inch superior and 1 inch anterior to the profile of the heel."[33]

In the insertion of Steinmann pins, the skin must be prepared as one would in any surgical procedure. Gloves are worn; the area is isolated with towels, and sterile precautions are observed.

Frequently, the patient will be under general or spinal anesthesia; but there is no reason why the pins cannot be inserted under local infiltration anesthesia, provided care is taken to infiltrate the periosteum adequately.

In drilling the pin, particularly when a skin incision has not been used, the skin may be caught by the pin and be puckered. If left like this, it will slough; and tension should be relieved by nicking it with a knife at three points equidistant from each other.[33] The pin holes should be dressed by sponges impaled on the pins and soaked with tincture of benzoin or Ace adherent.

Traction for Femoral Fractures. Traction as a means of immobilization of fractures is most often used in fractures of the femur. Although these fractures may be treated by traction alone in the 90-90 position (i.e., with both the hip and knee flexed to 90 degrees) or merely over a pillow as Perkins describes, most fractures of the femur are treated in some form of additional splintage.

The most popular method is balanced suspension in a Thomas splint or variant of it with a Pearson attachment (Fig. 1-39) and isotonic traction with weights. Commonly, the reduction of these fractures is achieved by the traction and the secondary use of pads, slings, or pushers. I much prefer, whenever possible, to reduce the fracture by gentle manipulation under anesthesia and hold the position gained by maintenance traction. This technique is also preferred by Charnley, who makes an excellent case for isometric traction in a straight Thomas splint.[33]

Charnley also advises the use of a "traction unit," which is a short-leg cast incorporating the tibial Steinmann pin.[33] Whenever a smooth Steinmann pin is used for traction, I believe it should be anchored in plaster. Other advantages claimed for this "traction unit" are: (1) it prevents equinus of the foot, (2) the popliteal nerve and calf muscles are protected from the pressure of the slings of the splint, (3) external rotation of the foot and distal femur is controlled, (4) the tendo calcaneus is protected from pressure, (5) it is comfortable, and (6) fractures of the tibia and ipsilateral femur can be treated in this way.

Hugh Owen Thomas personally made his bed-splints to fit the patient, but made-to-measure splints are a luxury not obtainable in many hospitals. In most institutions it is difficult to find a splint of exactly the right size. The leather covering the rings is often hard, dry, and cracked and, frequently, soiled by the last patient to use it. For this reason, I have converted to the Harris splint, which does not have a ring and can be adjusted to fit most of our patients. Although it may not be quite as good as the ideal Thomas splint, in our hands it has been completely satisfactory (Fig. 1-39).

Many hospitals utilize a variant of the Thomas splint with a half ring (Keller-Blake) which can be swivelled so that one splint can be used for both right and left extremities. When used with the ring posteriorly, the ring is uncomfortable and also tends to collapse. If one uses such a splint, it is better to place the solid half ring anteriorly and pass the webbing strap posteriorly over an abdominal pad.

In 1924, Hamilton Russell published a

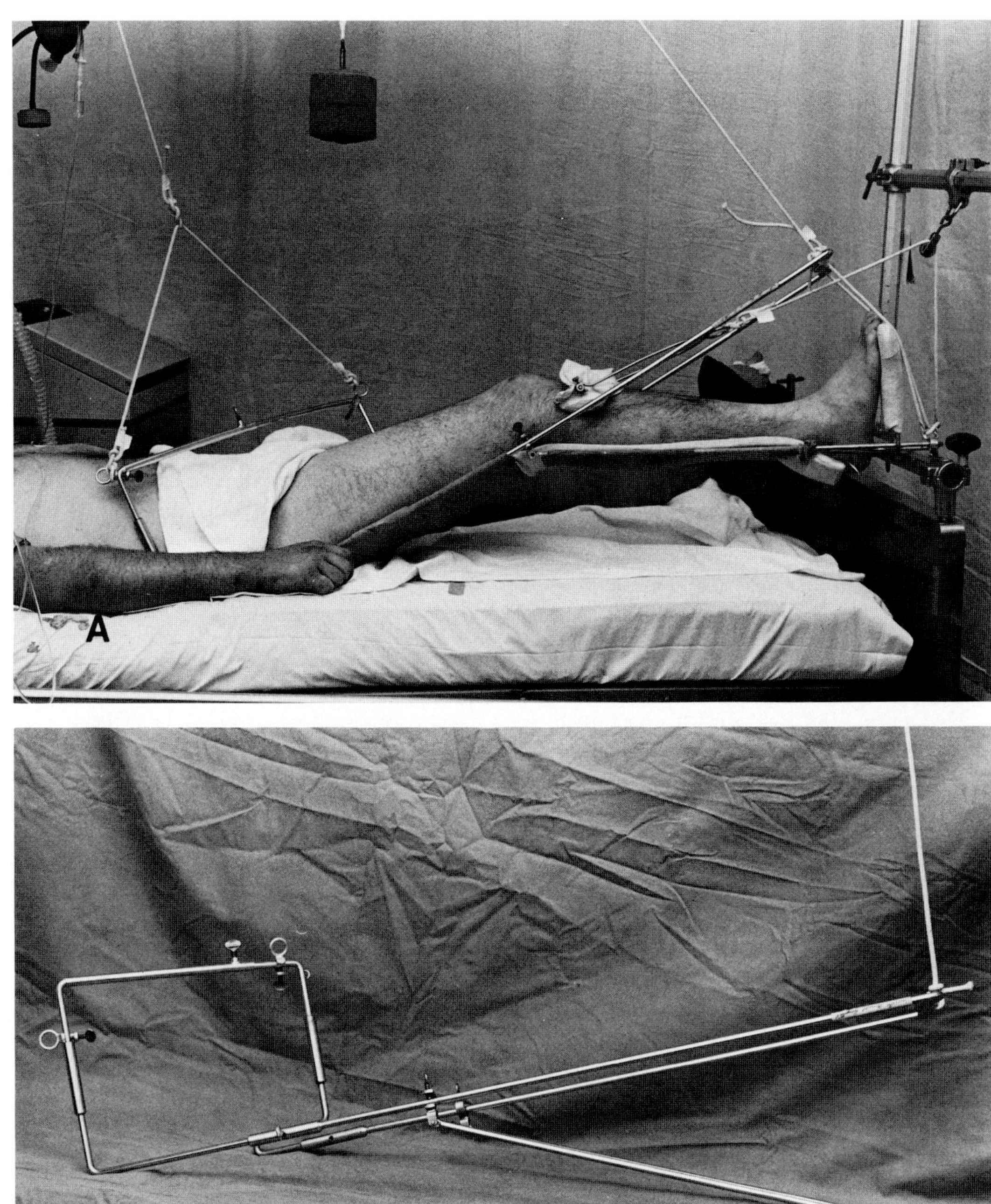

Fig. 1-39. Balanced traction in a Harris splint with Pearson attachment. The entire system is counterbalanced by a 10-pound weight. Longitudinal traction is applied to a pin through the tibia, and the foot is kept out of equinus position by a plantar support. Care must be taken to see that the tendocalcaneus is well-padded and that pressure over bony prominences or the peroneal nerve does not occur.

method of treating fractures of the femur.[145] In this method, a single rope is attached to a sling that supports the thigh and also exerts a longitudinal pull on a foot plate attached to the patient. The traction applied to the femur is the result of the forces acting at the thigh sling and on the foot. By an arrangement of pulleys at the distal end, a 10-pound weight can exert a 20-pound pull. I feel the reason for this method's popularity was the feeling that one was getting something for nothing—a 20-pound pull for 10! In practice, I find this traction a tedious business requiring continual readjustment and attention. However, a development of this traction is a method known as split Russell's, where traction is applied through both a supracondylar pin and an os calcis pin attached to separate weights. Again, the pull on the femur is the resultant of these two forces.

Another modification (Litchman and Duffy)[104] employs two slings: one has been added under the calf, and a constant-force spring has been substituted for weights. This arrangement dispenses with the pillow under the limb as described by Russell. Although the authors use this arrangement for children, it could easily be modified for adults by using a pin through the os calcis.

Recently, a most ingenious traction system has been invented by Neufeld which he has called the Dynamic Method[122] (see Chap. 15). A Steinmann pin is inserted through the proximal tibia, which is anchored in a plaster gaiter or below-knee cast. A half-ring Thomas splint with a Pearson splint is applied with the half-ring placed anteriorly. The distal end of the Thomas splint has been cut off, making the assembly very similar to a Fisk splint. The leg is now affixed to the Pearson attachment by more plaster-of-paris, and the leg and splint assembly is suspended by ropes attached to the splint at mid-leg and mid-thigh. These ropes are attached to each end of a crossbar, which is suspended by a single rope at its mid-point. This single rope runs over a nylon traction pulley which is free to run on an overhead bar. The weight for this traction is transmitted by this pulley over the foot of the bed and is between 10 and 20 pounds. Immediate knee motion is permitted by this apparatus, and in a short time the patient is able to stand up in bed. This traction has been used for all ages from 5 or 6 years to 80 or 90.

Traction has been shown to be a safe and dependable way of treating fractures for more than 100 years. It does, however, require constant care and vigilance, and it is costly, in terms of days in hospital. Posterior bowing and late varus deformities in fractures of the femur due to the pull of the adductors will plague the unwary, but the use of posterior pads and abduction of the hip do prevent these. Over-distraction of the fracture with consequent delayed union or nonunion is a major complication, and the method risks all the hazards of prolonged bed rest—thromboembolism, decubiti, pneumonia, and atelectasis.

Preliminary traction for short periods (10 to 14 days) followed by cast-bracing is rapidly becoming popular and is a safe and satisfactory method of treating most fractures of the femur.

Traction by Plaster. Traction may also be applied my means of plaster-of-paris casts. Fractures of the humerus may be treated by a hanging cast.[30,161] In this method, a very light cast is applied from the knuckles to a point no higher than 2.5 cm. above the fracture site and is suspended at the wrist by a string around the neck. The combined weight of the upper extremity and cast apply traction to the humeral fracture. Anteroposterior bowing may be corrected by shortening or lengthening the string, and varus or valgus angulation, by altering the suspension point at the wrist.

In very unstable fractures of the leg, particularly where there has been marked comminution, it may be impossible to prevent gross shortening in a conventional cast.

Under these circumstances, pins may be inserted through the proximal tibia and os calcis. Then the fracture is pulled out to length, and a cast is applied incorporating the pins. Thus, continuous traction or distraction is applied to the fracture.

There are a variety of apparatuses designed to hold the pins and fracture while the cast is being applied. In Louisville, we still use the device invented by Dr. Arnold Griswold, a former professor of surgery at the University of Louisville, which works extremely well (Fig. 1-40). After 3 or 4 weeks, when the fracture has gained some inherent stability, the pins are removed, and a walking cast is applied. Walking should not be allowed as long as the pins are *in situ,* due to the danger of breaking. This method of treatment is particularly useful in explosion fractures of the distal end of the tibia.

Complications of Plaster and Traction

A prime cause of successful malpractice suits against orthopaedists and fracture surgeons are complications of plaster and traction.

Plaster Sores. The skin is not designed to be compressed without relief over extended periods of time. When such pressure does occur—for as little as 2 hours—irreversible damage may occur. The skin and the underlying fat, which has a poor blood supply, may necrose, and a plaster sore—nasty-smelling and usually infected—occurs.

These unhappy events do not occur with-

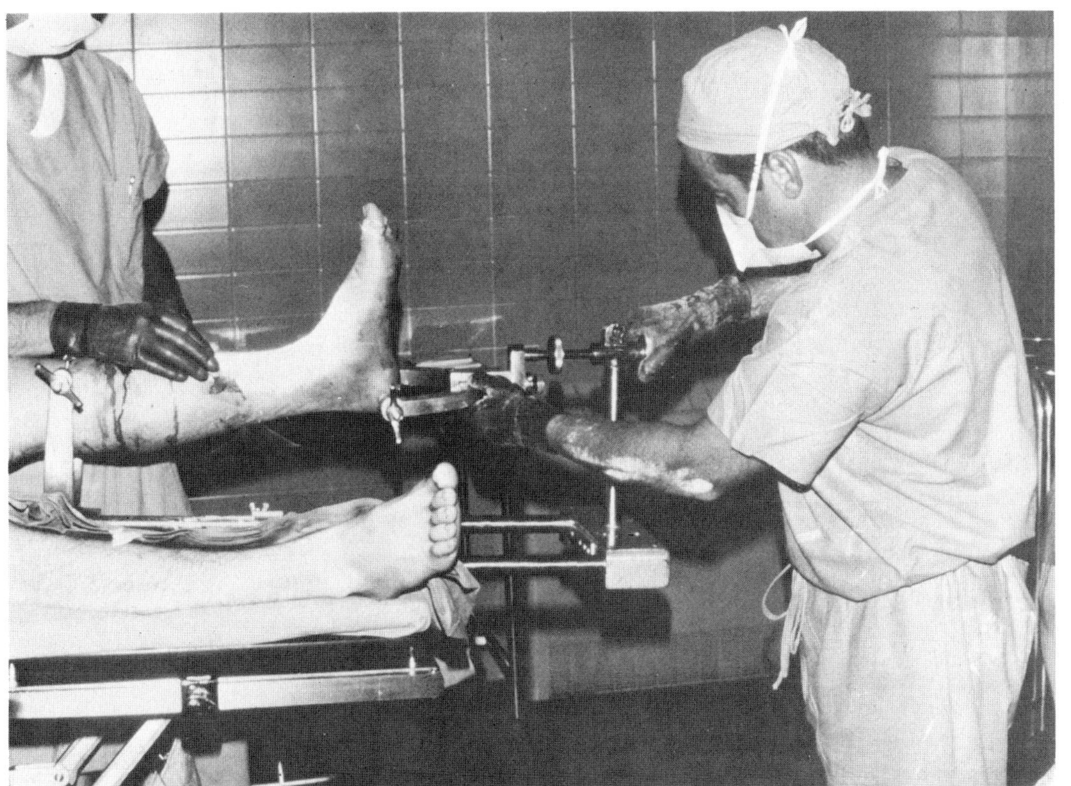

Fig. 1-40. Traction of the left tibia by the Griswold Distraction Machine. Pins have been applied to the proximal tibia and the os calcis, and the tibia was pulled out to length. Rotation and valgus and varus angulation may be adjusted by this machine, and when adequate reduction is achieved a plaster-of-paris cast is applied incorporating the Steinmann pins.

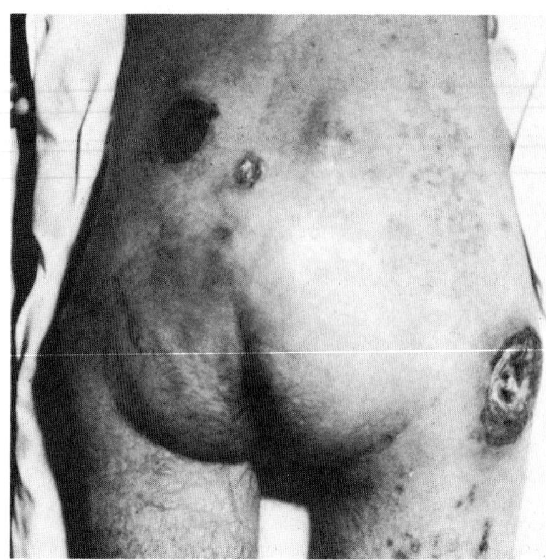

Fig. 1-41. This young man with multiple fractures was sent to convalesce at home in a plaster-of-paris spica. Although he did suffer some discomfort, his pain disappeared along with the skin over the trochanters, sacrum, and left posterior superior iliac spine. All complaints of pain under plaster-of-paris casts must be taken seriously.

out warning unless the patient is unconscious or insensitive. Circular casts should be shunned for paraplegics or those who have impaired sensation (Fig. 1-33). The patient harboring a potential plaster sore invariably complains of burning pain or discomfort, and these complaints must always be taken seriously. If neglected, the discomfort eventually disappears, but by then so has the skin and its nerve endings (Fig. 1-41). In all cases, the site of patient's complaints should be inspected without delay. Irritating trips to the hospital in the middle of the night and the mutilation of one's elegant plaster casts can be avoided to some extent by paying attention to minor details in the initial application of the cast.

It is not good practice, if you apply stockinette over the entire length of the lower limb, to have your assistant support the extremity by holding the stockinette while you plaster (Fig. 1-42). This creates pressure over the heel, which is enough to

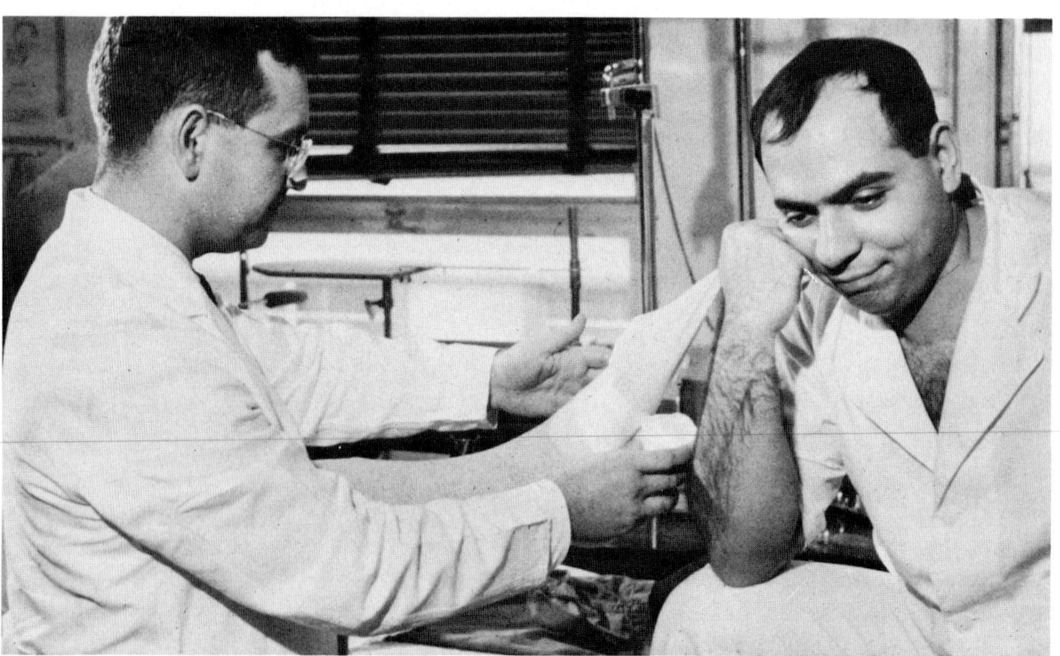

Fig. 1-42. It is not good practice to have the lower extremity supported by an assistant holding the stockinette. This inevitably causes undue pressure of the stockinette over the heel, and it may cause burning pain or even a sore. The same effect can be produced by pulling too vigorously on the stockinette when folding it over the sharp edges of the cast.

impair circulation and produce discomfort. Similarly, in finishing the cast, pulling too vigorously on the stockinette may cause pressure on bony pressure points.

Finger indentations on a cast produce high-pressure points to a much greater extent than do broad indentations made by the hand. In any case, indentations rarely occur when the cast is supported by the flat of the hand, and nurses and other helpers must be instructed accordingly (Fig. 1-43). After the cast is completed, it should not be allowed to rest on a sharp edge which will indent it but should be supported by a pillow or something soft.

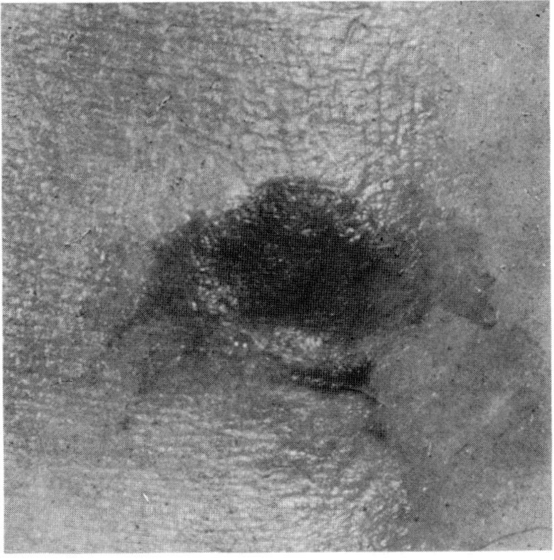

Fig. 1-43. The surgeon in this case inadvertently made an indentation with his thumb while molding the fractured ankle. The result was skin necrosis over the medial malleolus.

The upper end of a cast may be unduly sharp and cause an excoriation. This is particularly common in the fold of the buttock, especially in obese patients. It can be avoided by bending out the upper edge of the cast with the fingers so that it flares. Not infrequently the patient may compound the difficulty by inserting Kleenex tissues or something soft between the cast and the skin or by cutting away the offending plaster, often leaving a jagged edge that produces another sore. Patients should be told that if the cast cuts, the border should be

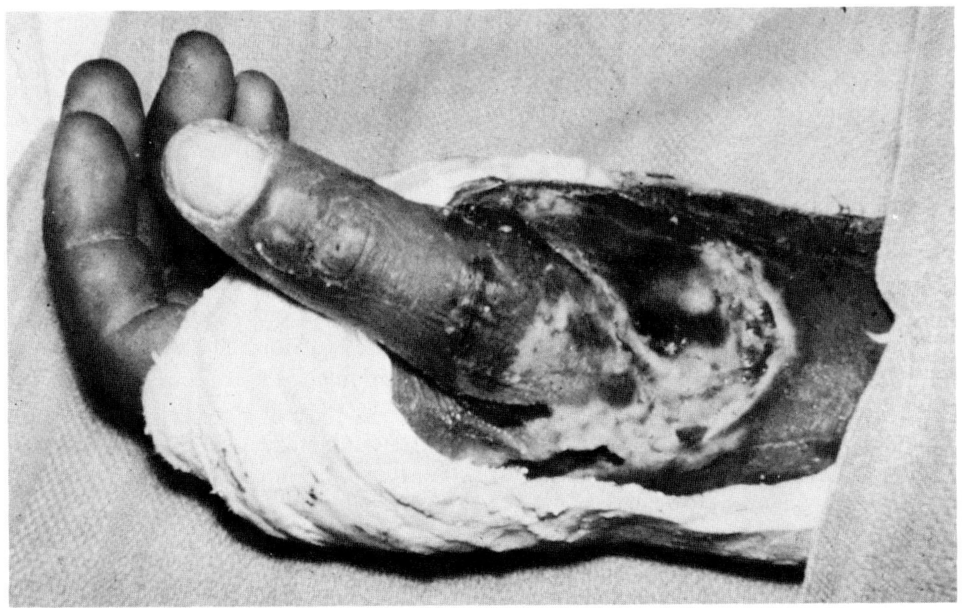

Fig. 1-44. This is the end result of pressure exerted by an improperly applied cast over the thumb metacarpal. The patient had a large, full-thickness skin slough and lost the abductor and extensor tendons of his thumb in the bargain. The sharp edges of the thumb hole must always be everted, and undue pressure over the base of the thumb metacarpal must be avoided.

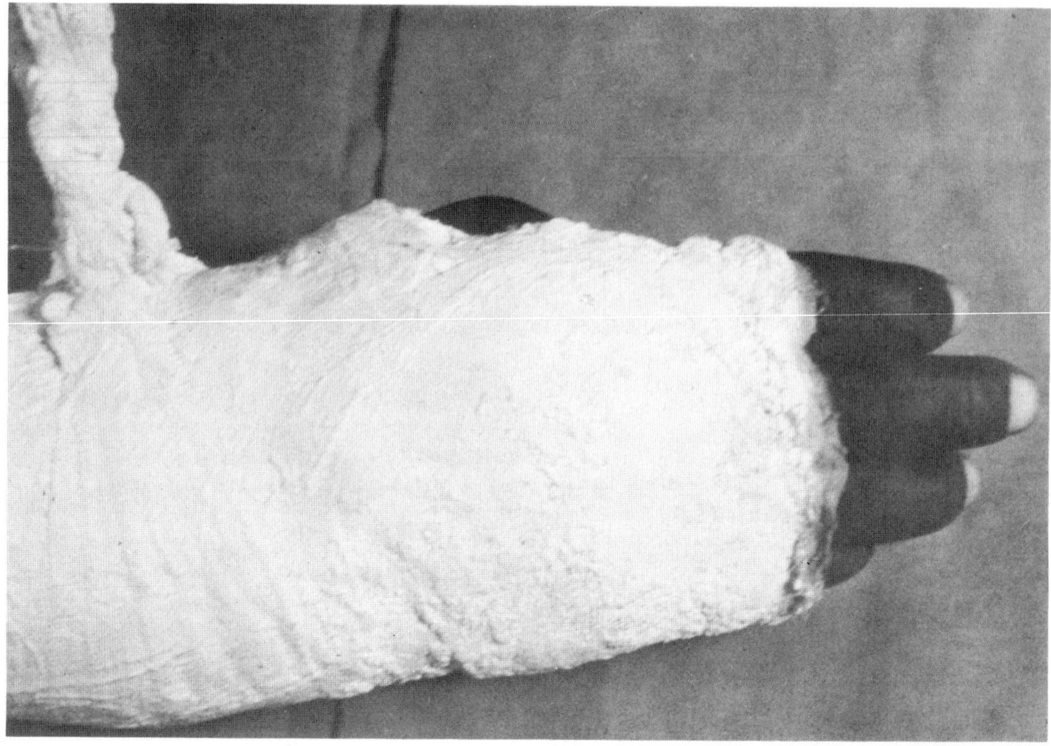

Fig. 1-45. This is the hand portion of a poorly applied hanging cast. Not only is this plaster rough and improperly applied, but extending over the fingers, it limits their motion and holds the metacarpophalangeal joint in extension. Such a monstrosity, applied for even a short time, can cripple a hand.

bent out with a pair of pliers. This also applies to the margins of the thumb hole (Fig. 1-44).

Immobilization of the metacarpophalangeal joints of the fingers, especially in extension, must be avoided like the plague, owing to the danger of permanent stiffness (Fig. 1-45; see Chap. 6).

On occasion, patients in casts will be seized by an uncontrollable itch. In their efforts to get relief, they commonly unravel a coat hanger and scratch under the cast with the wire. Not only do they scratch up their skin, but the padding may be wadded up and cause a pressure sore.

Felt pads placed over bony prominences may migrate and have the opposite effect from that intended. If they are applied as the last layer before the plaster, they will be anchored to the cast. They must never be placed between the layers of sheet wadding.

The Tight Cast. Care should always be taken not to wrap a plaster bandage too tightly. However, even when a cast was not tight when applied, if the limb swells, it may become tight later. Pain is the first and most constant complaint of the patient with a tight cast; and even when the peripheral circulation appears unimpaired, the prudent course is to split the cast (Fig. 1-46). It is not enough merely to split the plaster; the padding must be split to the skin too. Sheet wadding soaked in blood may be just as unyielding as the plaster itself. Circular bandages of gauze or encircling adhesive tape should never be applied under a cast, because these, too, may have a tourniquet effect (Fig. 1-47).

Wherever possible after internally fixing

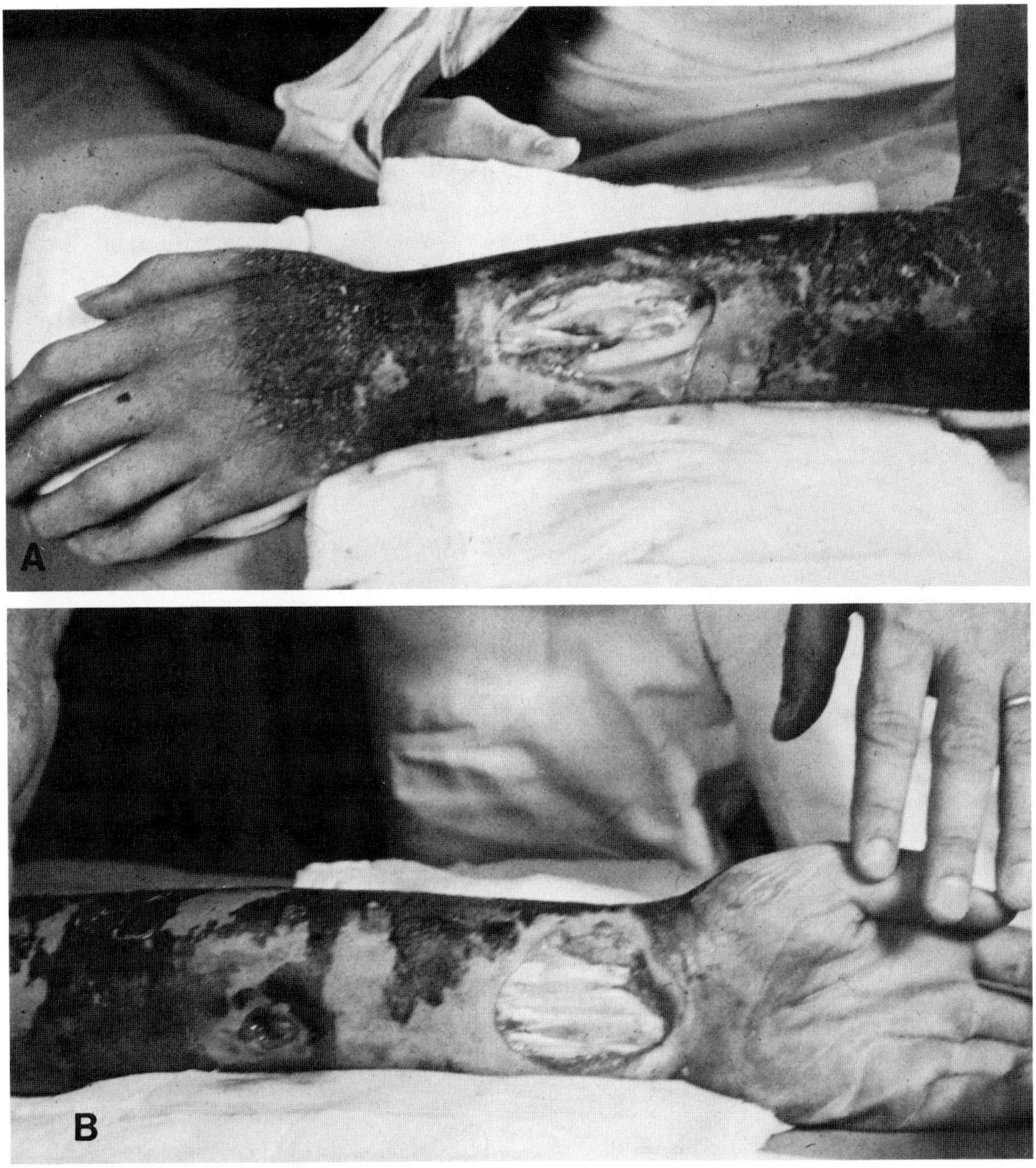

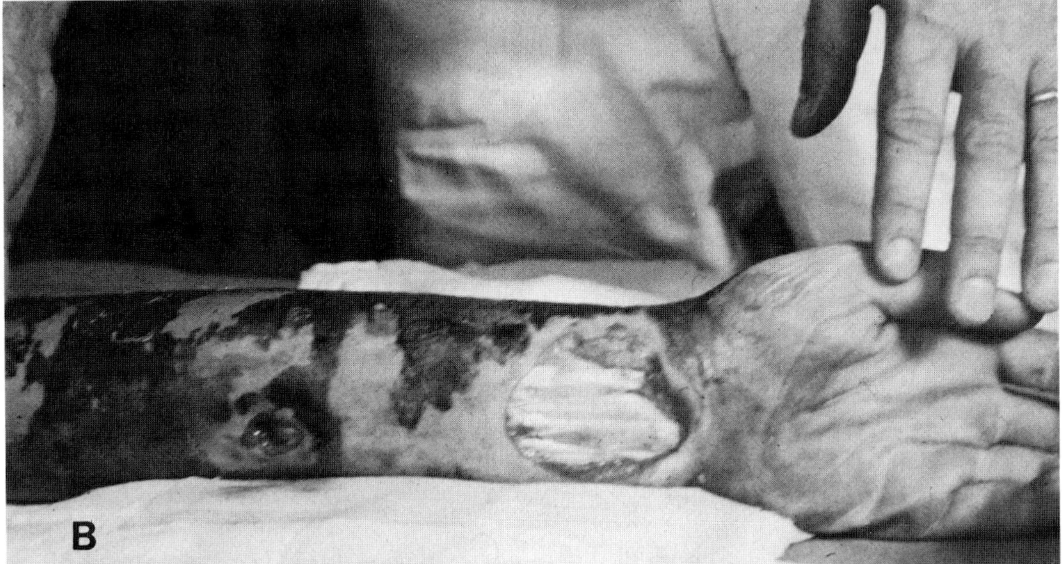

Fig. 1-46. (*A, B*) This young man had an open fracture of his left forearm treated by a plaster-of-paris cast. When, subsequently, the arm became infected and swollen, his complaints of pain were disregarded. Ultimately his entire forearm became necrotic. This is how it looked immediately prior to amputation.

fractures or where swelling is expected, I use a Jones type dressing, with or without plaster reinforcements. The Jones dressing is a bulky dressing usually applied after knee surgery. It consists of a thick layer of absorbent cotton bandage wrapped with domett or elastic bandages followed by two more layers of cotton and bandage. I have modified this by using Kling or Kerlex bandages and cheap cotton batting instead of absorbent cotton and finishing the last layer with an elastic bandage.

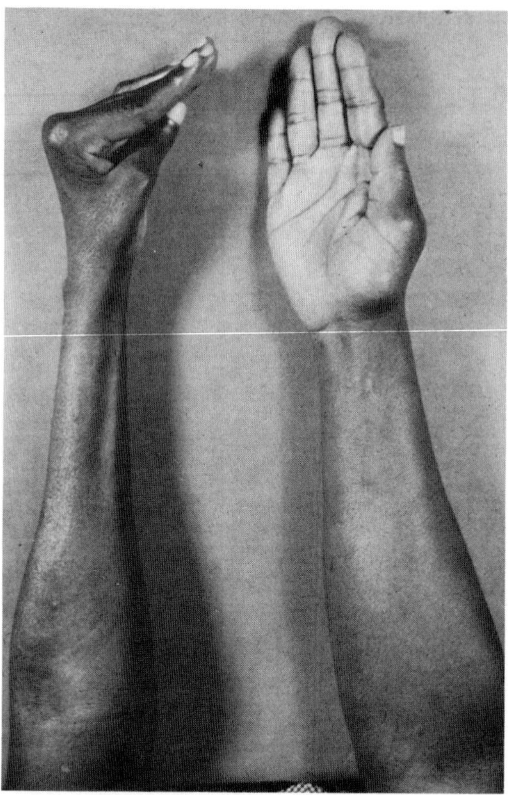

Fig. 1-47. The end result of circular constriction may be Volkmann's ischemic contracture, which in this case involved the intrinsic muscles of the left hand. This is the "main d'accoucheur." When a patient complains of pain, all encircling dressings and plaster-of-paris casts must be split.

Where additional stability is required, slabs of plaster are placed on the medial and lateral sides of the limb. A similar sort of bulky dressing may also be used in the upper limb. This should not be called a compression dressing, because then people will be encouraged to apply them too tightly. It should be applied without much tension and if too tight, it is easily removed with scissors in seconds.

The Cast Syndrome. In the past, compression fractures of the spine have been treated with hyperextension body jackets. Some patients treated in this way developed pernicious vomiting and electrolyte imbalance and even died. This "cast syndrome" is due to an obstruction of the third portion of the duodenum resulting from constriction by the superior mesenteric vessels.[121] Few people now believe that immobilization of stable compression fractures of the spine is necessary, and certainly the position of extreme hyperextension should be avoided.

Some nervous individuals feel unduly constricted by any type of cast that encloses the body, a condition akin to claustrophobia. They, too, are liable to vomit and have a variety of psychosomatic complaints, which lead to the cast having to be removed. The vomiting in such cases is rarely as severe and life-threatening as in the true cast syndrome.

Traction Hazards. Patients in traction develop pressure ulcers just as readily as those treated by plaster. The skin in contact with the ring of a Thomas splint, the sacrum, and other pressure areas must be inspected daily. In some of the high risk patients, the sacrum should be protected by an "antigravity pad." A sheepskin, real or synthetic, is also helpful to preserve the back of a patient who will be in traction for extended periods. The heels and heel cords are particularly liable to develop decubiti and should be protected by heel caps or sponge rubber pads.

If the foot is allowed to lie in the equinus position, a permanent drop-foot contracture may develop. This should be prevented by active exercise, and the provision of some type of device to hold up the foot.

Circular bandages should be checked and reapplied as necessary to prevent constriction of the circulation and to assure that the skin tapes are not slipping.

Under no circumstances, should the lower extremity be allowed to rotate externally in a Thomas splint. This may cause pressure on the common peroneal nerve with subsequent paralysis.

In the treatment of fractures of the cervical spine, traction by means of a head

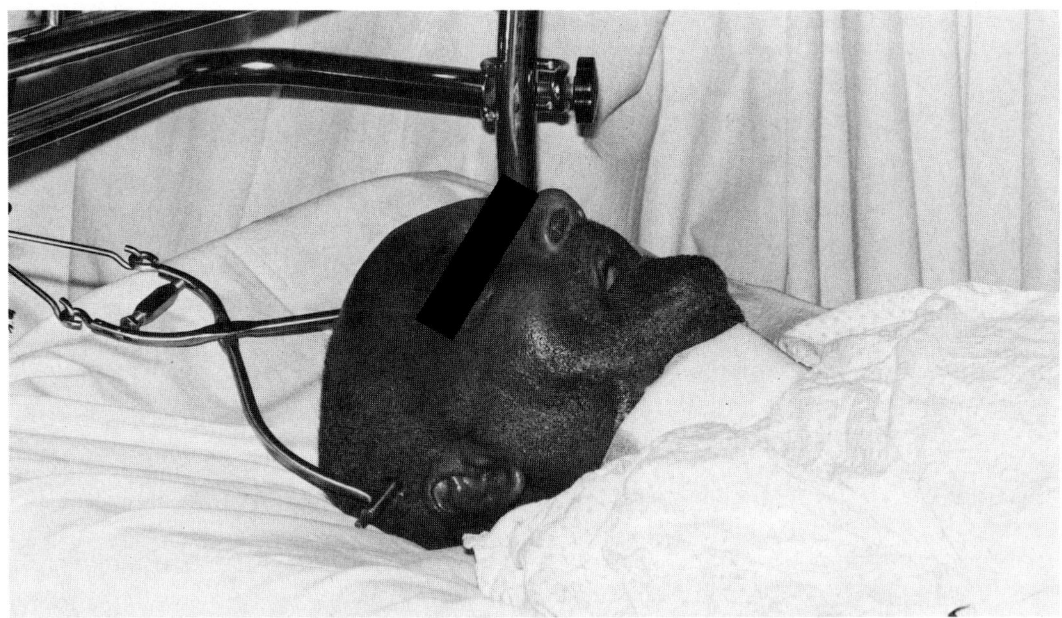

Fig. 1-48. Traction for injuries of the cervical spine should be by means of some type of skull tongs. The use of the head halter for more than a short period of time, especially if heavy weight is to be used, will give rise to excoriation of the skin over the chin.

halter should only be used for a short time, as sores develop readily over the chin. Skull tongs should be inserted as early as possible (Fig. 1-48).

INTERNAL FIXATION OF FRACTURES

Lord Lister repaired a fracture of the patella with silver wire, and Hugh Owen Thomas used silver wire ligatures in the treatment of open fractures of the mandible. However, it is probably true that the father of internal fixation of fractures was Sir Arbuthnot Lane.[79,102]

Initially, Lane used wire transfixion stitches or steel screws, but in 1907, he described the use of plates. These plates were made of German silver or steel in the beginning, but later he used only plates of steel. Unfortunately, the deleterious effects of metallic corrosion were not appreciated in those days; and loosened screws, broken plates, rarefying osteitis, and signs of inflammation were frequent. Lane himself ascribed these untoward complications to infection and incompetence on the part of the surgeon. To circumvent such infections, he invented his celebrated "No-Touch Technique," where instruments were used instead of fingers, and the business ends of instruments were never touched by hand.[79]

The fact that metal appeared to produce serious reactions in the tissues tempted surgeons to use as little as possible, and implants were made so skimpy that their mechanical effectiveness was impaired. As recently as 1952 Sir Reginald Watson-Jones was advocating the treatment of difficult comminuted fractures by the use of a single screw.[173] Sherman, in the United States, criticized Lane's plates because they broke too easily and invented this own plates which were much stronger.[155] Lane made his plates longer and stronger to take care of the serious fractures being sustained in World War I, but it was only after the introduction of stainless steel, by Lange, and

Vitallium, by Venable and Stuck[167] of San Antonio, that internal fixation came into its own.

Types of Internal Fixation

Wire Fixation. Although wire fixation was one of the earliest means of internally fixing fractures, it appears to be in disrepute in English-speaking countries. Charnley has decried the use of circumferential wiring.[33] The evil effects, he believes, are due to circumferential stripping of the periosteum and the encircling wire's obstructing the bridging of periosteal callus. Furthermore, he maintains that the fixation provided by wiring oblique fractures is vastly inferior to that obtained by screws, and the fact that such treatment is successful is "a tribute to the remarkable healing power of bone." In rebuttal of this view, Thunold has treated 18 oblique fractures of the tibia by cerclage, all of which went on to uncomplicated union without rarefaction or abnormal bone apposition around the wires.[167] Rhinelander, after making microcirculatory studies of the effects of cerclage, states, "This time-honored technique has been strongly condemned on the ground that a circumferential wire loop strangles bone. The periosteal blood supply, however, enters the cortex through innumerable small vessels. No periosteal arteries of the long bones run longitudinally to be pinched off with encircling wires. Callus grows abundantly over the wires, which are tight and hold the fracture reduced. It is only when the immobilization is insuffiicent that troubles arise."[140] It is generally agreed that Parham's bands, since they cover a much greater area, do significantly interfere with periosteal circulation, and they are best avoided.

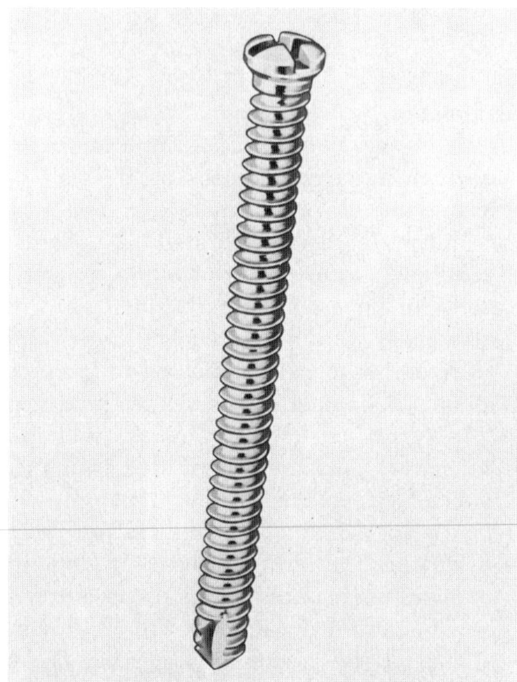

Fig. 1-49. This is a drawing of a typical machine screw. It is threaded from the head to the tip. The head is the cruciate or Woodruff type and there is a fluted end which indicates it is self-tapping. (Courtesy, Zimmer, U.S.A.)

In my own practice, I use cerclage sparingly but have found it useful in supplementing intramedullary nailing of the femur where there is a loose butterfly fragment. It is also an excellent method of treating transverse fractures of the patella and fractures of the olecranon. In the latter case, the wire is passed through a drill hole in the ulnar shaft, and a figure-of-eight rather than a simple loop is used to approximate the loose fragments.

Fixation by Screws and Plates. *Machine Screws.* The screw most commonly used in orthopaedics is the machine screw, threaded from head to tip and with a blunt end. To insert these screws in bone, a preliminary drill hole must be made. Following this, threads may be cut by a tap prior to the insertion of the screw, or the screw may be designed to cut its own path with a fluted tip (this is a self-tapping screw; Fig. 1-49). The head of a typical screw may have a single slot to accommodate the screwdriver, but more commonly screws now have a cruciate head.

The *pitch* of a screw is the distance between threads, and the *lead* is the distance

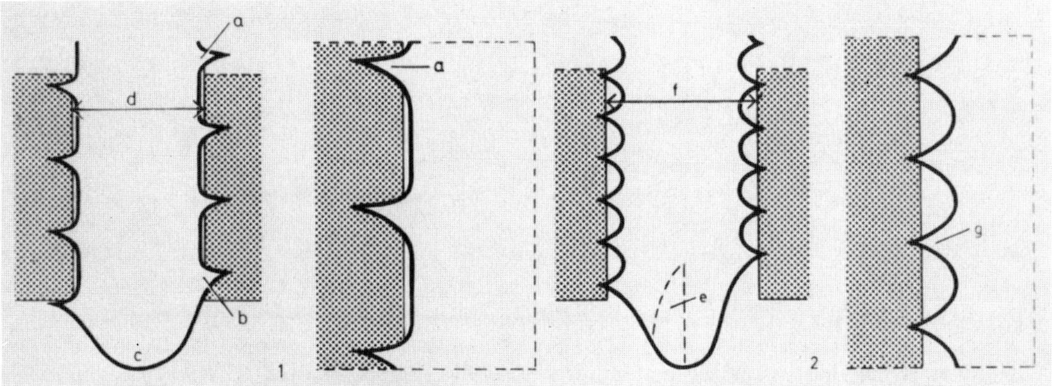

Fig. 1-50. (1) The thread of the AO screw, which is at right angles to the axis and has a greater purchase on the bone than the conventional self-tapping screw (2). (Müller, M. E., Allgöwer, M., and Willenegger, H.: Manual of Internal Fixation. New York, Springer-Verlag, 1970)

through which a screw advances with one turn. If the screw has only one thread, then the pitch and lead of the screw are identical. However, if there is more than one thread, then the lead of the screw is increased proportionately to the number of threads. A double-threaded screw has a lead of double the pitch, and this allows the screw to be tightened more rapidly.[63]

The tensile strength of a screw, or its resistance to breaking, depends on the root diameter of the screw (the minimum diameter between threads), while the pull-out strength depends on the outside diameter of the threads. The number of threads per inch has no effect on the pull-out strength of the screw, provided five or six threads are in the cortex. In very osteoporotic bone with thin cortices, this may be a factor, in addition to the diminished strength of the bone.

Although Bechtol and Lepper[12] feel that thread configuration is of very little importance, Frankel and Burstein disagree.[63] They say that the ability to resist stripping depends on the total cross-sectional area of material presented to the root of the thread (Fig. 1-50). Koryani *et al.* found no difference in the holding power of the V-threads of coarse and fine Sherman screws and the buttress threads of the ASIF screws, but in comparing the holding power of the fluted ends of the fine and coarse Sherman screws with the shank of the screw, they found a reduction of 17 per cent and 24 per cent, respectively.[97]

Fixation of fractures by screws alone is mechanically feasible only in long oblique and spiral fractures. To attempt to fix transverse or short oblique fractures with one or more screws is mechanically unsound. Although the medical literature is replete with roentgenograms showing fractures fixed by screws inserted at right angles to the fracture line, this is the least secure configuration. Arzimanoglou and Skiadaressis compared the results of fixing a standard fracture by screws inserted at right angles to the shaft, at right angles to the fracture line, and by a combination of the two.[5] The greatest stability in compression was obtained by screws inserted at right angles to the shaft, and the least by those inserted perpendicular to the fracture line. Müller *et al.* have endorsed this principle, but for treating spiral fractures with a loose butterfly fragment they recommend fixing the two major fragments with a transverse screw and inserting the remaining screws at an angle midway between the perpendiculars

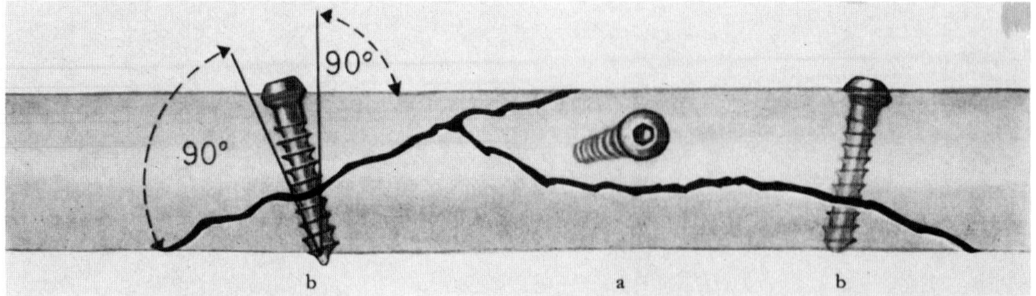

Fig. 1-51. This illustration demonstrates the AO method of fixing a spiral fracture by screws. The screw connecting the two major fragments is inserted at right angles to the long axis of the shaft while the remaining two screws holding the butterfly fragment in place are inserted at an angle bisecting the perpendiculars to the shaft and the fracture line. (Müller, M. E., Allgöwer, M., and Willenegger, H.: Manual of Internal Fixation. New York, Springer-Verlag, 1970)

to the shaft and the fracture line[117] (Fig. 1-51). Although transverse screws give the greatest stability against compression, the combination position gives more protection against bending in an axis perpendicular to the screws.[63]

There is general agreement that when machine screws are used in this manner, the near cortex should be over-drilled. This allows the screw head to be countersunk and, more importantly, produces a lag effect, which compresses the fracture line.

Wood Screws. Wood screws have a taper and a sharp point. The neck portion is unthreaded, and these screws force their way into bone without needing a preliminary drill hole. They are not suitable for use in cortical bone, because they tend to split it. They have been recommended for use in cancellous bone, although Venable states, "No screw holds well in cancellous bone. Wider threads to increase holding power intensify the concentration strain on the screw with an increasing absorption rate of calcium about the screw."[169] Other lag screws have been developed by the ASIF group for use in cancellous bone and to fix femoral condyles and tibial plateaus. I would much sooner use these or Knowles' pins than wood screws.

Plates. Short oblique and transverse fractures may be treated by plates and screws. The plates should be long and rigid enough to impart stability to the fracture, and preferably should be screwed to the bone extraperiosteally. Inevitably, the circulation of the periosteum under the plate will be impaired, but further damage should not be inflicted by wide periosteal stripping. Damage to the periosteal sleeve by stripping the end of the bone may produce a ring sequestrum and impede union.

Technically, several points need emphasizing.[133] The plate should not be scratched or treated roughly; the screw holes should be drilled using a drill guide to center the screw hole and direct it at right angles to the shaft. A screw centered incorrectly, so that it does not fit the well in the plate, has a great deal of unnecessary stress on the head and is liable to fail. The length of the screw should be accurately determined by a depth gauge, an instrument that looks like a crochet hook with a scale. The hook is caught on the far cortex, and the screw size is read from the scale. The screws should not be tightened all the way until the last screw is inserted, and the tension on the screws should be made as uniform as possible.

It is essential to use the correct diameter drill point. If the drill hole is too large, the screw will have no purchase; and if too small, the screw will bind and the cortex

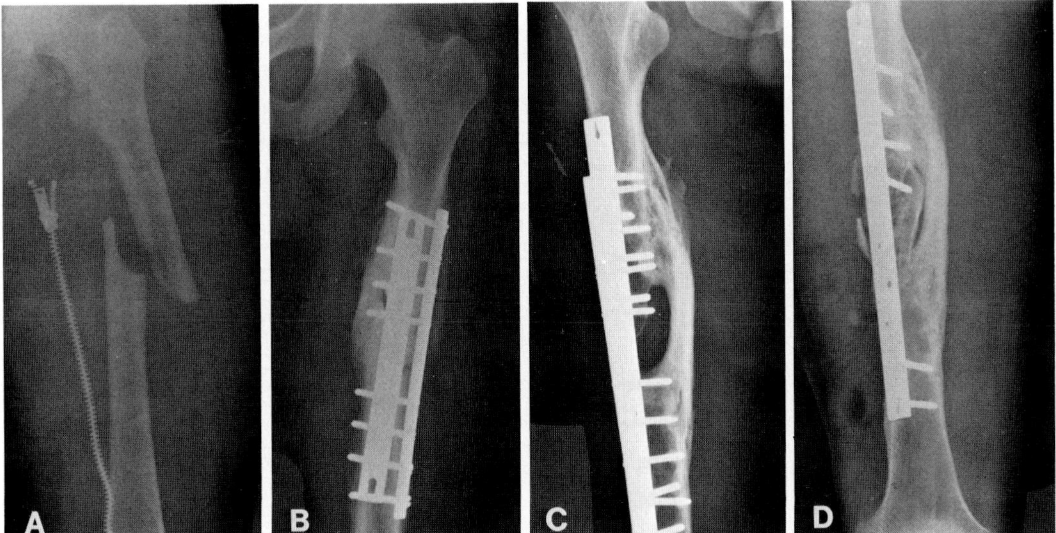

Fig. 1-52. (*A*) This spiral fracture of the femur was "immobilized" by an inflatable splint that barely reaches the fracture site. (*B*) End result after application of two plates at 90 degrees. Proponents of rigid plating would not be pleased by the obvious periosteal callus. (*C*) Another patient treated by this method had resorption of a butterfly fragment. The stability of these rigid plates maintained the femur while a periosteal "flying buttress" formed. (*D*) Same case after bone graft and the removal of one plate. If both plates are removed simultaneously there is serious danger of refracture through screw holes.

may split. Bechtol and Lepper advise that the diameter of the drill should be midway between that of the root of the screw and that of the thread.[12] They also state that the screw holds best when inserted by a torque equal to 75 per cent of that required to strip the screw.

Whether one uses hand tools or power equipment is a matter of personal choice, but care should be taken not to burn the bone. The risk is much greater when dull drill bits are used, so these should be discarded. Tungsten-steel drills are exceedingly sharp, but also brittle. If they are to be used, they must never be angulated or treated roughly; lest they snap off in the bone and become permanent monuments to one's surgical ineptitude.

If the plate has to be bent to make it conform to the contour of the bone, it should be done before it is applied. Otherwise, it will be bent by the insertion of the screws. This will give rise to unequal tension on the screws and a greater chance of screw failure.[133]

In general, the most secure fixation and the best results are obtained with the heavier, stronger plates. When a fracture is plated, the bone itself carries the majority of the compression load. The resistance of a plate assembly to bending depends on the strength of the screw fixation, and in torsion the load is transmitted as a bending moment to the screws. The most secure fixation of all would be that achieved by having two plates on opposite sides of the bone; but this, although mechanically sound, may be biologically disastrous. Plating of shafts by two plates at 90 degrees has been advocated by Murray *et al.* and gives excellent fixation but is open to criticism because it requires excessive soft-tissue dissection and periosteal stripping.[118,134] However, bone is quite capable of healing

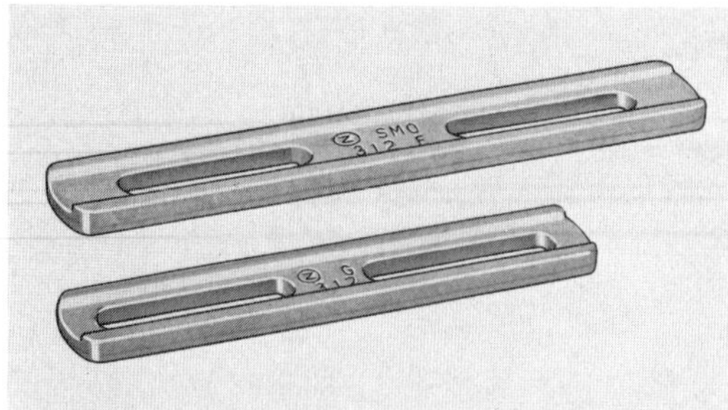

Fig. 1-53. Eggers compression plates with slots that allow impaction of the fracture prior to tightening the screws. (Courtesy, Zimmer, U.S.A.)

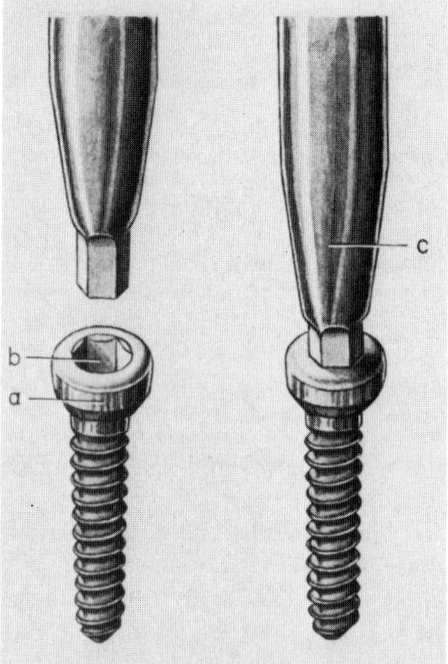

Fig. 1-54. The AO screw and screw driver. The screw head has a shallow cylindrical flank which gives better contact with the hole in the plate, and the hexagonal screw driver with matching recess in the screw gives a much larger surface area for transmission of the torque from the screw driver to the screw. (Müller, M. E., Allgöwer, M., and Willenegger, H.: Manual of Internal Fixation. New York, Springer-Verlag, 1970)

without periosteal callus, provided the endosteal circulation is intact, and these authors reported excellent results (Fig. 1-52).

While the purpose of plates is to hold fractures together, sometimes they succeed only in holding the fragments apart. Eggers invented slotted plates so that the fractures could be impacted at the time of surgery to prevent this difficulty[50] (Fig. 1-53). The belief that these plates allow the fractures to impact later, after resorption at the fracture site, is not well-founded.

Compression Plating.[117] The most dramatic innovation in the internal fixation of fractures has been the development of implants and instruments by the ASIF or AO (Swiss Association for the Study of Internal Fixation). The aims of the AO treatment are to secure anatomical reduction and, by providing rigid internal fixation, to allow "early, active, pain-free mobilization of the muscles and joints adjacent to the fracture, without interfering with bone union." Their system includes various types of intramedullary nails, blade-plates and lag screws, but the most significant contribution has been the use of heavy rigid plates and the enhancement of fixation by compressing the fracture site. Axial compression is achieved by means of a plate, often erroneously called a compression plate, but more correctly named a tension band. After the fracture is reduced, the tension band is applied to that aspect of the bone that will be in tension (i.e., the convexity of the fracture angulation or side opposite the soft-tissue hinge). The plate is then screwed to one fragment, and the tension device is applied to the opposite end. A guide is inserted into the last hole of the plate to determine where the hole should be drilled for the tension device. The tension device is a worm screw, which, when tightened, pulls the plate toward it, thereby compressing the fracture site. When sufficient pressure is applied to the fracture site, the remaining screws are inserted into the plate and

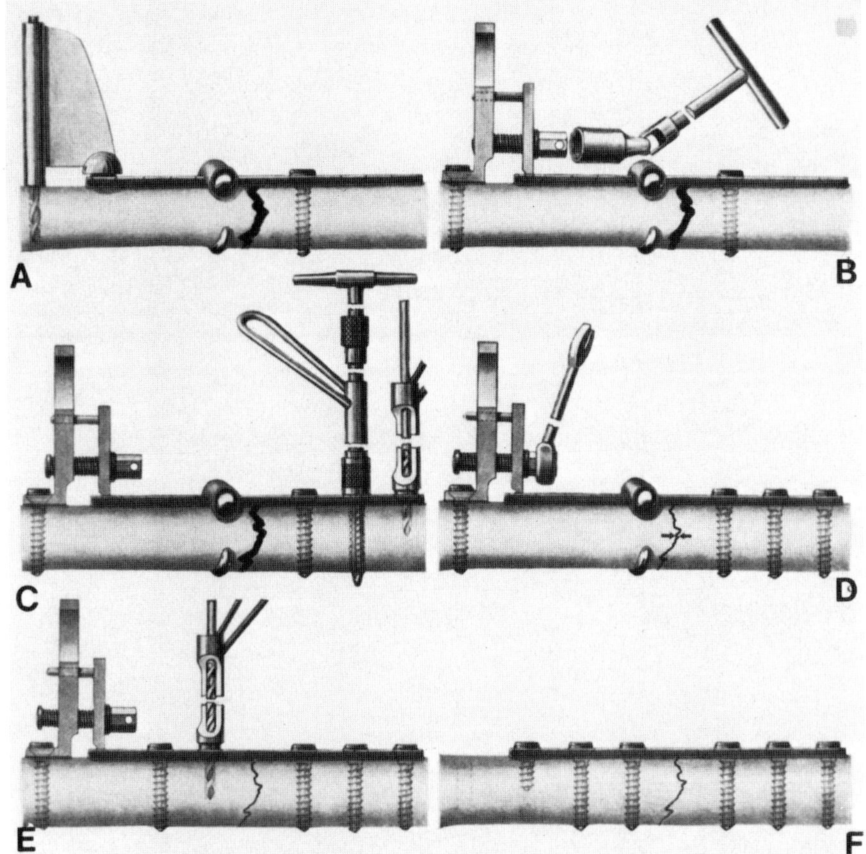

Fig. 1-55. These diagrams illustrate the steps in applying a straight tension band. (*A*) The plate is applied with a single screw and using a guide, a hole is drilled for anchoring the tension device. (*B*) The tension device is applied and tightened until the reduction is complete. (*C*) The remaining screws are replaced in one end of the plate. The holes are pre-drilled using a centering device, after which the threads are tapped and the screw is inserted. (*D*) Extra compression is applied by means of an open-ended wrench. (*E*) The remaining screws are inserted on the other side of the fracture line. (*F*) The completed compression plating. The short screw gripping only one cortex is said to smooth out the gradation between the normal elastic bone and the rigid segment deep to the plate. (Müller, M. E., Allgöwer, M., and Willenegger, H.: Manual of Internal Fixation. New York, Springer-Verlag, 1970)

the compression device is removed (Figs. 1-54, 1-55).

A second type of tension band is a plate similar to that described by Bagby, where axial compression is applied by inserting screws eccentrically into oval holes in a semitubular plate (Fig. 1-56). More recently this principle of applying compression by the insertion of screws into plates with slotted holes has been incorporated into the design of the Dynamic Compression Plate (DCP). This plate is made of titanium, and the slot for the screw has a sloping surface at one end on which a

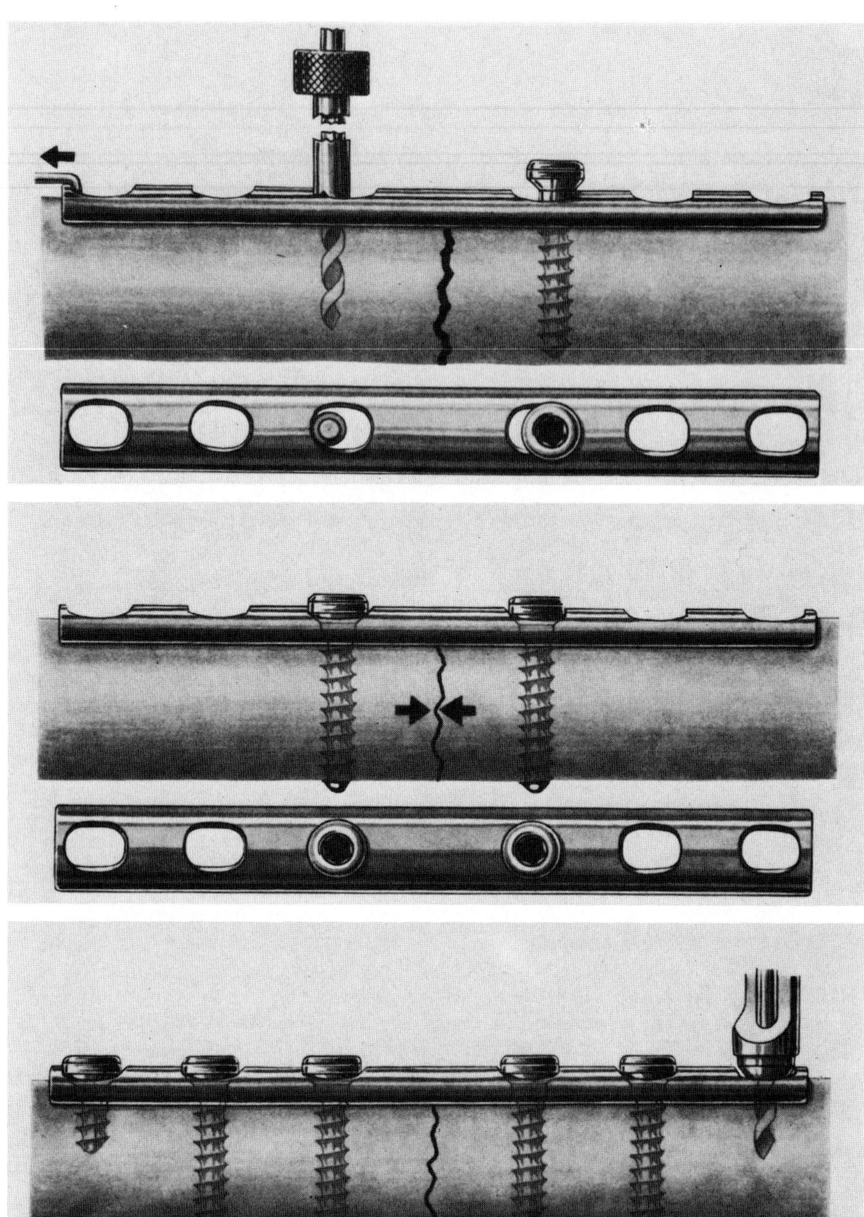

Fig. 1-56. This demonstrates the use of the semitubular plate of the AO system. The tightening up of eccentrically placed screws produces motion of plate and compression at the fracture site. (Müller, M. E., Allgöwer, M., and Willenegger, H.: Manual of Internal Fixation. New York, Springer-Verlag, 1970)

spherical screw head impinges to produce movement of the plate and compression of the fracture site.[2A] As the screws are tightened, the fracture site is compressed. The screws immediately proximal and distal to the fracture are inserted first and the others subsequently. The semitubular plates find their greatest use in fractures of the forearm, where it is difficult, especially in fractures of the proximal third, to employ the compression device, or in small bones such as the fibula or the fifth metatarsal.

Oblique and spiral fractures are treated by "interfragmental compression." The near cortex is over-drilled to produce a lag effect and compression of the fracture line. The large hole at the head of the screw has been called the "gliding hole," and the far one, the "thread hole."

In some comminuted fractures, especially in the tibia, where interfragmental compression does not provide sufficient stability, a neutralization plate is employed. This plate is narrower than a tension band but is also applied under axial compression. The compression may be applied in two ways. In the metaphysis, the plate is applied across a concavity, so that when the plate is screwed down, compression is produced. In the diaphysis, the neutralization plate is pre-bent, so that there is a gap of 1 or 2 mm. between the middle of the plate and the bone. One screw is applied to the middle of the plate into a major fragment, and the compression device is inserted into the other major fragment and compression is applied. The remaining screws are then inserted. Such neutralization plates are used most frequently in fractures of the tibia, where the plate is most commonly applied to the medial surface.

Double plating is never used in diaphyseal fractures but may be necessary in metaphyseal fractures.

The regular AO cortex screw has a thread diameter of 4.5 mm., and the head has a hexagonal recess that fits the screwdriver (Fig. 1-54). In attaching a plate, a 3.2-mm. drill bit is used with a drill guide to make sure the hole is accurately centered. The hole is then threaded with a tap, and the screw is inserted (Fig. 1-55). When the screws are used for interfragmental compression, a 4.5-mm. drill is used to make the gliding hole. A drill sleeve with an outer diameter of 4.5 mm. is inserted in the hole until it abuts on the opposite fragment. A 3.2-mm. drill is then used to make the thread hole, which is then tapped, and the screw is driven home.

The insertion of screws into a bone immediately reduces the breaking strength of the bone. Bechtol and Lepper state that, when the holes are placed in an area of tension, the weakening effect is greatest.[12] The size of the hole has little effect on the breaking strength, so long as it is less than 20 per cent of the diameter of the bone. When this size is exceeded, the degree of weakening is proportional to the size of the hole. The presence of a screw also weakens the bone to the same extent as an unfilled hole, but the effect diminishes with the production of new bone. Brooks *et al.* studied the influence of drill holes on torsional fractures in paired canine femora.[21] With a 2.8-mm. hole and a load applied for 0.1 seconds, the mean reduction in energy absorption was 58.5 per cent, and for 3.6-mm. holes, 51.9 per cent. Since the energy absorbed is reduced, these fractures have less comminution.[21]

Burstein and his associates at Case Western Reserve University also found that a fresh screw hole weakened bone in bending and torsional loading. Whereas Bechtol found 20 per cent to be the critical level, Burstein determined that the screw hole had no effect on breaking strength until it exceeded 30 per cent of the diameter of the bone. When torque was applied to the drilled bone, the stresses around the hole were 1.6 times greater than those over the remainder of the bone, and when failure occurred, the fracture line passed through the drill hole in over 90 per cent of the bones tested. With time, however, the strength of the bone increases even with the screw *in situ,* but after removal of the screw the bone is again unduly susceptible to fracture. However, rather surprisingly, in these cases the experimental fracture line passed through the screw hole in only six of 38 fractures.

The presence of a rigid plate changes the modulus of elasticity of the bone, and the

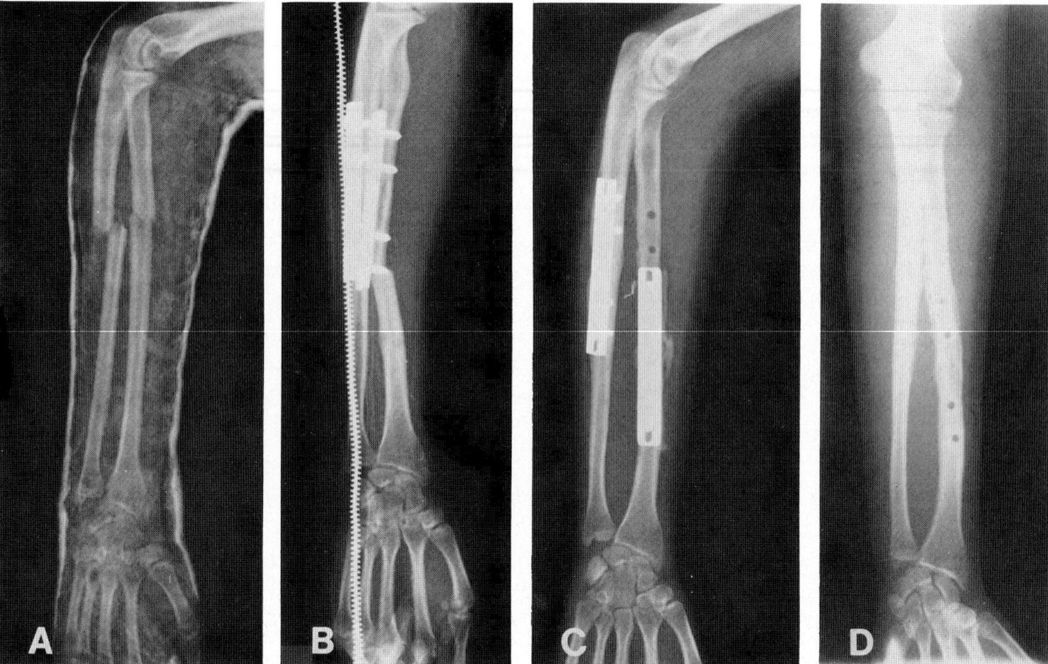

Fig. 1-57. (*A*) This 14-year-old girl sustained a fracture of both bones of the forearm. (*B*) Eight months after compression plating she refractured through the lower screw in the radius. (*C*) This fracture, too, was treated with a compression plate and the addition of an osteoperiosteal graft from her rib. (*D*) The appearance some 4 months later, after removal of both plates. The holes in the bone persist for some considerable time roentgenographically, but histologically the holes have healed by woven bone after 6 weeks in spite of their roentgenographic appearance.

sharp transition between plate and bone predisposes to fracture at the lower end of the plate. An attempt to decrease the magnitude of this change may be made by inserting the terminal screws through only one cortex. This problem may also be alleviated by the use of titanium alloy plates, which have greater flexibility. Yet another reason for removing plates is the inevitable corrosion, with time, between the plates and screw heads. This is more important in the lower extremity, where greater stresses are applied to the plates and the amplitude of motion between the plate and screw is correspondingly increased.

This has a therapeutic implication. Over a 2-year period at Louisville General Hospital, we had a 20-per-cent refracture rate in forearm fractures treated by compression plating. These fractures occurred through screw holes that were made either for attachment of the plate or the compression device (Figs. 1-57; 1-58). This encouraged us to switch to intramedullary Schneider nails, which are easier to remove and do not present this hazard.

After a fracture treated by compression plating heals it may be necessary to remove the internal fixation. These very rigid plates bypass the stress normally borne by the bone, so that atrophy occurs in that segment of the bone, making it more liable to refracture.

The holes left after removal of the screws are very obvious and are outlined by reactive bone. These holes are stress risers until healing occurs. Although these screw holes remain evident on roentgenograms for a long time, this does not mean that they have not healed. Histological examination

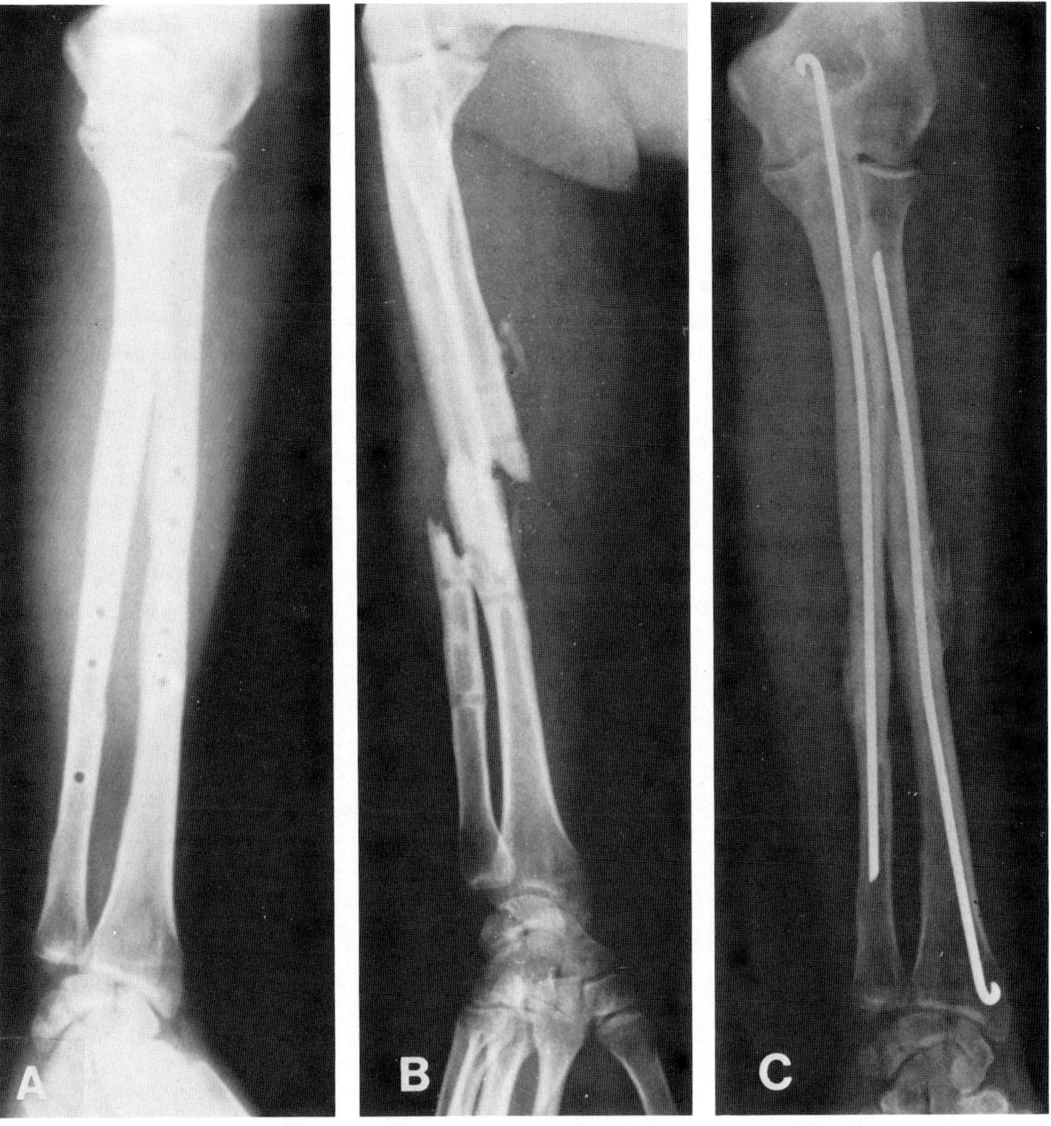

Fig. 1-58. (*A*) This young man had a fracture of both bones of the forearm treated by compression plates. It can be seen that there is some attenuation of the shaft of the radius where the plate has been. (*B*) Exactly two months later, following a trivial injury, he has refractured through the upper screw hole in the ulna and through the attenuated area of the radius. (*C*) The appearance of the forearm 11 months later, after the insertion of Rush nails and the addition of osteoperiosteal grafts from the rib.

has shown that they are filled by woven bone 6 weeks after removal of the screws. Reaming of the holes after removal of the screws is not helpful, because it does nothing to enhance the rate of healing.[27] Our high refracture rate was due, at least partially, to our not protecting the forearms after removing the plates. We now protect the forearm with a cast for 4 to 6 weeks after removal of the hardware.

The treatment of fractures by screws alone is unlikely to provide enough fixation to dispense with external immobilization, since such fixation is very vulnerable to torque. The addition of a plate may provide the additional stability to obviate a cast and allow active exercise.

Bynum *et al.* studied compression plating in horse metacarpals and found that in flexural loading the worst configuration was where the plate was under compression, and the best, where the bone was loaded from the side opposite the plate.[29] In the first case, the whole load was borne by the plate, and in the second, where the plate was under tension, the bone sustained some of the weight. In compression, transverse fractures did well, but when a cut was made at 45 degrees to the fracture a serious weakening resulted. Oblique fractures fared better than transverse fractures when torsional loads were applied, but in no case was the strength of the plated metacarpal adequate to sustain the stresses imposed by unrestricted weight bearing.

Laurence *et al.* compared the efficacy of various plates in the fixation of tibial fractures.[103] In both bending and torsion, a combination of two Venable plates was stronger than a 13-cm. Campbell plate, an 11-cm. "heavy duty Swiss-type plate," a 15-cm. Hicks plate, and the 14-cm. Stamm plate. A single Venable plate, however, was the weakest of all. The Stamm plate was strongest in compression; the Hicks, in torsion.

In this study, the bending moment required to fracture an intact tibia varied from 59 to 226 Newton-meters (mean = 137). However, tibias with 3-mm. drill holes fractured with 29 to 147 Newton-meters (mean = 98), and the Stamm plated tibia failed at 24 Newton-meters. Since quiet walking imposes 80 Newton-meters bending moment on the tibia, it is obvious that unrestricted weight bearing would not be feasible in plated tibias. Similar findings resulted in a study of torsion moments. Hicks feels that his lug plate is just as efficient in the treatment of tibial fractures as the AO (ASIF) plates.

Clinically, the ideal end result of rigid plating is what Danis calls "soudure autogene" (i.e., primary endosteal healing without perceptible periosteal callus).[125] The degree to which external callus forms is an index of the amount of motion at the fracture site. When ideal fixation is attained, there is no resorption of bone ends, and the fracture heals by revascularization of the bone ends and endosteal callus. Olerud and Dankwardt-Lilliestrom studied healing in dog tibias where a double osteotomy had been performed with removal of the loose segment to ensure its complete avascularity.[125] When this loose fragment was replaced and fixed by a compression plate, they found that within 2 weeks ⅕ of the intermediate fragment had vessels in the Haversian canals which were derived from the endosteal circulation. Both the intermediate fragment and the bone ends were being remodelled by simultaneous bone resorption and new bone formation in the Haversian systems.

Intramedullary Nailing. Hey Groves inserted the first intramedullary nail in a femur during the First World War,[76] and writing in 1921 on ununited fractures he states:

> It occurred to me therefore to use a long internal peg or strut, such as would render unnecessary any further fixation and would afford absolute rigidity. I have used pegs of various shapes, cylindrical, cross-sectional, and solid rods; and I am inclined to think that the last named are the best, because they give maximum strength, and there is an avoidance of hollows and crevices which form dead spaces.

His description of the operative technique could be as easily applied to the insertion of a present-day Schneider or Hansen-Street nail.

Hey Groves was defeated by inadequacies in metal, and it remained for Gerhardt Küntscher to rediscover, refine, and popularize intramedullary nailing.[98-101] Since that time, a variety of nails have been designed, and every long bone in the body has been treated in this manner (Fig. 1-59). The

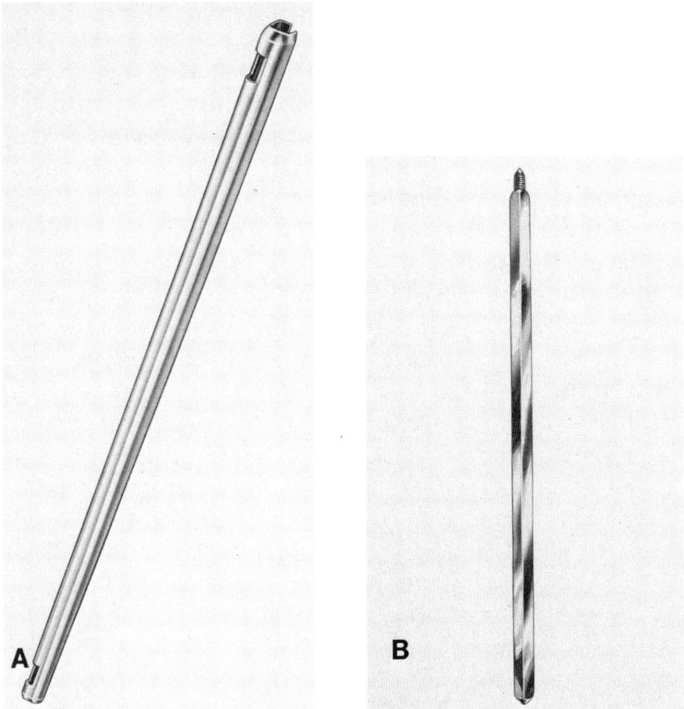

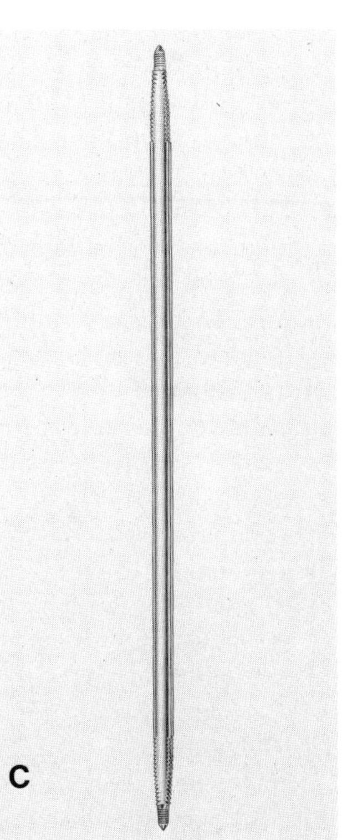

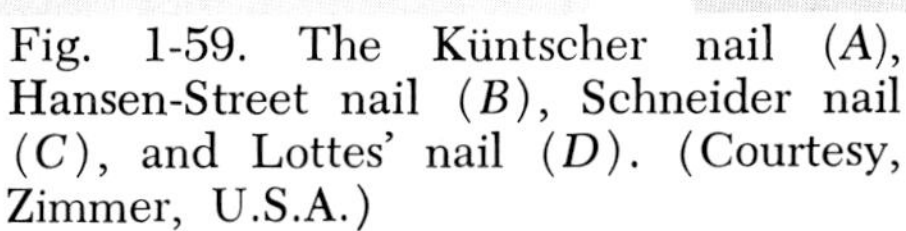

Fig. 1-59. The Küntscher nail (*A*), Hansen-Street nail (*B*), Schneider nail (*C*), and Lottes' nail (*D*). (Courtesy, Zimmer, U.S.A.)

nails may be inserted by open operation or blindly, under roentgenographic control.[14,15,37,100] The invention of the image intensifier and flexible reamers have made the latter technique much easier and less time-consuming. Küntscher's blind reaming of the medullary cavity and the insertion of very thick nails for all types of femoral shaft fractures has been endorsed by Clawson; but in general, surgeons in the United States tend to believe that open nailing is safer and that the results are as good.[37]

Biomechanically, intramedullary nails provide excellent protection against angulatory stresses but are very poor in resisting torque.[2] They function best in transverse, midshaft fractures, but almost every type of diaphyseal fracture has been treated by this method, with or without modifications.

The *Küntscher nail* is shaped like a cloverleaf in cross section and is designed to be introduced into the bone over a guide

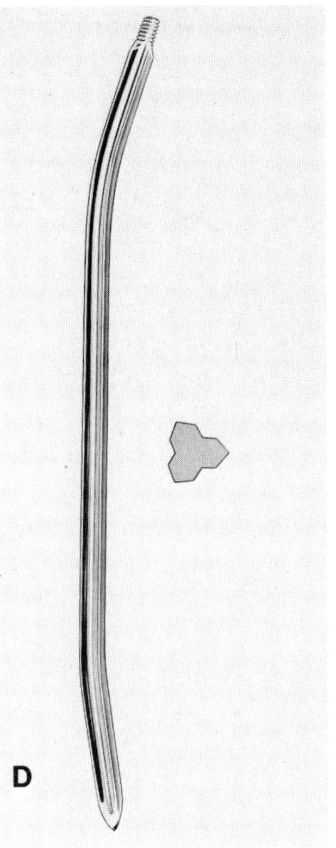

wire after preliminary reaming of the medullary cavity (Fig. 1-59). There is an open section in the nail which allows it to be compressed. Küntscher emphasized that this is an essential feature, since it allows compression of the nail by the isthmus of the medullary cavity, which he felt prevents the nail from loosening and helps to control rotation. The disadvantage is that the nail is a great deal weaker because of this open section. When inserted, the strongest configuration for the nail is to have the slot on the tension side (i.e., pointing away from the soft-tissue bridge). If placed in the reverse configuration, the nail tends to buckle when subjected to high load.

The greatest usefulness of the Küntscher nail is in fractures of the femur, and it is the only nail that lends itself easily to blind nailing. The greater the diameter of the nail, the greater its strength. For this reason, the femoral shaft should be reamed to allow the passage of as large a nail as possible, and the reamer should be 1 mm. larger than the diameter of the nail. No more than 4 mm. should be removed, nor should the cortex be reamed to less than half its original thickness.[37]

Inevitably, this medullary reaming destroys the endosteal circulation. It follows, therefore, that healing must of necessity be by periosteal callus. This is confirmed by roentgenograms of healed fractures, which show enormous wads of callus around the fracture. The exhaustive experimental work of Dankwardt-Lilliestrom and Olerud confirms this, and in addition, they have shown that the cortex is also infarcted by marrow forced into the cortex under pressure.[42] Under these circumstances, it would appear that the less the periosteum is damaged, the better will it be for healing. This is another incentive to perform this procedure by closed methods.

The two other most commonly used nails are the *Hansen-Street*[162,163] and *Schneider nails* (Fig. 1-59).[154] The Hansen-Street nail is diamond-shaped on cross section, while the Schneider, the strongest of all the nails in common use, is square with flanges. Since the Schneider is a self-broaching nail, no preliminary reaming is necessary.

Intramedullary nails have great resistance to bending moments but carry little, if any, of the compression load. If there is good gripping between the nail and the bone, torsional forces are transmitted to the nail, but in this regard, the open section of the cloverleaf nail makes it inferior to the others.

The working length of a nail is that portion of the nail that is left unprotected by intact bone. This varies from a few millimeters in transverse fractures to several centimeters in comminuted fractures. The greater the working length, the less rigid is the fixation. Burstein and Frankel have shown that the rigidity of the nail with ¼-inch working length is 16 times that of a nail with a working length of one inch. Another factor of importance is the area of contact between the nail and the bone. This, of course, is enhanced by reaming, and Clawson recommends each fragment have 2.5 cm. of total contact.

Intramedullary nailing is said to be particularly indicated in transverse or oblique fractures of the upper two-thirds of the femoral shaft, provided they are not higher than 5 cm. distal to the lesser trochanter. However, spiral and comminuted fractures are commonly treated by intramedullary fixation, often supplemented by circumferential wires or screws. The addition of a plate enhances the stability of the fracture to torque and has been recommended by Burwell for use in femoral fractures and by Massie in fractures of the tibia.[28,65,111]

Fractures below the flare of the femur are not immobilized well by intramedullary nails alone, because the distal fragment can rotate easily on the nail. One solution to this problem is the Vesely-Street split diamond nail, which exerts a much better grip on the distal fragment.[171] Another means of increasing resistance to torque is to embed the nail in methyl methacrylate.

Fractures of the tibia are also amenable to treatment by intramedullary nails (curved Lottes' nails[107,108] (Fig. 1-59) or a variety of straight nails). Fractures in the distal third of the tibia are similar to distal fractures of the femur, in that it is difficult to protect them from torque. In the forearm, nails to fix radial fractures must be prebent, and intramedullary nailing and plaster-of-paris casts to control rotational stresses are excellent methods of treatment.

Most intramedullary nails act by filling the medullary cavity. *Rush nails* (Fig. 1-58), however, are much smaller, with a round cross section, and have a hook at one end and a sled-point runner at the other. These nails are inserted with a curve under tension and immobilize by three-point fixation (i.e., the ends of the nail and where the curve of the nail is in contact with the opposite cortex). These nails have the advantage of being inserted blind or with a very small exposure, and they do not interfere drastically with the endosteal circulation. The technique of inserting these nails is demanding, and I do not believe the fixation is as good as that obtained with other nails.[143] However, Rush has reported a large series of femurs treated in this manner with admirable results,[144] and Holst-Nielson, in a smaller series, confirms the efficacy of this treatment.[84]

Complications of Intramedullary Nailing. The main hazards of intramedullary nailing are those due to trying to drive a nail down a medullary cavity that is too small. Excessively vigorous efforts in this direction may split the shaft longitudinally, or the nail may hang up so that it cannot be driven onward or easily retracted. This, of course, may be avoided by adequate reaming.

Not infrequently, subsidiary fractures that have not been conspicuous on the preoperative roentgenograms may separate. If these fragments are of considerable size, some form of subsidiary fixation may be required.

It is important to select a nail of the proper length and diameter. Preoperative scanograms (spot orthoroentgenograms) of the intact opposite extremity is the method I prefer for determining the length, although measuring with a tape measure may be accurate enough. If the nail is too long, it is liable to transgress the adjacent joint, or its proximal end will be prominent and give rise to discomfort and an adventitious bursa. A nail that is too short may not stabilize the fracture, or, even worse, may become completely intramedullary giving rise to considerable difficulties in retrieval. The latter complication is most likely to occur in the tibia.

A nail that is small in diameter is most likely to bend or break and will not adequately immobilize the fracture. With motion at the fracture-site, there will be rarefaction around the lower end of the nail where the cancellous bone has been resorbed—the windshield wiper sign (Fig. 1-60). In femoral fractures, when this happens, the nail frequently extrudes in the buttock. When a reinjury occurs in the femur with angulation at the fracture site, Küntscher nails often break; and this usually presents no great difficulty in removal. The solid Hansen-Street and Schneider nails tend to bend rather than break, and this presents a most difficult problem. The nail may be straightened before removal, but this is hazardous and may cause catastrophic fracture. In my experience, it has been impossible to straighten such nails completely. "Straightened" nails should always be removed, because once they have been bent, it is easier to deform or break them. The best solution, I believe, is to cut the angulated nail with a carborundum wheel in which diamond chips are embedded. Such a wheel on a power saw cuts the nail with astonishing ease. If a deformed

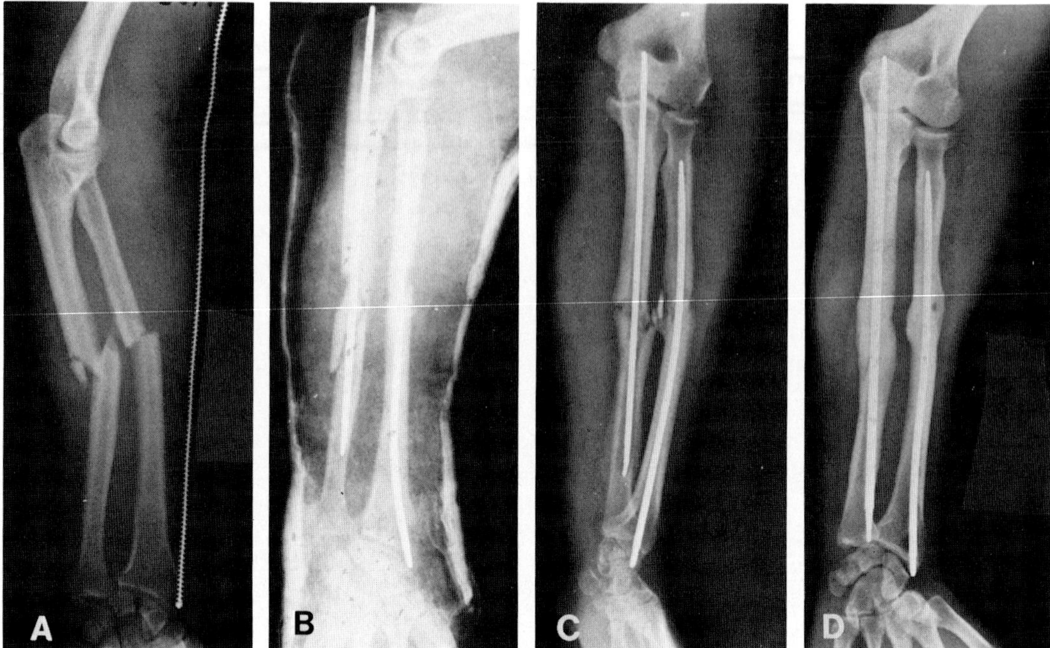

Fig. 1-60. (*A*) This patient sustained a fracture of both bones of the forearm. (*B*) There is an obvious loose butterfly fragment in the ulna, and the intramedullary nail used is too short to maintain stability. (*C*) Three months later there is an obvious nonunion of the ulna and motion of the lower end of the nail has eroded the bone, giving rise to the "windshield wiper sign." (*D*) After this nail was removed and replaced by a larger, longer nail, a solid union was obtained.

nail is left *in situ* and the fracture heals, it may be impossible to remove. This can be very embarrassing for the surgeon.

In the early days, there was considerable apprehension that the displacement of marrow fat during nailing would give rise to fat embolization. This has not proven to be a significant danger, although a circumspect surgeon will delay such operations for 10 days, or at least until the patient is out of shock and stabilized for several days.

Corrosion of Implants[19,32,71]

When two dissimilar metals are in contact with each other in an electrolyte solution, one of these metals will be positive relative to the other, according to their positions in the electromotive series. Atoms from the anode go into solution as positively charged ions, leaving the anode negatively charged. Were there no cathode, the negative charge on the anode would tend to attract these metallic ions back. However, at the cathode another reaction is going on, which takes electrons from the cathode metal surface: $4e^- + O_2 + 2H_2O = 4OH^-$. With contact of the metal surfaces, there is a flow of electrons (i.e., an electric current is produced, and the negative charge is reduced on the anode so that the attack on the anode continues). This is sometimes called a battery effect, as it is essentially the same process that goes on in an electric cell. Even in a single metal, a battery effect can be produced. If a strip of iron is immersed in a salt solution, the portion nearest the surface, where the oxygen tension is greatest, becomes the cathode; the anode is a zone at a deeper level. Where the cathode is large and the anode small, the corrosion is greatest. If the cathode is a plate and the anode a screw, severe corrosion takes place. For this reason, different metals should not be used in the same assembly, especially when they are far apart in the electromotive series. However, Hicks and Cater[82] have shown that mixing of plates and screws made of the more inert metals such as Vitallium and titanium does not give rise to significant corrosion.

If a layer of oxide is present on the surface of the metals, it acts as a block to the passage of ions. The presence of molybdenum in an alloy is a help in the formation of a passive oxide barrier, and stainless steel used in the manufacture of implants should contain 2.5 to 3.5 per cent molybdenum. The oxide layer can be thickened artificially by treating it with nitric acid (passivation) or electrochemically (anodizing).

In spite of the improvements in stainless steels, corrosion still occurs, and some of the mechanisms postulated to explain these cases are:

Transfer of Metals from Tools to Implant. Using radioactive tracer techniques, Bowden, Williamson, and Laing showed that significant amounts of metal were transferred from screwdrivers to screw heads and from drills to plates.[16] This difficulty could be solved by using tools made from the same material as the implant, by making the screwdrivers harder, and by using drill guides to prevent contact between drill and plate. Hicks and Cater,[82] however, did not believe that this transfer of metal was of any clinical significance.

Crevice Corrosion. Differences in oxygen tension or concentrations of electrolytes or changes in pH in a confined space, such as in the crevices between a screw and a plate, may result in local corrosion called crevice corrosion or "contact" corrosion.[58]

Fretting Corrosion. Cohen subjected plate-and-screw assemblies to cyclic stress in saline solutions and found the greatest corrosion in the screw assemblies where the heads rubbed on the plate and where the nuts and washers were in contact.[39] He felt this was most probably due to abrasion of the metal surfaces removing the protective oxide coating (i.e., fretting). Similar assemblies not subjected to the cyclical stresses did not show this marked effect.

Stress-Corrosion Cracking. Stress-corrosion cracking is a phenomenon in which a metal in certain environments, especially those rich in chlorides, is subjected to stress and fails at a much lower level than usual as a result of corrosion.

In austenitic steels a process called sensitization may result when implants are subjected to heat treatments during manufacture. It is believed that some of the chromium becomes converted to chromium carbide, so that the grain boundaries of the metal lose their protective coating of chromium. This gives rise to increased corrosion because (1) the metallic grains lose the passivation effect of chromium oxide and (2) a galvanic effect accentuates corrosion because of differences in the composition of the grain itself and its boundary region. Stress accentuates this destructive effect, giving rise to failure.[71]

Choice of Metals for Surgical Implants

If one were to be able to create the ideal implant material, it would be inert, nontoxic to the body, and absolutely corrosion proof. It would be cheap, easily worked, and capable of being wrought in a variety of shapes without expensive manufacturing techniques. It would have great strength and high resistance to fatigue.

Unfortunately, this material is not available at the present time. Implants are made of stainless steel; cobalt, chromium, and molybdenum alloys (e.g., Vitallium); and titanium. The characteristics of these materials have been detailed by Brettle in his excellent reviews of this subject.[18,19]

Of the materials available, stainless steel

has the best mechanical properties. It is stronger and has better fatigue resistance. It is easily worked and cheap to manufacture, but it has the serious drawback of corrodibility.

Vitallium has much better corrosion resistance than stainless steel, but it is in every way mechanically inferior. It has to be cast by the very complicated and expensive lost-wax process, and quality control is harder to achieve than with stainless steel. Vitallium also has a low ductility, and screws made of this material bond quite securely to bone. In removing screws that have become securely anchored, it is easy to screw the head off. Wrought Vitallium is a cobalt, chromium, nickel, and tungsten alloy with much more desirable mechanical properties than Vitallium, but no one has yet established whether its corrosion resistance is as good.

Titanium is the most inert of all. It is easily worked, and 1/16-inch plates are radiolucent. Unfortunately, this admirable metal has an extremely low modulus of elasticity (15×10^6 p.s.i., which is much less than the 28 to 30×10^6 p.s.i. for Vitallium and stainless steel). Although titanium alloys eventually may be used instead of titanium alone, it is Brettles' opinion that its modulus of elasticity will not be appreciably altered. Titanium plates and implants will, therefore, have to be bulkier in order to provide adequate rigidity.

Although titanium has been used in the manufacture of implants in Great Britain, it has not been available in the United States. Recently, however, the Zimmer (U.S.A.) Company has announced that it will be manufacturing implants from a titanium alloy (titanium 6AL4V), which they have named Tivanium. These implants will have a surface treatment that will make them gold-colored for easy identification. This alloy is said to have a greater tensile strength than either stainless steel or the chrome-cobalt alloys and almost twice the fatigue strength of these materials. Its ductility is equal to that of stainless steel. The modulus of elasticity is much closer to that of bone than the other implant materials, which may conceivably reduce the load on the implant.

METHOD OF SELECTION OF TREATMENT

The question before the modern surgeon is not whether operative treatment is to supersede manipulative treatment. The problem before each of us is how can we improve our skill and technique in both manipulative and operative treatment and what means we must adopt in each individual case to give to our patients the surest, safest, and most complete restoration of function.

Those who have a large and varied experience of the manipulative treatment of deformity will probably have greater confidence in their ability to deal with deformities resulting from fractures by manipulation and external splinting. They will reserve direct operation for those cases in which they have found that their manipulative skill has not proved equal to returning the limb in a correct position until union of the fragments has taken place.[87] *Sir Robert Jones; An Orthopaedic View of the Treatment of Fractures,* 1913.

The crying evil of our art in these times is the fact that much of our surgery is too mechanical, our medical practice too chemical, and there is a hankering to interfere, which thwarts the inherent tendency to recovery possessed by all persons not actually dying. *H. O. Thomas,* 1833.

The case that starts botched up stays botched up. *Michael Rosco,* 1967.

In the closed treatment of fractures an attempt is made to achieve adequate alignment of the fracture fragments. It is neither necessary, nor, in some cases, desirable to achieve an anatomical reduction. Lloyd Griffiths gives the reasons for reducing a fracture:[72]

1. To insure recovery of function of the limb where that is threatened by displacement of the fracture.

2. To prevent or to delay degenerative

changes in joints, and particularly weight-bearing joints, which will result from persisting deformity.

3. To minimize the deforming effect of injury.

If closed reduction is unsuccessful, Griffiths states, "the wrong technique may have been employed, or the fracture was unsuitable for closed reduction."

THE CHOICE OF OPERATIVE TREATMENT

With the advent of improved metals and better-designed implants, there has been an increasing trend, especially in continental Europe, to open reduction and internal fixation of fractures. The possible indications for such open reductions are:

When Closed Methods Have Failed

This failure, as Lloyd Griffiths has pointed out, may be due to the ineptitude of the surgeon, but undoubtedly, closed reduction will fail in the hands of even the most expert if the fragments of bone are impaled in soft tissues or if an otherwise suitable fracture for closed manipulation has been seen too late. If bony apposition and adequate alignment cannot be achieved, then open operation is indicated.

When It Is Known from Experience that Closed Methods Will Be Ineffective

Few would disagree that fractures of both bones of the forearm in adults or Monteggia and Galeazzi fractures are unlikely to be handled adequately by closed methods, so that open reduction and internal fixation is the method of choice. Similarly, fractures of the femoral neck would be poorly treated by traction or plaster immobilization.

When Articular Surfaces Are Fractured and Displaced

Even minor incongruities in the articular surfaces of joints will result in derangements of function and the eventual appearance of degenerative arthritis. This is particularly so in the joints of the lower extremities. In studying the end results of tibial condylar fractures, Rasmussen found that 4 to 11 years after injury 21 per cent of his patients had demonstrable osteoarthritis of the affected knees, while the same patients had an incidence of two per cent[137] in their uninjured knees.

Not all of this, however, could be ascribed to articular injury alone. Although bicondylar fractures gave the worst results, and poor results were associated with persistent condylar widening, other factors, such as valgus and (even more so) varus deformity and instability were also important. Rather surprisingly neither age, *per se,* nor localized joint depression appeared to affect the end result significantly.

Proponents of open reduction of T-shaped fractures of the lower end of the humerus and fractures involving the knee joint claim better results in their series than could be obtained by closed methods,[31,55,66,90] while proponents of early motion without operation contend the reverse[4,92,131] (Figs. 1-61, 1-62). By and large, it seems to me that the operative treatment of these injuries is difficult but when performed well, gives the best results (Fig. 1-13). On the other hand, the end results of poorly conceived and executed surgery are disastrous. Occasionally unstable fractures of articular surfaces may be reduced by manipulation and fixed percutaneously (Fig. 1-63). The choice of treatment must depend to some extent on the skill and experience of the surgeon.

In injuries to joints where loose fragments are knocked off, the tendency has been to remove them. When this is done in the hip joints, degenerative arthritis almost always supervenes early, so that primary arthroplasty has been recommended.[89] A review of fractures of the femoral head by Kelly has shown that the best results were

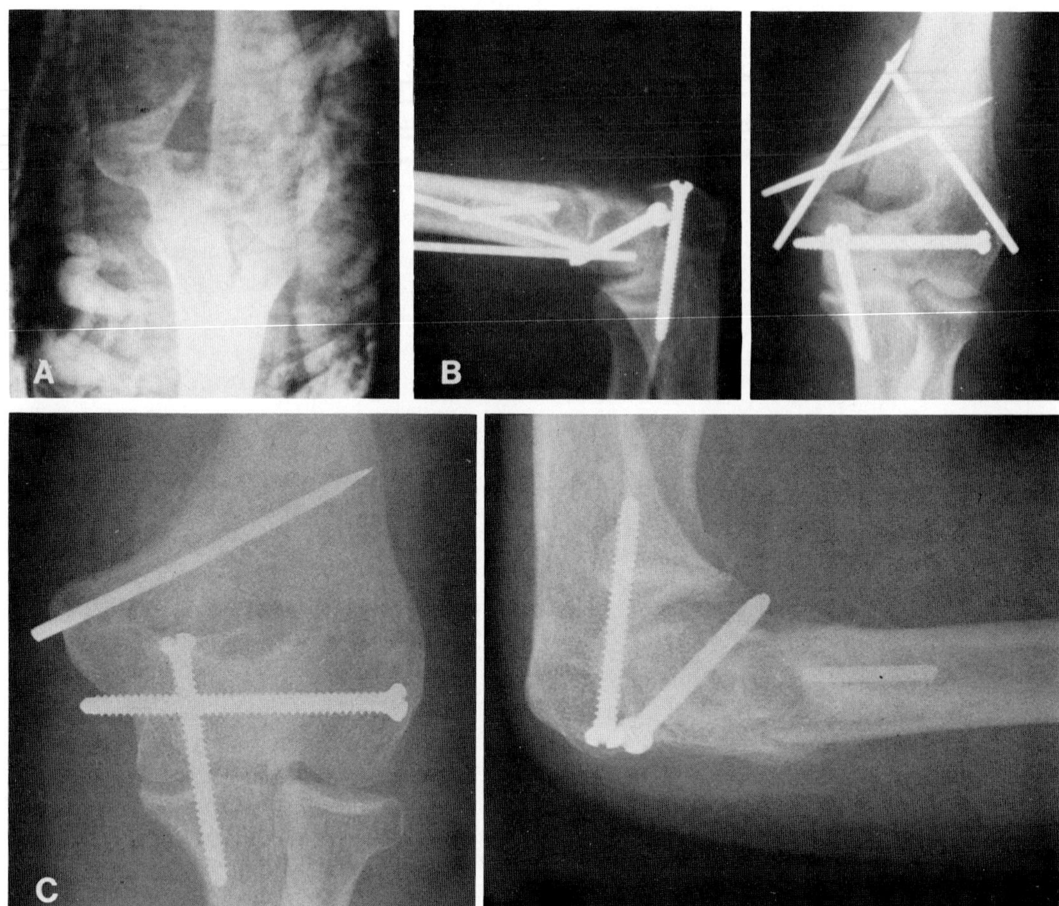

Fig. 1-61. (*A*) This 35-year-old woman fell on the point of her elbow, sustaining a comminuted **T**-shaped fracture of the lower end of the humerus. (*B*) The fracture was approached by osteotomizing the olecranon process, so that damage to the triceps muscle was minimized. The trochlea was reduced and fixed by a transverse screw, and the distal fragment was attached to the shaft by means of Steinmann pins. It would appear that one of the pins through the medial epicondyle is aberrant. (*C*) Two of the Steinmann pins were removed early because they presented under the skin and caused pain. The end result, however, was extremely good with almost a complete range of motion of the elbow.

obtained when the loose fragment was reduced by manipulation. When this could not be accomplished, open operation with internal fixation of the fragment gave an end result much superior to excision of the fragment (Fig. 1-64).[91]

When the Fracture Is Secondary to Tumor Metastasis

This subject is covered in Chapter 5. Internal fixation of such fractures relieves pain, makes nursing easier, and often allows the patient to return home and spend precious time with his family.

When There Is an Associated Arterial Injury

It has long been held that, where an arterial injury has been suffered in conjunction with a fracture, fixation of the fracture is mandatory in order to protect the arterial repair. Doubt is thrown on the concept by

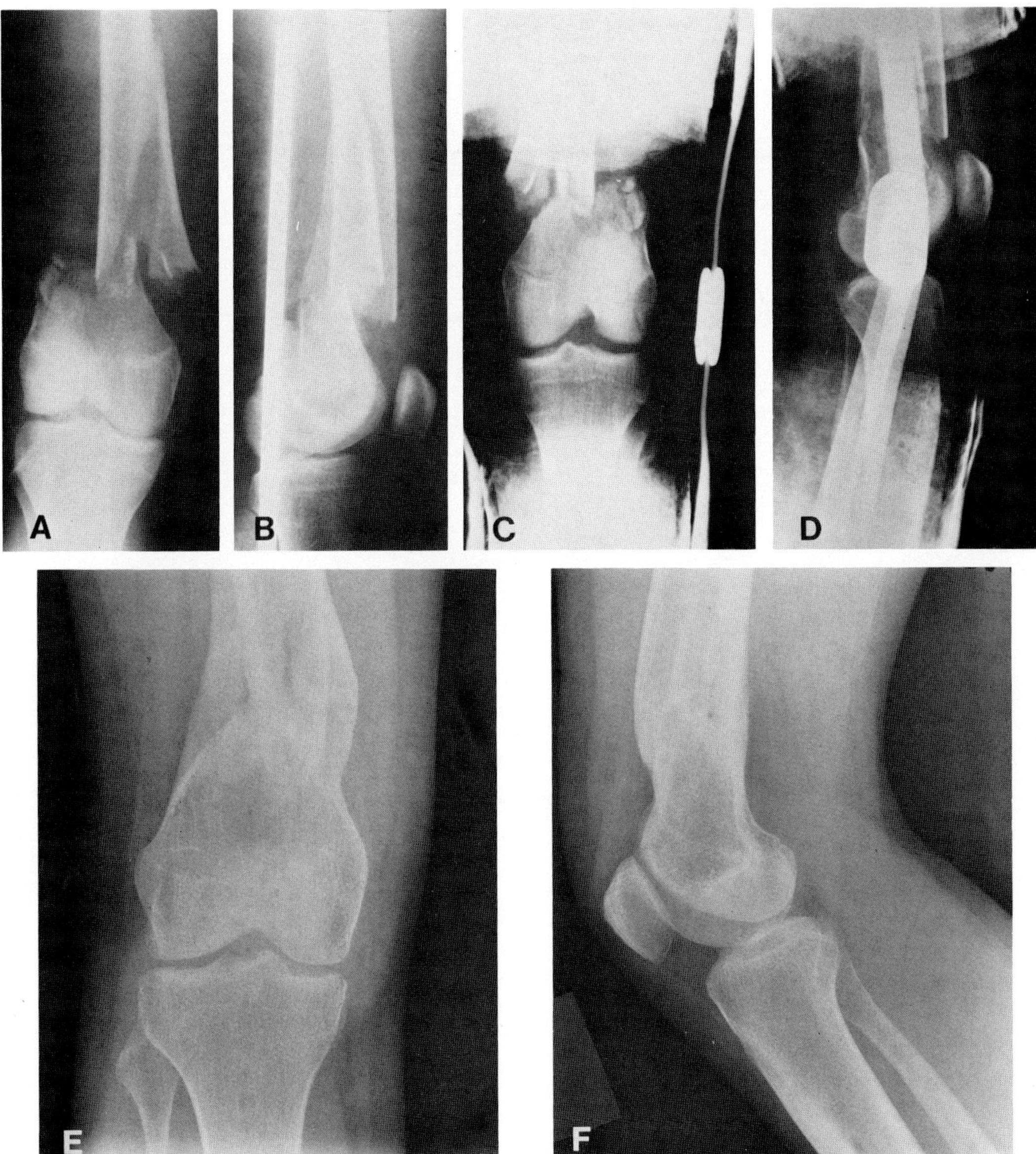

Fig. 1-62. (*A, B*) A 17-year-old girl sustained this fracture as the result of an accident on a motorcycle. In addition to the obvious fractures of the supracondylar region, she has an undisplaced fracture separating the condyles. (*C, D*) She was treated initially in traction followed by the application of a cast brace. (*E, F*) The final result; in spite of the fact that she does not have an anatomical reduction, she has a complete range of motion and no obvious cosmetic defect.

Rich *et al.* in their review of arterial injuries sustained in Vietnam.[141] Of 29 patients who had simultaneous arterial repair and internal fixation of the associated fracture, ten later came to amputation. Five of these amputations were directly due to infection of the fracture and the anastomosis, and half of the patients had complications from the intramedullary nail which dictated its removal. Although a series of

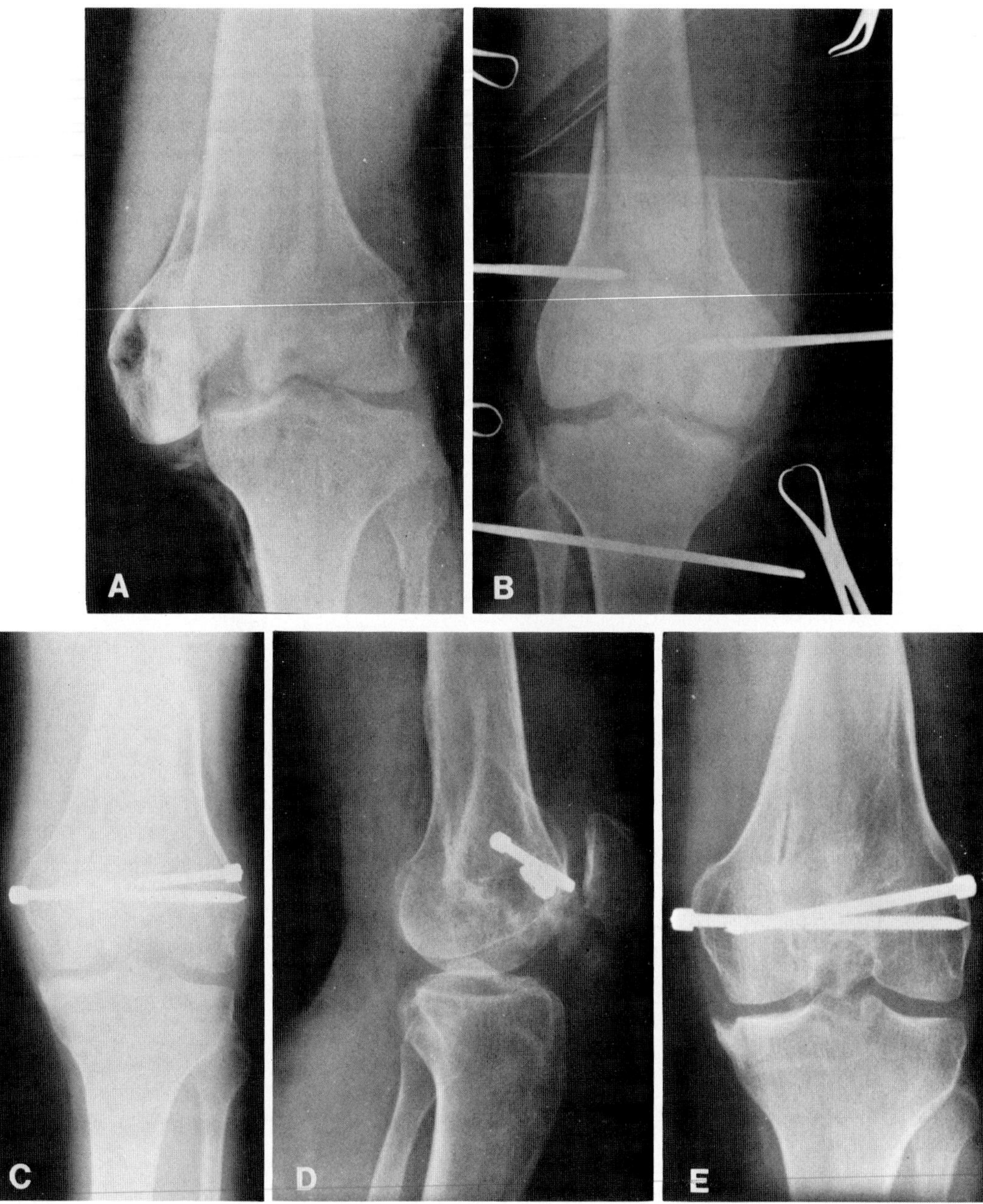

Fig. 1-63. (*A*) This unfortunate man had his right leg smashed between the bumpers of two cars when one ran into the back of the other. He sustained a large popliteal laceration with complete division of his popliteal vessels. The vessels were repaired and the popliteal laceration was grafted. Further operative treatment of his fractures was deemed unwise. (*B*) Since an adequate reduction could not be obtained by traction alone, the fragments were manipulated percutaneously by Knowles pins and when satisfactory alignment had been obtained, the pins were driven across the femur. (*C*) The appearance of the femur 4 months later. (*D*) A lateral view, however, shows a fragment anteriorly which united in malposition. (*E*) Seventeen months later there is an erosion of the medial plateau, but the patient has excellent range of motion and a painless joint. In spite of many invitations to have the aberrant fragment removed from his joint, he has steadfastly refused to have further surgery.

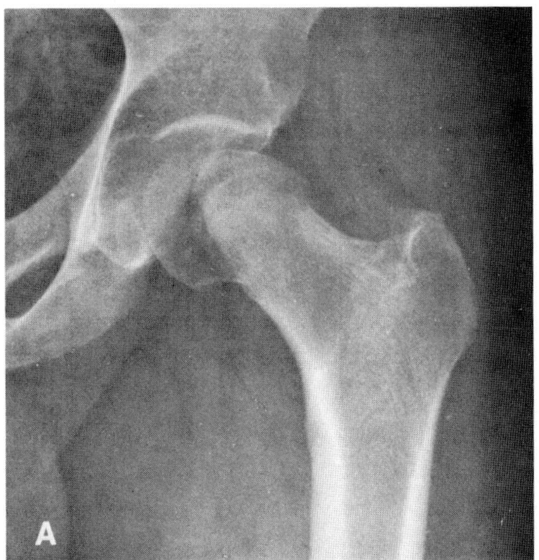

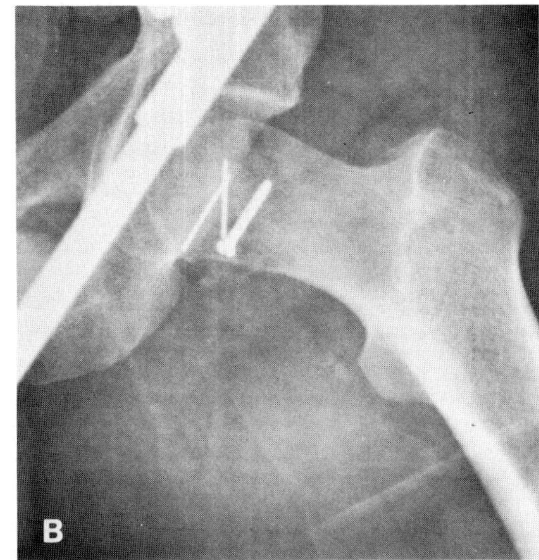

Fig. 1-64. (*A*) This policeman suffered a posterior dislocation of the hip with an associated fracture of the femoral head. After reduction of the hip, his femoral head fragment was not adequately reduced so that open reduction and internal fixation was undertaken. (*B*) The postoperative film shows the fragment reattached by means of a counter-sunk screw and two Smillie pins. A medial (Ludloff) approach was used.

29 patients is comparatively small, the amputation rate in these patients was 36 per cent—compared to an overall rate of 13.5 per cent in similar injuries treated without internal fixation—so that this must be considered significant.

Connolly carried out experiments on dogs where he fractured the femur, and after dividing the femoral artery, he repaired it with No. 6-0 silk. He found that an arterial anastomosis was able to withstand 40 lbs. of tibial traction without disruption.[40,41] Although one would expect traction to produce arterial spasm,[9,155] studies with flow meters showed that blood flow in a 3- to 4-mm. vessel was unaffected by 15 pounds traction, provided the postrepair flow was no less than 50 per cent of the original flow. From a review of the literature and 14 cases of popliteal artery injury associated with fracture from his own institution, he concluded, "This analysis . . . does not substantiate the need for internal fracture fixation. A satisfactory and practical method of immobilizing fractures associated with arterial injury was 4.5 to 6.8 kilograms of skeletal traction."

When Multiple Injuries Are Present

The association of several fractures makes it desirable to fix fractures internally for ease of nursing, for transportation, or to prevent joints from becoming stiff.[175] Bilateral femoral fractures treated by traction present problems in bedpanning and the prevention of decubiti. The common association of fractures of the femur and patella will almost certainly cause severe impairment of the knee when treated by traction, but early fixation or excision of the patella combined with intramedullary fixation of the femur gives much better results.[60]

Where Continued Confinement to Bed Is Undesirable

It is true that intertrochanteric fractures of the femur may be treated by traction with excellent healing of the fracture. However, this regimen requires skilled nursing if bed sores are to be avoided. Many of these old people have pulmonary emphysema, heart disease, hiatus hernias, and other ailments that make it mandatory for them to sit up. Satisfactory internal fixation under these circumstances would appear to be the treatment of choice, especially when it allows them to be transferred to an extended care facility.

When the Cost of Treatment May Be Substantially Reduced

It is easy to take a detached view of economics when the costs of treatment do not come out of one's own pocket. With the costs of hospital treatment rising daily, it makes good sense to keep patients in hospital for the shortest time compatible with their well-being and a good ultimate result. Furthermore, the sooner a man can return to a gainful occupation, the less financial strain will accrue to his family. If this can be achieved by intramedullary nailing of the femur, then it is a reasonable indication. The factors to be considered in the selection of treatment are the risks involved, the danger of infection, the ultimate functional result, and cosmesis.

CHOICE OF PLATES OR INTRAMEDULLARY NAILS

It seems irrelevant to me whether a fracture heals by endosteal or periosteal callus or a mixture of both. What is important is whether it heals or not. If open operation is decided upon, the best device for fixation of that fracture should be chosen rather than one selected on a basis of a particular dogma. By and large, treatment by closed methods skillfully applied would be my procedure of choice in all cases, except where operative methods are clearly shown to be superior. Whenever possible I use intramedullary fixation rather than plates, owing to the fact that intramedullary nails can be inserted through a more limited surgical approach and are more easily removed when their work is done. Compression devices have been most useful to me in the treatment of delayed union and nonunions. I use them sparingly in the management of acute injuries.

Before operating, the surgeon must have a clear plan of what he is going to do, based on sound mechanical principles. He should also have a contingency plan if his original one misfires, and he should not start until he has all the instruments and devices his strategies call for. Haphazard, ill-planned procedures are worse than no treatment at all (Figs. 1-65 to 1-67).

MATTERS RELATED TO FRACTURE CARE

JUDGING THE ADEQUACY OF REDUCTION

What constitutes adequate position must vary with the location of the fracture. Nothing short of anatomical restoration is adequate in the forearm, but in the humerus almost any position is compatible with good function. In general, one tries to line up the distal fragment so that it is in line with the proximal fragment (Fig. 1-64). An overlap of 2 centimeters in the femur or tibia can be compensated by pelvic tilt, but if it is greater than this, the shoe must be raised to avoid stress on the lumbar spine. Valgus or varus angulation must be no more than 5 degrees in the tibia, to avoid shear stresses on the knee and ankle. Late varus bow in the femur is not uncommon and gives surprisingly little trouble, but the upper limit of tolerance has not been established.

Malrotation of the tibia gives rise to perceptible deformity and ruins the alignment of the knee and ankle. According to Perkins, "When the joint above the fracture is a ball and socket joint, correction [of rota-

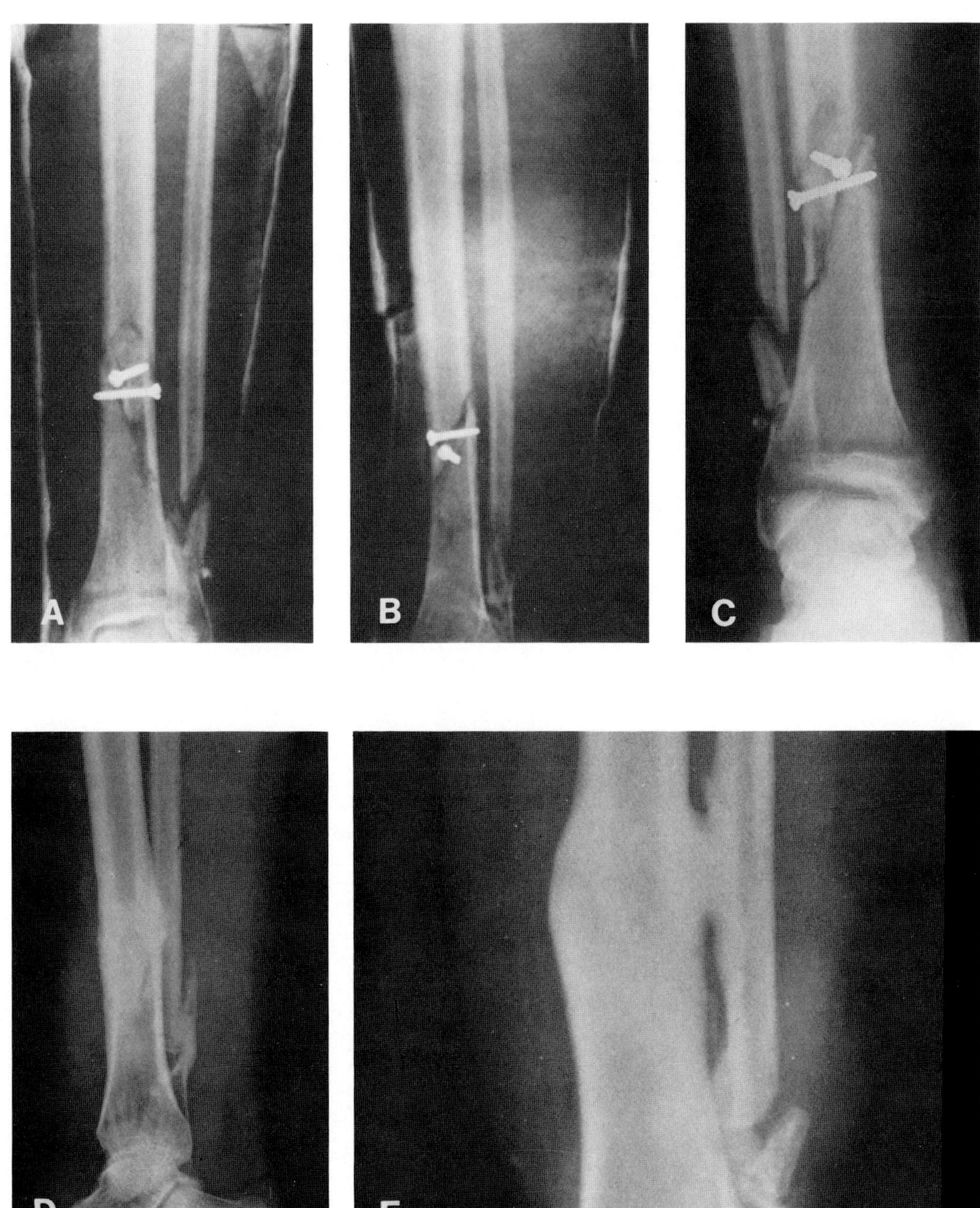

Fig. 1-65. (*A, B*) An oblique fracture of the right tibia was opened and inadequately fixed by two screws. (*C*) This subsequently became infected. (*D, E*) Before satisfactory union was obtained, some 2 years later, the patient had been subjected to several sequestrectomies and drainage procedures as well as bone grafting. This unhappy sequence could have been avoided by treating the patient with closed reduction and early weight bearing.

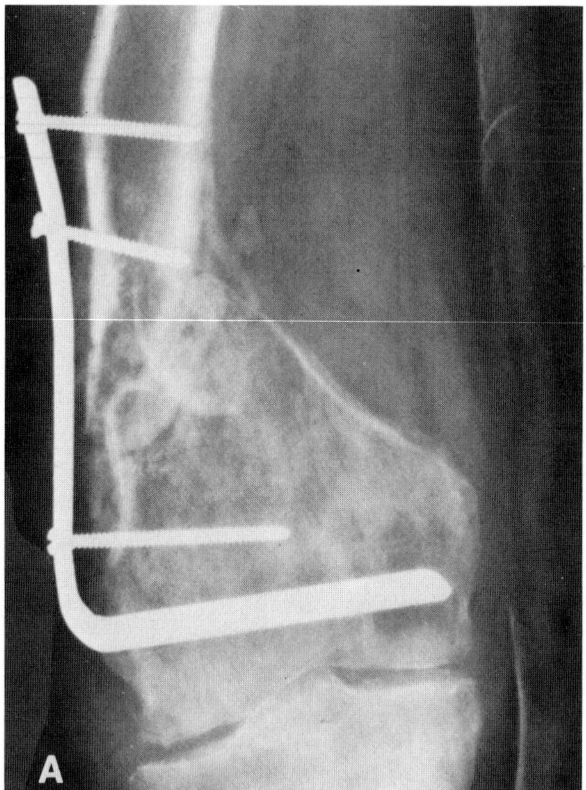

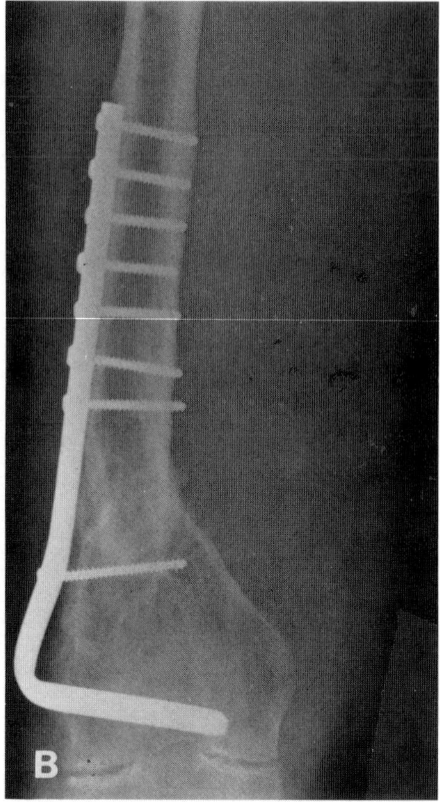

Fig. 1-66. (*A*) This middle-aged man with rheumatoid arthritis sustained a supracondylar fracture of his right femur. An inadequate operation was performed with inadequate fixation producing this result. (*B*) When adequate fixation was inserted and union obtained, he wound up with a completely ankylosed knee.

tion] is not essential. This is just as well, because one can only correct the rotation accurately at an operation where one can see exactly how the fragments fit and can maintain the reduction by a plate. Often, however, rotational deformity can be compensated for at the joint above and operation is not necessary. This is the case with two common fractures: fracture of the neck of the humerus and supracondylar fracture of the humerus."[131]

It would appear that some degree of malrotation occurs after both traction treatment and blind nailing of the femur. Ten degrees of malrotation is common and asymptomatic, but Sudman had one patient with 25 degrees of malrotation who walked with an obvious external rotation deformity and had pain, presumably on this account.[164]

Mayfield, in his review of 75 femoral shaft fractures, discovered that 31 patients had internal malrotation deformity.[114] Those with severe deformity manifested a Trendelenberg sign and a hip abductor weakness gait owing to the functional reduction of the lever arm of the femoral neck.

Anterior and posterior bowing are compensated by the hinge joints, which are contiguous. The main objection to such deformities is cosmesis.

THE PREVENTION OF INFECTION IN FRACTURES

When operation is undertaken, a closed fracture is converted into an open one with the potential danger of its becoming infected. This complication may be catas-

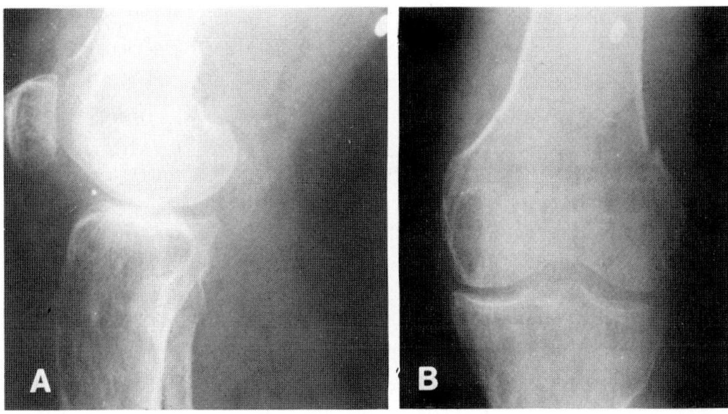

Fig. 1-67. (*A, B*) This patient, who lived an adventurous life, was admitted with a fracture produced by a .22-caliber bullet. (*C*) A roentgenogram of the ipsilateral hip demonstrated a nonunion of his shotgun fracture fixed by a blade-plate assembly. Nonunion had resulted with breakage of the plate through the first screw hole. This type of fixation is inadequate for subtrochanteric fractures and he would have been better treated by a Zickel nail. (*D*) This fracture went on to union after the insertion of a compression plate device.

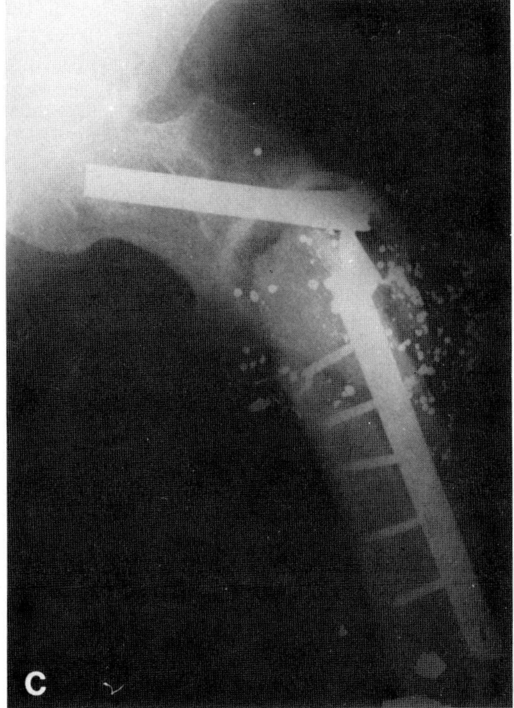

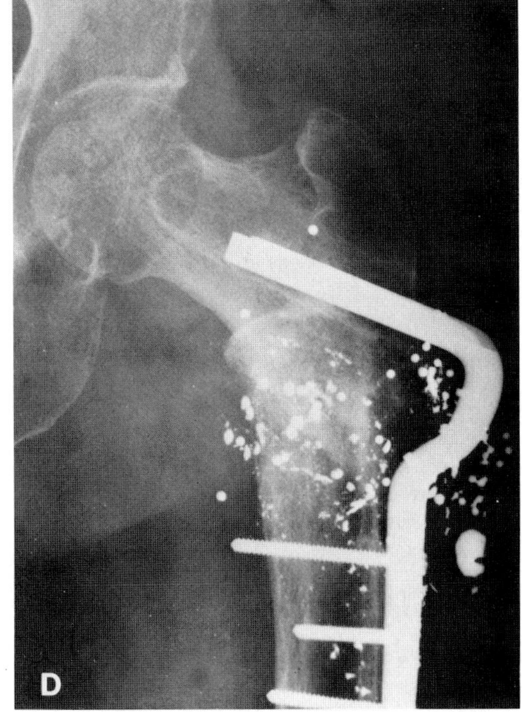

trophic—it can lead to the loss of the limb —or at best it prolongs the period of morbidity and may make more operations necessary and impair the quality of the final result. It follows, then, that every precaution must be taken to prevent this dismal series of events.

Care of the Soft Tissues

A fracture was defined, I believe, by Clay Ray Murray as "a soft-tissue injury complicated by a break in a bone." The most important single factor in the management of fractures is the treatment of the overlying soft tissues; in fractures of the tibia especially, it may determine the success or failure of treatment. Incisions made through traumatized, compromised skin may be the insult that causes its demise. Early open reduction of the tibia, even in highly skilled hands, is associated with skin breakdown, delayed healing, and infection.[80,126]

There is still a tremendous compulsion for surgeons to close wounds primarily, even though it has been shown quite conclusively that delayed primary closure or secondary closure by skin grafting is much safer.[23,24] Certainly in well-debrided wounds seen early where the soft-tissue damage and gross contamination have not been severe, it is permissible to suture primarily. On the other hand, ill-advised attempts to provide skin cover for fractured tibias by suturing wounds under tension, by making "relaxing" incisions, and by the rotation of flaps are so fraught with danger that they should never be done.[24] If cover is mandatory, Ger's technique, in which the bone is covered by transposed muscle belly followed by skin grafting on the fifth postoperative day, is by far the best means of achieving it.[66,67] All would agree that the most important predisposing causes of infection are the presence of dead or devitalized tissue, hematomas, dead space, and foreign bodies. It follows, therefore, that these conditions must be eliminated or controlled as well as possible. The management of open fractures and these problems are discussed in Chapter 3.

Prophylactic Antibiotics

The use of prophylactic antibiotics is still very controversial, but interest in this subject has renewed in an effort to find means of averting the disaster of infected total hip and knee arthroplasties. If it can be shown that prophylactic antimicrobial therapy is efficacious, then its application to fracture surgery is no less important. Unfortunately, the literature on this subject presents conflicting views. Many of the clinical studies are retrospective and poorly controlled, and even the laboratory studies are no more helpful.[169]

Fogelberg *et al.*, in their review of the subject, found that most of the studies concluded that prophylactic antibiotics either were of no value or enhanced the likelihood of postoperative infection.[61] Stevens, reviewing postoperative infections in Lexington, Kentucky, found that the infection rate increased significantly after procedures lasting more than 90 minutes and that prophylactic antibiotics in clean cases increased the incidence of sepsis.[157]

In more recent studies by Scales *et al.*, 1,816 patients operated on at the Royal National Orthopaedic Hospital and the Queen Elizabeth II Hospital were reviewed.[152] There was no correlation between the infection rate and such factors as age, sex, vacuum drainage, site of implant, weight bearing, corrosion of metal, or chemical composition of the implant. Those patients given pre- and postoperative antibiotics for a total of 5 to 7 days had the lowest incidence of wound infection, while those given antibiotics only after the surgery was completed had the highest rate of infection for the group.

Fogelberg *et al.*, using pre- and postoperative penicillin for patients undergoing spinal surgery and mold arthroplasty of the hip were able to reduce the incidence of infection from 8.9 per cent in the control group to 1.7 per cent in the treated group.[61] Similarly, Nach and Keim found that prophylactic oxacillin, penicillin, or lincomycin given before, during and after surgery was effective in reducing both major and minor infections.[120] The treated group had an incidence of 1.6 per cent major infection, while the control group had 11.4 per cent major infections and 3.8 per cent minor infections.

The use of local irrigants or aerosols containing antibiotics has also been shown to be effective in reducing the rate of postoperative infections.[62,95,172] Gingrass *et al.*, in their experimental studies, found that gentle scrubbing of contaminated wounds and irrigation with neomycin solution was superior to irrigation with saline or scrubbing with pHiso-Hex, either alone or in combination, in preventing infection in the contaminated wounds. Parenteral neomycin, while ineffective by itself, did improve the results when complemented by gentle scrubbing and neomycin irrigation.

If antibiotics are to be effective in preventing infection, they should be given prior to the establishment of a "biochemical lesion" (i.e., within 3 hours of wounding).[26] In view of these studies, it is now my practice to give patients with open fractures 1 gram of cephalothin (Keflin) intravenously in the emergency room, if this can be done within this time limit. During surgery 2 to 4 g. are given intravenously in 500 ml. of saline. Following this loading dose, the patient is then given Keflin, 1 g. every 6 hours for 5 days. Keflex, an oral analogue of Keflin, may be substituted in the latter 2 or 3 days.

In operating on fractures after the healing of contaminated wounds where I feel there is a risk of reinfection, Keflin or another appropriate antibiotic is started the day before the projected surgery.

Internal Fixation and Infection

It used to be held that an internal fixation device (being a foreign body) in some way, merely by being there, enhanced the chances of wound infection and was absolutely proscribed in the treatment of open fractures. This contention is apparently borne out by published series. Gustilo *et al.* in analyzing 511 open fractures found that of the 112 fractures treated by primary fixation, 11.6 per cent became infected whereas in the 299 without primary internal fixation the infection rate was only 6.68 per cent.[73] When infection did occur following internal fixation, it was formerly advised that the metal should be removed in order to control the sepsis. The idea that metal *per se* is responsible for infection is open to serious doubt.

MacNeur has shown that both in war wounds and open fractures in civilians, adequate management of the soft-tissue wound and the use of antibiotics allows the use of primary internal fixation without incurring prohibitively high infection rates.[111] Of 145 cases treated at the Alfred Hospital, early skin healing was obtained in 125. Twelve patients had delayed wound healing and only five developed infection. In his total series, there were only six infected fractures (3.6 per cent), and in none of these was the metal removed early. Four of these fractures went on to union in spite of infection.

Recent experience seems to confirm that when internal fixation is secure, it should not be removed; and with debridement, irrigation, and antibiotic therapy, union will eventually occur.[80,94,109,110,126,176] It may be that the optimum management of an infected nonunion is to combine aggressive treatment of the infection with secure, rigid, internal fixation.[108]

ANESTHESIA IN FRACTURE TREATMENT

Most fracture work is carried out under general or spinal anesthesia administered by an anesthesiologist. The choice of method and agents under these circumstances must be left to the anesthesiologist and will be dictated by the age and condition of the patient as well as the judgement of the physician administering the anesthetic. It is axiomatic that the patient should be resuscitated and stabilized prior to the administration of anesthesia, and whenever possible anesthesia in a patient with a full stomach should be deferred to avoid the danger of aspiration pneumonia.

At Louisville General Hospital it is our practice, when anesthesia must be induced, to intubate the trachea with the patient awake. Spinal anesthesia in an acutely injured patient is hazardous and is best avoided.

On occasion the surgeon is obliged to work without the services of an anesthesiologist. Fractures of the tibia seen soon after injury may often be reduced and immobilized without anesthesia or under analgesics such as morphine or meperidine. When these drugs are used, I prefer to administer them intravenously (e.g., 8 to 10 mg. morphine or 75 to 100 mg. meperidine), since the action is produced rapidly and predictably. They should be given slowly and well diluted. In general, fractures reduced without the services of an anesthesiologist are minor ones in the upper extremity—especially the wrist and hand—and those of the foot.

The methods commonly used to provide analgesia are local infiltration of local anesthetics, intravenous regional anesthesia (Bier's Block), and regional nerve block. Hypnosis or the use of ataractic drugs may also be employed.

Local Infiltration. If a needle is introduced into a fracture hematoma, blood is easily aspirated, and analgesia may be obtained by injecting lidocaine, mepivacaine, or some similar drug into the hematoma.[48] This method is most frequently used in the treatment of Colles' fracture. The fracture is palpated and 10 ml. of 1 per cent lidocaine or a similar agent is injected into the hematoma. Another 5 ml. must be injected around the ulnar styloid, or analgesia will be incomplete. Furthermore, at least 10 or 15 minutes should be allowed before starting to manipulate. Theoretically, this method would seem to carry the risk of infecting the hematoma, but in practice this rarely occurs. I do not use local infiltration for the reduction of fractures, nor do I recommend its use; it is mentioned only for the sake of completeness.

Intravenous Regional Anesthesia (Bier's Block). This technique originally described by Bier has been revived and may be used for minor surgery in the forearm and hand, as well as in the leg and foot. A needle or venous catheter is inserted into a convenient superficial vein. The arm or leg is then elevated and exsanguinated by wrapping with an elastic bandage—an Esmarch or an Ace bandage. A pneumatic tourniquet is inflated (250 mm. Hg in the arm; 400 mm. in the leg) and the bandage is removed. In the arm 20 to 40 ml. of 0.5 per cent lidocaine is injected into the vein (for larger volumes, 0.25 per cent solution can be used) and in the foot and leg 40 to 80 ml. is required. Atkinson *et al.* recommended that no more than 50 ml. of 0.5 per cent lidocaine should be used in the arm, and they use an average dose of 224 mg. of lidocaine.[8] Sorbie and Aracha use no more than 200 mg. in the arm and 400 mg. in the leg.[159] After this injection, anesthesia is usually produced within 5 minutes. At this point a second tourniquet is inflated distal to the first, and the original tourniquet, which is on unanesthetized skin, is deflated.

This method gives excellent anesthesia for an hour or more, although some patients complain of tourniquet pain. Should the tourniquet become deflated prior to 20 minutes after the injection, a toxic dose of lidocaine may be released into the general circulation. Great care should be taken to ensure that this does not happen, and drugs and equipment for dealing with reactions to local anesthetics must be on hand. No type of anesthetic should be undertaken without having another person in the room or at least within easy earshot. It goes without saying that no patient with a history of idiosyncrasy to local anesthetic agents should be treated by this method.

Regional Block. Excellent anesthesia of the upper extremity can be produced by interscalene or supraclavicular brachial block.[1] Since there is some danger inherent in both of these techniques, and because pneumothorax has been reported in up to 10 per cent of supraclavicular blocks, I believe that these methods are best left to those skilled in their use. Brachial block by the axillary route, on the other hand, is a simple, efficient, and risk-free means of producing upper extremity anesthesia. This technique has been described well by Burnham, de Long, and others.[20,45,177] Kleinert *et al.* reported the results of 647 blocks in 1963, and since that time axillary block has become our anesthetic of choice.[96] More than 90 per cent of the hands operated on in Louisville are anesthetized in this manner, as well as Colles' fractures and other minor injuries in the upper extremity. A subsequent paper from the same authors reported their experience with more than 10,000 cases.[88]

Technique. The patient lies in the supine position, and the shoulder is externally rotated and abducted to 90 degrees. The elbow is also flexed to a right angle, and the patient is placed in a comfortable position. After preparing the skin the axillary artery is palpated where it lies under the cover of the pectoralis major. Using a 10-ml. syringe and a ⅝-inch, 25-gauge needle, a wheal is raised in the skin overlying the artery, as high in the axilla as possible, and the needle is inserted into the neurovascular sheath (Fig. 1-68). A distinct sensation is felt as the sheath is pierced, and after detaching the syringe, the needle can be seen to pulsate due to the proximity of the artery. At this point the patient should be questioned regarding paresthesias in the limb, which confirms that the sheath has been entered. To avert the hazard of intravascular injection, the needle should be aspirated before the anesthetic agent is injected. The duration of the block is enhanced by the addition of epinephrine, 1:200,000, to the anesthetic agent. If lidocaine is used, 20 ml. of 1 per cent solution may be adequate to produce anesthesia of the hand and forearm, and where more extensive anesthesia of the extremity is required, the dosage may be increased to 40 ml. It is said that smaller doses may suffice if a tourniquet is placed around the arm prior to the insertion of the needle (Erickson technique) (Fig. 1-69). This tourniquet prevents peripheral leakage and diffusion of the agent.

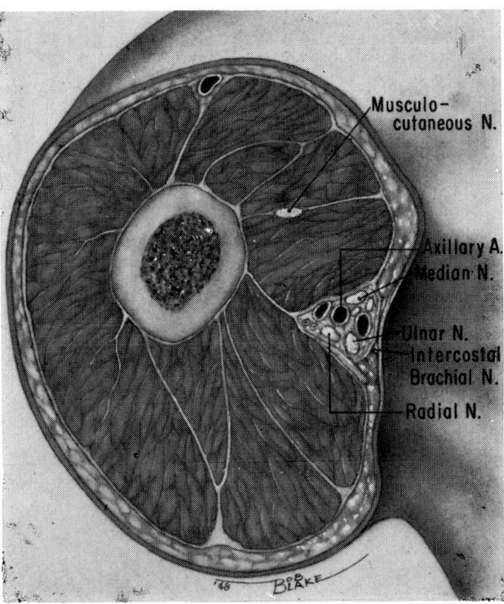

Fig. 1-68. A cross-section of the axilla demonstrating the superficial position of the neurovascular bundle. (Kasdan, M. L., *et al.*: Plast. Reconstr. Surg., *46*: 256, 1970)

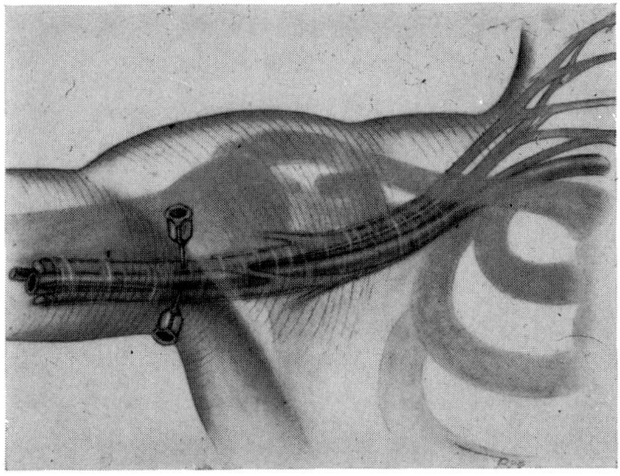

Fig. 1-69. The injection should be high in the axilla and a two-needle technique may be used to make sure that all three nerves are blocked. (Kasdan, M. L., *et al.*: Plast. Reconstr. Surg., *46*:256, 1970)

To make sure that all three cords are blocked, two needles may be inserted, one above and one below the artery, but in gen-

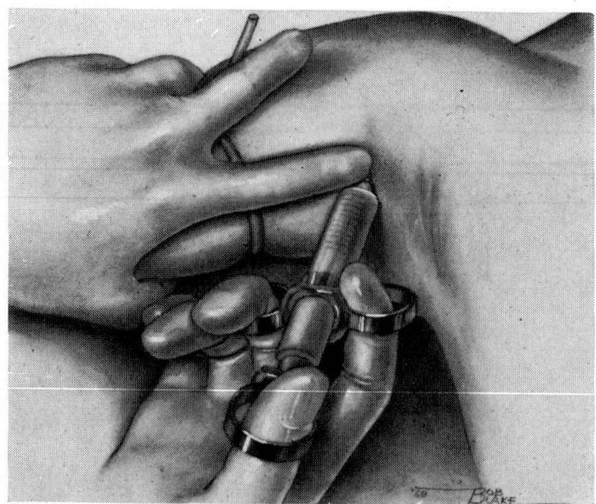

Fig. 1-70. The artery is palpated in the axilla, and the needle is passed close to the fingertips. A tourniquet prevents peripheral leakage and diffusion of the agent and allows the block to be produced by smaller dosages of local anesthetic. (Kasdan, M. L., *et al.*: Plast. Reconstr. Surg., *46*: 256, 1970)

eral one needle is sufficient (Fig. 1-70). A ⅝-inch needle is adequate for all but the most gargantuan arms, owing to the superficial location of the neurovascular bundle. If a longer needle is used, it is possible to inject the coracobrachialis muscle and produce no block at all. While inevitably, there will be a small percentage of unsuccessful blocks (Kasdan *et al.* reported 90 per cent success),[88] the commonest cause of failure is impatience. Although profound anesthesia may occur within 10 minutes, it may take 30 minutes. On occasion the patient awakes from general anesthesia with an excellent block because the surgeon was unwilling to wait.

Intravenous Diazepam. Diazepam (Valium) is a benzodiazepine derivative that has ataractic and muscle relaxant properties. It is recommended by its manufacturer (Roche) for the treatment of anxiety and tension states. Valium is also used for the relief of skeletal muscle spasm such as in cerebral palsy, athetosis, and the stiff-man syndrome. This drug is contraindicated in acute, narrow angle glaucoma and should not be administered to patients in shock, coma, or acute alcohol intoxication with depression of vital signs.

Bultitude *et al.* reported on the use of intravenous diazepam as the sole anesthetic agent for the reduction of Colles' fractures.[25] They advise a dose of 20 mg. given intravenously, or 30 mg. in heavy adults, administered over a period of seconds equal to twice the number of milligrams given (e.g., 20 mg. over 40 seconds). In their experience this was a useful anesthetic. They felt that the drug had little or no analgesic action but did induce transient amnesia. (One of my anesthesiologist friends has described this method as being the pharmacological equivalent of biting on a bullet.) Their patients were quick to recover, could sit up in 5 minutes, and were able to return home in 2 hours.

Of the 71 patients treated, only two 85-year-olds became unrousable for 2 minutes, and one of them had a fall in blood pressure for 10 minutes after the injection. Both of these patients made a full recovery. The only other complications reported in this study were pain at the injection site and thrombophlebitis. Others have noted respiratory depression following intravenous diazepam.

We have used this technique too but have given somewhat smaller doses (10 to 20 mg.). It has been useful in reducing dislocations of the shoulder and elbow as well as in minor fractures. Care must be taken with inebriated patients, since alcohol and diazepam appear to have a synergistic action. Diazepam or regional block should never be used where there is no one to help or if oxygen and means of ventilating the patient are not easily available.

Choice of Agent. Most of the commonly used local anesthetic agents are effective but bupivicaine (Marcaine) has the advantage of being extremely long-acting.[116] It lasts two to three times as long as lidocaine (Xylocaine) or mepivacaine (Carbocaine) and 20 to 25 per cent longer than tetracaine (Pontocaine). It is relatively less toxic than other similar drugs, and in our hands 0.5 per cent solutions have been excellent for both local infiltration and nerve blocks.

REHABILITATION FOLLOWING FRACTURES

The concept that rehabilitation is a process that should start after the healing of a fracture and may safely be delegated to physical therapists and physiatrists is fallacious. Rehabilitation is the business of the entire medical team, and it should start the minute the patient is admitted to hospital.

The prime goals of rehabilitation in the fracture patient are: (1) to maintain or restore the range of motion of joints, (2) to preserve muscle strength and endurance, (3) to enhance the rate of fracture healing by activity, and (4) to return the patient to function at the earliest juncture.

Maintenance of Joint Motion

The stiffness that results following immobilization of a joint is proportional to the length of time involved. The main factor in the production of this contracture is shortening of the surrounding musculature and, to a lesser degree, changes in the joint capsule. Intraarticular changes also occur—proliferation of the subsynovial fatty tissue which encroaches on and may obliterate the synovial cleft. In time this soft-tissue overgrowth may cover the articular cartilage and become confluent with it.[53,56] Where articular surfaces are in contact, especially under pressure, fibrillation and degeneration occur, and fibrous adhesions or even bony fusion may result. The articular cartilage must depend on synovial fluid for its nutrition. The obliteration of the joint and the lack of motion to "pump" the fluid in and out may also add to the decrease in thickness of the cartilage.[22,51]

It follows that no joint should be immobilized unnecessarily and all joints should be put through a full range of motion every day. The old woman with a Colles' fracture should never be left to vegetate in a sling and develop a frozen shoulder and stiff fingers. Proper exercise is as much a part of her treatment as the application of the cast.

The shoulder is particularly liable to develop stiffness in people who are middle-aged and older, and circumduction exercises must be started as soon as they can be tolerated by patients with fractures of the humeral neck. When a frozen shoulder does develop, an active program of exercises using overhead pulleys, large wheels, and wall-climbing exercises may mobilize the shoulder. In recalcitrant cases, gentle manipulation under general anesthesia may be tried, keeping in mind the danger of fracturing an osteoporotic humerus. The manipulation is best carried out by stabilizing the scapula and abducting the shoulder by pressure on the proximal third of the humerus. No sudden stress should be applied, and on no account must the whole lever-arm of the humerus be used by grasping the elbow, nor should rotational stress be applied.

The elbow does not tolerate injury well and frequently becomes stiff. Early active motion in these injuries is also indicated, and any attempt to force motion by passive manipulation is liable to defeat its own ends by inciting myositis ossificans.

Limitation of knee motion following fractures of the femur is not infrequently due to scarring down of the quadriceps to the underlying bone. Charnley advises that this may be prevented by the early use of isometric quadriceps exercises, and others have devised means of starting active knee motion during treatment by traction.[33] Nichols has shown that in the Royal Air Force the average time off-duty following a fractured femoral shaft is 26 weeks when treated by early intramedullary nailing and 32 weeks after treatment by skeletal traction.[123] This is due, at least to some extent, to earlier resumption of knee motion. In

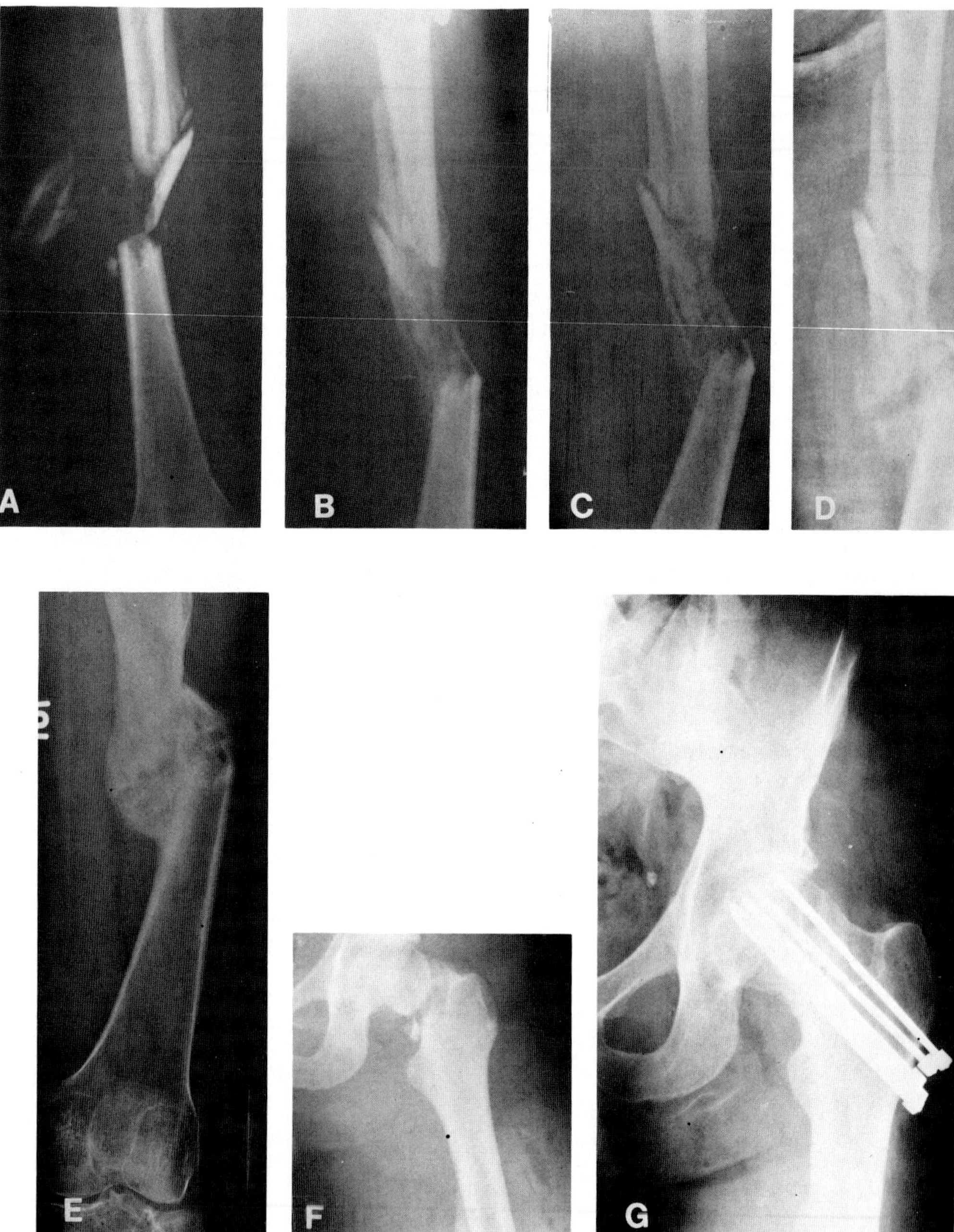

Fig. 1-71. (*A*) Open comminuted fracture of femoral shaft in young man with head injury, ruptured liver and spleen, fractured cervical spine, as well as ipsilateral fractures of the femoral neck and proximal tibia. (*B*) Healing by periosteal new bone after 4 months in traction and spica. (*C*) One month later a spontaneous fracture occurred during quadriceps exercises. (*D*) After application of cast brace. (*E*) End result 11 months after original injury. Knee flexion 0 to 110 degrees. (*F*) Original view of fractured hip—transcervical fracture with comminution of inferior neck. This is characteristic of high-energy fractures of the hip due to automobile accidents. (*G*) Open reduction was delayed more than a month. End result after opening the hip capsule and reducing fracture under vision with five Knowles' pins.

comparing the results of intramedullary nailing with traction, Rokkanen found that ultimately there was no significant difference in the range of knee motion in young people.[142] However, those over the age of 35 who had been treated by intramedullary nails had significantly better motion than the traction group. Vigorous attempts to regain knee motion after femoral fracture may result in refracture (Fig. 1-71). Reviewing the literature O'Brien found incidences ranging from 4 to 16.6 per cent in the published series.[124] One of the most attractive features of cast bracing fractures of the femur is the early resumption of knee movement, and it might well compare favorably in this regard with intramedullary fixation. I have not found passive manipulation to be rewarding in restoring motion to stiff knees after fractures of the femur, and the procedure of choice where more motion is needed is a quadricepsplasty.

Muscle Exercises

Muscle exercises may be isometric or isotonic. In isometric exercise the length of the muscle does not change, the joint on which it acts does not move, but the tension of its muscle fibers increases (e.g., quadriceps setting). Isotonic exercise, on the other hand, involves motion of the joint and shortening of the muscle fibers. The former are said to be more efficient in developing strength and are also indicated where joint motion causes pain and therefore secondary inhibition of the muscle. The latter is used to regain range of motion and to regain strength and endurance where the joint is not irritable. Either type of exercise may be modified by increasing the load against which the muscle must act as it grows stronger—progressive resistance exercises (PRE). To increase a muscle's strength it is necessary to make it contract with its maximum power daily without overloading it. Endurance, on the other hand, is achieved by repetitive exercise stopping short of fatigue.

The strength of a muscle contraction is proportional to the starting length of its fibers. The therapist should use this principle by fully extending the muscle and even applying gentle passive stretch. Greater power will also be gained by preceding the exercise by a maximal contraction of the muscle's antagonist and by recruitment of additional anterior horn cells by contracting additional muscles innervated by the same segment of the cord (e.g., by dorsiflexing the ankle [L 4.5] while exercising the quadriceps [L 3.4]). Where muscles are so weak as to be nonfunctional the exercises have to be assisted by the therapist or by eliminating gravity by hydrotherapy or supportive devices. At all costs a weak or partially innervated muscle should be protected from overstretching, since this greatly retards its recovery.

Gait Training

The cast-brace treatment of femoral fractures and early weight bearing in closed treatment of tibial fractures are firmly established in contemporary practice. However, if some supervision is not exerted many patients develop undesirable gait patterns which persist even after the removal of immobilization.

It is best if the patient be started standing in parallel bars to achieve standing balance equally distributed between the two feet. When this has been achieved he should then practice weight transfer from one foot to the other. He must achieve balance on each foot before walking is commenced. From the parallel bars he should graduate to crutches or canes and eventually, in some cases, to independent ambulation.

An even gait is impossible when there is marked discrepancy between leg lengths. For this reason I prefer an overshoe rather than a walking heel. This has the additional advantage of keeping the cast clean and dry. Alternatively, the shoe on the contralateral foot may be raised. This is particularly valuable in cast bracing for femoral fractures, where it prevents late varus bowing. The patient should never be allowed to swivel on his walking foot externally rotating at the hip but should be encouraged to walk as closely as possible to a normal heel-and-toe gait.

Ambulation Aids

Most patients with lower extremity fractures require some form of ambulation aid. While most rehabilitation centers appear to prefer other than simple axillary crutches, they have the advantage of being cheap and readily available. Since the large majority of patients use them for only a short time, the expense of providing more sophisticated crutches does not seem reasonable. In adjusting these crutches there should be a handsbreadth between the pad of the crutch and the axilla. The pad is designed to take pressure on the lateral side of the chest and not in the axilla, where pressure on the brachial plexus produces a "crutch palsy." The handpiece should allow the elbow to be flexed comfortably while bearing weight. In order to be able to use axillary crutches the patient must have strong triceps, and preparatory exercises with dumbbells to strengthen these muscles while the patient is still confined to bed is useful. For comfort the axillary portion and the handpiece should be padded with sponge rubber and, for safety, the largest size rubber tips should be added.

Crutch Gaits. After having prescribed crutches, the most appropriate gait should be taught.

Swing-To and Swing-Through. In this type of gait both crutches are placed forward and the patient either pulls his body to the crutches or propels his body through them so that his feet are now ahead of the crutch tips. The weight can be borne on both feet, as a paraplegic would, or on only one foot when weight bearing is proscribed for the fractured side. This is by far the most rapid means of progression on crutches and the most vigorous.

Three-Point. In this method the two crutches and the injured extremity are advanced together and bear weight simultaneously while the sound leg is advanced. The degree of weight bearing on the injured extremity is controlled by the amount of weight borne by the hands.

Two-Point. In an alternating two-point gait the crutch is advanced with the contralateral foot. This method would be used in bilateral injuries where partial weight bearing is desired.

Four-Point. This is similar to the two-point but one crutch is advanced first, then the contralateral foot, followed by the second crutch, and lastly the second foot. This is reserved for the most severely impaired or elderly patients.

Walkers. It is quite unrealistic to expect old ladies and indeed many old men to walk with crutches, since they have neither the strength nor the agility and coordination to use them. In such cases a simple walker made from tubular aluminum that they can lift up and place before them is the most stable and foolproof device. It is also unreasonable to prescribe non-weight-bearing ambulation for old people with fractured hips, and indeed the work of Rydell and Frankel would seem to show that partial weight bearing is more benign than many maneuvers carried out in bed. For this reason, in stable, well-fixed fractures of the hip we now start partial weight bearing much earlier than before.

Canes. Canes are useful but less efficient than crutches for maintaining balance and relieving weight. The patient's natural tendency is to hold the cane with the hand on the side of the injury, which gives rise to a very awkward gait. He should be instructed to use the cane in the opposite hand and bear weight on the injured limb and cane simultaneously. The use of a solitary crutch should be discouraged, as it too gives rise to an ugly gait. By and large, if a patient needs one crutch, he needs two.

In most departments of physical medicine there are a number of expensive machines the main purpose of which is to supply some form of heat to the tissues. I am not aware of any evidence that heat *per se* has any beneficial effect in rehabilitation after injury. Ultrasound has been shown to be more efficient in the heating of deep tissues but the therapeutic benefits of this are somewhat nebulous. The daily application of ultrasound to neck injuries sustained in rear-end collisions seems to me to benefit mainly the owner of the machine.

The application of heat to painful joints and muscles does relieve pain and discomfort and is a useful preliminary to active exercises. In this regard, one method does not appear to be superior to another. Hot packs or immersion in warm water are as good as more sophisticated methods and have the advantage of being available at home. If short-wave diathermy is used, it must never be applied over implants, since it induces high temperatures in the metal with damage to the tissues.

Cold applications may also be used as a means of reducing pain prior to exercise, but my own preference is for heat and, where applicable, to immersion in a Hubbard tank.

Exercise is dull, and most people prefer carrying out purposeful tasks. This fact is utilized by devising projects for patients that utilize the motion desired, e.g., using a screwdriver to gain supination range and power. Such therapy not only achieves a therapeutic aim but is a diversion for the patient that breaks the tedium of a stay in hospital.

Somewhat along the same lines, it is important to make the patient as self-sufficient as possible before he returns home. The use of the occupational therapist in supervising activities of daily living (ADL) is extremely helpful, but unfortunately these functions are rarely to be found outside rehabilitation centers and almost never in general or community hospitals.

Massage

Massage is a time-honored treatment, but the laying on of hands has little place in the rehabilitation of patients with fractures, except as a means of softening up and mobilizing scars that are impeding joint motion. It is extremely unlikely that massage will dissipate edema or improve circulation to an extremity.

Braces

Conventional bracing has very little place in the treatment of fractures. Long-leg braces with ischial seats or quadrilateral sockets and pelvis bands are sometimes prescribed to "protect" fractures of the femur or even, indeed, fractures of the hip. Mechanically, such braces are ineffective and much inferior to cast braces. Recent work has shown that even subtrochanteric fractures may be treated by a skillfully applied cast brace, but this certainly would not be true of a long-leg caliper.

Sarmiento has shown that fractures of the tibia may be managed with a patellar-bearing cast with a free ankle joint, and he has taken the process one step further by replacing the plaster-of-paris with Orthoplast, a plastic material that can be molded after heating. Such braces applied by an experienced orthotist are efficient, but such factors as cost and the availability of skilled orthotists make plaster casts the treatment of choice for most surgeons.

The major application for bracing in the treatment of fractures is to compensate for associated nerve injuries such as dropfoot secondary to peroneal palsy. Dynamic bracing is frequently used also in the after treatment of hand injuries, both to compensate for nerve deficits and to stretch out contractures gently and restore joint motion.

INJURY AND THE LAW

A surgeon treating fractures must inevitably become involved with the law. On occasion patients sue for disabilities incurred; those injured at work are entitled to benefits under Workmen's Compensation Laws; and unhappily, some patients, discontented with the results of his ministrations may sue the surgeon for malpractice. In addition, he will also be asked to render independent medical opinions on patients treated by other surgeons.

Most physicians do not enjoy giving testimony in court and resent the time and effort in writing legal reports or even, indeed, filling out the routine reports for insurance companies. These duties can only be performed by physicians, and should they be carried out in a perfunctory manner, the patient will suffer, and the physician's professional competency may be brought into question in any ensuing litigation.

THE MEDICAL REPORT

For a variety of legal purposes a medical report is necessary. Some examples of them do not support the contention that medicine is a learned profession. R. M. Fox, a personal injury attorney who has a somewhat slanted view of these matters, makes a valid criticism, "No medical school in the United States today offers a course in medicolegal report writing, in spite of its obvious socioeconomic importance and the billions of dollars in the type of claim. Little, if any, postgraduate medical education on this subject is available."[64]

A few words on the preparation of such reports seems to be in order. If the report is on a patient other than my own, I make a practice of prefacing the report by naming the party who has requested the examination and the date on which this examination was performed. When the report is on a patient of one's own, permission to release this information must be given by the patient.

History

Although the patient may give a lengthy account of the circumstances of the accident, only that which is germane to the assessment of his injury should be included in the report, and certainly no judgment as to culpability should appear in the medical report. Although the patient's account to a physician of the circumstances of the accident is inadmissible as evidence bearing on the actionable event itself, it will be admissible to the extent it is relevant in establishing the basis upon which the physician's ultimate opinion is based. If, in some way, these notes are erroneous, they may damage the credibility of the patient or in some way influence the outcome of the case.

The past history of the patient must be recorded, especially where previous injury or disease is directly concerned in the production or aggravation of the disability being assessed. If the report is on a patient whom you have treated yourself, then a detailed report of the initial examination and subsequent events should be included. The patient should be questioned regarding his current condition, and the nature, severity, duration, and frequency of his specific complaints should be listed and described.

Clinical Examination

The clinical examination is carried out in a meticulous manner. Notes are taken during the examination rather than depending on memory; care is taken to differentiate left from right. In many jurisdictions, the medical witness is permitted to refer to these notes to refresh his recollection, provided the notes were made contemporaneously with the examination or shortly thereafter. Thorough notes can be invaluable for responding intelligently and consistently in the event of a far-reaching, extended cross-examination. The sooner the formal report is dictated, the more accurate it will be. That which can be measured should be, with tape or goniometer. Scars should be noted, especially where they interfere with function or where cosmesis is important. Negative findings, where indicated, should also be noted.

Medical Assessment

After describing the medical findings in technical terms, I generally give a resume of the findings in nontechnical, lay terms or translate the technical language as I go, depending on the complexity of the case. This is very helpful to the recipient of the report if he be a lawyer or other lay person. In the summation of the report the diagnoses should be listed, some opinion should be expressed regarding the compatibility of the patient's injuries with the patient's history of how they were incurred, and whether the complaints are consonant with the physical findings. There is no place, however, for gratuitous and unnecessarily pejorative remarks regarding the patient.

The prognosis should be discussed when it can be reasonably determined. No one can expect an absolutely accurate forecast of events, but an educated guess is much more helpful than saying the prognosis is undetermined. The possible and probable end results and the length of time the patient is liable to be incapacitated should be estimated. If further surgery or rehabilitative treatment is necessary, this should be listed and justified.

Physical Impairment and Disability

In the event that the patient's condition is stable and no further treatment is indicated, many agencies and insurance companies will ask for an estimate of permanent disability, or permanent physical impairment expressed as a percentage. There is a distinction between these two terms. Disability is a measure of the loss of a person's ability to engage in his occupation or earn a living and therefore is not a purely medical determination. Physical impairment is a measure of loss of function or assessment of anatomical defect, which is the same for all similar patients, irrespective of how they earned their living. To quote a hackneyed example: If two men lost their left fifth fingers, their physical impairment would be identical. Were one a concert violinist and the other a manual laborer, their permanent disability would be vastly different. Obviously, disability has to be predicated on physical impairment, but the former is a legal determination and the latter, medical.

The physician is the final arbiter of physical impairment. He will be helped in this task by the use of various tables that have been devised by the American Medical Association as well as other publications by authorities in the field.[10,93,138]

TESTIMONY IN COURT

The large majority of personal injury claims are settled out of court, and this process is facilitated in many instances by a comprehensive and lucid medical report. In those cases where settlement cannot be reached amicably, the surgeon will usually be asked to give a deposition prior to the formal trial. A deposition is a pre-trial examination of a witness by the opposing attorneys without the presence of a judge. The proceedings are recorded by a court stenographer, and the evidence is given under oath. If the case goes to trial, the surgeon will answer the same or similar questions in more formal circumstances, or in the event that he is unable to attend in person, the deposition may be entered as evidence. Should the medical witness give substantially different replies in court to similar questions asked in a deposition, one or either of the attorneys will pick up the discrepancy, and this will inevitably vitiate his testimony.

The attorney and physician who are brought together in litigation should have a common goal—to assist the court or jury in arriving at the truth. While this is a time-consuming and occasionally frustrating experience, it is absolutely necessary for the physician to educate the lawyer regarding the medical aspects of the case. Failure to do so may do a great disservice to the patient, since the lawyer may never ask the questions most pertinent to the case. Particularly close cooperation is essential when the physician's opinion, as is often the case, is based upon a hypothetical question. The lawyer, in asking the hypothetical question upon which the medical opinion will be based, must include all relevant, material findings, including essential negative findings. Upon that assumed set of facts, the medical witness is asked, "Do you have an opinion and if so, what is that opinion?" The most frequently encountered gambit in cross-examination of the physician is to rephrase the hypothetical question with some omissions or possibly new inclusions. The experienced physician generally avoids these traps by paraphrasing the question by way of clarification (e.g., "Are you asking if my opinion would be different had the patient complained of sciatica at the time of my examination?").

As a witness, one should testify to that which he believes to be true and if he does not know the answer to the question or if it is beyond the area of his expertise, he should say so. Prior to a deposition the prudent physician refreshes his memory of the pertinent literature. While quotations from the medical texts or papers as such are not admissible as evidence, lawyers in many jurisdictions introduce such material in the process of cross-examination and ask the medical witness if the authors are recognized authorities and if he agrees with the opinions they have expressed. The surgeon should be at least as well-read as the attorney.

Not infrequently the attorney who has requested the surgeon to testify asks for a pre-trial or pre-deposition conference in which he goes over the evidence, asks for clarifications, and reviews the questions he will ask. There is nothing unethical in such conferences, but the surgeon should not lose his objectivity and become a partisan for one side or the other. He is a witness, not an advocate.

In the adversary system of justice each attorney attempts to dispose of his opponent's arguments and this may extend to discrediting the medical testimony too. A lawyer is duty-bound to try to throw doubt on all evidence inimical to his case. This should not be construed as a personal attack on the medical witness.

It is sometimes said that lawyers try to make fools out of doctors on the witness stand. This they cannot do without generous help from the doctor himself. If he sticks to the facts of which he is sure, no lawyer will be able to shake his testimony. Many physicians go wrong by becoming advocates; they become emotionally involved. After losing their *sangfroid* on the witness stand, not only is their testimony suspect, but they look foolish, too. The duty of the medical witness is to state the facts of the case as he knows them, to offer his best medical opinion where he has sufficient grounds to formulate one, and to confine his testimony to what he is asked. Since juries are laymen, explanations should be as simple and straightforward as possible with a minimum of medical jargon. The witness's remarks should be addressed to the jury, since they, not the attorneys, are charged with the duty of determining the facts of the case and assessing the credibility of witnesses. In the rare event that a lawyer harries a medical witness, the opposing attorney or the judge will invariably intervene. To lose one's temper or argue with counsel is unprofessional and diminishes the value of one's testimony. At all times the medical witness should speak up clearly and distinctly and act like a member of a learned profession.

WORKMEN'S COMPENSATION

Workmen's Compensation statutes vary from state to state, and the practicing physician should acquaint himself with the law of his own state. In essence, these laws have been enacted to compensate employees injured while at work for loss of earnings and for permanent disability. This compensation is paid by the employer or his insurance carrier, whether or not the employer was in any way negligent or whether the employee contributed to the accident by his own negligence. There is no attempt to compensate the employee for pain and suffering, but only for loss of earnings. Since Workmen's Compensation claims are usually settled by a referee and the physician is normally not present at these hearings, the quality of the medical report is of major importance in the settlement of these claims.

PHYSICIAN'S LIABILITY

A physician is liable to be sued whenever a patient believes his treatment has been inadequate. Whether these complaints have any substance is immaterial, and even the most careful and competent surgeon may be sued. It is commonly held by physicians that the present unhappy situation is due to the pernicious system of contingency payments to attorneys but this overlooks the fact that the suit must be brought in the first place by a disgruntled patient. It seems to me that the causes for such actions are as follows:

That the surgeon has indeed been negligent. Many of these suits are due to the complications of tight or improperly applied casts, and precedents are so well established in such cases that the surgeon who does not take appropriate steps when a patient complains of pain under a cast is not only negligent, he is stupid. It is a pity that the five p's of impending Volkman's ischemia (pallor, pulselessness, pain, paresthesia and paralysis) have been taught so well. The only one that is universally reliable is pain. Unreasonable pain in a limb immobilized by a cast must be investigated by splitting cast and dressings to the skin, so that no element of constriction can remain, and further decompression, fasciotomy, etc., must be undertaken as necessary. Another potent source of trouble is neglecting to make a roentgenographic examination of a painful area, so that a fracture goes undetected. The desire to spare the patient expense is a false economy, and the prudent surgeon makes such examinations even though he is reasonably sure that no fracture is present. He also must make sure that the examination is complete (e.g., the hip and knee must be x-rayed in fractures of the femur to rule out coexisting injuries of these joints). Furthermore, if the quality of the films is unsatisfactory, he must ensure that the examination be repeated and better films obtained. When a case is not progressing satisfactorily the surgeon should not hesitate to call for assistance from more experienced or knowledgeable colleagues.

That the patient is unhappy with the cosmetic or functional result. Even with the most assiduous care, it is impossible in all cases to restore an injured person to a condition comparable to that which he or she was prior to the accident. The surgeon should make a realistic prognosis early on in his management so that no unrealistic expectations will be entertained by the patient or the patient's relatives. All operative procedures other than those life-saving measures that require action without delay should be discussed frankly with the patient and with the appropriate members of his family. The scope and aim of the procedure and a frank appraisal of the inherent risks should be explained, and this should be reflected in the operative permit which the patient signs.

That there has been a breakdown in the rapport between doctor and patient. Many suits, perhaps the majority, are engendered when a patient becomes angry because his doctor belittles or berates him or in some way shows a lack of concern, unapproachability, or off-handedness in his treatment. This may be of no importance when the result is good, but when the result is poor, it may be the factor that precipitates a suit.

That the surgeon, another physician, or ancillary personnel make remarks that can be construed as being critical of the treatment received. It goes without saying that everything that is said regarding treatment, especially that given by someone else, should be carefully worded, so that no pejorative inference may be picked up by the patient. Criticism of another without knowing all the circumstances is unfair and unjust, and the instigation of a law suit against another physician, unethical.

The best defense a surgeon has against groundless suits is obviously to give his patients competent, assiduous, and courteous service. The only way that this can be documented for legal purposes is by the completeness of the patient's records, both those in the hospital and in the surgeon's office. Voluminous notes may not prove the treatment has been excellent, but a paucity of records does suggest a lack of care. In any case, the medical record may be the only evidence to corroborate the doctor's story. The sooner these notes are written or dictated after the events they describe, the greater is their value. In many hospitals the dates of dictation and transcription appear on such documents as operative reports. Obviously an operative report dictated 3 months after the event does not carry as much weight in a court of law as one dictated immediately after surgery.

After a suit has been initiated some misguided physicians attempt to doctor the record by additions or alterations. Almost always this is picked up by an alert attorney, and it damages the physician's case irreparably. Inevitably, errors creep into hospital records, owing to mistakes in transcription. When such errors are corrected or when anything is added to the record, these additions should be dated and initialled. Considerable caution should be exercised where operative notes are dictated by an assistant. These should be read carefully, countersigned, and amended where necessary. It is even more prudent, however, for the surgeon to do his own dictation.

Good Samaritan Laws

Some states have seen fit to enact legislation that exempts physicians from legal action as a result of their having given emergency medical treatment at the scene of an accident. Opinions vary as to whether such laws are really necessary. There is no legal compulsion for a physician to stop at any accident and give aid; but if he does so, he establishes a doctor-patient relationship and his conduct is then governed by what a reasonably prudent physician would do under similar circumstances. Suit being brought under these circumstances is highly unlikely and is even less likely to be sustained in a court of law, unless there has been gross mismanagement. The remote threat of a possible malpractice suit, at any rate, is a rather poor excuse for not carrying out one's obvious duty, and I feel that few physicians would refuse to render aid on this account.

GLOSSARY

Dyne. That force which, if applied to 1 gram mass, gives it an acceleration of 1 cm. per second per second (cm./sec.^{2})

Poundal. That force which, if applied to 1 pound mass, gives it an acceleration of 1 foot per second per second (ft./sec.^{2})

Newton. That force which, if applied to 1 kilogram mass, gives it an acceleration of 1 meter per second per second (m./sec.^{2})

Kilopond (Kp). The most recent unit of force, is the force required to give 1 kilogram mass an acceleration of 9.80665 meters per second per second (9.8m./sec.^{2}) or a force of 9.80665 Newtons. "This force is equivalent to the weight of one kilogram mass under standard earth gravity; it represents the force with which this mass is attracted toward the center of the earth."[38]

REFERENCES

1. Adams, J., Kenmore, P. J., Russel, P. H., and Hass, S. S.: Regional anesthesia in the upper limb. *In* Adams, J. P. (ed.): Current Practice in Orthopaedic Surgery. vol. 4. St. Louis, C. V. Mosby, 1969.
2. Allen, W. C., Plotrowski, M. S., Burstein, A. H., and Frankel, V. H.: Biomechanical principles of intramedullary fixation. Clin. Orthop., *60*:13-20, 1968.

2A. Allgöwer, M., Perren, S., and Malter, P.: A new plate for internal fixation—the dynamic compression plate (DCP). Injury, *2*:40-47, 1970.

3. Alms, M.: Fracture mechanics. J. Bone Joint Surg., *43B*:162-166, 1961.
4. Apley, A. G.: Fractures of the lateral tibial condyle treated by skeletal traction and early mobilisation. J. Bone Joint Surg., *38B*:699-708, 1956.
5. Arzimanoglou, A., and Skiadaressis, G.: Study of internal fixation by screws of oblique fractures in long bones. J. Bone Joint Surg., *34A*:219-223, 1952.
6. Ash, A.: Medicolegal aspects of traumatic neurosis. Ind. Med. Surg., *37*:30-36, 1968.
7. Ashton, H.: Effects of inflatable plastic splints on blood flow. Brit. Med. J., *2*: 1427-1430, 1966.
8. Atkinson, D. J., Modell, J., and Moya, F.: Intravenous regional anesthesia. Anesth. Analg., *44*:313-317, 1965.
9. Bagby, G. W., and Janes, J. M.: The effect of compression on the rate of fracture healing using a special plate. Am. J. Surg., *95*:761-771, 1958.
10. Baker, J., Frankel, V. H., and Burstein, A.: Fatigue fractures: biomechanical considerations. J. Bone Joint Surg., *54A*:1345-1346, 1972.
11. Bateman, J. E.: An introduction to disability evaluation of the extremities. AAOS Instructional Course Lectures, *17*: 332-336, 1960.
12. Bechtol, C. O., and Lepper, H.: Fundamental studies in the design of metal screws for internal fixation of bone. J. Bone Joint Surg., *38A*:1385, 1956.

12A. Berger, J. C. (ed.): Wound Ballistics. Washington, D.C., Office of the Surgeon General, 1962.

13. Blockey, N. J.: An observation concerning the flexor muscles during recovery of function after dislocation of the elbow. J. Bone Joint Surg., *36A*:833-840, 1954.
14. Böhler, J.: Percutaneous internal fixation utilizing the x-ray image amplifier. J. Trauma, *5*:150-161, 1965.
15. ———: Closed intramedullary nailing of the femur. Clin. Orthop., *60*:51-67, 1968.
16. Bowden, F. P., Williamson, J. B. P., and Laing, P. G.: The significance of metallic transfer in orthopaedic surgery. J. Bone Joint Surg., *37B*:676-689, 1955.
17. Brav, E. A.: Intramedullary nailing for non-union of the femur. Clin. Orthop., *60*:69-75, 1968.
18. Brettle, J.: A survey of the literature on metallic surgical implants. Injury, *2*:26-39, 1970.
19. Brettle, J., Hughes, A. N., and Jordan, B. A.: Metallurgical aspects of surgical implant materials. Injury, *2*:225-234, 1971.
20. Bromage, P. R.: Local anesthetic procedures for arm and hand. Surg. Clin. N. Amer., *44*:919-923, 1964.
21. Brooks, D. B., Burstein, A. H., and Frankel, V.: Biomechanics of torsional fractures: stress concentration effect of a drill hole. J. Bone Joint Surg., *52A*:507-514, 1970.
22. Brower, T. D., Akahoshi, Y., and Orlic, P.: Diffusion of dyes through articular cartilage in vivo. J. Bone Joint Surg., *44A*:456-463, 1962.
23. Brown, P. W., and Urban, J. G.: Early weightbearing treatment of open fractures of the tibia: end results study of 63 cases. J. Bone Joint Surg., *51A*:59-75, 1969.
24. Brown, R. F.: Compound fractures of the tibia—the soft tissue defect. Proc. R. Soc. Med., *65*:625-626, 1972.
25. Bultitude, M. I., Wellwood, J. M., and Hollingsworth, R. P.: Intravenous diazepam: its use in the reduction of fractures of the lower end of the radius. Injury, *3*:249-253, 1972.
26. Burke, J. F.: The effective period of preventive antibiotic action in experimental incisions and dermal lesions. Surgery, *50*: 161-168, 1961.
27. Burstein, A. J., Currey, J., Frankel, V. H., Heiple, K. A., Lunset, P., and Vessely, J. C.: Bone strength, the effect of screw holes. J. Bone Joint Surg., *54A*:1143-1156, 1972.
28. Burwell, H. N.: Internal fixation in the treatment of fractures of the femoral shaft. Injury, *2*:235-244, 1971.

29. Bynum, D., Jr., Ray, D. R., Boyd, C. L., and Ledbetter, W. B.: Capacity of installed commercial bone fixation plates. Amer. J. Vet. Res., *32*:783-791, 1971.
30. Caldwell, J. A.: Treatment of fractures of the shaft of the humerus by hanging cast. Surg. Gynecol. Obstet., *70*:421-425, 1940.
31. Cassebaum, W. H.: Open reduction of **T** and **Y** fractures of the lower end of the humerus. J. Trauma, 9:915-925, 1969.
32. Cater, W. H., and Hicks, J. H.: The recent history of corrosion in metal used for internal fixation. Lancet, *2*:871-873, 1956.
33. Charnley, J.: The Closed Treatment of Common Fractures. ed. 3. Edinburg, E. & S. Livingstone, Ltd., 1968.
34. Clarke, R.: Assessment of blood loss following injury. Brit. J. Clin. Pract., *10*:746-769, 1956.
35. Clarke, R., Topley, E., and Flear, C. T. G.: Assessment of blood loss in civilian trauma. Lancet, *1*:629-638, 1955.
36. Clarke, R., Fisher, M. R., Topley, E., and Davies, J. W. L.: Extent and time of blood loss after civilian injury. Lancet, *2*:381-385, 1961.
37. Clawson, D. K., Smith, R. F., and Hensen, S. T.: Closed intramedullary nailing of the femur. J. Bone Joint Surg., *53A*: 681-692, 1971.
38. Cochran, G. van B.: Kilograms and kiloponds: mass force or weight? J. Bone Joint Surg., *53A*:181-182, 1971.
39. Cohen, J.: Corrosion testing of orthopaedic implants. J. Bone Joint Surg., *44A*:307, 1962.
40. Connolly, J.: Management of fractures associated with arterial injuries. Amer. J. Surg., *120*:331, 1970.
41. Connolly, J. F., Whittaker, D., and Williams, E.: Femoral and tibial fractures combined with injuries to the femoral or popliteal artery. J. Bone Joint Surg., *53A*: 56-67, 1971.
42. Danckwardt-Lilliestrom, G.: Reaming of the medullary cavity and its effect on diaphyseal bone. Acta Orthop. Scand. [Suppl.]:128, 1969.
43. Dehne, E.: Treatment of fractures of the tibial shaft. Clin. Orthop., *66*:159-173, 1969.
44. Dehne, E., Deffer, P. A., Hall, R. M., Brown, P. W., and Johnson, E. V.: The natural history of the fractured tibia. Surg. Clin. N. Amer., *41*:1495-1513, 1961.
45. DeJong, R. H.: Axillary block of the brachial plexus. Anesthesiology, *22*:215-225, 1961.
45A. DeMuth, W. E., and Smith, J. M.: High velocity bullet wounds of muscle and bone. The basis of rational early treatment. J. Trauma, *6*:744-755, 1966.
46. Devas, M. B.: Compression stress fractures in man and greyhound. J. Bone Joint Surg., *43B*:540-551, 1961.
47. ———: Stress fractures. Practitioner, *197*:70-76, 1966.
47A. Dimond, F. C., and Rich, N. M.: M-16 rifle wounds in Vietnam. J. Trauma, *7*: 619-625, 1967.
48. Dinley, R. J., and Michelinakis, E.: Local anesthesia in the reduction of Colles' fracture. Injury, *4*:345-346, 1973.
49. Dodge, H. S., and Cady, G. W.: Treatment of fractures of the radius and ulna with compression plates. J. Bone Joint Surg., *54A*:1167-1176, 1972.
50. Eggers, B. W. N.: Internal contact splint. J. Bone Joint Surg., *30A*:40-52, 1948.
51. Ekholm, R.: Nutrition of articular cartilage. A radiographic study. Acta Anat., *24*:329-338, 1955.
52. Emergency War Surgery (NATO Handbook). Washington, D.C., United States Government Printing Office, 1958.
53. Enneking, W. F., and Horowitz, M.: The intra-articular effects of immobilization on the human knee. J. Bone Joint Surg., *54A*: 973-985, 1972.
54. Epps, C. H., and Adams, J. P.: Wound management in open fractures. Amer. Surgeon, *27*:766-769, 1961.
55. Evans, C. M.: Supracondylar **Y** fracture of the humerus. J. Bone Joint Surg., *35B*: 381-385, 1953.
56. Evans, E. B., Eggers, G. N. W., Butler, J. K., and Blumel, J.: Experimental immobilization of rat knee joints. J. Bone Joint Surg., *42A*:737-758, 1960.
57. Evans, F. G.: Relation of the physical properties of bone to fractures. AAOS Instructional Course Lectures, *17*:110-121, 1960.
58. Ferguson, A. B., and Laing, P. G.: Corrosion and corrosion resistant metals in orthopaedic surgery. AAOS Instructional Course Lectures, *15*:96-103, 1958.
59. Fisher, M. R.: Clinical signs following injury in relation to red cell and total blood volume. Clin. Sci., *17*:181-204, 1958.
60. Fitzgerald, J. A. W.: The management of fractures of the ipsilateral patella and femur. Injury, *1*:287-292, 1970.

61. Fogelberg, E. V., Zetzmann, E. K., and Stinchfield, F. E.: Prophylactic penicillin in orthopaedic surgery. J. Bone Joint Surg., *52A*:95-98, 1970.
62. Forbes, G. B.: Staphylococcal infection of operation wounds with special reference to topical antibiotic prophylaxis. Lancet, *2*:505-509, 1961.
63. Frankel, V. H., Burstein, A. H.: Orthopaedic biomechanics. Philadelphia, Lea & Febiger, 1970.
64. Fox, R. M.: The Medicolegal Report. Theory and Practice. Boston, Little, Brown, 1969.
65. Funk, R. J., Wells, R. E., and Street, D.: Supplementary fixation of femoral fractures. Clin. Orthop., *60*:41-49, 1968.
66. Ger, R.: The management of pretibial skin loss. Surgery, *63*:757-763, 1968.
67. ——: The management of open fractures of the tibia with skin loss. J. Trauma, *10*: 112-121, 1970.
68. Gingrass, R. P., Close, A. S., and Ellison, E.: The effect of various topical and parenteral agents on the prevention of infection in experimental contaminated wounds. J. Trauma, *4*:763-783, 1964.
69. Gissane, W.: Symposium on the treatment of fractures of the shafts of the long bones. Proc. Roy. Soc. Med., *52*:291-295, 1959.
70. Gottfries, A., Hagert, C. G., and Sorenson, S. E.: **T** and **Y** fractures of the tibial condyles. Injury, *3*:56-64, 1971.
71. Greener, E., and Lautenschlager, E.: Materials for bioengineering applications. Biomedical *In* Brown, J. H. V., Jacobs, J. E., and Stark, L. (eds.): Biomedical Engineering. Philadelphia, F. A. Davis, 1971.
72. Griffiths, D. L.: Hazards of closed reduction of fractures. Texas Med., *64*:46-50, October, 1968.
73. Gustilo, R. B., Simpson, L., Nixon, R., Ruiz, A., and Indeck, W.: Analysis of 511 open fractures. Clin. Orthop., *66*:148-154, 1969.
74. Hassard, H.: Medical Malpractice: Risks, Protection, Prevention. Oradell, New Jersey, Medical Economics Book Division Inc., 1966.
75. Heutschenreuter, P., Perren, S. M., Steinemann, S., Geret, V., and Klebl, M.: Some effects of rigidity of internal fixation on the healing pattern of osteotomies. Injury, *1*:77-81, 1969.
76. Hey Groves, E. H.: Methods and Results of transplantation of bone in the repair of defects caused by injury or disease. Brit. J. Surg., *5*:185-242, 1918.
77. Hicks, J. H.: The fallacy of the fractured clavicle. Lancet, *1*:131-132, 1958.
78. ———: External splintage as a cause of movement in fractures. Lancet, *1*:667-670, 1960.
79. ———: The influence of Arbuthnot Lane on fracture treatment. Injury, *1*:314-316, 1970.
80. ———: High rigidity in fractures of the tibia. Injury, *3*:121-134, 1971.
81. ———: [Letter to the editor.] Injury, *4*: 361, 1973.
82. Hicks, J. H., and Cater, W. H.: Minor reactions due to modern metals. J. Bone Joint Surg., *44B*:122-128, 1962.
83. Holden, C. E. A.: The role of blood supply to soft tissue in the healing of diaphyseal fractures. J. Bone Joint Surg., *54A*:993-1000, 1972.
84. Holst-Nielson, F.: Dynamic intramedullary osteosynthesis in fractures of the femoral shaft. Acta Orthop. Scand., *43*: 411-420, 1972.
85. Hubbard, M. J. S.: Experimental femoral shaft fractures. Acta Orthop. Scand., *44*: 55-61, 1973.
86. Hughston, J. C.: Fracture of the distal radial shaft—mistakes in management. J. Bone Joint Surg., *39A*:249-264, 1957.
87. Jones, Sir R.: An orthopaedic view of the treatment of fractures. Amer. J. Orthop. Surg., *11*:314-335, 1913.
88. Kasdan, M. L., Kleinert, H. E., Kasdan, A. P., and Kutz, J. E.: Axillary block anesthesia for surgery of the hand. Plast. Reconstr. Surg., *46*:256-261, 1970.
89. Kelly, P. J., and Lipscomb, P. R.: Primary Vitallium mold arthroplasty for posterior dislocation of the hip with fracture of the femoral head. J. Bone Joint Surg., *40A*: 675-680, 1958.
90. Kelly, R. P., and Griffin, T. W.: Open reduction of **T**-condylar fractures of the humerus through an anterior approach. J. Trauma, *9*:901-913, 1969.
91. Kelly, R. P., and Yarbrough, S. H., III: Posterior fracture dislocation of the femoral head with retained medial head fragment. J. Trauma, *11*:97-108, 1971.
92. Keon-Cohen, B. T.: Fractures at the elbow. J. Bone Joint Surg., *48A*:1623-1639, 1966.
93. Kessler, H. H.: Disability—Determination and Evaluation. Philadelphia, Lea & Febiger, 1970.

94. Key, J. A., and Reynolds, F. C.: The treatment of infection after medullary nailing. Surgery, *35*:749-757, 1954.
95. Kia, D., and Dragstedt, L. R., II: Prevention of likely wound infections. Arch. Surg., *100*:229-231, 1970.
96. Kleinert, H. E., DeSimone, K., Gaspar, H. E., Arnold, R. E., and Kasdan, M. L.: Regional anesthesia for upper extremity surgery. J. Trauma, *3*:3-11, 1963.
97. Koryani, E., Knecht, C. D., and Janssen, M.: Holding power of orthopaedic screws in bone. Clin. Orthop., *72*:285-286, 1970.
98. Küntscher, G.: Die Marknagelung von Knochenbruchen. Tierexperimentaller Teil. Klin. Wchn. Schr., *19*:6, 1940.
99. ———: The Küntscher method of intramedullary fixation. J. Bone Joint Surg., *40A*:17-26, 1958.
100. ———: Practice of Intramedullary Nailing. Springfield, Illinois, Charles C Thomas, 1967.
101. ———: The intramedullary nailing of fractures. Clin. Orthop., *60*:5-12, 1968.
102. Lane, Sir W. A.: The direct fixation of fractures. Tr. Clin. Soc. London, *27*:167, 1893-1894.
103. Laurence, M., Freeman, M. A. R., and Swanson, S. A. V.: Engineering considerations in the internal fixation of fractures of the tibial shaft. J. Bone Joint Surg., *51B*:754-768, 1969.
104. Litchman, H. M., and Duffy, J.: Lower extremity balanced traction. Clin. Orthop., *66*:159-173, 1969.
105. London, P. S.: Observations of the treatment of some fractures of the forearm by splintage that does not include the elbow. Injury, *2*:252-270, 1971.
106. ———: Observations of medical investigation of ambulance services. Injury, *3*: 225-238, 1972.
107. Lottes, J. O.: Intramedullary nailing of the tibia. AAOS Instructional Course Lectures, *15*:65-77, 1958.
108. ———: Medullary nailing of infected fractures. Clin. Orthop., *60*:99-101, 1968.
109. MacAusland, W. R.: Treatment of sepsis after intramedullary nailing of fractures of the femur. Clin. Orthop., *60*:87-94, 1968.
110. MacAusland, W. R., and Eaton, R. G.: Sepsis following fractures of the femur. J. Bone Joint Surg., *45A*:1643-1653, 1963.
111. McNeur, J. C.: Management of open skeletal trauma with particular reference to internal fixation. J. Bone Joint Surg., *52B*:54-60, 1970.
112. Massie, W. K.: Intramedullary fixation of tibial shaft fractures. Clin. Orthop., *2*:147-160, 1953.
113. Mathysen, A.: Plaster-of-paris in the treatment of fractures. Leige, Grandmont-Donders, 1852.
114. Mayfield, G. W.: Rotational malunion of femoral shaft fractures and its functional significance. J. Bone Joint Surg., *56A*: 1309, 1974.
115. Mooney, V., Nickel, V. L., Harvey, J. P., and Snelson, R.: Cast brace treatment for fractures of the distal part of the femur. J. Bone Joint Surg., *52A*:1563-1578, 1970.
116. Moore, D. C., Bridenbaugh, L. D., Bridenbaugh, P. O., and Tucker, G. T.: Bupivacaine. A review of 2,077 cases. J.A.M.A., *214*:713-718, 1970.
117. Müller, M. E., Allgöwer, M., and Willenegger, H.: Manual of Internal Fixation. New York, Springer-Verlag, 1970.
118. Murray, W. R., Lucas, D. B., and Inman, V. T.: Treatment of non-union of fractures of the long bone by the two plate method. J. Bone Joint Surg., *46A*:1027-1048, 1964.
119. Mustard, W. T., and Simmons, E. H.: Experimental arterial spasm in the lower extremities produced by traction. J. Bone Joint Surg., *35B*:437-441, 1953.
120. Nach, D. C., and Keim, H. A.: Prophylactic antibiotics in spinal surgery. Orthop. Rev., *2*:27-39, 1973.
121. Nelson, J. P., Ferris, D. O., and Ivins, J. C.: Cast syndrome: case report. Postgrad. Med., *42*:457-461, 1967.
122. Neufeld, A. J., Mays, J. J., and Naden, C. J.: A dynamic method of treating femoral shaft fractures. Orthop. Rev., *1*:19-21, 1972.
123. Nicholls, P. J. R.: Rehabilitation after fractures of the shaft of the femur. J. Bone Joint Surg., *45B*:96-102, 1963.
124. O'Brien, J. P.: Femoral shaft refracture. Aust. New Zealand J. Surgery, *39*:194-197, 1969.
125. Olerud, S., and Danckwardt-Lilliestrom, G.: Fracture healing in compression osteosynthesis. Acta Orthop. Scand. [Suppl.]: 137, 1971.
126. Olerud, S., and Karlstrom, G.: Tibial fractures treated by AO compression osteosynthesis. Acta Orthop. Scand. [Suppl.]: 140, 1972.
127. ———: Secondary intramedullary nailing of tibial fractures. J. Bone Joint Surg., *54A*:1419-1428, 1972.
128. Olix, M. L., Klug, T. J., Coleman, C. R.,

and Smith, W. S.: Prophylactic penicillin and streptomycin in elective operations on bone, joint and tendons. Surg. Forum, *10*:818-819, 1959.

129. Peltier, L. F.: A brief history of traction. J. Bone Joint Surg., *50A*:1603-1617, 1968.

130. Pentecost, R. L., Murray, R., and Brindley, H. H.: Insufficiency and pathologic fractures. J.A.M.A., *187*:1001-1004, 1964.

131. Perkins, G.: Fractures and Dislocations. London, The Athlone Press, 1958.

132. ———: The Ruminations of an Orthopaedic Surgeon. London, Butterworth, 1970.

133. Peterson, L. T.: Principles of internal fixation with plates and screws. Arch. Surg., *64*:345-354, 1947.

134. Peterson, L. T., and Reeder, O. S.: Dual slotted plates in fixation of fractures of the femoral shaft. J. Bone Joint Surg., *32A*:523-541, 1950.

135. Piekarski, K., Wiley, A. M., and Bartels, J. E.: The effect of delayed internal fixation on fracture healing. Acta Orthop. Scand., *40*:543-551, 1969.

136. Pruigle, R. A.: Missed fractures. Injury, *4*:311-316, 1973.

137. Rasmussen, P. S.: Tibial condylar fractures as a cause of degenerative arthritis. Acta Orthop. Scand., *43*:566-575, 1972.

138. Rattner, I. N.: Injury Ratings. How to Figure Dollar Values in the U.S.A. New York, Crescent Publishing Co., 1970.

139. Regan, L. J.: Doctor, Patient and the Law. ed. 3. St. Louis, C. V. Mosby, 1956.

140. Rhinelander, F. W.: Normal microcirculation of the cortex. J. Bone Joint Surg., *50A*:784-800, 1968.

141. Rich, N. M., Metz, C. W., Hutton, J. E., Baugh, J. H., and Hughes, C. W.: Internal versus external fixation of fractures with concomitant vascular injuries in Vietnam. J. Trauma, *11*:463-473, 1971.

142. Rokkanen, P., Slatis, P., and Vankka, E.: Closed or open intramedullary nailing of femoral shaft fractures? A comparison with conservatively treated cases. J. Bone Joint Surg., *51B*:313-323, 1969.

143. Rush, L. V.: Atlas of Rush Pin Technique. Meridian, Miss., Berwon, 1955.

144. ———: Dynamic intramedullary fracture fixation of the femur. Clin. Orthop., *60*: 21-27, 1968.

145. Russell, R. H.: Fracture of the femur: a clinical study. Brit. J. Surg., *11*:491-502, 1924.

146. St. Clair Strange, F. A.: The Hip. Baltimore, Williams & Wilkins, 1965.

147. Salter, R. B., and Field, P.: The effects of continuous compression on living articular cartilage. An experimental investigation. J. Bone Joint Surg., *42A*:31-49, 1960.

148. Sarmiento, A.: The brachioradialis as a deforming force in Colles' fracture. Clin. Orthop., *38*:86-92, 1965.

149. ———: A functional below-the-knee cast for tibial fractures. J. Bone Joint Surg., *49A*:855-875, 1967.

150. ———: Functional bracing of tibial and femoral shaft fractures. Clin. Orthop., *82*: 2-13, 1972.

151. ———: A functional treatment of forearm fractures—preliminary report. AAOS Annual Meeting, Dallas, 1974.

152. Scales, J. T., Towers, A. G., and Roantree, B. M.: The influence of antibiotic therapy on wound inflammation and sepsis associated with orthopaedic implants. Acta Orthop. Scand., *43*:85-100, 1972.

153. Scheinberg, S.: The SAM (structural aluminum malleable splint). [In press]

154. Schneider, H. W.: Use of the 4-flanged self-cutting intramedullary nail for fixation of femoral fractures. Clin. Orthop., *60*:29-39, 1968.

155. Sherman, W. O'N.: Vanadium steel bone plates and screws. Surg. Gynecol. Obstet., *14*:629-634, 1912.

156. Simmons, E. H.: An experimental and clinical study of vascular spasm. Arch. Surg., *73*:625-634, 1956.

157. Smith, J. E.: Internal fixation in the treatment of fractures of the shafts of radius and ulna in adults. J. Bone Joint Surg., *41B*:122-131, 1959.

158. Solheim, K.: Tibial fractures treated according to the AO method. Injury, *4*:213-220, 1973.

159. Sorbie, C., and Chacha, P.: Regional anesthesia by intravenous route. Brit. Med. J., *1*:957-960, 1965.

160. Stevens, D. B.: Postoperative orthopaedic infections. J. Bone Joint Surg., *46A*:96-102, 1964.

161. Stewart, M. J.: Fractures of the humeral shaft. Curr. Prac. Orthop. Surg., *2*:140-162, 1964.

162. Street, D. M.: One hundred fractures of the femur treated by means of a diamond-shaped medullary nail. J. Bone Joint Surg., *33A*:659-669, 1951.

163. Street, D. M., Hansen, H. H., and Brewer, B. J.: The medullary nail, presentation of a new type and report of a case. Arch. Surg., *55*:423-432, 1947.

164. Sudman, E.: Rotational displacements

after percutaneous intramedullary osteosynthesis of femoral shaft fractures. Acta Orthop. Scand., *44*:242-248, 1973.

165. Swanson, S. A. V.: Biomechanical characteristics of bone. *In* Kenedi, R. M. (ed.): Advances in Biomedical Engineering. vol. 1. New York, Academic Press, 1971.
166. Tachdjian, M. O., and Compere, E. L.: Postoperative wound infections in orthopaedic surgery. Evaluation of prophylactic antibiotics. J. Internat. Coll. Surgeons, *28*:797-805, 1957.
167. Thunold, J.: Fractura Cruris. Acta Chir. Scand., *135*:611-614, 1969.
168. Venable, C. S., and Stuck, W. G.: Electrolysis controlling factor in the use of metals in treating fractures. J.A.M.A., *111*:1349-1352, 1938.
169. ———: Results of recent studies and experiments concerning metals used in the internal fixation of fractures. J. Bone Joint Surg., *30A*:247-250, 1948.
170. Vere Nicholl, E. D.: Air splints for the emergency treatment of fractures. J. Bone Joint Surg., *46A*:1761-1764, 1964.
171. Vesely, D. G.: Technic for use of the single and the double split diamond nail for fractures of the femur. Clin. Orthop., *60*: 95-97, 1968.
172. Waterman, N. G., and Pollard, N. T.: Local antibiotic treatment of wounds. *In* Maibach, H. I., and Rovee, D. T. (eds.): Epidermal Wound Healing. Chicago, Year Book Medical Publishers, 1972.
173. Watson-Jones, R.: Fractures and Joint Injuries. Baltimore, Williams & Wilkins, 1952.
174. Weber, B. G.: Fractures of the femoral shaft in childhood. Injury, *1*:65-68, 1969.
175. Weissman, S. L., and Khermosh, O.: Orthopaedic aspects of multiple injuries. J. Trauma, *10*:377-385, 1970.
176. Wickstrom, J., Corban, M. S., and Vise, G. T.: Complications following intramedullary fixation. Clin. Orthop., *60*:103-113, 1968.
177. Winnie, A. P., and Collins, W. J.: Subclavian perivascular technique of brachial plexus anesthesia. Anesthesiology, *25*: 353-363, 1964.

2 Healing of Bone, Tendon, and Ligament

Richard L. Cruess, M.D., F.R.C.S. (C)
Jacques Dumont, M.D., F.R.C.S. (C)

The musculoskeletal system is an extremely complex and important part of the human body, and damage to it is seldom simple. The structures injured include bones, soft tissues, joints, muscles, tendons, ligaments, and blood vessels. Other organ systems may be involved, making repair complex. Through the millions of years of human evolution, repair processes have developed, which are extremely predictable and which assure survival of the species by returning individual members to useful, functional existence. A knowledge of these active repair processes is essential for any surgeon who would undertake the treatment of the musculoskeletal system. It would appear reasonable that wherever possible, the natural processes should be allowed to take their course and that interference with this normal course should only be attempted when there is demonstrable need or substantial benefit to the patient.

BASIC FRACTURE HEALING

As our knowledge has increased, our understanding of the sequence of events following a break in continuity of a bone has become clearer. Some concepts have been abandoned as basic knowledge of the cellular responses involved became more detailed.

Fracture healing can be divided conveniently into phases, but it must be stressed that events described in one phase persist into the next and that events that occur in subsequent phases begin in an earlier phase (Fig. 2-1). The arbitrary phase division makes the overall picture clearer. These events have been described through the years in investigative reports and review articles.[50,132]

Inflammatory Phase

After a fracture, the bone itself is dam-

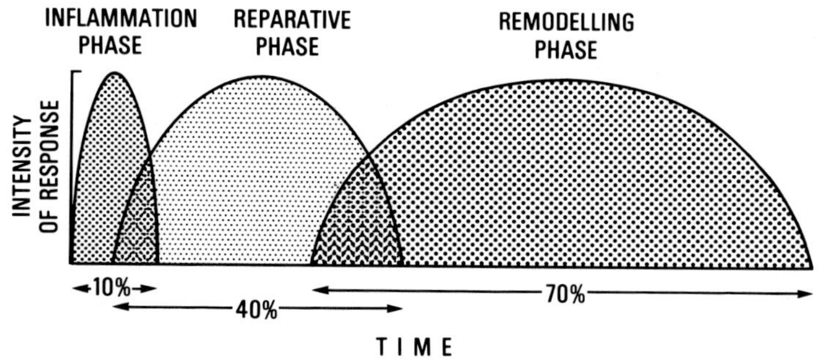

Fig. 2-1. An approximation of the relative amounts of time devoted to the inflammation, reparative, and remodelling phases in fracture healing.

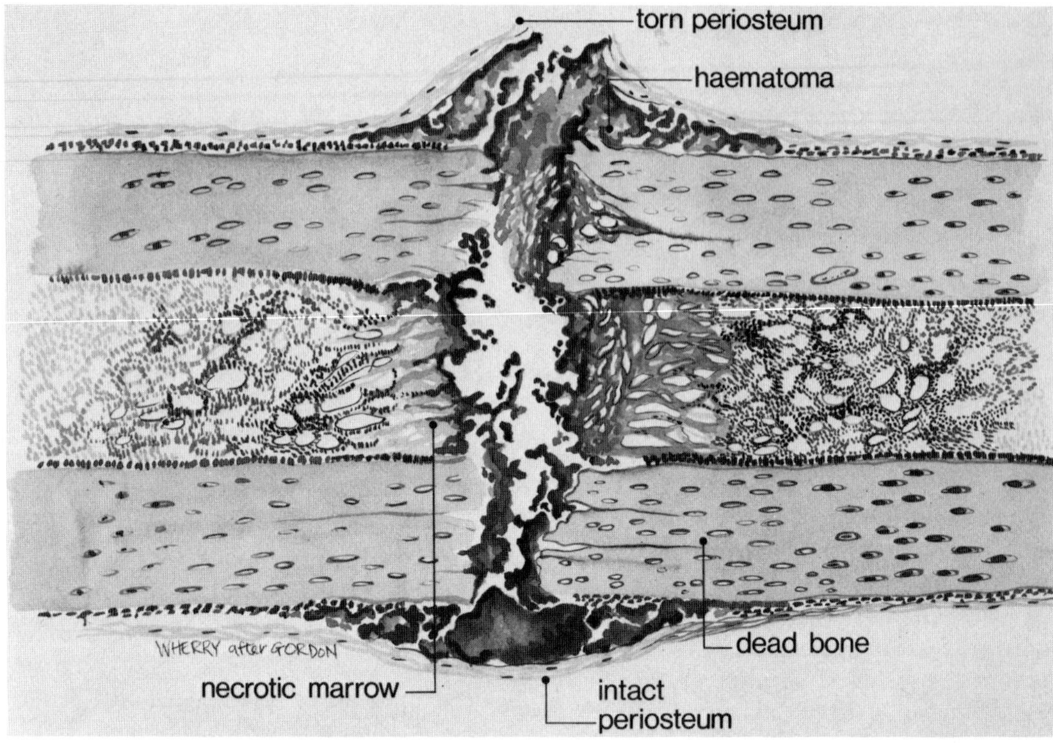

Fig. 2-2. The initial events involved in fracture healing of long bone. The periosteum is torn opposite the point of impact, and in many instances, is intact on the other side. There is an accumulation of hematoma beneath the periosteum and between the fracture ends. There is necrotic marrow and dead bone close to the fracture line.

aged (Fig. 2-2). The soft-tissue envelope, including the periosteum and surrounding muscles, is torn, and numerous blood vessels crossing the fracture line are ruptured. There is an accumulation of hematoma within the medullary canal, between the fracture ends, and beneath any elevated periosteum. This blood rapidly coagulates to form a clot. The effect of damage to the blood vessels is of paramount importance. Osteocytes are deprived of their nutrition and die as far back as the junction of collateral channels. Thus, the immediate ends of a fracture are dead—they contain no living cells. Severely damaged periosteum and marrow as well as other surrounding soft tissues may also contribute necrotic material to the region.[50]

The presence of so much necrotic material elicits an immediate and intense acute inflammatory response. There is widespread vasodilatation and plasma exudation, leading to the acute edema seen in the region of a fresh fracture. Acute inflammatory cells migrate to the region, as well as polymorphonuclear leukocytes followed by macrophages. As the acute inflammatory response subsides, the second phase begins to take over and gradually becomes the predominant pattern.

Reparative Phase

The first step in the reparative phase is identical with the repair process seen in other tissues. The hematoma is organized (Fig. 2-3), and while there is some controversy as to the necessity of this step, it seems unavoidable in the natural repair process.[2] This hematoma probably plays a very small mechanical role in immobilizing the fracture and serves primarily as a fibrin scaffold over which repair cells perform

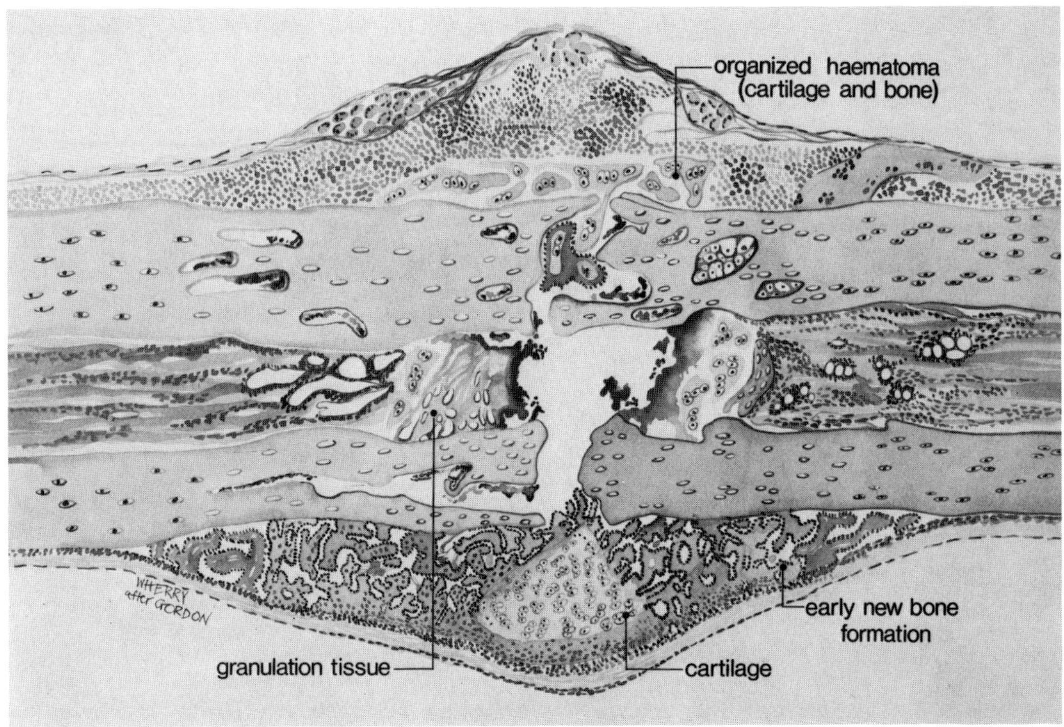

Fig. 2-3. Early repair. There is organization of the hematoma, early primary new bone formation in subperiosteal regions, and cartilage formation in other areas.

their function.[103] It has been known for some time that at this stage, the microenvironment about the fracture is acid,[120] which may well be an additional stimulus to cell behavior during the early phases of repair. During the repair process, the pH gradually returns to neutral and then to a slightly alkaline level.

The cells involved directly in the repair of fractures are of mesenchymal origin and are pluripotential. In the process of fracture healing, cells, probably of common origin, form collagen, cartilage, and bone. Small variations in their microenvironment and in the stresses to which they are subjected probably determine which behavior predominates.[6] Some cells are derived from the cambium layer of the periosteum and form the earliest bone, particularly in children, in whom this layer is active and important. Endosteal cells also participate. Surviving osteocytes do not take part in the repair process, as they are destroyed during resorption.[123] However, the majority of cells involved directly in fracture healing enter the fracture site with the granulation tissue, which invades the region from surrounding vessels.[125] Whether these reparative cells are derived directly from endothelium,[125] or are "wandering cells,"[142] or are derived from nucleated red cells[10] seems less important than the fact that repair is indivisably linked with the ingress of capillary buds. It is notable that the entire vascular bed of an extremity is increased shortly after fracture, but the osteogenic response is limited largely to the zones surrounding the fracture itself.[139] The principal origin of the blood vessels has been a subject of controversy in the past. It appears that under ordinary circumstances[107,108] the periosteal vessels contribute the majority of capillary buds early in normal bone healing, with the nutrient medullary artery becoming more important later in the process. When the surgeon interferes with this natural process, either by stripping the periosteum excessively or by destroying the

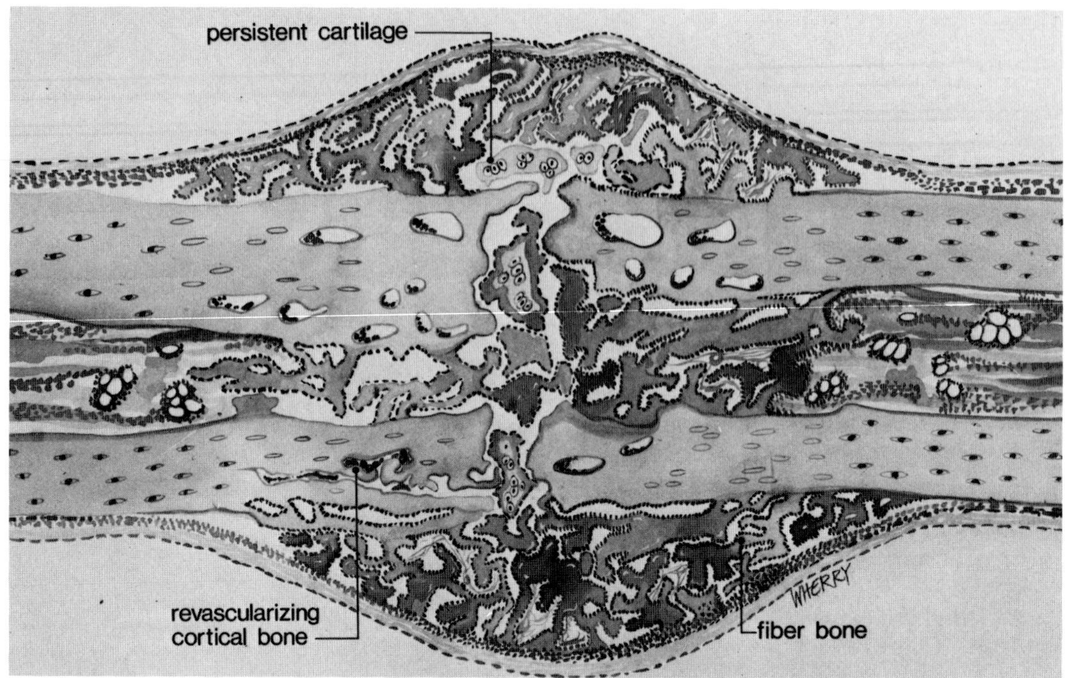

Fig. 2-4. At later stage in the repair, early immature fiber bone is bridging the fracture gap. Persistent cartilage is seen at points most distant from ingrowing capillary buds. In many instances, these are surrounded by young new bone.

intramedullary system through the use of medullary nails, repair must proceed with vessels derived from the surviving system.[31]

The cells invade the hematoma and begin rapidly producing the tissue known as callus, which is made up of fibrous tissue, cartilage, and young, immature fiber bone. This rapidly envelopes the bone ends and leads to a gradual increase in stability of the fracture fragments. The mechanisms that control the behavior of each individual cell at this stage of the repair process probably derive from the microenvironment in which the cell finds itself. Compression or the absence of tension discourages the formation of fibrous tissue. Variations in oxygen tension undoubtedly lead to the formation of either bone or cartilage, cartilage being formed where oxygen tensions are relatively low,[6] presumably owing to the distance of the cell from its blood supply.[107]

Cartilage, thus formed, is eventually resorbed by a process indistinguishable from endochondral bone formation, except for its lack of organization. Bone will be formed *per primam* by those cells that receive enough oxygen and are subjected to the proper mechanical stimuli. Early in the repair process, cartilage formation predominates, and glycosaminoglycans (mucopolysaccharides) are found in high concentrations. Later, bone formation is more obvious (Fig. 2-4).

The biochemical events follow a sequential pattern: a high level of glycosaminoglycans is present early in the repair process, followed by a gradual increase in the concentration of collagen, with accumulation of calcium hydroxyapatite crystals occurring as a third stage (Fig. 2-5). The collagen content by weight tends to return to normal levels after mineralization has occurred.[129]

Mineralized tissues are highly organized in their internal structure, and this organization occurs as the result of cellular activ-

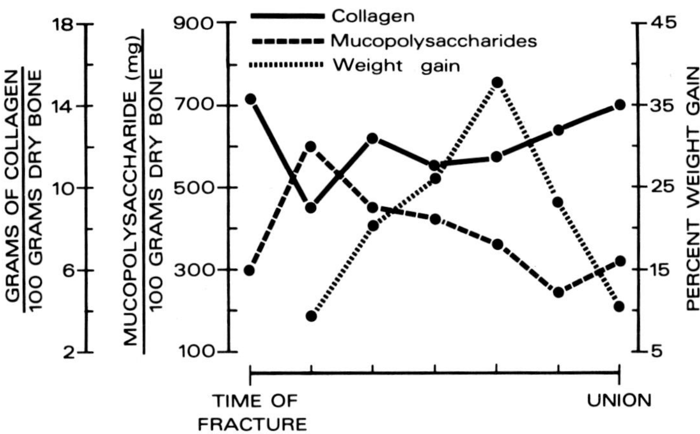

Fig. 2-5. A schematic representation of the biochemical events following a fracture. Collagen formation precedes significant accumulation of mineral, and mucopolysaccharide falls gradually as fracture healing progresses after an initial rise.

ity. The initial step is the formation by osteoblasts of tropocollagen, which moves from inside the cells to outside and polymerizes to form collagen fibrils.[49]

Collagen fibrils have their own internal organization, and within the substance of the fibrils are spaces.[56] These have been called hole zones, and they occur in regular fashion as the result of the internal structure of the collagen molecules (Fig. 2-6).

The initial appearance of mineral occurs in this region[43] as a result of an interaction between metastable solutions of calcium and phosphate and the groups of specific amino acid side chains within the holes.[47] The result of this is a series of organized collagen fibrils within and around which are clustered crystals of calcium hydroxyapatite.

As this phase of repair takes place, the bone ends gradually become enveloped in a fusiform mass of callus containing increasing amounts of bone. Immobilization of the fragments becomes more rigid because of this internal and external callus formation, and eventually clinical "union" is said to have occurred. Once more, however, it should be stressed, that union as an end point does not yet exist, because in the middle of the reparative phase, the remodelling phase begins with resorption of unneeded or inefficient portions of the callus and the laying down of trabecular bone along lines of stress.

Remodelling Phase

In 1892, Wolff,[138] recognizing that the architecture of the skeletal system corresponded to the mechanical need of this system, postulated his law. Remodelling about a fracture takes place for a prolonged period of time. Radio-isotope studies have showed that increased activity in a fractured bone lasts much longer than had previously been thought.[136] In humans, there is increased activity for 6 to 9 years after a tibial fracture.

Osteoclastic resorption of superfluous or poorly placed trabeculae occurs, and new struts of bone are laid down which correspond to lines of force. The control mechanism that modulates this cell behavior is now believed to be electrical. When a bone is subjected to stress, electropositivity occurs on the convex surface and electronegativity on the concave, this current having been produced by a piezoelectric effect.[8] Circumstantial evidence indicates that regions of electropositivity are associated with osteoclastic activity and regions of electronegativity with osteoblastic activity.[7] While the subject of biophysical principles affecting bone structure is extremely complex, it is apparent that this, at least, is established and that Wolff's law is explainable in terms of alterations in the electrical currents generated by crystalline structures within the bone which have a direct effect on cellular behavior. The cellular module

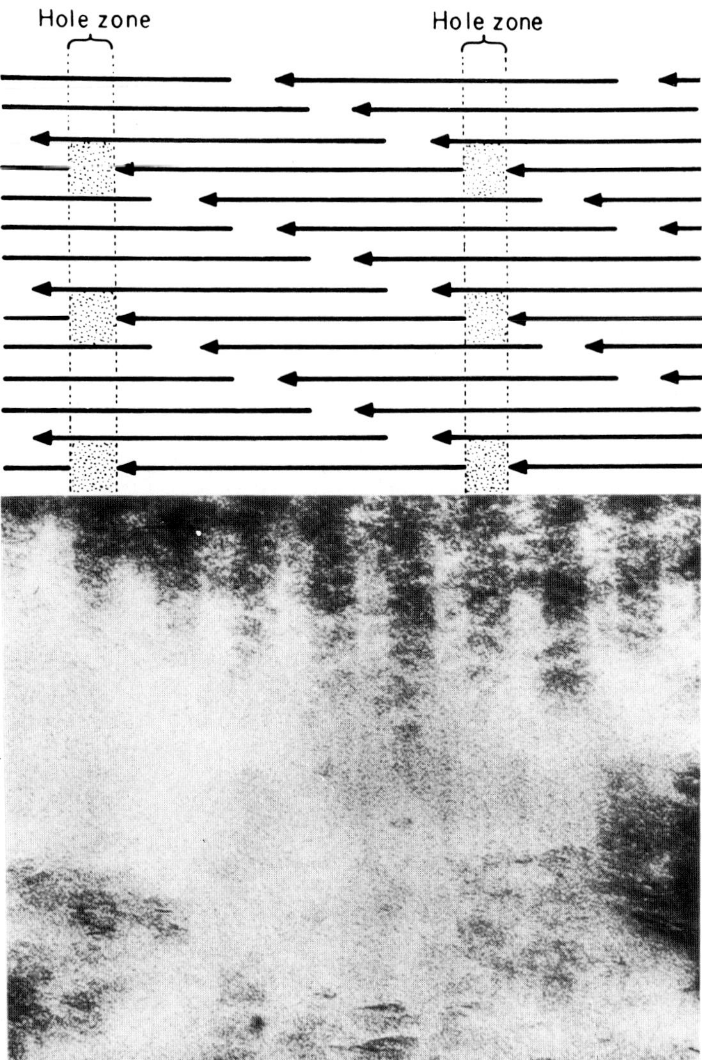

Fig. 2-6. Mineralization appears to occur in collagen with the first mineral appearing in the so-called hole zone. (Glimcher, M. J.: Clin. Orthop., *61*: 16-36, 1968)

that controls remodelling is the resorption unit, consisting of osteoclasts, which first resorb bone, followed by osteoblasts, which lay down new haversian systems.[46] The end result of remodelling is a bone that, if it has not returned to its original form, has been altered so that it may best perform the function demanded of it.

CONDITIONS INFLUENCING AND AFFECTING FRACTURE HEALING

Healing of a fracture in a living organism is carried out by cells, and so it can be modified by almost any endogenous or exogenous factor that has an influence on the metabolic function of cells. The literature abounds with reports of factors that can either promote or retard bone healing (Table 2-1).[96] While most of these factors do, in all probability, exert an influence that can be measured in the laboratory, in clinical practice fracture healing appears to proceed with a certain degree of predictability and is modified by relatively few influences.

Local Factors

The Degree of Local Trauma. Fracture

Table 2-1. Factors Influencing Bone Healing

Factors Claimed to Promote Bone Healing		Factors Claimed to Retard Bone Healing	
Factor	References	Factor	References
Growth hormone	58, 63, 65, 83, 88	Corticosteroids	39, 63, 67
Triiodothyronin	121	Alloxan diabetes	53, 54
Thyroxin	64	Castration	64
Thyrotropin	65	Vitamin A, high dose	128
Calcitonin	41, 143	Vitamin D, high dose	30
Insulin	116	Rachitis	30
Vitamin A	128	Anemia	110
Vitamin D	119	Aminoacetonitrile	66
Anabolic steroids	67	B-aminopropionitrile	137
Chondroitin sulphate	19, 55	Bone wax	57
Hyaluronidase	12	Delayed manipulation	92
Anticoagulants (Dicumarol)	109	Denervation	106
Ultrasonics	61	X-ray irradiation	5
Electric currents	10	Hyperbaric oxygenation 6 hr., 2 atm. daily	140
Hyperbaric oxygen 2 hr., 3 atm. daily	32, 141	Anticoagulants (Dicumarol)	33
Physical exercise	51		

healing has been described as involving differentiation of cells from a mesenchymal pool. It is well known that those fractures that are associated with more local trauma or trauma to the soft tissues surrounding the bone show retarded healing. This is undoubtedly due to a decrease in the rapidity of differentiation of the mesenchymal cells and in their total number. The soft-tissue envelope around the fracture, in addition to providing mesenchymal cells for fracture healing, must in this instance heal the soft tissues themselves. In addition, the hematoma escapes into the soft tissues, leading to a diffusion of mesenchymal cell effort. Finally, in simpler fractures a soft-tissue envelope is intact on at least the concave side of a fracture, providing both a ready source of mesenchymal cells and a tube that directs the repair efforts of these cells.[22] Of course, this tube also contributes to immobilization of the fragments. The differences in the repair process between undisplaced and displaced fractures are well documented.[107,108] They involve retardation of the rate as well as an increase in the amount of cartilage formed and a decrease in the amount of primary bone formation between the fracture ends.

The Degree of Bone Loss. The end result of any metabolic function depends upon the ability of the cells present to perform a given function. If the function exceeds their capacity, it is performed either slowly or not at all. Loss of bone substance or excessive distraction of the fragments leads to a condition in which the cells' ability to bridge the gap is compromised.

The Type of Bone Involved. Cortical and cancellous bone have been shown to respond in a somewhat different fashion to fracture. Cancellous bone unites very rapidly, but this occurs only at points of direct contact. Where cancellous bone is not in contact, the gap is filled by the spread of new bone from the points of contact.[22,23] Repair in cancellous bone is rapid, because there are many points of bone contact which are rich in cells and blood supply. Charnley has commented upon the lack of callus about fractures located primarily in cancellous regions.[22]

Cortical bone unites by two mechanisms, depending upon the local conditions. If exact apposition of cortical bone ends occurs and if immobilization is rigid, end-to-end healing takes place from the cortical surfaces with very little external callus.[85-97] If, on the other hand, wide displacement of the fragments occurs, or if immobilization is not rigid, the standard process of repair utilizing external callus is seen.

The Degree of Immobilization. This factor, along with the amount of soft-tissue trauma, probably is of paramount importance in fracture healing. Every clinician is aware of the fact that inadequate immobilization leads to delayed union or nonunion. Experimentally, repeated manipulation retards fracture healing.[92] It is probable that the initial fibrin scaffolding, which is the first step in fracture repair, is disrupted if immobilization is not adequate and the bony bridge of external callus fails to form properly. If inadequate immobilization continues throughout the repair process, a cleft forms between the fracture ends, and a false joint develops, leading to the classical pseudarthrosis.

Infections. For fracture healing to proceed at a satisfactory rate, the local resources must be devoted primarily to healing the break in bone continuity. If infection is superimposed upon a fracture or if the fracture occurs as a result of the infection, the local defenses are mobilized all or in part to attempt to wall off and eliminate the infection. Once more, healing will be retarded or may not occur at all.[4]

The Presence of Local Malignancy. Unless the malignancy itself is treated, fractures through bone involved with primary or secondary malignancies usually will not heal. Subperiosteal new bone formation and callus can be seen microscopically, but the presence of the malignant cells precludes effective immobilization of the fracture. This is particularly true if the malignant lesion is an expanding one in which the deposit actually extends into the areas from which healing must take place.

Other Local Pathological Conditions. Fractures through bones involved with nonmalignant conditions may heal in some instances,[86] but many conditions[87] such as Paget's disease or fibrous dysplasia heal slowly or not at all. Once more, the cause is a failure of normal differentiation of mesenchymal cells, and of ingrowth of capillaries from the surrounding tissues.

Radiation Necrosis of Bone. Bone that has been irradiated heals at a much slower rate, and in many instances nonunion results.[48] This is due to the patchy death of cells in the local region, to thrombosis of vessels, and to the fibrosis of the marrow, which once more interferes with the ingrowth of capillaries.

The Presence of Avascular Necrosis. Under ordinary circumstances, healing proceeds from both sides of a fracture with differentiation of healing cells occurring in approximately equal amounts. When one fracture fragment has been rendered avascular, the healing process depends entirely upon in-growth of capillaries from the living side. Fractures associated with avascular necrosis of one fragment will heal, but the rate is slower and the incidence is lower than in situations where this does occur.[13] If both fragments are avascular, the chances for union are very poor indeed.[22]

Intraarticular Fractures. Intraarticular fractures pose a more difficult problem to the normal healing processes. Synovial fluid contains fibrinolysins,[68] which have the capability of lysing the initial clot and thus retarding the first stage in fracture healing. As in the case of avascular necrosis, these fractures do heal, but the difficulties encountered in clinical situations are greater than in extraarticular fractures.

Systemic Factors

Age of the Patient. It is well known that young people's fractures heal very rapidly and that the closer to adult life an individual is, the more his rate resembles that of an adult. In addition, the rapid remodelling that accompanies growth allows correction of greater degrees of deformity in young persons. Experimental work in animals[124] utilizing tritiated thymidine shows that in the young there is more rapid differentiation of cells from the mesenchymal pool, which makes them available for the repair process. Among animals, elderly mature individuals heal at a slower rate than younger ones, but in clinical practice, this is difficult to document.

Hormones. *Corticosteroids.* In both experimental and clinical situations, corticosteroids are powerful inhibitors of the rate of fracture healing.[39] They have been shown to inhibit the differentiation of osteoblasts from mesenchymal cells[115] and to decrease the synthesis rates of the major components of bone matrix,[34] which are necessary for repair.

Growth Hormone. While alterations in the level of circulating growth hormone probably have very little effect on fracture healing at the clinical level, experimental work has shown that the rate of repair can be influenced profoundly by this substance.[58,65,83,88] Growth hormone is a potent stimulator of fracture healing.

Other Hormones. Thyroid hormone, calcitonin, insulin, vitamins A and D in physiologic dosages, and anabolic steroids have been reported in experimental situations to enhance the rate of fracture healing (Table 2-1). Diabetes, castration, hypervitaminosis D, hypervitaminosis A, as well as the rachitic state have been shown to retard fracture healing in experimental situations. Rarely in clinical practice do these substances or situations pose a serious problem.

Exercise and Local Stress About the Fracture. Denervation retards fracture healing, probably by diminishing the stress across the fracture site.[106] Exercise increases the rate of repair.[51] Clinicians have known that use of a fractured extremity promotes repair, and the recent development of weight-bearing techniques has confirmed this conviction.[38,84,112] It is probable that bone formation is stimulated by forces acting across the fracture site, perhaps by initiating piezoelectric effects that lead to accelerated bone formation.

Electric Currents. The application of local electric current can stimulate healing in a fracture that has previously failed to respond to adequate treatment.[45,75] This represents a clinical application of experimental work[8,9] and may prove to be an important factor in the future.

HISTORICAL REVIEW OF THE EFFECTS OF OPEN REDUCTION AND METALLIC IMPLANTS ON FRACTURE HEALING

Prior to the 20th century, sporadic attempts were made at internal fixation of fractures, but because of a poor understanding of metallurgy and poor aseptic techniques, uniform success was not achieved. Through the efforts of Lister and Cameron in Great Britain, and later of Langenbeck, Koenig,[62] and Gluck in Germany, internal fixation became an accepted method of fracture treatment. Lambotte[71-74] published a book on internal fixation of fractures in 1913 and was probably the first surgeon to advocate the use of external skeletal fixation of fractures. Simultaneously, Lane was developing his operative approach to fractures. Danis[36,37] studied the effects of axial compression and rigid immobilization in forearm fractures while Charnley[22] was investigating the effects of continuous compression on fractures to achieve bony union. As these principles became better understood and with improvements in metallurgy, internal fixation of fractures[102,108] became safer and more predictable. The failures of the pioneers in internal fixation were due primarily to galvanic corrosion,[133] which occurs when two pieces of metal in contact are of different molecular composition and thus have different electrical charges. Corrosion can also occur when the metal is in contact with various solutions. If the oxygen concentration[69] is not the same in all areas of the implant because of poor circulation of extracellular fluid, corrosion may also be seen. With the development of uniform material standards and especially through the work of the American Society for Testing and Materials (ASTM), implants manufactured now must meet precise criteria for composition and fabrication. In the current practice of fracture treatment, the implants used are made primarily of stainless steel, cobalt-base alloys, or titanium alloys.

Tissue Reaction to Implants

Following insertion of metallic implants in the tissues,[70] first there is a phase of acute and later of chronic inflammatory reaction. This is primarily a response to surgical trauma. Repair follows immediately with the production of fibrous tissue in a haphazard fashion, which later becomes organized. The cellular response in the early stage is not affected by the presence of large implants. Mature fibrous tissue seals the implant in place. If it is totally inert and remains passive in the organism, this may be the end of the reaction. However, since no metal is completely inert, ions are liberated from the metal. The typical response following the initial inflammatory reaction and formation of fibrous tissue, seen early after insertion of the implants, is modified in direct proportion to the degree of corrosion. There is phagocytosis of the metallic particles which are seen inside the cellular cytoplasm. The fibrous tissue starts to thicken and become more vascular, and in extreme cases giant cells are seen.

Table 2-2. ASTM Standard Composition for Stainless Steel Used in Surgical Implants

Element	Grade A %	Grade B %
Carbon	0.08 max.	0.03 max.
Manganese	2.00 max.	2.00 max.
Phosphorus	0.025 max.	0.025 max.
Sulfur	0.010 max.	0.010 max.
Silicon	0.75 max.	0.75 max.
Chromium	17.00–20.00	17.00–20.00
Nickel	10.00–14.00	10.00–14.00
Molybdenum	2.00–4.00	2.00–4.00

(Laing, P.: Orthop. Clin. N. Amer., *4*:249, 1973)

Stainless Steel. The ASTM standards[3] for stainless steel are the F-138 and the F-139. For the fabrication of stainless steel implants, the 316-L is used in North America. Its physical properties are given in Table 2-2.

316-L stainless steel is susceptible to galvanic corrosion in the body when it is bathed in fluid resembling salt solution. While there is always corrosion in tissues, it is generally minimal if the implants have been made well and used properly.

Cobalt Alloys. Just as iron can be alloyed into a steel with a stable austenitic structure, so can cobalt. The most commonly used cobalt alloy is Vitallium (cobalt-chrome-molybdenum). Its typical composition is shown in Table 2-3.

Table 2-3. ASTM Standard Composition for Cobalt-Chrome-Molybdenum Alloys Used in Surgical Implants

Element	Minimum %	Maximum %
Chromium	27.0	30.0
Molybdenum	5.0	7.0
Nickel	—	2.5
Iron	—	0.75
Carbon	—	0.35
Silicon	—	1.00
Manganese	—	1.00
Cobalt	Balance	Balance

(Laing, P.: Orthop. Clin. N. Amer., *4*:249, 1973)

The implants are fabricated by the lost wax process. The tissue reaction to the long-term implantation of Vitallium is minimal.[26,42] Fibrous tissue formation around the implant is less profuse than with stainless steel, but corrosion may be seen. There are increased concentrations of cobalt and chromium in the blood, urine, and hair after the insertion of implants.[27] This indicates that the implants are not

Table 2-4. ASTM Standard Composition for Titanium

Element	Flat Product	Bar and Billett	Flat Product	Bar and Billett
Nitrogen, maximum	0.07	0.07	0.07	0.07
Carbon, maximum	0.10	0.10	0.10	0.15
Hydrogen, maximum	0.015	0.0125*	0.0150	0.0125
Iron, maximum	0.30	0.30	0.50	0.50
Oxygen, maximum	0.35	0.30	0.45	0.40
Titanium†	Remainder	Remainder	Remainder	Remainder

*Bar only: maximum hydrogen content for billet is 0.100 per cent.
†The titanium content is determined by difference.
(Laing, P.: Orthop. Clin. N. Amer., *4*:249, 1973)

completely inert in the body, but no detectable tissue damage has been reported.

Titanium and Alloys. Titanium and its alloys are used mainly in a chloride environment and have good corrosion resistance. Implants made of titanium have been used in patients in the form of concentric cups, plates, and screws. The ASTM standard[3] composition for titanium is shown in Table 2-4.

Very little tissue reaction can be observed in the body when titanium is used.[69] It is thus an excellent material for orthopaedic implants.

Mechanical Behavior of Biological and Implant Structures

When an implant is placed in the human body, it modifies the skeleton significantly. The strength of a metal is important in preventing its failure, but is different from that of bone. The ASTM standards[3] of ultimate strength (point of metal failure) and yield strength (point of permanent metal deformation) are given in Table 2-5.

Stiffness of a substance is indicated by its modulus of elasticity. Bone has a modulus of elasticity, when tested longitudinally, of 2×10^6 and of 1×10^6 when tested transversely. By comparison, steel has a modulus of elasticity of 30×10^6. Thus steel is more than ten times as stiff as bone.

When a fractured bone, fixed with an implant, is loaded, its biological behavior is altered, because Wolff's law does not operate normally since the bone is unloaded by the plate. Microscopic studies have described this phenomenon in detail[130] and have shown that the cortical bone under the implant is progressively replaced by cancellous bone. Thus, when an implant is removed it is mandatory to protect the bone against excessive loading which could cause a refracture. Progressive loading allows the bone to regain its strength rapidly.

Implant Failures[9,44,114]

Metal Behavior. The deformation of a substance by a load, following which the

Table 2-5. Ultimate and Yield Strengths of Materials

	Ultimate Strength	Minimum kgf/mm.^{2}	Yield Strength	Minimum kgf/mm.^{2}
Stainless steel	53.0	88.0	21.0	70.5
Titanium	45.0	56.0	38.5	49.5
Cast cobalt-chromium alloy	66.5		45.5	
Wrought cobalt-chromium alloy	88.0	91.4	31.6	38.7

(Annual Book of ASTM Standards. Philadelphia, American Soc. for Testing and Materials, 1973.)

substance returns to zero when the load is removed, is called elastic behavior. Plastic behavior refers to a deformation which does not return to zero when the load is removed. A brittle material breaks before any plastic deformation takes place. A ductile material has a plastic behavior before it breaks.

Metal Failure. *Fatigue failure* by fracture of the implant is caused by cyclic loading, with or without permanent deformation.

Ductile failure of an implant due to excessive plastic deformation results in permanent bending.

Brittle failure by fracture of the implant occurs before permanent deformation is seen. This can occur because of the effect of stress concentrations or cyclic loading. Stress concentrations may be the result of poor design of an implant or alteration during the insertion procedures by damaging the metal.

Thus a knowledge of the mechanical properties of both the metal and the bone is essential if implants are to function without failure.

DELAYED UNION AND NONUNION

Despite the best management,[22,33,60] some fractures heal slowly or do not heal at all. It is difficult to set arbitrarily the time at which a given fracture should be united. Delayed union indicates that it takes longer than the average for a given bone injury to heal. Nonunion refers to an arrest of the healing process and the formation of a typical pseudarthrosis or a fibrous union in which the bone ends are either osteoporotic and atrophied, or sclerotic.

Watson-Jones[134] refers to another condition called slow union. Here the fracture line is still clearly visible, but there is no undue separation of the fragments, no cavitation of the surfaces, no calcification, and no sclerosis. Indolence at the fracture site is due to its type, its blood supply, or the age and constitution of the patient. Union has not been unnecessarily delayed and it is not an un-united fracture. This is a well recognized phenomenon in fracture treatment and only a variation from normal.

The causes of delayed- or nonunion are open and comminuted fractures, infected fractures, segmental fractures, pathological fractures, fractures separated by soft-tissue interposition, fractures in an area with poor blood supply, and iatrogenic interference to healing fractures.

Open and Comminuted Fractures

Open fractures resulting from motor vehicle accidents and war wounds present serious problems in management. Associated with the bone injury there can be significant comminution and often bone loss as a result of the open wound. At the fracture site, there is extensive stripping of the soft tissue surrounding the fracture. Large areas of bone are deprived of their blood supply, and normal union may not occur.

Infected Fractures

Open fractures that are severely contaminated may become infected, thus creating a situation that is more difficult for adequate orthopaedic treatment. The other common cause of infected fractures is the tragedy of a postoperative infection following internal fixation.

The management of these complicated problems necessitates the treatment of the infection by removing the infected bone and soft tissue and by appropriate antibiotic treatment. Infected fractures do unite if they are immobilized well, sometimes before the infection has completely disappeared.

Segmental Fractures

A segmental fracture often has impaired blood supply, usually to its middle fragment. Because of this, delay of union can be seen proximally or distally in these fractures. If internal fixation is undertaken, it is often wise to do a primary bone graft to prevent nonunion.

Pathological Fractures

A pathological fracture takes place through diseased bone and generally requires less force to be produced. If the underlying cause of the pathological fracture is not treated, the fracture often does not heal. It is thus important to determine the cause of the bone pathology, so that appropriate therapy can be given.

Fractures Separated by Soft Tissues

Obviously, the interposition of soft tissue at a fracture prevents healing of the fracture. This can generally be detected during the initial reduction, because it is often impossible to achieve a satisfactory position. If this is strongly suspected and demonstrated, an open reduction should be carried out.

Fracture with Impaired Blood Supply

The poor blood supply of certain parts of the skeleton can sometimes delay fracture healing. The marginal vascularization of the femoral head, the carpal scaphoid, and also of the talus is well known, and in these particular instances unless a fracture is rigidly immobilized for a sufficient period of time, nonunion associated with avascular necrosis of the fragment may occur.

Iatrogenic Interference with Healing Fractures

Sound principles of treatment should be adhered to at all times to prevent delayed union and nonunion. For instance, if a fracture is inadequately immobilized in traction or in a cast that allows excessive motion, the fracture does not unite. If plaster immobilization is selected, the joint above and below the fracture should usually be incorporated in the cast to prevent excessive motion, except in special situations, such as with the use of cast braces. Similarly if an open reduction is carried out, one must avoid excessive periosteal stripping and also distraction of bone fragments by plates and screws. If a fracture is treated by conservative means, separation of the fracture site by excessive traction should be avoided, as it would undoubtedly delay union.

BONE GRAFTING IN THE TREATMENT OF FRACTURES

Bone grafts may be utilized in the treatment of delayed union or nonunion. The objectives in grafting are to stimulate bony union, to replace lost tissues, and to assist in the revascularization of avascular segments of bone.

Phemister[98] outlined the principles involved in the surgical management of nonunion. He established that the callus associated with an ununited fracture will ossify spontaneously when an adequate surgical procedure is performed. Resection of the nonunion was thus shown to be not only unnecessary but actually undesirable. If properly performed, a graft or stabilization of the fracture can induce union in a high percentage of cases.

There are four types of bone grafts:[111]

Autograft. Bone is taken from a donor site and placed in another site in the same individual

Isograft. Bone is transferred between individuals who are identical in histocompatibility antigens (identical twins)

Allograft. Bone is transferred between genetically dissimilar members of the same species

Xenograft. Bone is transferred from a member of one species to one of another species

The proper selection of a graft entails knowledge of the capacity of a graft to bring about union and of the host response to the grafted material. A graft promotes union by forming new bone itself or by inducing new bone formation in the recipient site.

The Mechanisms by Which Bone Grafts Bring About Union

Direct New Bone Formation by the Graft Cells. Properly utilized, bone can provide cells to the local area that are capable of forming new bone directly. In order for this to occur the cells must not be rejected by the recipient and must be kept alive prior to implantation. Thus bone grafts should not be dried, exposed to solutions that kill cells, or maintained out of the body for very long. In addition, they must have a ready route of nutrition following completion of the procedure. For all practical purposes, this limits direct new bone formation to cancellous or corticocancellous autografted bone, which has a large number of cells, many of which are on the surface. In addition, diffusion of nutrients into the bone graft can occur only if the particle size is not too large;[105] 5 mm. is the maximum thickness that can be nourished in this fashion.

Bone Induction. Cortical bone as well as all forms of frozen, irradiated, or preserved grafts provide no cells with immediate osteogenic capacity. Nevertheless, they possess the ability to induce local bone formation.[21] This capacity may well rest in the organic fraction of bone and be due to a protein.[131] This is the mechanism by which most bone grafts bring about union.

Immunologic Response to Bone Grafts

There is no immunologic response to autografts or isografts. Cells derived from an allograft[40] participate in the repair process for about 2 weeks, after which they invoke a major inflammatory response that obliterates the repair that has been effected until then. This is the classical rejection described for all tissues.[11,82]

For this reason, allografts in the fresh state are not useful and must be modified in order to alter their antigeniticity. While many methods have been utilized for this, in clinical practice frozen and freeze-dried bone are probably the most practical methods and appear to have the highest capacity to induce new bone.[20] These grafts may be taken and maintained under sterile conditions or sterilized with high energy radiation.[24,52,59,104,126,127]

The Fate of Bone Grafts

From a practical point of view, only surface cells of an autograft or an isograft survive and have any true osteogenic capacity. These surface cells may be either endosteal osteoblasts[1] or marrow cells, which apparently are capable of forming new bone.[20,35] Osteocytes in cortical bone and in the interior of cancellous bone are avascular and do not survive. The bone around these cells must be resorbed by creeping substitution. In the process, osteoclasts resorb the graft, bringing granulation tissue and osteoblasts which lay down new bone utilizing the graft material as a scaffold. This new bone probably arises as a result of induction.

Techniques of Grafting

Because there is no immunologic response on the part of the host, and because it does have the capacity to form new bone per primam, an autograft containing cancellous bone represents the ideal grafting material. When this is not feasible, a well-chosen allograft is preferred. A xenograft is not practical in clinical practice at the present time. Single- or double-onlay cortical grafts, inlay grafts, osteoperiosteal grafts, and corticocancellous chips are the commonly used techniques of grafting. The selection of the proper method depends upon a careful analysis of the needs of the patient and the anatomical region receiving the graft. Corticocancellous strips are used for osteogenesis; cortical bone is selected when deficient tissues must be replaced or when stability is required.

TENDON HEALING

The problem of tendon healing has concerned surgeons through the years. Sterling Bunnell,[16,17,18] his collaborators, and students directed their studies primarily toward the healing of flexor tendons divided in the canals of digits. The knowledge obtained from these classical experiments can be applied to tendon healing elsewhere in the body, whether one is dealing with a rupture of the tendo Achilles or of the patellar tendon.

Biomechanical analyses[135] have shown that in an intact musculotendinous system complete with its bony attachment, the muscle belly itself is the weakest point. In a tendon-bone preparation, the bone-tendon junction is the weakest point. Intact tendons fail at the point of clamping, the sites of maximal stress concentration. Of particular importance in considering the strength of a specimen is the dependence of the material on the rate at which it is loaded. When it is loaded rapidly, it behaves in a brittle fashion with high strength and low toughness. Loaded slowly its strength is lower, but its energy-absorbing capability is much greater. When a tendon is notched, it undergoes a disproportionate weakening.

It is now understood that the blood supply of tendon does not originate from its bony insertion or muscle origin, nor from the paratenon. Microdissections have shown[14,15,28,118] that there is a mesotenon on the tendon which brings to it a vascular network in an arcade comparable to the mesentery of the gut. In the digits the mesotenon is more important. It gives a short vincula at the level of the bony insertion of the tendons at the level of interphalangeal joints. This blood supply provides nutrition for the tendon to segments that do not exceed 2 or 3 cm. A tendon deprived of its blood supply degenerates and dies, as has been well demonstrated by wrapping tendon within an impermeable membrane.[99,100,101,117]

Our knowledge of tendon healing has been obtained primarily from animal experiments. It was previously believed[76-79] that the tenoblasts from the endo- and epitenon participated in tendon healing, or that the paratenon was the primary source of healing tissue. It is now known that the tendon itself does not take part in its own healing.[99-102] The essential source of new tissue is by fibroblastic infiltration from the surrounding soft tissues. Peacock[93,94,95] introduced the "one wound—one scar" concept in which the skin, the subcutaneous tissue, the tendons, and their sheaths are in continuity and take place in the same process of healing. Connective tissue proliferates from the outside, penetrating between the ends of sutured tendons and depositing collagen fibers which become progressively oriented and finally form tendon fibers identical with those of normal tendons (Fig. 2-7). It is the proliferating connective tissue from the surrounding area that becomes fixed on the exposed area of tendon.

The retraction of tendon ends within the sheath of a digit has shown that no healing process takes place directly from tendon ends. Similarly, tendon ruptures elsewhere in the body (e.g., biceps tendon, rotator cuff, and tendo Achillis), which have been completely separated will not heal unless they are approximated to allow collagenous tissue from the periphery to proliferate and repair the damaged tendon.

The end stage of tendon healing is difficult to determine. It has long been established[80,81] that early mobilization of a sutured tendon, instead of reducing adhesions, seems to contribute to hypertrophy of the tendon during the healing process. After the third week of immobilization, a finger tendon seems to be strong enough to resist rupture when gentle mobilization is begun. This applies to tendons in the hands, but obviously at 3 weeks, larger tendons will not be strong enough to allow unprotected use.

LIGAMENT HEALING

Anatomical studies of the repair of ligaments have shown that the most favorable condition for healing of a divided ligament is direct apposition of the surfaces. Such apposition minimizes scarring, accelerates repair, hastens collagenization, and comes closer to restoring normal ligamentous tissue. Ligaments[25,122] divided and immobil-

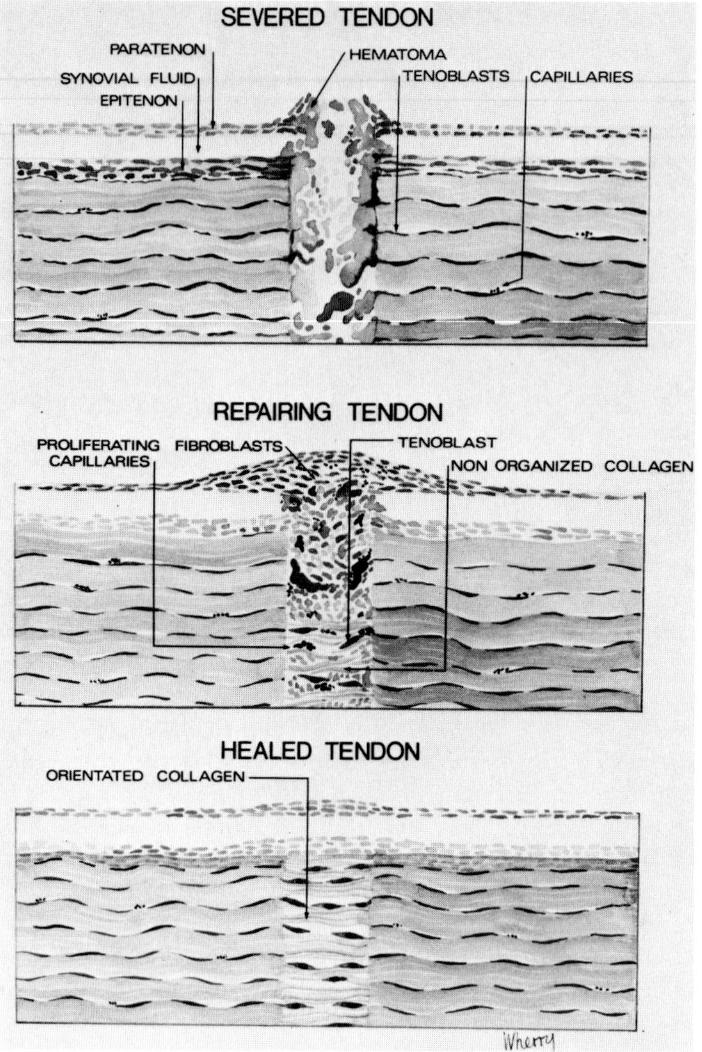

Fig. 2-7. The sequence of events following severing of a tendon is demonstrated. There is an initial hematoma between the tendon ends with an in-growth of fibroblasts from the surrounding tissue which gradually organizes the hematoma and leads to healing of the tendon.

ized heal with a gap of fibrous tissue between the cut ends. Ligaments that are sutured unite without formation of this gap.[89,90,91] When sutured ligaments are tested under tension, they are always stronger than the nonsutured ones, which fail in the area of scar tissue. Ligamentous instability may create serious problems in weight-bearing joints, namely the ankle and the knee, and restoration of normal anatomy should be the objective of treatment (Fig. 2-8). If excessive tension is placed on the suture line of a primarily repaired ligament, necrosis and failure of repair occur. If a ligament is left unsutured, it retracts, shortens, and becomes atrophic, making repair sometimes impossible after 2 weeks. At 10 weeks microscopic evidence of complete fibrous healing is demonstrated, but the tensile strength of the healed repaired ligament remains substantially less than that of a normal ligament.[91]

The histologic sequence of ligament healing is similar to the sequence of events that takes place in tendons. If the ends of the ligament are reattached to bone, collagen tissue will invade the end and attach the ligament firmly to periosteum and bone.[29]

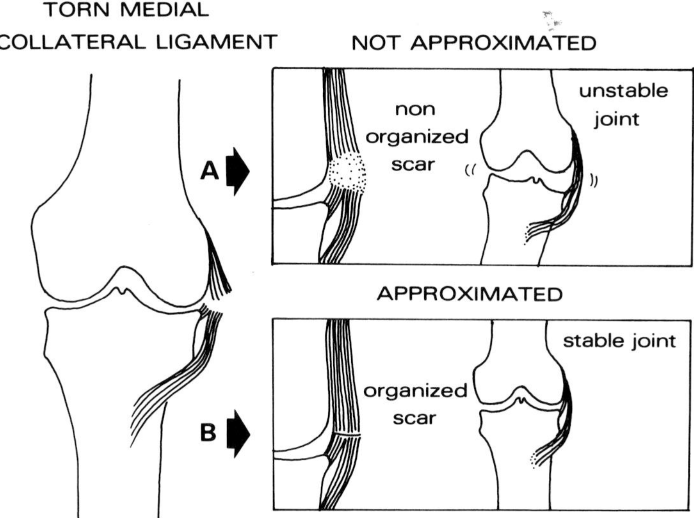

Fig. 2-8. Surgical approximation of a severed ligament leads to a ligament which more closely approximates the original structure and usually gives better function.

If the ligament has been ruptured in its substance, a careful suturing of the ligamentous end allows collagen to be formed and reoriented to reestablish the tensile strength of the ligament. Thus the fibroblastic activity comes from the ligament itself, and also from the tissues surrounding the ligament. The "one wound—one scar" concept applies here also. It appears evident that ruptured ligaments with separated ends should be sutured to allow restoration of normal function.

REFERENCES

1. Abbot, L. C., Schottsaedt, E. R., Saunders, J. B., and Bost, S. C.: The evaluation of cortical and cancellous bone as a grafting material. A clinical and experimental study. J. Bone Joint Surg., *29*: 381-414, 1947.
2. Aegerter, E., and Kirkpatrick, J. A., Jr.: Orthopaedic Diseases. Philadelphia, W. B. Saunders, 1968.
3. American Society for Testing and Materials. Annual Book of ASTM Standards. Philadelphia, 1973.
4. Andriole, V. T., Nago, B. A., and Southwick, W. O.: A paradigm for human chronic osteomyelitis. J. Bone Joint Surg., *55A*:1511-1515, 1973.
5. Aripow, U. A., Licmanowa, G. I., Saatow, C. I., and Chaitow, R. M.: Zu den Besonderheiten des Verlaufs der Reparationsprozesse bei der Einswirkung einiger physikalischer Faktoren auf den Organismus. Zentralbl. Chir., *92*:1097-1101, 1967.
6. Bassett, C. A. L.: Current concepts of bone formation. J. Bone Joint Surg., *44A*: 1217-1244, 1962.
7. ———: *In* Bourne, G. H. (ed.): Biochemistry and Physiology of Bone. Vol. 3. ed. 2. New York, Academic Press, 1971.
8. Bassett, C. A. L., and Becker, R. O.: Generation of electric potentials by bone in response to mechanical stress. Science, *137*:1063-1064, 1962.
9. Bechtol, C. O., Ferguson, A. B., and Laing, P. G.: Metals and Engineering in Bone and Joint Surgery. Baltimore, Williams & Wilkins, 1959.
10. Becker, R. O., and Murray, D. G.: The electrical control system regulating fracture healing in amphibians. Clin. Orthop., *73*:169-199, 1970.
11. Bonfiglio, M., Jeter, W. S., and Smith, C. L.: The immune concept. Its relation to bone transplantation. Ann. N. Y. Acad. Sci., *59*:417-432, 1955.
12. Boni, M., Lenzi, L., Silva, E., and Bolognani, L.: Action of testicular hyaluronidase administered in vivo on the mineralization of fracture callus in rats. Calcif. Tis. Res., *2*[Suppl.]:30-30A, 1968.
13. Boyd, H. B., and Salvatore, J. E.: Acute fracture of the femoral neck; internal fixation or prosthesis. J. Bone Joint Surg., *46A*:1066-1068, 1964.
14. Braithwaite, F., and Brockis, J.: The vas-

cularisation of a tendon graft. Brit. J. Plast. Surg., *2*:130-135, 1951.

15. Brockis, J. G.: The blood supply of the flexor and extensor tendons of the fingers in man. J. Bone Joint Surg., *35B*:131-138, 1953.
16. Bunnell, S.: Repair of tendons in the fingers and description of two new instruments. Surg. Gynecol. Obstet., *26*:103, 1918.
17. ———: Repair of tendons in the fingers. Surg. Gynecol. Obstet., *35*:88-97, 1922.
18. ———: Surgery of the hand. ed. 3. Philadelphia, J. B. Lippincott, 1956.
19. Burger, M., Sherman, B. S., and Sobel, A. E.: Observations on the influence of chonroitin sulphate on the rate of bone repair. J. Bone Joint Surg., *44B*:675-687, 1962.
20. Burwell, R. J.: Studies in the transplantation of bone VII. Fresh composite homograft—autograft of cancellous bone. J. Bone Joint Surg., *46B*:110-140, 1964.
21. Burwell, R. G.: Studies in the transplantation of bone. J. Bone Joint Surg., *48B*: 532-566, 1966.
22. Charnley, J.: The Closed Treatment of Common Fractures. Ed. 3. Edinburgh, E. & S. Livingstone, 1968.
23. Charnley, J., and Baker, S. L.: Compression arthrodesis of the knee. J. Bone Joint Surg., *34B*:187-199, 1952.
24. Chase, S. W., and Herndon, C. H.: The fate of autogenous and homogenous bone grafts; a historical review. J. Bone Joint Surg., *37A*:809-841, 1955.
25. Clayton, M. L., and Weir, G. L., Jr.: Experimental investigations of ligamentous healing. Amer. J. Surg., *98*:373-378, 1959.
26. Cohen, J., and Wulff, J.: Clinical failure caused by corrosion of a Vitallium plate. J. Bone Joint Surg., *54A*:617-628, 1972.
27. Coleman, R. F.: Concentration of implant corrosion products in the body. J. Bone Joint Surg., *55B*:422, 1973.
28. Colville, J., Callison, J. R., and White, W. L.: Role of the mesotendon in tendon blood supply. Plast. Reconst. Surg., *43*: 53-60, 1969.
29. Cooper, R. R., and Misol, S.: Tendon and ligament insertion. J. Bone Joint Surg., *52A*:1-20, 1970.
30. Copp, D. H., and Greenberg, D. M.: Studies on bone fracture healing. I. Effect of vitamins A and D. J. Nutr., *29*:261-267, 1945.
31. Cothman, L.: Vascular reaction in experimental fractures, microangiographic and radio-isotopic studies. Acta Chir. Scand., [Suppl.]:284, 1961.
32. Coulson, L. B., Ferguson, A. B., Jr., and Diehl, R. C., Jr.: Effect of hyperbaric oxygen on the healing femur of the rat. Surg. Forum, *17*:449-450, 1966.
33. Crenshaw, A. H.: Campbell's Operative Orthopedics. ed. 5. St. Louis, C. V. Mosby, 1971.
34. Cruess, R. L., and Sakai, T.: The effect of cortisone upon synthesis rates of some components of rat bone matrix. Clin. Orthop., *86*:253-259, 1972.
35. Danis, A.: Etude de l'ossification dans les greffes de moelle osseuse. Acta Chir. Belg., *3*:[Suppl.], 1-120, 1957.
36. Danis, R.: Théorie et Pratique de l'Ostéosynthèse. Paris, Masson & Cie, 1947.
37. ———: Le vrai but et les dangers de l'ostéosynthèse. Lyon Chir., *51*:740-743, 1956.
38. Dehne, E., Metz, C. W., Deffer, T. A., and Hall, R. M.: Non-operative treatment of the fractured tibia by immediate weight bearing. J. Trauma, *1*:514-535, 1961.
39. Duthie, R. B., and Barker, A. N.: The histochemistry of the pre-osseous stage of bone repair studied by autoradiography. J. Bone Joint Surg., *37B*:691-710, 1955.
40. Enneking, W. F.: Histological investigation of bone transplants in immunologically prepared animals. J. Bone Joint Surg., *39A*:597-615, 1957.
41. Ewald, F., and Tachdjian, M.D.: The effect of thyrocalcitonin on fractured humeri. Surg. Gynecol. Obstet., *125*: 1075-1080, 1967.
42. Ferguson, A. B., Jr., Laing, P. G., and Hodge, E. S.: The ionization of metal implants in living tissues. J. Bone Joint Surg., *42A*:77-90, 1960.
43. Fitton-Jackson, S.: The fine structure of developing bone in the embryonic fowl. Proc. Roy. Soc. Biol., *146*:270-280, 1956.
44. Frankel, V. H., and Burstein, A. H.: Orthopaedic Biomechanics. Philadelphia, Lea & Febiger, 1970.
45. Friedenberg, Z. B., and Brighton, C. T.: Feeling of non-union of medial malleolus by means of a direct current. A case report. J. Trauma, *11*:883-885, 1971.
46. Frost, H. M.: Laws of bone structure. Springfield, Charles C Thomas, 1964.
47. Glimcher, M. J.: A basic architectural principle in the organization of mineralized tissues. Clin. Orthop., *61*:16-36, 1968.

48. Goodman, A. H., and Sherman, M. S.: Post irradiation fractures of the femoral neck. J. Bone Joint Surg., *45A*:723-730, 1963.
49. Grant, M. E., and Prockop, D. J.: The biosynthesis of collagen. New Eng. J. Med., *286*:291-300, 1972.
50. Ham, A. W.: Histology. ed. 7. Philadelphia, J. B. Lippincott, 1974.
51. Heikkinen, E., Vihersaari, P., and Penttinen, R.: Effect of previous exercise on the development of experimental fractured callus in the mice. Scand. J. Clin. Lab. Invest., *25*[Suppl.]:113, 32, 1970.
52. Heiple, K. G., Chase, S. W., and Herndon, C. H.: Comparative study of the healing process following different types of bone transplantation. J. Bone Joint Surg., *45A*: 1593-1616, 1963.
53. Herbsman, H., Kwon, K., Shaftan, G. W., Gordon, B., Fox, L. M., and Enquist, I. F.: The influence of systemic factors on fracture healing. J. Trauma, *6*:75-85, 1966.
54. Herbsman, H., Powers, J. C., Hirschman, A., and Shaftan, G. W.: Retardation of fracture healing in experimental diabetes. J. Surg. Res., *8*:424-431, 1968.
55. Herold, H. Z., and Tadmor, A.: Chondroitin sulphate in treatment of experimental bone defects. Isr. J. Med. Sci., *5*:425-427, 1969.
56. Hodge, D. E., and Peturska, J. A.: *In* Ramachandran, G. N. (ed.): Aspects of Protein Structure. New York, Academic Press, 1963.
57. Howard, T. C., and Kelley, R. R.: The effect of bone wax on the healing of experimental rat tibial lesions. Clin. Orthop., *63*:226-232, 1969.
58. Hsu, J. D., and Robinson, R. A.: Studies on the healing of long bone fractures in hereditary pituitary insufficient mice. J. Surg. Res., *9*:535-536, 1969.
59. Hyatt, G. W., and Butler, M. C.: Bone grafting, the procurement, storage and clinical use of bone homografts. The American Academy of Orthopaedic Surgeons Instructional Course Lectures, *14*: 343-373, 1957.
60. Key, J. A.: Stainless steel and Vitallium in internal fixation of bone. Arch. Surg., *43*:615-626, 1941.
61. Knoch, H. G.: Der Einfluss von Nieder- und Hochfrequenz-schwingungen auf das Kallusgewebe im Tierexperiment. Zentralbl. Chir., *92*:1784-1799, 1967.
62. Koenig, F.: Moderne Behandlung der Frakturen der unterin Extremitäten. Z. Ärztl. Landpraxis, *3*:330-363, 1895.
63. Koskinen, E. V. S.: The repair of experimental fractures under the action of growth hormone, thyrotropin and cortisone. A tissue analytic, roentgenologic and autoradiographic study. Ann. Chir. Gynecol. Fenn., *48* [Suppl.]:90, 1-48, 1959.
64. ———: Effect of endocrine factors on callus development in experimental fractures. Symp. Biol. Hung., *7*:315-322, 1967.
65. Koskinen, E. V. S., Ryoppy, I., and Lindholm, T. S.: Bone formation by induction under the influence of growth hormone and cortisone. Isr. J. Med. Sci., *7*:378-380, 1971.
66. Kowalewski, K., Couves, C. M., and Lang, A.: Protective action of 17-ethyl-19-nortestosterone against the inhibition of bone repair in the lathyrus-fed rat. Acta Endocrinol., *30*:268-273, 1959.
67. Kowalewski, K., and Gort, J.: An anabolic androgen as a stimulant of bone healing in rats treated with cortisone. Acta Endocrinol., *30*:273-276, 1959.
68. Lack, C. H.: Proteolytic activity and connective tissue. Brit. Med. Bull., *20*:312-322, 1964.
69. Laing, P. G.: Compatibility of biomaterials. Orthop. Clin. N. Amer., *4*:249-273, 1973.
70. Laing, P. G., Ferguson, A. B., Jr., and Hodge, E. S.: Tissue reaction in rabbit muscle exposed to metallic implants. J. Biomed. Mat. Res., *1*:135-149, 1967.
71. Lambotte, A.: Notice sur l'emploi du fil de fer et de vis du même métal dans la suture osséuse. Presse Méd. Belge, *44*: 125-127, 1892.
72. ———: L'intervention Opératoire dans les Fractures. Paris, A. Maloine, 1907.
73. ———: Le Traitement des Fractures. Paris, Masson et Cie., 1907.
74. ———: Early Stages of Internal Fixation of Fractured Bones in Belgium. Société Belge de Chirurgie Orthopédique et de Traumatologie, 1971.
75. Lavine, L. S., and Shamos, M. H.: Electric enhancement of bone healing. Science, *175*:118-121, 1972.
76. Lindsay, W. K., and Birch, J. R.: The fibroblast in flexor tendon healing. Plast. and Reconst. Surg., *34*:223-232, 1964.
77. Lindsay, W. K., and McDougall, E. P.: Digital flexor tendons. An experimental study. Part III. The fate of autogenous

digital flexor tendon grafts. Brit. J. Plast. Surg., *13*:293-304, 1961.
78. Lindsay, W. K., and Thomson, H. G.: Digital flexor tendons. An experimental study. Part I. The significance of each component of the flexor mechanism in tendon healing. Brit. J. Plast. Surg., *12*: 289-316, 1960.
79. Lindsay, W. K., Thomson, H. G., and Walker, F. G.: Digital flexor tendons. An experimental study. Part II. The significance of a gap occurring at the line of suture. Brit. J. Plast. Surg., *13*:1-9, 1960.
80. Mason, M. L., and Allen, H. S.: The rate of healing of tendons. Ann. Surg., *113*: 424-459, 1941.
81. Mason, M. L., and Shearon, C. G.: The process of tendon repair. Arch. Surg., *25*:615-692, 1932.
82. Medawar, P. B.: Immunology of transplantation. Harvey Lectures Series 50, 114-146, 1957.
83. Misol, S., Samaan, N., and Ponsetti, I. V.: Growth hormone in delayed fracture healing. Clin. Orthop., *74*:206-208, 1971.
84. Mooney, V., Nickel, V., Harvey, J. P., Jr., and Snelson, R.: Cast brace treatment for fractures of the distal part of the femur. J. Bone Joint Surg., *52A*:1563-1578, 1970.
85. Müller, M. E., Allgower, M., and Willenegger, H.: Technique of Internal Fixation of Fractures. New York, Springer-Verlag, 1965.
86. Neer, C. S., Francis, K. C., Marcove, R. R. C., Terz, J., and Carbonara, P. N.: Treatment of unicameral bone cysts. J. Bone Joint Surg., *48A*:731-745, 1966.
87. Nicholas, J. A., and Killoran, P.: Fracture of the femur and patients with Paget's Disease. J. Bone Joint Surg., *47A*:450-461, 1965.
88. Nichols, J. T., Tot, P. D., and Chukos, N. C.: The proliferative capacity and DNA synthesis of osteoblasts during fracture repair in normal and hypophysectomized animals. Oral Surg., *25*:416-418, 1968.
89. O'Donoghue, D. H.: Surgical treatment of fresh injuries to the major ligaments of the knee. J. Bone Joint Surg., *32A*:721-738, 1950.
90. ———: An analysis of end results of surgical treatment of major injuries to the ligaments of the knee. J. Bone Joint Surg., *37A*:1-13, 1955.
91. O'Donoghue, D. H., Rockwood, C. A., Jr., Zaricznyj, B., and Kenyon, R.: Repair of knee ligaments in dogs. I. The lateral collateral ligament. J. Bone Joint Surg., *43A*: 1167-1178, 1961.
92. Pappas, A. N., and Radin, E.: The effect of delayed manipulation on the rate of fracture healing. Surg. Gynecol. Obstet., *126*:1287-1297, 1968.
93. Peacock, E. E.: A study of the circulation in normal tendons and healing grafts. Ann. Surg., *149*:415-428, 1959.
94. ———: Biological principles in the healing of long tendons. Surg. Clin. N. Amer., *45*:461-476, 1965.
95. Peacock, E. E., and Van Winkle, W.: Surgery and Biology of Wound Repair. Philadelphia, W. B. Saunders, 1970.
96. Penttinen, R.: Biochemical studies on fracture healing in the rat. Acta Chir. Scand., [Suppl.]:432, 1972.
97. Perren, S. M., Huggler, A., and Russenberger, S.: Cortical bone healing. Acta Orthop. Scand., [Suppl.]:125, 1965.
98. Phemister, D. B.: Treatment of ununited fractures by onlay bone grafts without screw or tie fixation and without breaking down of the fibrous union. J. Bone Joint Surg., *29*:946-960, 1947.
99. Potenza, A. D.: Tendon healing within the flexor digital sheath in the dog. J. Bone Joint Surg., *44A*:49-64, 1962.
100. ———: Critical evaluation of flexor tendon healing and adhesion formation within artificial digital sheaths. J. Bone Joint Surg., *45A*:1217-1233, 1963.
101. ———: The healing of autogenous tendon grafts within the flexor digital sheath in dogs. J. Bone Joint Surg., *46A*:1462-1484, 1964.
102. ———: Flexor Tendon Injuries. Orthop. Clin. N. Amer., *1*:355-373, 1970.
103. Potts, W. J.: The role of the hematoma in fracture healing. Surg. Gynecol. Obstet., *57*:318-324, 1933.
104. Ray, R. D.: Bone grafting: transplants and implants. American Academy of Orthopaedic Surgeons Instructional Course Lectures, *13*:177-186, 1956.
105. Ray, R. D., and Sabet, T.: Bone grafts, cellular survival D.S. induction. An experimental study in mice. J. Bone Joint Surg., *45A*:337-344, 1963.
106. Retief, D. H., and Dreyer, C. J.: Effects of neuro damage on the repair of bony defects in the rat. Arch. Biol., *12*:1035-1039, 1967.
107. Rhinelander, F. W., and Baragaray, R. W.: Microangiography in bone healing. Undisplaced closed fractures. J. Bone Joint Surg., *44A*:1273-1298, 1962.
108. Rhinelander, F. W., Phillips, R. S., Steel,

W. M., and Beer, J. C.: Microangiography and bone healing. II. Displaced closed fractures. J. Bone Joint Surg., *50A*:643-662, 1968.

109. Rokhanen, P., and Slatis, P.: The repair of experimental fractures during long-term anticoagulant treatment. Acta Orthop. Scand., *35*:21-38, 1964.
110. Rothman, R. H.: Effect of anemia on fracture healing. Surg. Forum, *19*:452-453, 1968.
111. Russell, P. S., and Monaco, A. P.: Biology of Tissue Transplantation. Boston, Little Brown, 1965.
112. Sarmiento, A.: A functional below-knee cast for tibial fractures. J. Bone Joint Surg., *49A*:855-875, 1967.
113. Scales, J. T.: Some biological and engineering aspects of surgical implants. J. Bone Joint Surg., *55B*:426, 1973.
114. Scales, J. T., Winter, G. D., and Shirley, H. T.: Corrosion of orthopaedic implants, screws, plates and femoral nail-plates. J. Bone Joint Surg., *41B*:810-820, 1959.
115. Simmons, D. J., and Kuvin, A. A.: Autoradiographic and biochemical investigations of the effect of cortisone on the bones of the rat. Clin. Orthop., *55*:201-212, 1967.
116. Singh, R. H., and Udupa, K. N.: Some investigations on the effect of insulin in healing of fractures. Ind. J. Med. Res., *54*:1071-1082, 1966.
117. Skoog, T., and Persson, B. H.: An experimental study of the early healing of tendons. Plast. Reconst. Surg., *13*:384-399, 1954.
118. Smith, J. W.: Blood supply of tendons. Amer. J. Surg., *109*:272-276, 1965.
119. Steier, A., Cedalia, I., Schwarz, A., and Rodan, A.: Effect of vitamin D_2 and fluoride on experimental bone fracture healing in rats. J. Dent. Res., *46*:675-680, 1967.
120. Stirling, R. I.: Healing of fractured bones. Trans. Roy. Med. Chir. Soc. Edinb., *46*: 203-209, 1931.
121. Tarsoly, E., Hájer, G., and Urbán, I.: Uber die Heilung von Knochenfrakturen bei hypo-bzw hyperthyreotischen Tieren. Acta Chir. Hung., *6*:435-445, 1965.
122. Tipton, C. M., Schild, R. J., and Flatt, A. E.: Measurement of ligamentous strength in rat knees. J. Bone Joint Surg., *49A*:63-72, 1967.
123. Tonna, E. A.: Electron microscopic study of osteocyte release during osteoclasis in mice of different ages. Clin. Orthop., *87*: 311-317, 1972.
124. Tonna, E. A., and Cronkite, E. T.: The periosteum; autoradiographic studies on cellular proliferation and transformation utilising tritiated thymidine. Clin. Orthop., *30*:218-233, 1963.
125. Trueta, J.: The role of the vessels in osteogenesis. J. Bone Joint Surg., *45B*: 402-418, 1963.
126. Turner, T. C., Bassett, C. A. L., Pate, J. W., and Sawyer, P. N.: Experimental comparison of freeze-dried and frozen cortical bone graft healing. J. Bone Joint Surg., *37A*:1197-1205, 1955.
127. Turner, T. C., Bassett, C. A. L., Pate, J. W., Sawyer, P. N., Trump, J. G., and Wright, K.: Sterilization of preserved bone grafts by high voltage cathode irradiation. J. Bone Joint Surg., *38A*:862-884, 1956.
128. Udupa, K. N., and Gupta, L. P.: Role of vitamin A in the repair of fracture. Ind. J. Med. Res., *54*:1122-1130, 1966.
129. Udupa, K. N., and Parsad, J. C.: Chemical and histochemical studies in the organic constituents in fracture repair in rats. J. Bone Joint Surg., *35B*:770-779, 1963.
130. Uhthoff, H. K., and Dubuc, F. L.: Bone structure changes in the dog under rigid internal fixation. Clin. Orthop., *81*:165-170, 1971.
131. Urist, M. R., Iwata, H., and Strates, B.: Bone morphogenetic protein and proteinase. Clin. Orthop., *85*:275-290, 1972.
132. Urist, M. R., and Johnson, R. W.: The healing of fractures in man under clinical conditions. J. Bone Joint Surg., *25*:375-426, 1943.
133. Venable, C. S., Stuck, W. G., and Beach, A.: The effects on bone of the presence of metals; based on electrolysis. Ann. Surg., *105*:917-938, 1932.
134. Watson-Jones, R.: Fractures and Joint Injuries. ed. 4. Edinburgh, E. & S. Livingstone, 1955.
135. Welsh, R. P., MacNab, I., and Riley, V.: Biochemical studies of rabbit tendon. Clin. Orthop., *81*:171-177, 1971.
136. Wendeberg, B.: Mineral metabolism of fractures of the tibia in man studied with external counting of strontium 85. Acta Orthop. Scand., *52*[Suppl.]:1-59, 1961.
137. Wiancko, K. B., and Kowalewski, K.: Strength of callus in fractured humerus of rat treated with anti-anabolic and anabolic compounds. Acta Endocrinol., *36*: 310-318, 1961.

138. Wolff, J.: Das Gaetz der Transformation. Transformation der Knochen. Berlin, Hirschwald, 1892.
139. Wray, J. B.: Vascular regeneration in the healing fracture. Angiology, *14*:134-138, 1963.
140. Wray, J. B., and Rogers, L. S.: Effect of hyperbaric oxygenation upon fracture healing in the rat. J. Surg. Res., *8*:373-378, 1968.
141. Yablon, I. G., and Cruess, R. L.: The effect of hyperbaric oxygenation on fracture healing in rats. J. Trauma, *8*:186-202, 1968.
142. Young, R. W.: Bone Biodynamics, edited by H. M. Frost, p. 117. Boston, Little Brown, 1964.
143. Ziegler, R., and Delling, G.: Effect of calcitonin on the regeneration of a circumscribed bone defect (bored hole in the rat tibia). Acta Endocrinol., *69*:497-506, 1972.

3 Open Fractures

Charles F. Gregory, M.D.

By definition, an open fracture is any in which a break in the integument and underlying soft tissue leads directly into the fracture and its hematoma. Depending upon the extent to which the soft tissues are injured, three specific consequences may be noted.

The first, and most significant, is the potential contamination of the area of injury by inoculation with bacteria from the external environment. Second, a greater or lesser degree of stripping of soft tissues renders both those tissues and the bone they cover more susceptible to the establishment of an active infection. Third, the destruction or loss of soft tissues that normally ensheathe bone may affect the methods by which the fracture can be effectively immobilized, and may deny the fracture site the usual contribution from overlying soft tissues in the bone repair effort (i.e., union and consolidation).

The first of these consequences is nearly universal. The other two vary with the extent of soft-tissue damage: a minor injury managed properly arouses no great concern; a major problem may even indicate immediate or early amputation. In any event, the problem of the open fracture is first the problem of the associated soft-tissue injury, and it is to this that we should initially direct our attention. The degree to which that can be effectively managed, may well determine the ultimate outcome for the bone, in the case of an open fracture, or the joint, in the case of an open dislocation.

HISTORICAL

Hippocrates, it is said, considered war the most appropriate training ground for surgeons. His greatest contribution in this regard lay in his recognition that surgeons can only facilitate healing, they cannot impose it. He recognized the need to accept certain consequences of injury, like swelling, as essential, and admonished against occlusive dressings before such swelling had occurred. He opposed frequent meddling with wounds, except to extrude purulent material, so long as the wound demonstrated progress in repairing itself. He further advocated "steel" or "iron" (actually the knife) in treating wounds that did not progress. His principal misconception is generally regarded as his aphorism, which held that diseases not curable by steel (knife) are curable by fire (cautery).

Galen and his followers also recognized purulence and admired it, considering it essential to the repair process. Frequent manipulations of a wound and a continuous search for medicaments that might be applied to enhance purulence were viewed as desirable to driving the wound to heal. Subsequently, most other schools represented one or the other of these viewpoints as a basis for their particular methods of treatment.

Brunschwig and Botello, in the 15th and 16th centuries, advocated the removal of nonvital tissue from wounds that did not progress properly. It remained for Desault, in the 18th century, to establish the making of a deep incision to explore a wound, remove dead tissue, and provide drainage. It was he who adopted the term debridement. His pupil, Larrey, extended the principle and included the issue of timing. The sooner debridement is done after wounding, he contended, the better the result.

Following Mathysen's development of plaster-of-paris bandages, the principle of occlusive dressings was reintroduced, only to lapse again because of untoward effects from misapplication.

Lister's introduction of carbolic acid dressings seemed the ultimate item in the Galenist search for a magic medication that would persuade wounds to heal. Seized with alacrity, it too proved disappointing, likely because the principles of debridement were too soon forgotten or abandoned —an episode destined to be repeated so many times thereafter.

The imperative of debridement of missile wounds was reestablished more firmly during World War I, first by the German army and subsequently by the Allies. Thereafter, Trueta brought together the combination of debridement and an occlusive dressing which also served as a splint (the plaster cast) in the treatment of wounded extremities during the Spanish Civil War. By contrast with prior experience, his vast number of examples demonstrated the virtues of this method when properly applied.

World War II began just after the start of the sulfa era. These agents supplanted antiseptic solutions, but like them were applied directly to injured tissues. Antibiotics were available during the Korean War. Yet in each of these military endeavors, the primacy of debridement and the Hippocratic precept of leaving the wound open had to be relearned and then reestablished by directive. The Galenist hope that medicines might circumvent the need to leave wounds open in order for them to heal uneventfully was dashed again. To be sure, failure was often the result of technically inadequate debridement. Yet the open wound may heal despite that, but a closed wound seldom can, even aided by antibiotics.

It seems now that the two major schools of thought can finally be brought together. For the wound that is inadequately debrided and is left open (Hippocratic) may benefit additionally from an appropriate antibiotic (Galenist) introduced at the proper time. Such wounds probably have the best prospect for healing uneventfully, whatever their subsequent management.

ETIOLOGY

The post-World War II era saw a gradual but distinct rise in the incidence of trauma in general until the mid-1960's, when it could be said to have reached a quasi-epidemic level. Open fractures have continued to constitute a significant proportion of the recorded injuries. Even as there was an absolute increase in the numbers of open fractures, so there has been an apparent increase in the magnitude of the injuries incurred.

Fractures occurring in two, three, or even all four limbs are no longer unusual. Moreover, one or more of the fractures is likely to be an open one.

Analyses of the patterns of injury that result from certain kinds of violence, plus some limited experimentation on the direct effects of controlled, violent forces have produced some useful information. Such knowledge of the mechanism of injury may alert the physician to seek evidence of obscure injury known to be associated with such mechanisms.

The essential equation underlying what is usually an unexpected application of a violent force to the human body is expressed as $K = \frac{MV^2}{2}$ where M represents mass and V the velocity of the wounding force. The contest thus arranged is a measure of how much kinetic energy (K) can be absorbed by the body's tissues before they are injured, or, how much injury occurs when the kinetic energy exceeds the ability of body tissues to resist, or absorb and disperse it. Moreover, the kinds of tissue injuries that occur vary in relation to the source of the kinetic energy. The converse holds equally true when the body itself is in motion and the offending or wounding agent is essentially stationary. Moreover, there are numerous examples of combinations of both.

Some of the common circumstances of injury can be measured fairly accurately. Others cannot. While the variety of conditions of injury are almost numberless, they fall in large measure into one of the following categories:

1. The body is stationary and struck by a moving object.
2. The body is in motion and strikes a stationary object.
3. The body is in motion and strikes another moving object or body.

In reviewing some examples of these three arrangements, certain other factors must be appreciated; among them, the actual kinetic energy of moving objects—be it the object striking the body or the body itself, the size of the area of impact, and the capacity of the impacted tissue to absorb and disperse energy. Analyzing a few examples may be useful.

Open fracture of the tibia is a common injury often produced when a car strikes a pedestrian. Not infrequently the initial contact is made over the posterior leg in the calf area. It is to be remembered that the force that remained great enough to fracture the tibia was transmitted first across the muscle bellies in the calf, even though the integument at that point had often remained intact. The muscles must have been damaged to some extent, and indeed we have found them on some occasions to be completely transected. The fractured bone ends are deflected anteriorly, against the rather thin overlying soft tissue and skin, which then ruptures, creating the open fracture. In the course of debridement, the surgeon who recognizes the potential damage to the posterior muscles may discover a communication between the fracture hematoma and the posterior compartment containing the damaged muscle. He must assume that contamination may have reached all parts of the wound, including the posterior compartment. He then faces a difficult decision. Should he confine his attentions to the anteriorly placed tissues, which are easily accessible, or should he consider entering the posterior compartment to deal with the injured tissue within?

In sharp contrast to the massive, relatively slow-moving car, which usually produces a broad area of impact when it strikes a body, a missile is a dense body of comparatively small mass. Yet, in accordance with the formula $\left(K = \frac{MV^2}{2}\right)$, the missile achieves a state in which it is highly freighted with kinetic energy. Moreover, it has a small impact area at contact, so that ordinarily its point of entry is small: approximately equal to its diameter. A number of factors enter into the pattern of subsequent effects, however, and they are worth a brief comment.

First, we must recall that gases are compressible and liquids are not. Should such a missile penetrate the chest wall and enter living tissue, it may pass through it, producing destruction only along its direct and immediate pathway (unless it should strike a bronchus or a large vessel). The air in the lung can be compressed momentarily as air in the flight path is pushed aside. On the contrary, when a rapidly moving missile strikes tissue with a high water content, such as the liver, it produces considerable displacement of the noncompressible liquid, creating in fact a significant momentary cavity.

An excellent illustration of this behavior can be easily contrived as follows: Make two targets, one a sealed can, empty except for atmosphere, and the other a sealed can of the same size, containing sauerkraut, which has a water content approximately equal to that of muscle or liver. Using a rifle with reasonably high-velocity bullets, hit each target from the same distance. If your marksmanship is equal to it, you will see the empty can jump from its resting place, and when it is examined, it will demonstrate small holes of entry and exit with little other distortion. Next hit the target can of sauerkraut, and you will note that it virtually explodes. Often its ends will be blown loose and its seam split, the whole greatly distorted. The sauerkraut will be widely spread about the area.

Muscle behaves in a similar fashion when struck by a high-velocity missile, except that the cavity that permanently disrupted the rigid can tends to be only a momentary cavity in an animal or human limb. The surrounding elastic tissue recollapses the cavity walls, leaving only the small pathway of destruction made by actual contact of the missile with tissue as the residual identifiable wound. Two corollary events may also occur, events that will not be noted unless one is aware of the foregoing mechanism. First, the fluid wave that displaces tissue as the momentary cavity comes into existence, may stretch or contuse adjacent nerves and blood vessels in the vicinity of the wave effect. Second, atmospheric air tends to rush into the momentary wound cavity in response to the rapidly produced vacuum and to sweep in with it whatever material lies adjacent to the wound of entry. The material thus introduced may well contain bacteria. We shall consider the clinical significance of these observations at a later point, when their importance will become evident.

Yet another example of the usefulness of knowledge regarding the etiology of an injury is the matter of close-range shotgun wounds. The shotgun shell usually contains a large number of small pellets. Though they are intended to scatter at target distance, initially they move from the gun barrel in a rather dense group called a shot cloud. If, while still quite closely packed, they strike a target, their collective impact may be somewhat like that of a bullet. However, each pellet has so much less kinetic energy than a bullet that they are soon expended. Thus, many such injuries are only penetrating ones. Occasionally some of the shot cloud emerges from the opposite side of the limb, producing thereby a perforating wound. The greatest danger is from the shell wadding, a bit of material, often made of jute and hair compressed with a binding agent. Wadding is impervious to gases and literally pushes the shot down the gun barrel ahead of it when the powder lying behind them is ignited. The wadding is less dense but has greater mass, and tends eventually to fall behind the shot cloud in flight, although remaining fairly close to the cloud and having the same trajectory for several feet. Thus not infrequently the wadding enters the wound with the shot cloud, particularly in close-range shotgun injuries. Wadding is extremely irritating to tissues and incites a severe inflammatory response. Thus it must be removed. Often it is difficult to locate even when its presence is suspected, and, indeed, all too frequently it has been overlooked—to the ultimate detriment of the wound and the patient.

Two other examples of somewhat special circumstances beset with hazards to the patient and surgeon are worth consideration. Not infrequently, a limb is caught in a violent compressive force, as often occurs when a motorcycle rider catches his leg between his machine and a car in a sideswipe collision. Sometimes the visible wound of the soft tissues is only modest, and the limb is not grossly deformed. Roentgenograms may confirm the diagnosis of fracture, but there is considerable increase in the separation between the tibia and fibula (Fig. 3-1). This is a sign of severe soft-tissue injury, which usually in-

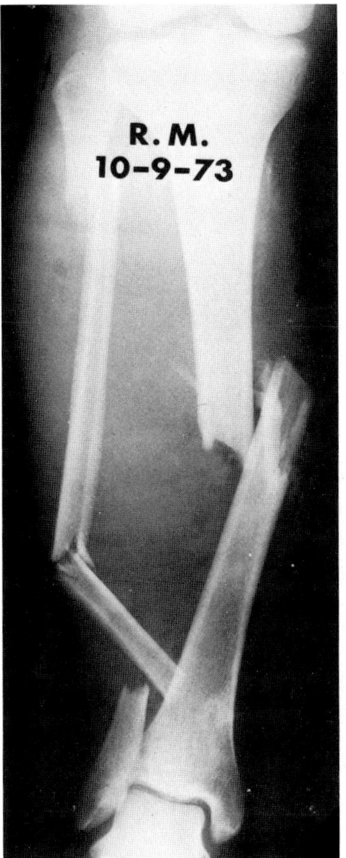

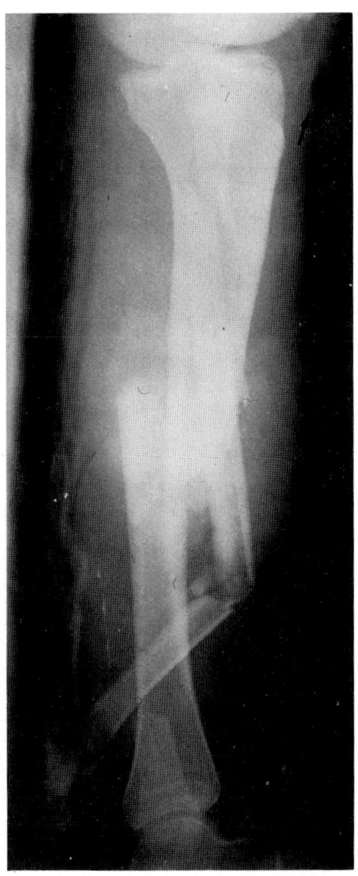

Fig. 3-1. The degree of "deep" soft-tissue injury is indicated by the wide separation of the tibial and fibular shafts. The extremely tough interosseous membrane, which normally binds them to one another, has been torn completely. The deep anterior and posterior tibial vessels lie nearby and are endangered.

cludes stripping of the extremely tough interosseous membrane. Intense swelling often follows, which, if it does not directly injure vessels, often produces compartment syndromes. Such swelling and its consequences can be anticipated by noting this tip-off in the roentgenograms, so that measures may be taken to prevent trouble.

Wounds incurred in a tornado are virtually always contaminated by finely dispersed soil, which literally fills the air in this awesome phenomenon. Importantly, such soil often carries a variety of usual and unusual pathogens, many anerobic. Recorded experience has indicated clearly that closing such wounds is very likely to lead to serious infections, including those produced by Clostridia.

Finally, injuries involving the rotary lawn mower are unique to our time. Though infrequent, individuals are sometimes struck by so unlikely a pseudo-missile as a bit of wire or other metal set in flight by contact with a mower blade. The wounds produced are usually small, yet the pseudo-missile may bury itself within a body cavity or even bone, which is some indication of the kinetic energy transferred to it by the mower blade. More importantly it is an indication of the energy contained in the whirling tip of the mower blade itself, which in high-speed machines develops a very significant sustained blade-tip velocity. Coupled with its mass, it is capable of producing a great deal of kinetic energy.

As noted earlier, experience has shown that there are rather unusual pathogenic bacteria to be found in the wounds incurred by tornado victims. And in a very real sense, a wound produced by a mower blade is created in a minor tornado. The normally earth-bound bacteria, afloat with the detritus in the vacuum created in a mower casing, may result in a wound inoculated by bacteria similar to those in a tornado. And for the same reasons we believe it wise never to close such wounds, but to debride them and leave them open.

These few major examples of the multiple and varying factors related to different kinds of injury were cited to illustrate the usefulness of knowing something about the "history" of how an injury was incurred. Though there are many others of course, those mentioned should make the point. Moreover, they underscore the need for further investigation about wounding mechanisms and their immediate and late effects upon tissues.

INITIAL MANAGEMENT

The initial assessment of the injured patient should, of course, be as comprehensive as his condition permits. In addition to identifying life-threatening conditions (e.g., airway obstruction, profound shock) and providing for their immediate relief, attention should be directed, as soon as practical, to detecting their causes and correcting them, including hemorrhage from an obviously injured limb. When threat to the patient's life has been relieved (or for the patient who was never in danger), nothing is acceptable other than a systematized examination of the whole patient. Consciousness and central nervous system function should be assessed. Next, the thorax, belly, and genitourinary systems should be appraised, followed by a careful examination of the apparently uninjured extremities. If one considers the head and neck a fifth extremity, it is logical to begin with the cervical spine. Undetected serious injury to the cervical spine, especially in the upper three vertebral units, still occurs too frequently, particularly in those patients who are unconscious when admitted. Next, the other apparently uninjured limbs may be examined and such injuries as may be found assessed and noted.

Examination of the Wound

After the measures outlined above have been taken, the obviously injured extremity may be approached deliberately, since the physician may then feel comfortable knowing that no other unrecognized or unassessed injury is likely to emerge suddenly or be further compromised by neglect or oversight. This plea for a deliberate and orderly assessment underscores the fundamental principle that, in dealing with the injured, one should take nothing for granted. To look offers the prospect to know—not to look is to guess. As an additional example, even now one of the well known triads of injury associated with fracture of the femoral shaft is still overlooked with distressing frequency: dislocation of the hip, fracture of the femoral neck, or rupture of a collateral knee ligament, on the same side as the fracture.

Several features of the obviously injured limb should be noted. The state of its blood supply as indicated by capillary blush, the filling of veins, and the state of peripheral pulses should be determined and recorded. Should circulation seem to be impaired, the same measures must be taken here as outlined elsewhere in this text. The integrity of the peripheral nerves must be determined, including both sensory and motor function for each major nerve, or branch of a nerve, which might be involved.

Specific to an open fracture is the general condition of the skin about the wounds. Has it been burned? Is it contaminated with usual or unusual agents—dirt, dust, petroleum products, paint, fertilizer? Any such contaminants that are obvious about the wound may also have invaded it. What are the dimensions of the wound? Is the surrounding tissue badly abraded, contused or flayed from its fascial bed? These points can be detected quite rapidly. However it is useful at some point to inspect that part of the limb, usually its posterior surface, which lies unseen against the splint or examining table. It is surprising how often significant wounds in that area are overlooked initially. The danger lies, of course, in not making provisions for dealing with them when formal treatment of the limb is undertaken.

Since formal debridement is indicated for obviously open fractures, there is not much justification for the digital exploration of such wounds in the emergency area. It usually provides little useful information, virtually always creates a new flush of bleeding, and may displace a large clot which can be followed by profuse bleeding at a time when little can be done to deal with it effectively. Dealing with large bleeding vessels requires good visualization and illumination. Therefore, deep exploration for the most part should be deferred until the time of formal debridement.

There remain a number of cases in which a small wound in the skin overlies a fracture, and immediately the question arises: does it communicate with the fracture site? Is it, therefore, an open fracture? In these circumstances it may be justifiable to invade the wound with a sterile, blunt probe. If bone is contacted, the answer is at hand. But if it is not, that may simply mean that the probe has followed the wrong pathway. It has been reported that saline can be injected through a prepared area of intact skin into the underlying hematoma, which, if it then escapes through the wound establishes the fact that an open fracture does exist. However, this maneuver carries the hazard of contaminating a closed fracture hematoma, and it must therefore be carried out with great care and antiseptic precautions. Where this basic problem exists with a large wound, it may serve as an exception to the gentle introduction of a sterile gloved finger for the purpose of establishing that the fracture is or is not an open one. Again however, chance may determine the plane taken by the exploring digit, and an open fracture may be overlooked or simply mistaken for a closed one. Even though failure to detect the communication between such minor wounds and a fracture is infrequent, as is infection in them, those infections that have been recorded are all too frequently disastrous clostridial gas gangrene. Therefore, if there is any suspicion at all that a wound may communicate with an adjacent fracture, it should be dealt with formally. The wound must be debrided under strict antiseptic precautions, so that its connection with the fracture may be determined. If there is no open fracture, nothing has been lost. But if the suspicion of open fracture is confirmed, a limb—even a life—may have been saved. The initial assessment of the open fracture having been carried as far as is safe or practical in the emergency room, the wound may then be dressed with a sterile cover and splinted, if that has not already been done.

The Patient's History

When there is no urgent need to proceed to surgical treatment at once, as much history as can be gleaned, both of a general medical nature and pertinent to the specific injury, should be obtained from the patient, relatives, witnesses, ambulance attendants, or whoever else may have information.

The status of the patient's immunity to tetanus should be determined if at all possible. If he knows the date of his last immunization, only toxoid may be needed as a booster. If it is uncertain, 250 to 500 units of immune globulin (human) should be given, especially when tetanus-prone wounds are present. It is also useful to initiate an active immunization for such patients at this time, but only for its usefulness in future injuries, not the one at hand.

Finally, all information gathered to this point, both historical and that derived by examination, should be carefully and accurately recorded. The record should also include all measures taken in treatment of the patient, the time they were carried out, and the patient's response to them. The results of pertinent laboratory work ought also to be recorded, of course.

While the use of antibiotics as a part of the initial treatment will be discussed later, if antibiotics are to be used, they should begin at the time of admission to the hospital, or at least as soon as the decision to use them has been made. Swabs for culture and sensitivity should be taken from the wound prior to the administration of any antibiotics.[17]

Roentgenographic Examination

A discussion of roentgenograms made of the open fracture has been delayed for the same reason that the taking of such x-ray films is usually delayed, but not because they are unimportant. They are important, but they are simply adjunctive.

Once the patient has been assessed (and, if necessary, revived and stabilized); all potential or probable injuries considered and listed; the wounds of open fractures inspected; and pertinent history elicited; all of the roentgenograms that may be needed can be taken at one time. To do so minimizes the extent to which the patient must be disturbed. Should some circumstance emerge such as suspicion of injury to the aortic arch or a tension pneumothorax, a chest roentgenogram may be made at once, of course. Treatment of these conditions is naturally assigned priority, because they do not tolerate well the more deliberate, systematic approach.

For patients with injuries in several systems, a considerable number of roentgenograms may be indicated. Cystograms, urethrograms, or excretory urograms, a good chest film, a KUB film, routine anteroposterior and lateral roentgenograms of the cervical spine as well as an anteroposterior and lateral roentgenograms of any part of a limb where a fracture or dislocation is known to exist or is suspected, might be properly included in such a list. The usefulness of roentgenograms is always proportionate to their quality, and quality films will more likely be produced if they are made deliberately and under the most favorable circumstances that can be arranged. Most open fractures are clearly obvious and need no roentgenograms to establish their presence. In such cases the roentgenogram may reveal a modest fracture line with essentially undisturbed fragments—but a fracture nonetheless. More frequently the extent of a fracture may be demonstrated as more than suspected, and even other unexpected fractures not related to the wound may be discovered. It is to be remembered that no roentgenographic examination of a bone may be considered as complete until all of the bone and the joints in which it participates have been demonstrated. Other useful findings sometimes emerge as well. Radiopaque foreign material may be revealed, alerting the surgeon to seek it during debridement. Not uncommonly, air trapped in tissue planes may be revealed. Of little initial importance, this finding may help interpret similar gas shadows found in a wound a few hours later, when gas-forming bacilli may be the only other logical explanation.

Finally, there is the usefulness of roentgenograms in deciding upon an appropriate method for dealing with the fractures *per se*. While knowledge of the pattern of the fractures may not alone determine what should be done with them, x-ray films can demonstrate which parts of the injured bone must be included in whatever form of treatment is finally selected.

The patient having been accurately assessed, his injuries documented, basic treatment instituted, and his response recorded, he is now ready for whatever surgical procedures may be required.

PREPARATION FOR DEBRIDEMENT

Not infrequently, more urgent injuries than open fractures properly take priority in the order of surgical treatment. When it is necessary to delay surgical attention to an open fracture, the wounds should be covered with sterile dressings, and the bones should be adequately splinted. Intermittent re-assessment of the circulation to the distal segment of the injured limb ought to be made and recorded.

It should be self-evident that even the most grossly contaminated open fracture usually is not really dirty in a bacteriologic sense. Yet, precisely because it is more susceptible to bacterial inoculation and colonization, it deserves the cleanest of surgical suites, and all of the antiseptic precautions ordinarily extended to elective surgical procedures. The I and D Room is not an acceptable location for treating open fractures! Even as the quarters for surgery must be clean, so also the approach of all involved personnel should be the same as for any operative procedure.

As a rule, an open fracture of average severity will require the same equipment as any elective open reduction. A full set of soft-tissue and bone instruments should be at hand or immediately available. A full assortment of fixation devices should also be available.

A fracture table that can serve as well as a standard operating table is often valuable. Lighting of the first quality is essential to facilitate the careful inspection of the numerous recesses so often encountered during debridement. And because these wounds must often be approached from a lateral aspect, a mobile operating room lamp may prove invaluable. A tourniquet with an accurately calibrated gauge should always be at hand. It is often wise to put the tourniquet in place (when space permits) even though it may never be inflated. Then if it is needed suddenly, its readiness may be life-saving.

Perhaps the most important item of supply is sterile normal saline, for certainly it is ordinarily used in greater quantities than any other supply. Often of use are detergents, organic solvents, soap, antiseptic solutions, shears, a razor, and even hair clippers. Less often required but at times indispensable are ring cutters, pliers, and on rare occasions even a hacksaw. A knowledge of where such items may be secured is a wise preparation.

Beyond this list, sooner or later some rare circumstance will require some unusual item such as a large, power metal saw. But one can neither anticipate nor provide for every contingency.

A good many open fractures occur in the night, leading Shires[17] to observe that the surgery of trauma is the surgery of inconvenience. Its relation to the matter of treating open fractures lies in the fact that many surgical facilities have only skeleton crews at night and for obvious reasons may choose to operate short-handed. Such practices are unsatisfactory.

The transport, prepping, and draping of seriously injured patients with wounded limbs requires at least a minimum number of skilled persons to carry them out effectively. To attempt their treatment with inadequate help is to compromise the prospect for properly executed initial care and thus the ultimate outcome as well.

Ideally the initial surgical treatment of severe open fractures in the lower extremity should enlist at least four persons to carry out the following assignments: (1) the surgeon, (2) an experienced anesthesiologist, (3) at least two additional persons to assist in positioning the patient, (4) at least two persons to conduct the preparation, (5) two persons to drape as a third person passes them sterile linen, (6) three persons to perform the debridement (including the scrub nurse), (7) two persons to apply the cast or arrange postoperative splinting, (8) as a rule, three persons (preferably four) to transfer the patient from table to bed.

Though four persons are really essential, five are even more desirable, as this provides a circulator. Less severe cases might be handled effectively with fewer, so long as the risk of compromising antisepsis is minimal.

While some injuries in the upper extremity may be managed by regional anesthesia, perhaps administered by the surgeon, those patients with multiple injuries or massive injuries of the lower extremities are best dealt with by an experienced anesthesiologist, well versed in the vagaries of trauma and its effects upon the patient. When the issue is compounded by alcohol or drug intoxication, his services may become virtually indispensable. Moreover, for some reason, most trauma patients have a full stomach!

Positioning requirements should be anticipated. The survey of the patient in the emergency room, if complete, will have revealed the more commonly obscured wounds, as well as the obvious ones, and may have suggested the most useful position of the patient for debridement. The position chosen should offer the most convenient possible approach to each wound, with the best advantage for illuminating them.

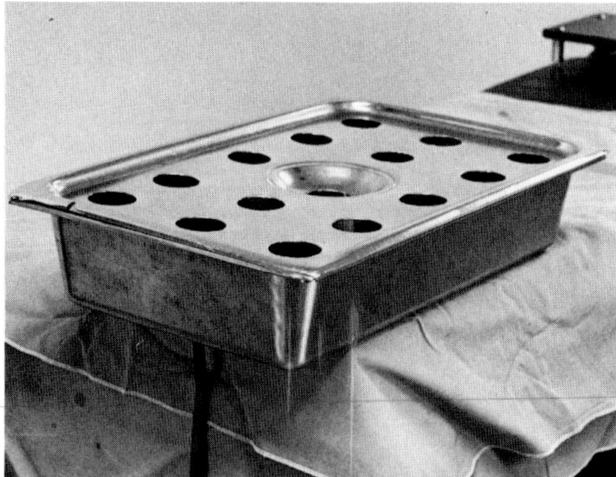

Fig. 3-2. When a limb is to be prepped or when debridement is to be performed, if the limb can be placed on the perforated surface of the pan illustrated, the necessary rinsing and sluicing with considerable quantities of fluid, can be carried out freely. Because a drainage tube vents the affluent into a pail on the floor, the operative field can be kept dry.

Prepping a limb that has an open fracture is properly biphasic. The first phase should cleanse the intact skin about and between wounds. Since harsh agents such as an organic solvent may be required, the open wounds should be protected throughout this phase by appropriate sterile dressings, changed as required. When the intact skin has been suitably cleansed, a new set-up should be available for dealing with the wound itself. It really requires only flushing unless it is unusually and grossly contaminated.

Scrubbing exposed tissues with detergents or agents such as pHisoHex for the purpose of sterilization is untenable. Additionally, the caustic effect of some prep solutions, plus the trauma to cells produced by scrubbing them, can only cause more of them to be destroyed. If gross and visible contaminants are present they are better plucked from the wound with an instrument, or if stuck, sheared away with some tissue. The formal debridement will eliminate the remainder more effectively than either scrubbing or sluicing. Unless there is an anticipated delay in the preparation and debridement of the wound, there seems little reason to lace it with antibiotic or antiseptic solutions. Placing the limb on a large pan with a perforated top (Fig. 3-2) while the original preparation is carried out can do much to keep the operative field, the patient, the personnel, and the floor dry without limiting the amount of rinsing solution used. The pan is fitted with an outlet spout from which a large-bore rubber hose can conduct effluent into a pail on the floor.

Draping should be carried out with at least two objectives in mind. First, the maintenance of a sterile field kept as free as possible of additional exogenous bacteria. Because drapes are likely to become wet in the course of debridement, it is useful first to cover the field (other than the limb to be treated) with a plastic or other moisture-proof drape. Second, the draping should be arranged so as to permit free manipulation of the limb, while providing access to whichever surfaces may require attention. Such maneuverability often tends to produce shifting of the drapes, and may dislodge a whole segment. Care plus ingenuity is often quite necessary to devise effective draping that will withstand these stresses. The wounds are now ready for debridement.

Until the first half of the 20th century, the surgery of open fractures was the surgery of osteomyelitis. Prepping and draping stand co-equal with debridement and medications in overturning this premise, making the uneventful healing of open fractures nearly equal in prospect to closed fractures treated by open reduction.

DEBRIDEMENT

Once employed only in the treatment of already infected wounds, debridement (literal translation: *unbridling*) was an incision to release the purulent content of an already infected wound. Gradually it was realized that adjacent bits of necrotic tissue could also be removed with benefit to the wound. Finally, it was learned that the removal of wound detritus, especially necrotic tissue and foreign material, achieves its best results when carried out immediately the patient comes under treatment.

The decision to carry out a debridement of some sort is not usually a difficult one. Yet some limbs are so badly mangled that, even with an intact neurovascular system, the prospect for salvaging the limb for any reasonable function is highly unlikely, so that primary amputation may be indicated. Totally mangled limbs are clearly to be dealt with only by amputation. Judgments concerning such matters are supported more frequently by experience than any reliable set of criteria available at this time.

There remains, at the other end of the spectrum, the small or minor wound—perhaps a puncture wound made from within outward by a displaced, slightly protruding bone end, or a low-velocity missile or other object. It may be forcefully argued that *no* wound is minor when it is directly associated with the fracture, for the wound makes the fracture an open fracture. Gas bacillus infections have proceeded too frequently from the first example, and organic foreign material found in the wound too often in the second. Further, it may be argued that the conservative approach to such wounds is to explore and debride them, while the radical approach is to simply dress them. This position can be supported in terms of relative morbidity. Even if only an occasional wound *not* treated by debridement becomes infected, when it does, the infection, always serious, may range from a chronic state, perhaps only compromising union, to the dreadfully serious, sometimes fatal gas gangrene. On the contrary, exploration produces but an extension of the initial wound, which rarely protracts or compromises the ultimate course and contributes little if any to its inherent morbidity.

The general objectives of the procedure identified as debridement can be stated:

1. The detection and removal of nonvital tissues.
2. The detection and removal of foreign material, especially organic foreign material.
3. The reduction of bacterial contamination.
4. The creation thereby of a wound whose viable tissue surfaces help render it capable of coping with residual bacterial contamination.

Skin and Subcutaneous Tissue

Incisions play a most important role in effective debridement. Small puncture wounds or holes may be elliptically excised (Fig. 3-3) and subsequently closed by suture, or may even close spontaneously, leaving a simple linear scar. The pernicious practice of coring a wound is to be deplored. It leaves a round hole that can only close by granulation and scar formation.

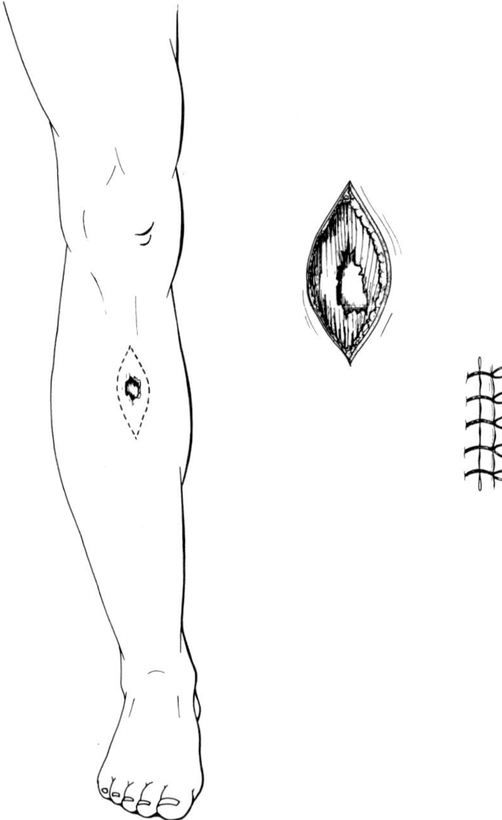

Fig. 3-3. An elliptical excision of the fracture wound permits proper inspection of the area of injury, as well as a better closure if the wound is sutured.

The cicatrix thus produced may create retraction and puckering in many instances.

Careful initial assessment of the wounds often permits planning the best additional incisions and the following points should always be considered:

1. The amount of gross loss of skin and subcutaneous tissue
2. The extent of flaying beneath remaining, apparently viable skin
3. The need to extend existing wounds for adequate inspection, and the best directions for such extensions
4. The usefulness of connecting adjacent yet separate wounds, or the dangers thereof
5. The prospect of survival for flaps created by injury or by planned incisions
6. The amount of skin that can be sacrificed, if any, to effect the most appropriate closure, should closure seem indicated
7. The usefulness of counterincisions to facilitate adequate debridement, arrange cover, or provide for wound drainage
8. The likelihood that a planned incision may transect a major superficial vein
9. The age of the patient and the state of his skin and subcutaneous tissues
10. The need to expose a wound widely enough to inspect its deeper recesses thoroughly

Generally the surgeon ought to be conservative in the excision of skin. Skin is tough and even though severely abraded, sufficient residual islands usually persist to produce a new epithelial layer. Care must be exercised in the amount of skin excised in those areas where it is not redundant, only just sufficient: the face, wrist, hand, ankle, and foot. An additional incision of adequate length to allow thorough exploration is often necessary for wounds created by objects that have high kinetic energy quotients and for those in which deep gross contamination is suspected. For example, a useful axiom for high-velocity missile wounds states that the wound and/or incision for exploration should equal in length the diameter of the limb at that level. Having removed the margins of damaged skin and extended the wound where necessary by carefully planned incisions, attention may next be directed to the deeper layers of tissue within the wound.

It seems much more satisfactory to proceed with debridement, layer by layer from the skin to the depths of the wound. Even where hemorrhage is troublesome, when it can be controlled by packing or a tourniquet if necessary, this orderly approach offers better assurance for thoroughness in the entire procedure. Damaged or contaminated subcutaneous tissue should be excised, but clean, intact tissue planes usually need not be opened, since the supporting circulation to skin is often transmitted across such planes. Damaged or contaminated fascia should be removed at least along the margins. The surgeon may be more generous in excising fascia than in excising skin.

Muscle

Whereas skin tends to tear or be punctured, and fascia to split or to shred, muscle, because of its high water content, is liable to damage by fluid waves when the offending agent producing the wound imparts sufficient kinetic energy to the area. It is easy, therefore, to overlook nonvital muscle, as it may not always provide immediate evidence that it has been disturbed or is damaged. Yet remnants of nonvital muscle within a wound offer a most salubrious pablum for bacterial growth. If the muscle is necrotic the greatest danger is posed by anerobes. Brav[2] for example, underscores a simple axiom: "When in doubt, take it out." To a degree this may be taken literally, unless a whole muscle lies in question, and even here that may be feasible if certain other criteria are fulfilled. Destruction of the major arterial supply of a severely damaged muscle is one of these. There are a few guiding points which, if observed during the debridement can assist the surgeon in his decisions about the viability of muscle. They are listed as an alliterative quartet: color, consistency, contractility, and capacity to bleed. However, there are some qualifications to be observed in their application.

Color can be misleading. What presents as dark, at times black muscle surfaces, may be only a thin layer of blood lying beneath the myonesium. When freed of this thin layer, the underlying muscle may be found normal in color.

Consistency is a subjective qualification and ranges from normal firm tissue to the stringy, friable, even mushy state of disintegrating tissue. The firmer the consistency, the more certainly the muscle is viable.

Contractility, when present, clearly establishes muscle viability. Muscle tissue that retreats from the incising edge of a scalpel or scissors is obviously very much alive.

Capacity to bleed must also be qualified. The presence of a spurter may simply mean that a conduit has been transected which was conveying blood to another remote part of a muscle and providing no capillary perfusion to the area under treatment. On the contrary, gentle persistent oozing from capillaries tends to demonstrate adequate local perfusion, indicating that the muscle is very probably viable.

Scully,[16] in an attempt to correlate these four features with histologic evidence of viability, concluded that consistency and capacity to bleed were very significant features for judging viability. Contractility is, of course, significant if present, yet not all noncontractile muscle is necessarily nonvital. Color is the least useful indicator of viability. Other circumstances may alter the state of the muscle tissue. Ischemia associated with shock may obscure bleeding, as may damage to a major vessel to the involved limb, or intrinsic vascular disease in the elderly patient.

Though serious effort should be made to remove all nonvital muscle tissue, there are many times when the surgeon is left uncertain that he has achieved his objective. In that circumstance (it often occurs when the wounding mechanism was a crushing injury or a high-velocity missile or a shotgun at close-range) a second look taken a day or two later may be wise. The wound will, of course, have been left open. The second inspection permits additional debridement if it is indicated, or at least permits the surgeon to know that the suspected wound is in no serious difficulty.

Bone

Whereas muscle tissue may mount a defense against invading bacteria, bone tissue is essentially defenseless. If judgments about muscle viability seem troublesome, judgments about what is to be done with bone fragments are perplexing. Generally speaking, small bits of bone free of any soft-tissue connection should be removed. It is the larger fragment, constituting a significant segment of the injured bone which, if removed, leaves a gap to be filled that causes consternation. If such a fragment has obvious soft-tissue connections, and especially if its small vessels bleed onto its exposed surface, it may be retained, even if that requires trimming the surfaces to eliminate minor contamination. Unless it is grossly contaminated the fragment probably should be preserved. The real problem in judgment lies with the fragment that has only a tenuous soft-tissue connection, or none at all. Its value as a bone graft, often naturally tailored to the defect, seems obvious. The question is, can it be sufficiently free of contamination that it will be tolerated? Or conversely, is the bed of viable tissue in which it is to be reimplanted capable of dealing with any residual contamination such a fragment may bear? There are no absolute criteria, and therefore such problems are decided arbitrarily on the basis of a judgment. Whether it is wiser to retain the prospect of earlier healing by eliminating a significant defect in bone, in spite of the hazard of infection, or, to better assure wound healing by taking the fragment out and risking a delayed or nonunion, seems to be the essence of the proposition. Since either pathway involves a risk or some vexing problem down the line, perhaps the inexperienced surgeon (if he cannot obtain consultation) should choose to risk the less serious complication: delayed union or nonunion. For there is a situation more difficult to deal with than nonunion. It is an *infected* nonunion.

Foreign Bodies

Foreign bodies, especially organic foreign bodies, often lead to so much morbidity if left in a wound that they should be sought. Fragments of wood are especially troublesome, for they are easily buried in tissue. Cloth and leather, on the other hand, often occupy tissue planes, and may find recesses remote from the site of injury. There is probably no material known to man that has not surprised one surgeon or another when encountered in a wound. A chewing gum wrapper does not often appear in an ankle joint, but at least one has been found there. The intrinsic recesses, pits, or crevices of the foreign material may harbor pathogenic organisms or their spores. And the foreign body itself, especially an organic foreign body, is likely to incite an inflammatory response. Even the sterile sponge inadvertently left during surgery is an example.

Hard material—metal, rocks and gravel, and some plastics—are hazards because of bacterial contamination. They should be recovered if they can be found. Bullets and especially pellets usually become buried. Unless easily detected, their recovery may entail more hazard by the tissue disturbed or destroyed in seeking them than they pose if left where they came to lie. Pellets ought to be removed only if they are casually encountered in debridement or if they have damaged a major blood vessel or nerve. (Bullets in veins have been reported on rare occasions to become emboli.) A singular exception to the matter of removing lead bullets relates to those that enter and lie, in whole or in part, within a joint. Joint fluid acting on lead tends to break it down, and as Leonard[9] has reported, can induce a serious synovitis, as well as low-grade lead poisoning. Therefore, lead bullets thought to lie inside a joint should be sought and removed. Close-range shotgun wounds are treacherous in this regard, because the wadding from a shell may enter the wound. It must be sought and removed, since the peculiar combination of materials of which it is made renders it extremely irritating to soft tissues. Those close range shotgun wounds that perforate and thereby

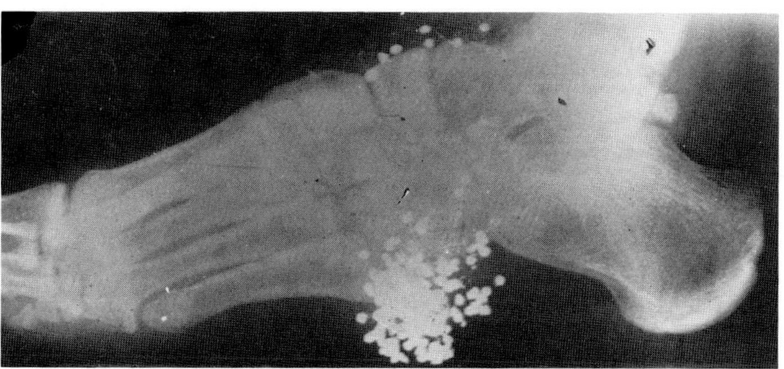

Fig. 3-4. The shot cloud has traversed this foot from its dorsal aspect, but it has come to lie on the deep aspect of the plantar fascia. It serves as a clue to the location of any associated shell wadding that may also have entered the wound.

create wounds of entrance and of exit, make access available to both wounds, and thus facilitate thorough inspection and debridement. But when the wound is simply penetrating, a thorough inspection is often difficult. Frequently, however, the shot cloud that creates the penetrating wound comes to lie against the fascia on the far side of the injured member (Fig. 3-4). Moreover, its wadding is often found with it. A counterincision is then justified, even mandatory. The counterincision facilitates the detection and removal of any wadding, along with the concentrated mass of easily accessible pellets.

Joints

Any wound that enters a joint mandates exploration. If it is simply a puncture wound, an arthrotomy of a conventional pattern may be performed. It should be generous enough to allow adequate exploration, including all those recesses where suspected or unsuspected foreign material might lurk. Debridement of the joints should otherwise follow the same postulates as debridement elsewhere.

Vessels

Brisk bleeders encountered during debridement should be ligated. Oozing generally abates gradually. Major vessel injury in conjunction with the open wound can usually be dealt with concomitantly with the debridement. It is generally agreed that both arteries and veins should be repaired if both have been injured. However it is because veins cannot always be repaired effectively that an admonition was offered earlier to spare the major superficial veins when extending incisions for debridement. That measure may preserve the only avenue for runoff of arterial inflow.

The matter of protecting an arterial repair when dealing with an adjacent fracture has elicited some sharply opposing viewpoints. Some argue that the critical matter of protecting the injured and repaired vessels regularly justifies internal fixation of open fractures in such situations. Others, notably Rich,[13] maintain that plaster casts with transfixing pins incorporated, or even the judicious application of traction and a splint do as well, with no real hazard to the vessel repair. Since the issue of internal fixation in open fractures will be dealt with later, the reader may withhold his opinion until that time.

Fasciotomy

Following arterial repair, massive swelling occurring distal to the site is not uncommon. It usually occurs in the forearm or leg. Fasciotomy may become necessary and is often urged as prophylaxis by some authors. Should there be any doubt about its indication it probably should be done. Moreover, it is better done too early than too late.

The forearm with its two major compartments can usually be relieved by two incisions 180 degrees from each other, one volar, the other dorsal. The leg, however, has four compartments: anterior, peroneal, superficial and deep posterior. Two incisions in corresponding locations on the leg may not achieve sufficient relief, especially of the deep posterior compartment which contains the extrinsic toe flexors. Patman[11] has suggested a means of relieving all four compartments by resecting the fibular shaft through a single incision. Occasionally a single compartment, such as the anterior tibial, is involved, and it may be sufficiently relieved by a single incision directly over it. Whether the simple technique of a short skin incision with extension of the fascial incision in both directions by scissors run subcutaneously, or extended incisions of both skin and fascia should be made, must be determined in part by the extent of the swelling present and what is required to relieve it completely. The contention that skin may be as constricting as fascia if the swelling is great enough is implicit. Not infrequently skin grafts may be required to provide eventual cover of such wounds, since swelling may recede too slowly to permit suturing of the wound in time. However, even this added morbidity pales in contrast with that visited upon the patient who needed a compartment decompression but did not receive it.

Use of a Tourniquet

In the business of debridement of open fractures, a tourniquet may be both useful and on occasions lifesaving, or it may not be required at all. If the injury lies far enough distal to the groin or axilla, it is useful at the outset of preparation to apply a tourniquet high on the thigh. It may then be inflated if needed to facilitate debridement or to control excessive bleeding, or it may be left uninflated if no indication arises which requires its use. If inflated, however, it may offer yet another advantage. When the tourniquet is released, the skin distal to the tourniquet usually undergoes an early and marked suffusion. Observation of the rate and extent of such suffusion, especially of flaps of skin considered to be in a precarious state, may provide useful evidence as to the adequacy of their blood supply and thus their prospect for survival. If the capillaries never fill, it may be wise to excise such areas rather than await the evidence of necrosis with its attendant hazards.

Irrigation

There is a constantly recurring theme in discussions of debridement, which holds that irrigation is the single most essential maneuver of the entire procedure. Indeed, this is one situation in which the adage, "if a little does some good, a lot will do a great deal more," seems generally accepted by most surgeons. Gustilo[7] has reported that a series of cases in which less than 10 l. of normal saline was used for irrigation showed a higher incidence of infection than a similar series in which more than 10 l. was used in each case. It would seem that his point is intended to emphasize the importance of thorough, or at least copious irrigation. But there are other considerations than the volume of irrigant used. Among the advantages of irrigation, the following may be listed:

1. Lavage, by flushing away blood, clears the area for inspection and thus facilitates the removal of foreign material.
2. Lavage may float otherwise undetected and often necrotic fronds of fascia, fat, or muscle into the field where they can be seen and removed.
3. Lavage may float contaminated blood clots and loose bits of tissue or debris from unseen recesses and tissue planes.
4. Lavage, by doing all these things, may help reduce the bacterial population.

Equally as important as the volume of irrigant used is the method of irrigating. Forcible streams, while they may loosen some clots and detritus, can also impact others farther into occult pockets, recesses, and tissue planes, where they can remain, undetected and dangerous residuals. On the contrary, the swirling movement of irrigating fluid gently instilled may, through its eddy currents, loosen, lift, and bring material into view. The newer jet-pulsed streams provided by a mechanical pump, if kept at low pressure, may, through their pulsations loosen and float to the surface detritus that otherwise might have remained within the wound. These devices are presently being evaluated, and some show considerable promise. Their rightful place remains to be established.

Having achieved a thorough debridement of the wound, and where possible leaving at its conclusion a bed of healthy viable tissue, a decision is now to be made as to the most appropriate method of definitive wound care.

DEFINITIVE WOUND MANAGEMENT

When attention can be safely focused upon a severely injured limb, a judgment is required at the outset: can it be salvaged or should it be amputated? When a decision to attempt salvage has been made, a debridement is required. When the debridement has been completed, two other decisions must be made: how shall the wound be further managed, and what shall be done with the fractured bone? The decision regarding definitive wound management usually permits the surgeon to choose from the following list of options:

I. Primary options for definitive wound management
  - A. Primary closure by suture
  - B. Primary closure with autogenous skin graft or flap graft
  - C. Wound left open
    1. Gauze dressings
    2. Biological dressings — homografts or heterografts

When option C is exercised, and the wound is left open, a series of secondary options must be exercised eventually.

II. Secondary options for definitive wound management
  - A. Delayed primary closure by suture
  - B. Delayed autogenous skin graft or flap graft
  - C. Secondary closure by suture or skin graft
  - D. Healing by secondary intention
  - E. Split-thickness skin graft with the intent of subsequent excision and closure by suture or with a flap graft

While the foregoing lists have included the majority of procedures that we have employed, they may at times be modified and are frequently combined for unusual situations.

PRIMARY CLOSURE

There seems little question that fractured bones in any case may heal most rapidly and effectively when they are ensheathed by infection-free, pliable, soft tissue. Thus as Brav[2] has pointed out, one of the early objectives of the treatment of the open fracture is converting it to a closed one. Clearly, healing might be expected more promptly if the wound is closed primarily by sutures —if no troubles occur. And therein lies the problem. When infection arises in the deep portions of a closed wound, it may not herald its appearance promptly, and it may be some time before the visible portion of the wound offers any indication of the presence of deep infection. During that interval, accumulating pus sealed from any exit at the surface behaves as an abscess, dissecting along tissue planes and usually around the fragments of the fractured bone. It is the specter of such an infection and its consequences that must be always in the mind of a surgeon contemplating primary closure by suture, by a primary flap, or even by a split-thickness autogenous graft which may completely seal the wound. Even in elective open reductions of closed fractures there seems to be an irreducible incidence of postoperative infection. The risk in open fractures closed primarily has been shown repeatedly to be even greater.

Still the wounds of many open fractures can be, and indeed often are, treated successfully by primary closure. What, then, are the proper circumstances, and can criteria be established that will aid in selecting those injuries in which primary closure may be expected to proceed to uneventful healing of the soft tissues? In theory at least, there is a list of criteria that ought always to be met if the surgeon decides upon primary closure.

1. All necrotic tissue and foreign material has been removed.
2. Circulation to the limb is essentially normal.
3. Nerve supply to the limb is intact.
4. The patient's general condition is satisfactory.
5. The wound can be closed without tension at its margins.
6. Closure of the wound will not create a dead space.
7. The patient does not have injuries in several systems.

Items 3, 5, 6 and 7 can be determined quite accurately. Items 2 and 4 are judgments and must be based upon assessments. Item 1 is always a speculation. While no mention is made of bacterial contamination in this list, it is assumed that there is always some residue of bacteria, even after thorough debridement and lavage.

When all seven factors have been judged favorably, the surgeon may assume that the wound has been converted to one that is free of necrotic tissue and foreign material, is comprised of viable, healthy soft tissues with a good blood supply that can deal effectively with the residual bacterial contamination. If any of the items listed is in question, in our view primary closure is countermanded. If one or more of the listed items seems to lie on a borderline, or whenever the surgeon is not quite certain, it seems wise to invoke the axiom: When in doubt, leave it open. Regarding those wounds that might qualify for closure, were it not for the hazard of tension at the suture line or the creation of a dead space, two alternatives remain: closure by split-thickness skin graft, or closure using a pedicle or flap graft.

Split Skin Grafts

Split-thickness skin grafts require support from host tissues upon which they are deposited. Pedicle- or flap grafts, since they carry their own blood supply, are not so dependent. Thus split grafts survive most predictably when placed upon host tissues that have a good, immediately available blood supply—usually muscle in fresh wounds, or granulation tissue in older ones. When split grafts are placed on tissues with a limited blood supply (periosteum, fascia, joint capsule), their prospect for survival is less certain, even without infection. Where a graft has prospect for taking promptly, it may serve as definitive closure. Or it may serve only as a temporary one, destined for later excision and closure of the wound by direct suture or replacement with a pedicle graft. When it appears that a prompt take of autogenous skin is unlikely, it is often better to leave the wound open, dressed with gauze or biological material until granulations appear that can support an autogenous split-thickness graft. Wounds that exhibit both kinds of surfaces, that is, muscle in some areas, periosteum in others, may be dealt with in stages. Autogenous split grafts may be put upon the muscle at once, while the remainder may be dressed with either gauze or biological dressings. Definitive autogenous split-thickness skin grafting of such areas may be delayed pending the appearance of granulation tissue.

Generally, relatively thin split-thickness skin grafts (0.010 to 0.012 inch) demonstrate greater survival. Random cuts placed in skin grafts to permit the escape of fluid or blood which might otherwise lift a graft from its bed seems sound, in principle. The danger seems greatest where there is a grossly uneven surface or when some degree of infection is either present or anticipated. The method of meshing the graft as described by Tanner[18] permits better contouring with less danger of surface displacement, as well as requiring considerably less skin. Though it requires a longer period of time to completely epithelialize an area covered by the extended meshed graft, it usually does occur rather evenly, because most such grafts tend to survive.

Only experience can teach which kinds of wounds and which kinds of grafts are liable to be displaced after their application and may therefore require frequent inspection. And experience also reveals to the surgeon the danger of inadvertently displacing a graft if it adheres to a dressing and is pulled away from its bed at the time the inspection is carried out. Forewarned by advice or experience, the surgeon learns to exercise care in this maneuver.

Flaps

The application of a pedicle- or flap graft to a wound immediately following debridement is in fact a form of primary closure. In theory, it too requires the retirement of the seven criteria previously listed. Should serious infection occur under such a flap or pedicled graft, there is danger not only to the wound proper but also to what may have been the only available source for such a graft. Ideally, the procedure has much to commend it. But like most ideal arrangements, its vulnerability is so great that it should be undertaken only by those surgeons who have had considerable experience with the wounds of open fractures and some experience with pedicle- or flap grafts generally. Whether the pedicle or flap is applied initially or delayed, the usual indications are a significant loss of soft tissue, especially over a bone that has a subcutaneous location. Such cover may be especially useful if some kind of surgical procedure is eventually required for a fracture located in such an area.

Closure Versus Cover

Before considering the issue of handling the wound which ought to be left open, it seems important to make a distinction between closure and cover. Closure implies sealing off the wound by sutures or by some form of graft. It assumes that nothing may enter the wound and also that nothing needs to escape from it. Cover in this context means simply to protect those tissues that cannot tolerate exposure to the atmosphere with some kind of tissue that can. Among the tissues that seem intolerant of the dessicating effect of the atmosphere are (1) bone void of its periosteum, (2) tendons void of their sheaths, (3) articulating cartilage, and to some degree, the following: (4) damaged ligaments, nerves and arteries.

Except for the subcutaneous surfaces of certain bones such as the tibia and ulna, the fragments of a reduced fracture are usually covered by their ensheathing muscles, unless there has been considerable muscle tissue loss. The bone that lies exposed through a simple gaping laceration over its surface is best covered by mobilizing surrounding muscle and remaining periosteum if there is any. If the wound is judged suitable for primary closure the problem has been resolved. But if the wound is considered unsuitable for primary closure, that portion of it that lies directly over the bone may be approximated, leaving unsutured the wound extensions, whether they were a part of the original wound or represent surgical extensions (Fig. 3-5). Such an arrangement can provide adequate drainage and yet satisfy the requirement for cover without closing the wound off.

Relaxing Incisions. A linearly disposed wound overlying a subcutaneous bone may

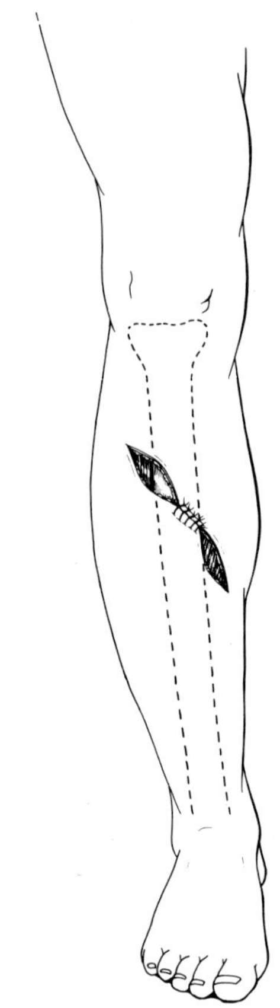

Fig. 3-5. A method of providing "cover" for an exposed medial surface of the tibial shaft while providing for drainage at either end of the wound. It is not suitable if very much skin has been lost, because tension may induce marginal necrosis of the distal edge at the sutured area.

pose a problem when closure which is sufficient to provide adequate cover also creates excessive tension at the suture line. In this circumstance relaxing incisions may be useful, both to relieve the tension on the suture line and to provide drainage from the fracture area proper (Fig. 3-6). However, care must be exercised in using such incisions, for they must be long enough to permit the desired effect of approximating the edges of the primary wound without tension and must therefore be at least as long as the wound itself. They should also be placed so that a natural plane leads from the relaxing incision into the fracture area if it is expected to facilitate drainage. Yet it must not be so close to the initial wound that it impairs the blood supply to the skin and underlying tissues located between the relaxing incision and the wound itself. This point is especially important, because the bridge of tissue created thereby is intended to be shifted toward the initial wound, and that may require undermining the bridge. Two points are to be borne in mind: first, rearrangement is hazardous if too large an area of tissue loss about the initial wound must be replaced; second, where such a problem exists, a rotational flap may be more suitable.

Finally, relaxing incisions are more suited to those areas in which there is some natural mobility of the skin and underlying tissue, such as the thigh and the proximal leg, but less so where mobility is limited, as in the lower leg and ankle region or about the wrist.

Muscle Transpositions. Ger[5] has described a considerable variety of muscle belly transpositions that may be used where the loss of skin and subcutaneous tissue is extensive and when suitable cover by the skin and subcutaneous tissues cannot be arranged. They are especially well suited for the leg, where the problem occurs most frequently. The soleus or deep flexor muscles are used most often, although other muscles whose vascular supply is suitably disposed may be utilized. The reader is referred to Ger's writings for a more extensive consideration of this technique, or to a standard anatomy text in an emergency.

Biological Dressings. While some similar mobilization of tissues is occasionaly required about a joint, or where tendons have been stripped of their sheaths, they usually overlie areas that have no easily available muscle or other tissue from which cover may be produced. They may be covered best with a biological dressing (homologous or heterologous skin). Such dressings should be changed frequently under aseptic

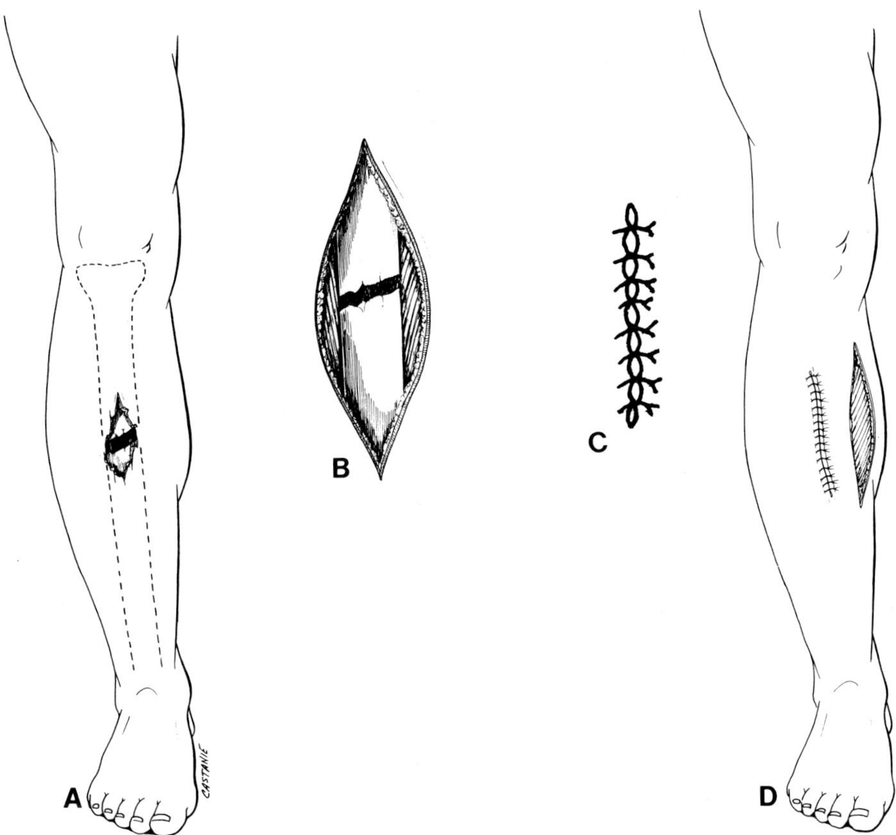

Fig. 3-6. (*A*) A rather significant loss of tissue directly over the crest of the tibia. (*B*) The degree of tissue loss after debridement. (*C*) The excessive tension at the wound margins which results when direct suture closure is attempted. (*D*) The principle of the relaxing incision. Care must be exercised to avoid making the interval bridge of skin (essentially a bi-pedicled flap graft) too narrow. The primary wound can now be closed for cover without tension at the suture line. The relaxing incision can communicate with the fracture in the interest of drainage.

conditions. Often, a skin dressing, by keeping the tendon in a tissue fluid environment, permits it to survive until enough granulations appear to support a definitive, autogenous graft, or until a pedicle or flap graft can be put down, if that alternative is considered more suitable. Of course, where cover can be provided by mobilizing adjacent muscle or periosteum, none of the aforementioned measures will be required. There remains, then, only the matter of the initial dressing for the wound that is to be left open.

LEAVING WOUNDS OPEN

There is a strong tendency for surgeons to put drains into wounds that have been left open, for whatever reasons. For draining an established abscess or tissue spaces that tend naturally to reseal themselves (e.g., the palmar space, subgluteal space) the reasons for and usefulness of such drains is acknowledged. However, mechanical drains of the usual variety, such as the Penrose, may by their presence irritate the tissues they contact and incite an innocent exudate. The trouble lies in the surgeon's uncertainty that such an exudate is in fact innocent. For major soft-tissue wounds that are to be left open after debridement, gauze dressings inserted to a point just beneath the fascia are sufficient, since it is the fascia and skin that usually create the most resistant barrier to the escape of accumulated purulent material. Therefore, the dressing ought to keep the fascial and skin edges separated. Such wounds should not be packed open, because such packing tends often to produce an obturator effect and thus retains the material that it seeks to release. Loosely arranged dressings may conduct small amounts of exudate or transudate by capillary action and simply guide larger volumes to the exterior. Unlike slippery drainage material, they usually remain where they are placed initially. When there is no drainage apart from the initial wound bleeding, the blood soaks into the dressing, coagulates, and may dry to a remarkable degree, leaving the dressing as a firm, rust-colored "blood shingle."

Should local symptoms of pain, odor, or obviously excessive drainage appear early on, or should more general signs of fever, leukocytosis, and so on be noted, early inspection is warranted. If the wound is indeed infected the dressing is usually at least wet if not saturated with identifiable purulence.

If there has been no indication for an early investigation of the wound, it is usually inspected between the fourth and sixth days. If the dressings are found to be wet, the wound is probably in some difficulty. The difficulty may be infection of varying degrees or simply remnants of necrotic tissue not removed at the time of the initial debridement. In either event, the wound is still unsuitable for any kind of closure. Cultures should be taken, obvious residual necrotic material should be removed, and inspection and exploration sufficient to confirm the adequacy of drainage should be carried out. The wound is then redressed until a future inspection. If there is strong evidence that infection is present, antibiotic treatment should be initiated. If there is no available information to identify the responsible organism, a broad-spectrum agent should be selected until cultures have established both the organism and its specific drug sensitivities.

Choosing 4 to 6 days as the appropriate time for removal of the first dressing is not entirely arbitrary. It is intended that the wound be inspected before granulation tissues make their appearance, for at that time the wound characteristics change. Granulating wounds tend to remain moist, owing, in part, to the normal transudate of granulating tissue. Moreover, they quickly evolve a surface flora of bacteria. Finally, as the granulations advance, the natural planes between tissues are sealed, thereby reducing tissue pliability.

If at early inspection a wound dressing is dry, even crusted to the quasi-solid "blood shingle," the wound generally has the healthy appearance of viable and vital tissues. At this point the surgeon must consider the second set of options:

1. Delayed primary closure by suture
2. Delayed primary closure by split-thickness skin graft, pedicle graft, or flap graft
3. Continuing to dress the wound open

DELAYED PRIMARY CLOSURE

For the most part, a wound left open initially can still be closed by procedures 1 or 2 at any time before granulation tissues appear. If edema has been controlled, the tissues are usually as pliable and as easily manipulated for suturing as at the initial debridement, perhaps even more so. Moreover, there is the further advantage that infection is less likely to emerge, since the wound has given evidence of its initial innocence. Similarly, if the wound is not suited to delayed primary closure because of tension at the suture line or the creation of a dead space, split-thickness, autogenous skin grafting can be carried out. Evidently clean wounds of this kind, free of residual necrotic material, are most receptive beds for autogenous skin grafts, since the early promise of granulation tissue creates an optimum circumstance for graft survival.

Although 4 to 6 days has been identified as the usual time for inspection, it should be noted that the aim is to inspect the wound and carry out the definitive procedure just prior to the emergence of granulation tissue. Since granulations may appear earlier in a child, a shorter period may be chosen. Contrarily, in some debilitated or elderly patients granulation tissue appears much later, and it may be wiser to defer the definitive delayed primary closure or split graft cover until 8 or 10 days have passed. Experience with these techniques eventually facilitates the surgeon's accuracy.

If the wound is left open after the first dressing, for whatever reason, it will eventually granulate. When that occurs the surgeon may again choose from the remaining options (although closure by any method at this time is viewed as secondary closure:

1. Secondary closure by suture
2. Secondary closure by split-thickness skin graft, pedicle graft, or flap graft
3. Continuing dressings and allowing the wound to close by secondary intention

SECONDARY CLOSURE

Secondary closure by suture may be more troublesome technically than either primary or delayed primary closure, since tissue pliability at that time is usually decreased. Good approximation may be difficult to achieve, if indeed it is even desirable. Granulation tissue surface transudate permits a kind of seroma to fill unevenly approximated wound surfaces. An avenue for their escape may be useful in facilitating wound healing.

Secondary split-thickness skin grafts usually take quite promptly on healthy granulation tissue. When the bed is uneven or some residual infection is demonstrated or suspected, the Tanner[18] meshed graft may again be more easily managed and produce a better take than solid sheets of skin. The perforations in the mesh permit the escape of surface drainage and minimize graft displacement by fluid collections beneath them. If granulations appear irregularly in some areas of the wound, that which is ready may be grafted while those areas not yet ready are left to improve their granulations. Flap grafts or pedicle grafts may also be put down on granulation tissue surfaces, although the same problems of accumulating fluid and minor degrees of infection, plus the loss of wound margin tissue mobility may offer some technical problems. If the wound is relatively small and located in an area of relative tissue abundance and natural mobility, the entire wound may be excised, granulations and all, and the new wound then closed by primary suture. That procedure is usually precluded for wounds about the wrist, hand, ankle, and foot (i.e., regions where primary closure by suture may produce too much tension on the wound margins).

There is much to be said in favor of option 3—continuing dressings and allowing the wound to close by secondary intention. Too often our judgments about wounds allowed to heal by secondary intention have been gained from inspecting wounds allowed to heal that way *because* they were in trouble, and the trouble was usually significant or serious infection. Or, they were the aftermath of inappropriate wound management, such as circular coring. Often such wounds have resulted in extensive cicatrix, puckering, and retraction. Few wounds that were properly debrided and showed no excess tissue loss and presented no evidence of infection have escaped either delayed primary or secondary closure by suture or grafts. Yet those accidents of omission, observed by many, frequently demonstrate the surprising ability of tissues to close large gaps spontaneously and produce a remarkably small scar. Where the laceration lies along natural skin lines of cleavage, the scar may be no greater than in lacerations closed by suture. The principal disadvantage of healing by secondary intention, if it can be called that, is the additional time required to achieve it. However, such wounds are rarely the prey of bacteria, which may invade them. On the contrary, they often seem able to handle such invasions much better for having been left open.

Dehne[4] and Brown,[3] have emphasized the facility with which open wounds may heal themselves quite satisfactorily by secondary intention, even as Trueta[12] so clearly demonstrated in the Spanish Civil War. And he without benefit of antibiotics.

BIOLOGICAL DRESSINGS

In those circumstances in which closure is not appropriate or cannot be carried out, and arrangements cannot be made for the covering of vulnerable tissues by the transposition of local tissues, biological dressings of skin are often of considerable value. Either homologous human skin harvested from cadavers, or heterologous porcine skin, which is prepared commercially and generally available will suffice. Such dressings are especially useful when wounds are not yet ready for delayed primary closure or graft and must be delayed beyond the appearance of granulation tissue. Baxter[1] has shown that such dressings have several advantages in the treatment of burned patients. Changing dressings is considerably less painful. They seem to be a deterrent to the development of infection, and there is some evidence that existing infection may be suppressed or controlled. Since host granulation tissue invades such grafts, allowing them to take for varying periods before an immune response later rejects them, biological dressings can give evidence of the readiness of a wound bed for definitive autogenous grafting. Because of this latter feature, such grafts should be changed frequently, for Salisbury[14] has shown that when granulation tissue from an autogenous graft donor site grows into an heterologous dressing, even though it be pulled away before any significant clinical take occurs, there remain in the host granulation tissue small bits of collagen from the "heterologous dressing tissue." This remnant collagen apparently tends to incite a rather chronic inflammatory response leading to some delay in epithelialization and an increase in cicatrix. The reader is referred to current literature on this rapidly advancing field.

ELEVATION

Perhaps there is no more critical point in the control of post-debridement swelling than the simple matter of elevation. Swelling that is aggravated or allowed to persist unnecessarily may keep tissues turgid and wound surfaces moist, and thereby prevent delayed primary closure, since edematous tissues tend to enhance tension at the suture line. Its other disadvantages include the enhancement of the prospect of infection, a loss of reduction of fractures, should swelling require a cast to be split and spread, and probably the hazard of thrombophlebitis.

While some swelling is inevitable in tissue injury, unnecessary additional swelling due to dependency cannot be tolerated.

Virtually every injured limb can be effectively and comfortably elevated. Such elevation should, moreover, be continuous. The usual method of propping up limbs in casts or splints is hazardous. They may fall off the prop (usually a stack of pillows) or be lifted off by the patient, especially during sleep. Limbs suspended from overhead frames by slings of muslin or even rope supports do not fall and are not easily removed from such suspension.

To realize its best effect elevation must

bring the suspended part above the heart and it must be continuous, at least until the initial swelling begins to subside. Yet some care is necessary in even so innocuous a measure as this. Older persons who have significant arterial disease may not tolerate elevation. In too high a position, blood may not be delivered to the elevated distal parts. They may even complain of the pain of ischemia. For such persons a more moderate degree of elevation must be arranged.

ANTIBIOTICS AND OPEN FRACTURES

At the outset it may be said that antibiotics cannot be given prophylactically for the average open fracture, since only rarely will a patient incurring an open fracture be taking an appropriate antibiotic at the time the injury is incurred. Thus antibiotic treatment cannot begin until after the injury. The debate then has evolved about two points: should antibiotics be used at all?, and if they are to be used, when should they be initiated? A secondary question arises regarding whether or not the antibiotics ought to be applied topically or given systemically, or both.

It should be said also at the outset (and it is worthy of frequent repetition) that antibiotics—by whatever method they are administered—cannot replace the fundamental measures of wound debridement and appropriate definitive wound care.

The author cannot speak authoritatively on the use of topical antibiotics. Yet it is doubtful that their use in the course of debridement affords any degree of protection, since the frequent and copious lavage which is urged as a regular part of debridement tends to dilute or sweep away any remnant of the agent that might be in the field. And it is generally considered that some quantum of time must be allowed for contact between the organisms and an antibiotic present in suitable concentration before any effect might reasonably be expected. Thus, when a surgeon anticipates dealing promptly with an open fracture, there probably is no merit in introducing topical antibiotics into the wound until it is prepped and debrided. If, on the other hand, mass casualties dictate that the treatment of wounds in some patients must be put off for an indefinite period of time, there may be merit in attempting to control the proliferation of bacteria within the necrotic tissue lying in such wounds. The reader is referred to the studies of Waterman[20] and Glotzer[6] for background of such considerations.

The issue of parenterally administered antibiotics seems now to have some better definition, although few studies have been carried out on a prospective bases. Moreover, the real value of antibiotics may be difficult to evaluate, since there is such a wide variety of open fracture patterns that no two seem alike. Thus fairly large numbers of cases are required to establish reliable data. Often treatment of associated injuries to other systems includes the use of antibiotics, though the agent selected may not be most suitable to the needs of the open fracture.

Theoretically, any antibiotic administered early in the treatment of an open fracture should have at least these characteristics: It should be bacteriocidal. It should be a broad-spectrum agent, active against both gram-positive and gram-negative organisms. It should be capable of producing suitable concentrations in blood, the extracellular fluids, and joint fluids. It should be given immediately when the patient is seen and prior to any surgical treatment. It should be as hypoallergenic as possible and be compatible with other antibiotics.

Our experience with 517 open fractures, of which 219 received some kind of antibiotic at some time after debridement, revealed that 18.9 per cent of those patients receiving antibiotics developed some degree of wound infection, while only 9.4 per cent of those *not* receiving antibiotics developed any significant infection. The lack of control invalidates any reliable conclusion, because it was also noted in the review that antibiotics were generally given to those patients who had the more severe open fractures and/or multiple injuries. The data may be used negatively, however, to point out that antibiotics used in this way cannot be relied upon to provide any protection against infection.

It has remained for Patzakis, Harvey, and Ivler[12] to present a controlled prospective study of antibiotic treatment used in conjunction with open fractures. Their data strongly support several useful points. First, a culture taken from the wound prior to any treatment is most likely to yield the organisms that will subsequently cause infection, although a given infection can occur in wounds where culture for that microbe was negative. Second, the commonest organism producing infection was a staphylococcus aureus (cultured from 11 of 22 wound infections), and most of these were penicillin-resistant. Third, the wound most susceptible to infection is the close-range shotgun wound. This is no surprise, because this wound regularly impels hard-to-locate organic, foreign material (wadding) into the wound, and it is difficult to determine on the initial debridement that all necrotic tissue has been removed.[10]

Patzakis and his associates concluded from their study that at that time Cephalothin was the most reliable of the antibiotics to be used in the initial treatment of the open fracture. Not only was it effective against coagulase-positive staphylococcus, it was also effective against some gram-negative organisms as well. Patients treated by the immediate administration of Cephalothin *and* adequate debridement had a far lower infection rate (2.3 per cent) than those in which a combination of penicillin-streptomycin was used which yielded an infection rate of 9.7 per cent. Where no antibiotic was employed the infection rate was recorded at 13.9 per cent.

It would appear from the work of Patzakis *et al.* that the use of Cephalothin as a part of the initial regimen in the management of open fractures has merit. Since they recorded the emergence of coagulase-positive staphylococcus aureus as a frequent offender, it would appear that those patients who also have multiple systems injuries, and may be receiving antibiotics to prevent infections in other systems from other organisms, receive in addition some agent specifically effective against penicillin-resistant staphylococcus.

Additional studies will likely clarify this issue and refine it in the future. But for the present it is essential to reiterate that antibiotics are not to be used in lieu of proper debridement and definitive wound care. They must remain, as always, an adjunct to the principle.

MANAGEMENT OF THE FRACTURE

Virtually all the methods presently employed in the management of closed fractures can be applied within certain limits to open fractures as well. However, in the open fracture, management of the bone fragments cannot logically be considered apart from the soft-tissue wound. If the wound is minor it is usually not much of a problem, but when the soft-tissue injury is extensive, often including significant loss of skin and ensheathing muscle, it may make management of the fracture most formidable. Thus what might be done with the fractured bone *per se* must often yield to what serves the best interest of the soft tissues—at least at the time of initial treatment. Whatever method of fracture treatment is chosen, it should fulfill certain criteria. Among them are the following:

1. The method should not compromise further the injured soft tissues.
2. The method should maintain length of the bone, especially in the lower extremity.
3. The method ought to produce alignment for the fragments but especially alignment of joints.

As in the treatment of closed fractures, no one technique seems clearly superior to any other, in *all* cases. Yet for the surgeon who deals with these problems only occasionally, or on a temporary basis, the simpler the method, the better. Such a policy usually creates fewer problems for the first surgeon, and provides greater latitude for definitive treatment by the last surgeon. However, the surgeon who treats such patients regularly should be aware of and consider all the usual range of available techniques and even combine them or, when indicated, improvise. A useful list of the usual methods for managing the bone fragments in open fractures follows:

1. Simple immobilization in cast or splint
2. Manipulation of fragments and the application of a cast or splint.
3. Transfixing bone pins incorporated in plaster
4. Walking casts and cast braces
5. Splint and/or traction
6. External skeletal fixation
7. Internal skeletal fixation

Some open fractures seem to be only technically "open." A small, almost unnoticeable wound may be associated with a minor fracture line in the underlying bone, whose fragments show no displacement on roentgenograms. Yet they are indeed open fractures. Such injuries are seductive in their appearance, and treacherous. The danger of serious, often fatal, infection proceeding from this circumstance has already been mentioned. The wound should receive the same consideration as any open fracture. The fracture as such may simply be splinted by a plaster slab or cast. When the wound has healed, a definitive cast may be applied until the fracture is sufficiently united.

Frequently larger wounds or those extended in the course of debridement and associated with displaced bone fragments, permit reduction under direct visualization. Yet such visualization is not always all that might be desired, for wounds, unlike incisions made for the purpose of exposure, are often neither appropriately located nor sufficiently extensive. At other times, of course, wounds are so large that the surgeon is distressed by how much of the fractured bone is so readily visible.

Immobilization in Plaster

For wounds of moderate dimensions and one in which a manipulative reduction of the fracture fragments to a stable acceptable position can be achieved, and where reasonable soft-tissue cover of the bone fragment results, a plaster-of-paris cast for immobilization is as appropriate here as for a closed fracture of similar pattern. And as with the latter, the cast should incorporate the joint above and below the fracture site. Depending somewhat upon the definitive management selected for the wound, it may be desirable or necessary to subsequently inspect that area. Such inspection is usually achieved by cutting a window in the cast. But there are sometimes technical difficulties with this simple procedure which can, with a little care, be circumvented. Creating a window for removing a dressing and inspecting a wound serves best when made directly over the wound, and it should be at least as large as the wound. Often the window is cut askew from the desired location, making the removal of dressings, inspection, or removal of sutures and redressing the wound difficult, or at least unsatisfactory. The alternative of enlarging the window to correct for the error only weakens the cast more. There are a few points that may simplify this procedure.

Upon completion of the debridement and at the time of wound dressing it is useful to add some more layers of gauze laid directly over the full extent of the wound. When a well-molded thin plaster cast is then applied, it will reveal a bulge on its external surface. A further check by measuring the location of the wound between adjacent joints, and noting its surface location at the same time, permits the surgeon to detect its location on the finished cast. An indelible marking pencil will effectively outline the area and signify the location for appropriate saw cuts when the window is finally to be made. Because the surgeon who must make the window may be someone other than he who applied the cast, these precautions may be invaluable. For that reason too, some additional information may be recorded indelibly on the cast and might include the date of injury, how the wound was left, the bones involved, and, if the surgeon has an artistic inclination, a drawing of the fragments and how they were disposed at the conclusion of the initial treatment. Since the cast is virtually always to be found with the patient, while his own medical record and roentgenograms may not be, these brief notations are often a great help.

After the window has been removed and whatever services the wound requires have been performed, there remains the matter of closing the aperture. If the limb is at all swollen, especially when the window was made on the posterior (dependent) surface of a limb, herniation of soft tissues followed in turn by constriction at the margins, aggravates the swelling and may create a serious, secondary problem. Clearly the plaster obturator should be reinserted. To avoid compression by its edge if it happened to be set into the fenestration unevenly, a layer of felt cut in the same shape and introduced atop the dressing before the plaster obturator is reinserted is helpful. When the window overlies some nondependent area the problem is less likely, unless that area of the limb is significantly swollen. Whether the obturator should be replaced permanently with additional plaster depends upon what was found at inspection and therefore what is planned for the wound. If reentry is anticipated, encircling turns of adhesive tape may be sufficient to hold the obturator in place. If reentry to the area is not anticipated, or when it appears the window may have weakened the cast significantly, it is wiser to secure the obturator and reinforce the cast with additional plaster.

Cutting windows in a cast may be scheduled or unscheduled. It may be the surgeon's plan to simply inspect the progress of a wound which has been closed primarily by suture or split-thickness skin graft, or to carry out a delayed primary closure. In the latter instance it is imperative that the exposure be adequate, and therefore the window must be placed accurately over the wound. Unscheduled entry is usually made in response to some indication that a wound is in difficulty. Local pain, distal swelling, odor, or evidence of unanticipated drainage, together with some general signals such as fever which cannot be explained otherwise are the more common ones. Ease of access for thorough inspection is no less critical here, because a serious judgment often has to be made. Where there are signs of trouble, we may again invoke the axiom: To look is to know; not to look is to guess.

Pins and Plaster

Not infrequently the bone fragments in open fractures, as in closed ones, cannot be manipulated into a stable position and tend to override, producing more shortening than is considered acceptable. When this circumstance occurs in the leg or forearm, the use of pins incorporated into a plaster cast may provide a suitable answer. Such casts can be windowed as easily as any other, though pin placement may occasionally interfere with or require some minor modification in placing windows. Moreover these casts may also be wedged, if that is required.

It should be remembered that a single pin placed in a bone fragment may prevent the fragment from moving along or about its own long axis, but the fragment can always move around the long axis of the pin itself. Thus, a single pin in a short proximal tibial fragment may control shortening and rotational deformity, but the pull of quadriceps can rotate the fragment around the long axis of the pin, allowing angular deformity to occur at the fracture site. This may be especially troublesome if the proximal tibial pin is utilized to effect traction for a fractured femoral shaft. Therefore, it is usually wise to place two pins in a proximal tibial fragment, while one may be sufficient for the distal fragment. Generally speaking, the same point applies for segmental fractures of the tibia or those fractures that show extensive comminution in the middle third of the shaft.

The problem of placing two pins close together in a very short proximal fragment, so that a firm grip can be taken on them by the plaster, may be solved by simply inserting the pins at diverging planes (Fig. 3-7). The pins are able to grasp the fragment effectively and satisfactorily prevent rotation.

Fractures in the radius and ulna pose a greater problem in locating appropriate points for pin placement. The distal end of the radius has its surface cluttered with essential tendons and sheaths, while its proximal end is hardly accessible at all. Because the interosseus membrane is sensitive to any intrusion, pins that transfix both bones in the region of that structure should be avoided. A pin may be passed through the olecranon area of the ulna (two pins if the proximal ulnar fragment is a short one), while a distal pin may be passed through the second or second and third metacarpals. After manipulative reduction has been carried out, a long-arm cast is applied, incorporating the two or three pins. While anatomical reductions are not easily achieved by this technique, at least length and often general linear alignment requirements can be satisfied until some other means of treatment or reconstruction can be applied.

As with any method of treatment there are certain technical points that must be acknowledged and fulfilled. In selecting a pin to be incorporated in plaster, it is to be remembered that the pin will have no linear tension applied to it to contribute to its rigidity. It must therefore have sufficient intrinsic rigidity to avoid bending (a complication illustrated in Fig. 3-8), which would effectively destroy the usefulness of the system and the objective it was designed to achieve. In the more heavily muscled leg this point is even more critical.

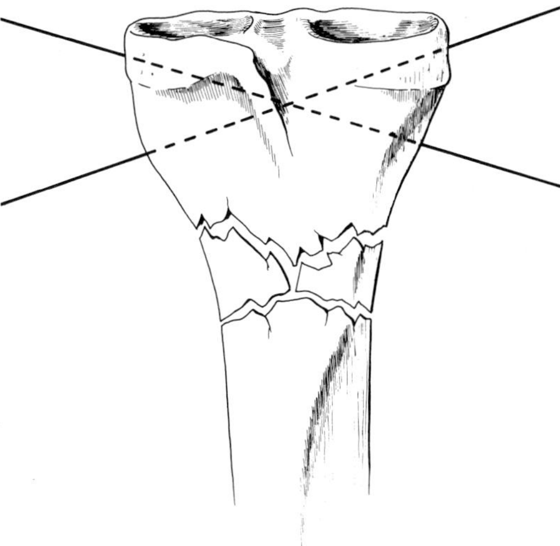

Fig. 3-7. A technique for introducing "two" pins across a short proximal tibial fragment for immobilization by incorporation in plaster. If traction must be applied through these pins, one of them should be in the coronal plane and the other, inclined at an angle to it.

Some fractures when reduced are quasi-stable, yet are so precariously arranged that reduction is apt to be lost during the application of a plaster cast. If the drifting fragments of the unreduced fracture are liable to compromise the soft-tissue injury, they had better be stabilized in some way, often by effectively used pins incorporated in plaster.

There is one such pattern that may permit the use of a transfixing pin and the application of a simple plaster cast. Mumford has pointed out that some mildly oblique fractures present a spike of cortex at one end that can be invaginated into the medullary canal of its opposing fragment. But the invagination is a short one, and it should be in order to minimize loss of length. It is therefore precarious. Such reductions may seem quite stable so long as

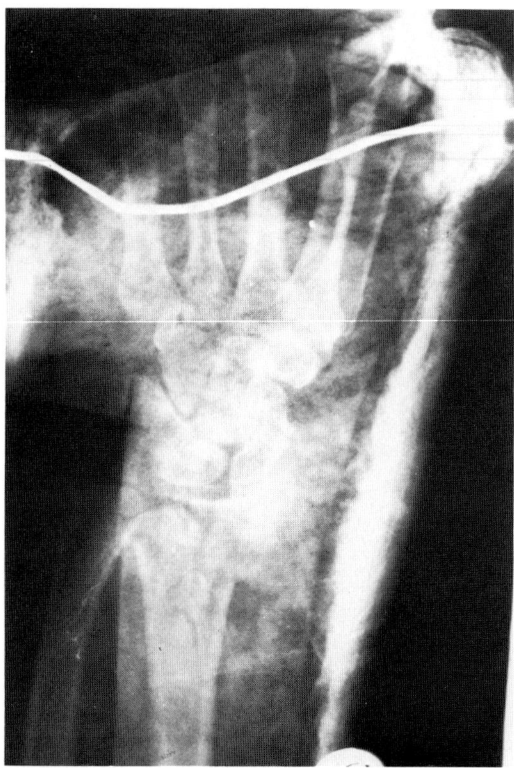

Fig. 3-8. The deflection of the pin placed in the metacarpals and incorporated in a plaster cast illustrates the need to utilize a pin sufficiently rigid to resist the pull of muscles attached to impaled fragments. In this example the reduction was lost owing to failure of the pin.

the parts are held in apposition, but reduction is likely to be lost during the application of the cast. If a transfixing pin is passed across both fragments assuring their position until the cast has been applied and is set, the reduction usually remains stable thereafter (Fig. 3-9). When the cast is set the pin may be withdrawn; but a note of caution: a smooth pin should be used. Its removal by simple half-turns sequentially in opposite directions permits the pin to emerge with little difficulty. A threaded pin, which must be turned continuously in a counterclockwise direction may ensnare itself in dressings and cast padding, disturbing them and making its recovery most troublesome. Withal, the stability of such a reduction often tolerates even the force of weight bearing without being disturbed.

Weight-Bearing Casts

For those fractures in the lower extremity that are sufficiently stable, the beneficial effect of continual compression forces upon the fracture produced by early weight bearing has been emphasized by Dehne[4] and reemphasized by Brown,[3] in the case of open fractures, and strongly emphasized by Sarmiento[15] in the case of closed ones. There are a few problems in the use of this method in either open or closed fractures, and a few points are not always made clear. First, unless a fracture is anatomically reduced and so maintained, some shortening is likely to ensue, regardless of the form of treatment employed. This is especially true if good compressive contact between adjacent fragments is to be regularly achieved. It is true that very little "additional" shortening is noted when this form of treatment is carried out properly. Certainly the shortening is generally not enough to disqualify the technique. Additionally in the open fracture the presence of a wound, especially a wound that is left open, tends to disturb total contact support and the effect imparted by the integrity of the various, quasi-fluid compartments with their supporting or splinting effect upon bone fragments. For this reason, application of the weight-bearing cast is sometimes delayed beyond the 10- to 14-day point generally advocated. When wounds can be appropriately and effectively closed before weight bearing is begun, one issue is resolved. If the wound is left open, arrangements for a window can be made, of course, yet this has the dual drawback of interrupting an area of surface contact useful to support and also of weakening the cast. Yet for many years it has been noted that wounds debrided properly may heal as well left undisturbed. Henry's[8] pungent observation —"Wounds may stink their way to health in plaster"—is clearly underscored by the

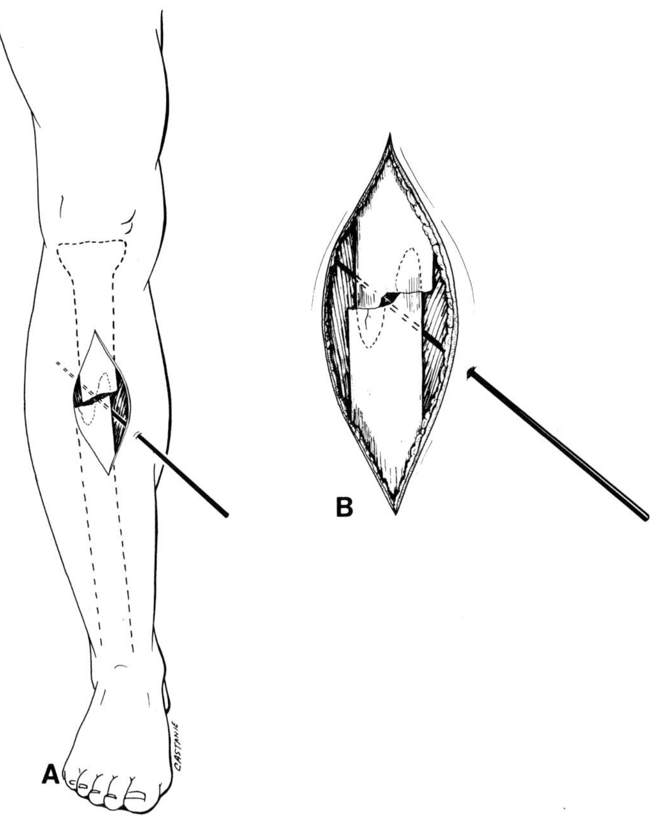

Fig. 3-9. (*A*) The general alignment that can be achieved by a temporary transfixing pin and (*B*) the features of reciprocal cortical invagination subsequently stabilized. When the plaster has set, the pin may be removed by the technique outlined in the text.

vast experience of Orr and his contemporaries in the treatment of chronic bone infection, but more so by the circumscribed, yet extensive experience of Trueta[19] in that method of management for fresh injuries in the Spanish Civil War. It was reemphasized by Brown and Urban[3] in the more recent Vietnam conflict. In all instances, principles of initial wound care were first served by the surgeon, after which the principles of wound healing served both the patient and his surgeon. The techniques are precise, and their successful application demands careful attention to details.

Consideration of the application of weight-bearing casts for treatment of open fractures after a wound has been skin grafted requires a note of caution. No matter that a cast has been skillfully fitted, some telescoping of the fragments occurs in any ununited fracture subjected to weight bearing. Such telescoping produces some friction between the skin and cast surfaces. Since not much padding is applied under such casts so that full firm contact with the limb surfaces may be realized, these same attritional forces act upon the skin or a skin graft.

Split-thickness skin grafts generally have two characteristics that may be detrimental to success. First, they are insensitive. Second, they have little mobility on their new bed, even if they are applied directly upon muscle. Where split-thickness grafts are applied over bone there is virtually no mobility. The hazard to the graft of course is the danger that attrition may bruise and blister it, which, because it is insensitive, may provide no notice that it is being disturbed. Irretrievable damage can occur before the trouble is discovered. The whole course of treatment of the injured limb may then be set back by the need to attend this complication.

What has been said of weight-bearing casts applies largely to injuries of the tibia and fibula, yet they apply also to the use of cast braces for fractures about the proximal tibia and distal half of the femur. Our experience has led us to treat these latter fractures by traction and splinting until 6 to 8 weeks, when some degree of intrinsic stability is manifest. When the limb is put into a cast brace at that time fewer troubles accrue. Moreover, in the case of open fractures, more time is allowed to achieve a well-healed wound which will require less attention when the cast brace is applied and produce fewer problems in and of itself. Where soft-tissue wounds are present about the knee, swelling in that area (always a problem in the employment of a cast brace) may be aggravated and in some instances may make the cast brace impractical if not impossible. The clear advantages in fracture healing which have been demonstrated for the weight-bearing cast techniques need not be denied the patient simply because he has an open fracture. The presence of soft-tissue wounds simply requires special attention, yet in many cases the wound is entirely compatible with the method. Indeed, some wounds may even progress more rapidly because of its use.

Skeletal Traction and Suspension

External splinting, with and without traction, is the most universal form of treatment in the initial and earlier phases of fracture management, whether the fracture is closed or open. Moreover, it may readily be continued as a definitive form of treatment in many of them. Indeed, certain open fractures may be managed better by one of these techniques than any other, because of associated soft-tissue wounds.

Conventional splints are generally more useful in the lower extremity, especially for the fractured femur, when they are combined with skeletal traction. The Thomas splint with Pearson leg attachment is the prototype. Not to be overlooked for certain fractures in the tibia is the Böhler-Braun frame, which also allows the application of skeletal traction. When such splints are properly constructed and applied, only the posterior surface of the limb is obscured from view by contact with the splint: the medial, lateral, and anterior surfaces are immediately available so that wounds involving only these surfaces can be easily attended when necessary. However, when wounds lie upon the posterior surface, especially in the upper half of the thigh, their status is difficult to determine, because inspection is often disturbingly painful to the patient, and at best the wound is poorly visualized. There are some useful alternatives for dealing with these and other similar problems.

If the surface wounds in the open fracture are extensive (circumferential), have loss of tissue along the posterior surface, or are burned, suspension without a splint can often be effectively arranged. There are two general techniques.

If a troublesome wound lies on the proximal and posterior aspect of the thigh and/or buttock, the limb may be comfortably suspended and the fracture effectively reduced by the so-called 90-90 attitude. That consists of suspending the lower limb so that the hip and knee are both flexed to 90 degrees, with 20 to 30 degrees of external rotation. It is achieved by passing a heavy Steinmann pin through the femur in the area immediately proximal to the femoral condyles. The femur is thus slung vertically from overhead (Fig. 3-10). Notice should be taken of the usefulness of a diversionary colostomy and urinary catheter for wounds extending into the perineal and rectal areas. The combination of these two methods of treatment markedly facilitates the care of such wounds. While this attitude of right-angle knee flexion is tolerated indefinitely by children under 12 years, it may become troublesome in the older patient and especially in adults. The continuous patellofemoral compression may make that

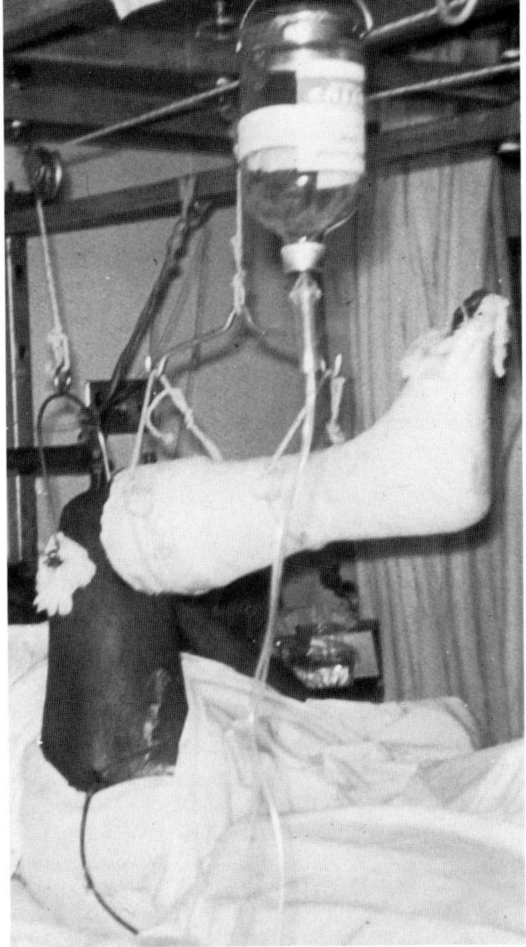

Fig. 3-10. Simple vertical traction on the femur (90°-90°, hip and knee) makes wounds located high on the posterior thigh or the buttock easier to attend. It must not be carried on longer than necessary in the adult because of its effect upon the patellofemoral joint.

joint painful, and postimmobilization stiffness can be a serious sequela. Thus, for the adult, the 90-90 position should be relieved as soon as the posterior wounds allow. If it is planned to treat the femur fracture definitively by traction, a Thomas splint may then be added and the knee and hip flexion reduced to something under 45 degrees. Once the fracture becomes stable, the limb may be easily and painlessly elevated for further inspection and additional management of the posterior wounds.

Restoration of a normal bowel pathway by closing the colostomy should await complete healing of perianal or perineal wounds, unless some problem arising from the colostomy itself should require its restoration at an earlier time.

Alternatively, a limb with a posterior wound, for example one rendered insensitive distal to the level of transection of the sciatic nerve, may be suspended as illustrated in (Fig. 3-11). In this example the

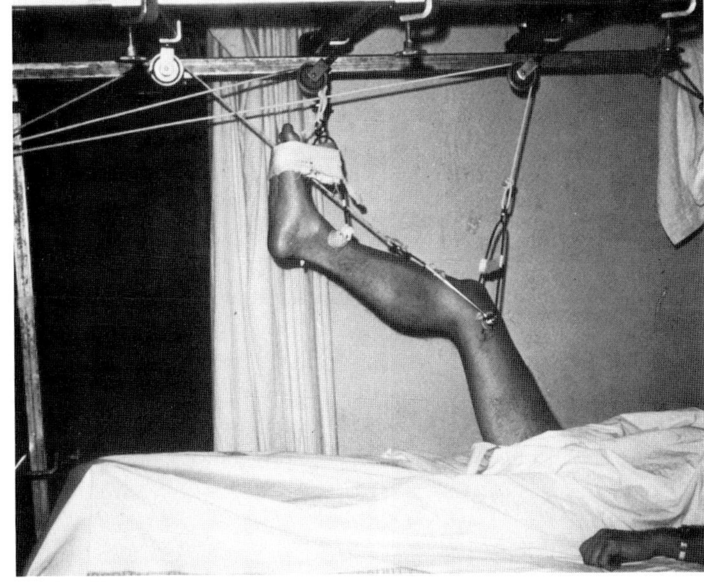

Fig. 3-11. Skeletal suspension of this kind can be rigged for insensitive limbs or those with extensive surface injury or burns. The combinations for such suspension are limitless, and the various necessary vectors of tension to achieve reduction of the fracture can be contrived to deal with most fracture patterns. This patient had a comminuted fracture of the femur and transection of his sciatic nerve.

usual posterior support of the leg in a Pearson attachment had resulted in an early pressure sore over the heel. The lesion was found during a routine daily inspection of the area (always essential in insensitive limbs); the patient was unaware of any difficulty there.

Other suspension arrangements designed to suit the needs of wounds and fractures may easily be arranged, but each should subserve the principles which have been identified and be mindful of the potential complications. Prominent among the latter are troubles with pins themselves.

Some care in the selection and placement of pins is imperative. The principal points may be listed as follows:

1. The pin should be large enough so that it will not deflect when put under stress during suspension.
2. The pin should be large enough so that it will not migrate due to traction tension, if placed in cancellous bone.
3. Large pins should be of the self-cutting type (diamond-shaped tip rather than trochar-shaped tip), and should be turned through the bone slowly enough to minimize heat generation.
4. Once the tip of a smooth pin has emerged from the outer surface of the far cortex, it should be driven by a mallet, rather than turned, to its final position to avoid soft-tissue damage by winding around the revolving pin.
5. The pin should be introduced across the skin through cruciate incisions (at both entrance and exit sites) to minimize skin tension.
6. Care must be exercised in making corrections for the shift in relationships between the point of entry across the skin and that in the underlying bone which will occur when the limb is placed in its definitive attitude and the overriding of fracture fragments is corrected as limb length is restored. The consequence is undue pin tension on skin, almost certain to create trouble. The problem may be circumvented by placing the limb in the intended definitive position when the pins are inserted, while as much length as possible is restored manually.

While these few points may not eliminate all pin problems, they serve to minimize them. Once a pin is in trouble, it can compromise the whole plan for treatment, if the plan is predicated on its continued use.

Skeletal traction in the upper extremity is usually necessary only for injuries that involve the arm or shoulder. As a rule the 90-90 attitude is tolerated easily there. Thus, a pin through the olecranon with overhead traction supporting the limb vertically reveals virtually all surfaces of the arm and shoulder and makes access to them convenient and free of major discomfort. Moreover, it usually achieves a satisfactory reduction of fractures. In this method the forearm is simply suspended horizontally in a simple sling arrangement and lies in a plane at right angles to the long axis of the trunk. It is rarely useful to suspend forearms in so formal a fashion, since many of these are managed adequately by a plaster cast or if necessary pins incorporated in plaster. Occasionally external skeletal fixation may be useful. Any of these methods are then amenable to suspension devices to maintain elevation.

External Skeletal Fixation

External skeletal fixation has appeared sporadically in one form or another over many years, but it was most recently popularized by Stader for the treatment of fractures in domestic animals. Again it enjoyed considerable popularity in military circles during World War II, emerged for a time as popular in civilian practice, then waned again and is currently applied sporadically, often as a solution for a difficult or unusual problem. Clearly problems with its use or some complication has reduced its popularity. Yet for certain circumstances, including some open fractures, it deserves consideration.

Its use in open fractures provides stabilization and additionally permits access to virtually the entire surface of the involved limb. Thus, accompanying wounds are never obscured but are easily available to direct vision, even if the patient must be turned. The variety of component parts of most of the commercially available skeletal fixation devices have the virtue of a kind of Tinkertoy versatility, which permits nearly unlimited patterns of arrangement to suit the needs of the widely varying fracture patterns encountered. In cases that pose unusual problems, both general access to the wounds and mobility of the patient unrestricted by fixed or suspended splints is often useful if not imperative. Once the advantages provided by the external skeletal fixation device are no longer required, it can be discontinued in favor of some other method of treatment of the fracture. But a word of caution is in order.

Unless the surgeon is experienced with this method or has access to some other surgeon who is, it may be wise to pay strict attention to the technical points recommended by its proponents and by the manufacturers of the devices to be used. Otherwise disappointment, frustration, and finally castigation may ensue, all of which are usually visited upon the system of treatment, when the cause of all the trouble may be *misuse* of the system. Moreover, even though the external fixation device may have been chosen in the interest of the soft-tissue problems or the patient generally, there is no reason that the very best effort possible should not be made to realize its most salutary effect upon the fractures themselves.

Internal Fixation

There are few more contentious issues currently at hand than the use of internal fixation in open fractures. Surgeons generally approve or disapprove of the method in the strongest terms. Few are ambivalent enough to be simply tolerant, and unfortunately there is usually more emotion than logic when the issue is raised for discussion. Though the negative dogma, forbidding the use of any internal fixation in open fractures, has long held sway, it is (in small degrees) being challenged effectively.

There can be no argument that innumerable cases of open fractures in which internal fixation was used have developed serious, even disastrous complications. But did the internal fixation alone account for the difficulty? The dogma against it implies that it did. Careful review of many such cases, plus experiences with others in which internal fixation was employed with an entirely satisfactory outcome, warrants a reconsideration of the entire question.

It is beyond the scope of this text to document the pros and cons of the argument, let alone settle the issue. Therefore only a few points will be offered in its consideration. First, internal fixation for open fractures generally should require the same indication as for similar closed fractures. Second, its use should not be undertaken by the surgeon who treats an open fracture only occasionally, and never by the physician who has had little or no experience at all with such fractures. Third, as a corollary to the axiom for soft-tissue wounds: "When in doubt, leave it open," the axiom for any surgeon with regard to the use of internal fixation should be: "When in doubt, leave it out." The author is convinced that on many occasions when an open fracture treated by internal fixation and primary wound closure subsequently became infected, the fault lay not necessarily with the use of internal fixation, but more frequently with the inappropriate primary closure of the wound.

MULTIPLE OPEN FRACTURES AND MULTIPLE SYSTEMS INJURY

While some single ideal form of treatment may be applied to the open fracture occurring in a limb as an isolated injury, in these days many patients suffer both open and closed fractures in several limbs and too frequently, serious or life-threatening injuries to other body systems. The

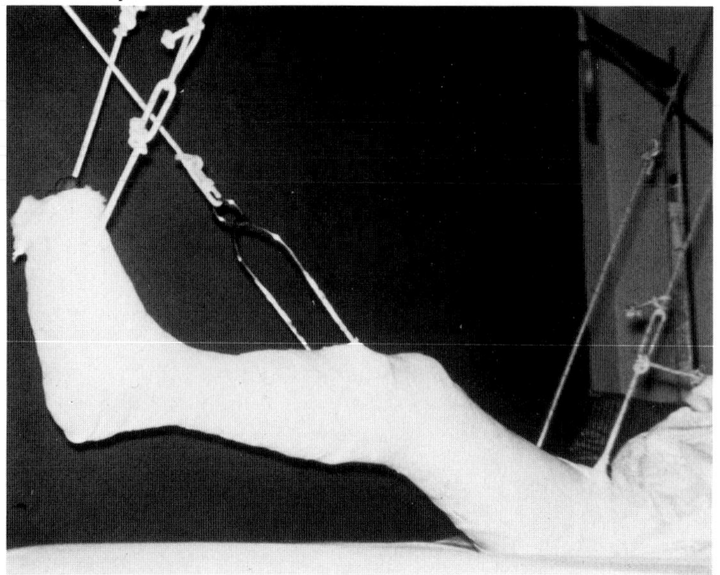

Fig. 3-12. A standard long-leg cast carried high on the thigh, with the ankle at neutral and the knee flexed 30 degrees, and incorporating a single tibial pin, makes a very satisfactory splint if slings of rope are incorporated during its construction. A traction bow may then be attached to the tibial pin. The technique is especially useful in bilateral shaft fractures, and in any patient who may require frequent or unusual transfers or manipulations.

combinations are almost limitless, so only a few of them may be considered here.

For the patient who has a straightforward open fracture of his femur, the thigh wound may be dealt with very promptly and the fracture may be effectively reduced and maintained by skeletal traction in a Thomas splint. But should the patient have incurred abdominal injury as well, or a chest injury that may compromise his respiration, the problem of his mobilization in the interest of his pulmonary problem may be seriously impeded by the Thomas splint and skeletal traction treatment of his fractured femur. It is in circumstances such as these that the judicious use of internal fixation of the fractured femur, in spite of the fact that it was open, may in fact be lifesaving. Alternatively, the limb might be placed in a long-leg cast with the tibial pin incorporated in the plaster. The cast can then be slung precisely as one suspends a Thomas splint, and the traction can continue through the tibial pin (Fig. 3-12). While the cast is not expected to provide definitive stability of the reduced femur fracture, it has, at least, the prospect of more easily transferring the patient from his bed to an operating table should that maneuver be necessary.

Similarly, for the patient who has incurred a combination of open and closed fractures in both lower extremities, and especially of both femurs, the irksome discomfort created by two Thomas splints applied to the same patient can be relieved, in part at least, by the use of long-leg casts as alternative kinds of splints while traction is continued as before.

Patients who have open fractures of extremities—or indeed extremity fractures of virtually any kind—associated with head injuries often pose a particularly difficult problem. Not infrequently the course of recovery from a head injury is attended by episodes of maniacal behavior and violent physical thrashing about, including the injured limbs. Proximal fragments are frequently activated violently by the muscles attached to them, producing at times unbelievable degrees of angular deformity. More importantly, overlying soft-tissue wounds may be equally disturbed, and on occasion, a closed fracture may be converted to an open one when the soft tisssues are compressed between an external constraining cast and the angulating fragments of an underlying bone under the influence of violent muscle spasm. When such fractures combined with head injury occur in the tibia and fibula for example, anticipating such events may permit the surgeon to provide protection against this complication by the incorporation of transfixing pins in plaster. Here again, bear in mind that the pin must be heavy enough to withstand the force it may encounter.

These few examples are offered simply to demonstrate the influence that factors external to the open fracture itself may have upon choosing a definitive form of management for them. From the wide armamentarium presently available to surgeons, some suitable means of management that takes into account all these factors can be found, or when necessary, invented.

REFERENCES

1. Baxter, C. R.: Homografts and heterografts as a biological dressing in the treatment of thermal injury. Paper presented at The First Annual Congress of the Society of German Plastic Surgeons. September 28, 1970.
2. Brav, E. A.: Open fractures: fundamentals of management. Postgrad. Med., *39*:11-17, 1966.
3. Brown, P. W., and Urban, J. G.: Early weight-bearing treatment of open fractures of the tibia. An end-result study of 63 cases. J. Bone Joint Surg., *51*:59-75, 1969.
4. Dehne, E.: Treatment of fractures of the tibial shaft. Clin. Orthop., *66*:159-173, Sept.-Oct., 1969.
5. Ger, R.: The management of open fractures of the tibia with skin loss. J. Trauma, *10*: 112-121, 1970.
6. Glotzer, D. J., Goodman, W. S., and Geronimus, L. H.: Topical antibiotic prophylaxsis in contaminated wounds. Experimental evaluation. Arch. Surg., *100*:589-593, 1970.
7. Gustilo, R. B., Simpson, L., Nixon, R., and Ruiz, A.: Analyses of 511 open fractures. Clin. Orthop., *66*:148-154, 1969.
8. Henry, A. K.: Extensive Exposure. ed. 1. Edinburgh, E. & S. Livingstone, 1952.
9. Leonard, M. H.: Solution of lead by synovial fluid. Clin. Orthop., *64*:255-261, 1969.
10. Paradies, L. H., and Gregory, C. F.: Early treatment of close-range shotgun wounds. J. Bone Joint Surg., *48A*:425-432, 1966.
11. Patman, R. D., and Thompson, J. E.: Fasciotomy in peripheral vascular surgery. Arch. Surg., *101*:663-672, 1970.
12. Patzakis, M., Harvey, J. I. P., and Ivler, D.: The role of antibiotics in the management of open fractures. J. Bone Joint Surg., *56A*: 532-541, 1974.
13. Rich, N. M., Baugh, J. H., and Hughes, C. W.: Acute arterial injuries in Viet Nam: 1000 cases. J. Trauma, *10*:359-367, 1970.
14. Salisbury, R.: Biological dressings for skin graft donor sites. Arch. Surg., *106*:705-706, 1973.
15. Sarmiento, A.: A functional below-the-knee cast for tibial fractures. J. Bone Joint Surg., *49*:855-875, 1967.
16. Scully, R. E., Artz, C. P., and Sako, Y.: An evaluation of the surgeon's criteria for determining muscle viability during debridement. Arch. Surg., *73*:1031-1035, 1956.
17. Shires, G. T.: Care of the Injured. The Surgeons Responsibility. Tenth Annual Scudder Oration. Bull. Amer. Col. Surgeons, Feb. 1973.
18. Tanner, J. C., Vanderput, J., and Alley, J. F.: The mesh skin graft. Plast. Reconstr. Surg., *34*:287-292, 1964.
19. Trueta, J.: Principles and Practice of War Surgery. St. Louis, C. V. Mosby, 1943.
20. Waterman, N. A., Howell, R. S., and Babich, M.: The effect of a prophylactic antibiotic (Cephalothin) on the incidence of wound infection. Arch. Surg., *97*:365-370, 1968.

4 Complications

C. McCollister Evarts, M.D.

SHOCK

The person with multiple fractures and with trauma to other organ systems is prone to develop shock. Treatment must be specific and prompt or the consequences may be disastrous. An understanding by the orthopaedic surgeon of the pathophysiology of the various types of shock is basic to appropriate therapy. It is difficult to offer a simple definition of shock because of the many factors involved in its production. Simeone[59] states that shock is "a clinical condition in which, because of insufficient effective circulating blood volume or because of abnormal partitioning of cardiac output, the capillary blood flow in vital tissues or in all tissues is reduced to levels below the minimum requirements for normal oxidative metabolism."

Although shock as a clinical entity has been recognized for several centuries, it has taken time to delineate the pathophysiology of various types of shock. In 1872, Gross[29] defined shock as a "manifestation of rude, unhinging of the machinery of life." Many investigators, including Crile,[22] Blalock,[7,8] and Wiggers,[66] have offered a variety of definitions for the state of shock. Many experimental studies have been performed to investigate the underlying pathophysiologic mechanisms.[12,15,17,23,31,34,39,44,47,49,62] All forms of shock ultimately relate to inadequate perfusion of oxygen to tissues in the vital organs. Continued studies of the underlying mechanisms of shock are in progress in special trauma units throughout the United States.

GENERAL PRINCIPLES

Classification

In 1937 Blalock[7] suggested four categories of shock: (1) hematogenic (oligemia); (2) neurogenic (caused primarily by nervous influences); (3) vasogenic (initially decreased vascular resistance and increased

Categories of Shock

I. Cardiogenic shock
   A. Myocardial dysfunction
      1. Myocardial infarction
      2. Cardiac arrhythmias
      3. Myocardial depression
   B. Mechanical restriction; venous obstruction
      1. Tension pneumothorax
      2. Vena caval obstruction
      3. Cardiac tamponade

II. Hypovolemic shock
   A. Blood loss
   B. Plasma loss
   C. Extracellular fluid changes

III. Resistance vessel (arteriolar) changes
   A. Neurogenic shock (decrease in resistance)
      1. Spinal anesthesia
      2. Neurogenic reflexes
      3. Hypovolemic shock
   B. Septic shock
      1. Peripheral arterial resistance changes
      2. Venous capacitance changes
      3. Peripheral arteriovenous shunting

vascular capacity); and (4) cardiogenic, due either to failure of the heart as a pump or to diminished cardiac output from various causes. Shires, Carrico, and Canizaro[56] believe that shock invariably results from the loss of function of one or more of four separate but interrelated functions (i.e., the heart, the volume of blood, the arteriolar resistance vessels, and the capacitance vessels). The categories of shock and their relation to function is outlined in the following list. The management of shock will obviously depend on the type or types of shock present in a patient who has sustained multiple injuries or undergone a complex, major operative procedure.

Pathophysiology

Shock, with its concomitant diminished tissue perfusion, leads to changes in the individual cells, organs, and systems (Fig. 4-1).[16]

Arterial blood pressure is maintained by cardiac output and peripheral vascular resistance; if the output is decreased, then the peripheral vascular resistance increases. Arterioles determine the outflow resistance from the heart, while capillaries and veins determine the intravascular volume to a large extent.[13] The resistance vessels contain receptors subject to various stimuli. A marked variation can occur in the distribution of total blood flow to the heart and brain, and, in certain states of shock, the mesenteric blood flow, along with the renal vessel and skeletal vessel flow, is markedly decreased. The maintenance of blood flow to the brain, heart, and liver takes precedence over blood flow to the other tissues and organs. It is obvious that such an adap-

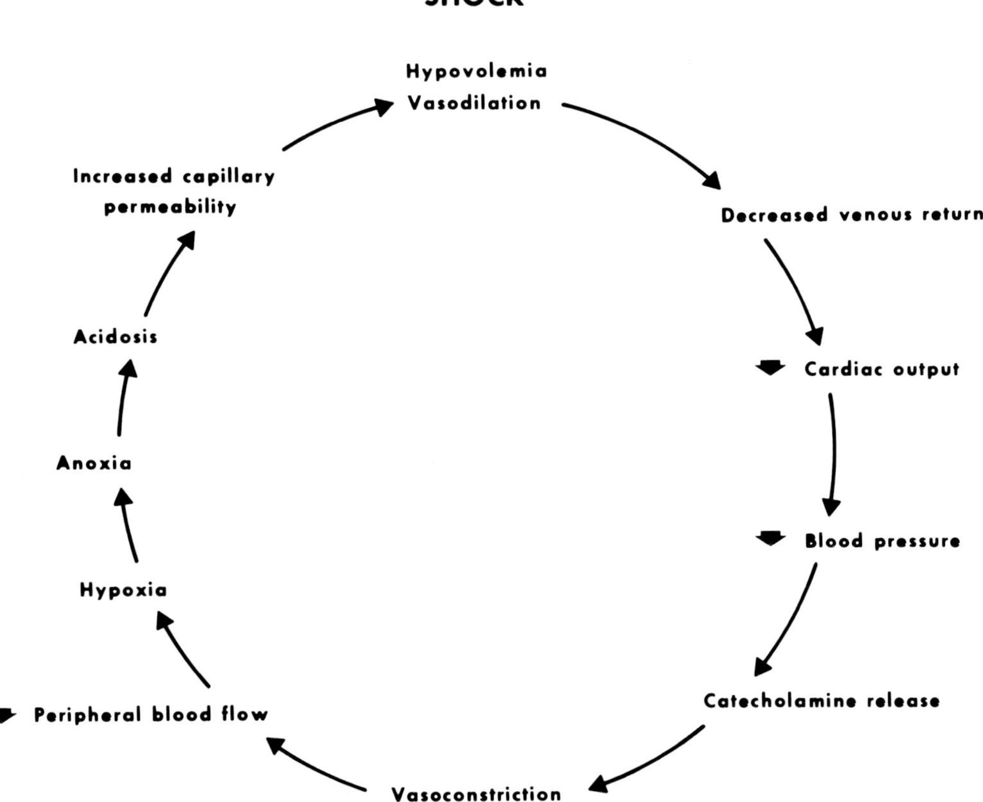

Fig. 4-1. The cycle of events in shock.

tive mechanism is reflected by the delay in the fall of blood pressure until the blood volume decrease is large enough to prohibit an effective response.[55] Immediately after the onset of hemorrhage, sympathetic adrenal medullary activity occurs. Serum catecholamine levels are elevated. Epinephrine and norepinephrine levels increase significantly following trauma, hemorrhage, or bacteremic shock.[64] The adrenergic beta receptors in the heart are stimulated, producing an increase in heart rate and contractility. A variety of forces—including metabolic, mechanical, or neural ones—may cause cardiac failure in shock states. This compensatory mechanism is influenced by the position of the patient. Shenkin *et al.*[54] in their studies of slow hemorrhage in normal volunteers, demonstrated that as much as 1000 ml. of blood may be lost without significant increase in the pulse rate. When observing a patient in shock the pulse rate must be monitored over a long period of time.

Moore[24] has described in detail the changes that occur in the adrenal cortex-pituitary axis following the onset of shock. He has discussed the sodium and water retention, potassium excretion, and negative nitrogen balance that occur after shock. Several authors have commented on the cytologic disorders that are associated with severe shock.[3,42,63] Recently, the changes that occur in the intracellular and extracellular fluid volumes in hemorrhagic shock have been the focus of several experimental and clinical studies.[21,24,50,57] It is felt that the extracellular fluid plays an important role in hemorrhagic shock. The reduction in extracellular fluid volume occurring with hemorrhagic shock must be reversed as part of the treatment of shock. Shires *et al.*[55,56,57] are of the opinion that a measurable reduction in interstitial fluid occurs in response to sustained hemorrhagic shock (Fig. 4-2). Also, the cellular response to hypovolemic hypotension demonstrates a consistent change in active ion transport. They have also suggested that sodium and water enter muscle cells, with resultant loss of cellular potassium to the extracellular fluid. The interstitial fluid holds the extruded potassium.

The effect of shock upon the kidney is to decrease renal function.[4,52,60] Such an effect is mediated by a decreased blood flow via the actions of antidiuretic hormone, aldosterone, and bacterial toxins. Progressive renal ischemia causes changes in the renal tubule and kidney function, leading to renal

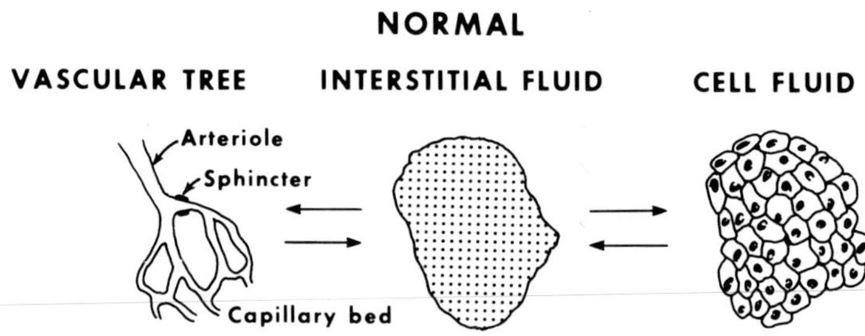

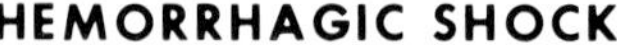

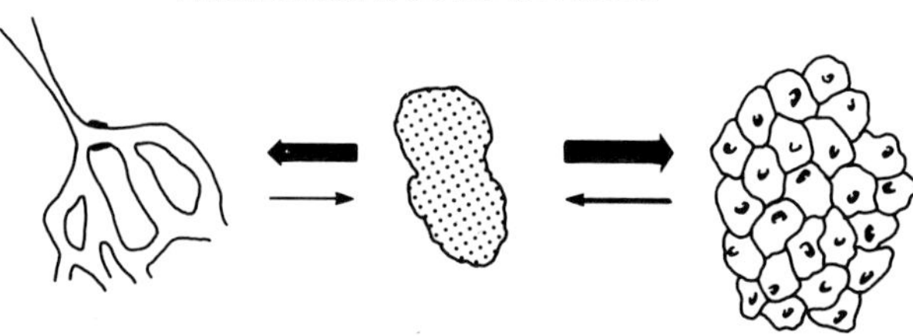

Fig. 4-2. A measurable reduction in interstitial fluid occurs in response to sustained hemorrhagic shock. (Modified from Shires, G. T., Carrico, C. J., and Canizaro, P. C.: Shock. p. 19. Philadelphia, W. B. Saunders, 1973.)

tubular necrosis. All the features involved in the production of acute renal failure following trauma are not completely understood, but it is thought that renal ischemia plays a key role. Proper management and attention to fluid and electrolyte administration early in the course of the shock state will aid in the prevention of renal insufficiency. Teschan[61] and others[9,26,38] have described the management of patients with posttraumatic renal insufficiency.

There has been considerable interest in the nature of respiratory insufficiency which follows trauma and shock.[10,36,41,59,68] Terms for the respiratory insufficiency—such as shock lung, pump lung, traumatic wet lung, respiratory distress syndrome, Da Nang lung—have been superseded by reports that identified and suggested treatment for the posttraumatic conditions of the lung frequently resulting in pulmonary insufficiency.[18,33] Blaisdell[6] has defined respiratory insufficiency as follows "Patients with pure respiratory insufficiency syndrome have respiratory insufficiency which is manifested initially by tachypnea and increased respiratory effort. Careful evaluation, including pulmonary function testing, reveals a progressive decrease in compliance, increased airway resistance, decreased arterial oxygen tension (PaO_2), and pulmonary arterial venous shunting. Pulmonary vascular resistance when measured is not increased until the terminal phases of this syndrome. The lungs sound dry to auscultation, and pulmonary secretions are minimal. The chest roentgenogram reveals diffuse alveolar infiltrates which may progress to complete consolidation." Moore *et al.*[48] divided the clinical picture into four phases:

Phase 1. Injury, resuscitation, and alkalosis. After the initial episode of injury, hemorrhagic shock and resuscitation of the patient, including multiple transfusions, intravenous fluid therapy, antibiotics, and surgery when indicated, the patient is often mildly alkalotic. There is a respiratory component due to spontaneous hyperventilation, but recovery frequently proceeds uneventfully.

Phase 2. Circulatory stabilization and beginning respiratory difficulty. This period is characterized by apparent stabilization of vital signs and adequate tissue perfusion. The arterial PO_2 may be below normal on room air.

Phase 3. Progressive pulmonary insufficiency. Increasing respiratory difficulty is apparent. The patient becomes dyspneic. Increased concentrations of inspired air do not change the level of hypoxemia. Endotracheal intubation and mechanical ventilatory assists are mandatory now, but they should be initiated before the patient reaches this advanced stage. The condition may stabilize, and the patient may begin to improve. A marked increase in inspired oxygen concentration is required to maintain the oxygen arterial tension value near normal. The blood pH becomes acidotic.

Phase 4. Terminal hypoxia and hypercarbia with asystole. As respiratory insufficiency progresses, an adequate arterial PO_2 cannot be obtained, tissue hypoxia becomes significant, and metabolic acidosis occurs. The urine output falls, coma and convulsions begin, and eventually bradycardia and asystole occur.

A partial list of the etiologic agents responsible for posttraumatic respiratory insufficiency are listed below.

Posttraumatic Respiratory Insufficiency

- Pulmonary injury (ischemic)
- Pulmonary infection
- Sepsis
- Embolic phenomena
    - Fat
    - Microembolism
    - Multiple blood transfusions
    - Intravascular coagulation
- Fluid overload
- Oxygen toxicity
- Pulmonary injury (direct)

Table 4-1. Grading of Shock

Degree of Shock	Blood Pressure (approx.)	Pulse Quality	Skin			Thirst	Mental State
			Temperature	Color	Circulation (response to pressure blanching)		
None	Normal	Normal	Normal	Normal	Normal	Normal	Clear
Slight	To 20% increase	Normal	Cool	Pale	Definite slowing	Normal	Clear and distressed
Moderate	Decreased 20%–40%	Definite decrease in volume	Cool	Pale	Definite slowing	Definite	Clear and some apathy unless stimulated
Severe	Decreased 40% to nonrecordable	Weak to imperceptible	Cold	Ashen to cyanotic (mottling)	Very sluggish	Severe	Apathetic to comatose, little distress except thirst

Beecher, H. K., *et al.*:[5] Surgery, 22:672, 1947.

The management of posttraumatic pulmonary insufficiency is well outlined by Shires, Carrico, and Canizaro.[56] They emphasize the importance of monitoring blood gas measurements, checking the pulmonary mechanisms, and assessing ventilatory efforts.

The normal blood gas values are as follows:

pH	A 7.40	7.35-7.45
	V 7.37	7.32-7.42
CO_2 Content (mEq./l.)	A 25	23-27
	V 27	25-29
CO_2 Tension (mm. Hg)	A 40	34-46
	V 46	42-55
Oxygen Tension (mm. Hg)	A 90	85-95
Oxygen Saturation (%)	A 95	95-98

Ventilatory supports consisting of an intermittent positive pressure apparatus employing an endotracheal tube or tracheostomy is vital to appropriate treatment. Occasionally continual positive pressure breathing becomes a necessity. Other means of treatment such as diuretics, steroids, and heparin, have been suggested.[14,51,67] The cornerstone of treatment of posttraumatic pulmonary insufficiency is ventilatory support in conjunction with the correction and management of the underlying disorders.

Clinical Characteristics

The classic clinical signs and symptoms of shock include those of peripheral circulatory failure (i.e., pallor, a cold, pale mottled skin, a thin thready pulse, low blood pressure, slow capillary return, and changes in the mental state). Beecher and coauthors[5] have discussed the signs and symptoms of shock in man (Table 4-1). Obviously the classic description of shock is subject to variations.[55] In hemorrhagic shock a cold, clammy skin is not as common as it is in septic shock or syncope secondary to neurogenic shock. Certain mental changes take place in shock. The sensory level may progress with increasing shock to an apathetic state and, finally, to coma. The patient may complain of thirst and demonstrate an increased respiratory rate. Nausea and vomiting from hypovolemic shock are common. Also, an increased initial response in the rate and depth of respiration occurs.

Treatment

The treatment of shock depends on early resuscitation of the patient and subsequent detection of the causative mechanism or mechanisms underlying the shock state. The clinical classifications that have been suggested are useful in determining causative factors. After identification of the type of shock the treatment of shock can proceed on a physiologic basis.

Immediate action must be instituted, and the early steps in the management of shock are as follows:[27] (1) Maintenance of the airway, especially in injuries about the head and neck. (2) Insertion of a large-bore venous cannula. Current evidence is that the side of the circulation into which the blood is transfused is not important, provided that a rapid rate of infusion can be assured.[32,35] (3) Maintenance of arterial blood pressure. Early infusion of 1,000 to 2,000 ml. Ringer's lactate solution should be given soon after arrival in the emergency room. Use of this balanced salt solution reduces the requirement of whole blood in the patient with hemorrhagic hypotension. (4) Insertion of nasogastric tube. (5) Bedside cardiac monitoring.

The measurement of the central venous pressure (normal pressure is 8 to 12 cm.) in patients with shock has extended the ability of the clinician to evaluate the clinical state.[28] The tip of a large catheter is inserted until it reaches the superior vena cava origin, and pressures are measured in centimeters of saline. The central venous pressure is used as a rough index of the degree of filling of the vascular tree and the ability of the heart to accommodate additional fluid volume loads. The value of central venous pressure monitoring of the patient in shock is that it is an indicator of the adequacy of intravascular volume.

HYPOVOLEMIC SHOCK

The treatment of hypovolemic shock consists of adequate volume replacement. Primary therapy consists of the administration of whole blood. Immediate steps should be taken to obtain proper types and cross-matched whole blood. If this is not available, low-molecular-weight dextran (with an average molecular weight of 40,000) can be substituted and has been shown to be effective in not only expanding plasma volume but in decreasing blood viscosity and increasing microcirculatory flow.[25] If a patient has a coexisting pulmonary contusion or pneumothorax, administration of oxygen by mask is indicated.

For the patient in hypovolemic shock with open fractures and large wounds, the administration of antibiotics (penicillin and tetracycline or ampicillin) is advisable.[37,43] Unless a patient has Addison's disease, has had an adrenalectomy, or has been receiving long-term corticosteroids, the use of steroids for the management of hypovolemic shock is contraindicated. The role of hypothermia in the treatment of hypovolemic shock is not yet clarified. The use of vasopressors in the treatment of this form of shock is rarely, if ever, indicated.[56] Several authors have investigated the use of vasodilators in the treatment of hemorrhagic shock.[2,11] The survival rates in experimental animals have been improved with the use of vasodilators. Chlorpromazine administration has resulted in a better survival rate in a clinical series.[19]

Renal function may be decreased by hemorrhagic shock, hyponatremia, urinary tract injury, or the use of pressor drugs. To determine whether the resultant oliguria is due to inadequate renal flow or to parenchymal damage, a rapid infusion of dextrose and water (500 ml. in 30 minutes) can be given. If the urine output promptly increases, the oliguria is most likely on the basis of decreased renal flow. If acute tubular necrosis has occurred, adequate renal flow will not occur after rapid infusion of water. If levels of azotemia, acidosis, or hyperkalemia increase, renal dialysis can be a life-saving procedure.

It is well to emphasize that the successful management of hemorrhagic shock is dependent upon constant monitoring of the patient in the first few hours after arrival at the hospital setting.

CARDIOGENIC SHOCK

The management of cardiogenic shock requires correction of the disorders of the cardiopulmonary pumping mechanism, repair of cardiac tamponade, digitalization for heart failure, the cardioversion of arrhythmias, and pulmonary embolectomy if necessary.[56]

Contractility of the cardiac musculature is improved with digitalization. Isoproterenol has a specific inotropic effect on cardiac musculature.[30] It can be useful for slow pulse rate, and should be administered by intravenous drip: 0.5 mg. in 250 ml. of 5-per cent glucose and water. Ganglionic blockade should be attempted only in special circumstances in the management of cardiogenic shock.[20] Abnormalities in cardiac rate occasionally respond to the administration of digoxin. On some occasions a continuous intravenous infusion of a vasoconstricting drug is helpful. Lidocaine or procainamide are given for premature ventricular contractions. The use of pacemakers for cardiogenic shock must be restricted at this time for specific circumstances and for patients who do not respond to more conventional therapy.[53]

SEPTIC SHOCK

Septic shock is a constant threat to the patient with multiple injuries and fractures. This kind of shock, being recognized with increasing frequency in surgical practice, is caused by gram-negative organisms that release endotoxin. The mortality is high if it is not diagnosed promptly and treated.[65] The clinical recognition of endotoxin shock depends on close observation of the patient. The genitourinary tract is the most frequent site of infection. Gram-positive cocci are the responsible agents in about one-third of the cases and gram-negative bacilli in two-thirds.[40] The patient may experience an abrupt onset of a shaking chill and demonstrate tachycardia. The skin is often cold and moist. The sensorium may be clouded, and lethargy may be attributed to the underlying infection *per se*. Hypotension is sometimes overlooked. One must always be concerned about the possibility of a gram-negative sepsis and subsequent endotoxic shock. No laboratory or roentgenographic procedure will establish the diagnosis. Rather, a high index of suspicion is required and the decision to begin treatment must be made early in the course of the disease.

The endotoxins of the gram-negative bacteria exert a powerful sympathomimetic effect upon smooth muscle and stimulate the production of massive amounts of catecholamine. The effect is intense vasoconstriction peripherally with accompanying ischemic anoxia. Metabolic acidosis and vasodilatation result, accompanied by stagnant anoxia and tissue necrosis. Fluid is lost in large quantities through the damaged capillary walls with subsequent hypovolemia. The sequence of events involves tissue anoxia, metabolic acidosis, vasodilatation, stasis, and profound hypovolemia with shock.

It is obvious that treatment must be directed to the elimination of the causal organism, to the correction of failure of the peripheral resistance, and to the replacement of an effective circulating blood volume. Eradication of the source of infection is essential, and abscesses should be surgically drained. One should not wait for positive cultural evidence of the offending bacterial organism but, rather, begin antibiotic therapy immediately. The common causative organisms, are *Escherichia coli, Klebsiella aerobacter, Proteus, Pseudomonas,* and *Bacteroides.* Combinations of antibiotics are given to the patient—cephalothin 8 g./24 hr. intravenously and gentamicin 1.5 mg./kg. body weight intramuscularly four times a day. Altemeier *et al.*[1] reported a mortality of 28 per cent, even when appropriate antibiotics were given to patients experiencing septic shock.

Fluid replacement is essential in the management of septic shock. If an hourly urinary output of 30 ml. or more can be maintained, this will provide some evidence of satisfactory renal perfusion. Ringer's lactate solution can be utilized for fluid replacement. Occasionally blood replacement is necessary. Monitoring of the fluid replacement by central venous pressure will provide guidelines for fluid administration. A patient will respond favorably to the administration of antibiotics and fluid with a rise in blood pressure, increase in urine output, clearing of the sensorium, and warming of the skin. The prevention or relief of the vasoconstricting effects of endotoxin and catecholamines is accomplished by the administration of corticosteroids such as methylprednisolone; 25 mg./kg. of body weight is given intravenously every 4 hours until beneficial effects are observed. The total dose is large, and tapering is not required. It should not be given for more than 24 to 48 hours.

NEUROGENIC SHOCK

This type of shock is associated with syncopal episodes in patients who are afraid of injections, have seen unpleasant sights, or have been given unpleasant news, and so forth. It is similar to the shock that is observed following high spinal anesthesia. It occurs because of interference with the balance between the vasodilator and vasoconstrictor controls of both arterioles and venules.

The treatment of neurogenic shock involves repositioning the patient and eliminating the offending stimuli. This type of shock is usually self-limiting and requires very little treatment. If the neurogenic shock is due to a high spinal anesthesia, a vasopressor drug can be given to increase the cardiac output and peripheral vasoconstriction.[46] If neurogenic shock is due to spinal cord transsection, fluid replacement may be necessary and central venous pressure monitoring is helpful.

SUMMARY

As the scope of orthopaedic surgery broadens, the necessity for a clear understanding of the recognition and treatment of all categories of shock is mandatory for the orthopaedic surgeon. The increasing number of trauma patients with associated shock requires greater involvement of the part of the orthopaedic surgeon.

CARDIAC ARREST

Attempts to treat cardiac arrest were recorded as long ago as biblical times, but only in the past few decades has it become a "treatable entity."[71,90] In 1960 closed chest cardiac massage was described,[77,80] and a new era in the management of cardiac arrest began. Many laymen have been instructed in the techniques of cardiopulmonary resuscitation and have used them successfully.

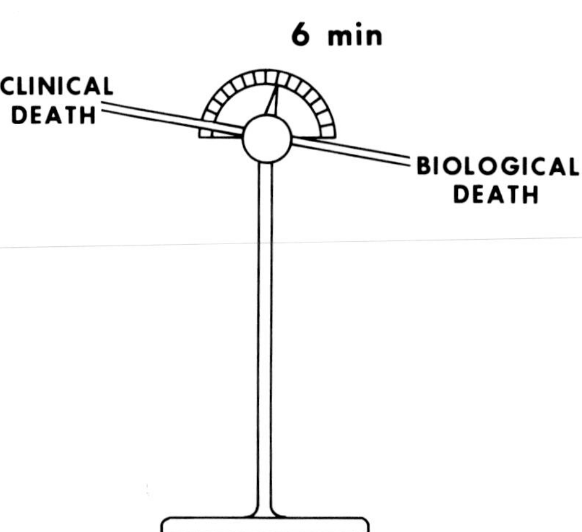

Fig. 4-3. Clinical death occurs at 0 minutes. Biological death occurs at 4 to 6 minutes.

Unfortunately, many physicians have not kept up with modern techniques. Too much reliance is placed upon the cardiopulmonary resuscitation team. This team is a medical necessity in a hospital, and definitive management of arrhythmia should be accomplished by the team upon their arrival at the scene. However, two features require emphasis. First, success is measured by adequate restoration of venilation and circulation in the first 4 to 6 minutes following cardiac arrest (Fig. 4-3).[69,73,79,92,94] Second, arrival of the resuscitation team may be delayed.

The practice of orthopaedic surgery includes numerous situations in which cardiac arrest can occur. Indeed, regardless of our definition of our individual roles in orthopaedics, juries in malpractice lawsuits have determined that all physicians should be capable of managing cardiac arrest.[72,81] The scope of orthopaedic surgery has changed and now includes the elderly patient with degenerative joint disease who may have accompanying cardiopulmonary and metabolic deterioration. Such patients are a greater risk in regard to cardiac arrest. The rheumatoid patient with physiologic aging —often steroid-dependent and occasionally receiving immunosuppressive drugs—is a potential candidate for cardiopulmonary arrest. An increase in highway accidents or in trauma of all forms adds to the number of patients who, for the orthopaedist, represent a specific risk for cardiopulmonary shutdown.

The widespread use of methyl methacrylate for fixation of component parts in artificial joints has been found to be associated with a fall in blood pressure because of the vasodilation effect of the monomer. Several reports of cardiac arrest have appeared in the literature.[74,86,88,91]

The incidence of pulmonary embolism is especially high in the orthopaedic patient, and in one series of 522 cardiac arrests, 52 were secondary to pulmonary embolization.[84]

In the overwhelming majority of patients who have experienced cardiac arrest, certain predisposing conditions (i.e., heart disease, respiratory dysfunction, hypoxia, shock, infection, metabolic acidosis, severe electrolyte imbalance, arrhythmias) are present. Prevention depends upon recognition of the potential problems with the disorders listed above. Early recognition and treatment of arrhythmias can also help to prevent cardiac arrest.[82,96] When arrest does occur, prompt recognition and treatment improve the chances of recovery. The severity of the underlying disorder often determines the outcome.[69,75,93]

Management

Cardiac arrest is defined as the sudden cessation of adequate circulation. A convulsion may mark its onset. This is followed by continued unconsciousness and absence of respiration. The pupils dilate about 30 to 60 seconds after cardiac arrest, and major arterial pulses are not palpable. No heartbeat can be heard. Once the diagnosis is made, immediate action must be taken. Opening the airway and restoring breathing are the basic steps of artificial ventilation. As irreparable brain damage occurs in 4 to 6 minutes after cardiac arrest, the time for institution of such action is short. The first step is to summon help immediately, and if in the hospital setting, alert another physician, an anesthesiologist, and the cardiac resuscitation team. After four quick respirations are given, check for the pulses. If there is no pulse and you were there when the arrest occurred, it is important to direct a sharp blow to the sternum with the fist. After two or three sharp blows over the precordium the heart may begin to beat spontaneously, and further treatment is not needed. If this maneuver is not successful, then external cardiac massage should be begun immediately in concert with restoration of ventilation.

Before ventilation can be restored the airway must be opened. The head should then be tilted back as far as possible with one hand on the forehead. Pinch the nostrils with the thumb and forefinger, applying extension force to the forehead with the hand. The opposite hand should be placed beneath the neck (Fig. 4-4). Inhale and give a short, forceful exhalation into the victim's mouth until the chest expands. If necessary, and respirations cannot be delivered, the mouth and pharynx should be cleaned out with the patient's head turned to the side. Repeat the exhalations rapidly

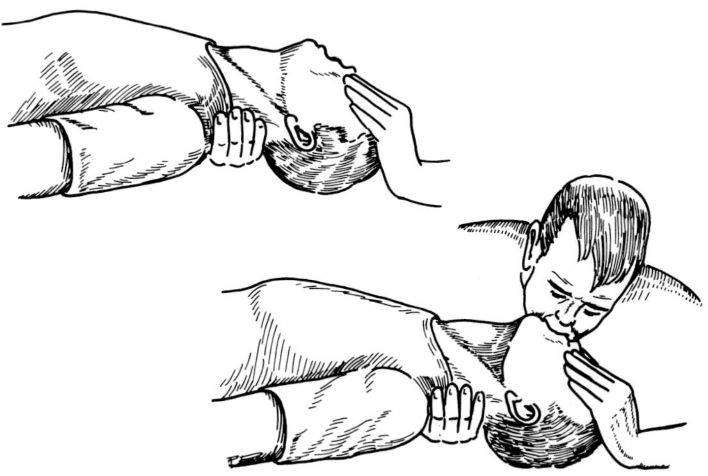

Fig. 4-4. Technique of mouth-to-mouth ventilation.

at first (three to four times) then 12 to 15 times per minute. Do not wait for the arrival of the anesthesiologist for intubation before beginning mouth-to-mouth resuscitation. Once an open airway has been obtained administration of oxygen can be begun effectively without intubation by mask for prolonged periods. Restoration of the open airway and respiration should precede cardiac resuscitation.

Closed heart compression is the accepted method for restoring circulation following cardiac arrest. It depends upon compression of the heart between the vertebral column and the sternum at 60 beats per minute. The compression rate for two rescuers is 60 per minute. This rate is practical because it avoids fatigue, facilitates timing on the basis of one compression per second, and allows optimum ventilation and circu-

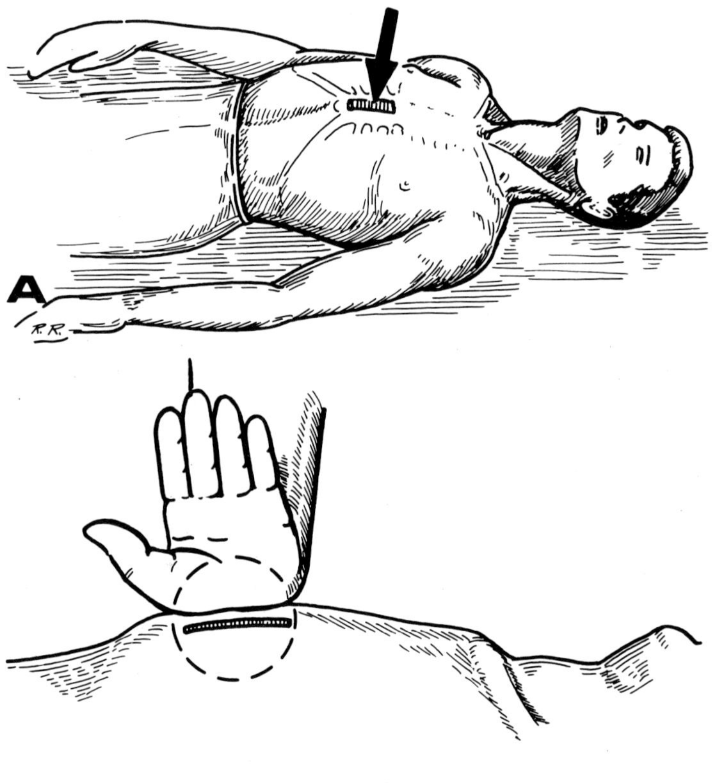

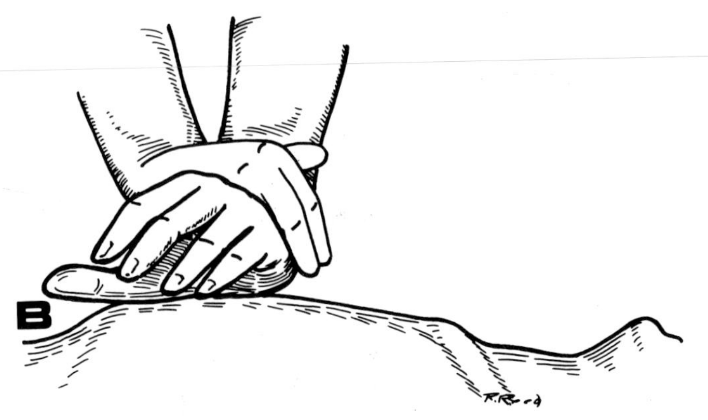

Fig. 4-5. (*A*) Site of application of pressure for external cardiac compression. (*B*) Technique of external cardiac compression. Place one hand on top; do not allow fingers to touch the chest wall.

lation to be achieved by quickly interposing one inflation after each five chest compressions without any pause in compressions (5:1 ratio).[94] However, even if performed properly only 30 to 50 per cent of the circulation is reestablished.[83] The patient must be placed on a firm surface. The heel of the hand is put over the lower half of the sternum but not over the xiphoid, the second hand being placed over the first. A firm surface, a board, or the floor provides resistance for effective external chest massage (Fig. 4-5). A thrust is made downward, displacing the sternum 3.8 to 5.1 cm. towards the spine, followed by a sharp release (Fig. 4-6). The hands must not leave the chest wall during this maneuver. Obviously, the size of the victim determines the amount of pressure. The effectiveness of the maneuver can be determined by the presence of a carotid or femoral pulse, constriction of the pupils, better skin color, and a return of spontaneous respiration.[78,89] It is easy to fracture ribs during this procedure and cause a pneumothorax, especially in an elderly person, as well as to separate the costochondral junction. Although rare, it is possible to fracture the sternum or cause direct trauma to the heart, lungs, spleen, or liver.

At this juncture it is imperative to consider the electrical activity in the heart. Arrhythmias are commonly associated with cardiac arrest, especially asystole and ventricular fibrillation. Both are easily recognized. If this occurs defibrillation can be accomplished sometimes with drugs, and normal rhythm results.[87,95] In the hospital setting, blind defibrillation should be tried in all arrests.

Certain drugs are used in the management of cardiac arrest. Epinephrine increases both the force of contractility and the heart rate. One ml. of 1:1000 or 10 ml. of 1:10,000 solution of epinephrine should be given intravenously or by direct intracardiac injection, and can be repeated every 3 to 5 minutes, as necessary. If the intracardiac route is used, the injection should be into a ventricle. A cardiac needle can be inserted into the left fourth or fifth interspace to enter the ventricle; however, the subxiphoid approach is recommended. If an overdose of epinephrine is given, ventricular fibrillation may occur. Another drug that has been administered for asystole is isoproterenol (Isuprel). It acts upon the beta adrenergic receptors and appears to stimulate the higher centers of the cardiac conduction system without producing ven-

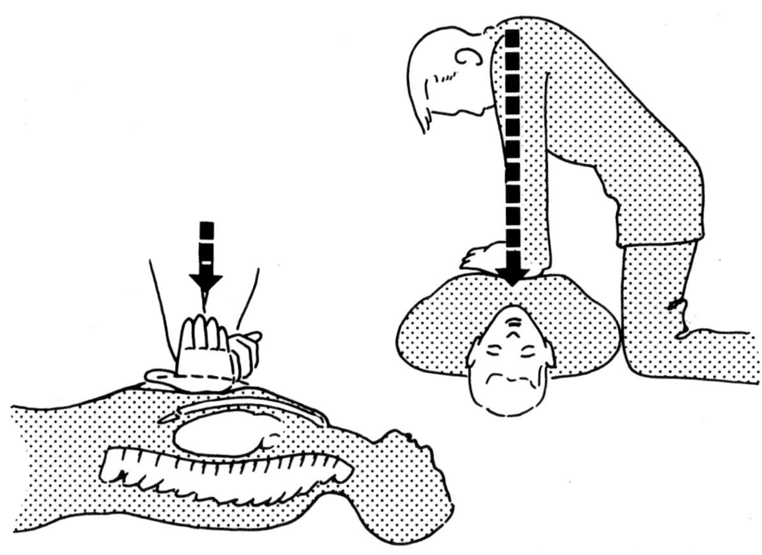

Fig. 4-6. External cardiac compression.

tricular irritability. One ml. is diluted with 9 ml. of saline solution and 1 or 2 ml. of the dilute solution is administered by direct intracardiac injection or intravenously. If no response is obtained with epinephrine or isoproterenol (Isuprel), 5 to 10 ml. of 10-per cent calcium chloride solution is given intravenously or by direct cardiac injection. Calcium can also be administered as calcium gluceptate in 5 ml. amounts. This non-specific cardiac stimulant may activate the heart.

Sodium bicarbonate is necessary to help treat metabolic acidosis. It is administered intravenously in an initial dose of 1 mEq./kg. by either bolus injection or continuous infusion over a 10-minute period. Once effective spontaneous circulation is restored, further administration of sodium bicarbonate may be harmful.[94]

If ventricular fibrillation has occurred, electrical defibrillation should be attempted.[97,98] It should never be delayed to give drugs. If defibrillation fails, then the use of bicarbonate and calcium is recommended. Occasionally 100 mg. of lidocaine is given slowly by the intravenous route. It should not be used initially. When defibrillation is necessary, the electrocardiograph (EKG) machine should be stopped. The defibrillator should deliver a 50-ohm load ranging from 0 to at least 250 watt-seconds; the EKG is reconnected and the result observed. Sinus rhythm may develop. Complex arrhythmias often follow attempts at defibrillation. If ventricular fibrillation is still present, resuscitation is continued, and two shocks of similar watt-seconds are given. It is important to continue cardio-respiratory resuscitation, as the anoxic myocardium is prone to fibrillate.[70,85] It is difficult to state the specifics of the length of resuscitation efforts; however, in a young person treatment should be continued for as long as 2 hours.

The aftercare of cardiopulmonary resuscitation requires immediate transportation to an intensive care unit and monitoring of the cardiac function. All modalities must be observed, and measurement of the arterial central venous pressure should be made, along with estimation of urinary output and observation of peripheral circulation. Close monitoring of the respiratory status must be maintained, including arterial blood gas determinations and careful maintenance of an open airway.

Summary

The success of cardiopulmonary arrest and its treatment is related directly to the clinical setting in which it occurs. Almost 100 per cent of the patients are resuscitated in the operating room or in a cardiac catheterization laboratory. The overall success rate is much lower if cardiopulmonary arrest occurs in a different setting. It is obvious that some patients will die following cardiopulmonary arrest. However, in the absence of a terminal illness, no effort should be spared in an attempt to save the patient. The orthopaedic surgeon must be prepared to swiftly and decisively begin cardiopulmonary resuscitation if arrest occurs, either at the office or in the operating room.[76] He must be aware of the high-risk patient and be ready to institute appropriate resuscitative measures should cardiopulmonary arrest occur.

HEMORRHAGIC COMPLICATIONS*

Hemorrhagic problems facing the orthopaedic surgeon usually fall into one of two categories. First are those related to the treatment, operative or conservative, of orthopaedic complications of lifelong bleeding disorders such as hemophilia. Second, there are those failures of the hemostatic mechanism that may arise during or after major surgical procedures or trauma. Each patient may present a unique problem, but certain generalizations can be made, and in this outline four main topics will be discussed: the normal hemostatic mechanism,

* This section was contributed by George C. Hoffman, M.B., B.Ch., M.R.C. Path., Dept. of Laboratory Hematology, Cleveland Clinic Foundation.

disorders of hemostasis, the diagnosis of these disorders, and the treatment of these disorders.

NORMAL HEMOSTASIS

When a blood vessel wall is pierced or damaged, a series of events occurs aimed at preventing loss of blood and repairing the wound. These consist of the aggregation of platelets at the site of the puncture; the formation of fibrin among the platelets; retraction of the clot to form an impervious barrier; the removal of the clot and reconstruction of the damaged vessel wall. The events are described sequentially, but they overlap considerably. There is, of course, a limit to the size of wound and size of vessel beyond which the normal mechanism is ineffective without the added support of local pressure or mechanical closure.

Platelet and Vascular Phase[101]

Platelets aggregate promptly at the point of damage in the vessel wall. These platelets release adenosine diphosphate (ADP), which causes more platelets to aggregate. The nature of the "message" that induces the first platelets to adhere to the damaged endothelial surface is not known, but collagen, which causes platelet aggregation, and the plasma factor missing in patients with von Willebrand's disease may be involved.

Local vascular constriction occurs and may play a role in slowing blood flow locally, thus enhancing the tendency to clot formation.

Blood Coagulation[99]

During this phase fibrin strands are laid down amongst the aggregated platelets. Thrombin, a proteolytic enzyme, converts soluble fibrinogen to an insoluble fibrin clot. There are two pathways that lead to conversion of prothrombin, an inactive precursor, to thrombin. Since blood drawn directly into a test tube forms a clot, everything necessary for fibrin formation is present in blood (or plasma) alone. This represents the intrinsic clotting pathway and it is activated by contact with a surface other than normal endothelium. The process of fibrin formation is accelerated by the addition of tissue of any sort, and under these circumstances the extrinsic pathway comes into play. The factors involved in these pathways are shown in Figure 4-7. Both pathways must be functioning for normal hemostasis to occur; this is evident from the fact that a hemophiliac (Factor VIII deficiency) bleeds despite having a normal extrinsic pathway and, conversely, a patient with Factor VII deficiency has a hemorrhagic diathesis, despite having a normal intrinsic pathway. As can be seen from the diagram,

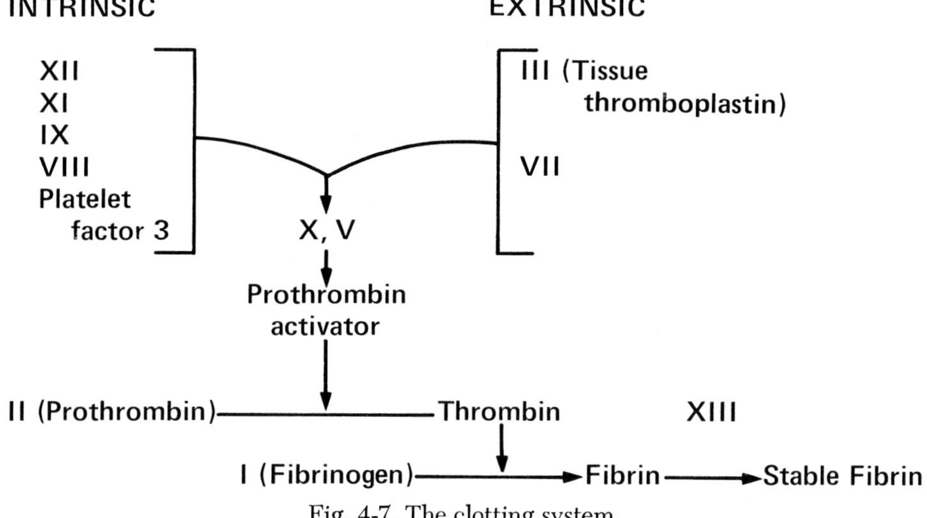

Fig. 4-7. The clotting system.

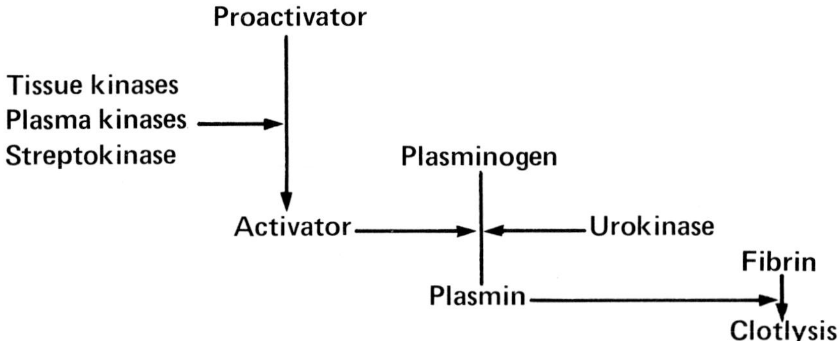

Fig. 4-8. A diagrammatic representation of the fibrinolytic system.

there is a final common pathway beyond Factor V.

Clot Retraction

Once fibrin strands have been laid down, the retractile protein within the platelets, sometimes referred to as thrombasthenin, pulls the strands together to form a firm clot. There is evidence that the retractile protein is actomyosin—identical to that found in muscle.

Fibrinolysis and Repair[105]

After the leak has been stopped the process of repair begins. The clot must first be removed by the fibrinolytic system (Fig. 4-8). Fibrinolysis has a similar basic framework to coagulation, namely an inactive precursor (plasminogen) which is converted by various activators and proactivators to an active enzyme (plasmin). Plasmin is a proteolytic enzyme, which can act on many substrates including fibrin, fibrinogen, Factor V, and other clotting factors. The process of repair of the vessel wall also involves the coagulation mechanism. It appears that Factor XIII (fibrin stabilizing factor) not only converts fibrin to a "stable" form but may also play a role in the laying down of fibroblasts.

HEMORRHAGIC DISORDERS AND LABORATORY TESTING

A derangement of any of the phases of hemostasis may lead to a hemorrhagic diathesis. It is important to bear this in mind when considering the possible cause of a hemorrhagic diathesis and the laboratory tests that may be used to elucidate it. In view of the complexity of the hemostatic process, the length of the list of causes of excessive bleeding should not be surprising. Discussion of each entity is beyond the scope of this brief outline. The commoner causes of hemorrhage and the more useful laboratory tests will be considered as they relate to the several phases of hemostasis.

Platelet and Vascular Phase

The commonest cause of a defect in the platelet and vascular phase is thrombocytopenia. There is no direct correlation between the platelet count and the occurrence of hemorrhage, but in general, bleeding may occur when the platelet count is less than 50,000/cu. mm. Typically, such bleeding occurs in skin and mucous membranes as petechiae, purpura, and bruising—a picture usually distinguishable from the hemophilia-like bleeding seen in abnormalities of the clotting system. Thrombocytopenia seldom causes, and is seldom associated with, orthopaedic disease. Whenever large amounts of blood over 3 days old are transfused, the platelet count may fall to critical levels; should this occur during surgery, a generalized oozing from the wound surfaces is seen.

On rare occasions vascular abnormalities (e.g., amyloid deposition) or qualitative platelet abnormalities (e.g., uremia) may affect this phase. One relatively common inherited disease, von Willebrand's disease, is associated with a prolonged bleeding time and is discussed later.

Tests of the vascular-platelet phase include a platelet count (or a platelet estimate from examination of the blood smear) and a bleeding time. The bleeding time is designed to test this phase by causing hemorrhage from small blood vessels and removing the blood as it exudes, thus limiting the effect of blood coagulation and testing the ability of the platelet plug to staunch the blood flow. If it is known that the platelet count is low or if petechiae are present, a bleeding time or tourniquet test is not indicated.

Blood Coagulation

Defects in the clotting mechanism may result either from the deficiency of one or more factors or from the presence of an anticoagulant (inhibitor) interfering with the action of one or more factors.

Factor deficiencies may be inherited or acquired. Inherited deficiencies usually involve only one factor. Hemophilia is the commonest and is a sex-linked disorder resulting in the production of a defective Factor VIII (antihemophilic factor, AHF) molecule.[107] The disease may be severe (less than 1 per cent Factor VIII activity), moderate (1 to 5 per cent Factor VIII activity) or mild (more than 5 per cent Factor VIII activity). Hemorrhage into deep tissues rather than into skin and mucous membrane is characteristic of hemophilia. Trauma underlies each episode but may be so slight that the bleeding appears to be spontaneous. Hemarthrosis is the major orthopaedic complication and occurs almost invariably in the severe, frequently in the moderate, but rarely in the mild form of the disease. Why hemarthrosis is such a common complication is not clearly understood. Christmas disease (Factor IX deficiency) is much less common than hemophilia, but is genetically and clinically similar. Von Willebrand's disease[107] is the second commonest inherited hemorrhagic disorder. This disease is a dominant trait and has two facets, deficiency of Factor VIII and a long bleeding time. The long bleeding time results from a deficiency of a plasma factor as yet not clearly defined but apparently not identical to Factor VIII. The platelet count is normal, but the ability of the platelets to adhere to foreign surfaces, such as glass beads, is less than normal.

Acquired deficiencies of clotting factors are usually multiple and arise most commonly from a deficiency of the vitamin K-dependent factors: II (prothrombin), VII, IX, and X. Lack of intake of vitamin K (newborn children), malabsorption, liver disease, or administration of coumarin drugs may underlie such a deficiency. Orthopaedic complications are rare. Deficiencies of several clotting factors, notably platelets and fibrinogen, may result from diffuse intravascular coagulation (DIC).[104] This alarming situation may arise when thromboplastic substances enter the bloodstream (postpartum, metastatic carcinoma of prostate, etc.), when widespread vascular damage activates the clotting mechanism, and as a rare complication of major surgery. This subject is dealt with in more detail in another section.

Endogenous circulating anticoagulants (inhibitors) cause a hemorrhagic diathesis by interfering with the action of one or more coagulation factors. The commonest is the anticoagulant (anti-Factor VIII) that develops in approximately 20 per cent of hemophiliacs. Other circulating anticoagulants include those found in some cases of lupus erythematosus. Hemorrhagic problems resulting from circulating anticoagulants do not differ clinically from deficiency states, but since they can seldom be corrected by replacement therapy, they are difficult to treat, and surgical intervention is fraught with danger. From a laboratory point of view, the commonest "circulating anticoagulant" is heparin. Its use results in one of the commonest "hemorrhagic disorders" (or non-disease) seen in hospital practice, since it is so commonly used for keeping intravenous tubes open.

Laboratory investigation of the clotting system involves answering four questions:

1. Is anything wrong?
2. Is something missing or is there an anticoagulant?
3. Is the intrinsic or extrinsic pathway affected?
4. Which specific factors are involved?

Numerous laboratory tests of the clotting system are available, from screening tests to specific assays of individual factors. The choice depends on the objective of the investigation and, to a certain extent, on personal preference.

Among the screening tests are the whole blood clotting time, the partial thromboplastin time (PTT), and the one-stage prothrombin time (PT). Whole blood clotting time is a measure of the whole intrinsic pathway. However, as a test it is time-consuming, insensitive, and difficult to standardize. The PTT involves the addition of a contact or activating substance (kaolin, celite, etc.) and a platelet Factor III substitute (partial thromboplastin) to the patient's plasma and measuring the clotting time of the mixture after adding calcium. The PTT tests the whole intrinsic pathway, except for platelet Factor III. The PT requires the addition of tissue thromboplastin (Factor III) to the patient's plasma and measuring the clotting time after adding calcium. The PT tests the whole of the extrinsic pathway. These two tests cover both coagulation pathways and are sensitive to clinically significant abnormalities. Various correction studies *in vitro* are required to distinguish between a deficiency and an anticoagulant; they may also be used to indicate the nature of a deficiency and the point of action of an anticoagulant.

Many other tests of the clotting phase are available; their use is usually predicated on the results of preliminary studies. Fibrinogen may be measured by specific chemical tests, and assays for the other plasma clotting factors are available.

Clot Retraction

The only common cause of failure of clot retraction is thrombocytopenia. Retraction may be estimated by observing a clot 1 hour after it has formed; there are also methods for measuring the activity, but clot retraction is usually an all-or-none phenomenon.

Fibrinolysis and Repair

Excessive fibrinolysis is almost always preceded by coagulation, usually of the diffuse intravascular type. Primary fibrinolysis is a rare disorder, if, indeed, it ever occurs. The hemorrhagic diathesis produced by fibrinolysis is often severe and may be life-threatening. Since fibrinolysis is preceded by DIC, laboratory studies should be aimed at demonstrating (1) a deficiency of factors utilized during hemostasis (platelets and fibrinogen in particular), (2) evidence of excessive fibrinolysis by various clot lysis techniques, and (3) the presence of fibrin and fibrinogen-split products produced by the action of plasmin. Numerous tests are available for detecting the latter.

Factor XIII (fibrin stabilizing factor) deficiency is a rare inherited disorder. Acquired Factor XIII deficiency is seldom, if ever, a clinically significant problem. Laboratory tests for Factor XIII are simple to perform and involve the solubility of "unstable" clots in monochloracetic acid.

Treatment

Hemorrhagic problems and orthopaedic disorders are most frequently associated in two situations; first, the orthopaedic problems associated with hemophilia and hemophilia-like diseases, and secondly, as a complication of operative procedures. In either situation, treatment may be local and systemic. Local therapy is easily forgotten—pressure and topical thrombin may be effective in a hemophiliac as they are in a normal individual!

Systemic therapy in a hemophiliac who has no circulating anti-Factor VIII complicating his disease revolves around the use of various concentrates of Factor VIII.[102,103] Cryoprecipitate from normal plasma contains the Factor VIII from about 250 ml. plasma in about 5 ml. of concentrate and is available from the Red Cross or most blood banks. Commercial concentrates are now comparable in price and efficacy. Replacement therapy with these concentrates enables one to obtain and maintain normal levels of Factor VIII with relative ease, and are used under three main circumstances: (1) prophylactically (a subject still being argued); (2) therapeutically as soon as significant hemorrhage occurs (home care may be used to advantage); and (3) before, during, and after surgical procedures.[100] In the latter, a Factor VIII level close to 100 per cent should be maintained during the operation and for 3 or more days after.

In hemophiliacs with circulating anti-Factor VIII, replacement therapy is often ineffective, and attempts may be made to treat the anti-coagulant with immunosuppressive or cytotoxic drugs.

Von Willebrand's disease is treated like hemophilia, but less concentrate is required to maintain a normal Factor VIII level.

Replacement therapy in other congenital deficiencies is less satisfactory, since many of the concentrates—especially those of vitamin K-dependent Factors (II, VII, IX and X)—contain hepatitis virus.[105] Fresh-frozen plasma or fresh plasma may be required. Acquired deficiencies involving vitamin K-dependent factors should be treated with vitamin K; however, the response may be poor if liver disease is the underlying cause.

Diffuse intravascular coagulation should be treated with heparin if the patient has active bleeding. The fibrinogen and platelet levels usually respond within 24 hours. Epsilon aminocaproic acid (EACA) which inhibits the action of plasmin and therefore might be considered in the treatment of fibrinolysis, should be used with the utmost caution.

Factor XIII deficiency is simply treated by transfusion of 1 or 2 units of plasma. Since the half-life of the factor is very long, the effect of such infusions lasts 2 weeks or more.

Thrombocytopenia severe enough to cause hemorrhage may be temporarily alleviated by platelet concentrates. The platelets from 4 to 8 units of blood are usually required for an adult, and this dose may have to be repeated until hemorrhage ceases or the underlying cause of the thrombocytopenia has been cured.

Summary

This brief review of hemostasis should indicate the complexities that may underlie the diagnosis and treatment of a hemorrhagic diathesis. This very complexity necessitates that a logical approach be developed. The days of "routine bleeding and coag time" are long gone. The choice of the best screening and diagnostic procedures to be used is, to some degree, a matter of personal preference, but certain principles should be kept in mind. From a diagnostic point of view, the history is of paramount importance; leading questions are needed and should cover such aspects as the nature and cause of any bleeding episodes, previous surgery, and a family history. When considering a battery of laboratory tests it must be remembered that a bleeding disorder is not synonymous with a coagulation defect, and the tests should cover the various phases of hemostasis. At a minimum the battery should include a study of the peripheral blood, with emphasis on the platelets (or a platelet count), a PTT and a PT. A logical sequence of investigation beyond the screening studies is best arrived at by close consultation between the laboratory and the clinician. If the patient gives a clear-cut history of excessive bleeding, then further studies should be carried out, even if the results of the screening tests are normal.

In emergency situations the distinction between local anatomic and generalized causes of hemorrhage may not be immediately obvious to the observer. This makes it even more important that sensitive and rapid screening tests should be employed.

THROMBOEMBOLISM

Thromboembolic disease is one of the most common and dangerous of all complications occurring in the orthopaedic patient, not only after skeletal trauma but also after elective major surgery.[135,143,184] Pulmonary emboli were the leading cause of death on the orthopaedic service at Massachusetts General Hospital from 1960 to 1965, excluding those patients who died within a week after severe trauma.[143] Evidence is accumulating that the incidence of pulmonary embolism is actually increasing and that a genuine rise in fatal pulmonary emboli has occurred.[154,163] Pulmonary emboli are now the leading cause of hospital admissions for respiratory disease, excluding pneumonia. The threat of thromboembolism increases with the age of patients, the extent and duration of the surgical procedure, the degree and length of immobilization, and the severity of the underlying systemic disease.[121,122] As the number of older patients undergoing major joint replacement increases, the incidence of the disease will rise.

It is difficult to ascertain the true incidence of thromboembolic disease. It is probably higher in most European countries and North America than in Africa, Asia, and South America.[177] Clinical investigators and, in particular, those using retrospective analysis, have grossly underestimated the incidence of thromboembolic disease. Orthopaedic surgeons have tended to deny that thromboembolic disease is a major problem. Such an outlook is not only incorrect but dangerous. In one autopsy study of 161 patients who died after hip fractures, 38 per cent died from pulmonary emboli.[135] In direct contrast, pulmonary embolism was thought to be the cause of death in only 2 per cent of 87 patients with hip fractures, but without an autopsy. Table 4-2 illustrates the high incidence of thromboembolism associated with fractures of the hip or lower extremities and pelvis. It is important to recognize that general

Table 4-2. Thromboembolism Associated with Fractures of the Hip or Lower Extremities or Pelvis

Author	Injury	Number of Patients	Thromboembolism (per cent)
Sevitt and Gallagher[178]	Hip fractures	319	39.3
Tubiana and Duparc[184]	Hip fractures	389	15.0
Fagan[134]	Hip fractures	162	28.7
Solonen[183]	Fractures of lower extremities	178	21.3
Neu and associates[166]	Fractures of pelvis, lower extremities	100	20.0
Salzman and associates[175]	Hip fractures	184	26.0
Freeark and associates[137]	Hip fractures	70	42.0*
Hamilton and associates[142]	Hip fractures	38	48.0*
Sevitt and Gallagher[179]	Fractures	468	20.3
Golodner and associates[140]	Hip fractures	25	36.0

* Diagnosis of venous thrombosis confirmed by venography

surgical patients are at less risk of thromboembolic disease than orthopaedic patients. Any study undertaken on the incidence, treatment, and prophylaxis of thromboembolic disease must be prospective, and the diagnosis must be established by phlebography or I^{125} fibrinogen uptake studies. The magnitude of the problem is such that at least 50 per cent of patients undergoing elective major joint replacement surgery, or sustaining fractures, develop deep venous thrombosis. Ten per cent of these patients run the risk of pulmonary emboli, and unless adequate protection is provided 2 per cent will die from fatal pulmonary emboli.[144]

Preventing thromboembolism is much preferred to treating it, as anticoagulation therapy beginning after the diagnosis of deep venous thrombosis has been made may *not* significantly decrease the incidence of pulmonary emboli.[157] The most effective treatment is prophylactic rather than therapeutic.

Thrombogenesis

Historically the basis for understanding thrombosis began more than a century ago when Virchow[185] provided a conceptual framework of thrombogenesis, Virchow's triad, that still remains valid. He stated that thrombosis may result from (1) changes in the vessel wall, (2) changes in the blood composition, or (3) changes in blood flow or stasis. Early research placed emphasis upon the role of plasma coagulation factors in thrombus formation.[126] Two types of thrombi were proposed, each with a different pathogenesis: first, the red thrombus composed primarily of erythrocytes and fibrin and characteristically forming in areas of venous stasis or retarded flow; second, the white thrombus—composed primarily of leukocytes and fibrin, relatively poor in erythrocytes, and found almost exclusively in areas adjacent to injured vessel wall or in areas of rapid arterial flow. The role of the platelet was thought to be secondary in the formation of a red (venous) thrombus. Controversy existed as to whether the activation of a clotting mechanism preceded or followed the development of a mural platelet thrombus as the first stage of thrombus formation, not only in the arterial but also in the venous system.[130] In addition a number of studies have demonstrated abnormalities of platelet adhesiveness and survival time and alteration in fibrinolysis in patients in whom postoperative thromboembolism develops.[120,146,156] The available evidence suggests that the activation of the venous thrombus may follow the formation of a small platelet nidus, thereby providing a common pathogenesis with its arterial counterpart.[147]

The cascade or waterfall mechanism for thrombus formation (Fig. 4-9) begins with adhesion of platelets to the exposed collagen in the damaged vessel wall. A series of morphological and biochemical changes occur via a chain of enzymatic steps. Adenosine diphosphate is released, causing platelet aggregation, and the thromboplastic vasolipid lipoprotein compound is activated. The clotting process then proceeds to thrombus formation (Fig. 4-9).

The exact sequence of events leading to thrombus formation after skeletal trauma or orthopaedic surgical procedures is not completely understood. Little is known about the types of thrombi that are prone to pulmonary emboli or that cause valvular damage and the postphlebitic syndrome. The pathogenesis of thrombosis remains elusive, despite extensive experimental work. More inquiry is required into the dynamics of peripheral clot formation.[111] In a study of 132 patients undergoing elective surgery, postoperative venous thrombosis developed in 40 patients.[150] Fourteen of the 40 clots disappeared within 72 hours of surgery; 17 of the 40 were localized in the calf veins, nine of the 40 showed extension, and four of the 40 (or 10 per cent) resulted in pulmonary emboli. Venography, autopsy studies, and I^{125}-labeled fibrinogen studies helped substantiate the viewpoint that thromboses primarily begin in the calf

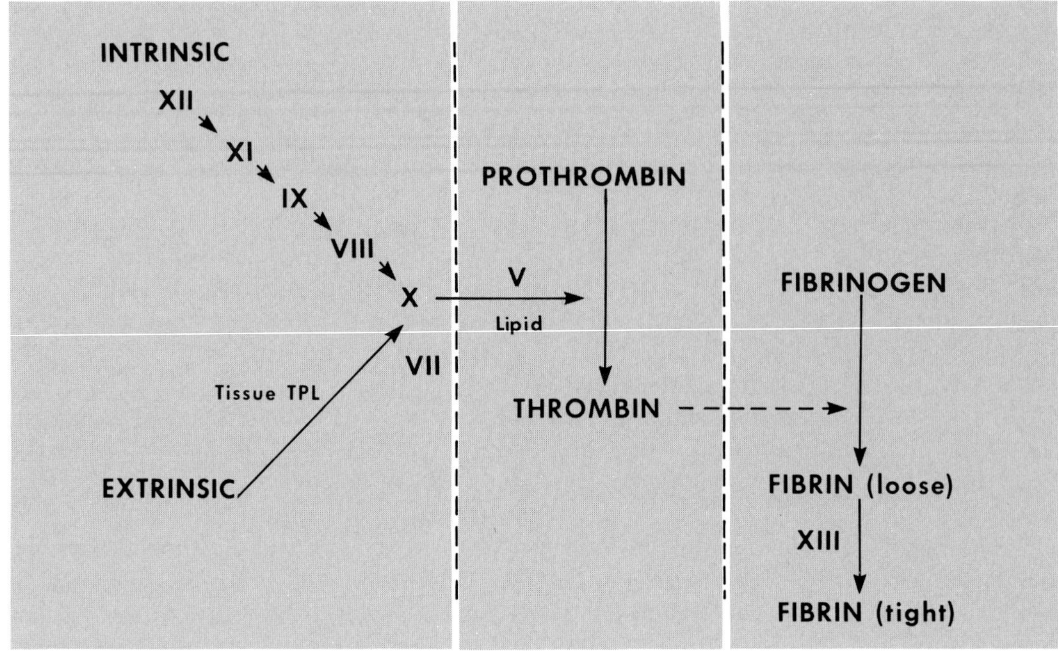

Fig. 4-9. Blood coagulation mechanism.

and later propagate into the popliteal and femoral veins. It is of great interest that Flanc and his associates[136] have shown that venous thrombosis is present in patients returning from elective surgery, strongly suggesting that the thrombotic process actually begins during surgery. In their study of 96 patients the I^{125}-labeled fibrinogen technique was employed for diagnosis, and the results were confirmed by venography. Thromboses developed in 35 per cent of patients; 50 per cent of the thromboses first developed during the operative procedure. This indicates that greater attention should be given to the administration of prophylactic agents before—and certainly during—the operative procedure. It is known that changes in platelet adhesiveness occur after elective hip surgery as well as after trauma. In view of the primary role of platelet adhesion and aggregation in thrombosis formation, an attempt can be made to alter these factors and suppress the development of thrombi. The usual anticoagulants, heparin and dicumarol, do not effectively suppress platelet surface reactions or ADP-induced platelet aggregation. These agents are effective only in preventing the growth phase of the thrombus and in decreasing the diffuse clotting effect.[110,112,138,164]

Diagnosis

Because the clinical signs and symptoms of deep venous thrombosis are notoriously unreliable, the detection of venous thrombosis cannot be based on clinical findings alone.[133] However, accurate evaluation of possible clot formation requires careful clinical observation, checking the calf and the remainder of the lower extremity daily for pain, swelling, and tenderness, accompanied by an increase in temperature and pulse rate. Such signs, if present, cannot be ignored but rather are an indication for further investigation of the possibility of deep venous thrombosis. At least one-half of the patients who develop deep venous thrombosis cannot be diagnosed clinically.[123]

Venography remains the standard of detection.[124] The lesser saphenous veins or subcutaneous veins of the foot provide excellent portals of entry to the venous system for the injection of the opaque medium used in venography. Current techniques allow for the identification of the soleal veins as well as the other calf veins and vessels of the lower extremity. The diagnosis of venous thrombosis depends upon certain signs: (1) constant filling defects, (2) abrupt termination of the opaque contrast medium column occurring at a constant site, (3) nonfilling defects of the entire deep system, and (4) diversion of flow.[168] Rabinov and Paulin[173] believe that the most direct sign of thrombosis is demonstration of the thrombus itself. The other three signs (i.e., abrupt termination of the opaque column, the nonfilling, and flow diversion) reflect obstruction to venous flow and are indirect signs.[125] The artifacts that occur with phlebography include underfilling, dilution, and streamlining. It is thought that a loose, potentially removable thrombus produces a ground-glass type of shadow and the contrast medium can be seen between the thrombus and the vein wall. If the thrombus is older and fixed, the affected vein disappears on roentgenography, and often dilated collateral veins appear more prominent. In one study, despite careful clinical examination by members of the peripheral vascular disease department, 30 of 37 cases (81 per cent) of postoperative venous thromboses were overlooked.[133] It remained for venography to demonstrate the presence of venous thrombosis in these patients.

Another technique for the detection of venous thrombosis in the lower extremity employs radioactive iodine-labeled fibrinogen.[109,149,165,170] This method is based on the principle that if labeled fibrinogen is injected intravenously it behaves *in vivo* as unlabeled fibrinogen and is converted into fibrin in any thrombotic process. The I^{125}-labeled fibrinogen accumulates in the thrombus and can be detected by a scintillation counter placed over the affected area. However, this technique may give false positive or false negative results in the area of a femoral artery or venous pooling in the calf. It cannot be used in the vicinity of a large wound and, hence, is impractical following major hip surgery. It cannot detect thrombosis in the upper thigh or iliac or deep pelvic veins, which represents a significant drawback. The human fibrinogen used in this procedure has the risk of transmitting serum hepatitis. This is avoided in part by obtaining the human fibrinogen from a restricted pool of donors who are screened by laboratory testing (including Australia antigens) to eliminate the possibility of the presence of viral hepatitis.[116] The accuracy of the method in detecting thrombi in the legs compares favorably to that of venography—90 to 95 per cent. It has been used widely in Great Britain for the detection of venous thrombosis.

Another screening test for the detection of deep venous thrombosis is based upon the use of an ultrasound flowmeter utilizing the Doppler effect, a noninvasive technique for detecting blood flow.[180,181] The patency of major veins can be examined. However, the obvious disadvantage is that small thrombi beginning in the calf or extending to the thigh veins cannot be detected. The test is inaccurate also for diagnosis in a large hip wound. Great sophistication is required in the technical aspects of its use, and the good results obtained by certain authors are not easily duplicated. The ultrasound technique is 76 to 93 per cent accurate as recorded by various studies.

Impedance phlebography is another method that has been suggested for the diagnosis of deep venous thrombosis.[189] This technique has been found to be quite inaccurate when compared with venography. It is technically difficult to perform on patients with hip pain and with a restricted range of hip motion. The impedance technique is only 53 to 88 per cent accurate.

As the techniques for the diagnosis for deep venous thrombosis have become more sophisticated it has been recognized that the detection of pulmonary embolism is equally inaccurate when based on the usual clinical roentgenographic, biochemical, and electrocardiographic criteria.[171,186] The diagnosis of pulmonary embolism during life is often impossible because of the absence of characteristic signs and symptoms or the explanation of certain signs and symptoms by alternative diagnosis. Smith, Dammin, and Dexter[182] estimated that pulmonary embolism is diagnosed before death in less than 50 per cent of cases. A retrospective study showed that many deaths occurred from pulmonary embolism which could have been prevented by anticoagulation.[172] Results of retrospective studies on pulmonary embolism are grossly inaccurate because of the inaccurate methods of routine autopsy. In 136 cases, Morrell and Dunnill[162] reported a 52 per cent incidence of pulmonary emboli in 263 right lungs. In the same study they found that the incidence of pulmonary embolism increased with age and that there was a distinct association between pulmonary embolism and the operation. In 14 per cent of the total number, death was entirely attributable to the embolism. The reported incidence in retrospective studies is approximately 10 to 18 per cent. Hildner and Ormand[145] stated that the majority of cases of pulmonary embolism were not identified by symptoms, physical findings, electrocardiographic examination, serum enzyme determinations, or chest roentgenography. A catheter technique of interruption of the inferior vena cava has been employed for prevention of pulmonary embolism.[161]

Radioisotope lung scanning has been employed to investigate the regional pulmonary blood flow to help determine the presence of perfusion defects.[160] However, it is difficult to differentiate the causes of such perfusion defects. If one combines a perfusion defect with a normal plain chest roentgenogram, along with the symptoms and signs of dyspnea, tachypnea, chest pain, cough, hemoptysis, cyanosis, tachycardia, fever, and early heart failure, the combination is highly suggestive of pulmonary embolism.

Pulmonary angiography is the most accurate diagnostic method of detecting pulmonary embolism.[114] The primary positive signs are the trailing edges of vascular occlusions within an arterial network of the lung and intraluminal defects outlined by a contrast material within the lung. There are associated secondary signs, nonfilling of vessels, areas of slow perfusion, vascular tortuosity, and delay in the clearance of contrast medium. Most orthopaedic services do not routinely employ these more sophisticated techniques in the diagnosis of pulmonary embolism.

Greater emphasis must be placed on the identification of the presence of a pulmonary embolus. Chest roentgenograms are obtained on all patients suspected of having a deep venous thrombosis or on patients with positive venograms or fibrinogen scans. If the chest roentgenograms are normal, scintograms of the lungs are obtained in an attempt to detect silent pulmonary emboli. If the diagnosis of pulmonary embolism can be made from the clinical picture, no further testing is necessary. If the chest roentgenograms are abnormal, pulmonary angiography may be requested to detect the presence of pulmonary emboli. Angiography and lung scanning are complementary studies; both should be performed when necessary and correlated with the plain chest roentgenogram.

Treatment

The hallmark of the treatment of thromboembolic disease is prevention. To approach the problem by beginning treatment after the fact is inappropriate. Rather, a profile of the orthopaedic patient in whom thromboembolic disease is likely to develop should be established. The archetype is an obese, elderly person with multiple injuries or operations and a history of associated cardiovascular or pulmonary disease who is about to undergo major operation. It has been statistically proved that two agents, crystalline sodium warfarin (Coumadin), an anticoagulant, and low-molecular-weight dextran, an antiplatelet agent, reduce the risk of thromboembolic disease when given prophylactically.[133,144] Both regimens require meticulous attention to detail. Ten mg. of Coumadin should be administered the evening prior to surgery. The prothrombin time must be obtained after surgery, and Coumadin is given the night of surgery, the usual dose being 5 mg. The daily maintenance dose is from 5 to 7 mg. per day, administered intramuscularly until the patient is able to take it orally. The prothrombin time should be maintained at 1½ times the control value. Harris and associates[144] in their studies of thromboembolic disease in orthopaedic surgery, have shown that this method is effective in the prevention of thromboembolic disease.

The use of Coumadin is contraindicated in patients with hemorrhagic disorders, peptic ulceration, active liver disease, hematuria, melena, hemoptysis, cerebral insufficiency, or a history of infarct. Certain drugs might decrease the effectiveness of Coumadin, for instance, aspirin, phenylbutazone, and barbiturates. After administration of Coumadin it is essential to obtain stool guaiac examinations periodically, hematocrit values three times per week, and prothrombin times daily.

Complications such as hemorrhage at the wound site, gastrointestinal bleeding, renal bleeding, and cerebral bleeding have occurred, along with the difficulty in administration and control of Coumadin anticoagulation.

The primary role of platelet adhesiveness and aggregation of thrombus formation has been emphasized previously. There is much to suggest that platelet activity underlies the initiation and propagation of venous thrombi.[127] In a search for safer and more reliable agents to prevent thromboembolism attention was directed toward the dextran solutions. In 1944 Gronwall and Ingleman[141] developed fractionate dextran as a plasma volume expander. Bull and associates[117] confirmed the clinical value of dextran and Bloom[113] prepared the first dextran in America and demonstrated its value as a blood volume expander. The dextrans represented a group of polysaccharides containing D-glucose units with predominantly 1:6 linkage. Clinical dextrans are glucose polymers containing a broad molecular weight distribution composed of the average molecular weight fractions, either low molecular dextran (average molecular weight 40,000) or clinical dextran (average molecular weight 70,000).

The antithrombotic actions of dextran have been studied extensively, both experimentally[108,115,129,148] and clinically.[152,174,190] Dextrans decreased thrombus formation after arterial surgery. In experimentally damaged large veins, dextran decreased the incidence of thrombosis.[148] The effects of dextran on the behavior of platelets were investigated with a ruby biolaser in the arterioles in the chambers of rabbits' ears.[108] It has been demonstrated that low-molecular-weight dextran increases cardiac output and reduces the mean transit time.[131] These changes are the result of plasma volume expansion and the reduction of blood viscosity due to hemodilution. Low-molecular-weight dextran causes a significant reduction in platelet adhesiveness, in part due to absorption on platelets and the alteration of their membranes, interaction of the plasma proteins, and coating of the endothelial walls. Following intravenous administration of low-molecular-weight dextran a change in electrophoretic mobility of the platelet occurs.[118,119] There appears to be no difference between antithrombotic effects of low-molecular-weight dextran in comparison with clinical dextran.

The efficacy of low-molecular-weight dextran as a prophylactic against thromboemboli has been demonstrated in clinical studies (Table 4-3).[133,153,176]

Low-molecular-weight dextran should be administered at least 2 to 4 hours before surgery and continued during and after surgery. One liter should be given on the day of surgery and for the next 2 days by continuous intravenous infusion. The dosage is then reduced to 500 ml. per day to

Table 4-3. Prevention of Thromboembolism

	Total Cases	No. Cases LMWD	Deep Venous Thrombosis	Pulmonary Embolus
Evarts, 1971[133]*	106	50	7	2
Langsjoen, 1971[153]	73	37	0	0
Salzman and associates, 1971[176]	169	49	5	2
Harris and associates, 1972[144]	227	113	7	2
Evarts, 1974	500	500	22	5†
	1075	749	41 (5.7%)	11 (1.5%)

* Detection of deep venous thrombosis by venography. Control incidence of 53.6 per cent of venous thrombosis.

† None fatal.

be given by continuous intravenous infusion until the patient is fully ambulatory.

Contraindications to the use of low-molecular-weight dextran are pulmonary edema, congestive heart failure, renal failure, severe dehydration, and allergic manifestations. Hypersensitivity reactions can range from mild cutaneous eruptions to generalized urticaria, nausea and vomiting, wheezing, and (rarely) to anaphylactic shock. Such reactions almost always develop in the first few minutes following initiation of therapy. Therefore, the patient should be observed closely during the initial infusion. If any of the above adverse symptoms or signs appear, the infusion should be stopped immediately. Therapy to counteract anaphylactoid shock, including epinephrine, steroids, and antihistamines, should be started promptly. Problems can occur with fluid overload following dextran administration. The cardiac status should be evaluated carefully before operation and should be monitored during surgery and postoperatively. Fluid and electrolyte balance must be maintained with the administration of low-molecular-weight dextran. If large amounts are given in the face of decreased urinary output, congestive heart failure and pulmonary edema may occur. A renal profile must be obtained preoperatively, and if chronic renal dysfunction is suspected its administration should be avoided. Renal failure has occurred after the administration of low-molecular-weight dextran, and renal dialysis has been required to save some patients.[133] Other complications are those of anaphylactoid reactions and congestive heart failure. Although other antiplatelet agents, such as aspirin and glyceryl glycolate, have been suggested for the prevention of thromboembolic disease, further proof is needed to substantiate their effectiveness. [128,169,187]

Recently much attention has been given to the role of minidose heparin in the prevention of thromboembolic disease.[139,151,167] Following the identification of a potent, naturally occurring inhibitor to activated Factor X and the recognition of the response by such a factor to minidose heparin, it was suggested that minidose heparin might prevent thrombus formation.[188] The anticoagulant effect of the inhibitor to activated Factor X is markedly influenced by trace amounts of heparin *in vitro*. One μg. of the inhibitor, by neutralizing 32 units of activated Factor X, indirectly prevents the generation of 1600 NIH units of thrombin. Activated Factor X may be a more potent thrombogenic agent than thrombin itself. However, in a study in which 5,000 international units (IU) of heparin were given subcutaneously 2 hours preoperatively, 5,000 IU postoperatively the night of surgery, and every 12 hours for the next 7 to 10 days, venous thrombosis developed in 7 of 25 patients.[132] Pulmonary embolism occurred in 6 of these patients undergoing total hip reconstruction. Apparently the blood levels of heparin were not sufficiently high to exert a prophylactic effect. It may be that the increased trauma of surgery in total hip reconstruction requires higher levels of minidose heparin in the blood. Further controlled studies with varying dosage and including the measurements of heparin levels *in vitro* are required before the efficacy of low-dose heparin in the prevention of thromboembolism will be proved.

As soon as the diagnosis of pulmonary embolism is established, treatment should begin with 10,000 to 15,000 IU of heparin (aqueous heparin sodium injection administered intravenously every 4 to 6 hours for 24 hours). The dosage of heparin is then decreased to 5,000 to 10,000 IU administered intravenously every 4 to 6 hours for 48 hours. The dosage of heparin is decreased during the next 72 hours, and Coumadin (10 to 20 mg. per day for 7 days) is begun. Coumadin is continued for 3 to 6 months. Infrequently, there may be certain indications for pulmonary embolectomy, namely, persistent hypotension, persistent cyanosis, and pulmonary arteriographic evidence of massive pulmonary embolism.[155] The initial treatment of an acute pulmonary embolism involves closed chest cardiac massage, the immediate administration of heparin, positive pressure ventilation, and vasopressors. If the patient survives, then pulmonary embolectomy may be indicated. Again, although infrequently, there are certain indications for surgical venous interruption.[158,159] These involve suppurative venous thromboembolism, microembolic clots with cor pulmonale, failure of anticoagulants to control thromboembolic episodes, and, in certain instances, when anticoagulants and antiplatelet agents are contraindicated.

Summary

It is imperative that the orthopaedic surgeon dealing with skeletal trauma and disorders recognizes the magnitude of the problem of thromboembolic disease. It is the most common disease following trauma or surgical procedures. It has been shown that at least 50 per cent of patients develop deep venous thrombosis and that 2 per cent of all untreated patients die from pulmonary embolism following elective hip surgery, including total hip reconstruction. A much higher percentage die from pulmonary embolism following trauma. A diagnosis of thromboembolism can be confirmed by venography or I^{125}-labeled fibrinogen scans.

Prophylaxis remains the cornerstone of treatment. The prevention of thromboembolism depends upon maintaining mobility and activity in the injured patient or the patient who has undergone operation, using elastic compression, elevating the lower limbs, prescribing anticoagulant therapy given orally, and the antiplatelet agent, low-molecular-weight dextran.

The severity of the problem of thromboembolism is of great concern. The search continues for the ideal oral agent to eliminate the disease.

DISSEMINATED INTRAVASCULAR COAGULATION

Disseminated intravascular coagulation is the term given to a group of bleeding states of diverse etiology. It frequently represents an acute bleeding state (the consequence of an extremely complex disarray of the hemostatic mechanism) in which acceleration, coagulation, and activation of the fibrinolytic system functioning in a patient result in varying degrees of thrombosis and bleeding.[193] It has been implicated in the causes of unexplained bleeding in a variety of clinical syndromes.[191,196,197,199,203,204,206,210] It has been called the defibrination syndrome, the fibrination syndrome, and consumption coagulopathy,[200] primarily because of the many ways in which the disorder presents to the clinician.

Disseminated intravascular coagulation may occur as a consequence of cardiac arrest, the fat embolism syndrome, sepsis, thromboembolic disease, neoplastic disease, mismatched blood, or after massive blood transfusions. In the orthopaedic patient, its manifestations may be obscured, making the diagnosis difficult to establish. With an increase in the frequency and complexity of certain orthopaedic procedures and the increase in patients with multiple injuries, the orthopaedic surgeon should be familiar with this syndrome.

Clinical Conditions Associated with Disseminated Intravascular Coagulation

A. Acute
  1. Shock
     Hemorrhagic
     Cardiogenic
     Neurogenic
     Septic
  2. Acute intravascular hemolysis
     Incompatible blood transfusion
     Hemoglobinuria
  3. Acute pulmonary embolism
  4. Burns
  5. Snake bites
  6. Transplant rejection

B. Subacute
  1. Malignancy
  2. Obstetrical
  3. Local thrombosis

C. Chronic
  1. Giant hemangioma
  2. Cavernous vessel transformation

(Merskey, C.: Clinical conditions associated with defibrination. *In* Biggs, R. (ed.): Human Blood Coagulation, Hemostasis, and Thrombosis. Oxford, Blackwell Scientific Publications, 1972)

Pathogenesis

Deykin[193] believes that the central pathologic process is a response to an underlying disorder resulting in a generalized activation of the hemostatic mechanism. The activation extends beyond that expected with local vascular injury.[192] Changes occur in the fibrinogen and other clotting factors to activate the fibrinolytic system. A striking feature of disseminated intravascular coagulation is the reduced level of plasma fibrinogen. Two proteolytic enzymes derived from plasma—thrombin and plasmin—act upon fibrinogen. Plasmin digests fibrinogen, fibrin, and certain intermediate products forming the fibrin degradation products (FDP). These products interfere with hemostasis in a number of ways causing abnormal results in blood coagulation.[194,208,209] As a result of the complex interaction of the many factors involved with disseminated intravascular coagulation, a variable amount of thrombin and plasmin may be produced and thrombocytopenia may occur.

Clinical Characteristics

The clinical characteristics are those of the underlying disorder with superimposed thrombosis, hemorrhage, and anemia. Ecchymosis and severe bleeding may be present. Excessive bleeding from nonoperative sites may provide a clue to the diagnosis. If unexpected bleeding occurs during or after surgery, disseminated intravascular coagulation might have occurred. It should be suspected if unexplained respiratory or renal failure occurs immediately after injury or during the postoperative period.

Laboratory Studies

The laboratory tests that aid in the diagnosis of disseminated intravascular coagulation have been divided into three categories by Deykin:[193] (1) clotting assays, (2) cellular studies, and (3) fibrinolytic studies (Table 4-4).

The prothrombin and activated partial prothrombin times are usually abnormal, and a small, fragile clot may be present in disseminated intravascular coagulation. The assay of the plasmin fibrinogen level is subject to many difficulties. If measurable it is usually depressed. The thrombin clotting time is one of the most valuable diagnostic tests in disseminated intravascular coagulation and is generally prolonged.[193] The coagulation factor levels tend to be reduced,

Table 4-4. Basic Tests for Disseminated Intravascular Coagulation

Test	Positive Result
Clotting assays	
Prothrombin time	Minimally to grossly prolonged
Activated partial thromboplastin time	Variable (short, normal, long)
Fibrinogen*	Usually depressed
Thrombin time*	Usually prolonged
Factor analysis	Variable (low, normal, elevated)
Cellular	
Platelet count*	Usually depressed
Red cell morphology	Often abnormal
Fibrinolytic	
Fibrinogen-degradation products*	Usually present
Plasminogen	Usually depressed
Euglobulin lysis time	Variable (often long, sometimes short)
Serial thrombin time	Variable (often prolonged)
Paracoagulation	Often positive (low specificity)

* Rapid, usually diagnostic, but may be result of liver disease

(Merskey, C.: Clinical conditions associated with defibrination. *In* Biggs, R. (ed.): Human Blood Coagulation, Hemostasis, and Thrombosis. Oxford, Blackwell Scientific Publications, 1972)

but in some instances elevated levels can occur. Factors V and VIII are reduced in severe cases of disseminated intravascular coagulation. Platelet counts are often depressed, and red blood cell morphology may be disrupted, resulting in the presence of histiocytes. In many cases plasminogen levels are depressed and fibrinogen degradation products are present.[198] Numerous tests are available for detecting the latter, including a protamine paracoagulation test and immunologic latex aggregation test.

In certain cases diagnostic problems are encountered in patients with little change in fibrinogen levels or other blood coagulation factors. In this situation the diagnosis of disseminated intravascular coagulation may have to be made in the presence of a prolonged clotting time, FDP in the serum, and the response to heparin therapy.

The differential diagnosis rests with distinguishing disseminated intravascular coagulation from acute hypofibrinogenemia secondary to severe hepatocellular disease or idiopathic pathologic fibrinolysis.[202]

In a series of twelve patients in whom unexplained bleeding developed during or after a surgical procedure, disseminated intravascular coagulation was thought to have occurred.[191] The overall mortality was 83 per cent. The coagulopathy that occurred was characterized by thrombocytopenia in 11 patients, fibrinogenemia in seven patients. Also, fibrinogen levels, the prothrombin activity, and clotting Factors II, V, VII, VIII, IX, and X were reduced. Fibrin degradation products were present in 11 patients. Postmortem examination showed macrothromboemboli, microthromboemboli, bronchopneumonia, and acute tubular necrosis of the kidneys.

Treatment

The treatment of disseminated intravascular coagulation must be directed primarily at the intravascular coagulation. The treatment of choice is the administration of heparin.[193,195,201,202,205] It has been shown to cause a rapid return to normal of the clotting mechanism abnormalities with the cessation of severe bleeding. In some instances the use of heparin has been life-saving. An initial dose of 50 to 100 units per kg. of body weight and a maintenance dose of 10 to 15 units per kg. per hour should be given by intravenous drip. The diagnosis of disseminated intravascular coagulation must be accurate, since heparin is harmful to patients in shock who do not have disseminated intravascular coagulation. The use of fibrinolytic inhibitors, such as epsilon aminocaproic acid, appears to be contraindicated in the management of disseminated intravascular coagulation, because intravascular thrombosis may result.[207] Therapy can be monitored by laboratory studies early in the course of treatment. Less fibrinogen degradation will be present, and the prothrombin time will return toward normal. As treatment continues an increase in platelets and fibrinogen levels may be found.

Summary

The diagnosis of disseminated intravascular coagulation is being made with greater frequency in the orthopaedic patient. In certain victims of massive trauma or in patients who have undergone major surgical procedures, disseminated intravascular coagulation may occur. The orthopaedic surgeon should be aware of its diagnosis and management. Currently, heparin is a potent but effective therapy.

FAT EMBOLISM

The fat embolism syndrome is one of the important causes of morbidity and mortality following fractures in the patient with multiple injuries. For more than a century the puzzling features of this entity have interested many. The relatively recent increase in highway accidents has resulted in an increasing number of patients with the fat embolism syndrome. Its relationship to skeletal and soft-tissue injury is well recognized, and many cases have been reported.[269] However, the fat embolism syndrome is not always a sequela of trauma. It has been reported in association with a variety of nontraumatic entities including hemoglobinopathy,[243] collagen disease,[248] diabetes,[229] burns,[231] severe infection,[259] inhalation anesthesia,[292] metabolic disorders,[249] neoplasms, osteomyelitis,[223,238] blood transfusion,[258] cardiopulmonary bypass,[264] renal infarction,[225] decompression due to altitude,[247] and renal homotransplantation.[251] In the past 15 years a better understanding of the underlying pathophysiologic mechanisms of the fat embolism syndrome has developed.[234]

Much attention has been given recently to the observations of Sproule, Brady, and Gilbert,[282] who identified the role of fat embolism in posttraumatic respiratory insufficiency. They have established that fat embolism must be recognized as one of the respiratory distress syndromes. With prompt recognition the treatment of the fat embolism syndrome has become more specific and less empiric, resulting in a decrease in morbidity and mortality.

Historical Aspects

In 1862 Zenker[296] described fat droplets in the lung capillaries of a railroad worker who sustained a fatal thoracoabdominal crush injury. In 1865 Wagner[288] described the pathologic features of fat embolism. However, in 1873 Bergmann[219] was the first to establish the clinical diagnosis of fat embolism in a 38-year-old patient who sustained a comminuted fracture of the distal femur. Postmortem examination revealed a large amount of pulmonary fat. In 1875 Czerny[230] called attention to the symptoms associated with cerebral fat embolism and noted the importance of a funduscopic examination. In 1879 Fenger and Salisbury[237] from Cook County Hospital made the first clinical diagnosis of fat embolism syndrome in the United States in a patient who had a proximal femoral fracture. Autopsy examination revealed massive fat emboli in the lungs and brain.

In 1879 Scriba[276] reviewed and correlated the clinical, pathologic, and experimental observations of the fat embolism syndrome. In 1911 Benestad[216] and Grondahl[244] first described a petechial rash seen with fat embolism syndrome. Warthin,[290] in 1913; Gauss,[240] in 1916; Lehman and Moore,[255] in 1927; Vance,[287] in 1931; and Scuder,[277] in 1941, presented review papers and experimental evidence on the origin and nature of intravenous fat globules, the frequency and importance of fat embolism, and the clinical entity of cerebral fat embolism. In 1957, 1969, and 1971 Peltier[268,270,271] appraised the problem of fat embolism and has continued his investigations and established the importance of pulmonary fat embolism. Sproule, Brady, and Gilbert[282] were the first to report severe arterial hypoxemia in three patients with the fat embolism syndrome. Ashbaugh and Petty,[214] in 1963, described the respiratory distress syndrome and emphasized the use of corticosteroids in the treatment of the respiratory complications of fat embolism syndrome.

Incidence

The exact incidence and mortality of the fat embolism syndrome is not known. It is difficult to assemble a statistically significant controlled study on the factors. Sutton[283] stated that 10 per cent of battle casualties in World War I suffered fat emboli. In World War II a postmortem study of 60 patients who died from battle wounds revealed a 65 per cent incidence of fat emboli.[295] In a study of 5,245 civilian accident victims, fat emboli occurred in 855 and contributed to death in over half.[239] It has been estimated that 800 deaths as a result of highway accidents in Britain occur because of the fat embolism syndrome.[266] Recent clinical studies,[211,220,222,260,265,274,286,294] including a review of posttraumatic fat embolism in children,[232,293] have served to document the frequent occurrence of this syndrome as a sequela to trauma, especially in patients with multiple fractures. It is apparent that increases in auto accidents, motorcycle accidents, snowmobile accidents, and other types of trauma, will lead to an increased frequency of the fat embolism syndrome. Also, the greatest risk of the fat embolism syndrome occurs with multiple fractures.[233] The mortality has been estimated to be as high as 50 per cent. The fat embolism syndrome has become a frequent, serious, and often fatal complication of trauma, both on the battlefield and in civilian life.

Pathogenesis

The pathogenesis of the fat embolism syndrome continues to be the subject of conjecture and controversy. The source of the embolic fat is thought by some to be the bone marrow.[241] The early German writers believed that the fat originated at the site of skeletal injury where free fat was liberated and forced into the vascular channels by the increased interstitial pressure.[240] Bone marrow or fragments have been demonstrated in lung sections indicating that mechanical fat embolization does indeed occur.[213,246,263,291] Fat globules and free fatty acids have been demonstrated intravascularly after skeletal trauma.[250,285,289] Experimental fat emboli following skeletal trauma appear to contain material similar to marrow fat.[221]

However, there is more recent evidence that the fat embolism syndrome can occur via other mechanisms in the absence of skeletal trauma.[218] The blood lipid changes during stress in combination with the changes that occur in the blood coagulation system may result in coalescence of chylomicrons into larger fat droplets.[253,275,281] The physiochemical theory of fat embolism postulates that the changes that occur in lipid stability after trauma and the alteration of the microcirculatory flow patterns combine to result in inadequate tissue perfusion, subsequent tissue hypoxia, and the fat embolism syndrome.[256,257] More than one possibility exists for the source of the embolic fat and the causes *are not* mutually exclusive.

Clinical Manifestations

The most common etiologic factor associated with the fat embolism syndrome is a long-bone fracture in a patient in the second or third decade, when tibial or femoral fractures are likely to occur, and in the patient in the sixth or seventh decade, when fractures of the hip are frequent. The onset of the clinical symptoms may be immediate or may not occur for 2 or 3 days following trauma.[236] Sevitt[278] stated that 25 of 100 patients with fat embolism showed symptoms within the first 12 hours after injury; by 36 hours, 75, and within 48 hours after injury 85 patients demonstrated symptoms. In the earlier literature, however, emphasis was placed upon the lucid interval; this in-

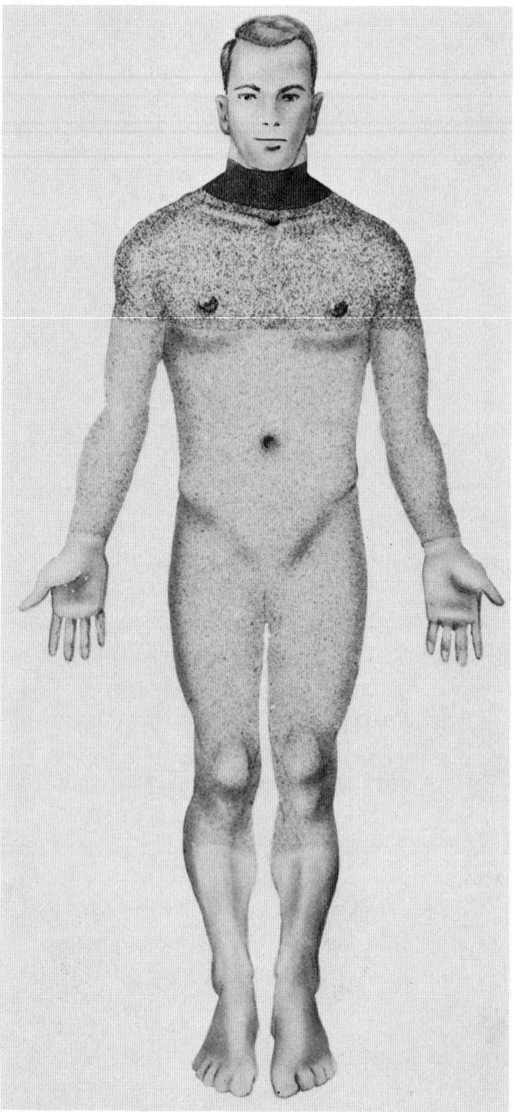

Fig. 4-10. Sites of petechial rash in the fat embolism syndrome. (Evarts, C. M.: Surg. Clin. N. Amer., *50*:493-507, 1970)

terval may be more apparent than real. It is difficult to diagnose a fulminating and rapidly progressing case that terminates in death and is associated with multiple fractures. Coma develops rapidly and is accompanied by marked respiratory distress. Occasionally the patient may demonstrate hemoptysis, and pulmonary edema may become manifest. Often the symptoms and signs of fat embolism syndrome are masked by shock, coma, or by an anesthetized state in a patient undergoing early operative treatment.

On the other hand, it is also likely that many cases of mild fat embolism syndrome are overlooked. The phenomenon called fracture fever, or hematoma fever, in the early postinjury state may be an unrecognized, mild variety of fat embolism syndrome.[236]

Certain features about fat embolism syndrome allow its early clinical recognition. Symptoms are shortness of breath, which may begin relatively suddenly, followed by restlessness and confusion. The patient often becomes obstreperous and difficult to manage. The clinical signs associated with the fat embolism syndrome involve temperature elevation to 39 or 40 degrees C; tachypnea, with rates of 30/minute or higher reflecting the hypoxia that is occurring within the pulmonary bed; and tachycardia with rates of 140/minute or higher. Blood pressure does not vary widely and usually remains within normal limits. Another striking feature or clinical sign of fat embolism syndrome is that of the changing neurological symptoms; the onset of restlessness, disorientation followed by marked confusion, stupor, or coma.[254] Long tract signs may be present with occasional extensor posturing and decerebrate rigidity. These neurological signs may change rapidly. Urinary incontinence may occur despite the patient's apparent well-being. In a young, healthy patient with a fracture such a situation may indicate the onset of the fat embolism syndrome. Recovery may take several months, and permanent neurological deficits have been reported, including severe mental retardation.

The second or third day after injury, petechiae may be seen and are characteristically located across the chest, the axilla and the root of the neck, and in the conjunctiva (Fig. 4-10). This is in contrast to the petechial rash seen in patients with subacute bacterial endocarditis. The petechial rash is fleeting and may last only a short while, fading rapidly (Fig. 4-11). It may occur periodically with accompanying attacks of coma. The conjunctival lesions are sharp and distinct and can be seen by rolling back the eyelids (Fig. 4-12). Retinal lesions can be identified by funduscopic examination and appear as microinfarcts at the ends of the retinal arterioles.[252] There may be permanent changes in the optic nerve center following the fat embolism syndrome.

The clinical manifestations as described result from a reduced blood flow to vital organs such as the lungs, demonstrating dyspnea and cyanosis; the cerebral cortex, with dyspnea, disorientation and restlessness; and occasionally the kidneys, with a resultant oliguria. If one maintains a high index of suspicion, the presumptive diagnosis of fat embolism syndrome can be made early after injury. There are many injuries other than multiple fractures that are associated with the fat embolism syndrome. The more frequent are intrathoracic, intra-abdominal, intracranial, and major arterial injuries. It is most important to identify all associated injuries, to institute corrective measures for their treatment, and not to overlook the blood loss that occurs with an associated injury as well as with the fracture.

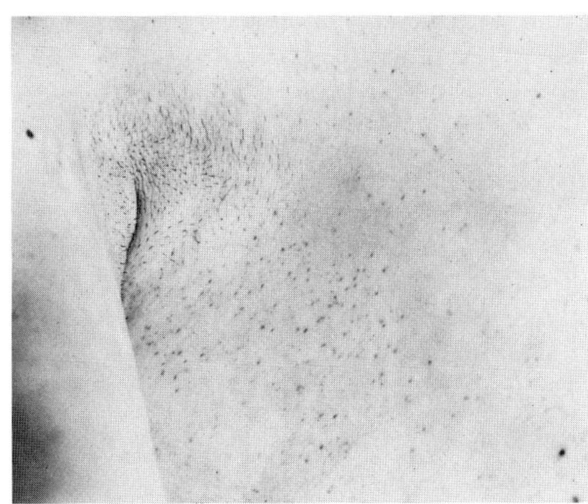

Fig. 4-11. Axillary petechiae. (Evarts, C. M.: Surg. Clin. N. Amer., *50*:493-507, 1970)

Laboratory Findings

Unfortunately a pathognomonic laboratory test for fat embolism syndrome does not exist. The diagnosis is mainly "clinical," based upon the characteristic clinical manifestations. Perhaps the most important de-

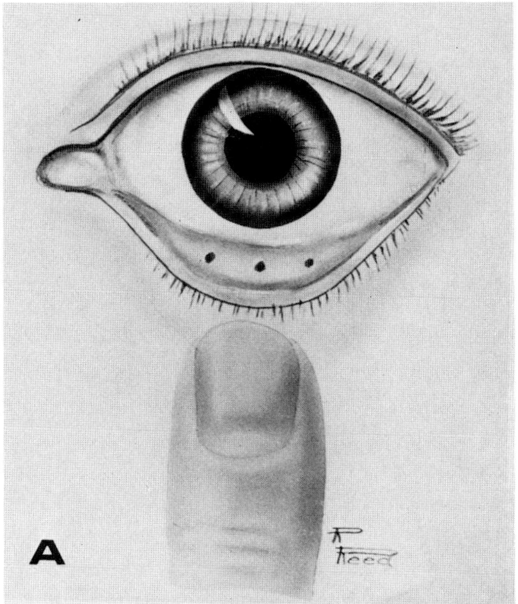

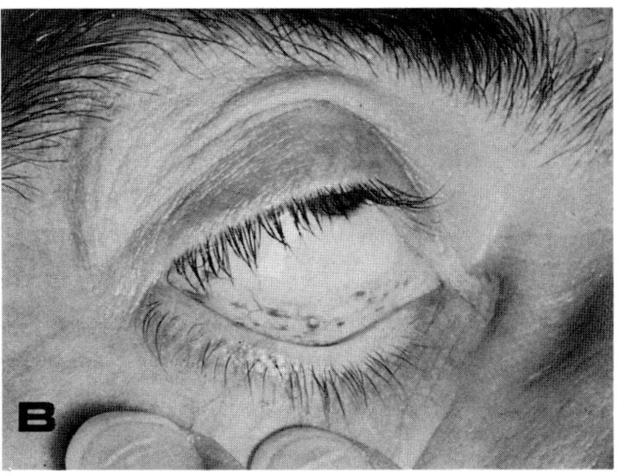

Fig. 4-12. (*A*) Diagram of conjunctival petechiae. (*B*) Clinical appearance of conjunctival petechiae. (Evarts, C. M.: Surg. Clin. N. Amer., *50*:493-507, 1970)

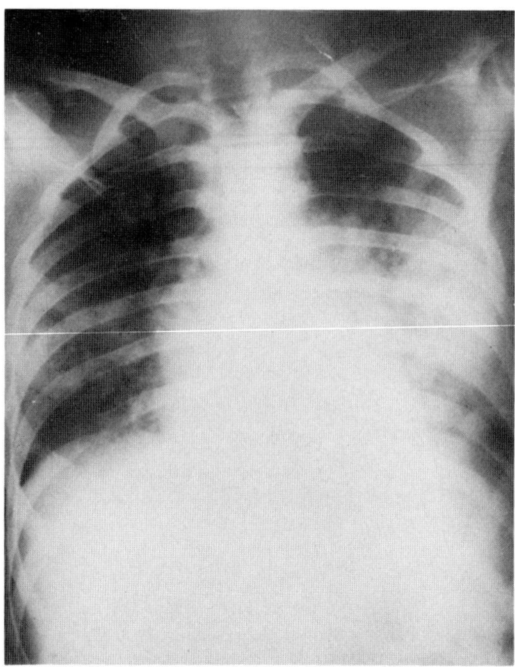

Fig. 4-13. Roentgenogram showing pulmonary infiltrate in a patient with the fat embolism syndrome.

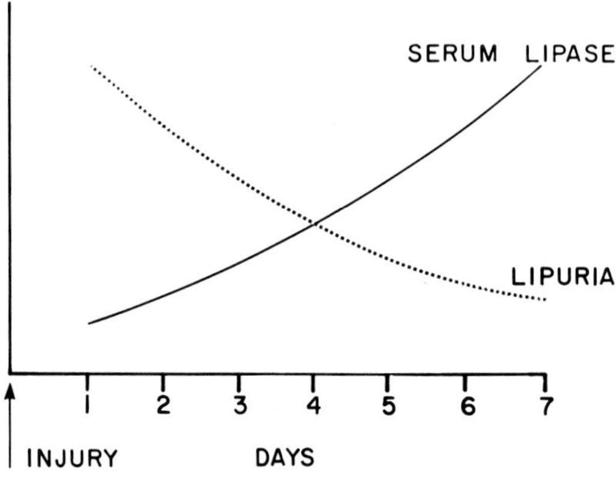

Fig. 4-14. Laboratory findings in the fat embolism syndrome.

velopment in the identification of the fat embolism syndrome, as well as in its management, has been the emphasis on the importance of testing pulmonary function in patients suspected of having fat embolism syndrome with pulmonary insufficiency.[215,217,224,267] The measurement of arterial hypoxemia is a sensitive index of the degree of pulmonary fat embolism and monitors the response to treatment. PO_2 values of less than 60 mm. Hg indicate significant pulmonary hypoxemia. More sophisticated studies, such as the alveolar arterial oxygen differences ($A - a\ DO_2$) measured after inhalation of 100 per cent oxygen for 10 minutes help determine physiologic shunting and also help identify the presence of pulmonary embolization. Serial determinations of the arterial PO_2 values can provide an index of the effectiveness of the treatment of the hypoxic state associated with pulmonary insufficiency accompanying the fat embolism syndrome. It has become clear that inapparent hypoxemia can occur in the patient without the clinical aspects of fat embolism.

In the early stages thrombocytopenia may occur with platelet values less than 150,000/mm.^{3} The hematocrit value often decreases, sometimes with startling drops.[273] Fat in the urine in the form of triglycerides occurs in about 50 per cent of patients within the first 3 days after injury.[212] Care must be used in identification of the free fat in the urine. The collecting apparatus must be fat-free. The supernatant fluid must be stained with freshly filtered Sudan 3 or oral Red O and examined for fat droplets.

Serial chest roentgenograms should be obtained as they demonstrate progressive snowstorm-like pulmonary infiltrations in patients with fat embolism syndrome. The changes in chest roentgenograms are characteristic but not specific (Fig. 4-13).[262] They frequently occur after the fat embolism syndrome is well underway. About 3 to 4 days following injury, serum lipase values may be elevated in about 50 per cent of cases.[272] However, by this time the fat embolism syndrome is full-blown (Fig. 4-14).

Electrocardiographic changes may occur, demonstrating prominent S waves, arrhythmias, inversion of T waves, and a right bundle branch block. However, these changes are not specific and reflect cardiac strain. Another helpful laboratory technique used for the identification of fat embolism syndrome is that of a cryostat frozen section of clotted blood, which reveals the presence of fat. Pathological fat in the venous circulating blood can be measured by filtering the blood through a microfilter with a pore size of 10μ, allowing filtration of smaller fat globules but retaining the larger fat globules for staining. Gurd[245] reported that his test is of some value in the identification of the fat embolism syndrome.

If coma persists and there is no means of identifying the patient's problem, one author has suggested renal biopsy as a diagnostic aid in differentiating between coma that has occurred from cerebral trauma and coma secondary to fat embolism.[278] Lung biopsy has been suggested for the same reason. It is unlikely that the risk will justify its widespread use. Biopsy of a skin petechial lesion can reveal the presence of embolic intravascular fat.[280] Analysis of the sputum for fat has not proved to be an accurate method, nor has the sizzle test of Scuderi.[277] Spinal fluid examination is not specifically diagnostic for fat embolism nor is the electroencephalogram.[284] The exact role of the elevated free fatty acids and serum triglycerides in fat embolism in patients with major surgery is not clear.[261]

Differential Diagnosis

When confronted with the symptoms and signs of the fat embolism syndrome involving the respiratory system, it is necessary to differentiate posttraumatic pulmonary insufficiency due to shock lung, pulmonary contusion, diffuse intravascular coagulation, or overhydration from pulmonary insufficiency due to fat embolism. This may be accomplished by demonstration of certain features of the fat embolism syndrome (i.e., tachycardia, tachypnea, confusion, and petechial rash). The most significant laboratory finding is a decreased arterial oxygen tension value. Also, the demonstration of a fat globule on cryostat frozen section of clotted blood can help in the differential diagnosis.

Pulmonary insufficiency associated with fat embolism is related to both the mechanical and chemical effects of the fat globules and their breakdown products, fatty acids. Initially, the agglomerated fat globules obstruct small capillaries, in turn leading to an increase in blood viscosity, reduction of intercapillary blood flow, and hyperpermeability of the basement membranes of the lung tissues. Hydrolysis of the embolic neutral fat leads to the release of free fatty acids which accumulate in the lung parenchyma producing toxic effects upon the alveolar lining cells. The overall effect is to produce edema, hemorrhage, and atelectasis with its attendant pulmonary insufficiency.[270] This type of pulmonary insufficiency is reflected by a decreasing lung compliance, increasing physiologic shunting, alveolar capillary blocks, and alveolar edema. The other causes of pulmonary insufficiency have salient features of their own that would exclude fat embolism as a cause.

Delirium tremens is another disease state in which fat embolism might be a factor. A differentiate can be established by a history of alcoholism as well as the absence of the clinical manifestation and laboratory studies commonly associated with fat embolism.

It is most difficult to differentiate certain cases of cerebral fat embolism from cases of severe craniocerebral trauma. Certain features are common to both states but are manifested in different ways (Table 4-5).

Treatment

Many different forms of treatment have been suggested for patients with the fat embolism syndrome.[236,270,271,279] Treatment can be considered in two categories: nonspecific, general measures, and specific measures. As with all patients who have sustained multiple injuries, the following general management principles should be followed: the airway must be maintained, blood volume should be restored, fluid and electrolyte balance must be maintained, and unnecessary transportation should be avoided. The injured part or parts should be immobilized before any transportation is

Table 4-5. Comparison of Features of Cerebral Fat Embolism and Craniocerebral Trauma

Signs and Symptoms	Cerebral Fat Embolism	Craniocerebral Trauma
Lucid interval	18 to 24 hours	6 to 10 hours
Confusion	Severe	Moderate
Pulse rate	Rapid (140 to 160)	Slow
Respiration rate	Rapid	Slow
Onset of coma	Rapid	Slow
Localizing signs	Usually absent	Usually present
Decerebrate rigidity	Early	Terminal

(Evarts, C. M.: J.A.M.A., *194*:899-901, 1965)

considered, as excess movement might cause further fat embolization.

The initial (and perhaps only specific) treatment of fat embolism is directed at decreasing the hypoxemia that occurs as a result of the fat emboli. Oxygen should be administered by face mask or nasal tubing immediately on admission to the emergency ward. It should be reemphasized that the respiratory failure is the most common cause of death in the fat embolism syndrome.[227,228] The need for ventilatory assistance is indicated by the presence of a tachypnea, a CO_2 retention with a PCO_2 greater than 50 mm. Hg in combination with a PO_2 of less than 60 mm. Hg. Accurate monitoring of blood gases is obviously critical in the management of pulmonary insufficiency. The arterial oxygen tension should be maintained at 70 mm. Hg or higher. If the degree of hypoxemia is relatively mild, oxygen can be given by mask or nasal catheter, but this can be expected to deliver only 40 to 50 per cent oxygen concentration. If the degree of hypoxemia is severe and respiratory failure is current, prompt mechanical ventilatory assistance is mandatory. Endotracheal intubation is the preferred method, as it provides suctioning and prevents aspiration. It has the disadvantage of causing tracheal necrosis when required for long-term use (more than 1 week). It is better to use a volume cycled ventilator for mechanical ventilatory support. The utmost caution should be given in the management of such patients; vigilance and meticulous attention to details are required if treatment is to be successful.

The use of massive intravenous steroid therapy has been suggested in the treatment of posttraumatic pulmonary insufficiency secondary to the fat embolism syndrome.[214] Methylprednisolone sodium succinate is given intravenously in divided doses of 600 to 1200 mg. every 24 hours. Reports have suggested that the steroids have improved gas exchange by decreasing the inflammation in the alveolar membranes.

Other modes of treatment have been introduced in an attempt to lower the plasma lipid content and to improve microcirculatory blood flow. Heparin has been suggested for the treatment of the fat embolism syndrome for two reasons: (1) It is a lipolytic agent that increases the serum lipase action and hastens the intravascular hydrolysis of ventral fat. (2) It is an anticoagulant and functions as an antiplatelet agent helping to prevent platelet aggregation.[226] It should be administered intravenously every 6 to 8 hours in dosages of 2500 units. Such a dosage schedule is not anticoagulant, but rather will elevate the clotting time slightly above normal levels. If heparin is to be effective it must be given early in the course of the fat embolism syndrome.

Low-molecular-weight dextran improves microcirculatory flow.[235] Also, the other effects of dextran, including expansion of the plasma volume, formation of a dextran-fibrinogen complex, alteration of the surface charges of erythrocytes, and a decrease in platelet adhesiveness and agglutination are thought to be helpful in the treatment of fat embolism.[242] Five hundred milliliters of low-molecular-weight dextran should be given every 12 to 24 hours by slow intravenous infusion. There are certain contraindications to the use of low-molecular weight dextran: pulmonary edema, congestive heart failure, renal failure, severe dehydration, hypofibrinogenemia, and a localized septic process.

The use of alcohol intravenously is not universally advocated in the treatment of fat embolism syndrome. It has been demonstrated that neither the emulsification nor the hydrolysis of fats is improved by alcohol.[226]

Prognosis

The prognosis for recovery of patients with fat embolism is poor in those who have marked pulmonary failure and coma. Mortality is high with these complications. Mild cases often go undetected, and mortality is low in patients without severe pulmonary insufficiency or cerebral manifestations. It is virtually impossible to perform a controlled prospective study to determine true mortality and morbidity rates. In the patient with a severe fulminating and progressive fat embolism syndrome, the treatment as outlined should be begun early and promptly. If not, the patient is likely to die. At the present time, fat embolism cannot be prevented. Its effects can be lessened by a high index of suspicion, prompt recognition, and early treatment consisting of oxygen therapy and administration of heparin, corticosteroids, and low-molecular-weight dextran as necessary.

Summary

Fat embolism syndrome is a frequent complication of multiple skeletal injuries. It produces a clinical syndrome with characteristic clinical manifestations and a few pertinent laboratory findings. Treatment must be prompt and, in light of our current knowledge, consists primarily of the administration of oxygen, either by mask or by mechanical ventilatory assistance followed by the use of heparin, low-molecular-weight dextran and steroids as outlined.

GAS GANGRENE

Gas gangrene is one of the most serious complications of traumatic wounds. Generally regarded as a disease associated with battlefield casualties, the recent increase in highway accidents has refocused the attention of the orthopaedic surgeon upon this devastating problem. MacLennan[332] has stated, "While true gas gangrene is an uncommon disease in civilian life, it is by no means so rare as is generally believed." Recently, several authors have described the recognition and management of gas gangrene and have commented upon the use of hyperbaric oxygen as an adjunct in the treatment of anaerobic infections.[308,342] Also, postoperative clostridial infections are being reported with increasing frequency.[312,315] It is becoming evident that many anaerobic bacteria thought to be commensals have become invasive and produce gas gangrene in the face of host changes induced by extensive surgery or therapy with corticosteroids, cytotoxic agents, or antibiotics.[305]

Although the historical accounts of gas gangrene date to the middle ages, accurate descriptions of this entity became available beginning in the 18th century.[325] In 1871 Bottini[306] recognized the bacterial nature of the disease but did not isolate the invading organism. Further descriptions separated the various disease states, but these were somewhat ignored until World War I. World War II brought forth the recognition that the term gas gangrene should be limited to those invasive anaerobic infections of muscle characterized by profound toxemia, extensive edema, massive tissue death, and gas production.[330] Robb-Smith,[338] in 1945, proposed the name anaerobic myonecrosis to emphasize that the basic lesion is necrotic rather than inflammatory.

Bacteriology

Clostridial Species Capable of Producing Gas Gangrene

C. perfringens (C. welchii)
C. novyi
C. septicum
C. histolyticum
C. bifermentans
C. fallax

The most important species in the list above is *Clostridium perfringens.* Identification is made on the basis of the morphology, the patterns of fermentation, and toxin production and its neutralization.[344] *C. perfringens* is a nonmotile, gram-positive, anaerobic bacillus without spores that produces marked milk fermentation with a lecithinase activity inhibited by *C. perfringens* antitoxin on a Nagler plate.[322,343] Such organisms are obligate anaerobes and cannot multiply in healthy tissues with high oxygen reduction potentials. Clostridia are found widely distributed in the fecal matter. *C. perfringens* is regarded as an ubiquitous organism also found in operating rooms, emergency wards, hospital corridors, cart wheels, and on shoes. It is a saprophytic commensal of the alimentary tract and can be isolated from skin in approximately 20 per cent of patients.[336] The risk of clostridial contamination is always present in the operating room. The significant toxins associated with the Clostridia are listed in the next column. When the cell wall (a lipoprotein complex containing a lecithin) is attacked by the alpha toxin, a dermonecrotizing lecithinase, cell wall destruction, and cell death occur.

It is well to remember that clostridial infections are not caused by the "extra virulence" of the organism but rather by unique local conditions. Oakley[334] discussed the factors required to establish a clostridial infection and pointed out that with ischemia and necrosis of muscle a decreased oxidation reduction potential promoted rapid advance of a highly lethal infection. The exact mechanism that converts the saprophytic state to the fulminating gangrenous state is not known. An unidentified lethal factor may contribute to the invasiveness and the toxemia that accompany gas gangrene.[333]

Histotoxins

1. Lecithinase (α toxin)
2. Collagenase
3. Hyaluronidase
4. Leukocidin
5. Deoxyribonuclease
6. Protease
7. Lipase

It is easy to understand how trauma from the injury itself, surgery, tight casts, etc. can lower the oxidation reduction potential values and create the proper environment for clostridial infection. Dirty wounds, especially those closed primarily without appropriate debridement, provide an ideal setting for the onset of gas gangrene.

The clinical infection of gas gangrene depends upon the spread of lethal toxins produced by clostridial organisms in a local

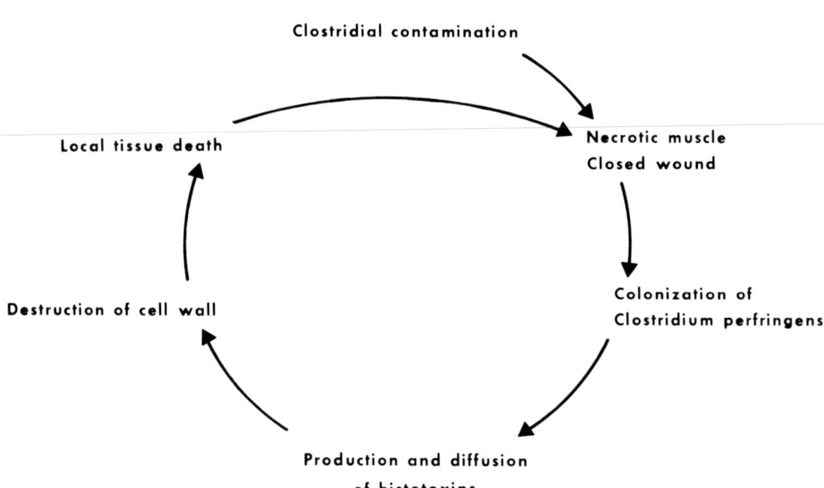

Fig. 4-15. Pathogenesis of clostridial myonecrosis.

lesion of dead tissue. The local lesion arises when toxigenic Clostridia are introduced into a deep wound of muscle, where under favorable conditions they multiply and produce toxins that diffuse into the surrounding tissues and devitalize them, allowing further colonization by the clostridial organisms.[309] Figure 4-15 illustrates the mode of action of Clostridia with the production and diffusion of the histotoxins. This vicious cycle promotes an astonishingly rapid rate of growth of the organisms and diffusion of the toxins. The toxemia associated with gas gangrene is not clearly understood. The circulating alpha toxins are extremely potent (intravenous injection results in intravascular hemolysis, jaundice, fever, hemoglobinuria, renal failure, and death).[324]

Classification

MacLennan[332] has provided a classification of the histotoxic infections of man:

Histotoxic Infections

I. Traumatic wound infections
   A. Simple contamination
   B. Anaerobic cellulitis
   C. Anaerobic myonecrosis
      1. Clostridial myonecrosis
      2. Streptococcal myonecrosis

II. Nontraumatic infections
   A. Idiopathic
   B. Infected vascular gangrene

It is important to recognize the different categories of traumatic wound infections. The mere presence of anaerobic organisms in the wound and their multiplication does not cause pain or a systemic reaction, and such an infection is not often recognized. In a few instances the wound appears ragged and deep with a watery, brown, seropurulent discharge. This represents a simple contamination of a wound, and the surgeon need only remove the necrotic debris.

Anaerobic cellulitis is a clostridial infection of ischemic tissue usually occurring after several days in an inadequately debrided wound. Altemeier and Culbertson[297] commented on the rapidly spreading emphysematous infection along the fascial planes with extensive gas formation. Altemeier and Fullen[298] outlined the causes of crepitation in a wound (see below):

Crepitant Nonclostridial Lesions

I. Bacterial
   A. Aerobic aerogenic infections
      1. Coliform
      2. Mixed
   B. Hemolytic staphylococcal fasciitis
   C. Hemolytic streptococcal gangrene
   D. Anaerobic streptococcal infections
   E. Infections with Bacteroides organism

II. Nonbacterial
   A. Mechanical effect of trauma
   B. Air hose injury
   C. Irrigation with hydrogen peroxide
   D. Benzine injection

(Altemeier, W. A., and Fullen, W. D.: J.A.M.A., *217*:806-813, 1971)

The other common gas forming organisms are the coliform bacteria, anaerobic Streptococci and the anaerobic Bacteroides. In anaerobic cellulitis the onset is gradual; the toxemia is slight. The exudate is brown and seropurulent.[305,315,332] The gas formation is foul smelling and abundant, but there remains no actual muscle invasion. There have been many needless amputations for anaerobic cellulitis, since it may be confused with gas gangrene. Table 4-6 presents the differential features.

The nontraumatic infections have been classified as idiopathic and infected vascular gangrene.[319] It is doubtful that true idiopathic gas gangrene occurs in man, although it is well documented in veterinary medicine. It is more likely that the Clostridia spores remain dormant in the scar tissues for years after the original injury.

Infected vascular gangrene represents a specific histotoxic infection of man in which gas-producing anaerobes are found proliferating in gangrenous but anatomically intact muscle.[309] The organisms are saprophytes, *not* invaders in a limb that is

Table 4-6. Histotoxic Infections—Differential Diagnosis

Features	Anaerobic Cellulitis	Streptococcal Myonecrosis	Clostridial Myonecrosis
Incubation	> 3 days	3 to 4 days	< 3 days
Onset	Gradual	Subacute	Acute
Toxemia	Slight	Severe (late)	Severe
Pain	Absent	Variable	Severe
Swelling	Slight	Severe	Severe
Skin	Little change	Tense, copper colored	Tense, white
Exudate	Slight	Seropurulent	Serous, hemorrhagic
Gas	Abundant	Slight	Rarely abundant
Smell	Foul	Slight	Variable, "mousy"
Muscle	No change	Moderate	Severe

(DeHaven, K., and Evarts, C.: J. Trauma, *11*:983-991, 1971)

ischemic. A "line of demarcation" is seen, and bacterial spread is limited. A foul smell and gas production occur, but rarely are the signs and symptoms of acute toxemia observed. Although a relatively benign form of infection, vascular gangrene, if neglected, can develop into a true clostridial myonecrosis.

Incidence

The incidence of gas gangrene is not known. Reports have emphasized the continuing problem of clostridial myonecrosis in civilian practice.[335,337] The presence of clostridial organisms in a wound has been reported as high as 18 to 46 per cent of cases.[340] Anaerobic cellulitis may develop in approximately 5 per cent of traumatic wounds. In a total series of 187,936 traumatic wounds, the overall incidence of gas gangrene was 1.76 per cent.[299] The incidence of gas gangrene is related to the lapse of time between injury and surgical treatment. Also, the site of injury is significant. Clostridial myonecrosis occurs most frequently in wounds of the buttocks and thigh, then in the shoulder and, finally, in the lower extremity. The mortality varied from more than 50 per cent in World War I to less than 25 per cent in World War II.[328] Treatment modalities, including the use of antibiotics and hyperbaric oxygen, have helped lower the morbidity and mortality.

Clinical Characteristics

The third category of traumatic wound infection in MacLennan's classification is anaerobic myonecrosis, separated into clostridial and streptococcal myonecrosis.[316,318] Almost without exception the original wound involves injury to muscle—a deep, penetrating wound sealed off from ready access to the surface. The incubation period of Clostridia is not long—12 to 24 hours after injury. The initial symptom is pain or a sense of heaviness in the affected area, followed by local edema and exudation of a thin, dark fluid. There is a dissociation between tachycardia and temperature elevation; the pulse rate is elevated but the temperature is not high initially. The progress of the disease is rapid and spectacular with an increase in toxemia and local spread of the infection. Profound shock may occur. The wound develops a peculiar bronze discoloration with a musty odor and a slight amount of gas production. A symptom characteristic of gas gangrene is the mental awareness marked by a terror of death in the face of a profound toxemia. Shortly before death the patient usually becomes apathetic and coma ensues. It is difficult to determine the actual extent of muscle invasion and necrosis without surgical exploration. When examined the muscle appears edematous, grey or dark red, and ischemic. Contractility is absent, and gas bubbles forth from the muscle fiber bundles.[317] Muscle involvement is invariably greater than the skin changes might indicate.

The other form of anaerobic myonecrosis is secondary to anaerobic streptococcal infection.[318,331] The majority of streptococcal myonecrosis infections have been located either in the perirectal or inguinal regions. Superficially this infection resembles clostridial gas gangrene, however, there is a slightly longer incubation period and the characteristic pain of clostridial myonecrosis is not present. Gas formation is slight, but there is a large amount of seropurulent discharge—in direct contrast to the discharge found in clostridial myonecrosis. Toxemia is less at the outset, and marked pain and septicemia do not occur except as terminal events. Certain differential features of anaerobic cellulitis, streptococcal myonecrosis, and clostridial myonecrosis are listed in Table 4-6.

Diagnosis

The diagnosis of clostridial myonecrosis can be made by its clinical features. The most important are severe local pain and swelling associated with severe tissue destruction and marked systemic toxemia. Gas formation is not a pathognomonic feature and in some instances may be scant.[301] Occasionally jaundice, hemoglobinemia and hemoglobinuria occur. Other differential features are listed in Table 4-13. Detection of gas may be obscured by the massive edema. Modern-day trauma can produce infections by other types of gas-forming organisms.[14]

The radiographic interpretation of gas in the tissues is not specific for clostridial myonecrosis. Obviously it can detect the presence of a gas-forming organism but it cannot identify it.[326]

The bacteriologic demonstration of pathogenic Clostridia in infected tissues is also of limited significance, because the organisms as previously mentioned, are commensal and widespread.[323] Type-specific identification takes a relatively long period of time—too long, in fact, for life-saving treatment to be delayed. However, a gram stain of the exudate should be made. The common identifying features are listed in Table 4-7.

Prophylaxis

The initial measure of prophylaxis is to recognize the predisposing causes of clostridial myonecrosis. These include deep penetrating wounds of the buttock and thigh, tight plaster casts, and loss of blood supply. The greatest problem in prophylaxis is delay of effective treatment. The fact that clostridial infections are not due to uniquely pathologic strains but rather to uniquely local circumstances requires reemphasis. The most important prophylactic step is early surgical treatment, which consists of meticulous and complete removal of any necrotic tissue.[345] The nonviable muscle must be removed; tight packing should be avoided, as should immediate primary suture if any possibility of clostridial infection remains.

The use of antibiotics has been demonstrated to be of value in the prevention of gas gangrene, both in the laboratory animal and in humans.[300,311,314,320] Penicillin is the

Table 4-7. Analysis of Gram Stain of Exudate from Histotoxic Infections

Features	Anaerobic Cellulitis	Streptococcal Myonecrosis	Clostridial Myonecrosis
Leukocytes	Present	Present	±
Gram-positive Rods	Present	Absent	Present
Flora	Varied	Streptococcus	Varied

antibiotic of choice. There is no evidence that penicillin alone will prevent the onset of clostridial necrosis in man in the absence of proper surgical debridement and cleansing.

Although immunologic prophylaxis would be most desirable, no consistently effective preparation has been found for active immunization against *C. perfringens.* Further investigation is required in the identification of different strains of *C. perfringens,* the conversion of toxins to toxoids, and the fractionation of toxic compounds of *C. perfringens.*

In the absence of a satisfactory active immunization much has been written concerning passive immunization.[321,329,333] This subject is controversial and the use of polyvalent antitoxin is not without hazard, since marked sensitivity may occur and fatal anaphylaxis has been reported. The use of polyvalent antitoxin has been seriously questioned but it is still widely used. The Subcommittee on Trauma of the National Research Council has recommended that gas gangrene antitoxin *not* be given prophylactically at the time of injury.

Treatment

The success of the treatment of gas gangrene is dependent upon an early diagnosis and prompt surgical decompression and debridement. Surgery does remain the cornerstone of the treatment of clostridial myonecrosis.[309,324] Multiple incisions and fasciotomy for decompression and drainage of the fascial compartments, excision of the involved muscles, and open amputation, constitute appropriate operative management.[332] Arrest of the infection can be accomplished without amputation if the diagnosis has been made early in the course of the disease.

Resuscitation must include careful scrutiny of fluid, blood, and electrolyte requirements; prompt replacement is mandatory. Fluid loss is marked, more so than with third degree burns. Central venous pressure monitoring and urinary output measurements aid fluid replacement therapy.

Large intravenous doses of penicillin, 3 million units every 3 hours, should be administered. Tetracycline hydrochloride, 500 mg. intravenously every 6 hours, has been suggested by Altemeier and Fullen[298] if mixed flora is present within the wound. Vigorous antibiotic therapy is an important adjunct to operative treatment.

An exciting, relatively recent adjunct in the treatment of clostridial myonecrosis is the use of hyperbaric oxygen. In 1956 Boerema[304] developed a hyperbaric chamber and subsequently treated two patients with advanced gas gangrene who recovered dramatically. Then, Brummelkamp *et al.*[307] reported its use in gas gangrene. The mechanism underlying the action of oxygen at high pressure is not clear. From experimental studies *in vitro* it has been observed that the toxin actions of Clostridia are markedly decreased after exposure to high oxygen tension. It appears that the production of alpha toxin is inhibited but that the clostridial organisms are not killed. However, growth of the clostridial organisms may also be inhibited.[302,303] Three atmospheric pressures are recommended for obtaining arterial oxygen tensions from 1200 to 1700 mm. Hg PO_2. The patient should be placed in a hyperbaric chamber for 60 to 90 minutes every 8 to 12 hours as necessary. Usually four to six exposures result in maximum effect. There are distinct hazards in the use of hyperbaric oxygen therapy, including barotrauma, decompression sickness, convulsions, otitis media, claustrophobia, and oxygen poisoning.[341] Lung damage has been reported in animals. If a large hyperbaric oxygen chamber is available, the surgical treatment can be performed during the initial hyperbaric oxygen exposure. The patient should be ventilated with 98 per cent oxygen and 2 per cent halothane. Few such chambers are available in the United States, and for most hospitals the cost of such a large chamber is quite prohibitive. Vital time may be lost transferring patients to facilities with hyperbaric oxygen. The iron lung can be readily converted in an economical manner to a satisfactory hyperbaric oxygen chamber.[309] It has the disadvantage of not allowing an operation to be performed inside the chamber; however, treatment with hyperbaric oxygen can begin immediately after surgical debridement. Such a chamber makes it economically feasible for hyperbaric oxygen therapy to be available on a regional basis.

Several reports have illustrated the efficacy of hyperbaric oxygenation in the treatment of clostridial myonecrosis.[308,313,337,339] It has been found to be instrumental in arresting the progress of the clostridial infection and allows amputation at the lowest possible level. In patients with fulminating clostridial myonecrosis and those in whom ablative surgery is not feasible, the use of hyperbaric oxygen may be lifesaving.

The administration of polyvalent gas gangrene antitoxin for the treatment of clostridial myonecrosis remains controversial. MacLennan[332] and Altemeier and Fullen[298] state that the dose is 50,000 units of polyvalent antitoxin every 4 to 6 hours for 24 to 48 hours in patients with profound toxemia and hypotension. Others do not use it in the management of clostridial myonecrosis.

The treatment regimen consists of four phases beginning immediately after the clinical diagnosis is made: (1) fluid and electrolyte replacement, (2) antibiotic administration, (3) polyvalent antitoxin administration, (4) meticulous surgical debridement and decompression, and (5) hyperbaric oxygenation. This regimen has resulted in a striking reduction of morbidity and mortality.

Illustrative Case.[309] A 10-year-old girl, fell while horseback riding and sustained open fractures of both bones of her right forearm. Initial treatment consisted of blind surgical pinning of the ulna, primary suture of the open wound of the forearm, reduction, application of a long-arm cast, and administration of ampicillin and chloramphenicol.

Twenty-four hours after the injury, the patient began to have severe pain in the forearm, followed by swelling of the hand and low-grade fever. Splitting the cast gave no relief, and the cast was removed. The forearm wound was foul and discolored, and a hemorrhagic exudate was present. Smear of the exudate showed gram-positive rods. The patient was given a large dose of penicillin and was transferred to the Cleveland Clinic Hospital.

On admission to the hospital, 90 hours after injury, she was toxic, with a temperature of 105 degrees F, and tachycardia of 140. She was fearful of dying. Her right hand was white, swollen, anesthetic, and paralytic. The forearm wound was foul and necrotic, with a thin hemorrhagic exudate, and gas was bubbling up in the wound. Smear of the exudate again revealed gram-positive rods and cultures subsequently grew *C. perfringens.*

Treatment consisted of immediate debridement and decompression. There was extensive necrosis affecting all muscles of the volar aspect of the forearm, with associated thrombosis of major vessels, and there were pockets of gas within the muscle substance up to the level of the antecubital fossa. The wound was packed open, and the patient was placed in the hyperbaric oxygen chamber. In addition, she was receiving penicillin and polyvalent antitoxin intravenously. A total of three treatments with hyperbaric oxygen were given.

Within 6 hours the patient's temperature was essentially normal and the toxemia cleared. It was subsequently necessary to perform amputation below the elbow, after which she made an uneventful recovery.

The history of falling off a horse is very significant and must not be disregarded. Barnyard contamination represents a real threat. Internal fixation of a forearm fracture in a 10-year-old child is not indicated, especially when an open wound is grossly contaminated. There was inadequate debridement and drainage of the wound, and primary suturing of such a wound is ill-advised. Delayed primary suture is safer, and provides a satisfactory cosmetic result. A circular cast should be used during the first 48 to 72 hours only if absolutely necessary, and should be immediately bivalved to allow for swelling. There was only a slight delay in recognition of the development of gas gangrene, but there was a significant delay in definitive treatment because of geographic separation from a hyperbaric oxygen treatment facility.

Conclusions

The incidence of anaerobic infections ranging from simple contamination to massive necrotizing muscle involvement is significant and may be increasing. The orthopaedic surgeon must be familiar with the diagnosis and management of the infections caused by the histotoxic anaerobic bacteria.

TETANUS

Tetanus is a potentially fatal disease but, unlike gas gangrene, a preventable one. It is a severe, infectious complication of wounds, especially lacerations, abrasions, or open fractures. In contrast to clostridial myonecrosis, which occurs in the patient with the neglected deep wound, tetanus may occur in the patient with a very superficial wound or in patients with no demonstrable wound.[39] Tetanus toxin must be produced by *C. tetani* organisms for tetanus to occur. In contrast to clostridial myonecrosis, tetanus immunization is effective, and complete primary immunization with tetanus toxoid provides a long-lasting protective antitoxin level.

Accurate descriptions of tetanus (lockjaw) is found in the works of Hippocrates[363] and Aretaeus.[347] In 1884 Carle and Rattone[350] produced the disease in rabbits. In 1889 Kitasato[370] obtained a pure culture of *C. tetani* and in 1890 described the antitoxins produced by this organism. The concept and use of tetanus toxoid for active immunization was presented by Roman and Zoeller[382] in 1927. By 1946 tetanus immune globulin (human) was available from fractionated plasma. In 1966, 250 units of tetanus immune globulin (human)[373,376] was established as the routine prophylactic dose.

Bacteriology

C. tetani organisms are found widespread in fecal matter of both domestic animals and humans. Soil fertilized with manure contains these anaerobes, whose function is to convert organic waste material into fertile soil. *C. tetani* are resistant and may be dormant for years, sealed in scar tissue. With subsequent injury, infection may take place. In direct distinction to *C. perfringens,* the tetanus organism is noninvasive and tends to remain localized. *C. tetani* is a large, gram-positive, motile bacillus, strictly anaerobic.[393] Spores cannot germinate in the presence of small amounts of oxygen.[383] *C. tetani* produces two exotoxins (Table 4-8).[395] Tetanospasmin is extremely toxic and a very small amount can be lethal. Spores are quite resistant and 1 to 4 hours of boiling is necessary to kill the organism. Autoclaving for about 10 minutes at 120 degrees C provides satisfactory sterilization.

Table 4-8. *Clostridium Tetani* Exotoxins

Exotoxin	Action
Tetanospasmin	Neurotoxin
Tetanolysin	Cardiotoxin

The skin of humans, especially outdoor workers, is frequently contaminated, and any wound, however small, can carry *C. tetani* deep into the tissues. Three factors favor progression of the infection: (1) deep wounds without exposure to air; (2) wounds producing ischemic tissues; (3) wounds infected with other organisms. Once *C. tetani* begin to grow, the exotoxin tetanospasmin is produced and carried via the bloodstream and lymphatics to the nervous system. In both the central and peripheral nervous tissues the toxin is bound with high affinity to the gangliosides.[369] The exact mechanism and site of action is not known, but experimental studies in the mouse demonstrate that tetanus toxin causes a presynaptic block of neuromuscular transmission and "functional denervation" of muscle.[355] Voluntary muscle is more sensitive to the toxin effects than involuntary.

Muscle spasms in humans are due to hyperactivity of spinal motor neurons.[348] There is considerable evidence that tetanus toxin impairs cholinergic transmission in both the voluntary and autonomic nervous systems.[368,378,390] Morphologically, no tissue damage is done by the tetanus toxin; however, a critical feature of tetanus infection is the inability of the antitoxin to neutralize tissue-bound toxin.

Incidence

Tetanus has been a major problem during wars. Despite the availability and widespread use of a highly effective toxoid vaccine, tetanus continues to be a serious health problem in the United States.[356] Figure 4-16 shows the incidence and mortality from tetanus in the United States from 1954 to 1966. The incidence was highest in the lower Mississippi Valley and the Southeast. The case-to-fatality ratio has remained at about 65 per cent. The hands and feet are the most common sites of injury, and injuries occurring at home accounted for more than 50 per cent of all cases of tetanus infection.[372] The mean incubation period is about 1 week and, in one series of studies, 88 per cent of the cases began within 14 days of injury. The length of the incubation period has been considered an indication of the prognosis of tetanus—a short period indicating a poor prognosis.[387] Tetanus involved all age groups but is more serious, often fatal, in the neonate and the aged.

Clinical Characteristics

Frank Glenn[361] has stated, "In my clinical experience I have never seen such a terrifying disease as tetanus." Tetanus may appear either locally or in a general form. Local spasm at the site of injury may be the first sign associated with this infection. The local form tends to be less serious.

The symptoms of generalized involvement are most commonly trismus, risus sar-

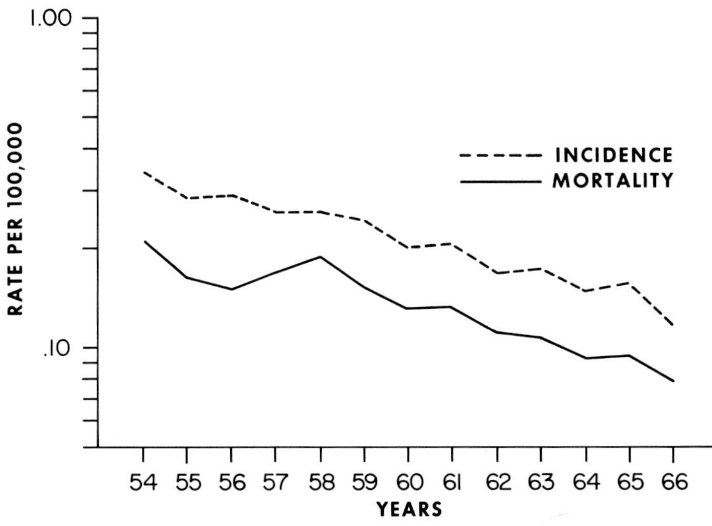

Fig. 4-16. Tetanus incidence and mortality in the United States.

donicus, and difficulty in swallowing. The trismus is caused by muscle spasm, and the sustained contraction of the facial muscles produces a wry expression. Some patients have prodromal symptoms of restlessness and headaches. If the pharyngeal muscles are in spasm, swallowing is difficult. Opisthotonos is very common, especially in patients with severe tetanus. Other muscle groups become progressively involved and muscle hyperirritability occurs. Frequent tonic convulsions are part of the picture of *C. tetani* infection and are produced by minimal stimuli.[360] Death in tetanus infection may occur from the asphyxia associated with unremitting spasm of the laryngeal and respiratory muscles. During the course of the disease the patient remains mentally clear. There is an associated tachycardia and often marked perspiration due to hyperparasympathetic activity. The deep tendon reflexes are hyperactive, but no sensory changes are observed in tetanus. Death usually occurs within 2 weeks of the onset of the *C. tetani* infection. The mortality, although difficult to determine, is about 50 per cent.

The diagnosis of *C. tetani* infection must be made from its clinical features. In one series of 160 cases only 32 per cent of the cultures were positive for *C. tetani*.[372] This finding is related to the very specific anaerobic growth requirements of *C. tetani*. Occasionally bacterial overgrowth is thought to decrease the chance of recovery of the organism. Despite the absence of bacteriologic confirmation, the dramatic and characteristic symptoms and signs of tetanus in the presence of a wound or site of infection make possible the diagnosis. Other common laboratory studies are nonspecific in establishing the diagnosis of tetanus.

Prophylaxis

Satisfactory active immunization exists for tetanus. The disease can be prevented. Progress has been made on an international basis to develop a standard tetanus toxoid.[367] Tetanus toxoid has been administered by intramuscular or subcutaneous injection. The experience in World War II demonstrates the efficacy of tetanus toxoid as a prophylactic agent.[374] No tetanus occurred in the United States Army from 1956 to 1971.* Once administered, the immune reactions are sensitized so that subsequent tetanus toxoid booster doses result in the production of circulating serum tetanus antitoxin. Allergic reactions to tetanus toxoid are rare but are manifest as serum sickness, as well as anaphylaxis and death.[371] Allergic reactions to injections of tetanus antitoxin have resulted in professional liability suits against both physicians and hospitals.[369] Generally, failure to administer a scratch test before the injection of full doses is now considered negligence. There are a few older professional liability cases allegeing missed diagnosis or negligent treatment of tetanus. Most decisions involving any aspect of the subject in later years, however, alleged negligent administration of tetanus antitoxin.[365]

Tetanus toxoid is highly effective and its administration results in excellent protection. The National Health Service Advisory Committee on Immunization Practice has suggested that primary immunization with DTP—diphtheria, tetanus toxoid, and pertussis vaccine—should be given to children 2 months to 6 years old. It should be given intramuscularly four times; 3 doses at 6-week intervals and a fourth dose 1 year after the first injection. For preschool children a single DTP injection is recommended. Following the initial immunization they recommend that one dose of adult tetanus-diphtheria toxoid be given every 10 years, provided wound management is not required.[357]

The success of the prophylaxis of tetanus depends on early recognition and prompt surgical wound management. All wounds must be meticulously debrided and cleansed. The tissue care should be gentle, and wounds should not be closed primarily if there are questions about anaerobic con-

* Neel, S. Personal communication.

ditions deep within the wound. The attending physician should determine for each patient with a wound what is required for adequate prophylaxis against tetanus.

The Committee on Trauma of the American College of Surgeons has published a guide to prophylaxis.[346]

PROPHYLAXIS AGAINST TETANUS IN WOUND MANAGEMENT

General Principles

I. The attending physician must determine for each patient with a wound, individually, what is required for adequate prophylaxis against tetanus.

II. Regardless of the active immunization status of the patient, meticulous surgical care, including removal of all devitalized tissue and foreign bodies, should be provided immediately for all wounds. Such care is essential as part of the prophylaxis against tetanus.

III. Each patient with a wound should receive adsorbed tetanus toxoid* intramuscularly at the time of injury, either as an initial immunizing dose, or as a booster for previous immunization, unless he has received a booster or has completed his initial immunization series within the past five (5) years. As the antigen concentration varies in different products, specific information on the volume of a single dose is provided on the label of the package.

IV. Whether or not to provide passive immunization with tetanus immune globulin (human) must be decided individually for each patient. The characteristics of the wound, conditions under which it was incurred, its treatment, its age, and the previous active immunization status of the patient must be considered.

V. To every wounded patient, give a written record of the immunization provided, instructing him to carry the record at all times, and, if indicated, to complete active immunization. For precise tetanus prophylaxis, an accurate and immediately available history regarding previous active immunization against tetanus is required.

VI. Basic immunization with adsorbed tetanus toxoid requires three injections. A booster of adsorbed tetanus toxoid is indicated 10 years after the third injection or 10† years after an intervening wound booster. All individuals, including pregnant women, should have basic immunization and indicated booster injections.

Specific Measures for Patients with Wounds

I. Previously immunized individuals
   A. When the patient has been actively immunized within the past 10† years:
      1. To the great majority, give 0.5 cc. of adsorbed tetanus toxoid* as a booster unless it is certain that the patient has received a booster within the previous 5 years.
      2. To those with severe, neglected, or old (more than 24 hours) tetanus-prone wounds, give 0.5 cc. of adsorbed tetanus toxoid,* unless it is certain that the patient has received a booster within the previous year.
   B. When the patient has been actively immunized more than 10† years previously:
      1. To the great majority, give 0.5 cc. of adsorbed tetanus toxoid.*
      2. To those with severe, neglected, or old (more than 24 hours) tetanus-prone wounds:
         a. Give 0.5 cc. of adsorbed tetanus toxoid*‡
         b. Give 250 units of tetanus immune globulin (human)‡
         c. Consider providing oxytetracycline or penicillin.

II. Individuals not previously immunized
   A. With clean minor wounds in which tetanus is most unlikely, give 0.5 cc. of adsorbed tetanus toxoid* (initial immunizing dose)
   B. With all other wounds:

* The Public Health Service Advisory Committee on Immunization Practices in 1972 recommended DTP (diphtheria and tetanus toxoids combined with pertussis vaccine) for basic immunization in infants and children from two months through the sixth year of age, and Td (combined tetanus and diphtheria toxoids: adult type) for basic immunization of those over six years of age. For the latter group, Td toxoid was recommended for routine or wound boosters; but, if there is any reason to suspect hypersensitivity to the diphtheria component, tetanus toxoid (T) should be substituted for Td. *(Morbidity and Mortality Weekly Report, Vol. 21, No. 25, National Communicable Disease Center)*

† Some authorities advise six rather than 10 years, particularly for patients with severe, neglected, or old (more than 24 hours) tetanus-prone wounds.

‡ Use different syringes, needles, and sites of injection.

1. Give 0.5 cc. of adsorbed tetanus toxoid* (initial immunizing dose) ‡
2. Give 250 units§ of tetanus immune globulin (human) ‡
3. Consider providing oxytetracycline or penicillin.

PRECAUTIONS regarding passive immunization with tetanus antitoxin (equine):

If the patient is not sensitive to tetanus antitoxin (equine), and if the decision is made to administer it for passive immunization, give at least 3000 units.

Do not administer tetanus antitoxin (equine) except when tetanus immune globulin (human) is not available within 24 hours, and only if the possibility of tetanus outweighs the danger of reaction to heterologous tetanus antitoxin.

Before using tetanus antitoxin (equine), question the patient for a history of allergy and test for sensitivity. If the patient is sensitive to tetanus antitoxin (equine), do not use it, as the danger of anaphylaxis probably outweighs the danger of tetanus; rely on penicillin or oxytetracycline. Do not attempt desensitization, as it is not worthwhile.

There is no absolute proof that the administration of antibiotics is effective in the prophylaxis of tetanus. Antibiotics are known to have no effect against the toxin produced.[380] Antibiotics, especially penicillin and tetracycline, given immediately after injury may have a deterrent action against *C. tetani* infection, by influencing the organisms that have not been removed surgically.[360] Antibiotics cannot be used as a substitute for active or passive immunization.

Treatment

The treatment of tetanus involves both general supportive therapy and the specifics of wound care, passive immunization, sedation, and pulmonary ventilation.[349,351,353,354,358,359,389]

The patients with marked hyperirritability should be kept in a quiet, dark room, avoiding as many external stimuli as possible. Intensive nursing care should be provided. Proper fluid and electrolyte balance must be maintained.

A combination of penicillin, 2,000,000 units intravenously every 6 hours, and streptomycin, 0.5 g. intramuscularly every 12 hours, helps decrease secondary invasive wound infections. The use of intrathecal injections of a mixture of antitoxin and prednisolone was suggested in 1967 and the clinical results were reported.[366]

The management of the wound is important. If the tissues have been crushed, they should be completely removed, and every attempt must be made to convert the wound from dirty to clean in every sense of the word.

Tetanus immune globulin (human) should be given early in doses of 500 to 1,000 units until 6,000 to 10,000 total dosage is received.[375,377,381] Sedation is one of the keystones in the management of tetanus. Mild cases can be treated with phenobarbital, secobarbital, or paraldehyde.[387] In more severe cases thiopental sodium should be given by intravenous drip to quiet the patient and to lessen the number of convulsive attacks. The administration of muscle relaxants (D-tubocurarine and succinylcholine) should be under the supervision of an anesthesiologist, as improper administration may result in respiratory arrest.[392,394]

Maintaining an open airway and avoiding the complications associated with tracheostomy are a challenge for the surgeon.[16] Proper emphasis upon the respiratory problems is a recent advance in the management of tetanus.[384-386] Smythe presented a series of infants in which the mortality was decreased to less than 20 per cent. The good results were thought to be due to the proper use of tracheostomy and detubation in the infant, the control of intermittent positive pressure respirations monitoring the CO_2, and the improvement in control of infection after instillation of penicillin and colistin into the tracheostomy tube.

If a patient develops pharyngeal or laryngeal spasm, tracheostomy should be promptly performed and assisted mechanical ventilation maintained. Careful, continuous observation and monitoring of blood gases is vital in the management and treatment of *C. tetani* infections.

§ In severe, neglected, or old (more than 24 hours) tetanus-prone wounds, 500 units of tetanus immune globulin (human) are advisable.

Other measures, such as hyperbaric oxygen, have been tried in the treatment of tetanus, but this has not been helpful in preventing the toxemic state of an acute *C. tetani* infection.[379]

Summary

Although the incidence of tetanus is gradually decreasing in the United States, it represents a potential major problem for the orthopaedic surgeon dealing with traumatic wounds.[352] Advances in the past century have made tetanus a preventable disease. It is the physician's responsibility to be aware of the prophylaxis and management of infections of all degrees caused by *C. tetani.*

OSTEOMYELITIS

Waldvogel, Medoff, and Swartz,[459] in a recent comprehensive review, suggested a marked change in the character of osteomyelitis. The majority of 248 cases reviewed were diagnosed as nonhematogenous osteomyelitis and occurred in an older age group, in contrast to a minority of cases of acute hematogenous osteomyelitis. The increase in injury to bone secondary to vehicular accident trauma with subsequent infection and the increase in major reconstructive orthopaedic surgical procedures have contributed to a definite rise in the incidence of nonhematogenous osteomyelitis.[404] The widespread use of antibiotics in the treatment of acute infections of bone has dramatically reduced the mortality from acute hematogenous osteomyelitis.[413,422,425,431]

Therefore, the orthopaedic surgeon is confronted not only with an increase in nonhematogenous osteomyelitis but also with different spectra of bacterial organisms causing bone infection.[427,445,452] There are fewer staphylococcal infections and more gram-negative and mixed infections. The bacteriologic identification of the infecting organisms is vital to the selection of the appropriate antibiotic. The techniques of obtaining material for culture, both soft tissue and bone, are of greater importance to the orthopaedic surgeon. He must face the complex management of open fractures, as well as the control of operating room environment and the possible selection and use of prophylactic antibiotics.[402,403,407,424]

Classification

Simply stated, osteomyelitis is a suppurative process in bone caused by a pyogenic organism. During the course of osteomyelitis, inflammation of the osteocytes and osteoblasts, their neurovascular components, and supportive connective tissues occurs within the confines of a mineral matrix. Bone matrix is destroyed by proteolytic enzymes, decalcified by hyperemia, and resorbed by osteoclasts.[398] Initially, osteomyelitis was classified acute or chronic, according to the duration and severity of the infection. Clinically, the distinction between acute and chronic osteomyelitis can be difficult. Patients with acute osteomyelitis may have indolent, subclinical, chronic bone infection; whereas, patients with chronic bone infections often experience actue exacerbations. Waldvogel and associates[459] have classified osteomyelitis into three categories on the basis of the pathogenesis of the lesion:

1. Hematogenous osteomyelitis
2. Osteomyelitis secondary to a contiguous focus of infection. (This form includes osteomyelitis secondary to trauma, open wounds, open fractures, postoperative wound infections or an extension of infection from an adjoining soft tissue focus.)
3. Osteomyelitis associated with peripheral vascular disease.

Incidence

Shortly after the widespread use of penicillin, the incidence of osteomyelitis secondary to staphylococcal organisms decreased.[421,431,433] The so-called golden era of antibiotics lasted from about 1944 to 1950. However, since 1951 pencillin-resis-

Table 4-9. Characteristics of Hematogenous Osteomyelitis at Various Ages

Characteristics	Infancy (< 1 yr.)	Childhood (1 to 16 yrs.)	Adult (> 16 yrs.)
Localization	Metaphysis	Metaphysis	Subchondral
Multiple foci	Frequent	Rare	——
Common organism	Streptococcus or Staphylococcus	Staphylococcus	Varied (Staphylococcus)
Spread	Joint space Epiphysis Subperiosteal Parosteal Diaphysis	Subperiosteal Diaphysis	Diaphysis Extraperiosteal Joint space
Fistula	Rare	Frequent	Frequent
Periosteal involucrum formation	Marked	Moderate	Weak

(Kahn, D. S., and Pritzker, K. P. H.: Clin. Orthop. *96*:13, 1973)

tant staphylococcal infections have become more prevalent.[425,448] Acquired resistance has become a problem associated with antibiotic therapy. New types or modifications of organisms develop according to the law of survival of the fittest. Certain chemotherapeutic agents permit enough growth of the resistant organism to allow the development of a resistant strain. The exact mechanism may involve genetic alteration. Ill-advised, small doses of chemotherapeutic agents contribute to the development of resistant pathogens. The orthopaedic surgeon continues to encounter an increase in penicillin-resistant staphylococcal infections. More cases of septicemia in acute hematogenous osteomyelitis with multiple involved sites have been observed. Fewer cases of hematogenous osteomyelitis have been reported, but osteomyelitis secondary to open fractures or major orthopaedic reconstructive procedures occurs more frequently. The mortality of osteomyelitis has decreased from 20 to 25 per cent before the chemotherapeutic era to approximately 2 per cent at the present time.[416,428,459]

Pathophysiology

Hematogenous Osteomyelitis. Acute bone infection is a complex process that depends upon many factors. It is recognized that the presence of the bacteria alone within bone is not sufficient to cause infection. The bacteria must be localized and the environment must support bacterial growth. The localization of acute hematogenous osteomyelitis has been outlined according to age by Kahn and Pritzker[437] (Table 4-9). In childhood the infectious process usually is localized in the metaphyseal portion of the long bones. Hobo[435] studied the vascularity adjacent to the metaphyseal side of the growth plate and demonstrated that branches of the nutrient arteries in the metaphyses have straight, narrow capillaries which, in turn, twist sharply back on themselves at the growth plate and terminate in veins with a much wider caliber than the capillaries. Trueta[458] felt that a decrease in blood flow occurred at the junction between the capillary side of the circulation and the larger-caliber veins on the venous side. He postulated that a relative stasis would increase the susceptibility to osteomylitis. Other factors determining the selection of the lower extremity for hematogenous osteomyelitis may involve the mechanical stresses and subsequent injury that occur at the epiphyseal growth plates in the growing child.[451,456] Metaphyseal hemorrhage and necrosis might occur, thereby providing a suitable environment for bacterial growth. A defective phagocytotic mechanism may exist in the metaphyseal region as compared with the diaphyseal areas.[435] Also, it is possible that rapid metaphyseal growth may provide a fertile area for the development of osteomyelitis. Once a focus of infection in bone is established the initial response is that of increased vascularity, leukocyte infiltration and edema of the surrounding tissues. The suppurative processes develop within a rigid-walled structure, and the resultant accumulation of pus exerts significant pressure on the surrounding tissues. The bacterial organisms liberate exotoxins causing cell death and necrosis; these necrotic tissues serve in turn as a culture medium.[441] The infection may spread from the metaphysis along the path of least resistance into either the medullary canal or the subperiosteal space.[434] The nutrient artery supplying the inner two-thirds of the cortex is compromised by the advancing infection. As the suppurative process spreads subperiosteally, the blood supply to the outer one-third of the cortex is destroyed. It can be appreciated that untreated acute hematogenous osteomyelitis can extend to involve the entire bone. If the anatomic location of the metaphysis is intracapsular, the infection can rapidly become intra-articular (e.g., the proximal femur).[437]

Nonhematogenous Osteomyelitis. As previously defined, nonhematogenous osteomyelitis is osteomyelitis secondary to a contiguous focus of infection.[459] The pathophysiology of this type of osteomyelitis is different from that of acute hematogenous osteomyelitis. The bacterial organisms gain entrance directly into the bone via interrupted tissue planes as a result of fractures or surgical procedures.[433,457] Initially, the bacterial organisms in these adjacent deep structures elicit no response. However, the original injury causes hematoma formation which, during the period of contamination, serves as a fertile culture medium. As the bacterial organisms multiply and the inflammatory response is evoked, the bacterial organisms often extend through the hematoma and along the vascular planes to contact the bony surfaces. The amount of soft-tissue damage, the extent of periosteal tearing and destruction, the amount of actual bone loss, and the degree of displacement of the fracture fragments influence the blood supply to the involved bone.[425,446] Internal fixation devices also change the blood supply. However, in nonhematogenous osteomyelitis the suppurative process is less confined than in acute hematogenous osteomyelitis. Less pressure develops, and the process is less likely to spread through the intramedullary canal or along the subperiosteal spaces. A common finding is a chronic draining wound with sinus formation. The presence of foreign materials—metal, plastic, or bone cement—contributes to the nature and extent of nonhematogenous osteomyelitis.

Clinical Characteristics

If a patient has severe pain, bone tenderness, high fever, headache, and vomiting, the diagnosis of this "classic form" of acute hematogenous osteomyelitis is not difficult.[425] However, this represents a clinical picture not frequently observed. Often patients have vague symptoms and signs with an insidious onset.[431] Slight fever, few constitutional symptoms, and minimal complaints of pain may be present. A history of upper respiratory tract infection or mild trauma may be elicited. If a high index of suspicion is not maintained, further examination of the musculoskeletal system will not be performed, and the diagnosis of osteomyelitis will be missed. Inappropriate use of antibiotics often obscures the clinical signs and symptoms, and the usual course of events associated with osteomyelitis is altered.

The erythrocyte sedimentation rate is consistently elevated, although the temperature may be normal. The leukocyte count may not be elevated, but there is a consistent shift to the left of the differential count.[409,411]

The clinical characteristics of osteomyelitis secondary to a direct infection occurring with an open fracture or a reconstructive orthopaedic procedure are somewhat different. The symptoms and signs are not those of severe sepsis. The patient may complain of pain or have a low-grade fever. The wound usually becomes edematous and erythematous. The wound drains in the majority of cases. The diagnosis is often obscure. Any attempt at aspiration of the involved area should be performed under sterile precautions and fluoroscopic control. If an early diagnosis of nonhematogenous osteomyelitis can be established rigid immobilization can be initiated in conjunction with specific antibiotic therapy.

Diagnostic roentgenography is not effective in the early management of osteomyelitis.[405] The bone changes seen on roentgenograms are delayed, appearing first 10 to 21 days after the onset of symptoms.[442] Soft-tissue swelling with a loss of well defined muscle planes and a diffuse haziness are usually the first roentgenographic signs. The earliest bone changes are hyperemia and demineralization. Actual changes in bone structure, such as lysis, are not visible on roentgenograms until 40 per cent of the bone substance has been destroyed. It is not common to observe massive periosteal reactive bone, although periosteal elevation appears simultaneously with the loss of bone. Bone sclerosis is a late roentgenographic sign and indicates chronicity of the osteomyelitis.[440] Antibiotic therapy given for the various forms of osteomyelitis has changed the roentgenographic features: the onset of bone changes is delayed; bone destruction is less; and multiple lytic defects are rare. The most common roentgenographic sign of early bone infection is rarefaction representing diffuse demineralization secondary to inflammatory hyperemia.

Bacteriology

The organism most frequently isolated from the bone of patients with hematogenous osteomyelitis is *Staphylococcus aureus*.[453,461] The presence of this organism as a causative agent for osteomyelitis suggests an inordinate virulence in bone. Notwithstanding the recent increase in the incidence of patients with nonhematogenous osteomyelitis who are potentially exposed to a large number of pathogens, S. *aureus* remains the most common infecting organism. Antimicrobial drugs have not eliminated staphylococci in recent bone infections.[423] Drug treatment has resulted in a decrease in clinical recurrence of osteomyelitis with organisms such as Streptococcus and Pneumococcus. The staphylococcal organism is different; it is somehow able to survive within contaminated bone for many years.[412,455] The individual, specific features of the staphylococcus providing for prolonged survival are not known. However, the prevalence of the S. *aureus* in osteomyelitis has decreased from an 85 to 95 per cent incidence in previous reports to 60 per cent in both hematogenous and nonhematogenous osteomyelitis.[459] More than one organism may cause nonhematogenous osteomyelitis, in part due to the exposure of a traumatic wound or surgical wound to an increased number of pathogens. The increased incidence of coagulase-negative staphylococcal infections as reported by culture has led some authors to suggest that this organism be considered pathogenic.[411,459] Cultures are reported as sterile or with "no growth" in several case studies. This may be the result of premature antibiotic therapy, or may represent the difficulty in the isolation of gram-negative bacteria or anaerobic pathogens. The S. *aureus* organism is becoming resistant to penicillin in 60 to 70 per cent of cases.[399] In recent years, bacteremic states due to gram-negative bacilli have occurred with greater frequency.[397] However, there has not been a parallel increase in the occurrence of osteomyelitis due to gram-negative bacilli. Table 4-10 lists the bacteriologic findings in 118

Table 4-10. Bacteriological Findings in Osteomyelitis

Organism	No. of Patients
S. *aureus* alone	65
S. *aureus* and other microorganisms	19
Proteus	5
S. *albus* or S. *epidermidis* with mixed gram-negative organisms	5
Pseudomonas	5
No growth	5
S. *epidermidis*	4
Aerobacter	3
Escherichia coli	2
Salmonella	2
Bacterioides	1
Beta streptococcus	1
Atypical mycobacterium	1

(Clawson, D. K., and Dunn, A. W.: J. Bone Joint Surg., *49A*:165, 1967)

cases of hematogenous osteomyelitis.[410] Kelly and co-workers[439] have listed the organisms cultured from chronic osteomyelitis of the tibia and femur in Table 4-11.

Treatment

The successful management of patients with osteomyelitis depends upon prompt, accurate, clinical and microbiological diagnosis followed by the institution of specific antibacterial therapy.[426] The orthopaedic surgeon must have available the information as to whether or not the infecting pathogen will be inhibited or killed by the antibiotic selected for use. The degree of susceptibility of various organisms to antibacterial drugs can be determined *in vitro* in the majority of cases. Certain test methods can be utilized in the selection of the "appropriate antibiotic."[400,418,450]

It is necessary in the treatment of bone and joint infections that a sufficient concentration of antibiotics reach the actual site of infection.[420,438] The antibiotic must penetrate joint fluid, hematoma, and infected bone.[396,460] Antimicrobial levels can be achieved in joint fluid with penicillin and its analogs. Chloramphenicol and tetracycline also provide satisfactory levels in joint fluid. Controversy exists as to the use of intraarticular antibiotic solutions. Since in the majority of cases adequate antibacterial levels are maintained in joint fluids with continuous intravenous administration, routine joint injections are not advised. However, the toxicity of certain antibiotic agents (kanamycin, gentamicin) is great enough to justify intraarticular injections. Kolczun has suggested the following dosage schedule for the intraarticular injection of antibiotics:*

penicillin G	100,000 mg./ml.
cloxacillin	100 mg./ml.
oxacillin	100 mg./ml.
cephaloridine	100 mg./ml.
kanamycin	50 mg./ml.
gentamicin	5 mg./ml.

Curtis[415] has urged drainage of the infected joint to eliminate the purulent exudate as well as the fibrin clots. He has questioned the use of joint irrigation with antibiotics.

A recent study[444] of antibiotic levels in bone has shown that there was no significant difference between the antibiotic concentrations in cortical and cancellous bone. Also, a constant intravenous infusion of antibiotics demonstrated that constant bone levels of antibiotics could be maintained as long as serum levels remained constant. Intravenous infusion was the best method of maintaining such serum levels. It was also demonstrated that satisfactory serum and bone antibiotic concentrations could be consistently achieved by the intravenous administration of antibiotics (on a mg./kg. body weight dosage schedule) ½ hour prior to surgery and followed by a continuous intravenous infusion.

It has been stated that all too often antibiotics are administered indiscriminately, routinely (rather than selectively), or hastily with an unrealistic sense of urgency.[443] Estimates indicate that up to 50 per cent of all drugs prescribed in the United States are antibiotics, that antibiotics are being

* Personal communication.

Table 4-11. Bacteriological Findings in Chronic Osteomyelitis of Tibia or Femur

	S. aureus Alone		*S. aureus* and Gram-negative Rods		Gram-negative Rods Alone		
Years	No. of Patients	%	No. of Patients	%	No. of Patients	%	Total*
1967-70†	35	41	18	21	33	38	86
1963-66	52	84	3	5	7	11	62
1959-62	37	74	3	6	10	20	50
1955-58	47	83	3	5	7	12	57

* Two cultures of Peptococcus not included.
† *S. aureus* was the predominant organism in all but four during this period.

(Kelly, P. J., Wilkowske, C. J., and Washington, J. A., II: Clin. Orthop. *96*:71, 1973)

prescribed without proper indication up to 90 per cent of the time, and that 50 to 60 per cent of the patients receiving antibiotics in hospitals do not have infections.[406] Certain principles of antibacterial therapy have been outlined by McHenry.[443]

Principles of Antibacterial Therapy

1. Select the drug most likely to be effective with the least side effects.
2. Administer the drug by an appropriate route for a sufficient time to eradicate or control infection.
3. Monitor the patient closely for a clinical and bacteriologic response and tolerance of the drug.
4. Modify the dosage when the circumstances indicate.
5. Discontinue the drug when infection is eradicated or controlled, when resistance emerges *in vitro* or *in vivo*, or when intolerable side effects develop.
6. Utilize adjunctive therapeutic measures including incision and drainage or removal of foreign materials whenever necessary.
7. Obtain follow-up studies including the appropriate cultures after therapy is terminated.

Specific problems relate to the use of implant devices and materials. Intraarticular infections and subsequent osteomyelitis are disastrous in the patient who has undergone reconstructive surgery of the hip or knee utilizing bone cement for fixation. It is equally devastating in the patient who has undergone intramedullary fixation for a long-bone fracture.

When a patient has sustained an open fracture it is mandatory to institute steps to prevent further contamination. The ends of bone fragments protruding from a wound should be covered with a sterile dressing. Reduction should not be accomplished by allowing the contaminated fracture fragments to be placed into the depths of a wound without previous cleansing. The cleansing and debridement of a contaminated open fracture should be performed in the operating room. It is a laborious, time-consuming process, but when finished all devitalized tissue should have been removed. Once such debridement and cleansing is finished then attention can be turned to reduction and immobilization of the fracture. Occasionally internal fixation devices are indicated under such circumstances. The use of suction-irrigation techniques frequently is indicated. Patzakis and Harvey[449] have recommended the use of cephalothin in the management of open fractures caused by direct trauma. In a study of 255 open fractures they have shown that the combined use of penicillin and streptomycin did not alter the rate of infection, while the rate of infection in the patients treated with cephalothin was 2.3 per cent (statistically significant with a p value of <0.05).

It is apparent that the treatment of osteomyelitis is based on the administration of systemic antibiotics in conjunction with surgery to drain abscesses or debride infective necrotic tissue. In early acute osteomyelitis antibiotic therapy without surgical intervention may result in cure. The blood supply has not yet been compromised, and adequate antibiotic levels in bone can be obtained. However, in subacute or chronic osteomyelitis, both antibiotics and surgery are necessary for adequate treatment. The surgical procedure often requires extensive debridement of the involved tissues and the removal of bone. The blood supply is such that its compromise prohibits delivery of the antibiotic to the bone surfaces.

Infection is a major hazard in the patient who has undergone internal fixation, endoprosthesis insertion, or joint replacement.

A common cause of pain following the use of an endoprosthesis is the presence of sepsis. If detected early, infection usually manifests itself as continued pain in the hip with characteristic wound changes accompanied by toxicity. The elderly patient may not have a significant rise in temperature or other signs of acute infection. It is necessary to aspirate the hip joint, to culture the infecting organisms, and to begin antibiotic therapy.[419] Usually removal of the implant devices along with meticulous debridement of involved tissues is necessary.

A number of reports have suggested the efficacy of closed suction-irrigation techniques for the treatment of chronic osteomyelitis.[409,414,417] Carefully planned surgery with debridement of all devitalized and infected tissues followed by closure of the wound with insertion of a suction-irrigation system is considered the treatment of choice by some authors. Jackson[436] has suggested the use of intermittent distention irrigation

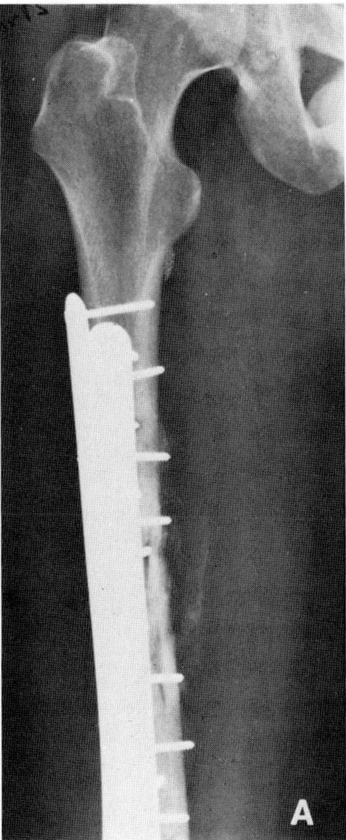

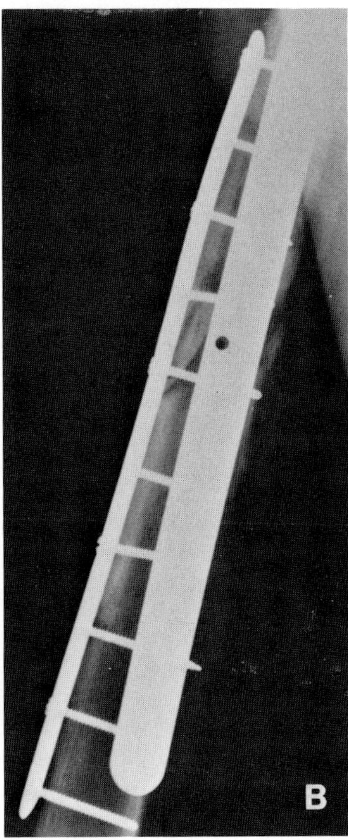

Fig. 4-17. (*A*) Anteroposterior and (*B*) lateral roentgenograms of the right femur with dual plates and early osteomyelitis.

in the management of septic joints. This form of treatment has added a new dimension to the management of osteomyelitis.

Many other forms of treatment including the use of regional perfusion,[430] hyperbaric oxygen,[401,429] saucerization, and immediate skin grafting,[454] and the use of pulverized bone[447] have been suggested for the management of chronic osteomyelitis.

A particularly difficult problem is that of chronic osteomyelitis in conjunction with an ununited fracture. It may be necessary to debride the involved tissues, provide rigid intramedullary fixation, use suction-irrigation and systemic antibiotics, and at a later date apply a bone graft to the fracture site.

Illustrative Case. Following a closed femoral shaft fracture sustained in an automobile accident in August 1968, a 21-year-old man underwent open reduction and internal fixation with plate application at another hospital. During the early postoperative period, purulent drainage from the wound and osteomyelitis of the fractured femur developed (Fig. 4-17). In November 1968 the plate and screws were removed and the patient was placed in a spica cast after 2 weeks of closed suction-irrigation treatment. He remained in the spica cast for 17 weeks, but the wound continued to drain and the culture was positive for Pseudomonas organisms (Fig. 4-18).

In April 1969 he was admitted to the Cleveland Clinic Hospital and underwent a massive sequestrectomy of the right femur that left a gap of 5 inches; a Küntscher rod

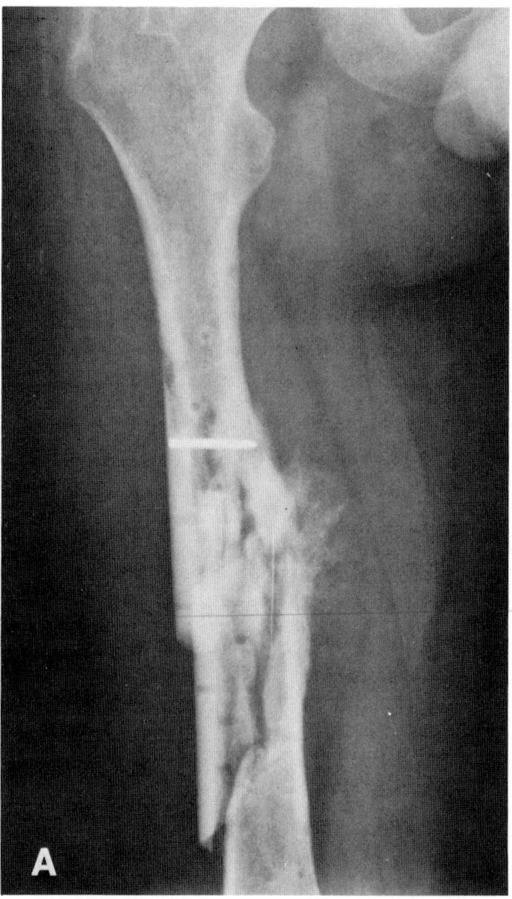

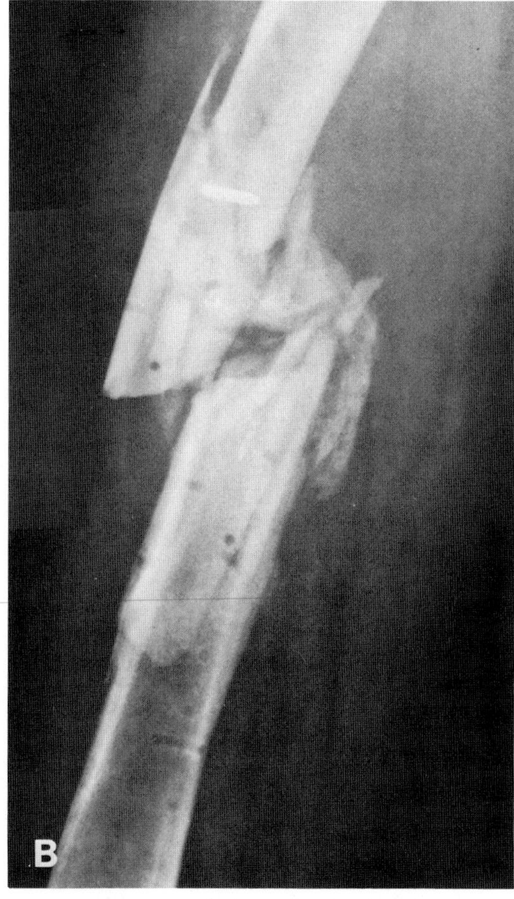

Fig. 4-18. Anteroposterior (*A*) and lateral (*B*) roentgenograms of the right femur showing chronic osteomyelitis with sequestra formation and nonunion.

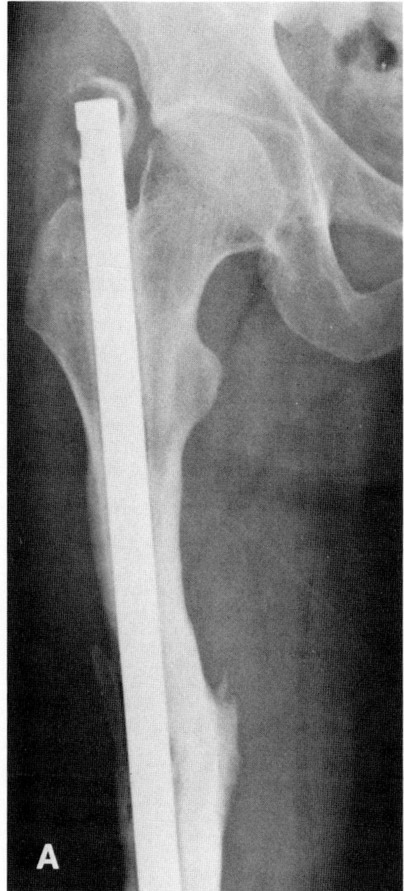

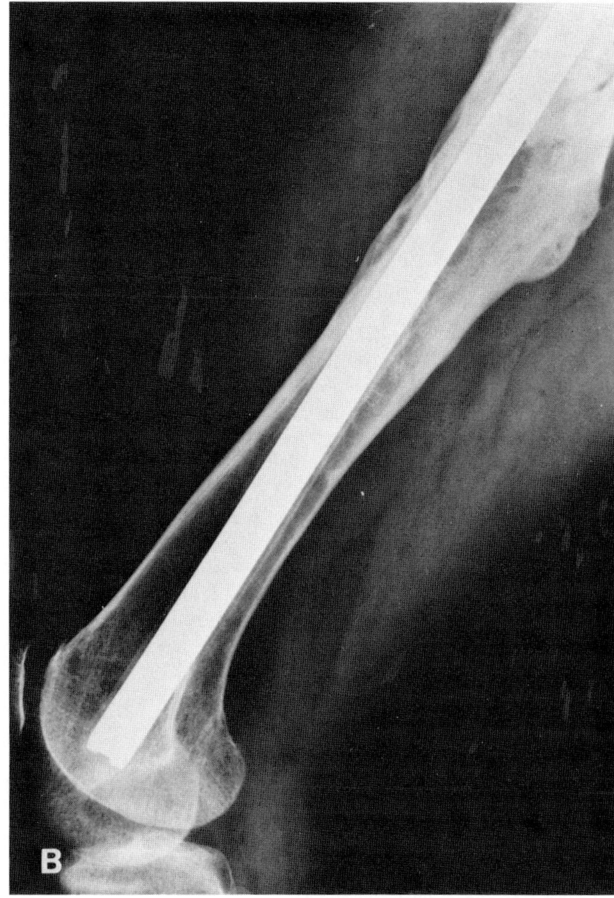

Fig. 4-19. Anteroposterior (*A*) and lateral (*B*) roentgenograms of the right femur showing union and resolution of osteomyelitis.

was inserted for stabilization and rigid fixation. The infecting organisms were *Proteus mirabilis* and staphylococcus, coagulase negative. Closed suction-irrigation was instituted, and ampicillin administered intravenously was begun. After a total of 4 weeks, suction-irrigation was discontinued, and the patient was given oral ampicillin.

In September 1969 the patient underwent autogenous iliac bone grafting to the involved femur. All cultures taken at surgery, both of bone and soft tissues, were sterile. Ampicillin was continued for 6 months.

Subsequently, the femur united, no drainage occurred, and the patient returned to work as a machinist (Fig. 4-19).

Summary

It is obvious that the orthopaedic surgeon must develop an increasing awareness of the management of acute hematogenous and nonhematogenous osteomyelitis. He must prepare himself for the complexities of the management of open fractures and postoperative infections and he needs to become knowledgeable in the selection and use of antibiotics.

POSTTRAUMATIC REFLEX DYSTROPHY

For many years certain vague, ill-defined, widespread, painful conditions have been observed following trauma, infection, or thrombophlebitis of the extremities.[467] A variety of terms such as minor causalgia,[476] causalgia-like states, posttraumatic painful osteoporosis, Sudeck's atrophy,[504] reflex dystrophy, posttraumatic dystrophy,[485] shoulder-hand syndrome,[503] and causalgia have been used to designate these conditions. Many theories regarding the pathogenesis of these conditions have been proposed, but no single theory has been proven. In this chapter the individual characteristics of reflex dystrophy, the shoulder-hand syndrome, and causalgia are considered. It is obvious that the orthopaedic surgeon is expected to manage these problems, which are often caused by fractures and dislocations with associated soft-tissue, nerve, and vascular injury.

Pathogenesis

DeTakats[467] has suggested a holistic concept under the heading of posttraumatic reflex dystrophy and has characterized this syndrome by (1) chronic sensory stimulus; (2) persistent vasomotor response; (3) motor response; (4) eventual atrophy of tissue, bone, tendon, and muscle, with joint contractures, chronic edema, and fibrosis. There has been no conclusive evidence to support the presence of sympathetic efferent fibers within the nervous system. It remains to be demonstrated how a minor injury can cause severe, persistent pain after the injured tissues have healed. A series of reflexes dependent upon cross-stimulation between sympathetic efferent and damaged demyelinated sensory fibers may account for the underlying pathophysiology.[468] Livingston[482] proposed that three factors caused a circle of reflexes. He believed that chronic irritation of a peripheral sensory nerve led to an abnormal state of activity in the internuncial neuron center, which in turn led to a continuum and increased stimulation of efferent motor and

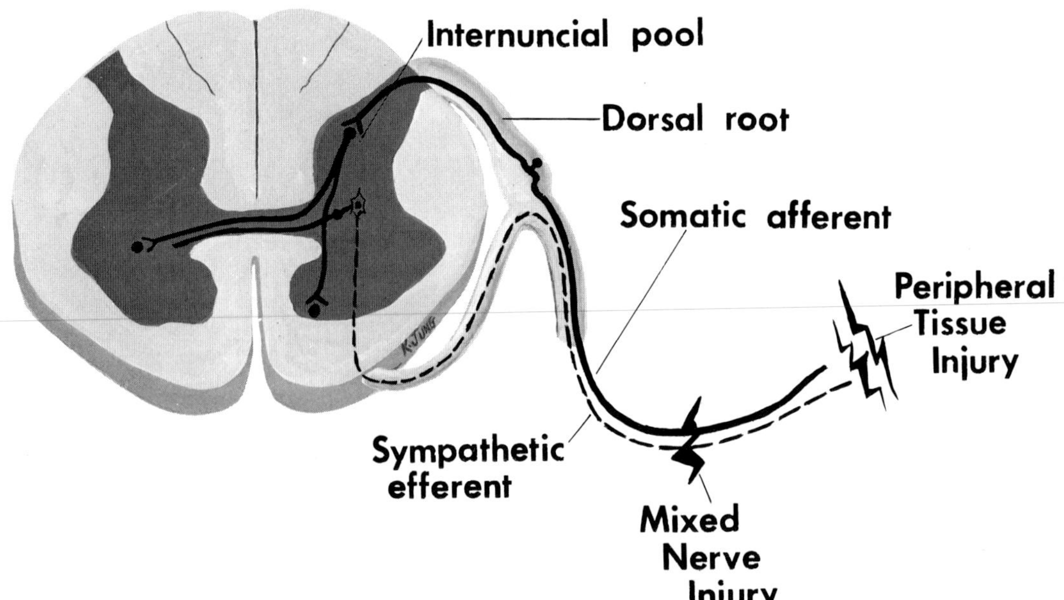

Fig. 4-20. Neural pathways in reflex dystrophy.

sympathetic neurons. Figure 4-20 illustrates the factors that may be involved in a reflex dystrophic state. No single concept of pathogenesis has been proven at this time.[465, 471,490,507,509]

REFLEX DYSTROPHY

Pain, hyperesthesia, and tenderness are the predominant features of a patient with reflex dystrophy. The pain can vary in severity and character and may be accompanied by swelling and decreased range of motion in the involved extremity. The skin color, texture, and temperature may vary. A clammy, cyanotic, cool, moist, painful, swollen extremity is a common finding[492] (Fig. 4-21).

Most authors have separated the clinical findings into three stages: (1) early, (2) dystrophic, and (3) atrophic. The first stage is identified by constant burning or aching pain in the extremity. The pain is increased by external stimuli or motion and is out of proportion to the severity of the injury. The stimuli that excite the pain response may vary from peculiar noises, height, excitement, emotional upset, vibration, arguments, deep breathing, laughter, or using certain words.[467,492]

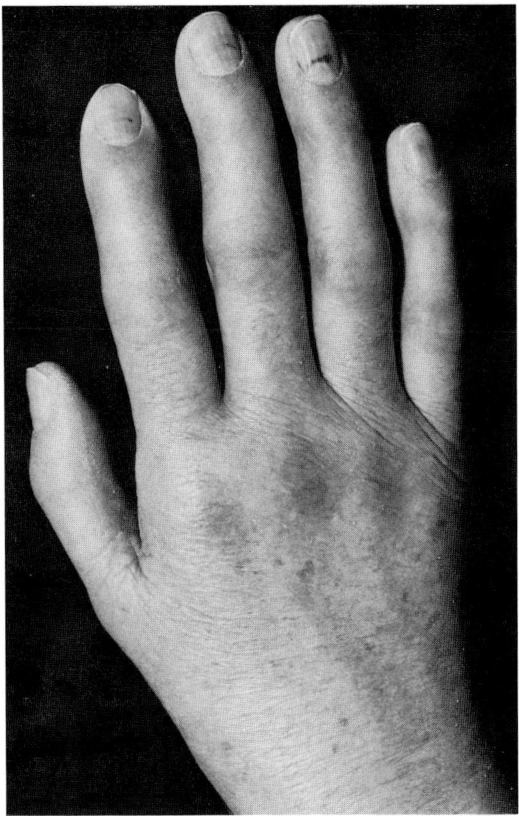

Fig. 4-21. Photograph showing swollen, pale, stiff fingers in patient with posttraumatic reflex dystrophy.

The second stage develops in approximately 3 months. At this stage most patients have cold, glossy skin and a limited range of joint motion. Roentgenograms often reveal a diffuse osteoporosis.

The third, or atrophic, stage is marked by a progressive atrophy of the skin and muscle; joint motion is severely limited; and contractures occur which may be irreversible. Marked, diffuse osteoporosis is seen on the roentgenographs. The pain may involve the whole limb and approach intractability.

In 1900, Sudeck[504] described acute bone atrophy, relating the onset to "inflammation." Subsequently, Sudeck[505] expanded his concept to include trauma or infection as causes of bone atrophy. He believed that the clinical features of pain, muscle atrophy, cyanosis, and edema developed secondary to the bone atrophy. He also stated that the changes did not occur if a reflex arc was broken, as occurs in diseases such as syringomyelia or poliomyelitis. Lenggenhager[480] has suggested that aseptic inflammation around an involved joint is responsible for the mottled osteodystrophy and recommended forced mobilization under anesthesia of the stiffened joints.

The term Sudeck's atrophy should not be used if the characteristic roentgenographic appearance is not present (Fig. 4-22).[493] Spotty rarefaction, present in the involved bones, is different from the generalized "ground-glass" appearance seen with disuse atrophy of bone. The roentgenographic features occur approximately 6 to 8 weeks after the onset of symptoms.

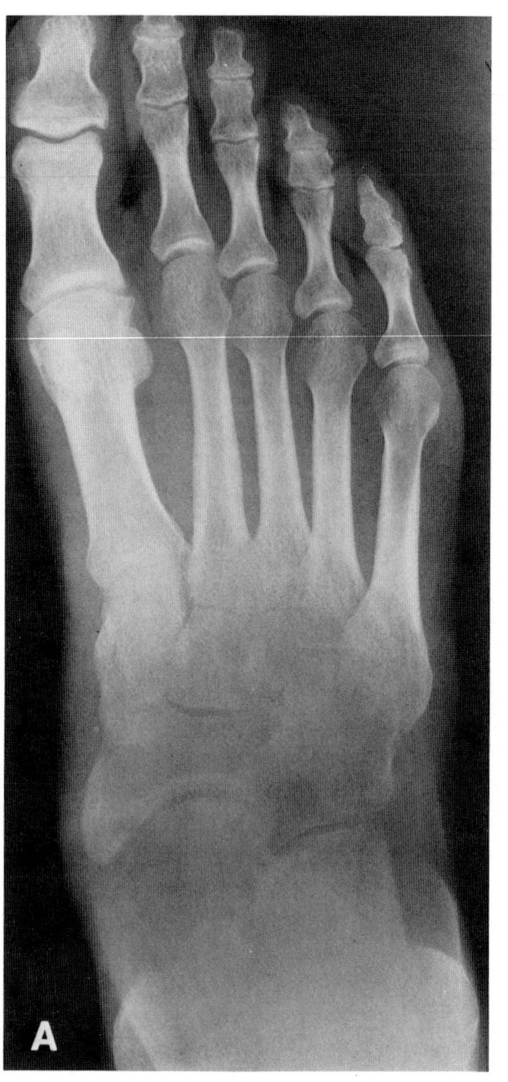

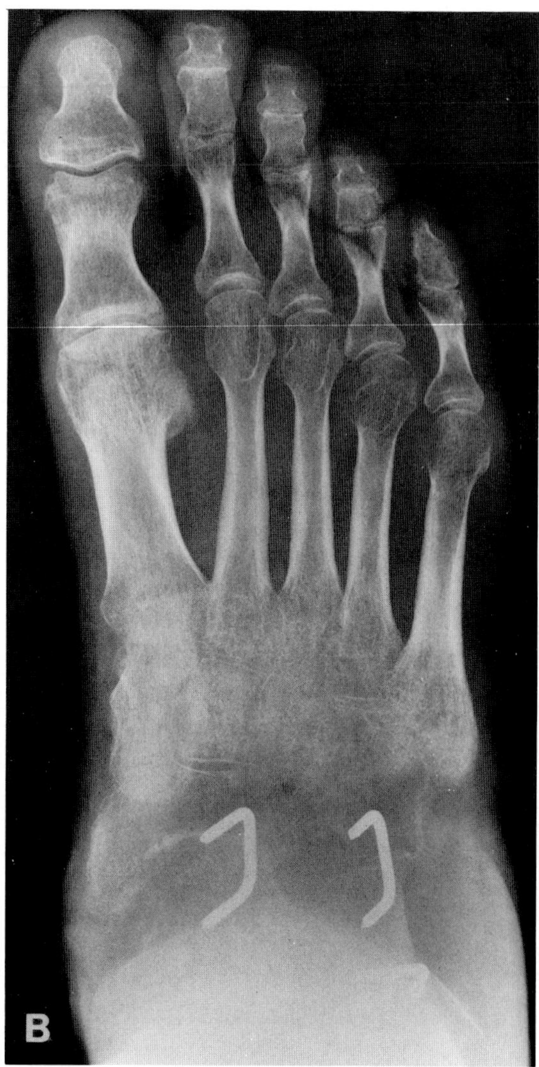

Fig. 4-22 (*A*) Anteroposterior roentgenogram of the right foot before operation. (*B*) Anteroposterior roentgenogram of the right foot after operation showing spotty rarefaction.

Hartley[472] lists several clinical entities that may cause confusion in the diagnosis of posttraumatic reflex dystrophy (e.g., tenosynovitis, disuse atrophy, senile osteoporosis, peripheral neuritis, and peripheral vascular disease states). It is often necessary to distinguish whether or not the patient's condition is due to a major functional overlay in conjunction with a minor organic problem. A procaine block of the appropriate sympathetic ganglia may relieve pain and aid in the diagnosis of reflex dystrophy.

Treatment

Many patients with mild forms of posttraumatic reflex dystrophy recover spontaneously. Prompt immobilization of the injured part may obviate further treatment.[478] It is important to provide emotional support for the patient with impending or early reflex dystrophy. If conservative measures fail, some form of sympathetic interruption is used.[485,492] Sympathetic blocks, occasionally multiple blocks, help a large number of patients.[559] If a causalgic state occurs, then regional sympathectomy is the treatment of choice.[466,470,498] Hermann *et al.*[473,474] have suggested that periarterial sympathectomy may provide considerable relief from the posttraumatic reflex dystrophy state.

A variety of medications including vasodilators, vegetable extracts, hormones, procaine injections, and corticosteroids have been used in the treatment of the problem.[464,469,483,495,496] No good evidence exists for their effectiveness.

SHOULDER-HAND SYNDROME

Steinbrocker and Argyros[501] have stated that the shoulder-hand syndrome is a distinctive and severe symptom complex with specific features that allow identification. It may result from external injuries or from internal disorders such as coronary occlusion or following a cerebrovascular accident. It is, however, a syndrome that can be classified as a form of reflex dystrophy.[477,489,491,497] The term shoulder-hand refers to the chief features of the syndrome—a painful disabled shoulder associated with painful disability of the hand and fingers.

The syndrome occurs more frequently in the older age groups and after cardiac dysfunction. It may follow cervical spondylitis, all types of fractures, a cerebrovascular accident, coronary occlusion, or any visceral, musculoskeletal, vascular, or neural processes that involve reflex neurovascular responses. This syndrome may evolve through three stages (Table 4-12).

The severity of the shoulder-hand syndrome is not proportional to the extent of the underlying disorder. A mild contusion of the shoulder might be followed by severe reflex dystrophy. Some authors feel that prompt recognition will lead to more effective treatment.[462,511] There is no specific drug for the treatment of the shoulder-hand syndrome. It is obvious that the underlying disorders need treatment before any resolution can be expected. Intramuscular in-

Table 4-12. Clinical Manifestations of Shoulder-Hand Syndrome

Changes	Shoulder	Hand	Fingers	Vasomotor Changes	Roentgenographic Changes
Stage I	Pain Limitation of motion Diffuse tenderness	Pain Diffuse marked tenderness Dorsal swelling	Swelling Incomplete painful flexion	Vasodilation Vasospasm (occasionally)	Spotty osteoporosis
Stage II	Pain Early atrophy	Induration of skin	Firm induration Shiny trophic skin	Vasospasm hyperhidrosis	Progressive diffuse osteoporosis
Stage III	Slight residual pain occurs Limitation of motion	Residual dystrophy and contractures	Diffuse atrophy Residual contractures	Usually absent with dystrophic changes	Generalized osteoporosis

(Modified from Steinbrocker, O., and Argyros, T. G.: Med. Clin. North Amer., *42*:1533-1553, 1958)

jections with lidocaine (Xylocaine) and corticosteroids may help to resolve the symptoms.[463,502]

It is not advisable to manipulate the shoulder under anesthesia. Gentle but progressive exercises of the shoulder and hand have been the most helpful. Contractures are gradually lessened and pain is decreased. Repeated sympathetic blocks may be effective. The administration of oral corticosteroids is of indefinite value in the management of shoulder-hand syndrome.

It may be possible to prevent the shoulder-hand syndrome by early recognition.[501] Casts and manipulation should be avoided, and gentle, graduated exercises should be encouraged. Injection of "trigger" points with lidocaine may prove to be of some benefit.

CAUSALGIA

Causalgia, by definition, means burning pain. In 1864, Mitchell, Morehouse, and Keen were the first to describe this clinical syndrome.[487] It is associated with a lesion of a peripheral nerve containing sensory fibers and is characterized by extreme pain in the affected extremity. Richards[494] has listed the features of causalgic pain: spontaneous, hot, burning, intense, diffuse, persistent, intermittent; elicited by stimuli that do not necessarily produce physical change. It leads to profound changes in the mental state of the patient. "We consider causalgia to be a clinical syndrome associated with a lesion of a peripheral nerve containing sensory fibers manifested by pain in the affected extremity. This pain is usually of a burning character and is usually located in an area corresponding to the cutaneous distribution of the involved nerve. An integral characteristic of this pain, one whose presence is necessary in order to make the diagnosis, is its accentuation by certain disturbing features of the affected individual's environment."[479]

The incidence of causalgia depends upon the criteria accepted for diagnosis. In the Civil War it was estimated to occur in 38 per cent of patients with nerve injuries.[499] White *et al.*[510] stated that causalgia occurs in about 5 per cent of wounds of major nerves, especially in those associated with injuries to the median and sciatic nerves. It is seen most frequently after a high-velocity missile injury with incomplete division of the tibial portion of the sciatic. Incised or lacerated wounds of nerves are rarely complicated by causalgia. It is not a frequent problem in civilian practice.

The exact etiology of causalgia remains uncertain, but it appears that there are crossover effects at the areas of injury that permit interaction between efferent sympathetic and afferent sensory fibers.[484,494]

The clinical picture is one of excruciating, unbearable pain with superimposed, stabbing, knife-like, crushing sensations. In about one third of cases the pain begins immediately after injury; in the remaining cases, within a week. The duration of pain is extremely variable, reaching maximum intensity within a month or two after injury and, in some cases, persisting for 20 years or more. The pain may regress spontaneously. The area of sensory involvement is usually more than the continuous distribution of a single nerve. The extreme guarding of the patient against external stimuli makes motor evaluation of the involved limb very difficult, but if the pain is relieved temporarily the extent of sensory and motor involvement appears to be no greater than that expected from a peripheral nerve lesion without causalgia.[494] Many different stimuli aggravate the pain—among them: movement, examination, dependence, noise, excitement, touching dry objects, hearing certain words, and laughter. Often the patients are referred for psychological evaluation and are thought to be emotionally unstable. The image of the patient with severe causalgia holding his involved limb wrapped in a moist towel, anxiously avoiding all contact with external forces, is dramatic and not easily forgotten. The presence of skin changes such as glossiness, atrophy, moistness, and mottling reflect the underlying vasoconstriction or dilatation.

Operation on the peripheral nerve or its scar has not been effective treatment.[486] Neurolysis does not provide relief of pain. Alcohol injections have been tried to no avail.[481] Other operations such as periarterial sympathetic section of the posterior nerve roots and arterial ligation have not proved helpful in the management of causalgia. In 1930 Spurling[500] described a complete cure of causalgia by cervical thoracic sympathetic ganglionectomy. The World War II experience with this lesion showed that interruption of the appropriate sympathetic nerve fibers is almost always successful in the treatment of causalgia. Sympathetic blocks often provide temporary relief—and in some instances, complete relief following a series of sympathetic blocks.[494] If a sympathetic block is to be done, it should be performed soon after the injury and the onset of symptoms.

Richards[494] in his centennial review of causalgia stated that certain facts are well established in regard to this syndrome: "(1) true causalgia is rarely seen, except in missile wounds; (2) the nerve injury is usually proximal in the limb and is multiple; (3) the nerve injury is usually incomplete; (4) the anatomic lesions of the nerve are similar to noncausalgic nerve lesions; (5) surgical removal of the involved sympathetic ganglion is an effective mode of treatment."

Although rare, this syndrome represents a challenge when encountered by the orthopaedic surgeon.

VOLKMANN'S ISCHEMIC CONTRACTURE

One of the most devastating complications following a limb injury is ischemic muscle necrosis and subsequent contracture. Classically, the supracondylar fracture of the humerus has been associated with Volkmann's ischemic contracture. However, this form of contracture has been observed following other fractures, not only in the elbow but in the clavicle, forearm, wrist, femur, tibia, and fibula.[525,537,557] It has also been noted after high-velocity missile injuries, wringer injuries, burns, drug overdose, soft-tissue contusion, arterial catheterization, and in patients with hemophilia.[527,535,540] It occurs predominantly in childhood when the incidence of supracondylar fractures is higher than in adults.

Despite a relatively small incidence of Volkmann's ischemic contracture after trauma, the orthopaedic surgeon must be equipped to recognize and effectively treat this complication, whether early or late in the course of events.

Historical Aspects

In the early 1800's most muscle contractures that occurred after a limb injury were thought to be caused by nerve paralysis. In 1872 Volkmann[558] reported the first account of a posttraumatic muscle contracture of acute onset which increased despite splinting and passive exercises. In 1875 he regarded this condition as "inflammatory myositis." However, in 1881 he[559] stated that:

> The paralysis and contractures following tightly applied bandages, chiefly on the forearm and hand and less often in the lower extremity, are viewed as ischemic. They arise from the arterial blood supply being interrupted for too long. Venous stasis, though occurring at the same time, does seem to accelerate the onset of the paralysis . . . Necrosis of the contractile substance is followed by reactive and regenerative processes of which the latter always remain very incomplete in man; the affected muscles become more unyielding and the contracture increases still further by cicatricial shrinkage. The prognosis of ischemic muscle paralysis and contracture will therefore depend upon the number of fibers which have necrosed or disintegrated. The severest cases affecting the hand and fingers are to be considered absolutely incurable. The prognosis is better in the lower extremity because here the main symptoms, i.e. muscular shortening, can easily be removed

by tenotomy. The milder cases are improved and cured only by the most energetic and consistent treatment.

The term Volkmann's contracture was first coined by Hildebrand[534] in 1890. Leser[541] ascribed the necrosis of muscle to ischemia produced by compression of arteries by compressive dressings. By 1914 more than 100 cases of Volkmann's ischemic contracture had been reported.[548] Further cases were accumulated in which constrictive casts or dressings were not used, leading to questioning the hypothesis that ischemic necrosis was produced solely by venous obstruction. However, in 1922 Brooks[516] advanced his concept of Volkmann's ischemic contracture following experimental studies on the pathologic changes in muscle as a result of circulatory disturbances. He and his associates[517] believed that venous obstruction caused the ischemic necrosis.

In 1940 Griffiths,[529] in The Hunterian Lecture to The Royal College of Surgeons of England, delivered a masterful paper on Volkmann's ischemic contracture in which he stated that arterial injury and the accompanying spasm of the collateral circulation was the cause of ischemic necrosis of muscle. He pointed out that many previously reported cases did not result from external limb pressure and that the pathologic changes of denervated muscle were interfibrillary necrosis, while the pathologic changes following arterial injury were fibrosis surrounding necrotic muscle fibers. He recognized that in Volkmann's ischemic contracture, necrotic muscle, and fibrosis are commonly found. Other authors have supported his conclusions.[526,529,550,555]

The acute anterior tibial compartment syndrome described by Severin[554] has become a well-established entity.[523,528,536,539] A unified concept of pathogenesis has been suggested by Bradley,[515] who felt that the decreased arterial perfusion is the primary initiating factor in this syndrome of increased presence and decreased perfusion resulting in a synergistic, vicious cycle terminating in ischemic necrosis.

Etiology

Volkmann's ischemic contracture is an uncommon complication of a small number of limb injuries; however, it should be reemphasized that many types of extremity injuries can result in circulatory insufficiency. It is not confined to supracondylar fractures of the humerus in children and has been reported in association with fractures of all the limb bones. The severity of the initial limb trauma is an important determinant, and contusions as well as crush injuries have resulted in ischemic contracture. Occasionally direct injury to the arterial system, the brachial artery or axillary artery, by gunshot or embolus, has eventuated in Volkmann's ischemic contracture.[537] Less common causes include carbon monoxide poisoning, regional perfusion with one of the nitrogen mustards, exposure to cold, and snakebites.[556]

The early descriptions of Volkmann's ischemic contracture implicated constrictive dressings or casts as the etiologic agent. However, further investigations have shown that external constriction is a secondary cause. It is of interest that 68 cases of Volkmann's ischemic contracture reported in 1967 were apparently a consequence of the tight splinting of fractures applied by bone setters in India.[512]

Occasionally a surgical procedure such as high tibial osteotomy can result in ischemic muscle contracture.[538] Arthroplasty of the

Causes of Anterior Tibial Compartment Syndrome

Exercise	Arterial bypass
Fractures	Inguinal herniorrhaphy
Arterial embolism	Regional intravenous infusion
Arterial injuries	Sprains
Buerger's disease	Bowleg brace
Periarteritis nodosa	Penetrating leg wounds
	Lumbar sympathectomy

elbow, open reduction of the forearm, humeral shaft fractures, and supracondylar fractures have caused Volkmann's ischemic contracture in a small number of cases.

Much has been written about the anterior tibial compartment syndrome, which characteristically follows vigorous exercise; however, a variety of other causes have resulted in this problem.[515,518,547,560,561]

Pathophysiology

As previously mentioned, conditions of different etiologies and pathologic findings were grouped together on the basis that they produced contracture in voluntary muscles. From the histologic studies of the areas of infarction, it was found that the lesions caused by temporary arterial occlusion are different from the lesions caused by venous occlusion.[514,519,531] The first is a central mass of yellow necrotic tissue composed of fibers separated into Bowman's discs around which lies a zone of fibroplastic connective tissue (muscle infarct). The lesion caused by venous occlusion has no sequestrum but rather a scattering of atrophic muscle fibers widely separated by dense fibrous tissue (diffuse interstitial fibrosis with normal muscle bundles). From this histologic evidence Harman[532] felt that venous obstruction played no part in the pathogenesis of experimental or clinical ischemic necrosis of skeletal muscle.

Although it appears irrefutable that arterial occlusion initiates the process of ischemic necrosis in muscle, other pathways are involved in the extension of the process. Foisie[526] stated that Volkmann's contracture is the key factor in the development of the loss of collateral circulation.

Bloomfield[513] demonstrated several types of intramuscular vascular patterns in humans. There are peculiarities of the vascularity of specific muscle groups, and the anastomatic pathways are such that whole muscles or segments can be affected by vascular occlusion in the face of absent distal signs of ischemia.[524,546] Hughes[536] showed that the anterior tibial artery may be functionally classified as an end artery. There appears to be a susceptibility of certain muscles of the forearm (the flexors) in which vascular injury can cause profound damage. The vulnerability of a muscle to vascular injury is determined by the specific pattern and the efficiency of intramuscular anastomoses and the relationship between the volume of muscle and the size of the main nutrient vessels. The course of the brachial artery makes it susceptible to injury and compression at several levels. A supracondylar fracture may lacerate, contuse, or compress the artery. The lacertus fibrosis fascia serves to fix the brachial artery distally. The sole blood supply to the flexor digitorum profundus and flexor pollicis longus muscles is the anterior interosseous artery.

It is of interest to note the anatomic location of the median nerve. It is vulnerable to compression as it actually lies on the undersurface and *within* the investing fascia of the flexor sublimis muscle. Peacock and associates[551] have emphasized that the median nerve in the proximal half of the forearm is located within a tunnel of investing fascia surrounding the flexor sublimis muscle.

It is an established fact that the peripheral nerves require a continuous and adequate supply of oxygen. Recent experimental studies on the effects of temporary ischemia with special reference to intraneural microvascular pathophysiology show that the microvessels of nerves possess an excellent capacity to recover function, even after long periods of ischemia.[545]

When muscle becomes anoxic, histamine-like substances are released which dilate the capillary bed and increase the endothelial permeability. Subsequently, intramuscular transudation of plasma occurs with erythrocyte sludging and a decrease of the microcirculatory flow.[533] The muscle gains in weight in proportion to the duration of ischemia and has been observed to increase as much as 30 to 50 per cent.[532] The necrosis of muscle is not immediate as some arterial blood flow often continues, but the intramuscular edema is progressive. Eaton

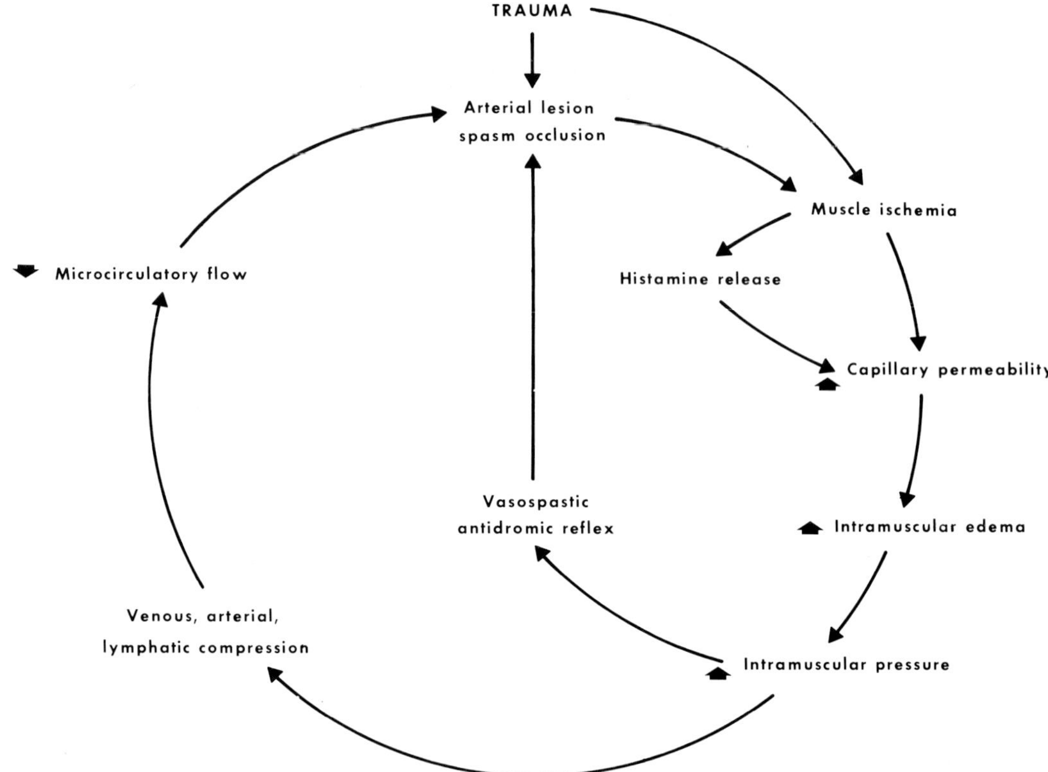

Fig. 4-23. Traumatic ischemia-edema cycle. The initial nonspecific arterial lesion results in muscle ischemia, anoxia, and release of histamine-like substances. Capillary permeability increases, and intramuscular plasma transudation occurs with an increase intramuscular edema and pressure. Subsequent venous, arterial, and lymphatic compression leads to a decrease in microcirculatory flow and eventually the cycle is completed with a further increase in the vascular lesion. Also, with an increase in intramuscular pressure, receptors initiating a proximal reflex vasospasm are activated and arterial spasm is furthered. (Modified from Eaton, R. G., and Green, W. T.: Orthop. Clin. North Amer., 3:175-186, 1972)

and Green[521] have described a traumatic ischemia-edema cycle which depends in part on a vasospastic antidromic reflex precipitating increased pressure within a restricted space (progressive muscle edema confined by a fascia[537] envelope with pressor receptors in muscles causing proximal arterial spasm (Fig. 4-23). Thus, a cycle of trauma-spasm-ischemia-edema-reflex arterial spasm occurs in the development of Volkmann's ischemia and continues until the arterial lesion is relieved and internal constricting forces are decreased. If external constriction is also present, muscle expansion is limited and the internal pressures are increased. Venous occlusion occurs and intramuscular edema increases.

Clinical Characteristics

The classic signs of impending Volkmann's ischemia are pain, pallor, paralysis, and pulselessness. However, each sign must be evaluated separately and interpreted with the overall clinical picture.[537] Pain is perhaps the most important sign. It is characterized as deep, unremitting, and poorly localized. It is not the type of pain usually associated with a fracture and is difficult to control with the usual analgesic measures. In upper extremity fractures, passive finger extension causes an exacerbation of the pain and is an early physical finding. Following satisfactory fracture reduction in a child, one should be alerted if restlessness and pain continue.[556]

Although pallor has been considered a sign, the extremity may appear cyanotic or mottled early in the course of events. Cyanosis is present early, while marked pallor of the distal extremity occurs late, after major arterial occlusion has occurred.

It is common to demonstrate some degree of sensory loss in the involved extremity, but not necessarily in an anatomic distribution. The loss may begin distally and extend proximally as the syndrome worsens. The median nerve deficit is consistent, and an ulnar deficit can be found in most instances.[521] It is difficult to identify the exact paralysis in face of the pain occurring with Volkmann's ischemia. The paralysis may involve a specific muscle group, such as the flexor profundus.

The presence or absence of a radial pulse has been emphasized in the evaluation of impending ischemic necrosis. However, the presence of a radial pulse is not always a reliable sign, as the radial artery may be patent in the face of significant forearm muscle ischemia. It may not disappear until the entire vascular system is in spasm. The color and capillary circulation of the nailbeds and fingertips are more accurate indices of peripheral circulation. It is important to reemphasize that all signs must be carefully evaluated; if changes are observed prompt surgical decompression is indicated.

Treatment

The syndrome of Volkmann's ischemia is progressive and requires prompt recognition and early action. If circulation of the extremity is occluded for more than 12 hours, it is possible that the ischemia will lead to severe muscle contractures.

It is imperative to reduce the fracture, elevate the limb, remove all circular and constrictive dressings or casts, and relieve elbow flexion. The use of skeletal traction for immobilization is recommended, especially in unreduced or partially reduced supracondylar fractures.[522,530,542]

The next phase of early treatment is the interruption of the sympathetic reflex arc. Sympathetic block of the stellate ganglion in the neck or of the lumbar paravertebral plexus has been suggested. If circulatory improvement does not occur within 30 minutes after sympathetic block, surgical intervention is indicated.[526]

If the physical findings of pain, inability to passively extend the fingers, a sensory deficit, and loss of radial pulse are present, there should be no hesitation in proceeding with fasciotomy, epimysiotomy, and exploration of the brachial artery. When there is any evidence that the ischemic process is progressing, surgery should be considered. It is far better to proceed than to procrastinate and adopt the policy of watchful waiting.[520,552]

The technique suggested by Eaton and Green[521] is described as follows. A longitudinal incision is made medial to the biceps tendon, extended down the mid-flexor surface of the forearm to the flexor crease of the wrist. It can be extended for brachial artery exploration or carpal tunnel decompression avoiding longitudinal incisions across the flexor creases. The antibrachial fascia must be resected longitudinally for its full length. The epimysium involved muscles should be sectioned from distal to proximal aspects avoiding direct damage to the muscle. The return of circulation may be marked following fasciotomy and epimysiotomy. Following decompression of this nature the pulse should return, but if it does not, exploration of the brachial artery proximally should be performed. The fascia should not be closed, and occasionally the entire wound should be left open and covered with nonadherent dressings. A delayed closure can be accomplished in 48 to 72 hours when edema subsides. Proper attention to postoperative splinting is vital, and systematic exercises are essential.

Peacock, Madden, and Trier[551] have emphasized the anatomic location of the median nerve in the proximal half of the forearm. They also have felt that if a sensory loss or intrinsic paralysis follows an upper-arm forearm injury, emergency exploration on the brachial artery and the median and ulnar nerves is indicated. They emphasized that the median and ulnar nerves should be transferred to a subcutaneous position following excision of all ischemic muscles if these nerves do not lie in normally perfused tissue.

Lipscomb and Burleson[543] have stated that early and adequate treatment of the acute vascular complication of supracondylar fractures of the humerus is necessary, even though it means surgical exploration of the antecubital fossa and resection of the injured segment of the brachial artery. In eight patients resection of the damaged section of artery helped to prevent the Volkmann's ischemia. They also felt that nerve palsy should be observed for a few weeks after fracture reduction, but that surgical exploration was indicated if no improvement in nerve function was observed in this time interval. *The goal of early treatment is to restore adequate circulation before irreparable damage is done.*

A subacute stage of ischemic necrosis occurs when the ischemia-edema cycle evolves gradually. The process is not always rapidly progressive but may take up to 16 weeks. Despite early evidence that some of the antebrachial musculature is involved, during the subacute phase the ischemic process may extend to involve all of the antebrachial muscle. The findings are those of wrist and finger contractures, nerve palsies, and induration in the forearm muscles Eaton and Green[521] feel that as long as the induration is present, fasciotomy will provide some benefit.

The treatment of severe established Volkmann's ischemic contracture demands special knowledge in the reconstructive surgery of the extremities (Fig. 4-24). Seddon[553] has stated, "The lesion is a massive infarct. The treatment is, briefly, excision of all irreparably damaged muscle and nerves followed by such reconstructive procedures as may be required to minimize the deficiency."

In the upper extremity the infarct may take the form of an ellipsoid with the greatest damage in the flexor digitorium profundus or flexor pollicis longus. The superficial muscles and deep extensors may also be fibrotic.

Littler[544] has emphasized that there are three elements to Volkmann's ischemic muscle fibrosis: (1) intrinsic muscle paralysis (but not fibrosis), (2) loss of sensibility of the hand, and (3) contracture producing pronation of the forearm with wrist and digital flexion. He condemned carpectomy and radioulnar resection and felt that the whole length of the forearm must be exposed to excise the functionless and contracted muscle mass completely. Both median and ulnar nerves should be dissected free. With return of sensibility and intrinsic muscle action, extrinsic flexor power can be restored by synergistic tendon transfer. The muscle slide procedure advocated by Page[549] produces a dynamic tenodesis in a less severe case.

In the lower extremity the goal is a stable, plantigrade foot. Tendon transfers can restore dorsiflexion, and occasionally mid- and hind-foot fusions are necessary.

Summary

The management of Volkmann's ischemic

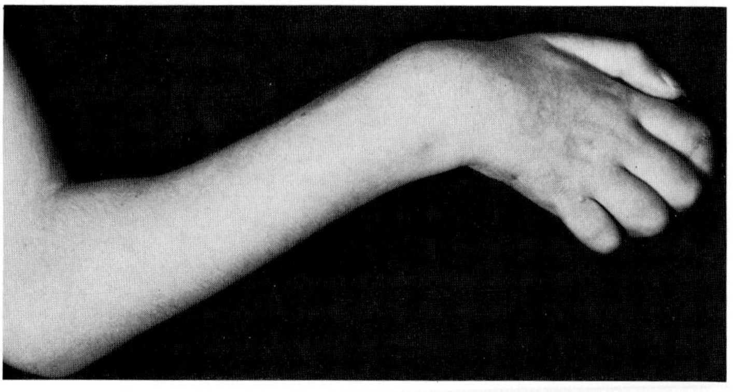

Fig. 4-24. Photograph of the forearm and hand in a patient with late Volkmann's ischemic contracture.

contracture—including its prevention, early recognition, prompt treatment, as well as the reconstruction of established contractures—requires great skill on the part of the orthopaedic surgeon. He must be familiar with all phases of care.

I thank Mrs. Marilyn Williams for her assistance in the preparation of this chapter and Miss Rita Feran for editorial assistance.

REFERENCES

Shock

1. Altemeier, W. A., Todd, J. C., and Inge, W. W.: Gram-negative septicemia: a growing threat. Ann. Surg., *166*:530-542, 1967.
2. Aviado, D. M.: Pharmacologic approach to the treatment of shock. Ann. Intern. Med., *62*:1050-1059, 1965.
3. Baue, A. E., Wurth, M. A., and Sayeed, M. M.: The dynamics of altered ATP-dependent and ATP-yielding cell processes in shock. Surgery, *72*:94-101, 1972.
4. Baxter, C. R., Zedlitz, W. H., and Shires, G. T.: High output acute renal failure complicating traumatic injury. J. Trauma, *4*:567-580, 1964.
5. Beecher, H. K., Simeone, F. A., Burnett, C. H., Shapiro, S. L., Sullivan, E. R., and Mallory, T.B.: The internal state of the severely wounded man on entry to the most forward hospital. Surgery, *22*:672-711, 1947.
6. Blaisdell, F. W.: Respiratory insufficiency syndrome: clinical and pathological definition. J. Trauma, *13*:195-199, 1973.
7. Blalock, A.: Shock. Further studies with particular reference to the effects of hemorrhage. Arch. Surg., *29*:837-857, 1937.
8. ———: Principles of Surgical Care, Shock, and Other Problems. St. Louis, C. V. Mosby, 1940.
9. Bluemle, L. W., Jr., Webster, G. D., Jr., and Elkinton, J. R.: Acute tubular necrosis; analysis of 100 cases with respect to mortality, complications and treatment with and without dialysis. Arch. Intern. Med., *104*:180-197, 1959.
10. Bredenberg, C. E., James, P. M., Collins, J., Anderson, R. W., Martin, A. M., Jr., and Hardaway, R. M.: Respiratory failure in shock. Ann. Surg., *169*:392-403, 1969.
11. Boba, A., and Converse, J. G.: Ganglionic blockage and its protective action in hemorrhage: a review. Anesthesiology, *18*: 559-572, 1957.
12. Byrne, J. J.: Symposium on Shock. Am. J. Surg., *110*:293-297, 1965.
13. Byrne, J. J.: Shock. N. Engel. J. Med., *275*:543-546, 1966.
14. Cafferata, H. T., Aggeler, D. M., Robinson, A. J., and Blaisdell, F. W.: Intravascular coagulation in the surgical patient. Am. J. Surg., *118*:281-291, 1969.
15. Cahill, J. M., Jouasset-Strieder, D., and Byrne, J. J.: Lung function in shock. Am. J. Surg., *110*:324-329, 1965.
16. Carey, L. C., Lowery, B. D., and Cloutier, C. T.: Hemorrhagic shock in current problems in surgery. Chicago, Year Book Medical Publishers, 1971.
17. Cloutier, Lcdr. C. T., Lowery, Lcdr. B. D., and Carey, L. C.: Acid-base disturbances in hemorrhagic shock. In 66 severely wounded patients prior to treatment. Arch Surg., *98*:551-557, 1969.
18. Collins, J. A.: The causes of progressive pulmonary insufficiency in surgical patients. J. Surg. Res., *9*:685-704, 1969.
19. Collins, V. J., Jaffee, R., and Zahony, I.: Shock. A different approach to therapy. Ill. Med. J., *122*:350-353, 1962.
20. Cook, W. A., Schwartz, D. L., and Bass, B. G.: Arfonad therapy. Hemodynamic responses and control. Ann. Thorac. Surg., *7*:322-332, 1969.
21. Crenshaw, C. A., Canizaro, P. C., Shires, G. T., and Allsman, A.: Changes in extracellular fluid during acute hemorrhagic shock in man. Surg. Forum, *13*:6-7, 1962.
22. Crile, G. W.: Blood Pressure in Surgery: An Experimental and Clinical Research. Philadelphia, J. B. Lippincott, 1903.
23. Duff, J. H., Scott, H. M., Peretz, D. I., Mulligan, G. W., and MacLean, L. D.: The diagnosis and treatment of shock in man based on hemodynamic and metabolic measurements. J. Trauma, *6*:145-156, 1966.

24. Essiet, G. S., and Stahl, W. M.: Water and electrolyte content of tissues in hemorrhagic shock and surgical trauma. Surg. Gynecol. Obstet., *137*:11-14, 1973.
25. Evarts, C. M.: Low molecular weight dextran. Med. Clin. North Amer., *51*: 1285-1299, 1967.
26. Franklin, S. S., and Merrill, J. P.: Acute renal failure. N. Engl. J. Med., *262*:711-718, 1960.
27. Friedman, E. W., and Frank, E. D.: Management of traumatic shock in man. Orthop. Clin. North Amer., *1*:3-11, 1970.
28. Friedman, E., Grable, E., and Fine, J.: Central venous pressure and direct serial measurements as guides in blood-volume replacement. Lancet, *2*:609-614, 1966.
29. Gross, S. G.: A System of Surgery: Pathological, Diagnostic, Therapeutique, and Operative. Philadelphia, Lea & Febiger, 1872.
30. Gunnar, R. M., and Loeb, H. S.: Use of drugs in cardiogenic shock due to acute myocardial infarction. Circulation, *45*: 1111-1124, 1972.
31. Hamit, H. F.: Current trends of therapy and research in shock. Surg. Gynecol. Obstet., *120*:835-854, 1965.
32. Hampson, L. G., Scott, H. J., and Gurd, F. N.: A comparison of intraarterial and intravenous transfusion in normal dogs and in dogs with experimental myocardial infarction. Ann. Surg., *140*:56-66, 1954.
33. Hankins, J. R., Attar, S., Turney, S. Z., Cowley, R. A., and McLaughlin, J. S.: Differential diagnosis in pulmonary parenchymal changes in thoracic trauma. Amer. Surg., *39*:309-318, 1973.
34. Hardaway, R. M.: Microcoagulation in shock. Amer. J. Surg., *110*:298-301, 1965.
35. Harkins, H. N.: Shock, Surgery: Principles and Practice. Philadelphia, J. B. Lippincott, 1961.
36. Henry, J. N.: The effect of shock on pulmonary alveolar surfactant. Its role in refractory respiratory insufficiency of the critically ill or severely injured patient. J. Trauma, *8*:756-773, 1968.
37. Jones, R. C., and Blotcky, M. J.: Initial management of the severely injured patient. South Med. J., *62*:260-265, 1969.
38. Kiley, J. E., Powers, S. R., Jr., and Beebe, R. T.: Acute renal failure; eighty cases of renal tubular necrosis. N. Engl. J. Med., *262*:481-486, 1960.
39. Litwin, M. S.: Blood viscosity in shock. Amer. J. Surg., *110*:313-316, 1965.
40. Maclean, L. D.: Shock due to sepsis—a summary of current concepts of pathogenesis and treatment. J. Trauma, *2*:412-423, 1962.
41. Martin, A. M., Jr., Soloway, H. B., and Simmons, R. L.: Pathologic anatomy of the lungs following shock and trauma. J. Trauma, *8*:687-699, 1968.
42. Mela, L. M., Miller, L. D., and Nicholas, G. G.: Influence of cellular acidosis and altered cation concentrations on shock-induced mitochondrial damage. Surgery, *72*:102-110, 1972.
43. Miller, R. M., Polakavetz, S. H., Hornick, R. B., and Cowley, R. A.: Analysis of infections acquired by the severely injured patient. Surg. Gynecol. Obstet., *137*:7-10, 1973.
44. Moncrief, J. A.: Shock in the multiple-injury patient. J. Bone Joint Surg., *49A*: 540-546, 1967.
45. Moore, D. C.: Complications of regional anesthesia. *In:* Clinical Anesthesia, Bonica, J. J., (ed.). Philadelphia, F. A. Davis, 1969.
46. Moore, F. D.: Metabolic Care of the Surgical Patient. Philadelphia, W. B. Saunders, 1959.
47. ———: Terminal mechanisms in human injury. Amer. J. Surg., *110*:317-323, 1965.
48. Moore, F. D., *et al.*: Post-traumatic Pulmonary Insufficiency. Philadelphia, W. B. Saunders, 1969.
49. Ollodart, R., and Mansberger, A. R.: The effect of hypovolemic shock on bacterial defense. Amer. J. Surg., *110*:302-307, 1965.
50. Peterson, R. E., O'Toole, J. J., and Kirkendall, W. M.: The variability of extracellular fluid space (sucrose) in man during a 24 hour period. J. Clin. Invest., *38*:1644, 1959.
51. Pontoppidan, H., Geffin, B., and Lowenstein, E.: Acute respiratory failure in the adult. N. Engl. J. Med., *287*:690-698, 1972.
52. Powers, S. R.: The maintenance of renal function following massive trauma. J. Trauma, *10*:554-564, 1970.
53. Saunders, C. A., Buckley, J. J., Leinbach, R. C., Mundth, E. D., and Austen, W. G., *et al.*: Mechanical circulatory assistance. Current status and experience with combining circulatory assistance, emergency coronary angiography, and acute myocardial revascularization. Circulation, *45*: 1292-1313, 1972.

54. Shenkin, H. A., Cheney, R. H., Gorons, S. R., Hardy, J. D., Fletcher, A. G. Jr., and Starr, I.: On the diagnosis of hemorrhage in man: a study of volunteers bled large amounts. Amer. J. Med. Sci., *208*: 421-436, 1944.
55. Shires, T., and Carrico, C. J.: Current Status of the Shock Problem. *In* Current Problems in Surgery. Chicago, Year Book Medical Publishers, 1966.
56. Shires, G. T., Carrico, L. J., and Canizaro, P. C.: Shock. Major Problems in Clinical Surgery. Philadelphia, W. B. Saunders, 1973.
57. Shires, G. T., Cunningham, J. N., Baker, C. R. F., Reeder, S. F., Illner, H., Wagner, I. Y., and Maher, J.: Alterations in cellular membrane function during hemorrhagic shock in primates. Ann. Surg., *176*:288-295, 1972.
58. Simeone, F. A.: Shock. *In* Davis, L. (ed.): Christopher's Textbook of Surgery. Philadelphia, W. B. Saunders, 1964.
59. ———: Pulmonary complications of nonthoracic wounds; a historical perspective. J. Trauma, *8*:625-648, 1968.
60. Tanner, G. A., and Selkurt, E. E.: Kidney function in the squirrel monkey before and after hemorrhagic hypotension. Amer. J. Physiol., *219*:597-603, 1970.
61. Teschan, P. E.: Management of patients with posttraumatic renal insufficiency. J. Trauma, *3*:181-188, 1963.
62. Thal, A. P., and Sardesai, V. M.: Shock and the circulating polypeptides. Amer. J. Surg., *110*:308-312, 1965.
63. Thal, A. D., and Wilson, R. F.: Shock. Current Problems in Surgery. Chicago, Year Book Medical Publishers, 1965.
64. Watts, D. T.: Arterial blood epinephrine levels during hemorrhagic hypotension in dogs. Amer. J. Physiol., *184*:271-274, 1956.
65. Weinstein, L., and Klainer, A. S.: Management of emergencies. IV. Septic shock —pathogenesis and treatment. N. Engl. J. Med., *274*:950-953, 1966.
66. Wiggers, C. J.: The present status of the shock problem. Physiol Rev., *22*:74-123, 1942.
67. Wilson J. W.: Treatment or prevention of pulmonary cellular damage with pharmacologic doses of corticosteroid. Surg. Gynecol. Obstet., *134*:675-681, 1972.
68. Wilson, R. F., Kafi, A., Asuncion, Z., and Walt, A. J.: Clinical respiratory faliure after shock or trauma. Prognosis and methods of diagnosis. Arch. Surg., *98*: 539-550, 1969.

Cardiac Arrest

69. Baringer, J. R., Salzman, E. W., Jones, W. A., and Friedlich, A. L.: External cardiac massage. N. Engl. J. Med., *265*:62-65, 1961.
70. Beck, C. S., Pritchard, W. H., and Feil, S. H.: Ventricular fibrillation of long duration abolished by electric shock. J.A.M.A., *135*:985-986, 1947.
71. Boehm, R.: V. Arbeiten aus dem pharmakologischen Institut der Universitat Dorpat: 13, Ueber Weiderbelebung nach Vergiftungen und Asphyxie. Arch. Exper. Path., *8*:68-101, 1878.
72. The closed-chest method of cardiopulmonary resuscitation—revised statement. Circulation, *31*:641-643, 1965.
73. Cole, S. L., and Corday, E.: Four-minute limit for cardiac resuscitation. J.A.M.A., *161*:1454-1458, 1956.
74. Gresham, G. A., Kuczynski, D., and Rosborough, D.: Fatal fat embolism following replacement arthroplasty for transcervical fractures of femur. Brit. Med. J., *2*:617-619, 1971.
75. Himmelhoch, S. R., Dekker, A., Gazzaniga, A. B., and Like, A. A.: Closed-chest cardiac resuscitation; a prospective clinical and pathological study. N. Engl. J. Med., *270*:118-122, 1964.
76. Johnson, J. D.: A plan of action in cardiac arrest. J.A.M.A., *186*:468-472, 1963.
77. Jude, J. R., Kouwenhoven, W. B., and Knickerbocker, G. G.: Clinical and experimental application of a new treatment for cardiac arrest. Surg. Forum, *11*:252-254, 1960.
78. ———: A new approach to cardiac resuscitation. Ann. Surg., *154*:311-319, 1961.
79. Klassen, G. A., Broadhurst, C., Peretz, D. I., and Johnson, A. L.: Cardiac resuscitation in 126 medical patients using external cardiac massage. Lancet, *1*:1290-1292, 1963.
80. Kouwenhoven, W. B., Jude, J. R., and Knickerbocker, G. G.: Closed-chest cardiac massage. J.A.M.A., *173*:1064-1067, 1960.
81. Landau, I.: New legal risks in cardiac arrest. Hospital Physician, *2*:80-91, 1966.
82. Lown, B., Amarasingham, R., and Neuman, J.: New method for terminating cardiac arrhythmias; use of synchronized

capacitor discharge. J.A.M.A., *182*:548-555, 1967.
83. MacKenzie, G. J., Taylor, S. H., McDonald, A. H., and McDonald, K. W.: Haemondynamic effects of external cardiac compression. Lancet, *1*:1342-1345, 1964.
84. Messer, J. V.: Cardiac arrest. N. Engl. J. Med., *275*:35-39, 1966.
85. Nachlas, M. M., and Miller, D. I.; Closed-chest cardiac resuscitation in patients with myocardial infarction. Amer. Heart J., *69*:448-459, 1965.
86. Newens, A. F., and Volz, R. G.: Severe hypotension during prosthetic hip surgery with acrylic bone cement. Anesthesiology, *36*:298-300, 1972.
87. Phillips, J. H., and Burch, G. E.: Management of cardiac arrest. Amer. Heart J., *67*:265-277, 1964.
88. Powell, J. N., McGrath, D. J., Lahiri, S. K., and Hill, P.: Cardiac arrest associated with bone cement. Brit. Med. J., *3*:326, 1970.
89. Safar, P., Brown, T. C., Holtey, W. J., and Wilder, R. J.: Ventilation and circulation with closed-chest cardiac massage in man. J.A.M.A., *176*:574-576, 1961.
90. Schiff, M.: Ueber direckte Reizung der Herzoberflache. Arch. ges. Physiol., *28*: 200-228, 1882.
91. Schuh, F. T., Schuh, S. M., Viguera, M. G., and Terry, R. N.: Circulatory changes following implantation of methyl methacrylate bone cement. Anesthesiology, *39*: 455-457, 1973.
92. Shohet, S. B., and Sweet, R. H.: Cardiac resuscitation; the combined use of external cardiac massage, external cardiac defibrillation and external cardiac stimulation. N. Engl. J. Med., *267*:976-977, 1962.
93. Stahlgren, L. H., and Angelchik, J.: Cardiac arrest: evaluation of cardiac massage in treatment of seventy patients with emphasis on cardiac arrests occurring outside the operating room. J.A.M.A., *174*:226-233, 1960.
94. Standards for Cardiopulmonary Resuscitation of Emergency Cardiac Care. J.A.M.A., *227* [Suppl.]:47, 1974.
95. Symposium on Emergency Resuscitation. Acta Anaesth. Scand., [Suppl.] 9:11-203, 1961.
96. Zoll, P. M., and Linenthal, A. J.: Termination of refractory tachycardia by external countershock. Circulation, *25*:596-603, 1962.
97. Zoll, P. M., Linenthal, A. J., Gibson, W., Paul, M. H., and Norman, L. R.: Termination of ventricular fibrillation in man by externally applied electric countershock. N. Engl. J. Med., *254*:727-732, 1956.
98. Zoll, P. M. Linenthal, A. J., and Zarsky, L. R. N.: Ventricular fibrillation; treatment and prevention by external electric currents. N. Engl. J. Med., *262*:105-112, 1960.

Hemostasis

99. Bennett, B., and Douglas, A. S.: Blood Coagulation Mechanism. Clin. Haematol., *2*:3-22, 1973.
100. Bennett, B., and Ratnoff, O. D.: Studies on the response of patients with classic hemophilia to transfusion with concentrates of antihemophilic factor. J. Clin. Invest., *51*:2593-2596, 1972.
101. Deykin, D.: Emerging concepts of platelet function. N. Engl. J. Med., *290*:144-151, 1974.
102. George, J. N., and Breckenridge, R.: The use of factor VIII and factor IX concentrates during surgery. J.A.M.A., *214*: 1673-1676, 1970.
103. Johnson, A. J., Karpatkin, M. H., and Newman, J.: Clinical investigation of intermediate and high-purity factor VIII concentrates. Brit. J. Haematol., *21*:21-41, 1971.
104. Kwaan, H. C.: Disseminated intravascular coagulation. Med. Clin. North Amer., *56*:177-191, 1972.
105. McNicol, G. P., and Davies, J. A.: Fibrinolytic enzyme system. Clin. Haematol., *2*:23-51, 1973.
106. Sandler, S. G., Rath, C. E., and Ruder, A.: Prothrombin complex concentrates in acquired hypoprothrombinemia. Ann. Intern. Med., *79*:485-491, 1973.
107. Zimmerman, T. S., Ratnoff, O. D., and Powell, A. E.: Immunologic differentiation of classic hemophilia (factor VIII deficiency) and von Willebrand's disease. J. Clin. Invest., *50*:244-254, 1971.

Thromboembolism

108. Arfors, K.-E., Hint, H. C., Dhall, D. P., and Matheson, N. A.: Counteraction of platelet activity at sites of laser-induced endothelial trauma. Brit. Med. J., *4*:430-431, 1968.
109. Atkins, P., and Hawkins, L. A.: The diagnosis of deep-vein thrombosis in the leg using ^{125}I-Fibrinogen. Brit. J. Surg., *55*: 825-830, 1968.

110. Bergentz, S. E., Gelin, L. E., and Rudenstam, C. M.: Fats and thrombus formation. An experimental study. Thromb. Diath. Haemorrh., *5*:474-479, 1961.
111. The Behavior of Thrombi. Arch Surg., *105*:681-682, 1972.
112. Berman, H. J.: Anticoagulant-induced alterations in hemostasis, platelet thrombosis, and vascular fragility in the peripheral vessels of the hamster cheek pouch. *In* Macmillan, R. L., and Msutard, J. F. (eds.): International Symposium: Anticoagulants and Fibrinolysins. Philadelphia, Lea & Febiger, 1961.
113. Bloom, W. L.: Present status of plasma volume expanders in the treatment of shock. Clinical laboratory studies. Arch. Surg., *63*:739-741, 1951.
114. Bookstein, J. J.: Segmental arteriography in pulmonary embolism. Radiology, *93*: 1007-1012, 1969.
115. Borgstrom, S., Gelin, L., and Zederfeldt, B.: The formation of vein thrombi following tissue injury; an experimental study in rabbits. Acta Chir. Scand., [Suppl.]: *247*:1-36, 1959.
116. Browse, N. L.: The ^{125}I fibrinogen uptake test. Arch. Surg., *104*:160-163, 1972.
117. Bull, J. P., Ricketts, C., Squire, J. R., Maycock, W. d'A., Spooner, S. J. L., Mollison, P. L., and Paterson, J. C. S.: Dextran as a plasma substitute. Lancet, *1*:134-143, 1949.
118. Bygdeman, S., and Eliasson, R.: Effect of dextrans on platelet adhesiveness and aggregation. Scand. J. Clin. Lab. Invest., *20*:17-23, 1967.
119. Bygdeman, S., Eliasson, R., and Gullbring, B.: Effect of dextran infusion on the adenosine diphosphate induced adhesiveness and the spreading capacity of human blood platelets. Thromb. Diath. Haemorrh., *15*:451-456, 1966.
120. Bygdeman, S., Eliasson, R., and Johnson, S. R.: Relationship between postoperative changes in adenosine-diphosphate induced platelet adhesiveness and venous thrombosis. Lancet, *1*:1301-1302, 1966.
121. Coon, W. W., and Coller, F. A.: Some epidemiologic considerations of thromboembolism. Surg. Gynecol. Obstet., *109*: 487-501, 1959.
122. Coon, W. W., and Willis, P. W., III: Deep venous thrombosis and pulmonary embolism. Prediction, prevention and treatment. Amer. J. Cardiol., *4*:611-621, 1959.
123. Couch, N. P.: Guest Editor's Introduction. A.M.A. Archives Symposium on Diagnostic Techniques in Phlebothrombosis. Arch. Surg., *104*:132-133, 1972.
124. Culver, D., Crawford, J. S., Gardiner, J. H., and Wiley, A. M.: Venous thrombosis after fractures of the upper end of the femur. A study of incidence and site. J. Bone Joint Surg., *52B*:61-69, 1970.
125. DeWeese, J. A., and Rogoff, S. M.: Clinical uses of functional ascending phlebography of the lower extremity. Angiology, *9*:268-278, 1958.
126. Deykin, D.: Thrombogenesis. N. Engl. J. Med., *276*:622-628, 1967.
127. ———: Emerging concepts of platelet function. N. Engl. J. Med., *290*:144-151, 1974.
128. [Research Council] Effect of aspirin on postoperative venous thrombosis. Lancet, *2*:441-444, 1972.
129. Ernst, C. B., Fry, W. J., Fraft, R. O., and DeWeese, M. S.: The role of low molecular weight dextran in the management of venous thrombosis. Surg. Gynecol. Obstet., *119*:1243-1247, 1964.
130. Evans, G., and Mustard, J. F.: Platelet-surface reaction and thrombosis. Surgery, *64*:273-280, 1968.
131. Evarts, C. M.: Low molecular weight dextran. Med. Clin. North Amer., *51*: 1285-1299, 1967.
132. Evarts, C. M., and Alfidi, R. J.: Thromboembolism after total hip reconstruction. Failure of low doses of heparin in prevention. J.A.M.A., *225*:515-516, 1973.
133. Evarts, C. M., and Feil, E. I.: Prevention of thromboembolic disease. J. Bone Joint Surg., *53A*:1271-1280, 1971.
134. Fagan, D. G.: Prevention of thromboembolic phenomena following operations on the neck of the femur. Lancet, *1*:846-848, 1964.
135. Fitts, W. T., Jr., Lehr, H. B., Bitner, R. L., and Spelman, J. W.: An analysis of 950 fatal injuries. Surgery, *56*:663-668, 1964.
136. Flanc, C., Kakkar, V. V., and Clarke, M. B.: The detection of venous thrombosis of the legs using ^{125}I-labeled fibrinogen. Brit. J. Surg., *55*:742-747, 1968.
137. Freeark, R. J., Bostwick, J., and Fardin, R.: Posttraumatic venous thrombosis. Arch. Surg., *95*:567-575, 1967.
138. Fulton, G. P., Akers, R. P., and Lutz, B. R.: White thromboembolism and vascular fragility in the hamster cheek pouch after anticoagulants. Blood, *8*:140-152, 1953.
139. Gallus, A. S., Hirsh, J., Tuttle, R. J., Trebilcock, R., O'Brien, S. E., Carroll, J. J.,

Minden, J. H., and Hudecki, S. M.: Small subcutaneous doses of heparin in prevention of venous thrombosis. N. Engl. J. Med., *288*:545-551, 1973.

140. Golodner, H., Morse, L. J., and Angrist, A.: Pulmonary embolism in fractures of the hip. Surgery, *18*:418-423, 1945.

141. Gronwall, A., and Ingleman, B.: Dextran as a volume expander. Acta Physiol. Scand., *7*:97-107, 1944.

142. Hamilton, H. W., Crawford, J. S., Gardiner, J. H., and Wiley, A. M.: Venous thrombosis in patients with fracture of the upper end of the femur. A phlebographic study of the effect of prophylactic anticoagulion. J. Bone Joint Surg., *52B*:268-289, 1970.

143. Harris, W. H., Salzman, E. W., and DeSanctis, R. W.: The prevention of thromboembolic disease by prophylactic anticoagulation. A controlled study in elective hip surgery. J. Bone Joint Surg., *49A*: 81-89, 1967.

144. Harris, W. H., Salzmann E. W., DeSanctis, R. W., and Coutts, R. D.: Prevention of venous thromboembolism following total hip replacement. J.A.M.A., *220*: 1319-1322, 1972.

145. Hildner, F. J., and Ormond, R. S.: Accuracy of the clinical diagnosis of pulmonary embolism. J.A.M.A., *202*:567-570, 1967.

146. Hirsch, J., and McBride, J. A.: Increased platelet adhesivesness in recurrent venous thrombosis and pulmonary embolism. Brit. Med. J., *2*:797-799, 1965.

147. Hume, M., Sevitt, S., and Thomas, D. P.: Venous Thrombosis and Pulmonary Embolism. Cambridge, Mass., Harvard University Press, 1970.

148. Just-Viera, J. O., and Yeager, G. H.: Protection from thrombosis in large veins. Surg. Gynecol. Obstet., *118*:354-360, 1964.

149. Kakkar, V.: The diagnosis of deep vein thrombosis using the ^{125}I fibrinogen test. Arch. Surg., *104*:152-159, 1972.

150. Kakkar, V. V., Howe, C. T., Flanc, C., and Clarke, M. B.: Natural history of postoperative deep-vein thrombosis. Lancet, *2*:230-232, 1969.

151. Kakkar, V. V., Spindler, J., Flute, P. T., Corrigan, T., Fossard, D. P., Crellin, R. Q., Wessler, S., and Yin, E. T.: Efficacy of low doses of heparin in prevention of deep-vein thrombosis after major surgery. Lancet, *2*:101-106, 1972.

152. Koekenberg, L. J. L.: Experimental use of macrodex as a prophylaxis against postoperative thrombo-embolism. Bull. Soc. Int. Chir., *21*:501-512, 1962.

153. Langsjoen, P., and Murray, R. A.: Treatment of postsurgical thromboembolic complications. J.A.M.A., *218*:855-860, 1971.

154. Laufman, H.: Deep vein thrombophlebitis. Current status of etiology and treatment. Arch. Surg., *99*:489-493, 1969.

155. MacLean, L. D., Shibata, H. R., McLean, A. P. H., Skinner, G. B., and Gutelius, J. R.: Pulmonary embolism; the value of bedside scanning, angiography and pulmonary embolectomy. Can. Med. Assoc. J., *97*:991-1000, 1967.

156. Mansfield, A. O.: Alteration in fibrinolysis associated with surgery and venous thrombosis. Brit. J. Surg., *59*:754-757, 1972.

157. Marks, J., Truscott, B. M., and Withycombe, J. F. R.: Treatment of venous thrombosis with anticoagulants. Review of 1135 cases. Lancet, *2*:787-791, 1954.

158. Mavor, G. E., and Galloway, J. M.: Iliofemoral venous thrombosis. Pathological considerations and surgical management. Brit. J. Surg., *56*:45-49, 1969.

159. Miller, G. A. H.: The diagnosis and management of massive pulmonary embolism. Brit. J. Surg., *59*:837-839, 1972.

160. Mishkin, F.: Lung scanning: its use in diagnosis of disorders of the pulmonary circulation. Arch. Inte Med., *118*:65-69, 1966.

161. Mobin-Uddin, K., McLean, R., Bolloki, H., and Jude, J. R.: Caval interruption for prevention of pulmonary embolism. Arch. Surg., *99*:711-715, 1969.

162. Morrell, M. T., and Dunnill, M. S.: The post-mortem incidence of pulmonary embolism in a hospital population. Brit. J. Surg., *55*:347-352, 1968.

163. Morrell, M. T., Truelove, S. C., and Barr, A.: Pulmonary embolism. Brit. Med. J. *2*:830-835, 1963.

164. Murphy, E. A., Mustard, J. F., Rowsell, H. C., and Downie, H. G.: Quantitative studies on the effect of dicumarol on experimental thrombosis. J. Lab. Clin. Med., *61*:935-943, 1963.

165. Negus, D., Pinto, D. J., LeQuesne, L. P., Brown, N., and Chapman, M.: ^{125}I-labelled fibrinogen in the diagnosis of deep-vein thrombosis and its correlation with phlebography. Brit. J. Surg., *55*:835-839, 1968.

166. Neu, L. T., Jr., Waterfield, J. R., and Ash, C. J.: Prophylactic anticoagulant therapy in the orthopaedic patient. Ann. Intern. Med., *62*:463-467, 1965.

167. Nicolaides, A. N., Desai, S., Douglas, J. N., Fourides, G., Dupont, P. A., Lewis,

J. D., Dodsworth, H., Luck, R. J., and Jamieson, C. W.: Small doses of subcutaneous sodium heparin in preventing deep venous thrombosis after major surgery. Lancet, *2*:890-893, 1972.

168. Nylander, G.: Phlebographic diagnosis of acute deep leg thrombosis. Acta Chir. Scandinav., *387* [Suppl.]:30-34, 1968.

169. O'Brien, J. R.: Effects of salicylates on human platelets. Lancet, *1*:779-783, 1968.

170. ———: Detection of thrombosis with Iodine^{125} fibrinogen. Data reassessed. Lancet, *2*:396-398, 1970.

171. Parker, B. M., and Smith, J. R.: Pulmonary embolism and infarction. A review of the physiologic consequences of pulmonary arterial obstruction. Amer. J. Med., *24*:402-427, 1958.

172. Pollak, E. W., Sparks, F. C., and Barker, W. F.: Pulmonary embolism. An appraisal of therapy in 516 cases. Arch. Surg., *107*: 66-68, 1973.

173. Rabinov, K., and Paulin, S.: Roentgen diagnosis of venous thrombosis in the leg. Arch. Surg., *104*:134-144, 1972.

174. Russell, H. E., Jr., Bradham, R. R., and Lee, W. H., Jr.: An evaluation of infusion therapy (including dextran) for venous thrombosis. Circulation, *33*:839-846, 1966.

175. Salzman, E. W., Harris, W. H., and DeSanctis, R. W.: Anticoagulation for prevention of thromboembolism following fractures of the hip. N. Engl. J. Med., *275*:122-130, 1966.

176. ———: Reduction in venous thromboembolism by agents affecting platelet function. N. Engl. J. Med., *284*:1287-1292, 1971.

177. Sandritter, W.: Die pathologische Anatomie der Thrombose und Lung en Embolie. Son Derdruck aus Behring-werk-Mitteilungen, *4*:37-54, 1962.

178. Sevitt, S., and Gallagher, N. G.: Prevention of venous thrombosis and pulmonary embolism in injured patients. A trial of anticoagulant prophylaxis with phenindione in middle-aged and elderly patients with fractured necks of femur. Lancet, *2*:981-989, 1959.

179. ———: Venous thrombosis and pulmonary embolism: a clinico-pathological study in injured and burned patients. Brit. J. Surg., *48*:475-489, 1961.

180. Sigel B., Popky, G. L., Mapp, E. M., Feigl, P., Felix, W. R., Jr., and Ipsen, J.: Evaluation of Doppler ultrasound examination. Its use in diagnosis of lower extremity venous disease. Arch. Surg., *100*: 535-540, 1970.

181. Sigel, B., Popky, G. L., Wagner, D. K., Boland, J. P., Mapp, E. M., and Feigl, P.: A Doppler ultrasound method for diagnosing lower extremity venous disease. Surg. Gynecol. Obstet. *127*:339-350, 1968.

182. Smith, G. T., Dammin, G. J., and Dexter, L.: Postmortem arteriographic studies of the human lung in pulmonary embolization. J.A.M.A., *188*:143-151, 1964.

183. Solonen, K. A.: Prophylactic anticoagulant therapy in the treatment of lower limb fractures. Acta Orthop. Scandinav., *33*:329-341, 1963.

184. Tubiana, R., and Duparc, J.: Prevention of thrombo-embolic complications in orthopaedic and accident surgery. J. Bone Joint Surg., *43B*:7-15, 1961.

185. Virchow, R.: Die verstopfung den lungenarterie und ihre folgen. Beitr. Exper. Path. Physiol., *2*:1-12, 1846.

186. Wacker, W. E. C., Rosenthal, M. Snodgrass, P. J., and Amador, E.: A triad for the diagnosis of pulmonary embolism and infarction. J.A.M.A., *178*:8-13, 1961.

187. Weiss, H. J., Aledort, L. M., and Kochwa, S.: The effect of salicylates on the hemostatic properties of platelets in man. J. Clin. Invest., *47*:2169-2180, 1968.

188. Wessler, S., and Yin, E. T.: Theory and practice of minidose heparin in surgical patients. Circulation, *47*:671-676, 1973.

189. Wheeler, H. B., Person, D., O'Connell, D., and Mullick, S. C.: Impedance phlebography. Technique, interpretation and results. Arch. Surg., *104*:164-169, 1972.

190. Winfrey, E. W., III, and Foster, J. H.: Low molecular weight dextran in small artery surgery. Antithrombogenic effect. Arch. Surg., *88*:78-82, 1964.

Disseminated Intravascular Coagulation

191. Cafferata, H. T., Aggeler, P. M., Robinson, A. J., and Blaisdell, F. W.: Intravascular coagulation in the surgical patient; its significance and diagnosis. Amer. J. Surg., *118*:281-291, 1969.

192. Deykin, D.: The role of the liver in serum-induced hypercoagulability. J. Clin. Invest., *45*:256-263, 1966.

193. ———: The clinical challenge of disseminated intravascular coagulation. N. Engl. J. Med., *283*:636-644, 1970.

194. Fischer, S., Fletcher, A. P., Alkjaersig, N., and Sherry, S.: Immunoelectrophoretic characterization of plasma fibrinogen derivatives in patients with pathological plasma proteolysis. J. Lab. Clin. Med., *70*:903-922, 1967.

195. von Francken, I., Johansson, L., Olsson,

P., and Zetterqvist, E.: Heparin treatment of bleeding. Lancet, *1*:70-73, 1963.

196. Hardaway, R. M.: Syndromes of Disseminated Intravascular Coagulation: with Special Reference to Shock and Hemorrhage. Springfield, Charles C Thomas, 1966.

197. Hardaway, R. M., James, P. M., Jr., Anderson, R. W., Bredenberg, C. E., and West, R. L.: Intensive study and treatment of shock in man. J.A.M.A., *199*:779-790, 1967.

198. Hawiger, J., Niewiarowski, S., Gurewich, V., and Thomas, D. P.: Measurements of fibrinogen and fibrin degradation products in serum by staphylococcal clumping test. J. Lab. Clin. Med., *75*:93-108, 1970.

199. Lasch, H. G., Heene, D. L., Huth, K., and Sandritter, W.: Pathophysiology; clinical manifestations and therapy of of consumption-coagulopathy ("Verbrauchokoagulopathy"). Amer. J. Cardiol., *20*:381-391, 1967.

200. Lasch, H. G., Róka, L., and Heene, D.: The defibrination syndrome. Throm. Diath. Haem., *20* [Suppl.]:97-105, 1966.

201. McKay, D. G., and Müller-Berghaus, G.: Therapeutic implications of disseminated intravascular coagulation. Amer. J. Cardiol., *20*:392-410, 1967.

202. Merskey, C.: Defibrination syndrome. *In* Biggs, R. (ed.): Human Blood Coagulation, Haemostasis, and Thrombosis. Blackwell Scientific Publications, Oxford, 1972.

203. Merskey, C., Lalezari, P., and Johnson, A. J.: A rapid simple sensitive method for measuring fibrinolytic split products in human serum. Proc. Soc. Exp. Biol. Med., *131*:871-875, 1969.

204. Merskey, C., Johnson, A. J., Kleiner, G. J., and Wohl, H.: The defibrination syndrome; clinical features and laboratory diagnosis. Brit. J. Haematol., *13*:528-549, 1967.

205. Merskey, C., Johnson, A. J., Pert, J. H., and Wohl, H.: Pathogenesis of fibrinolysis in defibrination syndrome; effect of heparin administration. Blood, *24*:701-715, 1964.

206. Phillips, L. L.: Alterations in the blood clotting system in disseminated intravascular coagulation. Ann. J. Cardiol., *21*: 174-184, 1967.

207. Ratnoff, O. D.: Epsilon aminocaproic acid—a dangerous weapon. New Eng. J. Med., *280*:1124-1225, 1969.

208. Sasaki, T., Page, I. H., and Shainoff, J. R.: Stable complex of fibrinogen and fibrin. Science, *152*:1069-1071, 1966.

209. Shainoff, J. R., and Page, I. H.: Significance of cryoprofibrin in fibrinogen-fibrin conversion. J. Exper. Med., *116*:687-707, 1962.

210. Verstraete, M., Vermylen, C., Vermylen, J., and Vandenbraucke, J.: Excessive consumption of blood coagulation components as cause of hemorrhagic diathesis. Amer. J. Med., *38*:899-908, 1965.

Fat Embolism

211. Aach, R., and Kissane, J. (eds. : Clinicopathologic conference. Fat embolism. Amer. J. Med., *51*:258-268, 1971.

212. Adler, F., and Peltier, L. F.: The laboratory diagnosis of fat embolism. Clin. Orthop., *21*:226-231, 1961.

213. Armin, J., and Grant, R. T.: Observations on gross pulmonary fat embolism in man and the rabbit. Clin. Sci., *10*:441-469, 1951.

214. Ashbaugh, D. G., and Petty, T. L.: The use of corticosteroids in the treatment of respiratory failure associated with massive fat embolism. Surg. Gynecol. Obstet., *123*:493-500, 1966.

215. Baker, P. L., Kuenzig, M. C., and Peltier, L. F.: Experimental fat embolism in dogs. J. Trauma, *9*:577-586, 1969.

216. Benestad, G.: Falle von Fettembolie mit punktformigen Blutungen in der Haut. Dsch. Z. Chir., *112*:194-205, 1911.

217. Benoit, P. R., Hampson, L. G., and Burgess, J. H.: Value of arterial hypoxemia in the diagnosis of pulmonary fat embolism. Ann. Surg., *175*:128-137, 1972.

218. Bergentz, S. E.: Studies on the genesis of posttraumatic fat embolism. Acta Chir. Scand., *282* [Suppl.]:1-72, 1961.

219. Bergmann, E. B.: Ein Fall todlicher Fettembolie. Klin. Wochenschr., *10*:385-387, 1873.

220. Bivins, B. A., Madauss, W. C., and Griffen, W. O., Jr.: Fat embolism syndrome: a clinical study. South. Med. J., *65*:937-940, 1972.

221. Blath, R. A., and Collins, J. A.: The relationship of lipuria to fat embolism in rabbits. J. Trauma, *10*:901-904, 1970.

222. Bradford, D. S., Foster, R. R., and Nossel, H. L.: Coagulation alterations, hypoxemia, and fat embolism in fracture patients. J. Trauma, *10*:307-321, 1970.

223. Broder, G., and Ruzumna, L.: Systemic fat embolism following acute primary osteomyelitis. J.A.M.A., *199*:1004-1006, 1967.

224. Cahill, J. M., Daly, B. F. T., and Byrne,

J. J.: Ventilatory and circulatory response to oleic acid embolus. J. Trauma, *14*:73-76, 1974.

225. Carver, G. M., Jr.: Traumatic renal infarction concurrent with massive fat embolism. J. Urol., *66*:331-339, 1951.

226. Cobb, C. A., Jr., and Hillman, J. W.: Fat embolism. American Academy of Orthopaedic Surgeons Instructional Course Lectures, *18*:122-129, 1961.

227. Collins, J. A., Gordon, W. C., Jr., Hudson, T. L., Irvin, R. W., Jr., Kelly, T., and Hardaway, R. M., III: Inapparent hypoxemia in casualties with wounded limbs: pulmonary fat embolism? Ann. Surg., *167*:511-520, 1968.

228. Collins, J. A., Hudson, T. L., Hamacher, W. R., Rokous, J., Williams, G., and Hardaway, R. M., III: Systemic fat embolism in four combat casualties. Ann. Surg., *167*:493-499, 1968.

229. Cuppage, F. E.: Fat embolism in diabetes mellitus. Amer. J. Clin. Pathol., *40*:270-275, 1963.

230. Czerny, V.: Ueber die klinische Bedeutung der Fettembolie. Klin. Wochenschr., *12*:593-595; 604-607, 1875.

231. Derian, P. S.: Fat embolization—current status. J. Trauma, *5*:580-586, 1965.

232. Drummond, D. S., Salter, R. B., and Boone, J.: Fat embolism in children: its frequency and relationships to collagen disease. Can. Med. Assoc. J., *101*:200-203, 1969.

233. Evarts, C. M.: Emerging concepts of fat embolism. Clin. Orthop., *33*:183-193, 1964.

234. ———: Diagnosis and treatment of fat embolism. J.A.M.A., *194*:899-901, 1965.

235. ———: Low molecular weight dextran. Med. Clin. North Amer., *51*:1285-1299, 1967.

236. ———: The fat embolism syndrome: a review. Surg. Clin. North Amer., *50*:493-507, 1970.

237. Fenger, G., and Salisbury, J. H.: Diffuse multiple capillary fat embolism of the lungs and brain in a fatal complication in common fractures; illustrated by a case. Chicago Med. J., *39*:587-595, 1879.

238. Field, M.: Fat embolism from a chronic osteomyelitis. J.A.M.A., *59*:2065-2066, 1912.

239. Fuschsig, P., Brücke, P., Blümel, G., and Gottlob, R.: A new clinical and experimental concept on fat metabolism. N. Engl. J. Med., *276*:1192-1193, 1967.

240. Gauss, H.: Studies in cerebral fat embolism: with reference to the pathology of delirium and coma. Arch. Intern. Med., *18*:76-102, 1916.

241. ———: The pathology of fat embolism. Arch. Surg., *9*:593-605, 1924.

242. Gerbershagen, H. U.: Fettembolie: Therapie mit niedrig viscösem Dextran. Anaesthesist (Berlin), *21*:23-25, 1972.

243. Graber, S.: Fat embolization associated with sickle cell crisis. South. Med. J., *54*:1395-1398, 1961.

244. Grondahl, N. B.: Utersuchungen über Fettembolie. Dtsch. Z. Chir., *111*:56-124, 1911.

245. Gurd, A. R.: Fat embolism: an aid to diagnosis. J. Bone Joint Surg., *52B*:732-737, 1970.

246. Hausberger, F. X., and Whitenack, S. H.: Effect of pressure on intravasation of fat from the bone marrow cavity. Surg. Gynecol. Obstet., *134*:931-936, 1972.

247. Haymaker, W., and Davison, C.: Fatalities resulting from exposure to simulated high altitudes in decompression chambers; clinicopathologic study of 5 cases. J. Neuropathol. Exp. Neurol., *9*:29-59, 1950.

248. Hill, R. B., Jr.: Fatal fat embolism from steroid-induced fatty liver. N. Engl. J. Med., *265*:318-320, 1961.

249. Immelman, E. J., Bank, S., Krige, H., and Marks, I. N.: Roentgenologic and clinical features of intramedullary fat necrosis in bones in acute and chronic pancreatitis. Amer. J. Med., *36*:96-105, 1964.

250. Jacobs, R. R., Wheeler, E. J., Jelenko, C., III, McDonald, T. F., and Bliven, F. E.: Fat embolism: a microscopic and ultrastructure evaluation of two animal models. J. Trauma, *13*:980-993, 1973.

251. Jones, J. P., Jr., Engleman, E. P., and Najarian, J. S.: Systemic fat embolism after renal homotransplantation and treatment with corticosteroids. N. Engl. J. Med., *273*:1453-1458, 1965.

252. Kearns, T. P.: Fat embolism of the retina; demonstrated by flat retinal preparation. Amer. J. Ophthalmol., *41*:1-2, 1956.

253. King, E. G., Weily, H. S., Genton, E., and Ashbaugh, D. G.: Consumption coagulopathy in the canine oleic acid model of fat embolism. Surgery, *69*:533-541, 1971.

254. Kraus, K. A.: Ueber Fettembolie des Gehirns nach Unfallen. Monatsschr. Unfallheilkd., *58*:353-361, 1955.

255. Lehman, E. P., and Moore, R. M.: Fat embolism; including experimental production without trauma. Arch. Surg., *14*:621-662, 1927.

256. LeQuire, V. S., Hillman, J. W., Gray, M.

E., and Snowden, R. T.: Clinical and pathologic studies of fat embolism. American Academy of Orthopaedic Surgeons Instructional Course Lectures, *19*:12-35, 1970.

257. LeQuire, V. S., Shapiro, J. L., LeQuire, C. B., Cobb, C. A., Jr., and Fleet, W. F., Jr.: A study of the pathogenesis of fat embolism based on human necropsy material and animal experiments. Amer. J. Pathol., *35*:999-1016, 1959.
258. Love, J., and Stryker, W. S.: Fat embolism; a problem of increasing importance to the orthopedist and the internist. Ann. Intern. Med., *46*:342-351, 1957.
259. Lynch, M. J.: Nephrosis and fat embolism in acute hemorrhagic pancreatitis. Arch. Intern. Med., *94*:709-717, 1964.
260. McCarthy, B., Mammen, E., Leblanc, L. P., and Wilson, R. F.: Sublinical fat embolism; a prospective study of 50 patients with extremity fractures. J. Trauma, *13*: 9-16, 1973.
261. McNamara, J. J., Molot, M., Dunn, R., Burran, E. L., and Stremple, J. F.: Lipid metabolism after trauma. Role in the pathogenesis of fat embolism. J. Thorac. Cardiovasc. Surg., *63*:968-972, 1972.
262. Maruyama, Y., and Little, J. B.: Roentgen manifestations of traumatic pulmonary fat embolism. Radiology, *79*:945-952, 1962.
263. Meek, R. N., Woodruff, B., and Allardyce, D. B.: Source of fat macroglobules in fractures of the lower extremity. J. Trauma, *12*:432-434, 1972.
264. Miller, J. A., Fonkalsrud, E. W., Latta, H. L., and Maloney, J. V., Jr.: Fat embolism associated with extra-corporeal circulation and blood transfusion. Surgery, *51*:448-451, 1962.
265. Motamed, H. A.: Fundamental aspects of post-multiple injury fat embolism. Clin. Orthop., *82*:169-181, 1972.
266. O'Driscoll, M., and Powell, F. J.: Injury, serum lipids, fat embolism, and clofibrinate. Brit. Med. J., *4*:149-151, 1967.
267. Parker, F. B., Jr., Wax, S. D., Kusajima, K., and Webb, W. R.: Hemodynamic and pathological findings in experimental fat embolism. Arch. Surg., *108*:70-74, 1974.
268. Peltier, L. F.: Collective review: an appraisal of the problem of fat embolism. Int. Abstr. Surg., *104*:313-324, 1957.
269. ———: The diagnosis of fat embolism. Surg. Gynecol. Obstet., *121*:371-379, 1965.
270. ———: Fat embolism. A current concept. Clin. Orthop., *66*:241-253, 1969.
271. ———: The diagnosis and treatment of fat embolism. J. Trauma, *11*:661-667, 1971.
272. Peltier, L. F., Adler, R., and Lai, S. P.: Fat embolism: the significance of an elevated serum lipase after trauma to bone. Amer. J. Surg., *99*:821-826, 1960.
273. Pipkin, G.: The early diagnosis and treatment of fat embolism. Clin. Orthop., *12*: 171-182, 1958.
274. Rokkanen, P., Lahdensuu, M., Kataja, J., and Julkunen, H.: The syndrome of fat embolism; analysis of thirty consecutive cases compared to trauma patients with similar injuries. J. Trauma, *10*:299-306, 1970.
275. Saldeen, T.: Fat embolism and signs of intravascular coagulation in a posttraumatic autopsy material. J. Trauma, *10*: 273-286, 1970.
276. Scriba, J.: Untersuchungen uber die Fettembolie. Leipzig J. B. Hirschfeld, 1879.
277. Scuderi, C. S.: Fat embolism; a clinical and experimental study. Surg. Gynecol. Obstet., *72*:732-746, 1941.
278. Sevitt, S.: The significance and classification of fat-embolism. Lancet, *2*:825-828, 1960.
279. ———: Fat Embolism. London, Butterworth, 1962.
280. Sevitt, S., Clarke, R., and Badger, F. G.: Modern Trends in Accident Surgery and Medicine. London, Butterworth, 1959.
281. Soloway, H. B., and Robinson, E. F.: The coagulation mechanism in experimental pulmonary fat embolism. J. Trauma, *12*: 630-631, 1972.
282. Sproule, B. J., Brady, J. L., and Gilbert, J. A. L.: Studies on the syndrome of fat embolization. Can. Med. Assoc. J., *90*: 1243-1247, 1964.
283. Sutton, G. E.: Pulmonary fat embolism and its relation to traumatic shock. Brit. Med. J., *2*:368-370, 1918.
284. Tedeschi, C. G., Walter, C. E., Lepore, T., and Tedeschi, L. G.: An assessment of the cerebrospinal fluid and choroid plexus in relation to systemic fat embolism. Neurology, *19*:586-590, 1969.
285. Tedeschi, C. G., Walter, C. E., and Tedeschi, L. G.: Shock and fat embolism; an appraisal. Surg. Clin. North Amer., *48*: 431-452, 1968.
286. Thomas, J. E., and Ayyar, D. R.: Systemic fat embolism. A diagnostic profile in 24 patients. Arch. Neurol., *26*:517-523, 1972.
287. Vance, B. M.: The significance of fat embolism. Arch. Surg., *23*:426-465, 1931.
288. Wagner, E.: Die Fettembolie der Lungencapillaren. Arch. Heilk., *6*:369-381, 1865.

289. Warner, W. A.: Release of free fatty acids following trauma. J. Trauma, *9*:692-699, 1969.
290. Warthin, A. S.: Traumatic lipaemia and fatty embolism. Int. Clin., *4*:171-227, 1913.
291. Weinberg, H., and Finsterbush, A.: Fat embolism; vascular damage to bone due to blunt trauma. Intraosseous phlebography study. Clin. Orthop., *83*:273-278, 1972.
292. Weisz, G. M., and Barellai, A.: Nonfulminant fat embolism: review of concepts on its genesis and orthophysiology. Anesth. Analg., *52*:303-309, 1973.
293. Weisz, G. M., Rang, M., and Salter, R. B.: Posttraumatic fat embolism in children: review of the literature and of experience in The Hospital for Sick Children, Toronto. J. Trauma, *13*:529-534, 1973.
294. Weisz, G. M., and Steiner, E.: The cause of death in fat embolism. Chest, *59*:511-516, 1971.
295. Wilson, J. V., and Salisbury, C. V.: Fat embolism in war surgery. Brit. J. Surg., *31*:384-392, 1944.
296. Zenker, F. A.: Beitrage zur Anatomie und Physiologie der Lunge. Dresden, J. Braunsdorf, 1861.

Gas Gangrene

297. Altemeier, W. A., and Culbertson, W. R.: Acute non-clostridial crepitant cellulitis. Surg. Gynecol. Obstet., *87*:206-212, 1948.
298. Altemeier, W. A., and Fullen, W. D.: Prevention and treatment of gas gangrene. J.A.M.A., *217*:806-813, 1971.
299. Altemeier, W. A., and Furste, W. L.: Studies in virulence of *Clostridium welchii*. Surgery, *25*:12-19, 1949.
300. Altemeier, W. A., Furste, W. L., and Culbertson, W. R.: Chemotherapy in gas gangrene; experimental study. Arch. Surg., *55*:668-680, 1947.
301. Aufranc, O. E., Jones, W. N., and Bierbaum, B. E.: Gas gangrene complicating fracture of the tibia. J.A.M.A., *209*:2045-2047, 1969.
302. Behnke, A. R., and Saltzman, H. A.: Medical progress. Hyperbaric oxygenation. N. Engl. J. Med., *276*:1423-1429, 1967.
303. ———: Medical progress. Hyperbaric oxygenation (concluded). N. Engl. J. Med., *276*:1478-1484, 1967.
304. Boerema, I.: An operating room with high atmospheric pressure. Surgery, *49*:291-298, 1961.
305. Bornstein, D. L., Weinberg, N., Swartz, M. N., and Kunz, L. J.: Anaerobic infections; review of current experience. Medicine, *43*:207-232, 1964.
306. Bottini, E.: La Gangrena traumatica invadente. Contribuzione sperimentali ed Illustrazioni cliniche. Giorn. Reale Accad. Med., *10*:1121-1138, 1871.
307. Brummelkamp, W. H., Boerema, I., and Hoogendyk, L.: Treatment of clostridial infections with hyperbaric oxygen drenching; a report of 26 cases. Lancet, *1*:235-238, 1963.
308. Colwill, M. R., and Maudsley, R. H.: The management of gas gangrene with hyperbaric oxygen therapy. J. Bone Joint Surg., *50B*:732-742, 1968.
309. DeHaven, K. E., and Evarts, C. M.: The continuing problem of gas gangrene; a review and report of illustrative cases. J. Trauma, *11*:983-991, 1971.
310. Doty, D. B., Treiman, R. L., Rothschild, P. D., and Gaspar, M. R.: Prevention of gangrene due to fractures. Surg. Gynecol. Obstet., *125*:284-288, 1967.
311. Dowdy, A. H., Sewell, R. L., and Vincent, J. G.: Prophylaxis and therapeusis of clostridial infections (gas gangrene). N. Y. State J. Med., *44*:1890-1896, 1944.
312. Eickhoff, T. C.: An outbreak of surgical wound infections due to Clostridium perfringens. Surg. Gynecol. Obstet., *114*:102-108, 1962.
313. Eraklis, A. J., Filler, R. M., Pappas, A. M., and Bernhard, W. F.: Evaluation of hyperbaric oxygen as an adjunct in the treatment of anaerobic infections. Amer. J. Surg., *117*:485-492, 1969.
314. Eveland, W. C., Newton, A., Pohutsky, E. R., Purdy, D. S., and Frick, L. P.: Effects of combinations of antibiotics on Clostridia in vitro. Antibiot. Chemother., *5*:470-473, 1955.
315. Filler, R. M., Griscom, N. T., and Pappas, A.: Posttraumatic crepitation falsely suggesting gas gangrene. N. Engl. J. Med., *278*:758-761, 1968.
316. Fisher, A. M., and McKusick, V. A.: Bacteroides infections; clinical, bacteriological and therapeutic features of 14 cases. Amer. J. Med. Sci., *225*:253-273, 1953.
317. Govan, A. D. T.: Account of pathology in some cases of Cl. welchii infection. J. Pathol. Bacteriol., *58*:423-430, 1946.
318. Grossman, M., and Silen, W.: Serious post traumatic infections with special reference to gas gangrene, tetanus, and necrotizing facitis. Postgrad. Med., *32*:110-118, 1962.
319. Gye, R., Rountree, P. M., and Lowenthal, J.: Infection of surgical wounds with

Clostridium welchii. Med. J. Austral., *48*: 761-764, 1961.
320. Hac, L. R., and Hubert, A. C.: Experimental *Cl. welchii* infections IV. Penicillin therapy. J. Infect. Dis., *74*:164-172, 1944.
321. Hall, I. C.: The ambiguity of international toxic units. Science, *103*:423-424, 1946.
322. Hayward, N. J.: The rapid identification of *Clostridium welchii* by Nagler tests in plate cultures. J. Pathol. Bacteriol., *55*: 285-293, 1943.
323. Hayward, N. J., and Gray, J. A. B.: Haemolysin tests for rapid identification of *Cl. oedematiens* and *Cl. septicum*. J. Pathol. Bacteriol., *58*:11-20, 1946.
324. Jeffrey, J. S., and Thomson, S.: Gas gangrene in Italy; a study of 33 cases treated with penicillin. Brit. J. Surg., *32*:159-167, 1944.
325. Kellett, C. E.: The early history of gas gangrene. Ann. Med. Hist., *1*:452-459, 1939.
326. Kemp, F. H.: X-rays in diagnosis and localization of gas gangrene. Lancet, *1*: 332-336, 1945.
327. Keppie, J., and Robertson, M.: The in vitro toxigenicity and other characteristics of strains of the Clostridium welchii type A from various sources. J. Pathol. Bacteriol., *56*:123-132, 1944.
328. Langley, F. H., and Winkelstein, L. B.: Gas gangrene; a study of 96 cases treated in an evacuation hospital. J.A.M.A., *128*: 783-792, 1945.
329. MacFarlane, M. G.: The therapeutic value of gas gangrene antitoxin. Brit. Med. J., *2*:636-640, 1943.
330. MacLennan, J. D.: Anaerobic infections of war wounds in the Middle East. Lancet, *2*:63, 1943.
331. ———: Streptococcal infection of muscle. Lancet, *1*:582-584, 1943.
332. ———: Histotoxic clostridial infections in man. Bacteriol. Rev., *26*:177-276, 1962.
333. MacLennan, J. D., and MacFarlane, R. G.: Toxin and antitoxin studies of gas gangrene in man. Lancet, *2*:301-305, 1945.
334. Oakley, C. L.: Gas gangrene. Brit. Med. Bull., *10*:52-58, 1954.
335. Pappas, A. M., Filler, R. M., Eraklis, A. J., and Bernhard, W. F.: Clostridial infections (gas gangrene). Diagnosis and early treatment. Clin. Orthop., *76*:177-184, 1971.
336. Qvist, G.: Anaerobic cellulitis and gas gangrene. Brit. Med. J., *2*:217-221, 1941.
337. Rifkind, D.: The diagnosis and treatment of gas gangrene. Surg. Clin. North Amer., *43*:511-517, 1963.
338. Robb-Smith, A. H. T.: Tissue changes induced by Clostridium welchii type A filtrates. Lancet, *2*:362-368, 1945.
339. Smart, J. F., Homi, J., Bobb, J. R. R., and Wasmuth, C. E.: Gas gangrene treated with hyperbaric oxygenation: report of a case. Cleve. Clin. Q., *32*:57-60, 1965.
340. Smith, L. DeS.: Clostridia in gas gangrene. Bacteriol. Rev., *13*:233-254, 1949.
341. Trippel, O. H., Ruggie, A. N., Staley, C. J., and van Elk, J.: Hyperbaric oxygenation in the management of gas gangrene. Surg. Clin. North Amer., *47*:17-27, 1967.
342. Van Unnik, A. J. M.: Inhibition of toxin production in Clostridium perfringens in vitro by hyperbaric oxygen. J. Microbiol. Serol., *31*:181-189, 1965.
343. Willis, A. T., and Gowland, G.: Some observations on the mechanism of the Nagler reaction. J. Pathol. Bacteriol., *83*:219-226, 1962.
344. Willis, A. T., and Hobbs, G.: Some new media for isolation and identification of Clostridia. J. Pathol. Bacteriol., *77*:511-521, 1959.
345. Wilson, T. S.: Significance of Clostridium welchii infections and their relationship to gas gangrene. Can. J. Surg., *4*:35-42, 1960.

Tetanus

346. American College of Surgeons Committee on Trauma. A guide to prophylaxis against tetanus in wound management. Bull. Amer. Coll. Surgeons, *57*:32-33, 1972.
347. Aretaeus the Cappadocian: On tetanus, *In* Adams, F. (ed.): The Extant Works, London, 1856.
348. Brooks, V. B., Curtis, D. R., and Eccles, J. C.: The action of tetanus toxin on the inhibition of motoneurones. J. Physiol., *135*:655-672, 1957.
349. Brown, H.: Tetanus. J.A.M.A., *204*:614-616, 1968.
350. Carle, A., and Rattone, G.: Studio experimentale sull' Eziologia del Tetano. Geordr. Accad. Med. Torino, *32*:174-180, 1884.
351. Christensen, M. A.: Important concepts of tetanus that form the basis for current treatment. *In* Eckmann, L. (ed.): Principles on Tetanus. 2d Proceedings of the International Conference on Tetanus. Bern, Hans Huber, 1967.

352. ———: [Editorial] Potential for tetanus unchanged; are your patients all properly immunized? J.A.M.A., *222*:578-579, 1972.
353. Christensen, N.: A treatment of the patient with severe tetanus. Surg. Clin. North Amer., *49*:1183-1193, 1969.
355. Cole, L., and Youngman, H.: Treatment of tetanus. Lancet, *1*:1017-1020, 1969.
355. Duchen, L. W., and Tonge, D. A.: The effects of tetanus toxin on neuromuscular transmission and on the morphology of motor end-plates to slow and fast skeletal muscle of the mouse. J. Physiol., *228*:157-172, 1973.
356. Eckmann, L. (ed.): International Conference on Tetanus, Principles of Tetanus. 2nd Proceedings. Bern, Hans Huber, 1967.
357. Edsall, G.: Specific prophylaxis of tetanus. J.A.M.A., *171*:417-427, 1959.
358. Forbes, G. B., and Auld, M.: Management of tetanus; report of fifteen consecutive cases with recovery. Amer. J. Med., *18*:947-960, 1955.
359. Furste, W.: Third International Conference on Tetanus; a report. J. Trauma, *11*: 721, 1971.
360. Furste, W., and Wheeler, W. L.: Tetanus: a team disease.
Current Problems in Surgery, 1972.
361. Glenn, F.: Tetanus—a preventable disease; including an experience with civilian casualties in the battle for Manila (1945). Ann. Surg., *124*:1030-1040, 1946.
362. Herzon, E., Killian, E., and Pearlman, S. J.: Tracheotomy in tetanus. Arch Otolaryngol., *54*:143-156, 1951.
363. Hippocrates: With an English translation by W. H. S. Jones, Cambridge, Mass.: Harvard University Press, 1923, Vol. 1, p. 165.
364. Holder, A. R.: Law and medicine. Tetanus antitoxin reactions. J.A.M.A., *224*: 559-560, 1973.
365. Holder, A. R.: Law and Medicine. Tetanus. J.A.M.A., *224*:659-660, 1973.
366. Ildirim, I.: A new treatment for neonatal tetanus. Antitetanic serum and prednisolone given together intrathecally. Turkish J. Pediat., *9*:89-95, 1967.
367. International Comments. Guide lines Regarding Tetanus. J.A.M.A., *198*:687-688, 1966.
368. Kaeser, H. E., and Saner, A.: The effect of tetanus toxin on neuromuscular transmission. Europ. Neurol., *3*:193-205, 1970.
369. Kerr, J. H., Corbett, J. L., Prys-Roberts, C., Smith, A. C., and Spalding, J. M. K.: Involvement of the sympathetic nervous system in tetanus. Studies on 82 cases. Lancet, *2*:236-241, 1968.
370. Kitasato, S.: Uber den Tetanuserreger. Ztschr. Hyg., *7*:225-234, 1889.
371. Kittler, F., Smith, P., Jr., Hefley, B. F., and Cazort, A.: Reactions to tetanus toxoid. South. Med. J., *59*:149-153, 1966.
372. La Force, F. M., Young, L. S., and Bennett, J. V.: Tetanus in the United States 1965-1966. Epidemiologic and clinical features. N. Engl. J. Med., *280*:569-574, 1969.
373. Levine, L., McComb, J. A., Dwyer, R. C., and Latham, W. C.: Active-passive tetanus immunization. Choice of toxoid, dose of tetanus immune globulin and timing of injections. N. Engl. J. Med., *274*:186-190, 1966.
374. Long, A.: The Army Immunization Program. Vol. III. Preventive Medicine in World War II. Washington, D.C., United States Government Printing Office, 1955.
375. McComb, J. A.: The Combined Use of Homologous Tetanus Immune Globulin and Toxoid in Man. *In* Eckmann, L. (ed.): Principles on Tetanus. Bern, Hans Huber, 1967.
376. McComb, J. A., and Dwyer, R. C.: Passive-active immunization with tetanus immune globulin (human). N. Engl. J. Med., *268*:857-862, 1963.
377. McCracken, G. H., Jr., Dowell, D. L., and Marshall, F. N.: Double-blind trial of equine antitoxin and human immune globulin in tetanus neonatorum. Lancet, *1*:1146-1149, 1971.
378. Mellanby, J. H.: Presynaptic effect of tetanus toxin at the neuromuscular junction. J. Physiol., *218*:68P-69P, 1971.
379. Milledge, J. S.: Hyperbaric oxygen therapy in tetanus. J.A.M.A., *203*:875-876, 1968.
380. Murphy, K. J.: Fatal tetanus with brainstem involvement and myocarditis in an ex-serviceman. Med. J. Austral., *2*:542-544, 1970.
381. Nation, N. S., Pierce, N. F., Adler, S. J., Chinnock, R. F., and Wehrle, P. F.: Tetanus; the use of human hyperimmune globulin in treatment. California Med., *98*:305-307, 1963.
382. Ramon, G., and Zoeller, C.: L'Anatoxine tétanique et l'Immunisation active de l'Homme vis-à-vis du Tétanos. Ann. Inst. Pasteur, *41*:803-833, 1927.
383. Smith, A.: Tetanus. *In* Beeson, P. B., and McDermott, W. (eds.), Cecil-Loeb Text-

book of Medicine, ed. 13. Philadelphia, W. B. Saunders, 1971.

384. Smythe, P. M.: Studies on neonatal tetanus, and on pulmonary compliance of the totally relaxed infant. Brit. Med. J., *1*:565-571, 1963.

385. ———: The problem of detubating an infant with a tracheostomy. J. Pediat., *65*: 446-453, 1964.

386. ———: Treatment of tetanus in neonates. Lancet, *1*:335, 1967.

387. Spaeth, R.: Therapy of tetanus. A study of two hundred and seventy-six cases. Arch. Intern. Med., *68*:1133-1160, 1941.

388. Tateno, I.: Incubation period and initial symptoms of tetanus: a clinical assessment of the problem of the passage of tetanus toxin to the central nervous system. Jap. J. Exper. Med., *33*:149-158, 1963.

389. Turner, V. C., and Galloway, T. C.: Tetanus treated as a respiratory problem. Arch. Surg., *58*:478-483, 1949.

390. Van Heyningen, W. E., and Messanby, J.: Tetanus toxin. *In* Kadis, S., Montie, T. C., and Ajl, S. J. (eds.): Microbial Toxins. Vol. 2A. New York, Academic Press, 1971.

391. Vinnard, R. T.: Three hundred fifty-two cases of tetanus. Surgery, *18*:482-492, 1945.

392. Weed, M. R., Purvis, D. F., and Warnke, R. D.: d-Tubocurarine in wax and oil; for control of muscle spasm in tetanus. J.A.M.A., *138*:1087-1090, 1948.

393. Wessler, S., and Avioli, L. A.: Tetanus. J.A.M.A., *207*:123-127, 1969.

394. Woolmer, R., and Cates, J. E.: Succinylcholine in the treatment of tetanus. Lancet, *2*:808-809, 1952.

395. Wright, G. P.: Neutrotoxins of *Clostridium botulinum* and *Clostridium tetani*. Pharmacol. Rev., *7*:413-465, 1955.

Osteomyelitis

396. Alexander, J. W., Sykes, N. S., Mitchell, M. M., and Fisher, M. W.: Concentration of selected intravenously administered antibiotics in experimental surgical wounds. J. Trauma, *13*:423-434, 1973.

397. Altemeier, W. A., Todd, J. C., and Inge, W. W.: Gram-negative septicemia. A growing threat. Ann. Surg., *166*:530-542, 1969.

398. Anderson, W. A. D.: Pathology. ed. 4. St. Louis, C. V. Mosby, 1961.

399. Barber, M., and Waterworth, D. M.: Penicillinase-resistant penicillins and cephalosporins. Brit. Med. J., *2*:344-349, 1965.

400. Barry, A. L., Garcia, F., and Thrupp, L. D.: An improved single-disk method for testing the antibiotic susceptibility of rapidly-growing pathogens. Amer. J. Clin. Pathol., *53*:149-158, 1970.

401. Bernhard, W. F., and Filler, R. M.: Hyperbaric oxygenation: current concepts. Amer. J. Surg., *115*:661-668, 1968.

402. Bowers, W. H., Wilson, F. C., and Greene, W. B.: Antibiotic prophylaxis in experimental bone infections. J. Bone Joint Surg., *55A*:795-807, 1973.

403. Boyd, R. J., Burke, J. F., and Colton, T.: A double blind clinical trial of prophylactic antibiotics and hip fractures. J. Bone Joint Surg., *55A*:1251-1259, 1973.

404. Brown, P. W.: The prevention of infection in open wounds. Clin. Orthop., *96*: 42-50, 1973.

405. Butt, W. P.: The radiology of infection. Clin. Orthop., *95*:20-30, 1973.

406. Caldwell, J. R., and Cluff, L. E.: The real and present danger of antibiotics. Ration. Drug Ther., *7*:1-6, 1973.

407. Charnley, J.: Postoperative infection after total hip replacement with special reference to air contamination in the operating room. Clin. Orthop., *87*:167-187, 1972.

408. Clawson, D. K.: Common bacterial infections of bone. G.P., *32*:125-133, 1965.

409. Clawson, D. K., David, F. J., and Hansen, S. T.: Treatment of chronic osteomyelitis with emphasis on closed suction-irrigation techniques. Clin. Orthop., *96*: 88-97, 1973.

410. Clawson, D. K., and Dunn, A. W.: Management of common bacterial infections of bones and joints. J. Bone Joint Surg., *49A*:164-182, 1967.

411. Cluff, L. E., and Reynolds, R. C.: Management of staphylococcal infections. Amer. J. Med., *39*:812-825, 1965.

412. Cluff, L. E., Reynolds, R. C., Page, D. L., and Breckenridge, J. L.: Staphylococcal bacteremia and altered host resistance. Ann. Intern. Med., *69*:859-873, 1968.

413. Collins, D. H.: *In* Dodge, O. G. (ed.): Pathology of Bone. London, Butterworth, 1966.

414. Compere, E. L., Metzger, W. I., and Mitra, R. N.: The treatment of pyogenic bone and joint infections by closed irrigation (circulation) with a non-toxic detergent and one or more antibiotics. J. Bone Joint Surg., *49A*:614-624, 1967.

415. Curtis, P.: The pathophysiology of joint infections. Clin. Orthop., *96*:129-135, 1973.

416. Dickson, C. D.: The clinical diagnosis,

prognosis, and treatment of acute hematogenous osteomyelitis. J.A.M.A., *127*: 212-217, 1945.

417. Dombrowski, E. T., and Dunn, A. W.: Treatment of osteomyelitis by debridement and closed wound irrigation-suction. Clin. Orthop., *43*:215-231, 1965.
418. Drew, W. L., Barry, A. L., O'Toole, R., and Sherris, J. C.: Reliability of the Kirby-Bauer disc diffusion method for detecting methicillin-resistant strains of Staphylococcus aureus. Appl. Microbiol., *24*:240-247, 1972.
419. Evarts, C. M.: Endoprosthesis as the primary treatment of femoral neck fractures. Clin. Orthop., *92*:69-76, 1973.
420. Evaskus, D. S., Laskin, D. M., and Kroeger, A. V.: Penetration of lincomycin, penicillin, and tetracycline into serum and bone. Proc. Soc. Exper. Biol. Med., *130*: 89-91, 1969.
421. Eyre-Brook, A. L.: Septic arthritis of the hip and osteomyelitis of the upper end of the femur in infants. J. Bone Joint Surg., *42B*: 11-20, 1960.
422. Ferguson, A. B.: Osteomyelitis in children. Clin. Orthop., *96*:51-56, 1973.
423. Finland, M., Jones, W. F., and Barnes, M. W.: Occurrence of serious bacterial infections since introduction of antibacterial agents. J.A.M.A., *170*:2188-2197, 1959.
424. Fogelberg, E. U., Zitzmann, E. K., and Stinchfield, F. E.: Prophylactic penicillin in orthopaedic surgery. J. Bone Joint Surg., *52A*:95-98, 1970.
425. Gilmour, W. N.: Acute haematogenous osteomyelitis. J. Bone Joint Surg., *44B*: 841-853, 1962.
426. Gledhill, R. B.: Subacute osteomyelitis in children. Clin. Orthop., *96*:57-69, 1973.
427. Gordon, S. L., Greer, R. B., and Craig, C. P.: Recurrent osteomyelitis. Report of four cases culturing L-form variants of staphylococci. J. Bone Joint Surg., *53A*: 1150-1156, 1971.
428. Green, W. T., and Shannon, J. G.: Osteomyelitis of infants. A disease different from osteomyelitis of older children. Arch. Surg., *32*:462-493, 1936.
429. Hamblen, D. L.: Hyperbaric oxygenation: its effect on experimental staphylococcal osteomyelitis in rats. J. Bone Joint Surg., *50A*:1129-1141, 1968.
430. Harley, J. D., Wilson, S. D., Worman, L. W., and Carey, L. C.: Chronic osteomyelitis; treatment by regional perfusion with antibiotics. Arch. Surg., *92*:548-553, 1966.
431. Harris, N. H.: Some problems in the diagnosis and treatment of acute osteomyelitis. J. Bone Joint Surg., *42B*:535-541, 1960.
432. Harris, N. H., and Kirkaldy-Willis, W. H.: Primary subacute pyogenic osteomyelitis. J. Bone Joint Surg., *47B*:526-532, 1965.
433. Harris, W. H.: Sinking prostheses. Surg. Gynecol. Obstet., *123*:1297-1302, 1966.
434. Hart, V. L.: Acute hematogenous osteomyelitis in children. J.A.M.A., *108*:524-528, 1937.
435. Hobo, T.: Zur Pathogenese der akuten haematogen Osteomyelitis, mit Berucksichtigung der Vitalfar beng Shehre. Acta Sch. Med. Univ. Kioto, *4*:1-29, 1921-1922.
436. Jackson, R. W., and Parsons, C. J.: Distention-irrigation treatment of major joint sepsis. Clin. Orthop., *96*:160-164, 1973.
437. Kahn, D. S., and Pritzker, P. H.: The pathophysiology of bone infection. Clin. Orthop., *96*:12-19, 1973.
438. Kanyuck, D. O., Welles, J. S., Emmerson, J. L., and Anderson, R. C.: The penetration of cephalosporin antibiotics into bone. Proc. Soc. Exp. Biol. Med., *136*: 997-999, 1971.
439. Kelly, P. J., Wilkowske, C. J., and Washington, J. A., II: Comparison of gram-negative bacillary and staphylococcal osteomyelitis of the femur and tibia. Clin. Orthop., *96*:70-75, 1973.
440. King, D. M., and Mayo, K. M.: Subacute hematogenous osteomyelitis. J. Bone Joint Surg., *51B*:458-463, 1969.
441. Lazarus, G. S., Brown, R. S., Daniels, J. R., and Fullmer, H. M.: Human granulocyte collagenase. Science, *159*:1483-1485, 1968.
442. Lodwick, G. S.: The Bones and Joints. Atlas of Tumour Radiology. Chicago, Year Book Medical Publishers, 1971.
443. McHenry, M. C.: Antibacterial therapy. Cleve. Clin. Q., *37*:43-58, 1970.
444. Nelson, C. A., Bergfeld, J. A., Schwartz, J., and Kolczun, M.: Antibiotics in human hematoma and wound fluid. J. Bone Joint Surg., [in press].
445. Nettles, J. L., Kelly, P. J., Martin, W. J., and Washington, J. A.: Musculoskeletal infections due to bacteroides. A study of eleven cases. J. Bone Joint Surg., *51A*: 230-238, 1969.
446. Niekerk, J. P. deV.: Hand infections: management and results based on a new classification. A study of more than 1,000 cases. S. Afr. Med. J., *40*:316-319, 1966.
447. Overton, L. M., and Tully, W. P.: Surgical treatment of chronic osteomyelitis in

long bones. Amer. J. Surg., *126*:736-741, 1973.

448. Paterson, D. C.: Suppurative arthritis in children. J. Bone Joint Surg., *48B*:586, 1966.
449. Patzakis, M. J., Harvey, J. P., Jr., and Ivler, D.: The role of prophylactic antibiotics in the management of open fractures. Los Angeles, University of Southern California Medical Center.
450. Petersdorf, R. G., and Sherris, J. C.: Methods and significance of in vitro testing of bacterial sensitivity to drugs. Amer. J. Med., *39*:766-779, 1965.
451. Robertson, D. E.: Acute hematogenous osteomyelitis. J. Bone Joint Surg., *9*:8-23, 1927.
452. Rosner, R.: Isolation of protoplasts of Staphylococcus aureus. From a case of recurrent acute osteomyelitis. Tech. Bull. Reg. Med. Tech., *38*:205-210, 1968.
453. Shandling, B.: Acute hematogenous osteomyelitis: a review of 300 cases treated during 1952-1859. S. Afr. Med. J., *34*: 520-524, 1960.
454. Shannon, J. B., Woolhouse, F. M., and Eisinger, P. J.: The treatment of chronic osteomyelitis by Saucerization and immediate skin grafting. Clin. Orthop., *96*:98-107, 1973.
455. Skinner, D., and Keefer, C. S.: Significance of bacteremia caused by staphylococcus aureus. Arch. Intern. Med., *68*: 851-875, 1941.
456. Starr, C. L.: Acute hematogenous osteomyelitis. Arch. Surg., *4*:567-587, 1922.
457. Stevens, D. B.: Postoperative orthopaedic infections; a study of etiological mechanisms. J. Bone Joint Surg., *46A*:96-102, 1964.
458. Trueta, J.: The three types of acute haematogenous osteomyelitis. A clinical and vascular study. J. Bone Joint Surg., *41B*:671-680, 1959.
459. Waldvogel, F. A., Medoff, G., and Swartz, M. N.: Osteomyelitis. Clinical Features, Therapeutic Consideration, and Unusual Aspects. Springfield, Illinois, Charles C Thomas, 1971.
460. Wilson, F. C., Worcester, J. N., Coleman, P. D., and Byrd, W. E.: Antibiotic penetration of experimental bone hematomas. J. Bone Joint Surg., *53A*:1622, 1971.
461. Winters, J. C., and Cahen, I.: Acute hematogenous osteomyelitis. A review of 66 cases. J. Bone Joint Surg., *42A*:691-704, 1960.

Posttraumatic Reflex Dystrophy

462. Bayles, T. B., Judson, W. E., and Potter, T. A.: Reflex sympathetic dystrophy of the upper extremity (hand-shoulder syndrome). J.A.M.A., *144*:537-542, 1950.
463. Berger, H.: The treatment of postmyocardial infarction shoulder-hand syndrome with local hydrocortisone. Postgrad. Med., *15*:508-511, 1954.
464. Birkenfeld, B.: Erfahrungen mit der Echinacin-Therapie beim Sudeckschen Syndrom. Ther. Ggw., *93*:425, 1954.
465. Collins, W. F., and Randt, C. T.: Evoked central nervous system activity to peripheral unmyelinated or "C" fibers in cat. J. Neurophysiol., *21*:345-352, 1958.
466. de Takats, G.: The technic of lumbar sympathectomy. Surg. Clin. North Amer., *26*:56-69, 1946.
467. ———: Sympathetic reflex dystrophy. Med. Clin. North Amer., *49*:117-129, 1965.
468. Drucker, W. R., Hubay, C. A., Holden, W. D., and Bukovnic, J. A.: Pathogenesis of posttraumatic sympathetic dystrophy. Amer. J. Surg., *97*:454-465, 1959.
469. Dwyer, A. F.: Sudeck's atrophy and cortisone. Med. J. Austral., *2*:265-268, 1952.
470. Evans, J. A.: Reflex sympathetic dystrophy. Surg. Gynecol. Obstet., *82*:36-43, 1946.
471. Granit, R., Leksell, L., and Skoglund, C. R.: Fibre interaction in injured or compressed region of nerve. Brain, *67*:125-140, 1944.
472. Hartley, J.: Reflex hyperemic deossification (Sudeck's atrophy). J. Mt. Sinai Hosp., *22*:268-277, 1955.
473. Herrmann, L. G., and Caldwell, J. A.: Diagnosis and treatment of posttraumatic osteoporosis. Amer. J. Surg., *51*:630-640, 1941.
474. Herrmann, L. G., Reineke, H. G., and Caldwell, J. A.: Posttraumatic painful osteoporosis. A clinical and roentgenological entity. Amer. J. Roentgenol., *47*:353-361, 1942.
475. Hilker, A. W.: The shoulder-hand syndrome. A complication of coronary artery disease. Ann. Intern. Med., *31*:303-311, 1949.
476. Homans, J.: Minor causalgia; a hyperesthetic neurovascular syndrome. N. Engl. J. Med., *222*:870-874, 1940.
477. Johnson, A. C.: Disabling changes in the

hand-resembling sclerodactylia following myocardial infarction. Ann. Intern. Med., *19*:433-456, 1943.
478. Johnson, E. W., and Pannozzo, A. N.: Management of shoulder-hand syndrome. J.A.M.A., *195*:108-110, 1966.
479. Kirklin, J. W., Chenoweth, A. I., and Murphey, F.: Causalgia; a review of its characteristics, diagnosis and treatment. Surgery, *21*:321-342, 1947.
480. Lenggenhager, K.: Sudeck's osteodystrophy; its pathogenesis, prophylaxis, and therapy. Minn. Med., *54*:967-972, 1971.
481. Lewis, D., and Gatewood, W.: Treatment of causalgia; results of intraneural injection of 60 per cent alcohol. J.A.M.A., *74*: 1-4, 1920.
482. Livingston, W. R.: Pain mechanisms; a physiologic interpretation of causalgia and its related states. New York, Macmillan, 1943.
483. Marti, T.: Wesen und Behandlung des Sudeckschen Syndroms. Praxis, *43*:742, 1954.
484. Mayfield, F. H., and Devine, J. W.: Causalgia. Surg. Gynecol. Obstet., *80*:631-635, 1945.
485. Miller, D. S., and deTakats, G.: Post-traumatic dystrophy of the extremities; Sudeck's atrophy. Surg. Gynecol. Obstet., *75*:558-582, 1942.
486. Mitchell, S. W.: The medical department in the Civil war. J.A.M.A., *62*:1445-1450, 1914.
487. Mitchell, S. W., Morehouse, G. R., and Keen, W. W.: Gunshot wounds and other injuries of nerves. Philadelphia, J. B. Lippincott, 1864.
488. Moberg, E.: The shoulder-hand-finger syndrome. Acta Chir. Scandinav., *109*: 284-292, 1955.
489. Munch-Peterson, C. J.: The so-called shoulder-hand syndrome. Nord. Med., *51*: 291-293, 1954.
490. Nathan, P. W.: On pathogenesis of causalgia in peripheral nerve injuries. Brain, *70*:145-170, 1947.
491. Oppenheimer, A.: The swollen atrophic hand. Surg. Gynecol. Obstet., *67*:446-454, 1938.
492. Pak, T. J., Martin, G. M., Magness, J. L., and Kavanaugh, G. J.: Reflex sympathetic dystrophy; review of 140 cases. Minn. Med., *53*:507-512, 1970.
493. Plewes, L. W.: Sudeck's atrophy in the hand. J. Bone Joint Surg., *38B*:195-203, 1956.
494. Richards, R. L.: Causalgia; a centennial review. Arch. Neurol., *16*:339-350, 1967.
495. Roland, O.: Unsere Erfahrungen mit Depot-Padutin. Zentralb. Chir., *77*:1, 147, 1952.
496. Rose, T. F.: Sudeck's post-traumatic osteodystrophy of limbs. Med. J. Austral., *1*:185-188, 1953.
497. Rosen, P. S., and Graham, W.: The shoulder-hand syndrome. Canad. Med. Assn. J., *77*:86-91, 1957.
498. Smithwick, R. H.: The value of sympathectomy in the treatment of vascular disease. N. Engl. J. Med., *216*:141-150, 1937.
499. Speigel, I. J., and Milowsky, J. L.: Causalgia. J.A.M.A., *127*:9-15, 1945.
500. Spurling, R. G.: Causalgia of the upper extremity; treatment by dorsal sympathetic ganglionectomy. Arch. Neurol. Psychiat., *23*:784-788, 1930.
501. Steinbrocker, O., and Argyros, T. G.: The shoulder-hand syndrome; present status as a diagnostic and therapeutic entity. Med. Clin. North Amer., *42*:1533-1553, 1958.
502. Steinbrocker, O., Neustadt, D., and Lapin, L.: The shoulder-hand syndrome. Sympathetic block compared with corticotropin and cortisone therapy. J.A.M.A., *153*:788-791, 1953.
503. Steinbrocker, O., Spitzer, N., and Friedman, H. H.: The shoulder-hand syndrome in reflex dystrophy of the upper extremity. Ann. Intern. Med., *29*:22-52, 1948.
504. Sudeck, P.: Ueber die acute entzundliche knocken Atrophie. Arch. Klin. Chir., *62*: 147-156, 1900.
505. ———: Ueber die akute (trophoneurotische) Knockenatrophie nach Entzundungen und Traumen der Extremitaten. Deutsche med. Wchuschr., *28*:336-338, 1902.
506. Swan, D. M.: Shoulder-hand syndrome following hemiplegia. Neurology, *4*:480-482, 1954.
507. Threadgill, F. D.: Afferent conduction via the sympathetic ganglia innervating the extremities. Surgery, *21*:569-594, 1947.
508. Toumey, J. W.: Occurrence and management of reflex sympathetic dystrophy (causalgia of the extremities). J. Bone Joint Surg., *30A*:883-894, 1948.
509. Walker, A. E., and Nulsen, F.: Electrical stimulation of the upper thoracic portion of the sympathetic chain in man. Arch. Neurol. Psychiat., *59*:559-560, 1948.

510. White, J. C., Heroy, W. W., and Goodman, E. N.: Causalgia following gunshot injuries of nerves. Ann. Surg., *128*:161-183, 1948.

511. Young, J. H., and Pearson, A. T.: The shoulder-hand syndrome. M. J. Austral., *1*:776-780, 1952.

Volkmann's Ischemic Contracture

512. Aggarwal, N. D.: Ischaemic contracture of limbs from tight splintage. J. Bone Joint Surg., *49B*:388, 1967.

513. Blomfield, L. B.: Intramuscular vascular patterns in man. Proc. Roy. Soc. Med., *38*:617-618, 1945.

514. Bowden, R. E. M., and Gutmann, E.: The fate of voluntary muscle after vascular injury in man. J. Bone Joint Surg., *31B*:356-368, 1949.

515. Bradley, E. L., III: The anterior tibial compartment syndrome. Surg. Gynecol. Obstet., *136*:289-297, 1973.

516. Brooks, B.: Pathologic changes in muscle as a result of disturbances of circulation. Arch. Surg., *5*:188-216, 1922.

517. Brooks, B., Johnson, G. S., and Kirtley, J. A., Jr.: Simultaneous vein ligation; an experimental study of the effect of ligation of the concomitant vein on the incidence of gangrene following arterial obstruction. Surg. Gynecol. Obstet., *59*:496-500, 1934.

518. Campbell, R. E., and van Wagoner, F. H.: Ischemic necrosis of the anterior tibial compartment musculature. Arch. Surg., *71*:662-668, 1955.

519. Clarke, W. T.: Volkmann's ischaemic contracture. Canad. Med. Assn. J., *54*:339-341, 1946.

520. Crystal, D. K., Burgess, E., and Wangeman, C.: Thrombectomy in Volkmann's contracture. N. Engl. J. Med., *247*:1015-1017, 1952.

521. Eaton, R. G., and Green, W. T.: Epimysiotomy and fasciotomy in the treatment of Volkmann's ischemic contracture. Orthop. Clin. North Amer., *3*:175-186, 1972.

522. Eaton, R. G., Green, W. T., and Stark, H. A.: Volkmann's ischemic contracture in children. J. Bone Joint Surg., *47A*: 1289, 1965.

523. Editorial: Anterior tibial syndrome. Brit. Med. J., *1*:1060-1061, 1966.

524. Edwards, E. A.: The anatomic basis for ischemia localized to certain muscles of the lower limb. Surg. Gynecol. Obstet., *97*:87-94, 1953.

525. Ellis, H.: Disabilities after tibial shaft fractures with special reference to Volkmann's ischemic contracture. J. Bone Joint Surg., *40B*:190-197, 1958.

526. Foisie, P. S.: Volkmann's ischemic contracture; an analysis of its proximate mechanism. N. Engl. J. Med., *226*:671-679, 1942.

527. Gage, M., and Ochsner, A.: Prevention of ischemic gangrene following surgical operations upon major peripheral arteries by chemical section of cervicodorsal and lumbar sympathetics. Ann. Surg., *112*: 938-959, 1940.

528. Getzen, L. C., and Carr, E. J.: Etiology of anterior tibial compartment syndrome. Surg. Gynecol. Obstet., *125*:347-350, 1967.

529. Griffiths, D. L.: Volkmann's ischemic contracture. Brit. J. Surg., *28*:239-260, 1940.

530. ———: Volkmann's ischaemic contracture. J. Bone Joint Surg., *33B*:299-300, 1951.

531. Harman, J. W.: A histological study of skeletal muscle in acute ischemia. Amer. J. Pathol., *23*:551-565, 1947.

532. ———: The significance of local vascular phenomena in the production of ischemic necrosis in skeletal muscle. Amer. J. Pathol., *24*:625-638, 1948.

533. Harman, J. W., and Gwinn, R. P.: Recovery of skeletal muscle fibers from acute ischemia as determined by histologic and chemical methods. Amer. J. Pathol., *25*: 741-755, 1949.

534. Hildebrand, O.: Ischaemische Muskelcontracturen. Deut. Z. Chir., *30*:98-101, 1890.

535. Hill, R. L., and Brooks, B.: Volkmann's contracture in hemophilia. Ann. Surg., *103*:444-449, 1936.

536. Hughes, J. R.: Ischaemic necrosis of the anterior tibial muscles due to fatigue. J. Bone Joint Surg., *30B*:581-594, 1948.

539. Jones, D. A.: Volkmann's ischemia. Surg. Clin. North Amer., *50*:329-342, 1970.

538. Larsen, I. J., Boone, E. W., Coles, E. L., and Civin, W. H.: Local ischemic necrosis of the leg. Clin. Orthop., *16*:272-283, 1960.

539. Leach, R. E., Hammond, G., and Stryker, W. S.: Anterior tibial compartment syndrome; acute and chronic. J. Bone Joint Surg., *49A*:451-462, 1967.

540. Leriche, R., Fontaine, R., and Dupertuis, S. M.: Arterectomy; with follow-up studies on 78 operations. Surg. Gynecol. Obstet., *64*:149-155, 1937.

541. Leser, E.: Untersuchungen über Ischae-

mische muskelähmungen und Muskelcontracturen. Samml. Klin. Vortr., *77*:2087-2114, 1884.

542. Lipscomb, P. R.: The etiology and prevention of Volkmann's ischaemic contracture. Surg. Gynecol. Obstet., *103*:353-361, 1956.
543. Lipscomb, P. R., and Burleson, R. J.: Vascular and neural complications in supracondylar fractures of the humerus in children. J. Bone Joint Surg., *37A*:487-492, 1955.
544. Littler, J. W.: Procedure for lengthening interosseous tendons. *In* Converse, J. M. (ed.): Reconstructive Plastic Surgery. vol. 4. Philadelphia, W. B. Saunders, 1964.
545. Lundborg, G.: Limb ischemia and nerve injury. Arch. Surg., *104*:631-632, 1972.
546. McQuillan, W. M., and Nolan, B.: Ischaemia complicating injury: a report of thirty-seven cases. J. Bone Joint Surg., *50B*:482-493, 1968.
547. Mavor, G. E.: The anterior tibial syndrome. J. Bone Joint Surg., *38B*:513-517, 1956.
548. Murphy, B. B.: Myositis. J.A.M.A., *63*: 1249-1255, 1914.
549. Page, C. M.: An operation for the relief of flexion-contracture in the forearm. J. Bone Joint Surg., *5*:233-234, 1924.
550. Parkes, A. R.: Traumatic ischaemia of peripheral nerves, with some observations on Volkmann's ischaemic contracture. Brit. J. Surg., *32*:403-414, 1945.
551. Peacock, E. E., Jr., Madden, J. W., and Trier, W. C.: Transfer of median and ulnar nerves during early treatment of forearm ischemia. Ann. Surg., *169*:748-756, 1969.
552. Pollock, G. A.: Early operation for Volkmann's ischaemic contracture. Brit. Med. J., *1*:783, 1944.
553. Seddon, H. J.: Volkmann's contracture: treatment by excision of the infarct. J. Bone Joint Surg., *38B*:152-174, 1956.
554. Severin, E.: Umwandlung des Musculus Tibialis Anterior in Narbengewebe nach Uberanstrengung. Acta Chir. Scandinav., *89*:426-432, 1943.
555. Stanford, S.: Traumatic ischaemia in the forearm and leg. Lancet, *1*:462-463, 1944.
556. Tachdjian, M. O.: Pediatric Orthopaedics. Chap. 8. Philadelphia, W. B. Saunders, 1972.
557. Thomson, S. A., and Mahoney, L. J.: Volkmann's ischemic contracture and its relationship to fracture of the femur. J. Bone Joint Surg., *33B*:336-347, 1951.
558. Volkmann, R.: Die Krankheiten der Bewegung surgane. *In* Pitha, R. V., and Billroth, W. M. (eds.): Handbuch der Chirurgie, vol. 2. Stuttgart, Ferdinand Enke, 1872.
559. Volkmann, R.: Die ischaemischem Muskellähmungen und Kontrakturen. Zbl. Chir., *8*:801-803, 1881.
560. Willhoite, D. R., and Moll, J. H.: Early recognition and treatment of impending Volkmann's ischemia in the lower extremity. Arch. Surg., *100*:11-16, 1970.
561. Zohn, D. A., and Leach, R. E.: The role of the electromyogram in the diagnosis and management of the anterior tibial compartment syndrome. Arch. Phys. Med., *45*:311-314, 1964.

5 Pathological Fractures

Thomas D. Brower, M.D.

A traumatic fracture of a bone is a pathological alteration requiring repair similar to that required by other injured tissues. A pathological fracture is a fracture of a bone with preexisting structural weakness. The treatment methods for pathological fractures are not profoundly different from the methods described elsewhere in this book. The patient with a pathological fracture, however, should evoke two responses in the surgeon.

The first is that the surgeon must be more inquisitive as to why the bone is broken. What is the underlying pathology? Why does the bone look abnormally radiolucent, deformed, or osteoporotic? Although the history of the cause of the usual traumatic fracture may be helpful, the roentgenographic diagnosis of traumatic fracture does not demand any intellectual gymnastics. The roentgenographic diagnosis of pathological fracture demands a search to explain the preexisting disease.

Second, the finding of pathological fracture should cause the surgeon to alter some of the usual goals of treatment. We like to believe that most patients with traumatic fractures can return to normal function. This is a desirable and usually obtainable goal. Patients suffering pathological fracture due to benign disease may likewise return to normal function, but those suffering from metastatic disease probably will not. In such patients, at present, we are frequently forced to aim at less dramatic objectives. These patients will be grateful for relief of pain, improved nursing care, and some restoration of function.

The suspicion of pathological fracture necessitates an attitudinal change in the surgeon. Traumatic fractures usually require some mechanical management. A pathological fracture requires the diagnostic approach of internal medicine, the mechanical management of orthopaedics, and a goodly knowledge of bone pathology.

DIAGNOSTIC APPROACH

The approach to the diagnostic problem presented by a patient suffering from a pathological fracture is not much different from the challenge of solving any clinical problem. The following is the usual sequence used in working up a patient, with emphasis on areas of importance in patients with pathological fractures.

History

Any fracture resulting from trivial trauma must be considered pathological. The patient may have noted preexisting pain accompanying an abrupt increase in activity, circumstances that suggest a stress fracture that has suddenly become complete. A long-noted painless enlargement of a metacarpal or phalanx would be helpful in diagnosing a pathological fracture through an enchondroma of the digit. Any preexisting angular deformity of a long bone

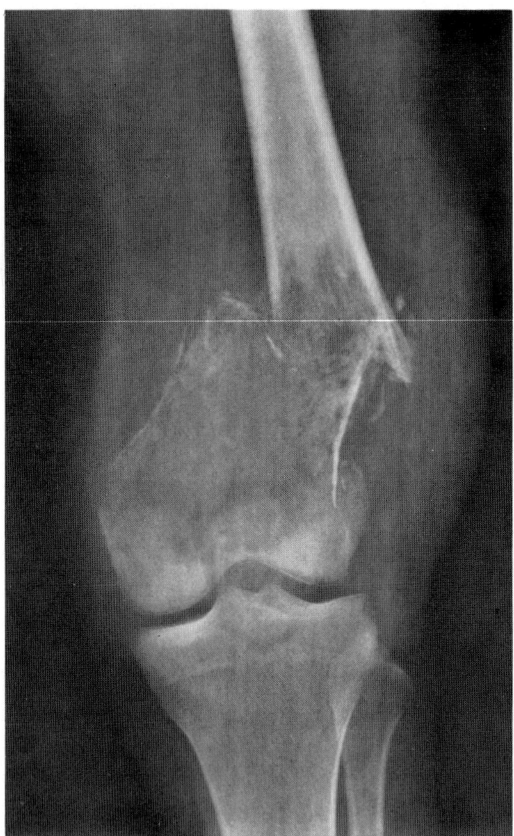

Fig. 5-1. A large destructive lesion in the distal femoral metaphysis through which a pathological fracture has occurred. There is a soft-tissue mass adjacent to the destructive area. The host bone has not reacted to the destructive process by forming either endosteal or periosteal bone. This indicates that the destructive process is more rapid than the bone's reparative ability. This pathological fracture has occurred through a squamous cell carcinoma in a chronic sinus tract.

with sudden onset of pain and instability would indicate a pathological fracture. Pain in the arm, thigh, hips, pelvis, or back may precede by a few days or a few weeks a pathological fracture due to metastatic disease, myeloma, or a sarcoma in Paget's disease of bone. A systems review may offer a clue as to the primary malignancy.

Physical Examination

The diagnostic signs of traumatic fracture are found in patients suffering from pathological fractures. However, any findings that confirm or support the suspicion of a preexisting abnormality are helpful: angular deformity, painless swelling, or generalized bone pain. General physical examination of the breast, in females, and

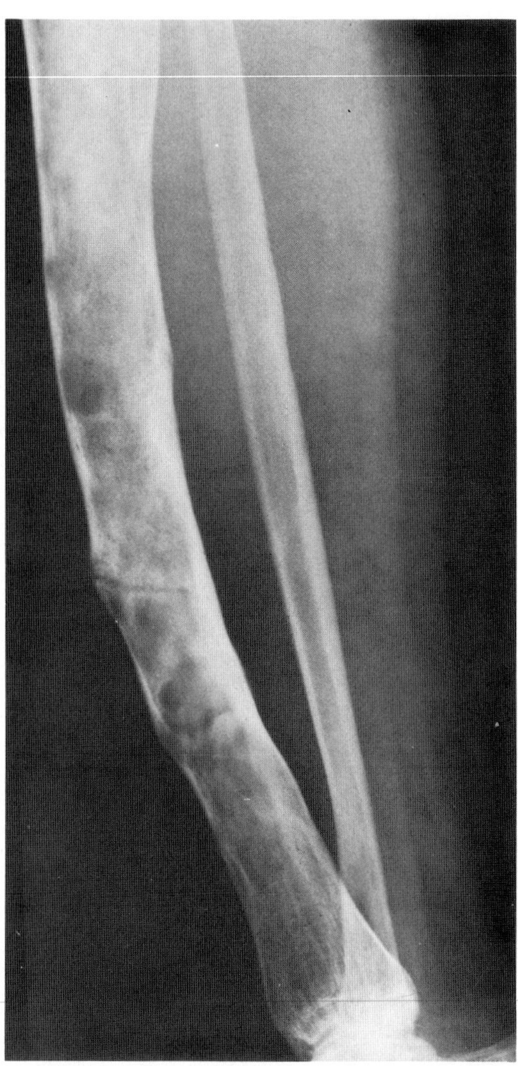

Fig. 5-2. The tibia of a 19-year-old girl who has noted anterior bowing of the tibia for many years and has had several stress fractures at the apex of the bow. One fracture is still visible. The scalloped cortices, the deformity, and the ground glass appearance of the intramedullary material suggest the basic pathology to be fibrous dysplasia. Biopsy confirmed the diagnosis.

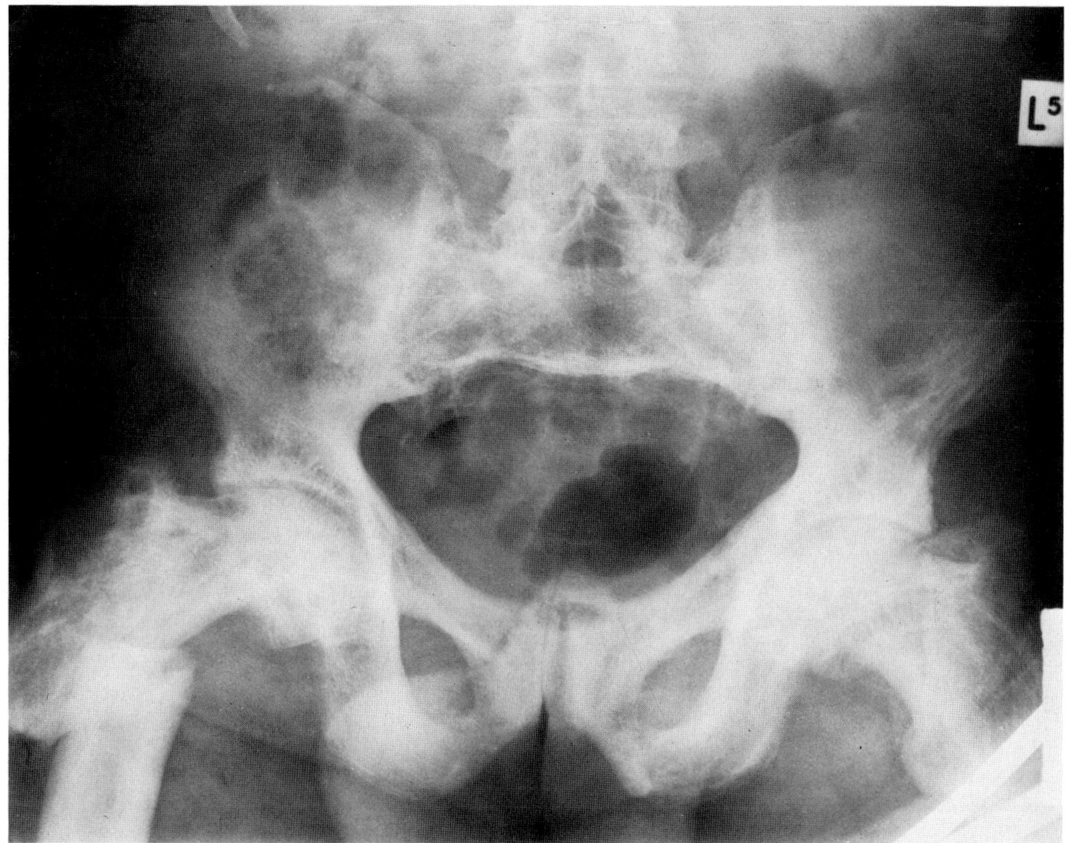

Fig. 5-3. The pelvis of a patient who has widespread Paget's disease of bone. The altered architecture of the trabeculae of bone is seen by the increase in size or coarseness of the trabeculae in the ischii, pubes, and proximal femora. The cortices of these bones are thickened. There are areas of radiolucency in the proximal right femur. There is a transverse subtrochanteric pathological fracture of the right femur. (Courtesy Dr. Hugh C. Barry)

the prostate, in males, may offer information regarding a primary malignancy.

Roentgenographic Diagnosis

The relative rarity of pathological fractures in the usual practice causes most surgeons to be caught off guard. The first evidence that a fracture is pathological is usually found on the roentgenogram. Certain bone changes are indicative of preexisting pathology.

Active Bone Destruction. The resorption of normal bone architecture by some process is referred to as active bone destruction. Figure 5-1 demonstrates a large destructive lesion in the distal femoral metaphysis through which a pathological fracture has occurred. There is a soft-tissue mass adjacent to the area in which destruction has occurred. The host bone has not reacted to the destructive process by forming endosteal or periosteal bone, which indicates that the bone is being destroyed faster than it can repair itself. This pathological fracture occurred through a squamous cell carcinoma arising in a chronic sinus.

Deformity. A 19-year-old girl had noted anterior bowing of the tibia for many years (Fig. 5-2). She had had several stress fractures at the apex of the bow. (One is still visible.) The scalloped cortices, the

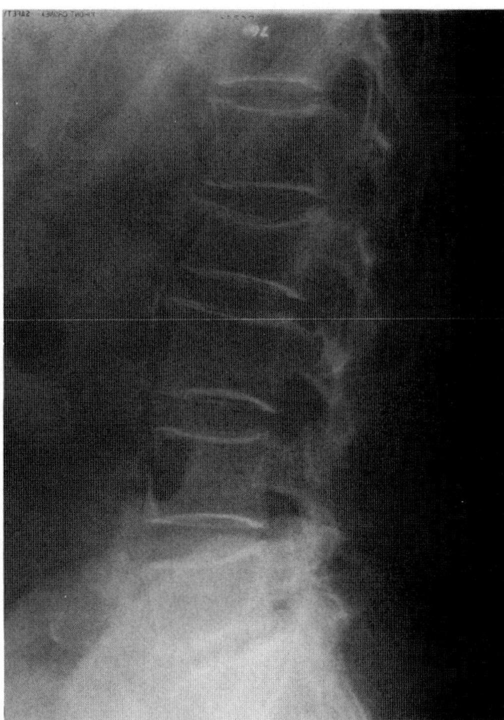

Fig. 5-4. A lateral projection of the lumbar spine in a 72-year-old man. The film demonstrates generalized osteoporosis of the bodies of the vertebrae with decreased density of the trabecular bone and stenciling of the cortices. There is a compression fracture of the body of L2 without any diminished height of the intervertebral disc. This is a classic compression fracture in senile osteoporosis.

deformity, and the ground-glass appearance of the intramedullary material suggested the basic pathology to be fibrous dysplasia. Biopsy confirmed the diagnosis.

Alteration of Architecture. Figure 5-3 is a roentgenogram of the pelvis of a patient who has widespread Paget's disease of bone. The altered architecture of the trabeculae of bone is seen by the increase in size or coarseness of the trabeculae in the ischii, pubes, and proximal femora. The cortices of these bones are thickened. There are areas of radiolucency in the proximal right femur. There is also a transverse subtrochanteric pathologic fracture of the right femur.

General Decreased Density of the Skeleton. Figure 5-4 is a roentgenogram of the spine in the lateral projection. The bodies of the vertebrae are less dense than normal. It is difficult to quantitate decreased density of bone by visual examination, but with experience one's judgment becomes rather accurate. The cortices of the vertebrae are thin. These changes suggest osteoporosis (i.e., less bone than normal). The bone that is present is normal. It is difficult roentgenographically to differentiate osteoporotic bone from osteomalacic bone.

Laboratory Examination

The initation of a number of laboratory investigations must be based on a reasonable expectation that the results will be helpful in reaching a diagnosis or in the management of the patient. The following is a list of laboratory tests I suggest with explanations of how I would expect the information to be used.

Complete Blood Count. Any new patient should have a CBC. The hemoglobin or hematocrit often shows an anemia of mild to moderate degree in the presence of malignancy. I do not find the white count very informative.

Sedimentation Rate. Many clinicians infer disease—malignancy, infection—from an elevated sedimentation rate. They conclude from a normal sedimentation rate that nothing terribly serious can be wrong with the patient. I, personally, have not found this determination to be very useful.

Calcium, Phosphorus, and Alkaline Phosphatase. These three determinations are used primarily to find evidence for systemic disease—primary or secondary hyperparathyroidism or osteomalacia. In the adult, one of the most common causes for elevation of the serum calcium is metastatic bone disease. Acid phosphatase is not routinely requested. If the patient has a blastic lesion in the lumbar spine, pelvis, or proximal femur, an acid phosphatase determination is indicated to help diagnose metastatic prostatic carcinoma. This blood sample must be drawn before digital examination of the prostate, because that examination causes an elevation of the acid phosphatase for 48 hours.

Serum Electrophoresis. About the only specific blood test for bone malignancy is the elevated abnormal globulin, which can indicate multiple myeloma. More than 80 per cent of all patients with multiple myeloma show an elevation of the M-component on the serum electrophoresis pattern. Since the roentgenographic alterations in this disease are not characteristic, it is wise to always obtain this determination when an adult has a pathological fracture.

Urinalysis. This classic laboratory examination is useful for obtaining leads to renal disease, genitourinary infection, and diabetes, and such information is helpful in patients with pathological fractures. Fifty to 60 per cent of all patients with multiple myeloma show Bence-Jones protein in the urine, so you should always test for it. Although not absolutely diagnostic, the presence of this abnormal protein in the urine is strongly suggestive of myeloma. The loss of the abnormal protein through the kidney may also give a false negative result in serum electrophoresis. Therefore, it is essential that both determinations be done in the diagnosis of myeloma.

Roentgenography. All patients suspected of having metastatic bone disease should have a roentgenographic chest examination.

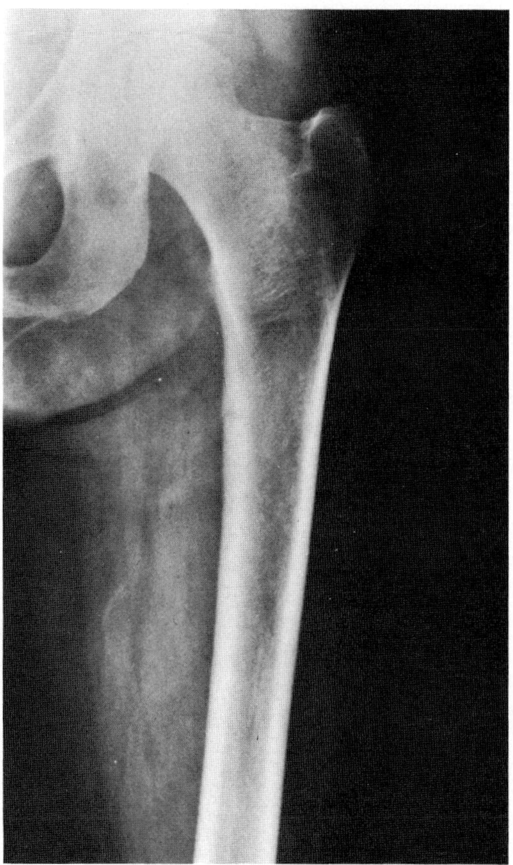

Fig. 5-5. The shaft of the femur of a 65-year-old woman who has osteomalacia due to a malabsorption syndrome. A small fracture is seen just distal to the lesser trochanter. The patient has complained of pain in the thighs, and she also has pain in one of her metatarsals due to a stress fracture. This roentgenogram reveals decrease of bone density with thinning of the cortices. There is some coarsening of the trabeculae in the proximal femur.

PATHOLOGICAL FRACTURES DUE TO SYSTEMIC BONE DISEASE

Osteoporosis

Caucasian adults beyond the age of 50 years have a higher incidence of fractures of the neck of the femur, intertrochanteric fractures, and fractures of the distal radius than adults of other races. Senile or postmenopausal osteoporosis seems to be a genetically controlled pathologic alteration of bone.[4] Therefore, such fractures could be interpreted as pathological, even though there is nothing pathological in the bone nor in its repair of the injury. (Osteoporotic fractures are covered in other chapters in this book. Pathological compression fractures of the vertebrae are a common manifestation of osteoporosis and are discussed in the section on pathological fractures of the spine.)

Osteomalacia

When the human skeleton loses the ability to mineralize osteoid, the bones become

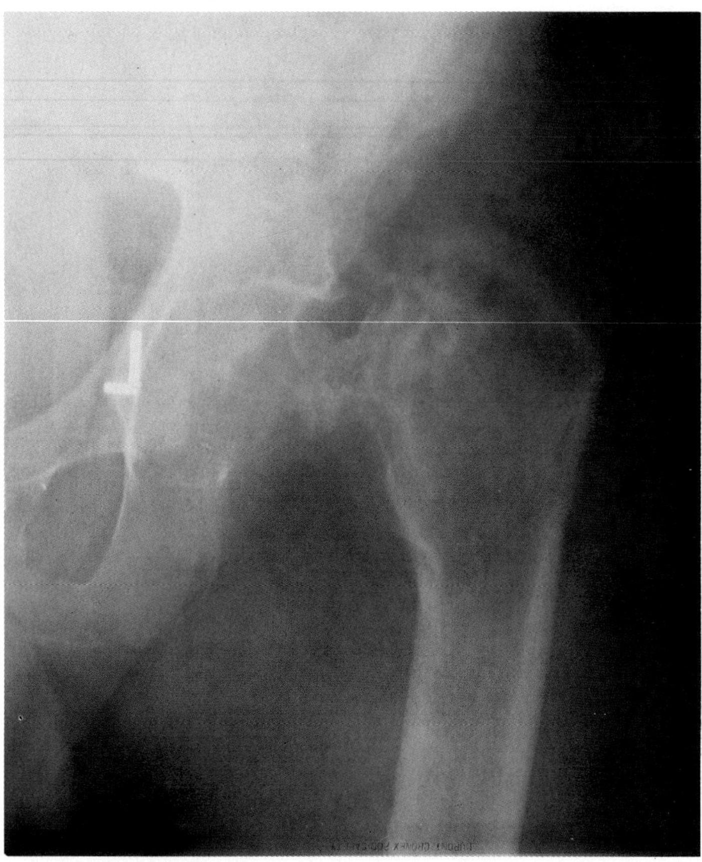

Fig. 5-6. The hip of a 60-year-old man who is suffering from secondary hyperparathyroidism. It demonstrates a very large destructive area in the intertrochanteric region and dissolution of the neck of the femur with a stress fracture at mid-neck. Biopsy of this area revealed that the large cavity was filled with fluid and there was some fibrous tissue at the periphery of the lesion. This fibrous tissue was similar to the material found in a "brown" tumor, and the bone showed advanced osteitis fibrosa cystica.

soft (a condition called osteomalacia). The causes of osteomalacia are many. Nutritional deficiencies, gastrointestinal absorption abnormalities, renal disease, and primary hyperparathyroidism are the most common. Regardless of the etiology of the disease, the effect on the adult skeleton is the same. Pathologically, there is an accumulation of osteoid that does not mineralize, and the result is a weakened skeleton. Roentgenographically, the skeleton appears less dense than normal. This roentgenographic appearance has provoked many vernacular terms for the description of such bone—"washed out," decalcified, demineralized. The term osteoporosis, as used in this discussion, means lessened density of bone on x-ray examination and does not imply the pathogenesis of the alteration; thus, osteomalacia is one subclass of osteoporosis.

Characteristically, the cortices are thin and the density decreased. In the advanced stage of the disease, there appears to be a change in the trabecular pattern of the bone. If osteomalacia has been present for a long time, the long bones of the adult may be deformed, owing to bending through small stress fractures.

The orthopaedist's first contact with these patients comes when a fracture occurs. Figure 5-5 shows a stress fracture through the proximal femur in a patient with osteomalacia due to a malabsorption problem. The patient complained of an ache in the thigh on weight bearing. Had she subjected this bone to a sudden stress, the probability is great that a displaced or angulated transverse fracture would have occurred. In 1934, Milkman[16] reported a case of "multiple spontaneous idiopathic symmetrical fractures" in a woman of 45 years. It seems

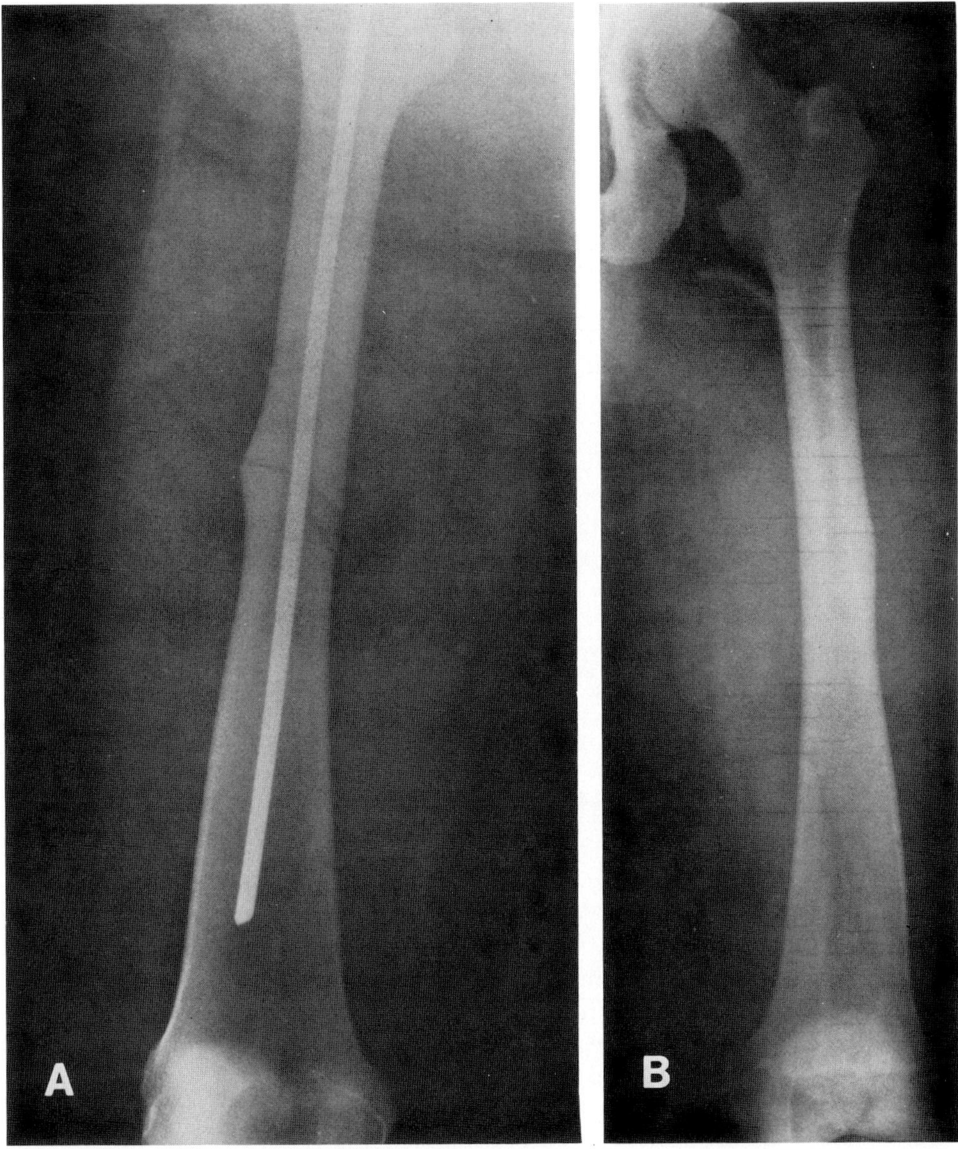

Fig. 5-7. (*A*) A 24-year-old man with pycnodysostosis and a pathological fracture in the mid-shaft of the femur. Note the increased density of the cortices and the very narrow intramedullary canal. The fracture was fixed with a Rush pin, because the canal measured only 4 mm. (*B*) The roentgenogram of the left femur taken to measure the length of the canal. Again it illustrates the narrow canal and the thick cortices with a little prominence in the mid-shaft of the femur. Three years later the patient returned with a fracture of the mid-shaft of this femur. The patient has also suffered pathological fractures of both tibiae in the last several years.

to be the consensus at this time that his patient had osteomalacia of unknown etiology. The importance of the report is that observation of multiple spontaneous stress fractures in an adult is almost diagnostic of osteomalacia and should force further evaluation to establish the diagnosis. The treatment of osteomalacic fractures requires protection of the bone as necessary until it heals, but more importantly, a search for the cause of the osteomalacia and its correction.

Generalized osteomalacia of hyperparathyroidism is not significantly different, histologically, from that of any other cause. Hyperparathyroidism does produce peculiar lytic tumors of bone, called "brown tumors." Should a brown tumor sufficiently weaken a bone, it may sustain a pathological fracture (Fig. 5-6). The author has seen one patient who had three pathological fractures treated over several years before someone thought to obtain blood calcium, phosphorus, and alkaline phosphatase determinations. The elevated serum calcium, depressed serum phosphorus, and markedly elevated alkaline phosphatase led to the diagnosis of hyperparathyroidism.

Osteogenesis Imperfecta Tarda

Rarely, a pathological fracture in adult life may be the first manifestation of osteogenesis imperfecta tarda. Family history indicating the genetic possibility of the disease and the presence of blue sclerae may be the only hints of the underlying pathology. Roentgenographic examination is not diagnostic, nor is the microscopic examination of the bone helpful in the adult form of the disease. No laboratory determination is specific for this disease. The treatment of the fracture is not significantly different from standard fracture care.

Pycnodysostosis

Pycnodysostosis is a rare form of dwarfism that is characterized by dysplasia of the skull, obtuse mandibular angle, dysplastic clavicles, partial or total aplasia of the terminal phalanges, and generalized increased roentgenographic density of the skeleton.[7] Patients are also subject to pathological fractures, which can occur in early childhood or in adult life. Figure 5-7A reveals a pathological fracture of the right femur that was fixed with a Rush pin. The intramedullary canal was so small that no other fixation device could be used. Figure 5-7B shows the roentgenogram of the left femur taken to measure the length of the intramedullary canal. Three years later, the patient suffered a similar fracture in this femur. He has also suffered fractures of both tibiae. In this disease, as in osteopetrosis, the dense bone is subject to pathological fracture. As bone healing seems not to be retarded, pathological fractures in pycnodysostosis should be treated by standard methods.

PATHOLOGICAL FRACTURE OF THE SPINE

Patients complaining of back pain constitute a large segment of an orthopaedist's practice. A very small but important portion of these patients have pathological fractures of the spine. Although such a fracture may occur in any of the vertebrae from the occiput to the sacrum, the majority occur at the lumbodorsal junction. It may involve a single vertebra, several consecutive ones, or several single vertebrae at different levels.

The patient's complaints usually start suddenly and dramatically after a minimal stress, such as bending over to make a bed, bending over in gardening, lifting a light object, or experiencing a sudden jolt. The rather severe pain is localized over the compressed vertebra. There may be radicular pain around the chest in the compression fracture of the thoracic spine. Most patients with pathological fractures are middle-aged or older. In these age groups, back pain is so frequent and thus so "normal" that the patient rests at home for a few days before seeking medical help.

The history of incapacitating pain, a severe "catching" in the back on rotational movements of the trunk, and the inability to flex the spine should distinguish fractures from chronic low back pain. Some patients will notice a transient ileus.

The physical examination definitely separates the patient with pathological vertebral fractures from the large number of patients with backache. The former holds the trunk rigid. Assuming a recumbent position is painful and is usually done sideways. Palpation of the spine reveals tenderness over the spinous process of the involved vertebra or vertebrae. Usually there are no neurologic deficits. Of course, pathological fractures of the spine due to metastatic malignancy may be accompanied by subtle neurologic changes or even obvious paraplegia.

The roentgenographic appearance of a pathological fracture of the veterbrae is shown in Figure 5-4. The roentgenogram shows an obvious fracture of L2 and a less obvious fracture of the upper cortical plate of L1 in an osteoporotic spine. Indeed, pathological fractures may occur in one to five consecutive vertebrae or may be seen at different levels of the spine. The vast majority of compression fractures in osteoporosis occur at the lumbodorsal junction. On occasion, serial roentgenograms may be required to reveal the injury, as deformity may develop only after days or weeks.

Thus far, I have presented an adult patient with the acute onset of back pain following insignificant trauma and roentgenographic evidence of two compression fractures of the vertebra in an osteoporotic spine—a pathological compression fracture of the spine. This clinical picture should cause the physician to quickly review all his knowledge of bone pathophysiology in an effort to arrive at a diagnosis. The most important clues are found in a painstakingly detailed history. I will present an outline of the possible causes of osteoporosis of the spine and then suggest a plan for investigations that should lead to a definitive diagnosis in almost all cases. In this context, I am using the term osteoporosis in a general descriptive sense to mean a roentgenographic appearance of less dense bone without reference to the pathogenesis of the alteration.

This rather imposing list of diseases may seem overwhelming at first glance. A review of 105 patients suffering from compression fractures of the spine by Nicholas, Wilson, and Freiberger[17] confirms my clinical impression and greatly helps in organizing logical approaches to this multifaceted problem. Patients suffering pathological fractures of the vertebrae may be separated into two groups, those over 55 years of age and those under 55.

Of the 105 patients, 78 patients were over age 55. Fifty of these had postmenopausal or senile osteoporosis; 14 had primary or metastatic disease; seven had hypercortisonism and rheumatoid arthritis; four had osteomalacia secondary to malabsorption; and three had vertebral hemangioma, polycythemia vera, or Gaucher's disease.

The 27 patients under the age of 55 revealed a somewhat different incident of pathology. Five were diagnosed as having osteoporosis. Eleven had malignancy of bone—four due to multiple myeloma, and

The Causes of Osteoporosis of the Spine

1. Atrophy
   Disuse atrophy—prolonged bed rest
2. Osteoporosis
   a. Postmenopausal
   b. Postsurgical menopausal
   c. Senile
3. Ingestive aberration
   a. Cortisone
   b. Diet
4. Gastrointestinal tract abnormalities
   a. Malabsorption
   b. Bile duct obstruction
5. Renal abnormalities
   a. Chronic glomerular disease
   b. Tubular disease
6. Endocrinologic abnormalities
   a. Hyperthyroidism
   b. Hyperparathyroidism
   c. Cushing's disease
   d. Hypogonadism
   e. Acromegaly
7. Malignancy
   a. Multiple myeloma
   b. Metastasis
8. Polycythemia vera

the others due to metastatic disease. The remaining patients had various diseases, including hypercortisonism, osteomalacia, and polycythemia vera.

From a comparison of these two groups, one can make the generalization that a pathological compression fracture in a patient over the age of 55 is most likely to be caused by senile or postmenopausal osteoporosis, although not always. The physician should suspect malignancy or some other systemic disease as the cause of the complaint in a patient under 55 years.

"Diagnostic Screen"

A general plan for investigation of the patient suffering from a pathological compression fracture of the vertebrae might include the following:

Medical History. After the patient has been allowed to present the description of the initial episode, a rather direct systemic review should be done. The following is a list of the more important questions to be explored:

Has the patient had prolonged bed rest?
Has an operation brought on menopause?
Has there been any decrease in height?
Is there progressive kyphosis?
Are gastrointestinal and genitourinary systems normal?

The physical examination is no different from the examination of any patient who complains of pain in the back, but the examining physician should emphasize, (1) a description of posture and motion of the spine, (2) an accurate record of the areas of tenderness, and (3) a neurologic examination.

The roentgenographic examination of the spine has been illustrated. The usual observations will be one or more compression fractures and an osteoporotic spine. Subsequent to this observation, roentgenographic examination of the chest, skull, and hands is helpful. As the work-up proceeds, others may be indicated, such as intravenous pyelogram or gastrointestinal examination.

Laboratory Investigation. Because of the multiplicity of possibilities, the laboratory determinations could conceivably be endless. If one considers the probabilities, however, a very logical "screen" presents itself, and the following are suggested: complete blood count, sedimentation rate, urinalysis (to include Bence-Jones determination), serum protein electrophoresis, serum calcium, phosphorus, and alkaline phosphatase. Should these investigations suggest the need for further inquiry, the physician may need medical consultation, special calcium metabolic studies, sternal or iliac marrow biopsy, and even biopsy of the involved vertebra. Griffiths,[11] reporting a large series of patients with myelomatosis, emphasized that one-third of all patients with this disease have the presenting complaint of back pain.

Treatment

The treatment of pathological compression fractures in an osteoporotic spine requires a common-sense approach. The patient desires relief of pain. This can be accomplished by a few days of bed rest. Ambulation should be encouraged as soon as possible to avoid further osteoporosis or disuse. The patient should be instructed not to flex the spine or do heavy lifting.

Braces. I have found that if the fracture is at the level of D10 or below, corsets, for women, and braces, for men, afford some relief and enable the patient to be mobile for longer periods of time. Fractures above D10 have not been successfully treated, in my experience, by any brace. I depend on the stabilizing effect of the rib cage and direct the patient to walk as soon as symptoms allow.

Medication. In 1942, Fuller Albright[1] described the clinical picture of postmenopausal osteoporosis and suggested estrogen therapy. I have used various estrogen substitutes to treat the back pain of osteoporosis for years, and in the past decade I have used anabolic agents. My clinical impression has been that somewhat less than half of these patients experienced significant symptomatic relief. Rose,[22] in an excellent review, records that placebos seemed to give equal symptomatic relief. High calcium, diet, vitamin D, and fluoride ingestion did not seem to have any beneficial effects. The cause and treatment of osteoporosis is a highly controversial subject, and an excellent review is given in a book titled *Osteoporosis,* edited by Barzel.[4]

Pathological compression fractures due to corticoid ingestion and rheumatoid arthritis are treated in the same manner as those that arise from postmenopausal osteoporosis. In the opinion of some, anabolic agents may be of help.

Pathological Fractures Due to Metastatic Malignancy. If malignant metastasis causes fractures in the area of the vertebral column that can be treated with a brace, such treatment may alleviate the pain sufficiently to allow some ambulation. In some instances, the patient's pain demands complete bed rest on a firm mattress.

Radiation Therapy. When the diagnosis of metastatic malignancy has been established, a radiotherapist should be consulted. Most metastatic disease to the spine can be treated by irradiation sufficiently to relieve the symptoms to some degree. The relief will probably be temporary but greatly appreciated by the patient.

Hormone Therapy. Almost half of the patients suffering pathological fracture of the spine due to metastatic disease have primary malignancy of the breast. Hormonal therapy and irradiation seem to give the best relief.

Paraplegia Due to Pathological Fractures

The patient who presents with partial or total paraplegia due to pathological fractures of the spine offers a profound therapeutic problem. Clain[6] sets the average life expectancy of such patients, without treatment, at a little over 4 months. In this series, radiotherapy with androgen therapy was the most effective treatment in patients whose primary disease was carcinoma of the breast. Only three patients out of 18 were improved by laminectomy. Martin and Williamson[15] propose that lateral rachiotomy may be more helpful than laminectomy in treating paraplegia due to pathological fracture. At the present time, the author would advise that the treatment of paraplegia due to pathological fracture of the spine must depend on the type of tumor. Obviously, radiosensitive tumors should be irradiated. If indicated, endocrine therapy may be helpful. At present, prospects for survival are so dismal that little enthusiasm is offered for surgical intervention. Laminectomy occasionally may cause improvement. More radical surgical decompression will be required if we really wish to improve the neurologic status and stabilize the spine.

PATHOLOGICAL FRACTURE DUE TO BENIGN TUMORS IN ADULTS

Benign tumors of bone are rare lesions in the adult. A pathological fracture through such a lesion is frequently the first indication that any disease exists.

Enchondromas of the Hand

Enchondromas of the metacarpals and phalanges are the most common sites of pathological fractures in benign tumors in the adult. The patient may be aware that a painless enlargement of one of the bones of the hand has been present for years before the fracture occurred. The acute episode, a fracture of the phalanx or metacarpal, however, may be the first evidence of disease. Figure 5-8 shows a fracture through a typical enchondroma. The lesion is well circumscribed by a zone of reactive bone of the phalanx, apparently an attempt to contain the lesion. The lesion in this illustration contains no roentgenographically detectable calcified cartilage.

Treatment of an enchondromatous fracture of a digit offers several alternatives. The fracture can be treated as a traumatic one and be immobilized for 3 weeks. After

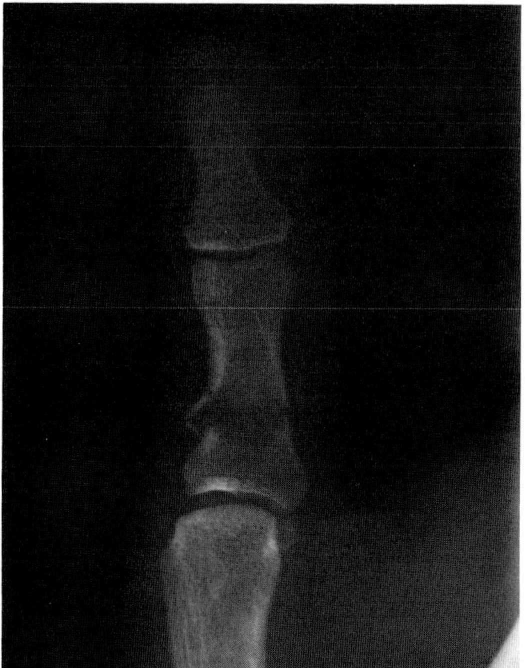
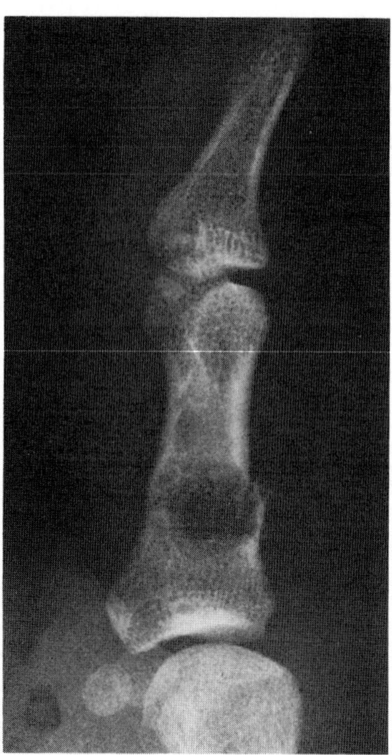

Fig. 5-8. Roentgenograms in two projections of the thumb of an adult. It shows a pathological fracture through a destructive lesion in the proximal phalanx. The lesion has not significantly interfered with the normal modeling of the thumb, but there is no distinct border at the endosteal surface of the lesion. However, the location, and age strongly suggest that this is an enchondroma of the phalanx.

it has healed and the digit has normal function, the decision can be made as to whether the lesion should be curetted. This rather conservative approach is the preferred treatment of pathological fractures through enchondromas of the hands and feet. It allows the fracture healing to offer stability to the bone, after which the enchondroma can be curetted completely. The digit is then immobilized for 10 to 14 days before motion is begun.

A second approach, curettage of the enchondroma in the presence of an acute fracture, has two disadvantages. First, curettage of any benign lesion of bone in the presence of an acute fracture is always a technically difficult and generally unsatisfying experience. Secondly, after the curettage, it will almost certainly be necessary to transfix the fracture in order to stabilize and reduce the digit. After having curetted the intramedullary portion of a phalanx of an enchondroma, transfixing the fracture with two Kirschner wires can be an exasperating experience.

Finally, rather large lesions sometimes involve the greater part of the proximal phalanx or metacarpal. These larger enchondromas may require resection, replacement of the defect with a properly fashioned bone graft, and internal fixation by Kirschner wires.

Benign Lesions of Long Bones

A pathological fracture through benign lesions of long bones in adults is a greater cause for concern than one through an enchondroma of the hand. The principal problem is that such lesions are frequently not benign. Figure 5-2 shows a stress fracture through the apex of a bowed tibia in a 19-year-old woman. The scalloped endosteal surfaces of the cortices of the tibia and multiloculated intramedullary lesion, with an ill-defined density of its own, strongly suggest fibrous dysplasia. Other similar lesions in the ipsilateral femur, and the skin pigmentation, support this diagnosis. Biopsy confirmed it. Biopsy in the presence of a stress fracture is not difficult if the surgeon takes the specimen from an area in which the cellular structure is not influenced by the fracture. Treatment of this fracture should be aimed at straightening the deformity to decrease the bending forces on structurally weakened bone. Pathological fractures through less well-defined lesions cause more problems. The diagnostic distinction of benign versus malignant bone tumors is fraught with pitfalls. Add to this the reparative process of a fracture, and the histologic picture can be terribly confusing. The biopsy should be done at the junction of normal bone and the lesion, as far from the fracture as possible.

Treatment

It is impossible to cover all the contingencies in the treatment of pathological fractures through benign tumors. I will, therefore, discuss some possibilities and approaches. Unicameral bone cysts may be seen in the long bones of an adult, but very, very rarely. Roentgenographically, they are not significantly different from those of children. The lesion is almost always away from the metaphysis. Should a fracture occur through a roentgenographically acceptable bone cyst, it could be treated by external immobilization; then the decision on further treatment could be deferred until after union. I, personally, could not pursue this course, for I would have to biopsy the lesion. Grossly, the lesion would be filled with bloody fluid because of the fracture. The biopsy should be taken at the junction of normal bone and the lesion, as far from the fracture as possible. If no neoplastic tissue is found, the fracture should be treated as one would treat any fracture at that site.

A pathological fracture through an intramedullary cartilaginous tumor of a long bone offers different problems. The roentgenographic appearance may be similar to that of a bone cyst. Flecks of calcification in the lesion on the roentgenogram may tip off the observer that the lesion is cartilaginous.

At biopsy the diagnosis of a cartilaginous tumor can and should be made grossly. The bluish white tissue is rarely confused with anything else. *Never trust an intramedullary cartilaginous tumor in the long bone or pelvis of an adult. Such tumors are always potentially malignant.* The microscopic examination of an intramedullary cartilaginous tumor merely confirms the diagnosis of cartilage. The differential diagnosis of enchondroma and chondrosarcoma by microscopic examination is not dependable. Resect the tumor if possible; curette the lesion if there is no better alternative immediately, but do not drive an intramedullary device down the canal. I have seen several cases in which intramedullary devices were driven through alleged enchondromas, which, a few months or years later, proved to be chondrosarcomas that had spread over the entire length of the long bone and encased the proximal protrusion of the intramedullary rod. In summary, should you be treating an adult patient with a pathological fracture through a cartilaginous lesion of a long bone (I avoid the term enchondroma), try to ablate the tumor and appose the remaining bone fragments without intramedullary fixation. Monitor the lesion rather closely by x-ray for many years.

PATHOLOGICAL FRACTURES IN PAGET'S DISEASE

One of the most prominent clinical features of Paget's disease of bone is pathological fracture. The femur and tibia are most commonly involved. Barry,[2] in a comprehensive monograph on Paget's disease of bone, states that while he was collecting a series of 70 cases of fractures of the femur

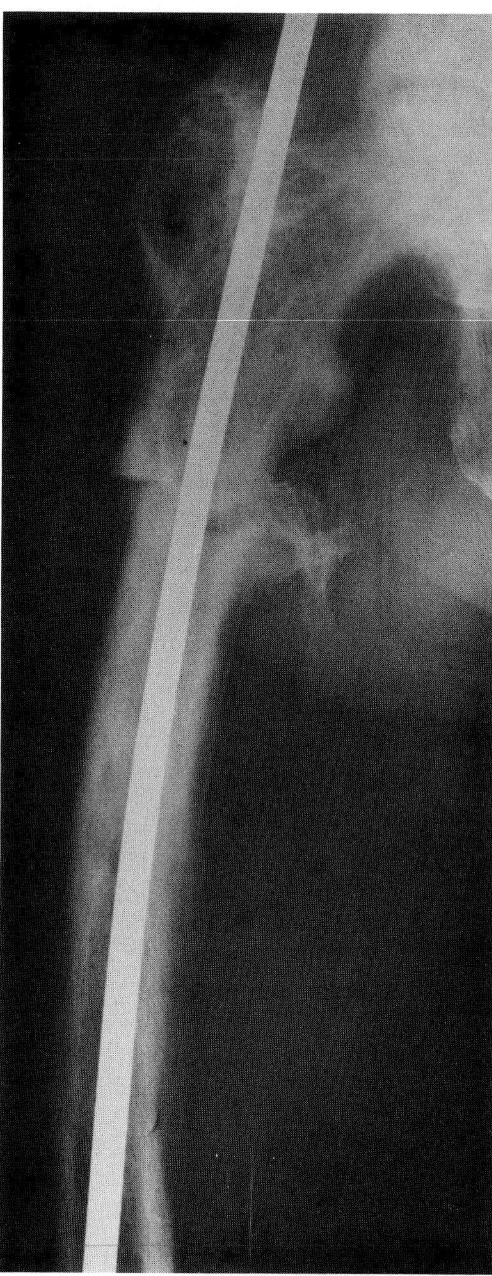

Fig. 5-9. A patient suffering from Paget's disease with a subtrochanteric fracture of the femur. The thickened cortices and coarse trabeculae are rather diagnostic of this disease. This patient has been treated by an intramedullary rod. The deformity of the femur was such that the rod had to be small enough to bend to the bow of the intramedullary canal. (Courtesy Dr. Hugh C. Barry)

in Paget's disease, he saw only seven fractures of the upper extremity due to the disease. Pathological fractures of the femur typically are transverse. The patient may complain of an ache in the region of the fracture for a short time before the bone fractures. Such symptoms may indicate a preexisting stress fracture or a sarcomatous change in the Paget bone. Barry's[3] later series of 90 pathological fractures of the femur showed 19 fractures in the proximal end, 30 subtrochanteric fractures, and the rest in the shaft.

Treatment

Pathological fractures of the femur in Paget's disease are treated in similar fashion to traumatic fractures. The author offers one admonition: have plenty of blood available for transfusion at operation. In my experience, I have been astounded at the vascularity of Paget bone. Bone in the osteoporotic or active stage of the disease seems to be the most vascular. Old, dense Paget bone may not bleed so alarmingly.

Pathological fractures of the neck of the femur may be treated by internal fixation. Paget bone tends to be brittle, and thus it may be wise to use a threaded device. An endoprosthetic replacement will also serve in the treatment of a fracture of the neck of the femur in this disease.

Intertrochanteric pathological fractures in Paget's disease should be treated by the standard methods for such fractures. In Barry's large series, the subtrochanteric area (Fig. 5-9) was a common area of fracture in the femur. Most of his patients were treated with skin traction, and quite successfully. The fracture line is always transverse, and the fracture can also be treated by an intramedullary nail or a Müller compression device.

Pathological fractures of the shaft of the femur were successfully treated, in Barry's series, with skin traction, skeletal traction, and intramedullary fixation. In this large series the healing time of the fractured femur was not significantly prolonged.

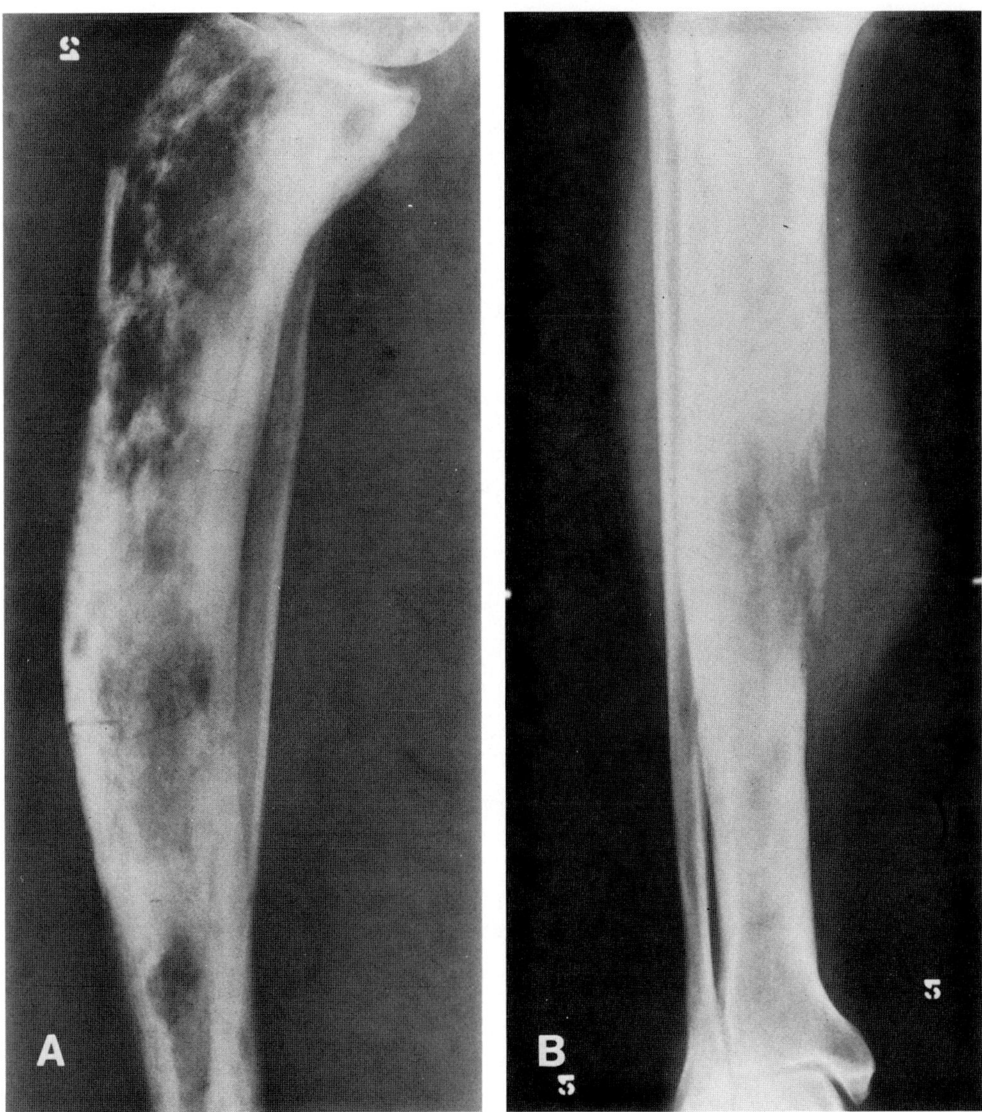

Fig. 5-10. The anteroposterior and lateral films of the tibia of a 76-year-old man who had been suffering from Paget's disease for some years. The roentgenogram shows the irregular destruction of a bone throughout the shaft and the thickened cortices and coarse trabeculae characteristic of Paget's disease. There is a pathological fracture at the apex of the bow seen in both projections. There is a soft-tissue mass, more visible on the anteroposterior than on the lateral projection, and there is active destruction of the Paget bone in the region of the pathological fracture. This man has a pathological fracture through a sarcoma in Paget's disease of the tibia.

Sometimes the bow in the femur is so severe that in addition to the fracture, one or more osteotomies are required to straighten the shaft sufficiently to allow intramedullary fixation.

Pathological fractures of the tibia usually do not offer much problem as far as treatment is concerned. The fracture is transverse, at or near the apex of the anterior bow of the Paget bone of the tibia without much displacement. The fibula is rarely involved in Paget's disease, so it can serve as

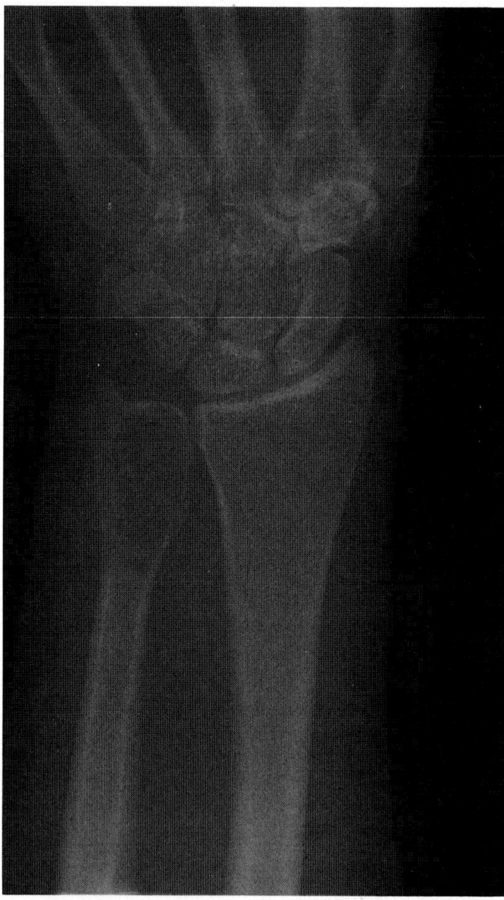

Fig. 5-11. The wrist of a 30-year-old housewife who complained of some swelling of the distal end of the ulna for several months. In the last week, she noted acute pain at the distal end of the ulna. It is apparent that she has a destructive lesion that has involved the epiphysis and metaphysis of the distal end of the ulna. The host bone has reacted by producing minimal periosteal new bone and no endosteum. On very close examination, a minute fracture is seen at the proximal end of this lesion. This is typical of the roentgenographic appearance of a giant cell tumor.

an internal splint. A patellar-tendon-bearing cast should be adequate treatment for this fracture.

Figure 5-10 shows a transverse pathological fracture through the mid-shaft of the tibia in Paget's disease. The important detail in this illustration, however, is the area of active destruction in the bone adjacent to the area of fracture. Such an alteration suggests a sarcomatous change in the Paget bone, and, indeed, this man had a fibrosarcoma. The clinician must be aware of the fact that a pathological fracture in Paget bone may be the first clinical indication of sarcoma in this disease. The treatment of a pathological fracture through a sarcoma in Paget's disease of bone should be amputation. The prognosis is dismal. Sarcomata arising in Paget bone are the most malignant of all primary bone tumors.

PATHOLOGICAL FRACTURES THROUGH GIANT CELL TUMOR

Giant cell tumors occur almost exclusively in skeletally mature individuals and usually in the ends of long bones. They probably arise in the epiphysis and extend into the metaphysis. Some time ago, such a tumor was called "benign giant cell tumor," but in recent years the word "benign" has been deleted. It is difficult to predict the clinical course of a giant cell tumor, and, therefore, the consensus at this time seems to be that the optimal treatment of this lesion is surgical ablation, if possible. Because the clinical course of this tumor is unpredictable, I have chosen to discuss pathological fractures occurring in this lesion in this section between pathological fractures in benign lesions of bone and pathological fractures occurring in metastatic bone disease.

Because giant cell tumors occur at the ends of long bones the fractures they cause are less obviously pathological fractures than are those through lesions in the bone shaft. Typically, the patient notes a gradual enlargement of the end of a long bone accompanied by some discomfort. These symptoms may not be severe enough to cause the patient to seek medical advice. Usually, he or she is forced to seek help when some minor trauma causes severe pain over the swollen part of the extremity. Motion of the adjacent joint accentuates the pain, but rarely does the patient note any deformity. This sequence of events usually indicates a small pathological fracture in a giant cell tumor.

The treatment of a pathological fracture through a giant cell tumor should aim at ablation of the primary tumor. Although the roentgenographic appearance of giant cell tumor, its location, and the age of the patient strongly support the diagnosis, the treatment plan should include a frozen section at the time of definitive surgery. There are several options available in the treatment of pathological fractures in giant cell tumors. A 30-year-old housewife had a minute fracture through a giant cell tumor in the distal end of the ulna (Fig. 5-11). The location of the tumor allowed total excision of the distal end of the ulna without any significant impairment of the function of the extremity. Were the pathological fracture and tumor in the distal end of the radius, resection could be done, and the defect could be bridged by a graft of the proximal end of the fibula.

Giant cell tumors arising in the distal end of the femur or the proximal end of the tibia are a greater challenge. Here again, the patient usually seeks medical advice because of a pathological fracture through one of the tibial plateaus or a femoral condyle (Fig. 5-12).

Ablation of giant cell tumors about the knee joint offers a major challenge to the surgeon. It is not within the scope of this chapter to discuss the treatment of giant cell tumors. Pathological fractures do occur in this lesion, however, and I will briefly outline the suggested methods of treatment. If a lesion is large enough to produce pathological fractures about the knee joint, local curettage may not excise it completely, though such treatment has had some success. More radical excision has a higher cure rate. Radical excision of the lesion and fusion of the knee afford a functional result. Parrish[18] has achieved some good results by resecting the distal end of the femur and transplanting a comparable section of homologous femur. All variations of these methods are available.

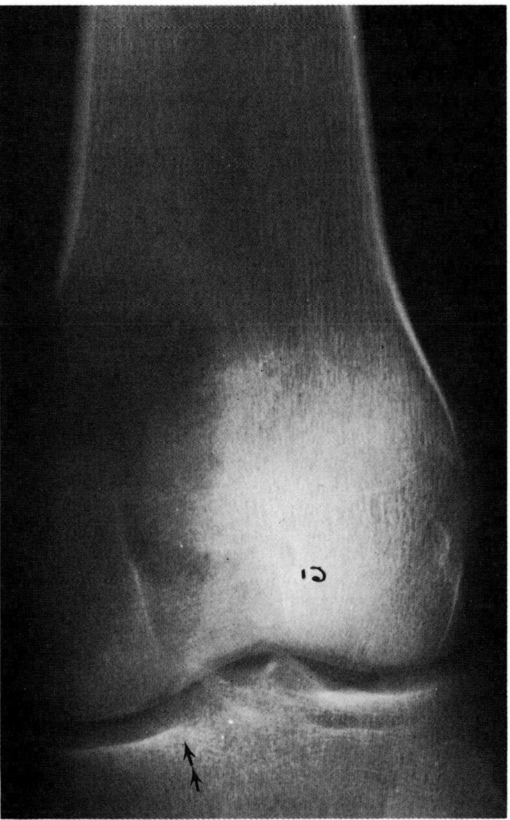

Fig. 5-12. The distal end of the femur of an adult with a destructive lesion involving the medial condyle of the femur and the medial side of the metaphysis. The destruction has involved the cortices and the cancellous bone of one-half of the femur. There is a very small fracture extending from the articular surface of the medial side of the medial condyle of the femur into the tumor. This is a giant cell tumor of the distal end of the femur. (Courtesy Dr. W. F. Enneking)

Pathological fracture through a giant cell tumor arising in the head and neck of the femur would best be treated by radical excision of the involved proximal end of the femur and replacement by an endoprosthetic device.

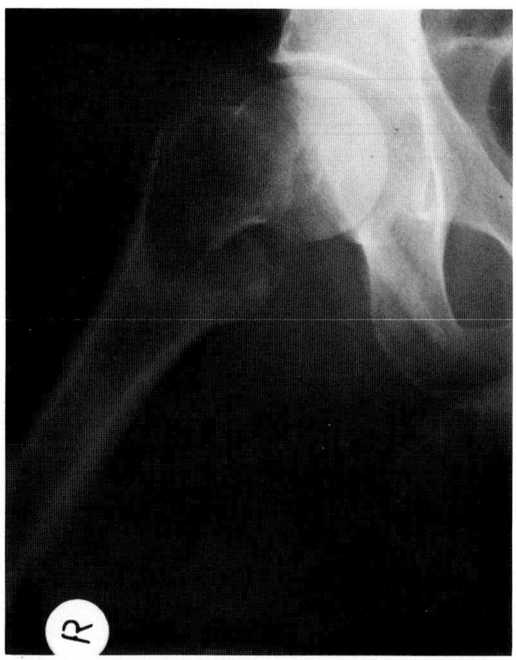

Fig. 5-13. The hip of a middle-aged man suffering from carcinoma of the lung. There is a very large destructive lesion involving the intertrochanteric area, and it has also destroyed a good portion of the neck of the femur. It is obvious that there is a fracture in the neck of the femur and that the host bone has not reacted to this destructive process. The location is very typical of a metastatic lesion to the proximal end of the femur with a pathological fracture.

PATHOLOGICAL FRACTURES IN METASTATIC MALIGNANCY OF LONG BONES

By far the most common pathological fractures in the adult occur through areas of metastatic malignancy in bone. Although metastasis to long bones is less common than metastasis to the pelvis, skull, and vertebral column, the orthopaedist is usually called when a pathological fracture has occurred in a long bone, because of the pain and problems with nursing care.[11] Over the past 2 decades, articles have appeared[5,9,13,19,20,21] pleading for aggressive treatment of patients suffering this tragedy. Orthopaedists now recognize that most of these patients can be offered relief of pain and great improvement of function by internal fixation of pathological fractures through a metastasis. This approach has two advantages. First, a biopsy can be obtained and secondly, internal fixation allows the patient better function and less pain and facilitates nursing care.

The vast majority of metastases to long bones occur proximal to the elbow and the knee. One-sixth of all fractures through long bone metastases occur in the proximal one-fourth of the femur. Clain[6] reports that only five per cent of fractures through metastases in the hip region will heal (Fig. 5-13). Francis, Higinbotham, Carroll, Jacobs, and Graham[10] have never noted union of such fractures.

Poingenfurst, Marcove, and Miller[21] reported on the results obtained in 110 operations for treatment of fractures through metastases in the femoral neck and the intertrochanteric region. They concluded that replacement of the femoral head was a reliable procedure. A long-stem prosthesis is more stable and may help fix any involved areas of the proximal femur. Should the patient have significant involvement of the ipsilateral ilium, head and neck resection should be performed in favor of endoprosthetic replacement. These authors state that internal fixation of these fractures leads to complications and unfavorable results more often than any other method. In my personal experience, internal fixation of pathological fractures through metastatic disease in the neck of the femur has never been successful.

The report by Harrington *et al.*[12] seems to offer more help in the treatment of pathological fractures in the proximal femur. They advocate the use of methylmethacrylate as an adjunct to prosthetic replacement of the proximal femur. Frequently the metastatic disease has destroyed some cortical bone on the medial aspect of the neck and/or the lesser trochanter, offering poor support for a prosthesis. These authors resect all involved cortical bone and, by

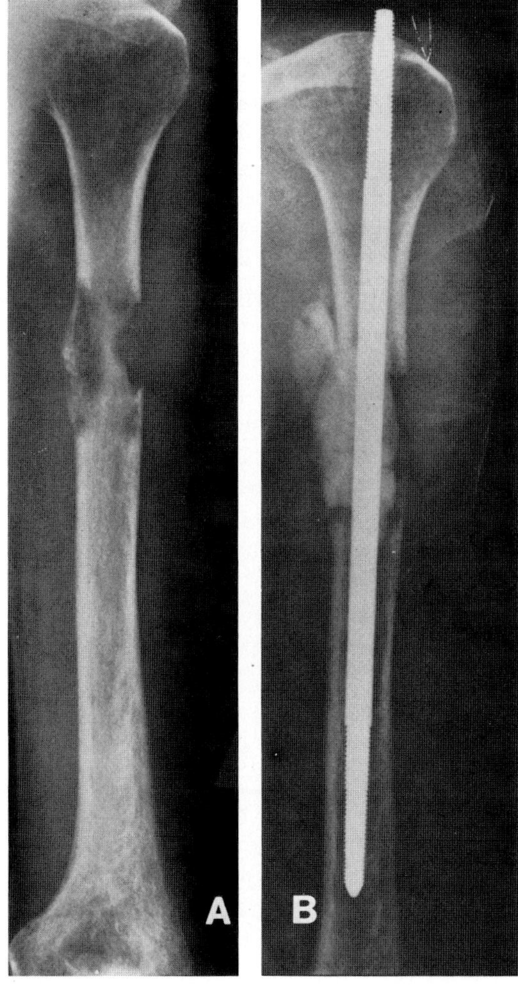

Fig. 5-14. (*A*) The left humerus of a 65-year-old man. The active destruction of the shaft of the humerus without any reaction suggests a malignant process, in all probability a metastatic lesion. This was another case of metastatic carcinoma of the lung. (*B*) The treatment was intramedullary rod fixation and methylmethacrylate cement to supplement the fixation and fill in the defect caused by the excisional biopsy.

properly molding cooled methylmethacrylate, fashion a substitute cortex to hold the prosthesis. It seems, therefore, that the endoprosthesis used in conjunction with methylmethacrylate allows more latitude in the treatment of fractures of the proximal femur. The more completely the metastatic disease is removed, the longer a functional result will last. For details of the method, the reader is referred to Harrington's article.[12]

Pathological fractures through metastases in the femoral shaft have been treated by intramedullary fixation since the introduction of the Küntscher rod. The results are usually quite gratifying. On rare occasions, however, the patient's disease progresses, destroying almost the entire shaft of the femur and causing loss of fixation. It is important to emphasize the advisability of prophylaxis by intramedullary fixation for metastatic lesions of the shaft of the femur. Should the surgeon be asked to biopsy a lesion in the shaft of the femur, concomitant direct intramedullary fixation is indicated. It may be necessary to convince the patient, the internist, and the radiotherapist that this is the wisest treatment. All too often, simple biopsy is looked upon as the conservative course. Most metastatic lesions that become clinically evident fracture spontaneously within days or, at most, a few weeks. Such a fracture requires another, somewhat more difficult operation; thus, the apparently conservative course becomes actually the more radical. Harrington *et al.*[12] also advocated the use of methylmethacrylate to replace segments of the femoral shaft destroyed by metastatic disease. Such treatment is an adjunct to intramedullary fixation.*

Pathological fractures through the humerus are managed as well as femur fractures with internal fixation for relief of pain and improvement of function. Although I have never treated a traumatic fracture of the humerus with an intramedullary rod, this method has been adequate for pathological fractures. More recently, the addition of methylmethacrylate has improved fixation of the fragments (Fig. 5-14).

When the intramedullary device became available, it was feared that its use in fractures due to metastatic disease would cause seeding of the neoplasm throughout the shaft of the long bone. Although this result seems logical, it rarely occurs. The possibility that the cancer might fungate from the operative wound was another concern, but this has not presented a problem. It is advised to close the wound in layers and avoid the use of drains. The author advises that before any biopsy or internal fixation is attempted in the presence of metastatic bone disease, several units of transfusible blood should be available. Most metastatic neoplasms do not bleed significantly at surgery, but occasionally bleeding can be catastrophic, particularly if the tumor is of renal origin.

Postoperative radiation therapy is frequently useful in controlling the patient's pain. Internal fixation devices do not interfere with radiotherapy. Such treatment may begin 3 to 5 days after surgery.

Rarely, a pathological fracture may be treated by amputation. I have done both forequarter and hindquarter amputation for such a problem. The patient who is confined to bed by a huge, weeping, edematous, painful extremity in which there is a pathological fracture can be relieved of pain and returned to some degree of mobility. Francis[9] also emphasizes that on rare occasions a solitary metastasis to bone from a renal carcinoma may present as a pathological fracture. If the renal lesion can be surgically removed, amputation of the involved extremity may effect a cure.

PATHOLOGICAL FRACTURE OF THE FEMORAL NECK AFTER IRRADIATION THERAPY

A very unusual pathological fracture is known to occur in the neck of the femur following irradiation therapy for carcinoma of the cervix. One of the largest series of patients with such fractures was reported by Leabhart and Bonfiglio.[14] They emphasized that the fracture had a high probability of union when treated by various modalities, but they advocated internal fixation. Leabhart and Bonfiglio reported on the pathological changes of the bone in postirradiation femoral neck fractures and felt the cause of these fractures to be a peculiar osteoporosis. The absence of total aseptic necrosis of the head of the femur would predispose a high union rate, if the fracture is properly immobilized.

REFERENCES

1. Albright, F.: Osteoporosis. Ann. Intern. Med., *27*:861-882, 1947.
2. Barry, H. C.: Paget's Disease of Bone. Edinburgh, E. & S. Livingstone, 1969.
3. ———: Fractures of the femur in Paget's disease of bone in Australia. J. Bone Joint Surg., *49A*:1359-1369, 1967.
4. Barzel, U. S.: Osteoporosis. New York, Grune & Stratton, 1970.

* Although at the time of this writing, an IND number was required for the use of methylmethacrylate in the treatment of pathological fractures other than in the region of the hip or knee, it is anticipated that the FDA will allow such use in the near future.

5. Bremner, R. A., and Jelliffe, A. M.: The management of pathological fracture of the major long bones from metastatic cancer. J. Bone Joint Surg., *40B*:652-659, 1958.
6. Clain, A.: Secondary malignant disease of bone. Brit. J. Cancer, *19*:15-30, 1965.
7. Elmore, S. M.: Pycnodysostosis: a review. J. Bone Joint Surg., *49A*:153-162, 1967.
8. Enneking, W. F.: Local resection of malignant lesions. J. Bone Joint Surg., *48A*:991-1007, 1966.
9. Francis, K. C.: The treatment of metastatic fractures with internal fixation. Am. J. Surg., *97*:484-487, 1959.
10. Francis, K. C., Higinbotham, N. L., Carroll, R. E., Jacobs, B., and Graham, W. D.: The treatment of pathological fractures of the femoral neck by resection. J. Trauma, *2*:465-473, 1962.
11. Griffiths, D. L.: Orthopedic aspects of myelomatosis. J. Bone Joint Surg., *48B*:703-728, 1966.
12. Harrington, K. D., Johnston, J. O., Turner, R. H., and Green, D. L.: The use of methylmethacrylate as an adjunct in the internal fixation of malignant neoplastic fractures. J. Bone Joint Surg., *54A*:1665-1676, 1972.
13. Higinbotham, N. L., and Marcove, R. C.: The management of pathological fractures. J. Trauma, *5*:792-798, 1965.
14. Leabhart, J. W., and Bonfiglio, M.: The treatment of irradiation fracture of the femoral neck. J. Bone Joint Surg., *43A*:1056-1067, 1961.
15. Martin, N. S., and Williamson, J.: The role of surgery in the treatment of malignant tumors of the spine. J. Bone Joint Surg., *52B*:227-237, 1970.
16. Milkman, L. A.: Multiple spontaneous idiopathic symmetrical fractures. Amer. J. Roentgenol., *32*:622-684, 1934.
17. Nicholas, J. A., Wilson, P. D., and Frieberger, R.: Pathological fractures of the spine: etiology and diagnosis. J. Bone Joint Surg., *42A*:127-137, 1960.
18. Parrish, F. F.: Treatment of bone tumors by total excision and replacement with massive autologous grafts. J. Bone Joint Surg., *48A*:968-990, 1966.
19. Parrish, F. F., and Murray, J. A.: Surgical treatment for secondary neoplastic fractures. J. Bone Joint Surg., *52A*:664-686, 1970.
20. Patterson, R. L., Jr., and Eichenholtz, W.: Management of patients with pathological fractures. J. Bone Joint Surg., *37A*:1119, 1955.
21. Poigenfurst, J., Marcove, R. C., and Miller, T. R.: Surgical treatment of fractures through metastases in the proximal femur. J. Bone Joint Surg., *50B*:743-756, 1968.
22. Rose, C. A.: A critique of modern methods of diagnosis and treatment of osteoporosis. Clin. Orthop. *35*:17-42, 1967.

6 Fractures and Dislocations in the Hand

David P. Green, M.D.
Spencer A. Rowland, M.D.

Although truly accurate figures of relative incidence are difficult to derive, it is likely that fractures of the metacarpals and phalanges are the most common fractures in the skeletal system. In 1962, Butt[34] reviewed 200,000 Workmen's Compensation injuries and noted that fractures of the hand accounted for 30 per cent of the cases settled and were the most frequently encountered fractures. Emmett and Breck,[46] in their comprehensive review of 11,000 consecutive fractures treated in a busy private practice, found that fractures of the phalanges and metacarpals accounted for 10 per cent of the total.

Perhaps because they are so common, and perhaps because they occur in small bones and are therefore considered minor injuries, these fractures are often relegated for treatment to the more inexperienced members of the medical team. Unfortunately, the results of treatment of fractures in the hand are not universally good, and indeed the incidence of stiffness, malunion, and prolonged functional disability and economic loss is rather striking. As Quigley and Urist[96] pointed out, nowhere else in the body are motion and function more closely related to anatomical structure than in the hand.

GENERAL PRINCIPLES OF MANAGEMENT

Initial Evaluation

The initial evaluation and primary care of an injured hand is critical, for at that time the surgeon has his best opportunity to assess accurately the extent of damage and to restore the altered anatomy. Many authors have observed that the fate of the hand largely depends upon the judgment of the doctor who first sees the patient.

Maximum functional recovery must be the goal in every hand injury, and this can be achieved only by considering the injury in relation to the patient's needs and life style. His age, hand dominance, and occupation are critical factors, and the opening sentence of the history of any patient with an injured hand should record this information: "A 45-year-old, right-handed electrician. . . ." Knowledge of the patient's avocations or hobbies is important as well, for a clerk or stockbroker may be an accomplished musician or an amateur carpenter.

Obtain precise details about the injury. *How* did it occur (i.e., what was the mechanism of injury)? Was it crushing, tearing, twisting, or a clean laceration? A human bite is a notoriously dangerous injury, and a short, curved laceration over a small joint in the hand must be immediately suspected of having been caused by a tooth. *Where* did the injury occur? Was it in a relatively clean environment, or was it in a stable or a greasy garage? Did it occur on the job or elsewhere; this has important financial implications to the patient and may have significant bearing on the outcome. How much time has elapsed since the injury? *What* has been done in the interim? Has any treatment been given and *by whom*?

Physical Examination

Some fractures and dislocations may be immediately obvious because of local swelling and deformity. Angulation and displacement are often readily apparent, but in fractures of the metacarpals and phalanges it is even more important to recognize rotational malalignment.

One of the greatest pitfalls in treating injuries of the hand is to focus on the obvious fracture and overlook more subtle, but often more significant, damage to soft tissues. One must always determine the precise area of tenderness, in order to accurately assess the damage to soft tissues as well as to bone. For example, if the patient has a swollen proximal interphalangeal joint, it is imperative to ascertain whether the maximum tenderness is over the collateral ligaments laterally, or dorsally, over the central slip insertion. Careful assessment must be made of an open wound with regard to its precise location, its relationship to skin creases, the direction and viability of skin flaps, the extent of actual skin loss, and the degree of contamination of the wound. An open wound should not be probed or handled excessively; gentle inspection with sterile instruments and gloves will give sufficient preliminary information until a thorough exploration can be done in the operating room. Damage to nerves and tendons can usually be determined by careful motor and sensory testing, rather than by probing the wound in the emergency room.

Both open and closed injuries must be examined meticulously for injury to adjacent tendons, nerves, and blood vessels. Precarious circulation may be particularly subtle in closed injuries and must be assessed by noting color and temperature, capillary filling, and patency of collateral circulation by Allen's test[1] at the wrist and in the digit itself.[80]

One always has reason to suspect the presence of foreign bodies in all open or penetrating wounds. Roentgenograms alone cannot be relied upon to uncover foreign bodies, because wood splinters, most types of glass, and many other foreign contaminants are not radiopaque.

Satisfactory physical examination may not be possible without local or regional anesthesia, but the block should be postponed until an initial assessment of nerves and blood vessels has been made in the unanesthetized hand.

Roentgenographic Examination

Roentgenograms are essential in virtually all injuries of the hand, even if no bone injury is obvious on clinical examination. Many significant fractures and joint injuries are missed simply because adequate roentgenograms were not taken on the day of injury. Three views are necessary: posteroanterior, lateral, and oblique. Oblique films are particularly helpful in accurately assessing intraarticular fractures. For injuries involving a finger, it is absolutely mandatory that a true lateral of the individual digit be obtained. Superimposition of the other fingers on a lateral view of the entire hand will obscure significant details that are easily seen on a lateral view of the single digit. Angulation in metacarpal fractures may be difficult to assess accurately on a true lateral film. We have found that added information can be obtained by including a lateral view in 10 degrees of supination (for the fourth and fifth metacarpals) or 10 degrees of pronation (for the second and third metacarpals).

Again, the temptation is great to concentrate on obvious abnormalities in the roentgenograph and overlook important but more obscure injuries. For example, one or more carpometacarpal joints may be subluxated or dislocated when there is a displaced or angulated fracture of an adjacent metacarpal.

Anesthesia for Hand Injuries

Hand injuries cannot be treated properly without adequate anesthesia. In some instances, it may be necessary to provide anesthesia in order to obtain a satisfactory examination, but in virtually all cases, manipulation or reduction requires muscle relaxation and relief of pain. General anesthesia is rarely necessary, unless the patient has concomitant injuries that require it. Axillary or brachial block provides excellent anesthesia, but this is more than is generally required. Intravenous lidocaine (Bier block) provides good muscle relaxation and relief of pain.

We prefer to do most of our fracture manipulations and reductions under regional or digital block. Perhaps the most useful of these is a median nerve block at the wrist combined with a radial wheal, which provides excellent anesthesia for the thumb, index, and long fingers. Ulnar nerve block can be performed at either the elbow or the wrist; if at the wrist, it is necessary to add a wheal to block the dorsal sensory branch. We prefer to block the ulnar nerve at the wrist. If anesthesia of an individual finger is desired, digital block is adequate. It should not be a ring block at the base of the finger because of the greater likelihood of vascular impairment. A metacarpal block at the level of the palmar crease or injection of the nerves in the web space is preferable. It is, of course, a well-established principle that epinephrine should never be used with any local anesthetic agent in the hand, for fear of vascular compromise. (Moore's[84] book on regional anesthesia is an excellent source of reference for reviewing the techniques mentioned above.)

Small wounds can be adequately anesthetized with local infiltration, but we prefer not to use it to manipulate closed fractures. When local anesthesia is employed, edema of the tissues can be minimized by adding one vial of hyaluronidase (Wydase) to each 30 ml. of anesthetic solution.

Proper Use of Facilities

Closed injuries in the hand are easily treated in the emergency room, plaster room, or office, provided the proper precautions are taken. If any type of intravenous or regional anesthesia is used, one must have immediately available resuscitation equipment such as an airway, Ambu bag, and intravenous drugs. Complications from the use of lidocaine and other local anesthetics are uncommon, but when they do occur, one must be prepared to deal with shock, seizures, and allergic reactions.

All open wounds except the most minor should be treated in an operating room or minor surgery suite. Open fractures and other injuries that require debridement or significant operative dissection should not be treated in the emergency room.

MASSIVE HAND TRAUMA AND MULTIPLE FRACTURES

Most of the discussions in this chapter deal with the specific management of individual fractures and dislocations in the hand, and little attention is directed towards the severely crushed or otherwise massively injured hand. In dealing with these difficult problems, one can apply the basic guidelines outlined throughout this section, but additional principles are pertinent to this type of injury as well.

The ultimate aims must be to return the patient to his usual activities as soon as possible and to restore the structure and function of the hand to as near normal as possible. To achieve these goals in the severely injured hand, the surgeon must often manage concomitant injuries that seem to demand diametrically opposed methods of treatment. For example, multiple displaced fractures may create marked instability of the entire hand skeleton, and yet prolonged immobilization can be disastrous. Soft-tissue damage accompanying fractures in the hand inevitably calls forth a tremendous accumulation of edema fluid. Tendons, ligaments, and intrinsic muscles become bathed in this protein-rich fluid, which gradually becomes transformed into tough, unyielding, fibrous tissue. A bulky compressive dressing properly applied minimizes the initial edema, and early movement helps pump the fluid out of the hand before it can become organized. Prolonged immobilization enhances its conversion into an inelastic encasement of scar.

The experience with massive hand wounds in Vietnam[29] demonstrated rather conclusively that all hand wounds do *not* require primary closure, and in fact, some wounds in the hand *should not* be closed at the time of initial debridement. High velocity missile wounds, severe crush injuries, human bites, and open wounds that have gone untreated for longer than 8 to 12 hours are all contraindications to primary wound closure in the hand. The risk of infection is minimized by careful and adequate debridement, copious irrigation, bulky sterile dressings, and a second look in the operating room 3 to 5 days later. At the time of the second operation, delayed primary closure or skin grafting can be done if the wound is surgically clean, or even further debridement with a third look several days hence may be necessary.

Early skeletal alignment is critical in the crushed or otherwise massively injured hand. Peacock[92] has shown how the strategic placement of a few small Kirschner wires at the time of the initial or subsequent operation can often provide enough stability to allow early motion and thereby minimize the stiffness that inevitably results from this type of injury. Finding the ideal compromise between stabilization and mobilization in the massively injured hand will often tax the ingenuity of even the most experienced hand surgeon.

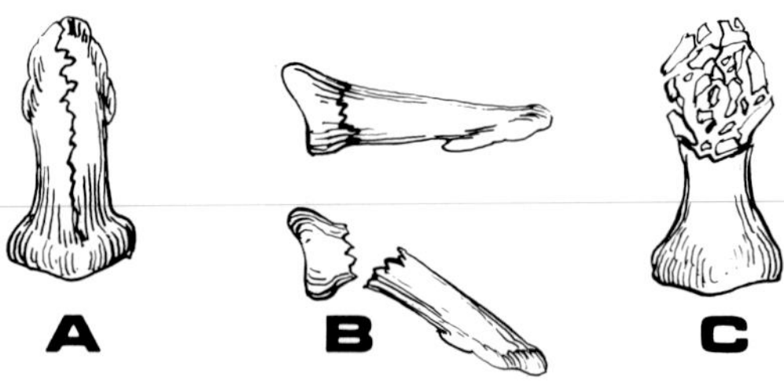

Fig. 6-1. The three general types of fractures of the distal phalanx. (*A*) Longitudinal fractures rarely show displacement. (*B*) A transverse fracture may show a marked degree of angulation and may require internal or external splinting. (*C*) The so-called crushed-egg-shell type of comminuted fracture.

FRACTURES OF THE DISTAL PHALANX

It is not surprising that fractures of the distal phalanx account for more than half of all hand fractures, as the distal portion of the hand is the most exposed to injury.[76,77,78] In Butt's[33] series of fractures, the distal phalanx of the long finger was injured more than twice as often as the distal phalanx of the thumb, which was next in frequency.

Anatomy

The extensor and flexor tendons that insert on the base of the distal phalanx play no role in displacing fractures of the distal phalanx, except for avulsion injuries (which are discussed in the following section). Fibrous septa, which radiate from bone to insert into the skin, form a dense meshwork and probably stabilize the fracture and prevent displacement.[97] Acute swelling and hematoma formation in these closed fibrous compartments undoubtedly account for the severe pain that often accompanies crushing injuries of the distal phalanx.

Etiology and Classification

The majority of distal phalangeal fractures are produced by crushing injuries, and, therefore, extensive soft-tissue damage and subungual hematomas are common. Kaplan[60] classified fractures of the distal phalanx into three general types: longitudinal, comminuted, and transverse (Fig. 6-1). Longitudinal fractures rarely show displacement; however, a transverse fracture close to the base of the phalanx may show a marked degree of angulation. The comminuted fracture usually involves the distal tuft of the phalanx and has been called the "crushed eggshell type."[97] In addition to being the most frequent type, the crushed, comminuted fracture is also most commonly associated with soft-tissue damage.

Treatment

Treatment of nondisplaced fractures should be directed toward the soft-tissue damage. Dorsal or volar splints, which are frequently used for immobilization, may cause severe pain if they are applied too tightly. A hairpin splint used initially allows swelling to occur without compressing tissues (Fig. 6-2).

Evacuation of the subungual hematoma will give marked relief of pain and is best done by burning a hole in the nail with a hot paper clip. Pressure caused by drilling a hole is unnecessarily painful. Theoretically, by evacuating the hematoma, the physician converts a closed fracture into an open one, although no infection has been reported following this common practice.

Transverse angulated fractures must be reduced and held with either an external splint or a smooth Kirschner wire. No attempt is made to reduce the displaced fragments of the tuft fractures, which resemble a "crushed eggshell." The fragments usually are not problematic, but the finger itself can remain painful for many months.

The majority of the fractures of the distal phalanx rarely require more than 3 to 4 weeks of protective splinting[35] even though, on the average, complete bone healing is not roentgenographically demonstrable for 5 months.[97]

One should keep in mind that the main reason for splinting fractures of the distal phalanx is to relieve pain. Except in the displaced, transverse variety, these fractures do not require immobilization to hold a reduction. Rather, the splint is provided to protect the tender fingertip from further external trauma.

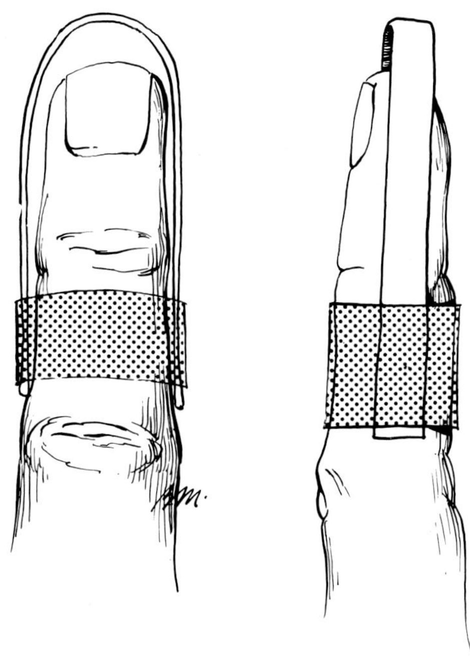

Fig. 6-2. A hairpin splint protects the fractured distal phalanx from further injury but allows swelling to occur without tissue compression.

MALLET FINGER OF TENDON ORIGIN

The term mallet finger, by common usage, has come to mean a particular deformity resulting from loss of extensor tendon continuity to the distal finger joint.[149] This tendinous injury must not be confused with an intraarticular fracture involving one third or more of the dorsal lip of the distal phalanx, which also causes a typical mallet deformity. (This troublesome fracture will be discussed under a separate heading, for it is a distinctly different entity.)

Mechanism of Injury and Classification

The deformity that results from the end of the finger being forcibly flexed has become known as the "mallet" or "baseball finger." It has been described, perhaps more accurately, by Bunnell[28] as "drop finger." The injury usually occurs when the extensor tendon is taut, as in catching a ball or striking an object with the extended finger. The deformity may result from relatively minor trauma or even after crush injuries of the distal joint.[149] With sudden forceful flexion, any of several pathological conditions may occur that result in mallet deformity.[138]

A. The extensor tendon fibers over the distal joint may be stretched without completely dividing the tendon. The degree of drop of the distal phalanx is usually not pronounced—a loss of perhaps 5 to 20 degrees of extension (Fig. 6-3A)—and the patient retains some weak active extension.

B. The extensor tendon may be ruptured or torn from its insertion into the proximal phalanx. In addition, the dorsal capsule, which is intimately associated with the tendon, may also be ruptured (Fig. 6-3B).[25,132] In this instance, there is a 40- to 45 degree loss of extension, and the patient has complete loss of active extension at the distal joint.

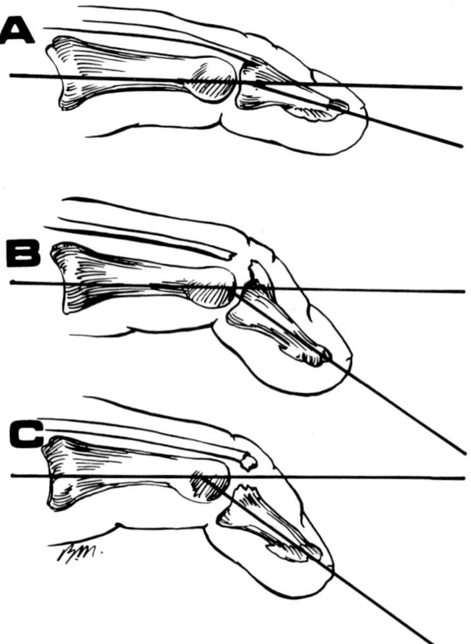

Fig. 6-3. The three types of injury that cause a mallet finger of tendon origin. (*A*) The extensor tendon fibers over the distal joint are stretched without complete division of the tendon. Although there is some drop of the distal phalanx, the patient retains weak active extension. (*B*) The extensor tendon is ruptured from its insertion on the distal phalanx. There is usually a 40- to 45-degree flexion deformity, and the patient has loss of active extension at the distal joint. (*C*) A small fragment of the distal phalanx is avulsed with the extensor tendon. This injury has the same clinical findings as that shown in B.

C. A small fragment of the distal phalanx may be avulsed with the extensor tendon. In this instance, the injury has the same characteristics as the tendon injuries mentioned above, and the degree of drop will depend not upon the small fragment, but rather upon the amount of loss of continuity of the tendon mechanism. These injuries should be treated as tendon injuries rather than fractures (Figs. 6-3C; 6-4). In Stark, Boyes, and Wilson's series,[149] 24 per cent of the injuries were associated with small bony avulsion fractures, but this finding had no effect on the final result.

In all of these different types of injuries, if the flexion deformity of the distal joint is severe, a secondary hyperextension deformity of the proximal interphalangeal joint may occur because of imbalance of the extensor mechanism (Fig. 6-5).

Methods of Treatment

Most of the methods used in the treatment of mallet deformity of tendon origin have aimed at hyperextending the distal joint and flexing the proximal interphalangeal joint. The rationale for this position is based on the fact that flexion of the proximal joint advances the central slip, causing an advancement of the lateral bands for a distance that, according to Bunnell,[28] amounts to 3 mm. Hence, any apparatus that holds the proximal joint in approximately 60 degrees of flexion and the distal finger joint in hyperextension allows for apposition of the torn extensor tendon at the distal joint or shortening of an attenuated extensor tendon (Fig. 6-6). Smillie (1937),[145] Bunnell (1944),[28] and Williams (1947)[152] accomplished this with plaster immobilization. Because many experienced difficulties in applying and maintaining the plaster,[115,139,144,152] various types of splints have been advocated.[121,127,128,130,134,147,151,152]

In 1952, Pratt[139] introduced a method he called an "internal splint." A medium caliber (0.045-inch) smooth Kirschner wire was introduced across the distal and middle finger joints, holding the distal joint in hyperextension and the proximal joint in 60 degrees flexion. The wire was cut off underneath the skin. Casscells and Strange[124,125] modified this technique because some of their patients developed painful and permanent limitation of motion of the proximal interphalangeal joint. They suggested that only the distal joint be fixed with a Kirschner wire and that the middle joint be maintained in 60 degrees of flexion by means of skin plaster.

Poor results after conservative treatment led some surgeons to carry out immediate operative repair of the torn tendon. As early as 1930, Mason[136] had recommended early operative repair of the ruptured extensor expansion. Operative treatment is aimed at freshening and approximating the edges of the tear; it is followed by immobilization of the distal and middle joints.[23] An avulsed bone fragment can be reattached with a pull-out wire, but, if small, it may be excised and the tendon reinserted by a pull-

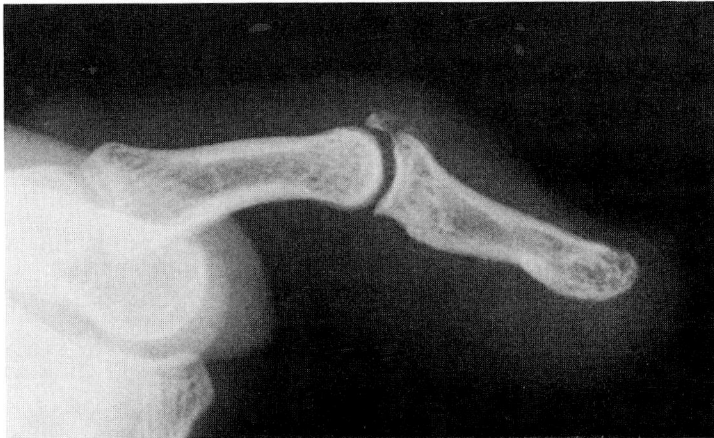

Fig. 6-4. Mallet finger deformities with small fragments such as this should be treated as tendon injuries rather than as fractures.

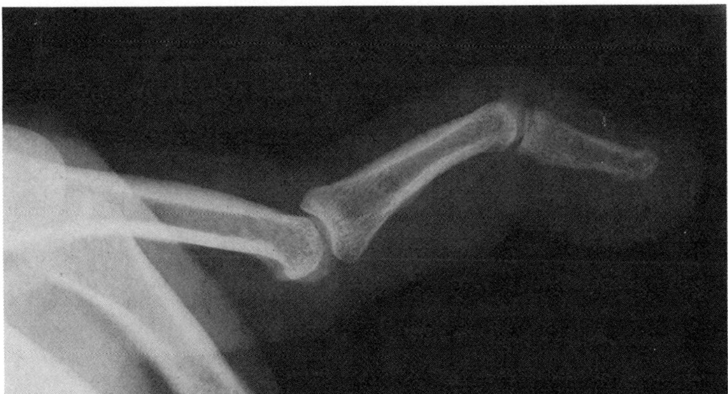

Fig. 6-5. With severe flexion deformity of the distal joint in mallet finger injury, a secondary hyperextension deformity of the proximal interphalangeal joint may occur because of imbalance of the extensor mechanism.

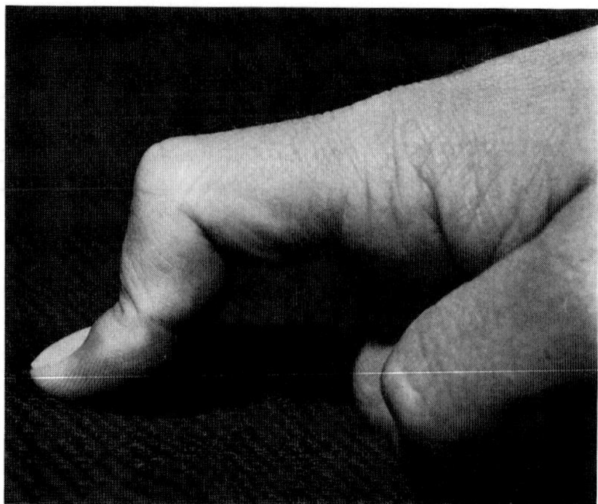

Fig. 6-6. The position of immobilization generally advocated for treatment of a mallet finger. The amount of hyperextension in this photograph is excessive. Skin slough over the dorsum of the distal joint is a possible complication if the joint is immobilized in extreme hyperextension. Although many types of splints have been devised to hold the proximal joint in flexion and the distal joint in extension, the authors believe that most mallet finger deformities in reliable patients can be treated by splinting only the distal joint (*see text*).

out wire through tiny drill holes.[23] The results of operative repair of the tendinous lesions are not always satisfactory. While they give good cosmetic results, flexion is often lost, owing to scarring on the dorsal aspect of the joint. The assessment of the late results in Robb's series[142] suggested that early operative repair was unnecessary, as was found to be true in other studies.[149]

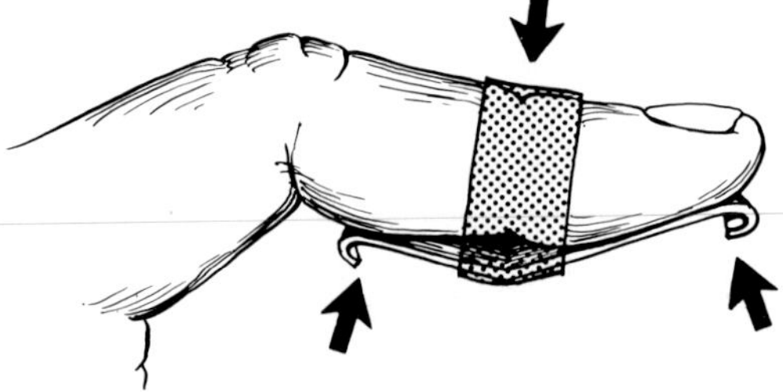

Fig. 6-7. Our usual method of immobilizing a mallet finger is with a simple volar unpadded aluminum splint which has been fashioned to allow three-point fixation of the distal joint only. Some prefer to apply the splint on the dorsum of the joint to allow better use of the finger during the period of immobilization.

The imperfect and often harmful results that followed both open and closed treatment led some to believe that the mallet deformity was being overtreated. Stiff proximal interphalangeal joints, Kirschner wire tract infections, and skin slough were severe penalties to pay for treatment of an injury that rarely caused any functional disability. Some authors[142,144] have stated that, in time, practically all of the mallet deformities of tendinous origin improve gradually to a satisfactory state of recovery without treatment. These authors believed that without treatment the extensor tendon healed in a lengthened state and that gradual contraction of the fibrous scar tissue took place over the ensuing 6 months, resulting in a satisfactory state of recovery. For this reason, Robb[142] felt that the only treatment necessary for most patients with mallet finger was the application of an elastic adhesive strapping or a straight spatula splint in order to relieve the initial discomfort from the injury. Others[20,121,123,135,148] have also advocated splinting only the distal joint.

Stark, Boyes, and Wilson[149] analyzed their results of 163 mallet fingers and concluded that all patients with mallet finger could not be treated in the same way. Treatment should depend on the elapsed time following injury, the previous treatment, the degree of loss of extension, the degree of functional disability, and the age of the patient. In their series, only four patients were treated by open surgery, and none by Kirschner were fixation.

Authors' Preferred Method of Treatment

Acute Mallet Finger. The authors' preferred treatment for acute mallet finger is based, in general, on the principles outlined by Stark, Boyes, and Wilson,[149] but the proximal interphalangeal joint is no longer immobilized routinely. Our results have been as satisfactory, and this method avoids the risk of proximal interphalangeal joint

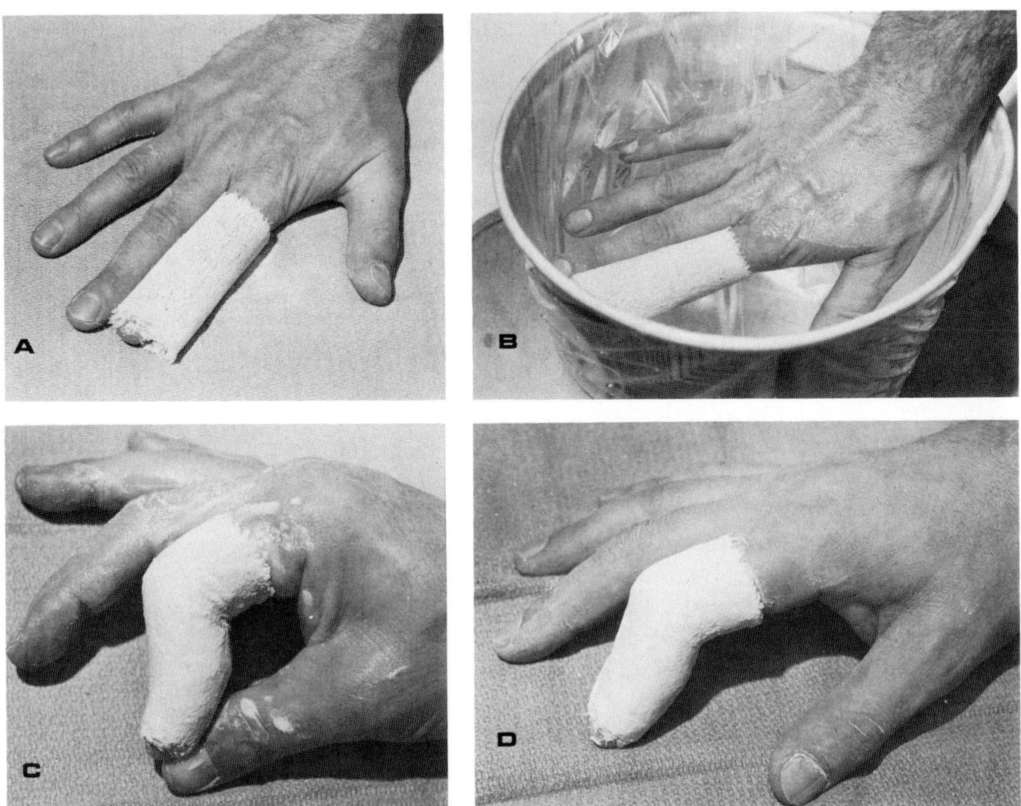

Fig. 6-8. Smillie[145] described a simple method of applying a mallet finger cast. (*A*) An 18-inch strip of 3- or 4-inch dry plaster is rolled into a tube and slipped over the end of the injured finger. No padding is used. (*B*) The patient dips his hand into a bucket of water, holding the tube of plaster in place over the finger. (*C*) The patient himself holds the finger in the correct position of immobilization while the physician smooths out the plaster. (*D*) The completed cast. Removal is facilitated by soaking the plaster.

stiffness. We have never opted for operative repair of the extensor tendon, and only rarely for percutaneous Kirschner wire fixation. Our usual method is to immobilize only the distal joint with a simple volar unpadded aluminum splint, which has been fashioned to allow three-point pressure (Fig. 6-7). There are two volar points of pressure—one distal and one proximal to the distal interphalangeal joint. The counterpoint of pressure is applied with adhesive tape over the dorsum of the joint. We attempt to put the distal joint in gentle hyperextension, but the degree depends on the mobility of the patient's joints and on the degree of discomfort. The splint should never cause pain. The patient is shown how to take it off and reapply it daily for the purpose of skin care. At no time is the patient to allow the distal phalanx to drop during this important procedure in the daily care of the skin. This method of treatment is successful only for patients who are reliable and reasonably intelligent, because it requires conscientiousness and cooperation. If there is doubt about the patient's reliability or ability to follow instructions, a more permanent form of immobilization must be used. For such patients, one of us (D. P. G.) prefers a plaster cast that immobilizes the proximal interphalangeal joint in flexion and the distal joint in neutral or mild hyperextension. The simplest method of applying such a cast is that described by

Smillie[145] in 1937 (Fig. 6-8). We prefer this over any of the commercially available mallet finger splints which are also easy for the unreliable patient to remove.

The period of immobilization varies according to the degree of extensor tendon tear. If only the distal joint is immobilized, the splint is worn 6 weeks for partial tears and 8 weeks for complete tears. An additional 4 weeks of immobilization at night only is also recommended.

If the proximal interphalangeal joint is immobilized, the cast should be worn for 5 to 6 weeks; after which the distal joint only should be splinted at night for 2 to 3 weeks more.

We want to emphasize that we prefer to treat acute mallet finger by immobilizing only the distal joint, but satisfactory results can be achieved with the Smillie cast.

Rarely, one sees a patient, such as a dentist or a surgeon, for whom external splinting for a prolonged period of time would be an economic hardship. In these patients, immobilizing only the distal joint in full extension with a 0.045-inch Kirschner wire is an acceptable method of treatment. The pin is cut off beneath the skin, and the patient can return to his usual activities almost immediately. Following removal of the wire at 6 weeks, an additional 4 weeks of night splinting is recommended.

Late Mallet Finger. A drop finger seen within 3 to 4 weeks should be treated as an acute injury, although the longer the delay, the less successful the result. Mallet deformities that were not seen until 2 to 3 months after injury have improved with 8 weeks' splinting of the distal joint.

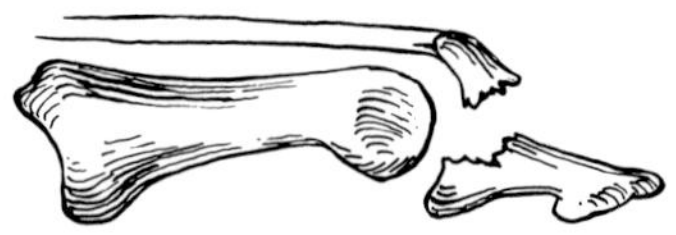

Fig. 6-9. The mallet finger originating from bone injury. The fracture fragment, which involves one-third or more of the dorsal articulation surface, is often tilted and malrotated, with the remainder of the distal phalanx subluxated volar to the condyles of the middle phalanx.

Harris[129] applied Fowler's concept of treating old mallet deformities that would not respond to the usual methods of treatment. In Fowler's technique, the central slip of the extensor tendon is cut as it inserts into the base of the middle phalanx, allowing the extensor apparatus along its entire length to glide proximalward further than normal, exerting increased tension on the extensor tendon at the distal joint. There are no reports on the long-term results of this technique.

It has been the authors' experience that the possible complications of this operation outweigh its advantages. Unless it is performed with extreme care by a skilled surgeon, the procedure can leave the proximal interphalangeal joint painful and stiff, or it may even cause a boutonniere deformity. We believe that no form of treatment for the relatively minor drop finger deformity should jeopardize the function of the extremely important proximal interphalangeal joint.

MALLET FINGER OF BONY ORIGIN

A fracture involving the dorsal articular surface of the distal phalanx produces a mallet deformity, because the extensor tendon, which is attached to the fractured fragment, loses its ability to extend the distal joint. Ordinarily, the fragment includes one third or more of the dorsal articular surface. The fragment is often tilted and malrotated, and the base of the distal phalanx may subluxate volar to the condyles of the middle phalanx (Fig. 6-9). Closed reduction is seldom successful, and open reduction to restore joint continuity is usually indicated (Fig. 6-10). A large dorsal fragment with its attached extensor tendon can be held with one or more Kirschner wires; a smaller fragment, with a pull-out wire. Open reduction is more difficult than one might anticipate because of the difficulty of handling a small frag-

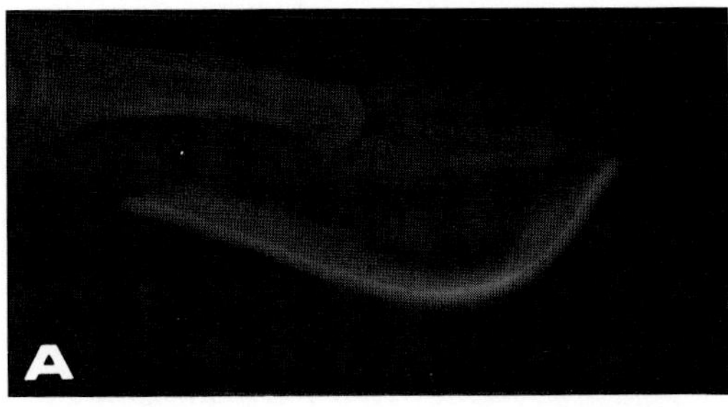

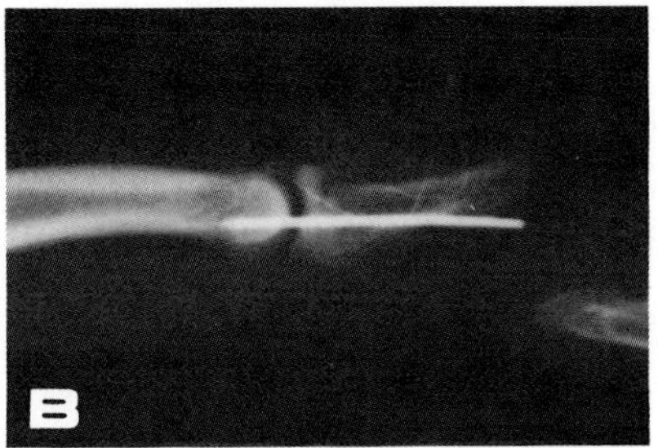

Fig. 6-10. A typical mallet finger of bone origin. (*A*) Note the displacement and rotation of the avulsed fragment and the volar subluxation of the distal phalanx. (*B*) The fragment has been reduced anatomically and a small Kirschner wire has been passed across the distal interphalangeal joint to protect the repair until it is completely healed. This is one of the few areas in the hand where we believe it is important to wait for roentgenographic evidence of bony union before removing the Kirschner wire, even though this may take 8 to 10 weeks. Earlier removal of the pin may result in loss of reduction and subluxation of the joint.

ment, the tendency for it to break up into smaller pieces when the Kirschner wires are introduced, and the difficulty of visualizing the articular surface. Cutting the ulnar collateral ligament, as suggested by Stark,[111] may help achieve anatomical reduction. Kirschner wire fixation, if possible, is probably better than a pull-out wire, because it may take considerably longer for the fragment to unite than the time that a pull-out wire may be safely left in place. Following reduction, immobilization of the proximal interphalangeal joint in 60 degrees of flexion minimizes the pull of the extensor tendon on the distal fragment. Motion of the proximal interphalangeal joint should be started at 3 weeks to prevent stiffness; the distal joint should be immobilized until roentgenographic evidence of bony union can be seen, even though this may take 8 to 10 weeks.

FLEXOR DIGITORUM PROFUNDUS AVULSION

Avulsion of the flexor digitorum profundus tendon from its insertion into the base of the distal phalanx is an uncommon injury and frequently missed. The literature[17,26,31,50,94] is scant regarding this injury, but the recent article by Carroll and Match[37] is an excellent summary of the problem.

Mechanism of Injury and Pathology

Flexor digitorum profundus avulsion is caused by forceful hyperextension of the distal interphalangeal joint while the flexor digitorum profundus is in maximum contraction. It is most commonly seen in athletics such as when a football player reaches out to tackle the ball carrier and grabs only a handful of jersey. The ring finger has been involved most frequently in those cases previously reported in the literature.

The tendon may rupture directly from its insertion on the bone, or it may avulse a fragment of variable size from the base of the distal phalanx. The degree of soft-tissue injury and hemorrhage is far greater than in a simple laceration of the profundus tendon, so there is extensive scarring within the flexor tendon sheath. As the avulsed end retracts proximally, it may become entrapped at the chiasma of the flexor digitorum sublimis in the region of the proximal interphalangeal joint, and subsequently a flexion contracture may develop at that level. Occasionally, the tendon retracts to the base of the finger or to the level of the lumbrical origin in the palm.

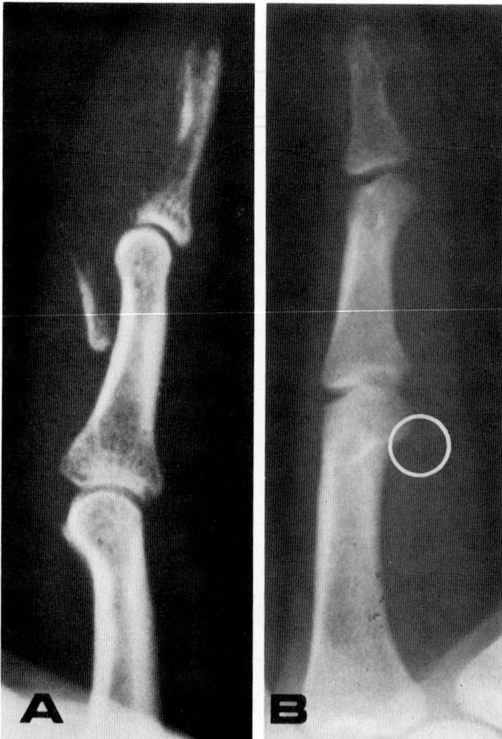

Fig. 6-11. Rupture of the flexor digitorum profundus from its insertion into the distal phalanx may be accompanied by an avulsion fragment from the distal phalanx. (*A*) An unusually large avulsion fragment. (*B*) A very tiny avulsion fragment is seen at the level of condyles of the proximal phalanx. Good quality roentgenograms in true lateral and oblique views are necessary to identify the fragment. In some cases, the injury is a pure rupture of the tendon from its insertion, and no fragment is seen. (*A* from Green, D. P.: Amer. Family Physician, 7:114, 1973)

Diagnosis

If the injury goes unnoticed by the patient, it may not come to a physician's attention for several days or several weeks. Even when the patient is seen immediately, the problem may not be obvious, as there is not a characteristic deformity. The diagnosis is readily made by demonstrating inability to actively flex the distal interphalangeal joint. Pain and local tenderness are usually more marked over the proximal interphalangeal joint, where the retracted end of the tendon has come to rest, than over the point of avulsion at the distal phalanx. If the tendon has retracted into the palm, there will be local tenderness there.

Lateral and oblique roentgenograms of the individual finger are mandatory to confirm the diagnosis if a fragment of bone has been torn loose from the distal phalanx by the tendon. The avulsed bone can range in size from a very large fragment to a tiny speck barely visible on the roentgenogram (Fig. 6-11). In some patients, the tendon ruptures directly from the bone, and no fragment is seen on the roentgenograms.

Treatment

Early operative repair to reinsert the avulsed tendon is mandatory to restore active flexion of the distal joint. The success of repair is directly related to the length of delay following injury, and the most satisfactory results are obtained with immediate open reduction. Carroll and Match[37] have noted that a successful result can be achieved up to 4 weeks after injury, but after that time, it is usually impossible to bring the contracted tendon back out to its insertion. Even if it can be accomplished that late, the finger may develop a severe flexion deformity because of muscle contracture and scarring in the sheath.

The patient with a late, untreated profundus avulsion presents a dilemma for the surgeon. Usually the deformity is painless, but the patient cannot flex the distal joint. In deciding upon the proper treatment, it is important to ascertain whether or not it is a handicap to that particular patient. The treatment chosen must not jeopardize the normal range of motion in the proximal interphalangeal joint. The choice—arthrodesis of the distal joint, free tendon grafting, or doing nothing—is one that demands mature clinical judgment and a recognition of the consequences of each.

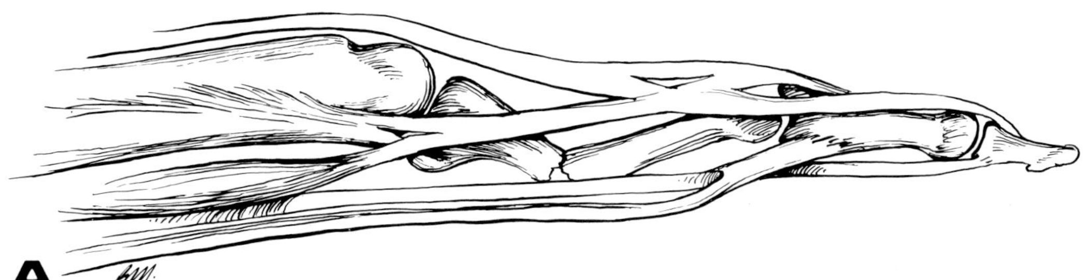

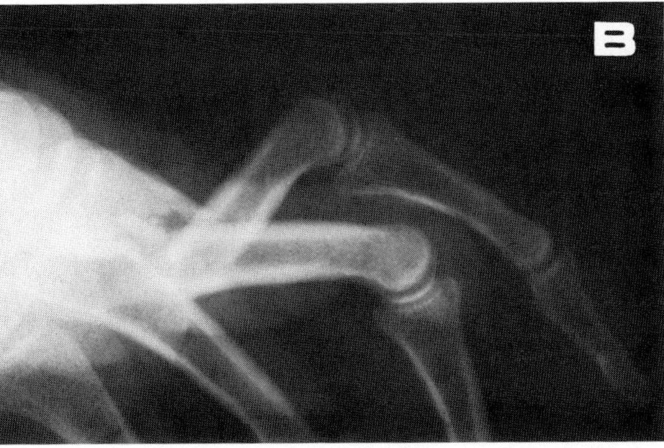

Fig. 6-12. Unstable fractures of the proximal phalanx typically present with volar angulation. (*A*) The proximal fragment is flexed by the bony insertion of the interossei into the base of the proximal phalanx. Once the stability of the proximal phalanx is lost, there is an accordionlike collapse at the fracture site, aggravated by further pull on the extensor hood by the extrinsic muscles. (*B*) A roentgenogram showing the typical, though somewhat exaggerated, volar angulation. More commonly, the angulation is 20 to 30 degrees.

FRACTURES OF THE PROXIMAL AND MIDDLE PHALANGES

There is an enormous divergence of opinion regarding the treatment of phalangeal fractures. An understanding of the rationale and principles underlying many different methods of treatment is important, not merely for their historical interest, but because not all fractures in the fingers can or should be treated in the same manner. Harrison McLaughlin,[74] many of whose tenets are reflected in these pages, used to say that one should not make a fracture fit a favorite treatment. Rather, the method of management should be tailored to the peculiarities of the given fracture and to the needs of the individual patient.

In the following section, we describe some of the many methods of treatment that have been advocated, and we attempt to put each in its proper perspective.

Anatomy

As in other long bone fractures, displacement and angulation in fractures of the phalanges are influenced by two factors: the mechanism of injury and the muscles acting as deforming forces on the fractured bone. The type of injury often determines the nature of the fracture; e.g., a direct blow is more likely to cause a transverse or comminuted fracture, while a twisting injury will more often result in an oblique or spiral fracture. The direction of angulation seen in fractures of the phalanges primarily depends on the muscles acting upon that bone.

Unstable fractures of the proximal phalanx typically present with volar angulation (Fig. 6-12). The proximal fragment is flexed by the bony insertions of the interossei into the base of the proximal phalanx. Although there are no tendons inserting on the distal fragment, it tends to be pulled into hyperextension by the central slip acting upon the base of the middle phalanx. Once the stability of the proximal phalanx is lost, there is an accordionlike collapse at the fracture site, aggravated by further pull on the extensor hood by the intrinsic muscles.

The middle phalanx is much less commonly fractured than the proximal phalanx, and muscle forces acting upon them are different. The important deforming forces to be considered are the insertion of the central slip into the dorsum of the base of the middle phalanx and the insertion of the flexor digitorum sublimis volarly. The central slip has a well defined area of insertion, and its action is to extend the middle phalanx. Although the action of the flexor sublimis is to flex the middle phalanx, its insertion is rather complex and is not confined

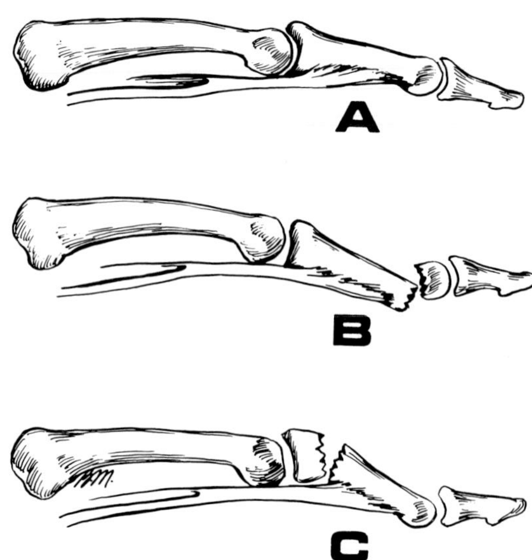

Fig. 6-14. (*A*) A lateral view showing the prolonged insertion of the sublimis tendon into the middle phalanx. (*B*) A fracture through the neck of the middle phalanx is likely to have a volar angulation, as the proximal fragment is flexed by the strong pull of the sublimis. (C) A fracture through the base of the middle phalanx is more likely to have a dorsal angulation due to the extension force of the central slip upon the proximal fragment and a flexion force on the distal fragment by the sublimis.

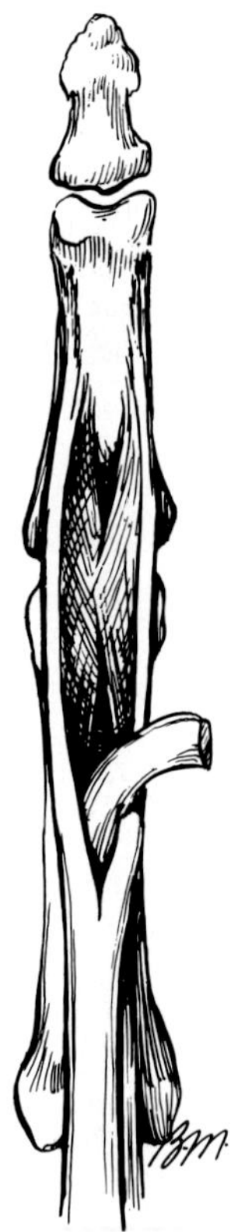

Fig. 6-13. The flexor digitorum sublimis has a complicated and extensive insertion into the middle phalanx. Each half of the tendon rotates a full 180 degrees to insert into nearly the entire volar surface of the middle phalanx. Note that fibers from each insertion also cross to the opposite side, forming a broad expanse of tendon beneath the profundus tendon. (Redrawn from Kaplan, E. B.: Functional and Surgical Anatomy of the Hand. ed. 2. Philadelphia, J. B. Lippincott, 1965)

to a short segment of the phalanx. Kaplan[10] has described in detail the decussation of the sublimis tendon to allow the profundus tendon to pass through its two slips, and the reader is referred to Kaplan's textbook for this detailed description. In essence, however, the sublimis divides into two halves, each half turning 90 degrees to allow the profundus to pass through and then completing another 90 degrees of rotation to insert into nearly the entire volar surface of the middle phalanx (Fig. 6-13). If one carefully examines a disarticulated middle phalanx, he will see that there is a narrow ridge along each side of the middle two thirds of the volar aspect of the bone, into which the sublimis inserts. In many textbooks one finds drawings that depict the sublimis insertion as a precise, fixed point on the volar aspect of the bone. A more accurate representation is illustrated in Figure 6-14A, which shows the very prolonged insertion of the sublimis, extending *from a point just distal to the flare of the base to a point only a few millimeters proximal to the neck.* A fracture through the neck of the middle phalanx is likely to have a volar angulation, as the proximal fragment tends to be flexed by the strong pull of the sublimis (Fig. 6-14B). A fracture through the base of the middle phalanx proximal to the insertion of the sublimis would be more likely to have a dorsal angulation due to the extending force of the central slip upon the proximal fragment and a flexing force on the distal fragment by the sublimis (Fig. 6-14C). Fractures through the middle two thirds of the bone, however, may be angulated in either direction or not at all, and the angulation cannot always be predicted with accuracy entirely on the basis of the tendon insertion.[91]

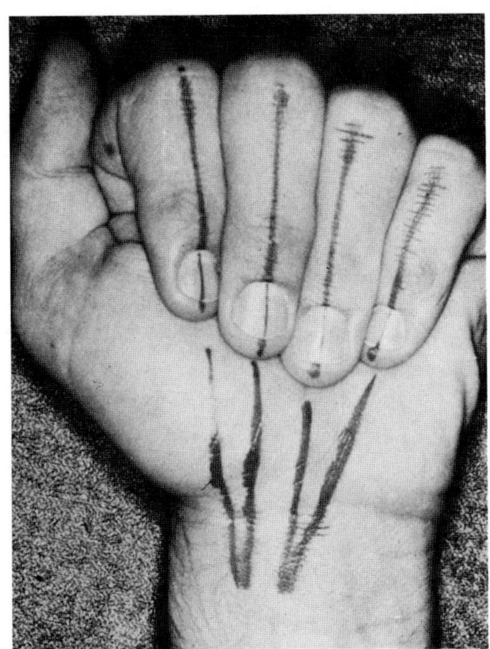

Fig. 6-15. Maintaining correct rotational alignment is one of the most difficult and subtle aspects of treating fractures of the phalanges. When the fingers are flexed, they do not remain parallel as they are in full extension. They point toward the region of the scaphoid, although they do not actually converge upon a single fixed point, as is sometimes depicted.

Malrotation at the fracture site is one of the most frequent complications of phalangeal fractures, and one that can be avoided only by careful attention to anatomical detail. When the fingers are flexed, they do not remain parallel, as they are in full extension. Rather, they point towards the region of the scaphoid tubercle, although they do not actually converge upon a single fixed point, as is sometimes depicted (Fig. 6-15). Thus it is relatively easy to detect malrotation when the fingers are in full flexion (Fig. 6-16). With the fingers only semiflexed, it is helpful to use the planes of the fingernails as an additional guide to correct rotation. The opposite hand must be checked for comparison, for often the border fingers lie in a slightly different plane of rotation as seen end-on (Fig. 6-17).

Methods of Treatment

Early Active Motion. The method that James[57] calls "garter strapping" others refer to as "buddy taping" or "dynamic splinting." The technique is simply to tape the injured finger to an adjacent normal digit and allow—in fact, encourage—the patient to move the finger and to use the hand as normally as possible while the fracture heals. The rationale is that early motion prevents stiffness in the small joints of the finger which almost invariably results from immobilization. In a large series of patients with finger fractures, Wright[120] discovered that those treated with early active motion had less stiffness and less economic disability than those treated by immobilization. We basically agree with the idea that stiffness can be minimized and the patient can return to his job sooner if the fracture is treated with dynamic splinting rather than immobilization. However, the method is *not* suitable for the treatment of *all* phalangeal fractures. Certain undisplaced fractures and impacted transverse fractures of

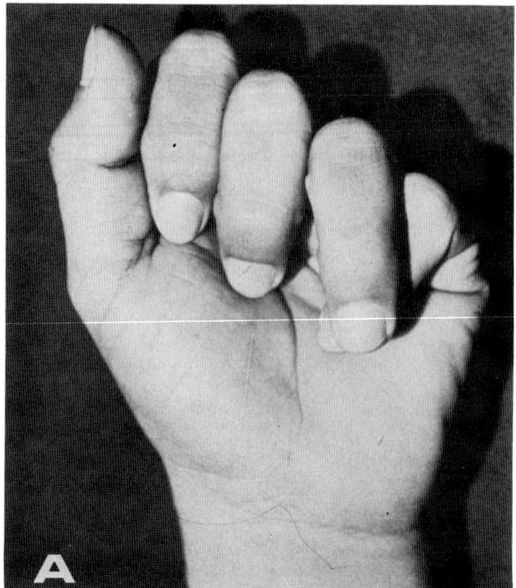

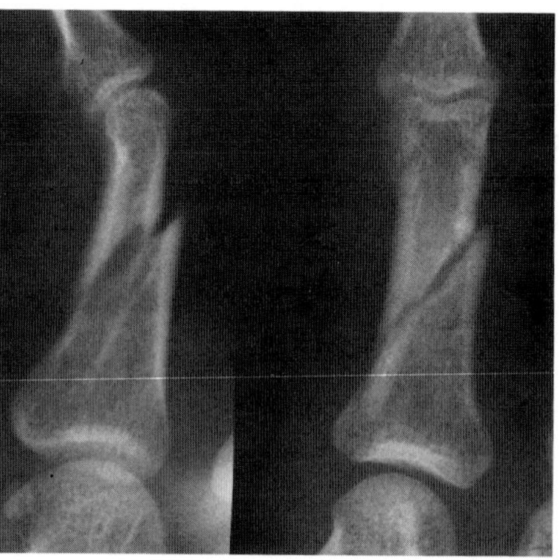

Fig. 6-16. (*A*) Gross malalignment of the ring finger seen in a patient in whom a fracture of the proximal phalanx was allowed to heal with rotational deformity. (*B*) Although subtle malalignment can be evaluated more critically by clinical means, rotational deformity may also be seen roentgenographically. The wide discrepancy in cross-sectional diameter of the proximal and distal fragments as seen on the lateral view clearly demonstrates a severe rotational deformity. On the anteroposterior view, the deformity is less obvious, although any discrepancy in diameter of the two fragments should alert the physician to the possibility of rotational deformity.

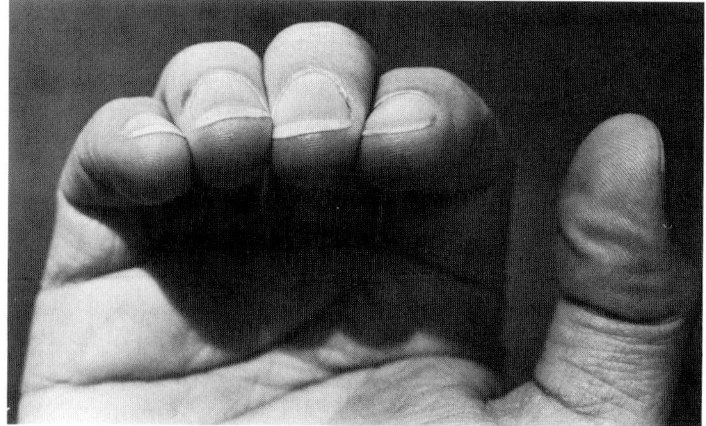

Fig. 6-17. With the fingers only semiflexed, it is helpful to use the planes of the fingernails as an additional guide to correct rotation. The opposite hand must be checked for comparison, for often the border fingers lie in a slightly different plane of rotation as seen end-on.

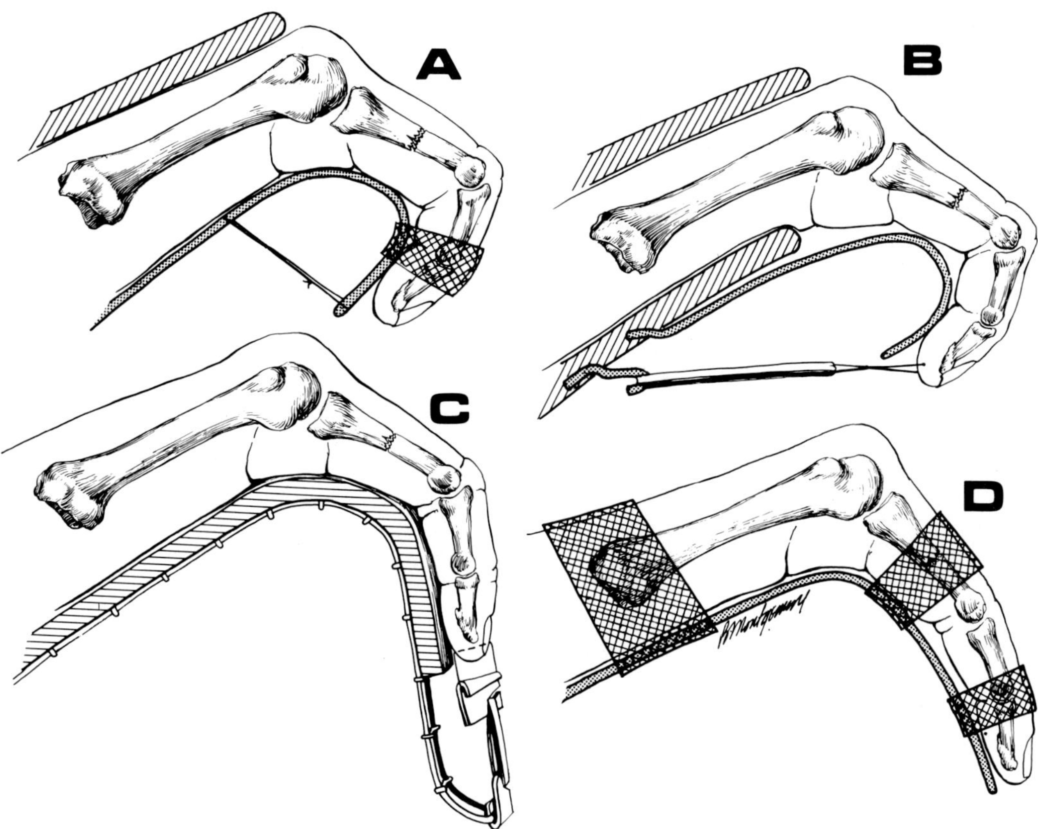

Fig. 6-18. Several types of splinting have been described for treating fractures of the phalanges. (*A*) Böhler described the use of a wire outrigger combined with a dorsal plaster slab which immobilized the wrist. The tip of the outrigger was wired to itself to hold the finger in rather acute flexion. (*B*) Bunnell, and later Boyes, used a modified Böhler splint together with pulp traction, applying just enough tension to maintain the position obtained by manipulation. (*C*) Moberg designed a padded wire ladder which is used widely in Sweden, but is not available in this country. This technique uses a specialized form of nail-pulp traction. (The illustration is slightly inaccurate, in that the wire should pass through the periosteum at the tip of the distal phalanx.) (*D*) James has advocated that fingers should not be immobilized in the position of function, but rather in a position that more nearly resembles the intrinsic plus position in which the metacarpophalangeal joints are immobilized in at least 70 degrees flexion, and the interphalangeal joints in minimal flexion (*see text*).

the phalanges are ideally managed with buddy taping, but *only* if two basic principles are observed. First, the fracture must truly be stable (i.e., undisplaced or impacted) with no angulation in any plane. Coonrad and Pohlman[41] have clearly illustrated the pitfall of misinterpreting an anteroposterior roentgenogram as showing an impacted fracture, when in fact the lateral view shows significant volar angulation. Such fractures must be immobilized in flexion and are not amenable to the dynamic splinting technique. Secondly, careful clinical and roentgenographic follow-up of the patient during the healing phase is imperative to immediately recognize displacement or angulation at the fracture site, should it occur.

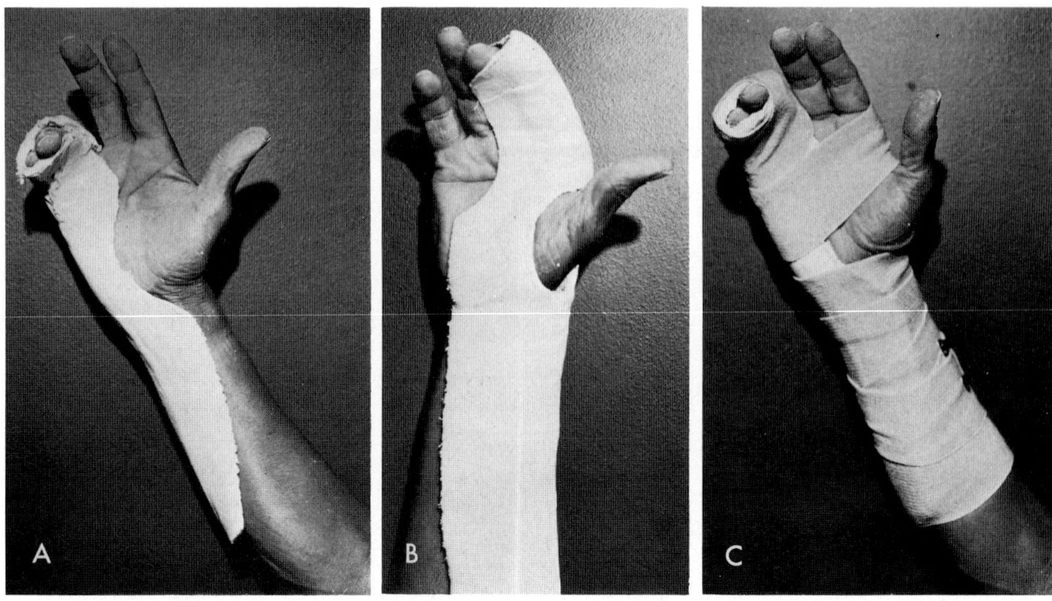

Fig. 6-19. We frequently use gutter plaster splints in the treatment of phalangeal and metacarpal fractures. (*A*) Fractures involving the ring- and small fingers can be adequately immobilized with an ulnar gutter splint, leaving the radial digits completely free. (*B*) A similar splint can be used on the radial side of the hand, cutting out a hole for the thumb. (*C*) The splint is held in place with an elastic bandage, wrapped securely but not tightly.

Closed Reduction and Immobilization. Most fractures of the phalanges can be adequately managed by closed reduction and external immobilization. A basic principle applicable to fractures in the hand, as well as those in other long bones, is that the controllable distal fragment must be brought into alignment with the uncontrollable proximal fragment.[43,66] It is important to emphasize also that definitive manipulative reduction must be performed before application of the external splint. The splint must not be relied upon to reduce the fracture.

The standard and most widely accepted method of immobilizing phalangeal fractures is with a short-arm cast to which some sort of outrigger support for the injured digit is incorporated. Since several muscles that act as deforming forces on the fracture originate in the forearm, it is advisable to immobilize the wrist as well as the injured finger. This eliminates the tenodesis effect of the extrinsic tendons upon the fracture caused by movements of the wrist. A well molded plaster gauntlet extends from the proximal forearm, near the elbow to the proximal palmar crease, immobilizing the wrist in 15 to 20 degrees extension.

Several types of outriggers can be used, most of which are modifications of the wire finger splint described by Böhler[19] (Fig. 6-18A). This should preferably be a wire loop with a felt pad or adhesive-tape sling upon which the finger lies without pressure or tension. Moberg[81,82] has designed a padded wire ladder, which is widely used in Sweden but is not available in this country. Because of its availability, many surgeons prefer to use a padded malleable aluminum splint, although this does not stabilize the finger as securely as the wire loop does. An outrigger made entirely of plaster can be used, but this is more likely to crack or break and jeopardize the reduction. Fractures involving the ring or small finger can be adequately immobilized with an ulnar gutter plaster splint, leaving the radial digits completely free (Fig. 6-19A). A similar radial gutter splint, with a hole for the thumb, can be used for the index and long fingers (Fig. 6-19B).

As we noted in the previous section on anatomical considerations, most displaced fractures of the proximal phalanges have a volar angulation, which may be corrected by splinting the finger in flexion. In the Böhler splint, the hand is immobilized in the so-called position of function, in which the metacarpophalangeal joint is flexed approximately 45 degrees, the proximal interphalangeal joint at least 50 to 70 degrees, and the distal interphalangeal joint 10 to 20 degrees. Böhler[19] tied the tip of the outrigger to the mid-hand part of the splint to prevent its being bent upwards, noting that the distance between fingertip and distal palmar crease should be about 2 cm. One can easily see that this position places the proximal interphalangeal joint in rather severe flexion (Fig. 6-18A), and the desirability of this much flexion has been questioned by some authors.

In recent years, James[58] has advocated that fingers should *not* be immobilized in the position of function, but rather in a position more nearly resembling the "intrinsic plus" position, in which the metacarpophalangeal joints are immobilized in at least 70 degrees flexion, the proximal interphalangeal joints in no more than 15 to 20 degrees flexion, and the distal interphalangeal joints in approximately 5 to 10 degrees flexion (Fig. 6-18D). His reasoning regarding the preferred flexed position of the metacarpophalangeal joints is quite sound and is based upon tension in the collateral ligaments as affected by the cam effect of the metacarpal head (see p. 293). As James points out, the metacarpophalangeal joints almost never become stiff in flexion because in that position, the collateral ligaments are stretched to their maximum length, whereas stiffness in extension is common, because the collateral ligaments will contract if immobilized in their shortened position.

The proximal interphalangeal joints are more likely to become stiff in flexion, but the explanation for this is not so clear-cut, as James himself admits. Although the proximal interphalangeal joint can and does occasionally become stiff in extension, the fact that it is more likely to become stiff in flexion lends support to the contention that these joints should be immobilized in only a few degrees of flexion. We agree that James' arguments are valid and we do attempt to approach the position he advocates. However, *one must be certain that the finger is immobilized in sufficient flexion to correct the volar angulation usually present at the fracture site.*

Ordinarily it is sufficient to immobilize only the injured finger, but when there is rotational malalignment, often it is controlled more easily by taping the fractured digit to an adjacent normal finger and immobilizing both together on the outrigger.

There are several types of external immobilization that we feel are undesirable. Jahss[55] advocated treatment of fractured phalanges by taping the injured finger flat against the palm, a position that immobilizes the finger in maximum flexion. We think this method is not advisable, particularly in older patients, because the position of flexion is excessive and may lead to prolonged, if not permanent, stiffness.

Strapping the entire hand over a roller bandage was used for many years as a method of immobilizing fractures of the phalanges in flexion. This is generally considered to be a poor method because it immobilizes the entire hand unnecessarily.

For many years a favorite and convenient method of immobilizing finger fractures was with the ubiquitous tongue-depressor splint. Suffice it to say that the hand should never be immobilized with *all* joints of the finger in full extension. Not only does this lead to stiffness in the injured finger, but holding the distal joint in complete extension prevents full active flexion of the other digits and may make them stiffen as well. In avulsion fractures of the dorsum of the base of the middle or distal phalanx (boutonniere and mallet fractures, respectively) *only* the involved joint is immobilized in full extension. (These special situations are discussed elsewhere in this chapter.) Under no circumstances should the metacarpophalangeal and all the interphalangeal joints be immobilized simultaneously in full extension.

Traction. Although it is not particularly popular in the current American orthopaedic literature, traction (or extension, as it was often called) frequently has been advocated as the preferred method of treatment for finger fractures throughout the years.[51,79,81,83,86,97] Several different types have been described.

Skin Traction. Adhesive tape wrapped circumferentially or diagonally around a finger can provide adequate traction to hold a reduction, but its complications are both bothersome and potentially dangerous. Slipping of the adhesive is a common problem, and even with improved techniques such as that advocated by Schulze,[104] the danger of circulatory embarrassment is real enough to be of concern. Another disadvantage of skin traction is that it immobilizes the finger in full extension and virtually eliminates active motion of the interphalangeal joints while the fracture heals.

Pulp Traction. The major disadvantage of using a wire passed transversely across the pulp space for traction is the danger of pulp necrosis from squeezing the tip of the finger. Bunnell[28] and Boyes,[23] however, both used pulp traction in conjunction with a Böhler splint (Fig. 6-18B), applying just enough tension to maintain the position obtained by manipulation. Böhler, himself, originally used pulp traction,[19] but stopped because of complications from improper application.

Nail Traction. Pulling through the nail by means of a wire or silk suture has been advocated, but today it has few supporters. Boyes[23] says that nail traction tends to pull out the nail, and several authors[19,96] have noted that it is uncomfortable.

Nail-Pulp Traction. Moberg[81,82] has described extensive experience with a modified type of traction in which a stainless steel wire is passed vertically through the nail, the periosteum of the tip of the distal phalanx, and the pulp. He credits his success with this technique and absence of complications to the use of a spreading device, which prevents the wire from squeezing the fingertip (Fig. 6-18C). Since 1948 Moberg has made available throughout Sweden a kit that contains the materials for applying his special nail-pulp traction. Like Boyes, Moberg emphasizes that traction is used not to reduce a fracture, but only to maintain a reduced fracture in satisfactory position.

Skeletal Traction. Firm traction in the finger can be provided by means of a small Kirschner wire or needle passed transversely through the phalanx and attached to an outrigger by rubber bands in a variety of ways. Specially designed calipers have been used similarly,[36,83] with purchase provided by a tong-type mechanism, rather than passing a wire directly through the entire phalanx. For fractures of the proximal phalanx, it is desirable to have the wire as close to the fracture as possible; specifically, through the distal end of the proximal phalanx. The major disadvantage of this is that it is difficult (several authors say virtually impossible) to insert a wire transversely through the proximal phalanx without perforating some part of the extensor-hood complex. The major disadvantage of traction through the middle or distal phalanx is that it severely restricts or eliminates active motion in the proximal interphalangeal joint during the period of traction. Quigley and Urist[96] concluded that there is only one area in the finger where skin lies directly over fascia and bone, with no underlying tendons or neurovascular bundles; that is a triangular space on the dorsal surface of the middle phalanx, just distal to the insertion of the central slip.

They fashioned a traction hook from a Kirschner wire, and embedded it into bone in this location.

The banjo type of traction advocated many years ago is now universally condemned. The technique is improper for several reasons: rotation is difficult to control; the fingers are not truly supported; and most importantly, stiffness is enhanced by the position of full extension in all joints.

A serious and avoidable complication of traction is pressure necrosis of the volar skin caused by overzealous pull against an unyielding fulcrum. This can be prevented by observing several precautions: (1) padding the wire outrigger with a soft material; (2) never allowing the plaster gauntlet to extend far enough distally to touch the finger; (3) eliminating acute flexion of the proximal interphalangeal joint; and (4) avoiding excessive traction force.

If traction is used, it should never be continued for more than 3 weeks. The most important principle in the use of traction is that its purpose is to maintain a reduction, not to reduce the fracture.

Internal Fixation. Unstable fractures that cannot be reduced by closed manipulation and maintained with external splinting require internal fixation. Certain fractures can be reduced by closed manipulation and stabilized by percutaneous Kirschner wires. Vom Saal,[114] Clifford,[38] and Butt[32] have each described a method of closed reduction and percutaneous intramedullarily fixation of unstable fractures.

In most fractures that require internal fixation, open reduction is necessary to insure anatomical restoration of the fracture, especially in displaced intraarticular fractures.[87] Kirschner wires are the most versatile mode of fixation and the one most often used. Recently, however, advocates of the AO system[107] have used small screws and even tiny plates, but even they concede that such techniques are more amenable to metacarpal fractures than to fractures of the phalanges.[100]

One rationale for the use of internal fixation in phalangeal fractures is that stable fixation obviates external splinting, allows the patient early active motion during healing, and, it is hoped, prevents joint stiffness. However, the dissection and stripping of periosteum necessary to accomplish open reduction of a phalanx in itself creates adhesions, which, in turn, may contribute to joint stiffness. Open reduction of phalangeal fractures demands meticulous technique and precise dissection to minimize further scarring.

Amputation. An isolated fracture, is in itself, virtually never an indication for amputation. However, when severe crush in-

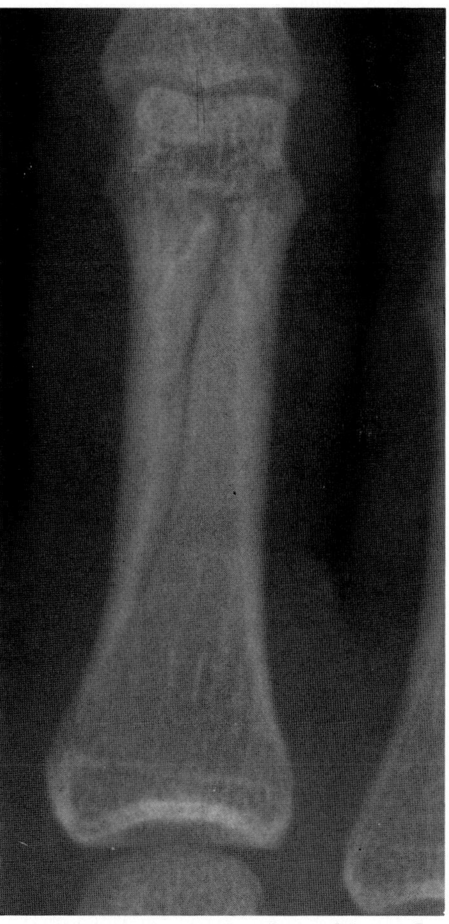

Fig. 6-20. An example of a stable, undisplaced fracture of the proximal phalanx which can be treated by buddy taping to an adjacent normal digit.

juries have damaged tendons, nerves, and blood vessels as well as bone, it may be the treatment of choice. The decision rests squarely on the judgment of the operating surgeon, although only the most obviously nonviable digits should be amputated as a primary procedure at the initial operation. If there is the slightest possibility of viability, it is wise to reconstruct the digit as well as possible and allow the natural course of events to help determine the necessity for amputation.

Authors' Preferred Method of Treatment

Extraarticular Fractures. Fractures of the proximal and middle phalanges can be divided into stable and unstable types.

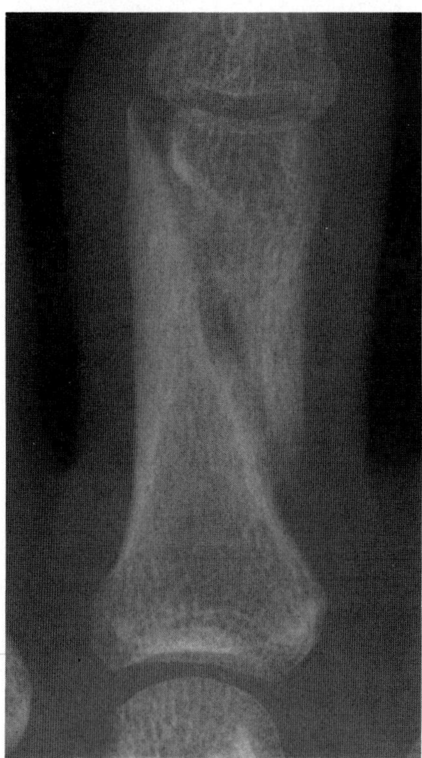

Fig. 6-21. The extraarticular fracture most likely to be unstable after closed reduction is a long oblique fracture of the proximal phalanx. This fracture often requires internal fixation. The surgeon has a choice between closed reduction and percutaneous pinning or open reduction and internal fixation (*see text*).

Stable fractures include undisplaced fractures (Fig. 6-20) and impacted transverse fractures. In the latter group, it is particularly important to be absolutely certain that there is neither rotation nor angulation at the fracture site. Rotation can be more readily appreciated by clinical examination than by roentgenography. It is determined by comparing the planes of the fingernails, as seen end-on, with those of the adjacent normal digits (Fig. 6-17), and by observing that the tips of the fingers converge toward the tubercle of the scaphoid as the patient actively flexes the digits (Fig. 6-16). Angulation can occur in any plane, but usually the apex is volar, and the distal fragment is dorsally displaced. It is easy to overlook significant angulation in this plane unless true lateral films of good quality are taken. Even a fracture that appears to be in excellent alignment in the anteroposterior view may have 25 to 30 degrees or more volar angulation.[41] The base of the proximal phalanx is often not well visualized in the lateral view, being obscured by superimposition of the other proximal phalanges. Careful and detailed interpretation of the roentgenograms is essential for accurate initial assessment of the degree of volar angulation in these fractures.

If one can be certain that the fracture is indeed stable and neither angulated nor rotated, then protection, but not immobilization, is required during the period of healing. For these fractures, we prefer to tape the injured finger to an adjacent normal digit and encourage active range of motion exercises from the outset. X-ray and clinical examinations should be done after approximately 1 week of such treatment to determine if there has been any change in the position of the reduced fracture, although if this method is reserved only for truly stable fractures, displacement is unlikely to occur during the period of healing. If there is any doubt about the stability of the fracture, the finger should have an initial 10- to 14-day period of splinting before the buddy taping system is instituted.

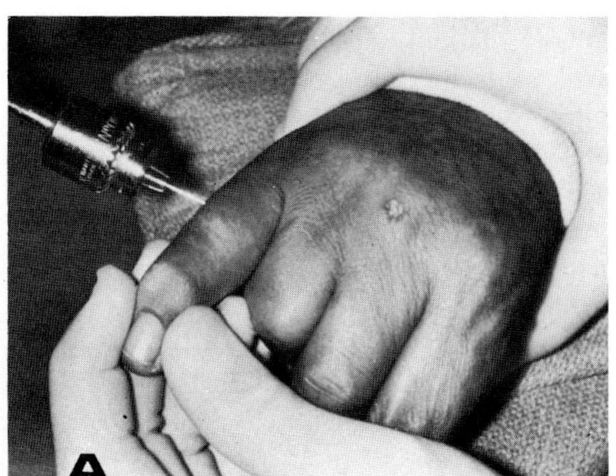

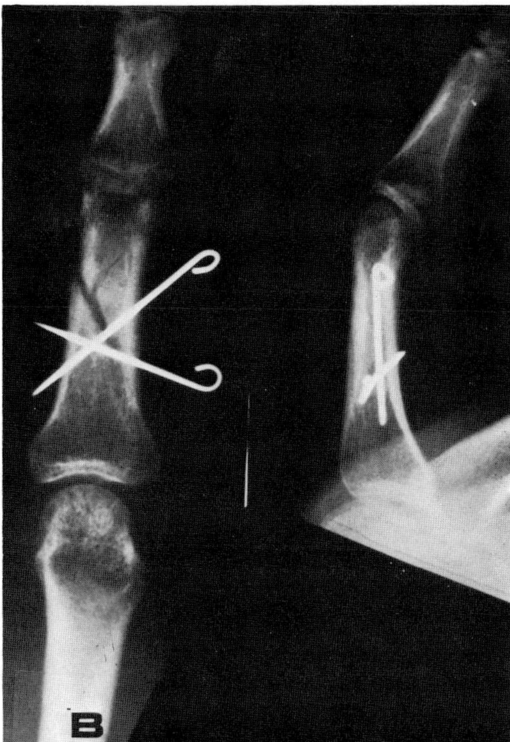

Fig. 6-22. Closed reduction and percutaneous pin fixation of unstable phalangeal fractures is a useful technique, but is not as easy to perform as one might anticipate. (*A*) Two knowledgeable surgeons are required. One must reduce and hold the fracture while the other simultaneously inserts the pins. (*B*) A typical oblique fracture of the proximal phalanx treated by closed reduction and percutaneous pin fixation. The pins may be cut off beneath the skin or left to protrude percutaneously and bent into a small loop to facilitate removal. (Green, D. P., and Anderson, J. R.: J. Bone Joint Surg., 55*A*:1652, 1973)

James[57] has pointed out that unstable fractures of the middle and proximal phalanges can be divided into those that are stable after reduction and those that require internal fixation. Most fractures of the phalanges can be reduced readily by closed manipulation and held by external immobilization with the finger in some degree of flexion. The metacarpophalangeal joint should be immobilized in at least 70 degrees flexion to prevent stiffness in extension, but the proximal interphalangeal joint should bė flexed only enough to prevent recurrence of the typical volar angulation. In some fractures, it may be possible to hold the fracture with the proximal interphalangeal joint in only 15 to 20 degrees flexion, as recommended by James (Fig. 6-18D), but in many others, more acute flexion may be necessary to stabilize the fracture. We prefer to immobilize the wrist in a short-arm plaster gauntlet, with the finger supported by a wire loop padded with soft felt, although any of the outriggers mentioned previously will provide satisfactory immobilization if used correctly. We frequently use an ulnar gutter splint to treat fractures in the ring- and small fingers. Traction generally is not necessary for extraarticular fractures in the phalanges, unless there is severe comminution and/or actual loss of bone substance, as occasionally occurs in gunshot wounds.

Rotational malalignment is the bane of existence to the surgeon treating phalangeal fractures. It may be extremely subtle to detect and equally difficult to control. Assuring precise rotational alignment with the single finger immobilized on an outrigger may be hazardous, and for this reason we often prefer to splint two digits together. By pairing up the fingers in this way, one can better compare the planes of the fingernails, which we find to be the best method of checking rotational alignment.

The extraarticular fracture most likely to be unstable after closed reduction is a long oblique fracture of the proximal phalanx (Fig. 6-21). This fracture often requires internal fixation, although a choice must be made between closed and open reduction. Open reduction and internal fixation of phalangeal fractures is, as was previously noted, an operation that demands precise and meticulous dissection in order to minimize the inevitable adhesions that develop between the extensor aponeurosis and the underlying disturbed periosteum. Pratt's[94] dorsal approach through an oblique skin incision and midline splitting of the extensor hood is preferred when open reduction is performed, as it provides the best exposure of the fracture.

In an attempt to avoid some of the complications persuant to open reduction of phalangeal fractures, we have used closed reduction and percutaneous pin fixation in certain selected cases.[49] The more oblique the fracture, the more ideally suited for closed reduction and pinning, but the procedure is not as easy to perform as one might anticipate. Two knowledgeable surgeons are required; one must reduce and hold the fracture while the other simultaneously inserts the pins (Fig. 6-22A). Accurate pin placement is essential to provide enough stability to allow early active motion. Using the lateral flare of the head of the phalanx as a guide, two or more pins are inserted perpendicular to the fracture line. These can be cut off beneath the skin or left to protrude if they are bent into a small loop or at a right angle (Fig. 6-22B). Although we have often seen mild drainage from percutaneous pin tracts, it promptly resolves after the pins are removed, and it has caused no significant residual problems. Dynamic splinting by taping the injured finger to an adjacent digit then permits immediate active range of motion and full use of the hand. The pins are removed after 3 weeks, but buddy taping is continued for another 3 weeks.

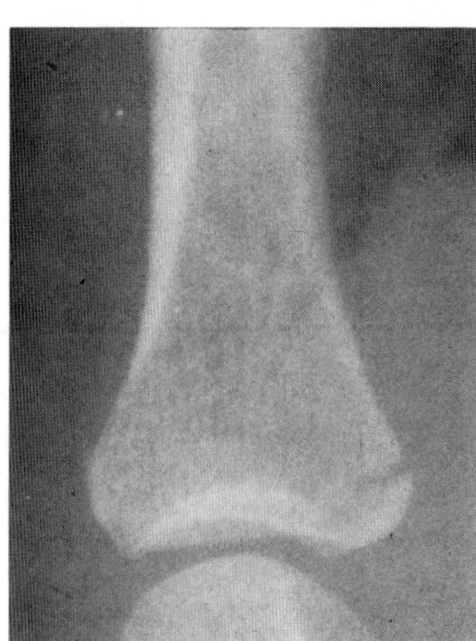

Fig. 6-23. Truly undisplaced intraarticular fractures of the phalanges are uncommon. They can be treated by carefully guarded and protected early range of motion using the buddy taping system.

Severely comminuted fractures of the phalanx are extremely difficult—often impossible—to restore satisfactorily by open reduction and internal fixation. Such fractures are better treated by traction, and if there is actual loss of bone, as in a gunshot wound, primary or secondary bone grafting may be required.

Intraarticular Fractures. Truly undisplaced intraarticular fractures are uncommon but do occur (Fig. 6-23). They are best treated by carefully guarded and protected early range of motion exercise using the buddy taping system. Immobilization of such fractures often leads to prolonged or even permanent stiffness due to intraarticular adhesions. Again, careful and frequent clinical and roentgenographic examinations are necessary to check for displacement of the fragments during the period of healing.

The goal of treatment in displaced, intraarticular fractures should be anatomical restoration of the joint surface by open reduction and internal fixation.

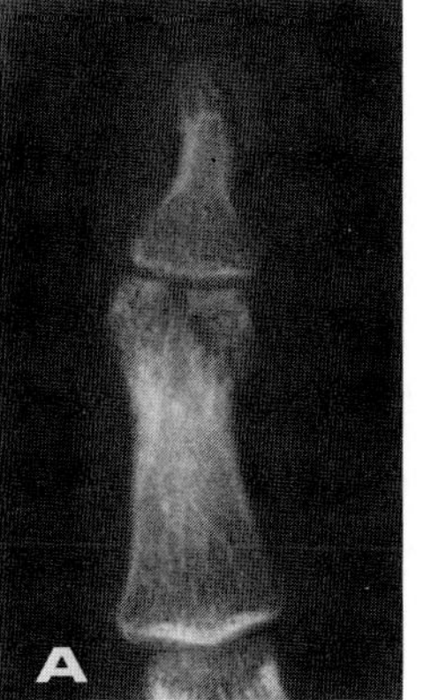

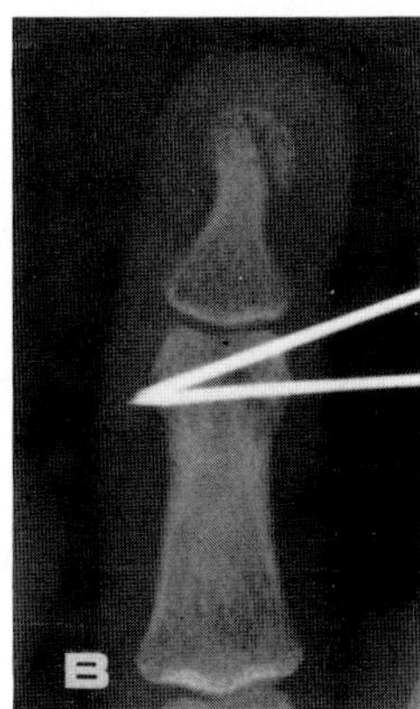

Fig. 6-24. A fracture that virtually always demands internal fixation is a displaced fracture of one or both condyles of the proximal phalanx. (*A*) This fracture most commonly splits off a single condyle, resulting in disruption of the joint and angular deformity of the finger. (*B*) This fracture should be treated with open reduction and exact anatomical restoration of the articular surface.

Condylar Fractures. A fracture that virtually always demands internal fixation is a displaced fracture of one or both condyles of the proximal phalanx; i.e., at the level of the proximal interphalangeal joint.[63] A similar fracture occurs at the distal joint, involving the middle phalanx. This fracture, somewhat analogous to a fracture of the distal humerus, most commonly splits off a single condyle (Fig. 6-24), but it may have a **Y** configuration, which displaces both condyles. Adequate operative exposure is the key to success, but it may be difficult to achieve. The surgeon must visualize the articular surface well enough to reduce the fracture anatomically, but at the same time he must not excessively strip away the vital soft-tissue structures attached to the fragment. We prefer a dorsal approach, splitting the central slip in the midline down to its bony insertion, but extreme care must be taken not to weaken or detach the insertion itself. A midlateral incision avoids the dorsal structures of the extensor aponeurosis, but adequate exposure of the articular surface is often difficult with this approach and may require cutting the collateral liga-

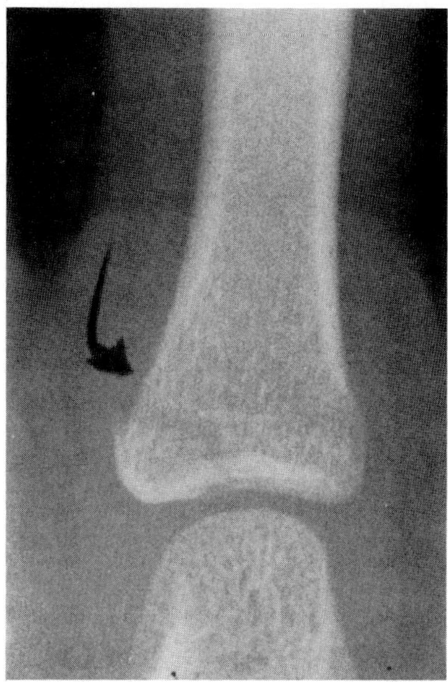

Fig. 6-25. Nondisplaced marginal fractures of the base of the proximal phalanx can be adequately managed by buddy taping.

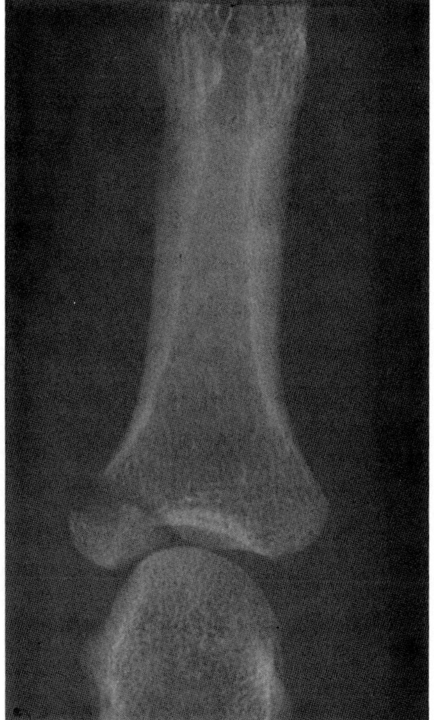

Fig. 6-26. Larger marginal fractures will result in incongruity of the articular surface if they are not reduced. They usually require open reduction and internal fixation.

ment to provide sufficient visualization to effect an anatomical reduction. Some permanent stiffness of the proximal interphalangeal joint is not uncommon following any type of treatment of this injury, but internal fixation stable enough to allow early protected range of motion is the best method of minimizing this.

Avulsion Fractures at the Base of the Proximal Phalanx. Marginal fractures of the base of the proximal phalanx involving the metacarpophalangeal joint usually represent avulsion fractures of the collateral ligament. Small or nondisplaced fragments (Fig. 6-25) can be adequately managed by dynamic splinting. Larger, displaced fractures of this type (Fig. 6-26) will result in incongruity of the articular surface if they are not restored by open reduction and internal fixation. A dorsal approach that splits the extensor hood is used, and the larger fragment is stabilized with small Kirschner wires. Placement of pins sometimes proves rather awkward because of the inaccessibility of the volar location of the fragment.

Boutonniere Injuries. Intraarticular fractures that involve the base of the middle phalanx are usually one of three types: (1) a dorsal chip fracture, which represents an avulsion of bone by the central slip of the extensor tendon, creating a boutonniere deformity; (2) a volar chip fracture, usually combined with a dorsal dislocation or subluxation of the middle phalanx—the so-called fracture-dislocation of the proximal interphalangeal joint (see p. 317); and (3) a lateral chip fracture representing avulsion of bone by the collateral ligament (see pp. 313, 331).

Boutonniere or buttonhole deformity is caused by disruption of the central slip of the extensor tendon combined with tearing of the triangular ligament on the dorsum of the middle phalanx, which allows the lateral bands to slip below the axis of proximal interphalangeal joint. Rupture of the central slip causes loss of active extension of the middle phalanx, leading to a flexion deformity of the proximal interphalangeal joint. This is further aggravated by

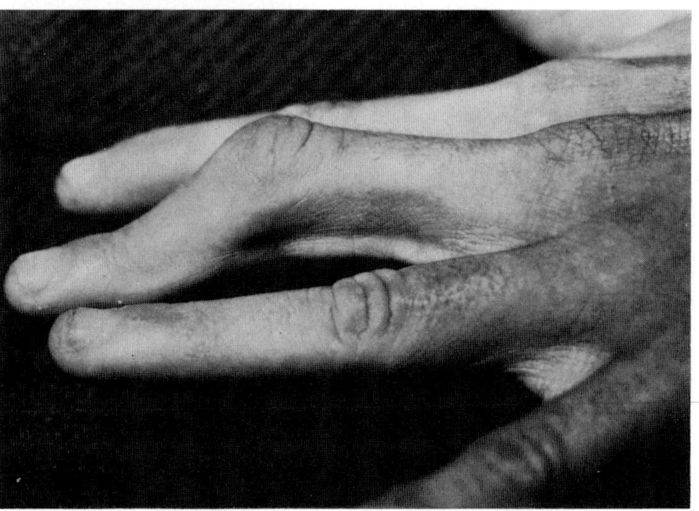

Fig. 6-27. A typical boutonniere deformity with flexion of the proximal interphalangeal joint and hyperextension of the distal interphalangeal joint. The acute boutonniere injury does not usually present with this typical deformity, but simply with a swollen, painful proximal interphalangeal joint. Early diagnosis is dependent upon careful clinical examination (*see text*).

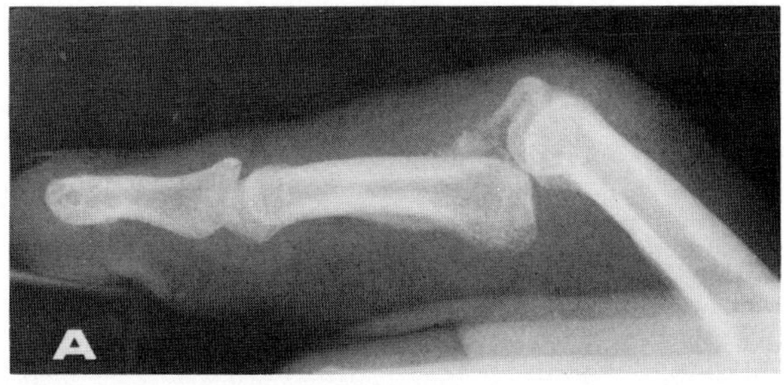

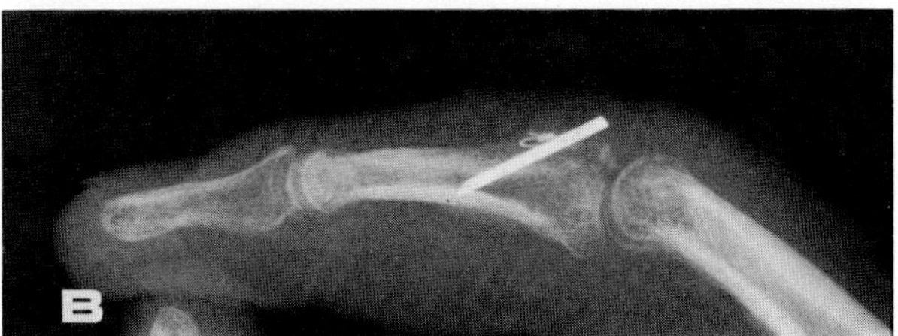

Fig. 6-28. Most boutonniere injuries are purely soft-tissue lesions that can be treated by closed methods (see text). (*A*) Occasionally there is a small fracture fragment avulsed by the central slip insertion into the base of the middle phalanx. (*B*) Open reduction and internal fixation of this fracture is usually necessary.

the pull of the lateral bands which have become flexors of the joint. The most disabling element of the boutonniere deformity, however, is the limitation of flexion, both passive and active, which develops in the distal interphalangeal joint. This results from the tenodesis effect of the displaced lateral bands, and in time may lead to the fixed hyperextension deformity of the distal joint seen in the classic boutonniere lesion (Fig. 6-27).

Most boutonniere deformities are caused by rupture of the central slip directly from its bony insertion; the diagnosis must be made by clinical examination. The acute injury docs not usually present with a typical boutonniere deformity, but simply with a swollen painful proximal interphalangeal joint. Rupture of the central slip is differentiated from the more common injury to the collateral ligament by the location of the maximum area of tenderness on the dorsum rather than the sides of the joint, and by the patient's inability to actively extend the proximal interphalangeal joint. If pain prevents active extension, it must be eliminated bý digital or metacarpal nerve block so that active motion can be tested. If a patient is suspected of having a ruptured central slip, roentgenograms of the involved finger should always be made, for in some instances, there will be an avulsion fracture arising from the dorsum of the base of the middle phalanx (Fig. 6-28).

A boutonniere lesion without a fracture should be treated closed, by splinting the proximal interphalangeal joint in full extension for 5 to 6 weeks.[138,146] Souter[146] has shown that successful results can be achieved in closed boutonniere lesions whose treatment is delayed up to 6 weeks after injury. It is extremely important that the distal joint not be immobilized; in fact, it must be actively and passively flexed during the period of treatment. After the initial period of immobilization, a removable splint that holds the proximal interphalangeal joint should be worn at night for an additional 4 weeks. During this period, the patient must be taught to actively bend the distal joint while holding the proximal interphalangeal joint in full extension. Treatment should not be considered complete until active flexion of the distal joint is equal to that in the opposite normal finger.

A boutonniere injury with a displaced avulsion fracture of significant size demands open reduction and internal fixation.

At the time of operation, it is important also to repair the triangular ligament to correct the volar subluxation of the lateral bands, although care must be taken not to reef these tendons dorsally under excessive tension as this will limit subsequent flexion of the joint. Postoperative immobilization should be limited to the proximal interphalangeal joint only (in full extension, by means of an external splint or with a smooth Kirschner wire passed obliquely across the joint), and the patient should be carefully instructed in active assisted flexion of the distal joint.

Comminuted Intraarticular Fractures. Severely comminuted intraarticular fractures that involve either the metacarpophalangeal or proximal interphalangeal joint are usually not amenable to internal fixation, and attempts to fix such fractures by open reduction are fraught with difficulty and frustration. We consider this type of injury to be the prime indication for traction in the fingers, and often reasonable restoration of the articular surface can be achieved by light skeletal traction to prevent shortening. For comminuted intraarticular fractures that involve the metacarpophalangeal joint, we prefer to use a small Kirschner wire passed transversely through the proximal phalanx near the flare of the head. This leaves the proximal interphalangeal joint free to move during the period of traction, while the proximal phalanx is supported lightly by a felt pad suspended between the arms of a wire outrigger. For comminuted intraarticular fractures involving the proximal interphalangeal joint, we use a transverse Kirschner wire through the center of the middle phalanx. Properly applied, it allows some motion in the proximal interphalangeal joint, although this will always be limited during the period of traction.

Follow-up Care and Healing Time of Phalangeal Fractures

There is, unfortunately, a disturbing tendency to regard fractures of the phalanges as minor injuries and to neglect the important follow-up care they require. Complications often result from finger fractures when an inexperienced surgeon reduces a phalangeal fracture, immobilizes the injured digit, and then tells the patient to return in 3 weeks to have the splint removed. No matter how accurate a reduction is achieved and how carefully the splint is applied, it is imperative that the patient be examined clinically and roentgenographically from time to time during the period of fracture healing. In particular, patients who are allowed early active motion should be seen periodically, to be instructed and encouraged in the performance of specific exercises to minimize joint stiffness and to regain full active motion.

Immobilization of an injured digit should not be continued until consolidation at the fracture line is visible on roentgenograms. Smith and Rider[109] demonstrated many years ago that the average "roentgenographic" healing time for fractures of the phalanges is 5 months, the range being 1 to 17 months. The important point is that "clinical" healing is evident in 3 to 4 weeks, and immobolization is not even required for the full extent of this time. With the exception of mallet and boutonniere chip fractures, is it rarely necessary to immobilize a closed fracture of a phalanx for longer than 3 weeks, and in fact it is usually detrimental. Some protection should be afforded the digit for 3 more weeks, however; it is easily accomplished by the buddy taping system, which allows the patient to move the joints actively, even in unstable fractures following the initial 3-week immobilization period.

A final point regarding the period of immobilization is that open fractures do not heal as rapidly as comparable closed fractures in the phalanges. Even in open fractures, however, external immobilization should rarely be continued longer than 4 weeks.

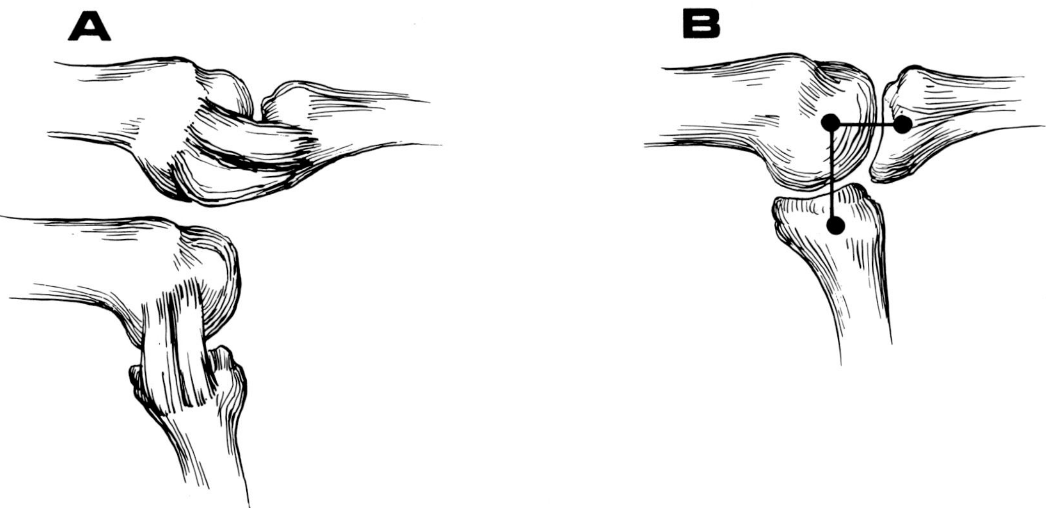

Fig. 6-29. The collateral ligaments of the metacarpophalangeal joints are relaxed in extension, permitting lateral motion, but become taut when the joint is fully flexed. This occurs because of the unique shape of the metacarpal head, which acts as a cam. The distance from the pivot point of the metacarpal to the phalanx in extension is less than the distance in flexion, so that the collateral ligament is tight when the joint is flexed.

METACARPAL FRACTURES (EXCLUDING THE THUMB)

Anatomy

The metacarpals are miniature long bones which are slightly arched in the long axis and concave on the palmar surface.[10,52] Their weakest point is just behind the head.[10]

The proximal ends of the index- and long-finger metacarpals articulate with the distal carpal row in practically immobile articulations, while those of the ring- and little fingers have approximately 15 and 25 degrees, respectively, of anteroposterior motion. The metacarpal shafts radiate like spokes of a wheel, terminating in the bulbous articular heads, which are weakly joined by transverse metacarpal ligaments. The collateral ligaments that join the metacarpal head to the proximal phalanx are relaxed in extension, permitting lateral motion, but become taut when the joint is fully flexed (Fig. 6-29A). This occurs because of the unique shape of the metacarpal head, which acts as a cam. The distance in extension from the pivot point of the metacarpal to the phalanx is less than the distance in flexion, so that the collateral ligament is tightened upon flexion of the metacarpophalangeal joint (Fig. 6-29B). This anatomical point explains why the metacarpophalangeal joints stiffen if the collateral ligaments are allowed to shorten, as they do when the metacarpophalangeal joints are immobilized in extension.[57,98,99]

The dorsal and volar interosseous muscles arise from the shafts of the metacarpals and act as flexors at the metacarpophalangeal joint. Their deforming force accounts for the dorsal angulation in metacarpal neck and shaft fractures.

Classification

Fractures of the metacarpals may be classified according to their anatomical location: (1) metacarpal head (i.e., distal to the insertion of the collateral ligaments); (2) metacarpal neck; (3) metacarpal shaft; and (4) base of the metacarpal.

Prior to 1932, according to Waugh and Ferrazzano,[117] practically all fractured metacarpals were treated by simple immobilization over a roller bandage, and there was little or no attempt to correct the displacement. In 1928, Magnuson[71] and, in 1932, McNealy and Lichtenstein[76] advocated treating all metacarpal fractures with a straight dorsal splint, holding the wrist and fingers in extension. The extension method of treatment, either with a straight dorsal splint or by a banjo splint, was recommended by Scudder,[106] Key and Conwell,[62] Cotton,[42] Owen,[91] and others. Neither method is currently considered acceptable for treating metacarpal fractures.

In 1935, Koch[65] wrote of the disabilities of the hand that resulted from stiffness when the metacarpophalangeal joints were immobilized in extension; he advocated immobilizing the hand in the functional position.

Currently, treatment of a metacarpal fracture is based on its anatomical location, whether it is stable or unstable, and the degree of comminution. The different forms of treatment commonly used today are: immobilization without reduction, closed reduction and immobilization, closed reduction and percutaneous wire fixation, and open reduction and internal fixation.

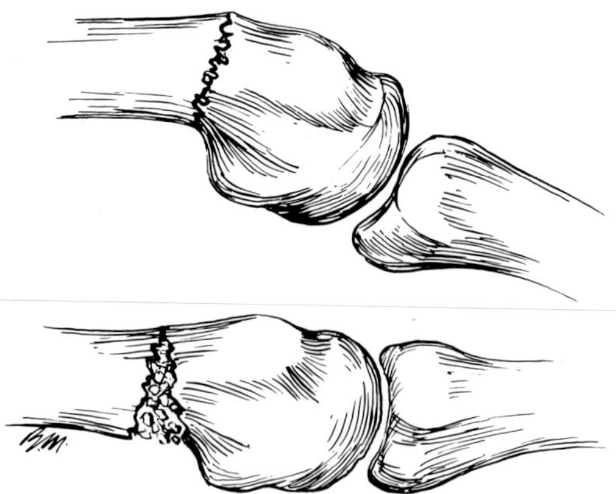

Fig. 6-30. Fractures of the metacarpal neck are basically unstable because of comminution of the volar cortex. For this reason, the reduced fracture tends to settle back to its original angulated position.

FRACTURES OF THE METACARPAL HEAD

Fractures involving the metacarpal head distal to the collateral ligament insertions are usually the result of crushing or missile injuries and often consist of many fragments. Attempts at open reduction of these severely comminuted fractures are futile. Rarely, one encounters a simple fracture of the metacarpal head in which a single large fragment has been displaced; in such cases, open reduction and internal fixation should be performed, although operative exposure and placement of the small Kirschner wires for fixation may be technically difficult.

For the more common comminuted fractures, we believe that prolonged immobilization should be avoided. A short period of splinting to alleviate pain should be followed by early active motion in the hope that the free fragments will be molded into some sort of acceptable articular surface. The end result, at best, will be loss of motion without disabling pain.

FRACTURES OF THE METACARPAL NECK

Fractures of the metacarpal neck are basically unstable because of comminution of the volar cortex (Fig. 6-30). For this reason, there is a tendency for the reduced fracture to settle back to its original angulated position. Because of this instability and the difficulties in maintaining reduction, many techniques of treatment have been proposed. It is important to separate the treatment of fractures involving the neck of the second or third metacarpal from those involving the fourth or fifth metacarpal. As mentioned previously, the ring and little fingers have approximately 15 and 25 degrees, respectively, of anteroposterior motion at the carpometacarpal joint, while the index and long fingers have practically none. Because of this mobility of the ring and little fingers, angular neck deformity can be accepted without a serious loss of hand function. This is not true of the more immobile second and third metacarpals, and their neck fractures should be reduced and held in anatomical alignment; otherwise, palmar angulation of the metacarpal head may produce a painful grip.

Methods of Treatment

Immobilization Without Reduction. Fractures of the neck of the fifth metacarpal (the so-called boxer's or fighter's fracture) account for the majority of all metacarpal neck fractures. This is indeed fortunate, because as noted above, greater degrees of residual angulation can be accepted in fractures of the fourth and fifth metacarpals. Eichenholtz[45] and Hunter and Cowen[54] have reported good functional results with significant angular deformities in the fifth metacarpal. In the latter's series[54] of 80 patients with fractures involving the neck of the fifth metacarpal, if the angulation was 40 degrees or less, the fracture was immediately splinted without reduction in a gutter-type splint from the proximal interphalangeal joint to the elbow, including the ring finger to prevent rotation. After 10 days of immobilization, the splint was removed twice a day for gentle motion. After 2½ weeks, the splint was discarded completely and the patient was encouraged to use his hand in more strenuous activities. At the end of 4 weeks, most of the patients were using their hands normally, and the majority returned to full activity. In this series of patients, if a fracture of the fifth metacarpal neck that had over 40 degrees angulation could not be reduced easily under local anesthesia, Hunter and Cowen accepted angulation up to 70 degrees, as long as rotational deformity was minimal.

Closed Reduction and Immobilization with Plaster. One of the earlier and most popular methods of treatment was that introduced by Jahss,[56] the so-called 90-90 method or the **C**-clamp treatment. This

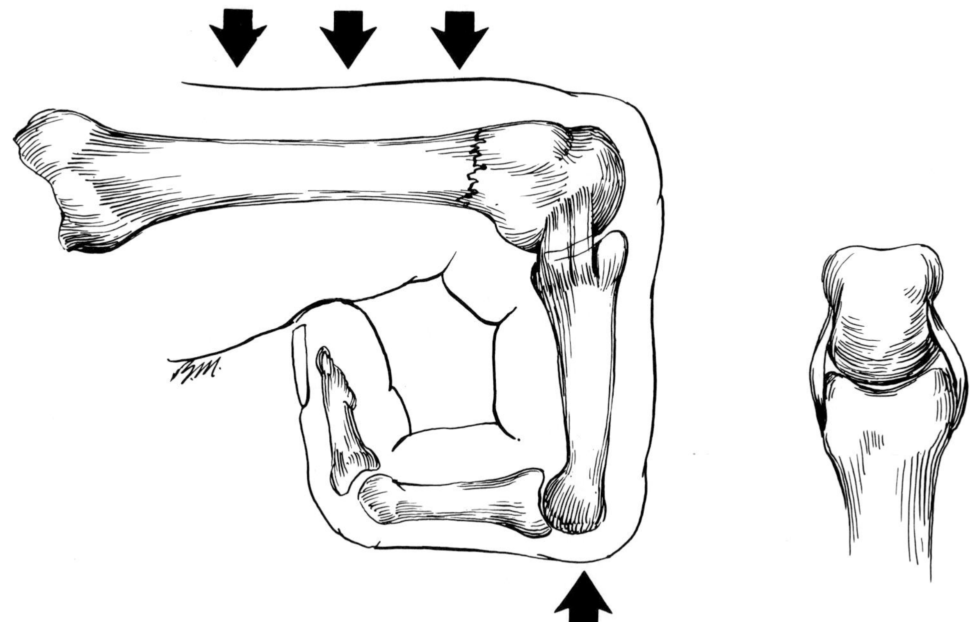

Fig. 6-31. The so-called 90-90 method of reducing a fracture of the metacarpal neck was introduced by Jahss (*see text*). Although this is the accepted method of reducing fractures of the metacarpal neck, it should never be used to immobilize a fracture because of possible stiffness of the proximal interphalangeal joint or skin slough over the dorsum of the joint.

method takes advantage of the anatomical fact that the collateral ligaments of the metacarpophalangeal joint are tight when the joint is flexed to 90 degrees.[73] With the tight collateral ligaments holding the loose metacarpal head, the proximal interphalangeal joint is flexed and the base of the proximal phalanx is used to push the metacarpal head back into position (Fig. 6-31). Because of the inherent instability of this fracture, Jahss maintained the reduction in plaster with the finger flexed 90 degrees at the metacarpophalangeal joint and 90 degrees at the proximal interphalangeal joint, the 90-90 position.

Jahss' method of *reducing* a metacarpal fracture is accepted by most authors, but the use of the 90-90 position to *hold* the reduction has been widely condemned. Even though loss of reduction can be prevented with this position, we feel strongly that it should never be used to immobilize a fracture. The possible complications of permanent stiffness of the proximal interphalangeal joint (Fig. 6-32) and skin slought over the dorsum of the proximal interphalangeal joint far outweigh any loss of function secondary to a malaligned fracture.

Closed Reduction and Percutaneous Pin Fixation. Because of the difficulty of holding a metacarpal fracture in plaster without using the 90-90 position, many authors[16,22,57,58,61,85,90,102,112,117] have advocated the use of percutaneous Kirschner wire fixation to hold the fracture after reduction. In 1936 Saypol[102] introduced a method of transfixing the reduced metacarpal to the adjacent normal metacarpal(s) with smooth Kirschner wires introduced transversely proximal and distal to the fracture site. He credited Lasher with originating the technique, and it was subsequently popularized in the late 1930's and early 1940's by Bosworth,[22] Waugh and Ferrazzano,[117] Berkan and Miles,[16] and others.

Vom Saal,[114] Butt,[32] Clifford,[38] and Lord[70] popularized the use of intramedullary pin fixation. This has the disadvantage of requiring passage of the pins through the extensor mechanism at the level of the metacarpophalangeal joint. Scarring of the extensor hood, with possible joint stiffness and loss of extension, is more likely to occur with this type of treatment.

The major advantage cited by most advocates of these percutaneous pin fixation techniques is that early motion can be started without external splinting. The pins are generally left in place for 3 to 4 weeks, during which time the patient may be allowed to use the hand.

There is a difference of opinion as to

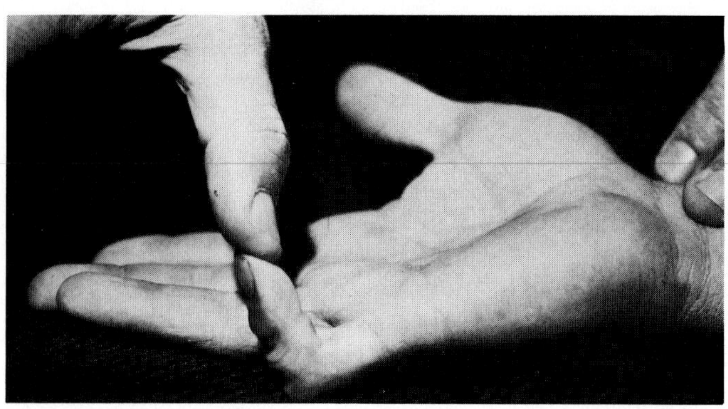

Fig. 6-32. A 90-degree fixed flexion contracture of the proximal interphalangeal joint in a 26-year-old man following treatment of a metacarpal neck fracture in the 90-90 position.

whether the pins should be cut off beneath the skin or left to protrude. The likelihood of pin traction infection is minimized by burying the wires, but many authors have reported leaving them out through the skin without serious problems from infection.[22,49,90,92,102,117]

Open Reduction and Internal Fixation. Open reduction and internal fixation is rarely indicated in acute neck fractures and is reserved for those unusual instances in which the metacarpal head and neck have been displaced entirely off the metacarpal shaft (Fig. 6-33).

Authors' Preferred Method of Treatment

In fractures of the fourth and fifth metacarpal necks, treatment by simple immobilization without reduction has been restricted to acute fractures with minimal angulation of less than 10 degrees, and fractures less than 7 to 10 days old that have angulation up to 40 degrees without clawing on finger extension (Fig. 6-34). Immobilization is in the form of an ulnar gutter splint extending from the distal interphalangeal joint of the ring and little fingers to the upper forearm, holding the hand and wrist in the functional position (Fig. 6-19A). As the purpose of the splint is simply to relieve pain, it is removed as soon as local tenderness has subsided, usually after 10 to 14 days. Protected gentle motion over the next few weeks is encouraged. When tenderness to firm palpation is no longer present, the patient may return to unprotected use of the hand.

Undisplaced fractures of the neck of the second or third metacarpal are also treated with gutter splints, immobilizing the index-

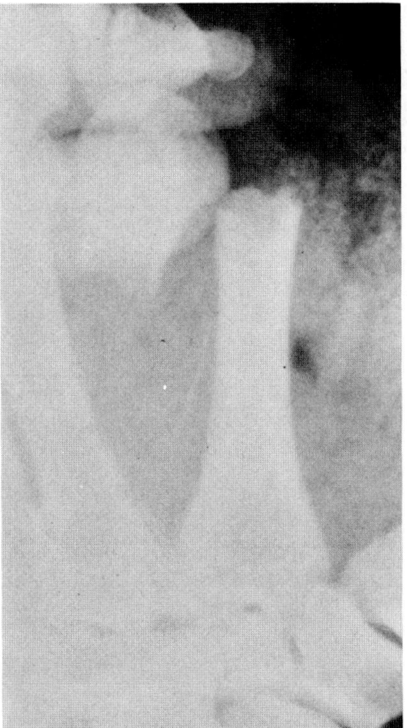
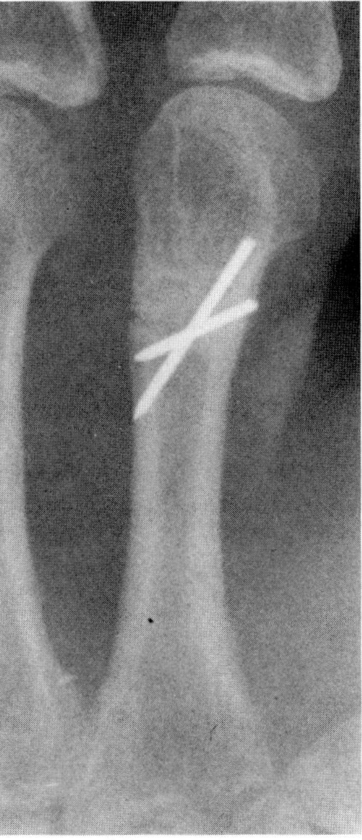

Fig. 6-33. Open reduction and internal fixation is rarely indicated in acute neck fractures and is reserved for those unusual instances in which the metacarpal head and neck have been displaced entirely off the metacarpal shaft, as in this patient.

and long fingers as described above, cutting a hole in the plaster for the thumb, as shown in Figure 6-19B. In neck fractures of the second and third metacarpals, it is extremely important that follow-up roentgenograms be taken on the fourth or fifth postfracture day. Any volar angulation must be corrected at this time, for further delay will make reduction impossible because of rapid bone healing.

It is our opinion that acute neck fractures of the fourth and fifth metacarpals with more than 10 degrees of angulation should be reduced. Reduction is generally done under ulnar block anesthesia, and may be facilitated by disimpacting the fracture with an initial five- to ten-minute period of finger trap traction. When the metacarpophalangeal joint is held at 90 degrees, the angulated metacarpal head can usually

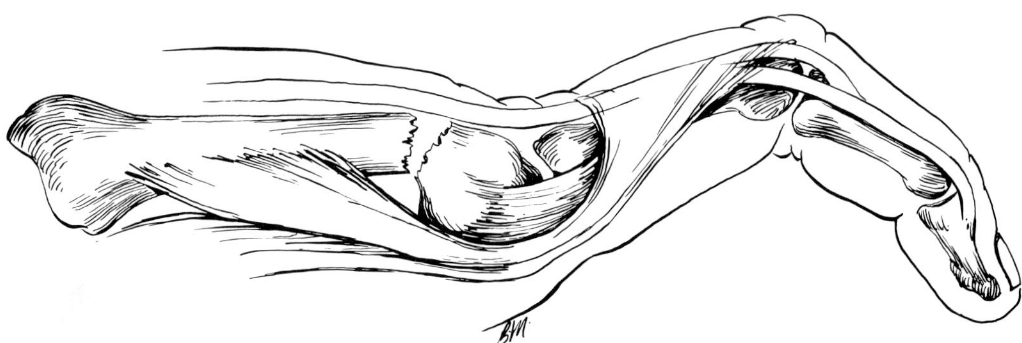

Fig. 6-34. If the angulation in a metacarpal neck fracture is severe, clawing may result when the patient attempts to extend the finger. We have found this to be a good clinical test to supplement the evaluation of the severity of the angulation as seen on roentgenograms.

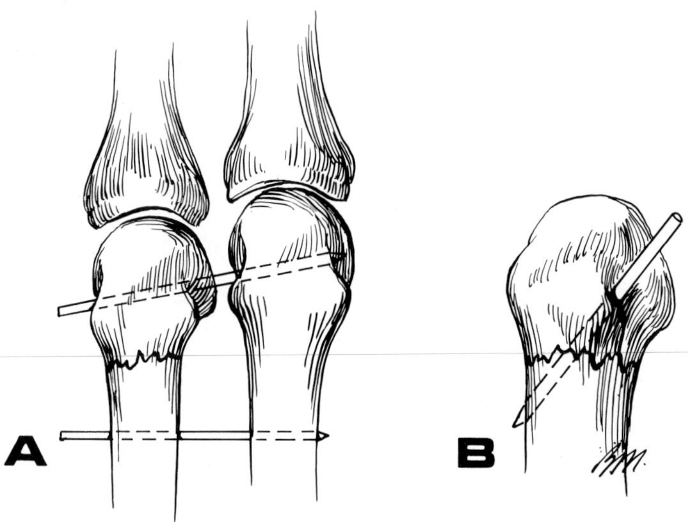

Fig. 6-35. In patients with excessive angulation and therefore more severe volar cortex comminution, we prefer closed reduction and percutaneous Kirschner wire fixation. The fracture may be held with either proximal and distal transverse pins into the adjacent metacarpal (*A*) or with an oblique Kirschner wire across the fracture site (*B*).

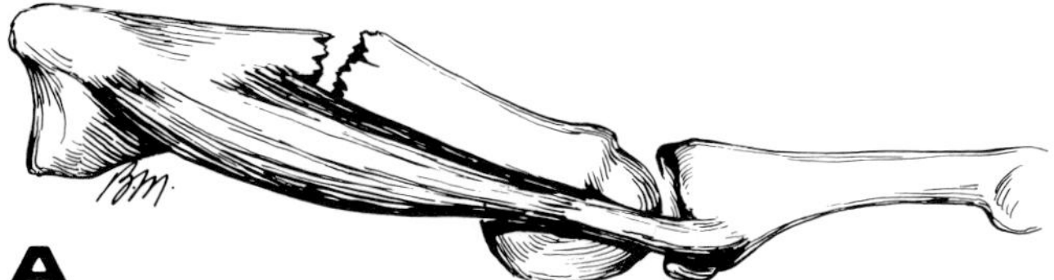

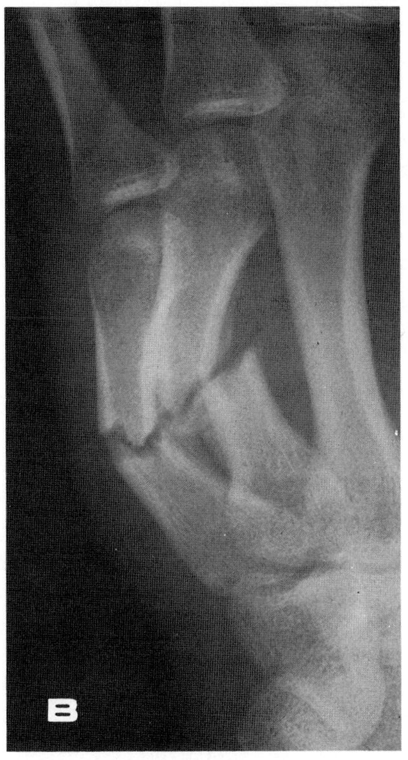

Fig. 6-36. Transverse fractures of the metacarpal are usually the result of a direct blow. (*A*) They generally angulate dorsally because of the interosseous muscles exerting a volar force. (*B*) A roentgenogram showing the typical dorsal angulation of fractures of the metacarpal shafts.

be pushed back easily into alignment with the Jahss[56] technique. The fourth and fifth metacarpals are then immobilized together in an ulnar gutter splint that extends from fingertips to the elbow, with the metacarpophalangeal joints in 45 to 70 degrees flexion, the proximal interphalangeal joints in 20 to 30 degrees flexion, and the distal joints in only a few degrees of flexion. Gentle pressure is applied over the dorsal aspect of the metacarpal just proximal to the fracture site and on the volar surface of the metacarpal head, using the proximal phalanx to help stabilize the metacarpal head. The splint is removed in 3 weeks, and protected motion is begun.

As noted previously, reduction of a metacarpal neck fracture is generally quite simple, but maintenance of that reduction may be difficult. The greater the initial angulation and the more severe the volar cortex comminution, the less likely it is that the reduction can be held with plaster immobilization alone. It has been our experience that functional loss is difficult to predict by measurement of roentgenograms alone and that a simple clinical test should be used in conjunction with them. If the patient is able to extend the fractured finger perfectly straight without clawing, then the fracture is treated by the closed reduction-immobilization method just described. If clawing is apparent with the finger in extension, we feel that the angle is excessive and the likelihood of significant reangulation in plaster is great (Fig. 6-34). For such patients, we prefer to use percutaneous Kirschner wire fixation to hold the reduction achieved by closed manipulation. The fracture may be held either with two transverse pins in the adjacent metacarpal (Fig. 6-35A) or with a Kirschner wire passed obliquely across the fracture site (Fig. 6-35B).

While this technique has been advocated by many authors as a method of allowing early motion, its primary goal in our hands is to stabilize a basically unstable fracture after reduction. If secure fixation is established, early protected use of the hand may be allowed, but equally satisfactory results can be achieved by having the patient wear a plaster gutter splint for 3 weeks until the wires are removed.

Virtually no angulation should be accepted in fractures of the second and third metacarpal necks. Since there is almost invariably some loss of alignment in plaster, we prefer to treat these fractures with closed reduction and percutaneous pin fixation. If a satisfactory reduction cannot be achieved with this method, then anatomical alignment should be restored with open reduction and internal fixation.

FRACTURES OF THE METACARPAL SHAFT

Fractures of the metacarpal shaft are of three types: transverse, oblique, and comminuted.

Transverse Fractures

Transverse fractures are usually the result of a direct blow, and they generally angulate dorsally because of the interosseous muscles exerting a volar force (Fig. 6-36). Following reduction, these fractures may be immobilized with volar and dorsal splints (or a gutter splint), applying three-point pressure to control the angulation. Rotational alignment is more easily maintained by extending the splints nearly to the tips of the fingers and by including an adjacent normal metacarpal. The same principles that apply to angular deformity of neck fractures apply to shaft fractures. No angulation can be accepted in the second and third metacarpals as there is no compensatory motion at the carpometacarpal joints. Some angulation of the fourth and fifth metacarpals may be accepted. The further the fracture is from the metacarpophalangeal joint, the more pronounced the dorsal angulation will appear. Therefore, less angulation can be accepted in mid-shaft fractures than in fractures through the neck (Fig. 6-37). If reduction is necessary, the authors prefer percutaneous fixation with nonthreaded Kirschner wires (0.045-inch), because there is a tendency for the deformity to recur with simple plaster immobilization. This may be accomplished in several different ways.

We prefer Saypool's[102] transverse pinning to an adjacent normal metacarpal, which is more applicable to the border metacarpals (second and fifth) but may also be used for the inner metacarpals (third and fourth). This technique has the advantage of controlling rotational as well as angular deformity.

An alternative method of percutaneous fixation is intramedullary pinning. Following closed reduction by the Jahss[56] method with the metacarpophalangeal joint flexed, a 0.045-inch smooth Kirschner wire is introduced percutaneously through the extensor hood into the metacarpal head and shaft. The wrist is then flexed, and the Kirschner wire is passed through the skin at the wrist level. The wire is then drilled retrograde until the distal end has passed out of the metacarpophalangeal joint, back into the metacarpal head. An intramedullary Kirschner wire such as this will control angulation but not rotation. Therefore, a modified

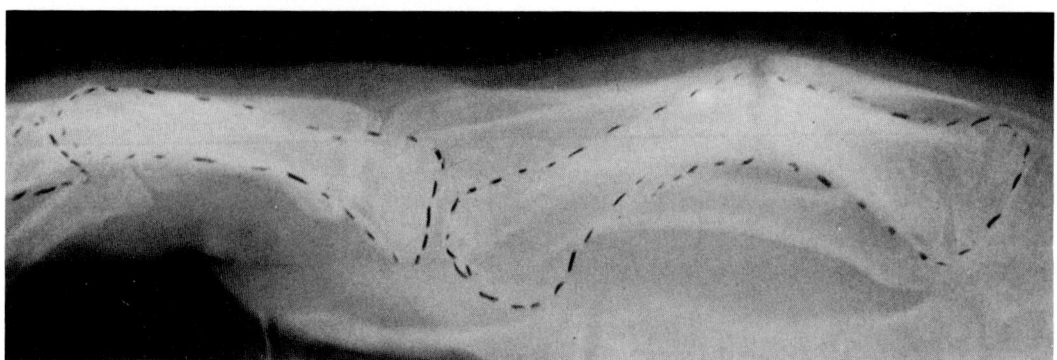

Fig. 6-37. The further the fracture is from the metacarpophalangeal joint the more pronounced the dorsal angulation will appear and the greater the clawing will be. Therefore, less angulation can be accepted in mid-shaft fractures than in fractures through the neck of the metacarpal.

Böhler splint incorporating two fingers should be used. The fingers are freed from the splint after 3 weeks, but the wrist is immobilized to prevent pin irritation at the wrist level until the pins are removed in 5 weeks.

If open reduction is necessary, internal fixation can be accomplished with an intramedullary pin, as described, or with crossed Kirschner wires at the fracture site. Except in grossly contaminated wounds, we generally prefer to use internal fixation in open fractures at the time of initial debridement, because the concomitant soft-tissue swelling usually present makes maintenance of reduction difficult in plaster. As mentioned in the section on phalangeal fractures, open fractures have delayed periods of healing, and therefore the pins should be left in place for at least 6 weeks following open fractures of the metacarpals. Immobilization of the entire hand during this time is not desirable, however, and sufficient stabilization should be established at operation to allow protected movement of the digit beginning at least by the third week.

Several authors have written about the use of small screws[64] and miniature plates[100] in the treatment of metacarpal fractures. We have had no experience with these, since stable internal fixation can usually be achieved with properly placed Kirschner wires.

Oblique Fractures

Oblique fractures of the metacarpal shafts result from a torque force with the finger acting as the long lever.[23] These fractures tend to shorten and rotate rather than angulate. The third and fourth metacarpals tend to shorten less because of the tethering effect of the deep transverse metacarpal ligament, while in the second and fifth metacarpals, shortening or rotation is more likely to be pronounced (Figs. 6-38, 6-39). Two to 3 mm. of shortening may be accepted without loss of function[18] as long as there is no angulation. If significant deformity is present, the fracture should be anatomically reduced and held with Kirschner wires. This is difficult to do without opening the fracture and directly visualizing the site. In oblique fractures, intramedullary wires will not prevent shortening or rotation, and transmetacarpal fixation, while it maintains length, may tend to hold the fracture apart and encourage delayed union. Therefore, oblique or crossed Kirschner wire fixation is preferred at the time of open reduction.

Comminuted Fractures

Comminuted fractures of the metacarpal shafts result from direct blows and frequently are nondisplaced fractures associated with a great deal of soft-tissue damage. A bulky compression dressing initially, to prevent the formation of edema, is adequate immobilization; this is followed by a modified Böhler splint, as described earlier. Discarding the finger outrigger in 3 weeks

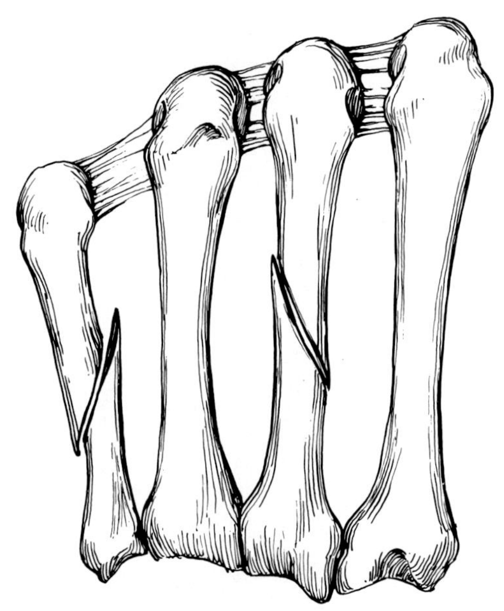

Fig. 6-38. Oblique fractures of the metacarpals tend to shorten and rotate rather than angulate. The third and fourth metacarpals tend to shorten less because of the tethering effect of the deep transverse metacarpal ligament. In the border second and fifth metacarpals, shortening and rotation are likely to be more pronounced.

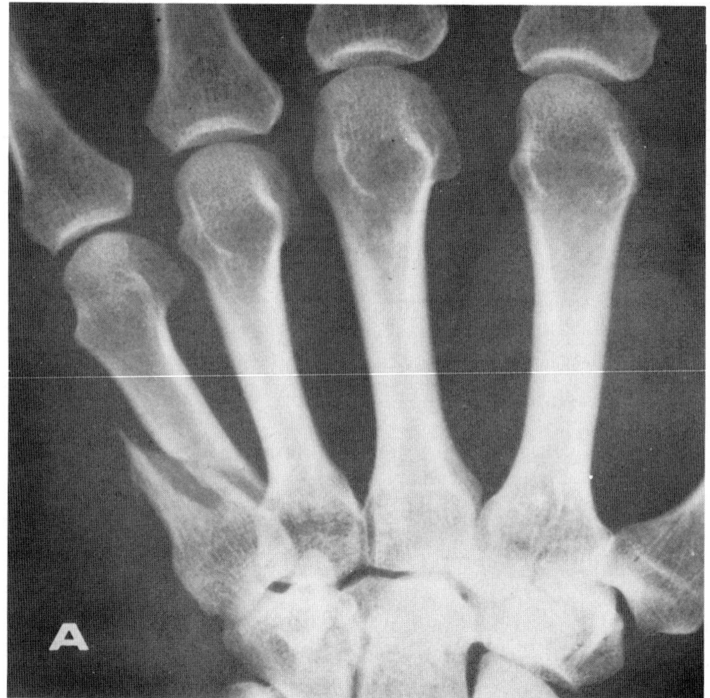

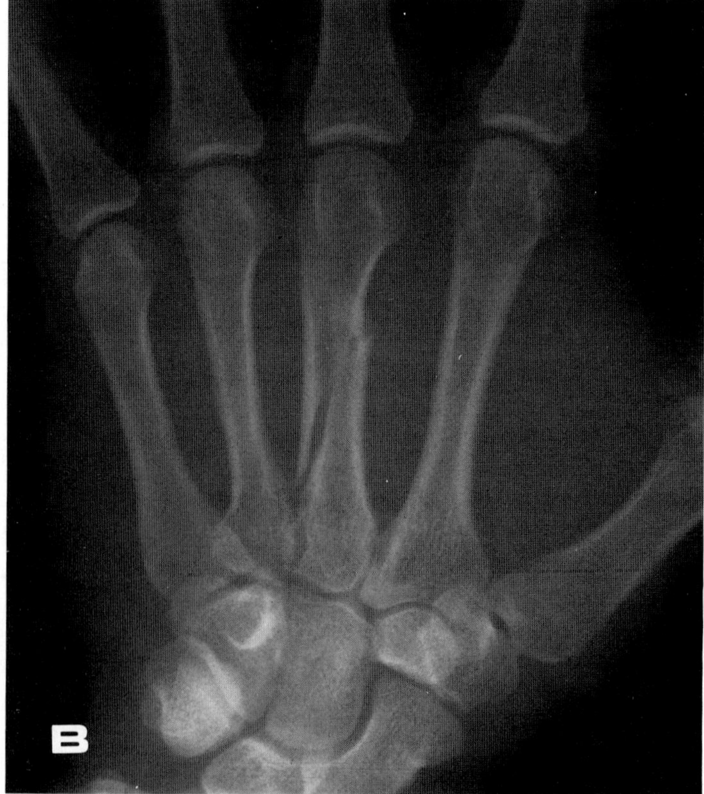

Fig. 6-39. (*A*) An oblique fracture of the proximal shaft of the fifth metacarpal. Note the significant shortening. (*B*) A long oblique fracture of the shaft of the third metacarpal. Note that only minimal shortening has occurred.

is important for early proximal interphalangeal joint motion, particularly if edema was present previously. The volar and dorsal splints can be discarded in 5 weeks, when clinical healing has occurred.

When displacement of bone fragments occurs, open reduction is difficult because of the degree of comminution. Because shortening of the bone tends to occur, transmetacarpal Kirschner wire fixation is the best form of treatment.

In gunshot wounds with bone loss, transmetacarpal Kirschner wire fixation into the adjacent normal metacarpal is an excellent way of maintaining bone length until bone grafting can be carried out.

FRACTURES AT THE BASE OF THE METACARPAL

Fractures at the base of the metacarpal are usually stable; however, one should not assume a complacent attitude regarding these fractures, as the slightest rotation will be greatly magnified at the fingertip. The patient's hand shown in Figure 6-40 demonstrates fractures at the base of the third, fourth, and fifth metacarpals with rotation in all three fingers, leaving a wide gap between the index and long fingers. Since this type of fracture is usually secondary to a crushing injury, the treatment as outlined for comminuted metacarpal shaft fractures should be used. If a fracture at the base of the metacarpal is intraarticular, arthrosis may develop, necessitating an arthrodesis or an arthroplasty of the carpometacarpal joint at a later date.

COMPLICATIONS OF METACARPAL FRACTURES

The complications seen following metacarpal fractures are related to concomitant soft-tissue injury, malunion, overzealous treatment, or improper treatment.

Fractures involving the shafts and bases of the metacarpals are most commonly due to crushing injuries, and the fractures frequently are open, involving several metacarpals. Frequently, there is soft-tissue damage followed by massive edema. Extensor and flexor tendons may be damaged or become adherent to the damaged bone. Interosseous muscles may be damaged, and scarring may result in an intrinsic contracture of the hand.

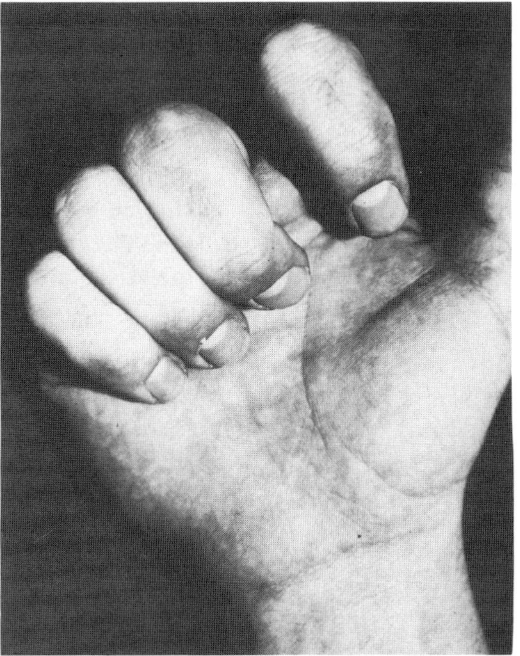

Fig. 6-40. This patient had fractures at the bases of the third, fourth, and fifth metacarpals. All three healed with rotational deformity, leaving a wide gap between the index and long fingers. Correct rotational alignment is particularly difficult to achieve with multiple metacarpal fractures.

Malunion of the metacarpal with the distal fragment angulated into the palm upsets the intrinsic and extrinsic muscle balance, causing a clawed finger and a painful grip.

Rotational malalignment is probably the most important complication of metacarpal fractures, and its prevention must be foremost in the mind of the physician managing these injuries. This problem is particularly likely to occur with fractures of the border metacarpals and is much more difficult to control when more than one metacarpal is fractured (Fig. 6-40). Malunion with rotational deformity may require a rotational osteotomy for correction.[39,93,118]

Stiffness of the proximal and middle finger joints is frequently the result of improper or overzealous treatment. Stiffness of the metacarpophalangeal joint is caused by treating the fracture with this joint in extension, allowing the collateral ligaments to shorten. Stiffness of the proximal interphalangeal joint is caused by holding the joint in acute flexion in the 90-90 position or by immobilizing the joint unnecessarily long.

Pin tract infection, although uncommon, is more apt to occur if the pins are left to protrude through the skin. The patient should be told how to recognize the infection early so that the wire may be removed.

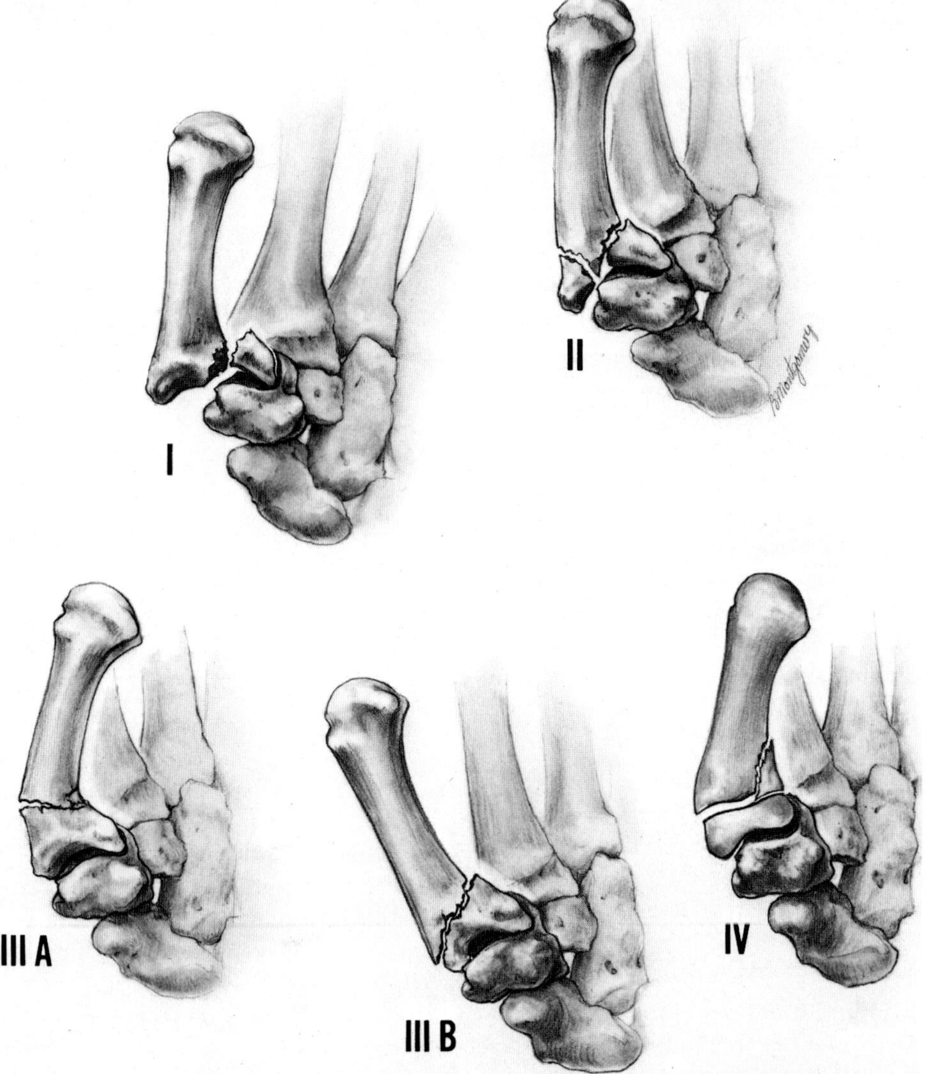

Fig. 6-41. Four distinct fracture patterns may involve the base of the thumb metacarpal. Type I (Bennett's fracture-dislocation) and Type II (Rolando's fracture) are intraarticular. These should be differentiated from the Type III extraarticular fractures, which may be either transverse or oblique. Type IV fractures are epiphyseal injuries seen in children. (Green, D. P. and O'Brien, E. T.: South. Med. J., 65:807, 1972)

FRACTURES OF THE THUMB METACARPAL

The thumb is a unique digit, and fractures of the thumb metacarpal are distinctively different from those in other metacarpals. Most thumb metacarpal fractures occur at or near the base, and therefore a thorough knowledge of the anatomy of the carpometacarpal joint is essential to understanding the mechanism of injury, the pathological anatomy, and the treatment of these fractures. (See p. 327 for a discussion of the pertinent anatomy.)

Classification

Four distinct fracture patterns may involve the base of the thumb metacarpal,[164,168,169] as illustrated in Figure 6-41. It is particularly important to differentiate the intraarticular fractures from the extraarticular types, for management of the two is quite different. Bennett's fracture-dislocation and Rolando's fracture are the intraarticular types, and the extraarticular fracture may have either a transverse or an oblique configuration. The epiphyseal fracture will be excluded from this discussion.

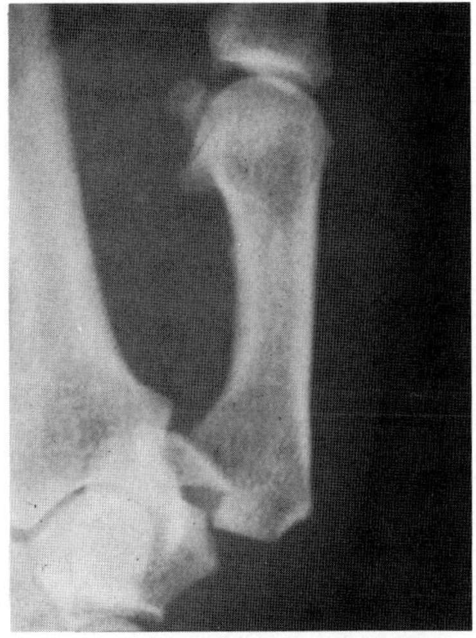

Fig. 6-42. A typical Bennett's fracture-dislocation. The small volar lip fragment remains attached to the anterior oblique ligament which anchors it to the tubercle of the trapezium.

BENNETT'S FRACTURE

More properly called a fracture-dislocation, this injury was first described by Edward Halloran Bennett[155] in 1882 and has been discussed exhaustively in the world literature since that time. The mechanism of injury is an axial blow directed against the partially flexed metacarpal, and not surprisingly, many of these injuries are sustained in fist fights. The fracture line characteristically separates the major part of the metacarpal from a small volar lip fragment, producing disruption of the carpometacarpal joint (Fig. 6-42). That an avulsion fracture occurs rather than a pure dislocation attests to the strength of the anterior oblique ligament, which anchors the volar lip of the metacarpal to the tubercle of the trapezium. The two primary variables of a Bennett's fracture are the size of the volar

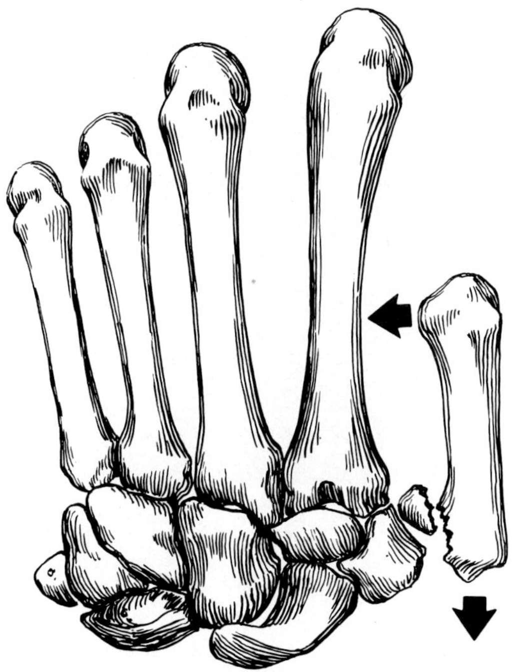

Fig. 6-43. In a Bennett's fracture, the base of the metacarpal is pulled dorsally and radially by the abductor pollicis longus, while the adductor further levers the base into abduction.

lip fragment and the amount of displacement of the shaft. The base of the metacarpal is pulled dorsally and radially by the abductor pollicis longus, while the distal attachment of the adductor further levers the base into abduction (Fig. 6-43).

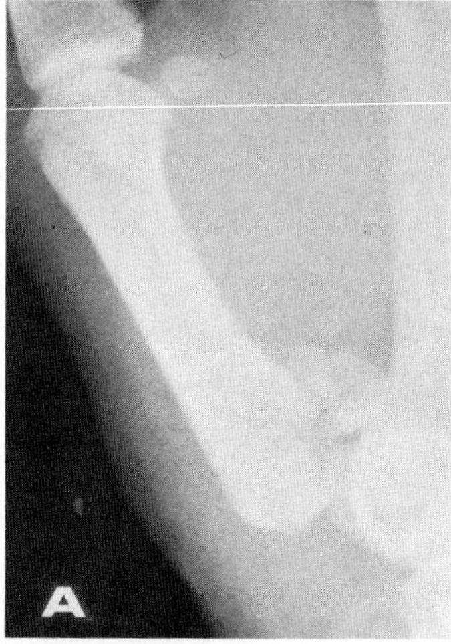

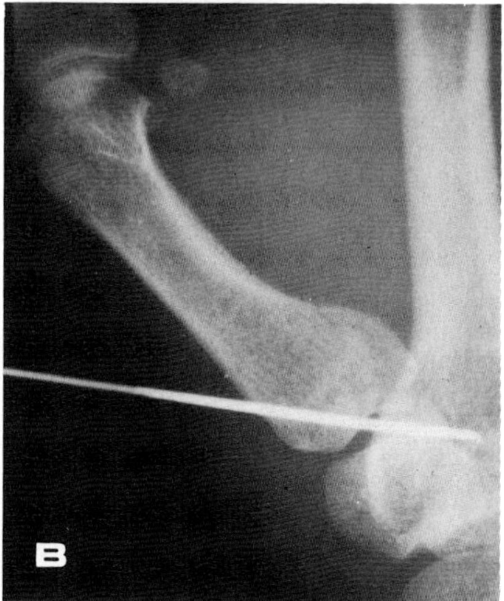

Fig. 6-44. Our preferred method of treatment for Bennett's fracture is an initial attempt at closed reduction and percutaneous pin fixation. (*A*) A typical Bennett's fracture-dislocation. (*B*) Anatomical reduction was achieved by closed reduction and percutaneous pinning. Note that no attempt is made to transfix the small volar fragment; rather the shaft of the metacarpal is held in the reduced position after a reduction has been achieved by closed manipulation.

Methods of Treatment

At least 18 different methods of treatment have been advocated for Bennett's fracture. At one end of the therapeutic spectrum is Blum,[157] who proposed that reduction of the fracture was not necessary and that good results could be achieved with early active motion. Charnley,[158] Roberts,[171] Böhler,[19] and Griffiths[165] separately advocated the use of a well-molded plaster cast. Griffiths[165] reported that even in unreduced Bennett's fractures, the results were not bad, noting that although these patients had some limitation of motion, they were generally free of pain. He concluded that the importance of the joint involvement in this fracture was generally overestimated.

Gibson and James[162] and Pollen[170] incorporated a felt pad into their casts to prevent the loss of reduction which frequently occurred with plaster alone. Robinson[172] and Watson-Jones[116] each advocated the use of continuous skin traction in addition to a cast, and Bunnell[28] described the method of skeletal traction that has been used rather extensively in the treatment of Bennett's fracture. Thoren[175,176,177] devised a unique method of applying oblique skeletal traction by means of a hook inserted into the base of the first metacarpal. He believed that traction should be applied in the direction of adduction and opposition rather than abduction to bring the displaced shaft back into alignment with the volar lip fragment.

Numerous types of external splints have been advocated, including the Goldthwaite splint[159] and Goldberg's felt pad[163] attached to an outrigger. Ross and Sinclair[174] treated a series of patients with the Stader splint, a forerunner of the Roger Anderson device. Closed reduction and percutaneous pin fixation was originally described by Johnson,[167] utilizing Waugh and Ferrazzano's[117] technique of transfixing a fractured metacarpal to an adjacent one. Wagner[178] later modified this method further by passing the pins from the shaft of the first metacarpal into the trapezium rather than into the second metacarpal. Wiggins, Bundens, and Park[179] used intramedullary wire fixation following closed reduction because of difficulty in positioning the wires in the manner described by Wagner.

Ellis,[160] in 1946, was apparently the first to advocate open reduction, although in his technique the fracture site was not actually exposed. Instead, he reduced the base of the metacarpal and passed small pins into the trapezium, leaving them protruding as a buttress to hold the reduction of the metacarpal. Gedda and Moberg[161] have been the prime advocates of open reduction and anatomical restoration of the fracture under direct vision. The results of Gedda's comprehensive study led him to conclude that exact open reduction produced results consistently superior to those achieved by simple plaster immobilization. Badger[153] used a small screw for fixation, obviating the need for plaster immobilization postoperatively.

Authors' Preferred Method of Treatment

The reports of good results from each of the above methods pose a perplexing dilemma for the surgeon choosing a plan of treatment for his patient with a Bennett's fracture. The very fact that so many different types of splinting, traction, and other methods of immobilization have been described implies that it is often difficult to achieve and maintain reduction of the articular surface by nonoperative means. Although some patients with malunited Bennett's fractures may indeed remain relatively asymptomatic despite the roentgenographic deformity, we believe that exact anatomical reduction of the fracture is the most reliable method of achieving consistently good results. A single attempt at closed manipulation and percutaneous pinning is usually performed (Fig. 6-44), but unless the roentgenogram reveals exact restoration of the articular surface, we believe that open reduction should be carried out (Fig. 6-45). Internal fixation under direct visualization is established with two fine Kirschner wires, and occasionally a separate pin is passed across the carpometacarpal joint for added support. A thumb plaster spica is worn for 4 to 6 weeks, after which the pin transfixing the joint is removed and active motion is begun. The wires holding the fracture are left in place for at least 6 to 8 weeks, because bony union of this intraarticular fracture is often slower than that of a fracture of the metacarpal shaft.

ROLANDO'S FRACTURE

In 1910, Silvio Rolando[172] described a fracture pattern that differed from the classic Bennett's fracture-dislocation. In the

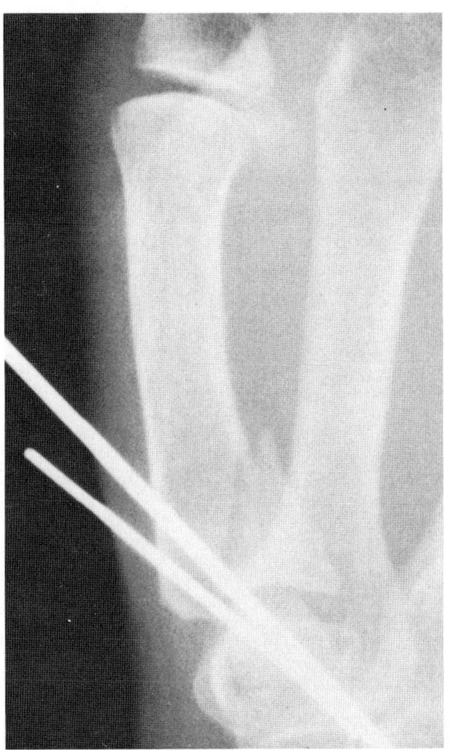

Fig. 6-45. A Bennett's fracture in which a successful reduction was not achieved by the closed method. We believe that inadequate reduction such as this should not be accepted. Either a second attempt at closed reduction or open reduction and internal fixation should be done.

fracture he reported, there was, in addition to the volar lip fragment, a large dorsal fragment, resulting in a **Y**- or **T**-shaped intraarticular fracture. Although the classic Rolando's fracture is that pictured in Figure 6-41, it should probably more properly be thought of as simply a *comminuted Bennett's* fracture, for in many instances instead of having the simple **Y**- or **T**-configuration, it may be severely comminuted. Rolando pointed out that the prognosis was poor following this injury, despite treatment either in a cast or with skin traction. More than 60 years later it remains a difficult fracture to treat, but fortunately it is the least common of the adult thumb metacarpal fractures.

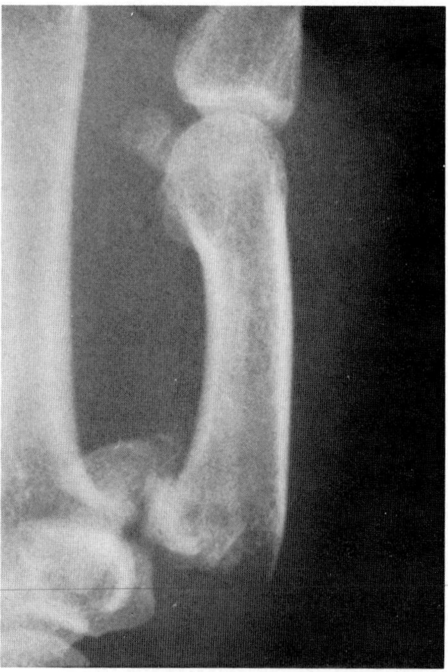

Fig. 6-46. A Rolando's fracture rarely has only the large dorsal and volar fragments. More commonly, it is severely comminuted, as illustrated here. In fractures such as this, open reduction and anatomical restoration of the articular surface is virtually impossible and should not be attempted. (Green, D. P. and O'Brien, E. T.: South. Med. J., *65*:807, 1972)

Methods of Treatment

The choice of treatment depends primarily on the severity of comminution of the fragments and, to a lesser extent, on the degree of displacement. Open reduction and internal fixation should be attempted *only* if the volar and dorsal components are single large fragments. More commonly, however, the base of the metacarpal is shattered into many fragments and attempts at operative restoration are frustrating, if not impossible (Fig. 6-46). In such severely comminuted fractures, some authors prefer the use of skeletal traction in an attempt to pull the articular surface back into some semblance of alignment. Before applying skeletal traction, however, it is advisable to take a roentgenogram while a longitudinal traction force is applied, to see if there has been any improvement in the articular surface. If the joint surface has been reasonably restored, a period of traction is justified, but if not, little will be gained from the use of traction. When the comminution is severe, we prefer to immobilize the thumb for a minimal period of time to relieve pain and then begin early active motion in an attempt to remold the badly distorted articular surface. Because of the infrequency of Rolando's fracture, no one has reported a series comparing the results of different forms of treatment. In our experience, the tendency in the past has been to err on the side of overtreatment (i.e., to attempt open reduction when it was virtually impossible to restore the articular surface). We repeat that significant comminution is a definite contraindication to operative treatment of this injury.

EXTRAARTICULAR FRACTURES

The extraarticular type is the most frequent fracture in the thumb metacarpal, and, fortunately, the simplest to treat. Two basic patterns are seen (Fig. 6-47): a transverse fracture and a less common oblique one. It is particularly important to distinguish these extraarticular fractures from the

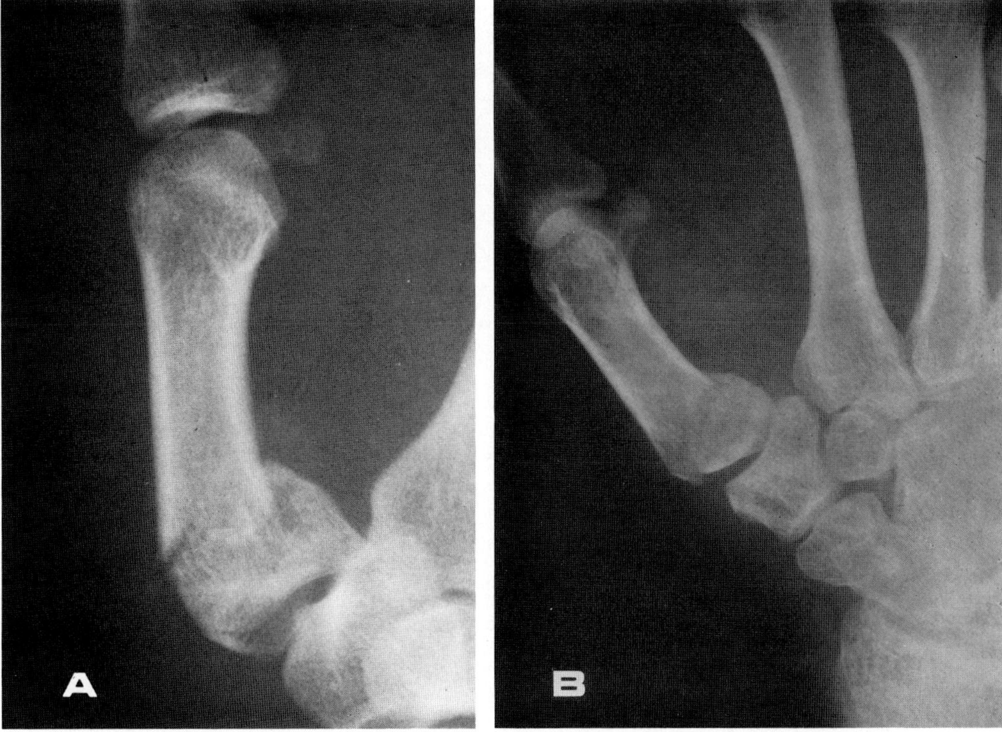

Fig. 6-47. It is particularly important to distinguish these extraarticular thumb metacarpal fractures from the intraarticular varieties. (*A*) The most common fracture of the thumb metacarpal is a transverse extraarticular type. (*B*) Less commonly seen is an oblique extraarticular fracture. This is the fracture that is most frequently confused with a Bennett's fracture. Careful examination of the roentgenogram reveals that the fracture line does not enter the joint.

more serious intraarticular Bennett's and Rolando's fractures, for rarely, if ever, is surgery indicated in the management of the extraarticular fractures. This differentiation is usually not difficult on careful study of the roentgenograms, although the oblique type may appear at first glance to be a Bennett's fracture. The distinguishing feature, of course, is that in the oblique extraarticular type, the fracture line does not enter the joint.

Treatment

One should resist the temptation to overtreat these extraarticular fractures. Anatomical reduction can usually be achieved readily by closed manipulation under regional or local anesthesia; the thumb is immobilized in a short-arm thumb spica for 4 weeks. Care must be taken to avoid hyperextension of the metacarpophalangeal joint in plaster. Failure to achieve exact alignment of the fracture should not be considered an indication for open reduction. At the very worst, the patient with an inadequately reduced transverse fracture is likely to have only a slight prominence at the base of the thumb and possibly some minimal limitation of thumb abduction. Even with 20 to 30 degrees of residual angulation, however, there is usually no detectable limitation of motion.

Occasionally the oblique type of extraarticular fracture may prove to be somewhat unstable, particularly if there is marked vertical inclination of the fracture line. Even in this type of fracture, however, open reduction is not warranted. If plaster immobilization is unsuccessful in holding the reduction, percutaneous pinning provides a simple method of securing the reduction achieved by closed manipulation.

DISLOCATIONS AND LIGAMENTOUS INJURIES OF THE INTERPHALANGEAL JOINTS

The proximal interphalangeal joint occupies a position of unique importance in the hand. Loss of motion in this joint severely restricts function. Conversely, if flexion and extension can be maintained in the proximal interphalangeal joint when there is significant damage in the other small joints of the same finger, satisfactory hand function can be preserved. Unfortunately, the propensity for stiffness in the proximal interphalangeal joint is great, not only following injury to the joint itself, but even after prolonged immobilization of an otherwise normal joint. For this reason, the utmost care and concern should be given to injuries involving the proximal interphalangeal joint, and unnecessary immobilization of this joint should be avoided when other injuries in the hand are treated.

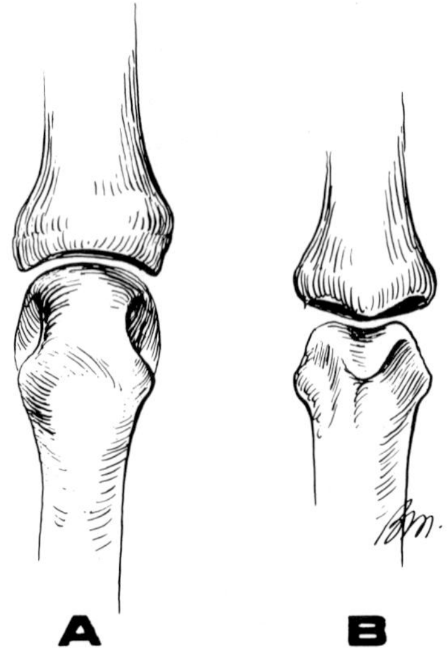

Fig. 6-48. Comparison of the metacarpophalangeal and proximal interphalangeal joints as seen in the anteroposterior view. (*A*) The metacarpophalangeal joint is a condyloid joint in which the globular head of the metacarpal articulates with the reciprocally concave base of the proximal phalanx. It allows flexion, extension, abduction, adduction, and a limited amount of circumduction. (*B*) The proximal interphalangeal joint is essentially a ginglymus or hinge joint, allowing only flexion and extension. It is inherently more stable than the metacarpophalangeal joint, by virtue of its bicondylar configuration, which gives it a modified tongue-in-groove appearance.

Anatomy

The proximal interphalangeal joint, although in some ways similar to the metacarpophalangeal joint, has numerous important differences which have been pointed out by Kuczynski.[11] The proximal interphalangeal joint is essentially a ginglymus or hinge joint, allowing only flexion and extension. It is inherently more stable than the metacarpophalangeal joint, by virtue of its bicondylar configuration, which gives it a modified tongue-in-groove appearance (Fig-6-48). The shape of the head of the proximal phalanx is less eccentric than that of the metacarpal head as seen in the lateral view, and, therefore, the cam effect is less significant (Fig. 6-49).

The collateral ligaments of the proximal interphalangeal joint are similar to those in the metacarpophalangeal joint, with a cord-like collateral ligament proper and a lower

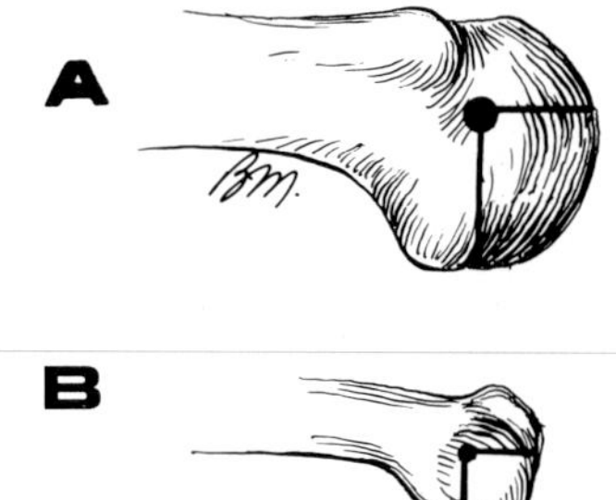

Fig. 6-49. Comparison of the metacarpophalangeal (*A*) and proximal interphalangeal (*B*) joints as seen in the lateral view. The shape of the head of the proximal phalanx is less eccentric than that of the metacarpal head as seen in the lateral view, and therefore, the cam effect is less significant in the interphalangeal joint.

accessory ligament (Fig. 6-50). The major difference lies in the fact that tension in these ligaments is essentially the same in flexion as it is in extension. This is due primarily to two factors: the absence of the cam effect and the parallel alignment of the collateral ligaments, as compared to the divergence of the ligaments in the metacarpophalangeal joint. The result of these anatomical peculiarities is that, while all parts of the collateral ligaments of the proximal interphalangeal joint are tight in flexion, the volar fibers of the ligament are also tight in extension.[3]

Range of motion in the proximal interphalangeal joint is usually from 0 to 105 degrees, and in many fingers flexion of 120 degrees is easily obtained. As in the metacarpophalangeal joint, the volar plate at this level has a firm distal attachment to the base of the middle phalanx and a more flexible proximal attachment to the neck of the proximal phalanx to allow folding with flexion of the joint. Kuczynski[11] has suggested that the volar plate is less mobile in the proximal interphalangeal joint than it is in the metacarpophalangeal joint.

Dorsally and dorsolaterally the extensor hood mechanism envelopes the joint, while on its volar aspect the volar plate separates the joint from the flexor tendons. (For more detailed descriptions of the ligamentous anatomy around the proximal interphalangeal joint, the reader is referred to the monograph by Milford[13] and the articles by Haines,[9] Landsmeer,[12] and Tubiana and Valentin.[15])

Classification

Injuries of the proximal interphalangeal joints may be classified as collateral ligament injuries, volar plate injuries, dislocations, and fracture-dislocations. In practice, the most important clinical consideration in these injuries is to distinguish between those that are stable and those that are unstable. As a general rule, those that are stable are easy to treat and have the best prognosis.

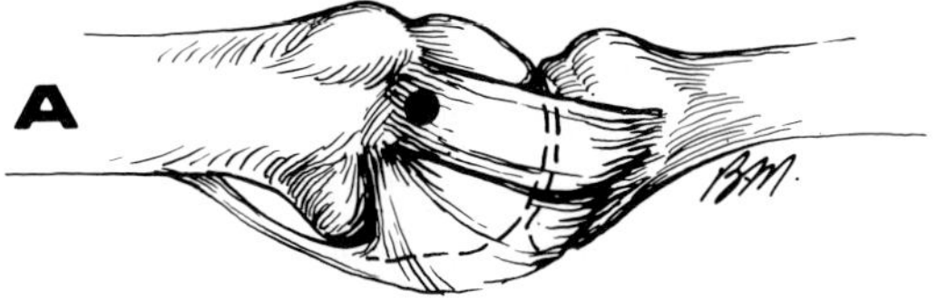

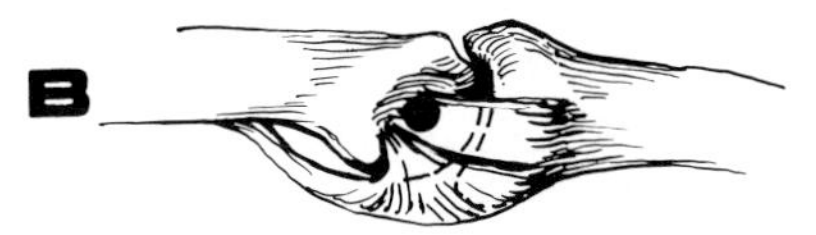

Fig. 6-50. The collateral ligaments of the metacarpophalangeal (*A*) and proximal interphalangeal (*B*) joints are similar. Both have a cordlike collateral ligament proper and a lower accessory ligament, which attaches directly into the volar plate.

COLLATERAL LIGAMENT INJURIES

Collateral ligament injuries are caused by abduction or adduction force applied to the finger, usually in the extended position.[196] Because of the long lever arm, the injury usually involves the proximal interphalangeal joint and is most frequently seen in sports as football, wrestling, baseball, and basketball. The injury is more common in the right hand and involves the radial collateral ligament more often than the ulnar collateral ligament.

Collateral ligament injuries may be classified as acute or chronic, and further subclassified as stable or unstable injuries. McCue and his colleagues[196] defined acute injuries in their series of patients as those diagnosed within 3 months of injury; the majority occurred within 3 weeks. It is the authors' opinion that any injury of the collateral ligament diagnosed after 6 weeks should be classified as an old or chronic injury and that the predictable results following collateral ligament repair are uncertain 3 weeks after injury.

Diagnosis

Apart from the initial pain, the symptoms following an acute injury are often mild, which explains why many patients seek medical attention late.[199] Well localized tenderness at the site of injury and pain on lateral stress are the usual findings. Lateral instability is demonstrable in patients with complete rupture and should be routinely tested for with the joint in extension in all patients with joint injuries.

In the patients with chronic or old collateral ligament injuries, where treatment has been ineffective or when no primary treatment was instituted, two signs are prominent: instability and swelling.[199] Instability may result from the ligament healing in elongation, or there may be total loss of continuity. Swelling at the site of collateral ligament injury is, at times, severe and quite painful, and it may be the patient's main complaint. This may be associated with limitation of joint motion. Swelling is due to excessive reparative connective tissue, which has been described by Moberg[199] as ligamentous callus.

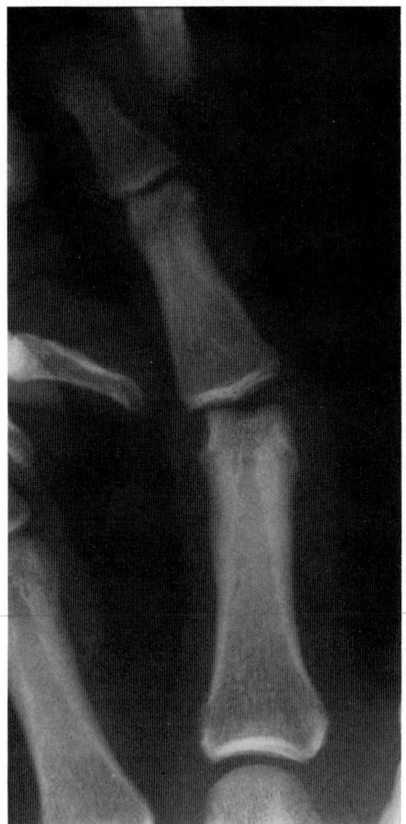

Fig. 6-51. A stress roentgenogram of the proximal interphalangeal joint, showing apparent rupture of the radial collateral ligament.

Partial tears of the collateral ligament can be difficult to differentiate from complete ruptures on clinical examination alone; therefore, when instability is suspected, stress roentgenograms should be compared with those of a finger of the opposite hand (Fig. 6-51).

Treatment

Acute Injuries with Partial Rupture. Most authors agree that incomplete tears of the collateral ligament should be treated with 2 to 5 weeks of dynamic splinting or immobilization,[196,199] depending on the degree of severity.

It has been our practice to grade incomplete collateral ligament injuries as follows: Grade I, local tenderness over the ligament but no instability; Grade II, mild instability; and Grade III, moderate instability but without evidence of complete rupture of the ligament. These are only subjective assessments of joint instability, but they are useful to us in planning treatment for individual patients. A Grade I collateral ligament injury is treated with the buddy system by taping the injured finger to the adjacent normal finger, maintaining and encouraging active joint motion. A Grade III collateral ligament injury is immobilized with a splint for 5 weeks with the joint flexed 35 degrees. Most ligamentous injuries are intermediate Grade II injuries and are immobilized for 3 weeks. Following the period of initial immobilization, guarded active motion is allowed with the buddy system, so that the joint is protected from further injury for a total of 6 weeks from the time treatment was instituted. No formal physical therapy is used other than active exercises. Occasionally, if persistent stiffness occurs, passive splinting to obtain a full range of motion may be necessary.

Acute Injuries with Complete Rupture. There is a difference of opinion concerning the treatment of complete ruptures of the collateral ligament. Some authors recommend splinting,[198,199] while others advise immediate surgical repair.[190,196,202] Still others[186] recommend that complete ruptures be treated with immobilization for 3 to 4 weeks and then be reevaluated. If there is instability, it is corrected operatively.

We agree with Redler[202] and McCue[196] that acute injuries with complete rupture of the collateral ligament should be operatively repaired at the time of injury, but only if complete rupture is unequivocally demonstrated by stress films or a displaced avulsion fracture. The most common lesion found at operation is separation of the collateral ligament from its proximal attachment. In half of Redler's patients, the retracted portion of the ligament was folded into the joint and had to be extracted at the time of surgery. A partial tear of the volar plate is usually associated with the injury.

Chronic or Old Complete Ruptures. Symptoms of pain and functional disability after a collateral ligament rupture are usually due to the ligament healing in an elongated state.[199] Moberg,[199] Redler,[202] and McCue[196] believe that without operation the prognosis of many total ruptures is poor and that operative procedures to correct the instability usually result in freedom from pain and satisfactory stability. The operative procedures recommended are reconstruction of a new ligament with a free graft, reattachment of the old ligament at the site of rupture, or shortening of the ligament if it healed in an elongated state.

The authors believe that asymptomatic instability or instability with minimal pain is not, in itself, an indication for operation. Late repair of old ruptures of the collateral ligament should be reserved for those patients with instability who also have significant pain or disability.

VOLAR PLATE INJURIES

Ruptures of the volar plate of the proximal interphalangeal joints are not uncommon and can produce a considerable degree of functional disturbance.[199] These ruptures usually result from a blow on the end of a finger causing a hyperextension force. The volar plate is usually torn from its distal attachment at the base of the middle phalanx,[196] and at times a small piece of bone may be avulsed by the volar plate.

Volar plate injuries may be grouped into acute injuries, which are usually seen within 6 weeks, and chronic or late injuries, which have not been treated or have not responded to conservative treatment.

Diagnosis. Hyperextension deformity of the proximal interphalangeal joint on extension of the finger associated with pain and catching or locking with flexion are the patient's usual complaints. If the hyperextension deformity is severe enough, the patient will have a compensatory flexion deformity of the distal interphalangeal joint secondary to the tenodesing effect of the flexor digitorum profundus tendon (Fig.

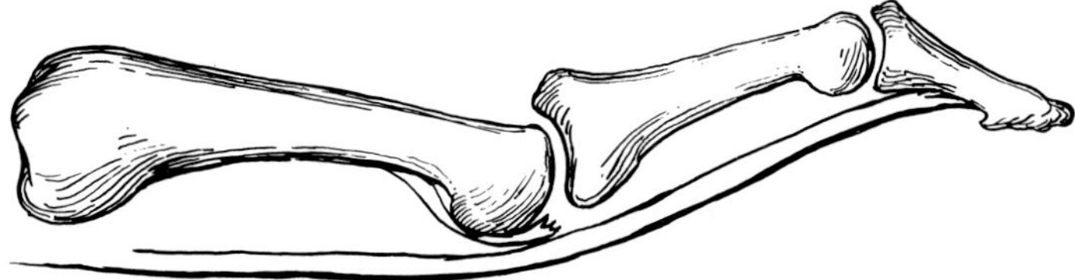

Fig. 6-52. Volar plate injuries of the proximal interphalangeal joint may result in hyperextension deformity of the joint. Some patients may also have a compensatory flexion deformity of the distal interphalangeal joint secondary to the tenodesing effect of the flexor digitorum profundus tendon.

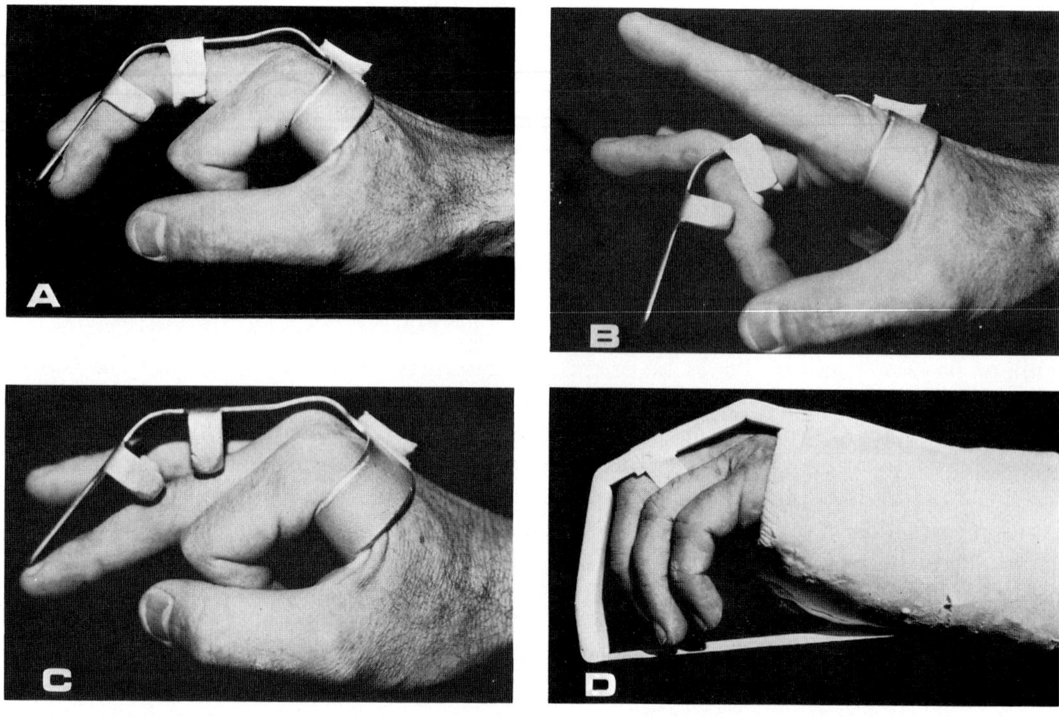

Fig. 6-53. The dorsal extension block splint is useful in treating some injuries of the proximal interphalangeal joint. Extension of the proximal interphalangeal joint can be limited to a predetermined angle (*A*), while at the same time active flexion can be carried out by the patient (*B*). It is particularly important to secure the proximal phalanx to the splint, for if this is not done, flexion of the metacarpophalangeal joint allows extension of the proximal interphalangeal joint, thereby negating the function of the splint (*C*). A custom-made orthosis is not necessary. The simplest way to construct the dorsal extension block splint is with a plaster gauntlet and a malleable outrigger which is firmly attached to the volar aspect of the cast to prevent bending in extension (*D*).

6-52). If the injury involves the index finger, the patient may also complain of loss of power of pinch. Examination of the finger reveals local tenderness over the volar aspect of the joint, pain on passive hyperextension with relief on passive flexion, and instability of the joint with loss of the normal checkrein effect of the volar plate on passive extension.

Roentgenographic examination taken with the finger in extension may reveal the abnormal hyperextension deformity of the proximal interphalangeal joint, particularly when compared with a normal finger. Small bone fragments avulsed from the base of the middle phalanx may be present, but usually early roentgenograms show no bone involvement. Late films may show fragments of periosteum that have calcified following the detachment.

Treatment. Following acute injuries, Moberg[199] recommends splinting the proximal interphalangeal joint in 30 degrees flexion for 3 to 5 weeks. It has been our policy to immobilize the joint in 30 degrees flexion for 3 weeks, followed by active flexion with an extension block splint set at 15 degrees of flexion for an additional 2 weeks (Fig. 6-53).

Chronic injuries with a persistent hyperextension deformity and disabling symptoms without joint arthrosis have been treated by most authors by reattaching the volar plate to the base of the proximal phalanx, reconstructing a volar checkrein, which prevents the last 15 degrees of extension of the proximal interphalangeal joint, or a combination of both.[28,180,182,184,194,199,201,204,208]

We have had occasion to reattach the volar plate and also to use one limb of the sublimis as a tenodesis of the proximal interphalangeal joint. Whatever procedure is used, as long as the joint is blocked in 10 to 15 degrees of flexion, the symptoms should be alleviated if there is no arthrosis in the joint.

DISLOCATIONS OF THE PROXIMAL INTERPHALANGEAL JOINT

Dislocations are of two types (Fig. 6-54), the common posterior dislocation and the rare anterior dislocation.

Posterior Dislocation

The frequency of posterior dislocation is unknown, as reduction is frequently accomplished at the time of injury by simple traction on the finger by a spectator, coach, trainer, or the patient himself. The mechanism of injury is hyperextension of the proximal interphalangeal joint. A frequent cause is when the outstretched finger is struck with a ball. Even though the majority of these injuries apparently "get well" by themselves, it is difficult to visualize how complete dislocation of the proximal interphalangeal joint can occur without rupture of a collateral ligament or of the volar plate. Moberg[199] states that a dislocation of any of the joints of the hand hardly ever occurs without total rupture of at least one ligament. This statement is further supported by McCue's[196] experience with open posterior dislocations of the proximal interphalangeal joint in 13 patients, all of whom were operated on immediately. All had complete ruptures of the volar plates.

Diagnosis. Acute swelling and pain accompanied by deformity are the characteristic findings. Posterior dislocation is confirmed by roentgenograms, which should be taken before reduction if possible. Follow-

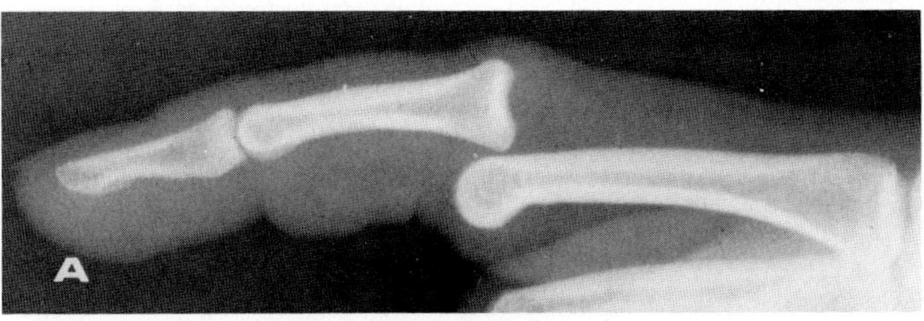

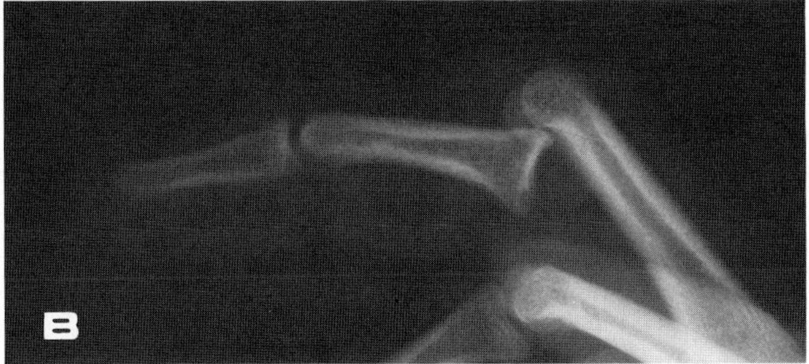

Fig. 6-54. Dislocations of the proximal interphalangeal joints are of two types: (*A*) the common posterior dislocation and (*B*) the rare anterior dislocation. Although both of these dislocations are easy to reduce, the anterior dislocation carries with it a far greater likelihood of permanent impairment because of rupture of the central slip (*see text*).

ing reduction, roentgenography should be repeated, because small avulsed fragments, which suggest complete ligament rupture, may not be visualized on the prereduction films. Following reduction, careful examination of the volar plate and collateral ligament stability is essential.

Treatment. Some authors treat acute dislocations by splinting with the proximal interphalangeal joint flexed approximately 15 degrees for 3 weeks, feeling that this will give the best opportunity for the injured volar plate to heal.

If the proximal interphalangeal joint is stable following dislocation, it has been our policy to start early motion but to protect the joint for 3 weeks by taping the injured finger to an adjacent normal finger. If, on the other hand, instability can be demonstrated, rigid splinting is carried out for 3 weeks with the proximal interphalangeal joint flexed 15 degrees. This is followed by active flexion with a dorsal splint blocking proximal interphalangeal joint extension 15 degrees short of full extension (Fig. 6-53) for an additional 3 weeks.

Associated collateral ligament injuries, although uncommon, should be diagnosed and treated as described on page 311.

Complications. Restricted joint motion, persistent thickening of the proximal interphalangeal joint, volar plate instability, associated collateral ligament instability, traumatic arthritis, and irreducible dislocations may result from posterior dislocation of the proximal interphalangeal joint.

One of the most common complaints following this injury is persistent thickening of the joint. Patients should be told that in all probability the joint will remain somewhat enlarged indefinitely, although that will not necessarily impair normal function of the finger.

Although most posterior dislocations of the proximal interphalangeal joint are easily reduced by closed methods, occasionally one is irreducible because of soft-tissue interposition. Tissues that sometimes have been found to prevent reduction are: a torn volar plate folded in the joint,[193,199] interposition of the profundus tendon, and interposition of a lateral band of the extensor apparatus.[192,200] In order to reduce these complex dislocations, the soft tissue must be removed operatively from the joint.

Anterior Dislocation

Anterior dislocations of the proximal interphalangeal joints are rare but important to recognize, as invariably the central slip of the extensor mechanism is torn from its insertion into the base of the middle phalanx. If the injury is not treated properly, a boutonniere deformity will develop.

In studying the pathogenesis of this injury on 30 fresh cadaver fingers, Spinner and Choi[205] found that anterior dislocation is caused by a combination of forces: a varus or valgus force producing a rupture of a collateral ligament and the volar plate, and an anteriorly directed force that displaces the base of the middle phalanx forward, rupturing the central slip of the extensor mechanism.

Treatment. Anterior dislocations are easily reduced and because of this, the important soft-tissue disruptions are occasionally missed and therefore inadequately treated. As previously mentioned, an ensuing boutonniere deformity will result unless the central slip heals satisfactorily. Operative repair of the central slip and collateral ligaments followed by immobilization of the joint in full extension with a small Kirschner wire for 3 weeks has been Spinner and Choi's[205] recommendation. We prefer to treat these injuries after reduction in the same manner as an acute closed boutonniere lesion (see p. 290); i.e., immobilization of the proximal interphalangeal joint in full extension for 5 weeks. Although we realize that there is greater propensity for stiffness following this injury because there is more extensive soft-tissue damage, a shorter period of immobilization is not sufficient to prevent a residual boutonniere deformity.

FRACTURE-DISLOCATION

Fracture-dislocation of the proximal interphalangeal joint is a relatively uncommon injury, which results from an extended finger being struck in such a fashion that longitudinal compression combined with hyperextension causes a fracture through the volar lip of the middle phalanx and a dorsal displacement of the middle phalanx and distal portion of the finger (Fig. 6-55). In over half the patients in one series[209] and in all of those of another,[203] the injury occurred as a result of an extended finger being struck by a ball.

Diagnosis

Acute swelling and pain are the usual findings following injury. Because of the degree of swelling, the deformity of the dorsal subluxation many times is not appreciated. Without roentgenograms, the diagnosis is often missed. The one constant physical finding is the inability of the patient to flex fully the middle joint of the finger.

Roentgenograms reveal a dorsal subluxation or dislocation of the middle phalanx on the proximal phalanx, associated with a fracture of the volar lip of the middle phalanx. The fractured fragment may be very small; however, in most instances it involves the volar one third of the articular surface of the middle phalanx. Roentgenograms fail to reveal the amount of cartilaginous damage, and therefore the size of the fracture cannot be used as the sole criterion for determining the future function of the joint.[209]

Methods of Treatment

Both closed and operative treatments have been advocated for the management of this difficult injury.

Robertson, Crawley, and Faris[203] used skeletal traction in a three-direction pull arranged on a banjo splint. Curtis[187,188] has stated that comminuted volar lip fracture-dislocations are best treated in this fashion. Schulze[204] reduced the fracture and the dislocation by traction and then immobilized the finger in acute flexion with a dorsal splint. At the end of a week or 10 days, the finger was gradually extended while immobilization continued. At the end of 3 weeks, the splint was removed, and active and passive exercises were started. Spray[206] described a similar technique wherein the finger is taped in extreme flexion. McElfresh, Dobyns, and O'Brien[197] modified the technique by using the extension block splint. These authors permit active flexion of the proximal interphalangeal joint immediately but block extension 10 to 15 degrees short of the demonstrated position of instability.

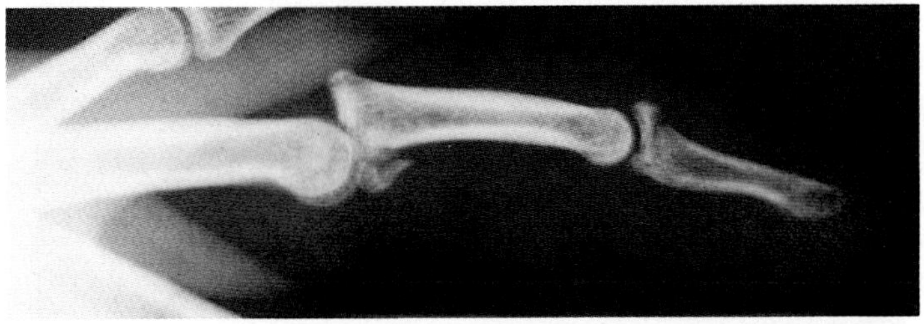

Fig. 6-55. A classic fracture-dislocation of the proximal interphalangeal joint. There is a volar lip fracture, which is frequently comminuted, as in this patient, and the middle phalanx subluxates dorsally on the proximal phalanx. The injury is frequently missed initially because of the lack of gross clinical deformity and the failure to take an isolated true lateral roentgenogram of the involved digit.

The angle of extension blocking is reduced about 25 per cent each week. Full extension is not permitted for 6 to 12 weeks.

Others[185,196,209] have advocated open reduction and internal fixation of the volar fragment, holding the reduced joint in place with a transarticular unthreaded Kirschner wire for 3 weeks, after which the wire is removed and joint motion is started. The Kirschner wire holding the volar fragment in place is removed once healing has taken place, usually in 6 to 8 weeks.

Authors' Preferred Method of Treatment

When the volar fragment is very small and the joint is stable, the injury is treated as a volar plate injury (see p. 313). The joint is splinted in flexion for 3 weeks, then in a dorsal extension block splint for 2 more, during which time the finger is allowed to extend progressively more each week. Use of the dorsal extension block splint from the outset is also an excellent method of treatment.[197]

In the unstable fracture-dislocation, if the volar fragment is a single large fragment, it is our feeling that open reduction and internal fixation best restores the articular joint surface and the buttressing effect of the volar lip, which assures joint stability. This is carried out as described by Wilson and Rowland.[209] It is a difficult operation; postoperative stiffness is common, and a long period of passive splinting is needed to restore maximum active range of motion.

If the volar lip is comminuted (Fig. 6-56), internal fixation is difficult or impossible. In such cases, we recommend the

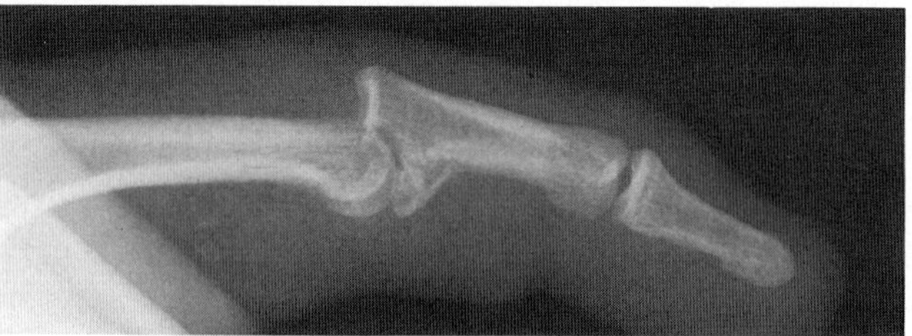

Fig. 6-56. If the volar lip fragment of a fracture-dislocation is severely comminuted and involves a large percentage of the articular surface as in this patient, internal fixation is difficult or impossible. In such cases we recommend the dorsal extension block splint method of treatment.

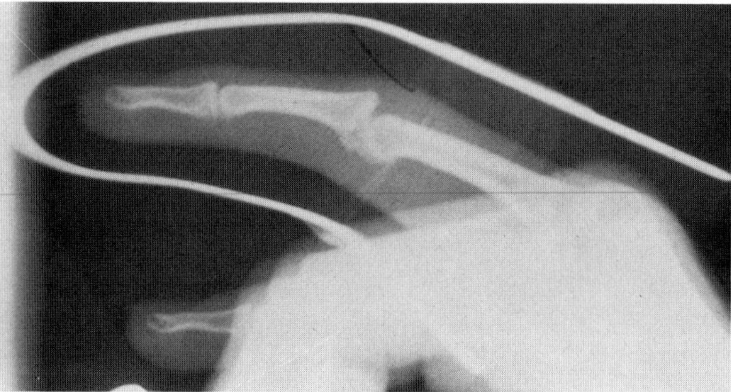

Fig. 6-57. A roentgenogram showing improper treatment of a fracture-dislocation of the proximal interphalangeal joint. There is insufficient flexion of the joint to maintain the reduction, and the middle phalanx has subluxated dorsal to the head of the proximal phalanx.

dorsal extension block splint described by McElfresh, Dobyns, and O'Brien (Fig. 6-53).[197] It should be emphasized that if nonoperative treatment is used, serial follow-up roentgenograms are mandatory during the first three weeks to insure maintenance of the reduction (Fig. 6-57).

DISLOCATIONS AND LIGAMENTOUS INJURIES OF THE METACARPOPHALANGEAL JOINTS (EXCLUDING THE THUMB)

Anatomy

The metacarpophalangeal joint is a condyloid joint that allows flexion, extension, abduction, adduction, and a limited amount of circumduction.[7] The globular head of the metacarpal articulates with the reciprocally concave base of the proximal phalanx, although the surface of the latter has a slightly less acute curve than the metacarpal head. The articular surface of the head is broader on its volar aspect than dorsally, allowing for the recesses in the dorsolateral aspects of both sides of the head to accommodate the collateral ligaments. The stability of the joint depends upon the col-

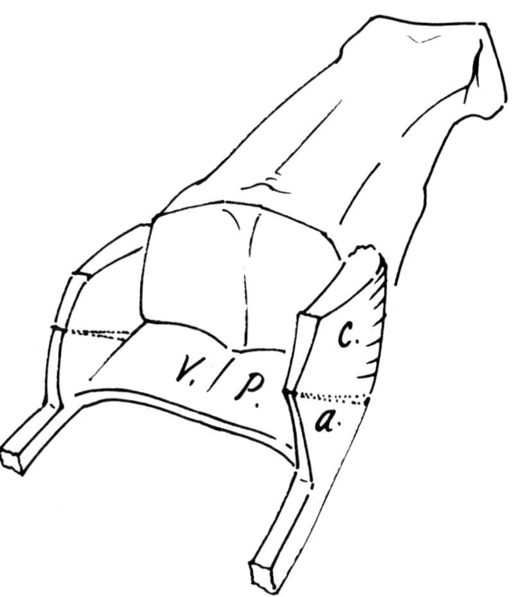

Fig. 6-58. The stability of the metacarpophalangeal joint depends, in large part, upon the collateral ligaments and volar plate, which together form a snug, boxlike configuration. (Eaton, R. G.: Joint Injuries of the Hand. Springfield, Charles C Thomas, 1970)

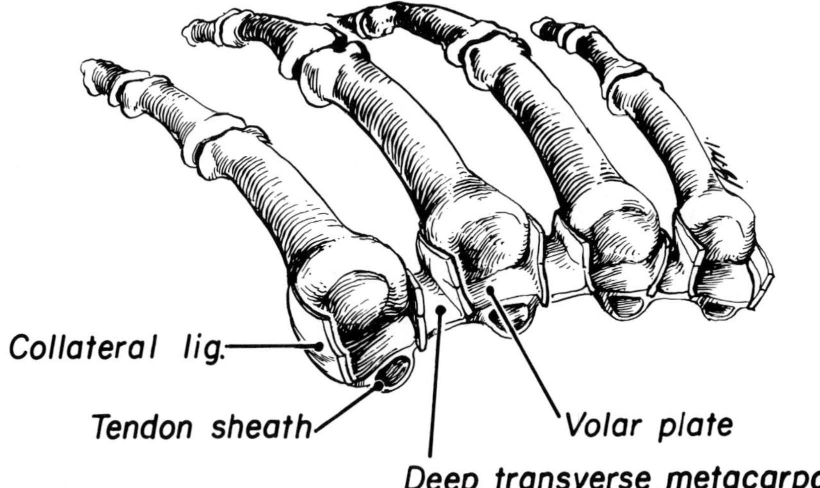

Fig. 6-59. The volar plates of the four palmar metacarpals are held together firmly by the deep transverse metacarpal ligament, which is, in fact, continuous with the volar plate.

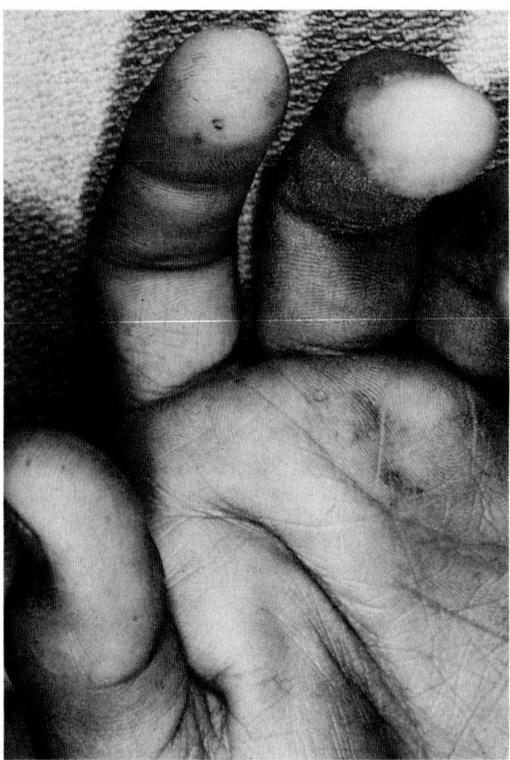

Fig. 6-60. A particularly important clinical sign, which is virtually pathognomonic of a complex dislocation of the index finger, is puckering of the skin in the proximal palmar crease.

lateral ligaments and volar plate, which together form a snug, box-like configuration as noted by Eaton[3] (Fig. 6-58).

Each collateral ligament has, essentially, two parts, an upper cordlike metacarpophalangeal ligament, and a lower accessory, or metacarpoglenoidal, ligament (Fig. 6-50). The latter, which attaches directly into the volar plate, is less rigid so that it can fold upon itself when the joint flexes. Lateral views show that the metacarpal head has an eccentric configuration: the distance from the center of rotation to the articular surface is greater in a volar direction than it is distally (Fig. 6-49). This produces a cam-like effect on the collateral ligaments, making them tight in flexion and loose in extension. One can readily demonstrate this in his own hand by noting that passive abduction and adduction are much more restricted with the joint held in maximum flexion than in full extension. This eccentricity of the metacarpal head is the major reason why the metacarpophalangeal joints are more likely to become stiff in extension than in flexion.

The volar plate of the metacarpophalangeal joint is a relatively thick, fibrocartilaginous condensation of the joint capsule forming the anterior wall of the joint. It is firmly attached distally to the base of the phalanx, but its proximal attachment to the neck of the metacarpal is more areolar and flexible, allowing passive hyperextension of the joint and permitting the volar plate to fold upon itself in flexion. The volar plates of the four palmar metacarpals are held together firmly by the deep transverse metacarpal ligament, which is, in fact, continuous with the volar plate (Fig. 6-59).

Classification and Mechanism of Injury

Dislocations of the metacarpophalangeal joint are of two types, simple and complex. Simple dislocations are those that can be reduced by closed manipulation; complex ones are irreducible.

Both injuries usually result from a fall on the outstretched hand that forces the metacarpophalangeal joint into hyperextension. The volar plate is torn loose from its membranous attachment at the neck of the metacarpal, allowing the proximal phalanx to be displaced dorsal to the head of the metacarpal.

Diagnosis

It is particularly important to differentiate between simple and complex dislocations of the metacarpophalangeal joint. This distinction can usually be made on the basis of clinical and roentgenographic findings, and the surgeon should not have to resort to multiple unsuccessful attempts at reduction to conclude that he is dealing with an irreducible dislocation. Although Farabeuf[215] described the complex dislocation in 1876 and Barnard[213] introduced this concept into the English literature in 1901, it was not until 1957 that the pathological anatomy became widely understood. In that year, Kaplan[220] published his now classic article in which he described the buttonholing of the metacarpal head into the palm and the anatomy of the constricting factors that prevent reduction by closed methods. Green and Terry[217] have recently correlated the pathological anatomy with the clinical and operative findings.

Dislocation of a metacarpophalangeal joint (excluding the thumb) virtually always involves the border digits (i.e., the index or little finger). There are no case reports in the literature of isolated dislocations in the ring or long fingers, although Wilhelmy and Hay[231] have reported a single case of simultaneous dislocation of the fourth and fifth metacarpophalangeal joints, and Moberg and Stener[262] described a patient with dislocation of all four metacarpophalangeal joints.

In a simple dislocation, the proximal phalanx is displaced dorsally at an angle approaching 90 degrees. In the typical complex dislocation, however, the proximal phalanx is only slightly hyperextended, resting on the dorsum of the metacarpal and partially overlapping the side of the adjacent finger. In both types, the metacarpal head lies prominently displaced in the palm. A particularly important clinical sign, which is virtually pathognomonic of a complex dislocation, is puckering of the skin in the proximal palmar crease (Fig. 6-60).

Roentgenograms of the complex dislocation usually show a widened joint space, indicative of interposition of the volar plate within the joint. A pathognomonic roentgenographic sign of a complex dislocation is the presence of a sesamoid within the widened joint space[217,225,229] (Fig. 6-61). In the thumb, the sesamoids lie in the lateral margins of the volar plate, but they are also incorporated into the tendons of the thenar intrinsic muscles. In the fingers, the sesamoids are likewise imbedded in the volar plate, but they are not associated in any way with the tendons of either the intrinsic muscles or the extrinsic flexors. Since in all the digits the sesamoids do lie within the volar plate of the metacarpophalangeal joint, the presence of a sesamoid within the joint space should be considered a sign of an irreducible dislocation. This finding must not be confused with a chip fracture of the metacarpal head, which may also occur but does not necessarily carry with it the same diagnostic significance.

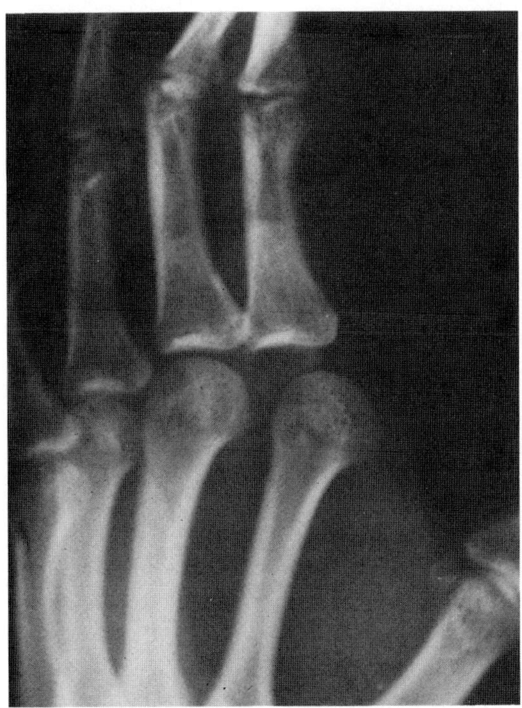

Fig. 6-61. A pathognomonic roentgenographic sign of a complex dislocation is the presence of a sesamoid within the widened joint space. Since the sesamoids reside in the volar plate, the presence of the sesamoid within the joint space is indicative of interposition of the volar plate within the joint. (Green, D. P. and Terry, G. C.: J. Bone Joint Surg., 55A: 1482, 1973)

Treatment

An attempt at closed reduction should be made in all dislocations of the metacarpophalangeal joint. Even if the pathognomonic signs of a complex dislocation are present,

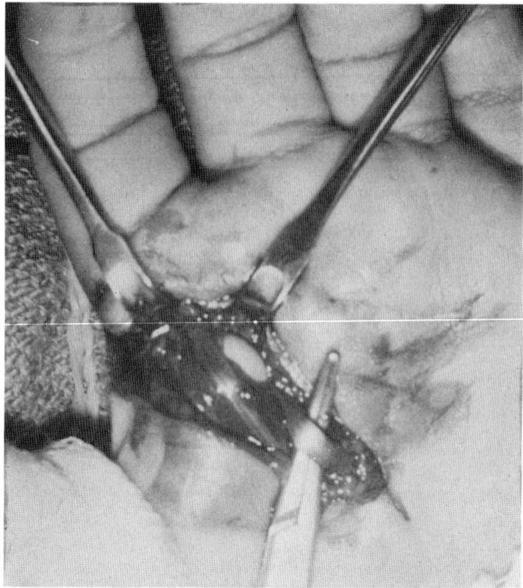

Fig. 6-62. Of extreme importance in the open reduction of a complex metacarpophalangeal dislocation is the vulnerable location of the neurovascular bundle caused by displacement of the metacarpal head into the palm. Invariably the digital nerve and artery are tented very tightly and superficially over the prominent metacarpal head, and lie immediately beneath the skin.

the surgeon is justified in making a single attempt at gentle reduction under adequate anesthesia, but he should be prepared to follow this with an immediate open reduction if the manipulation is unsuccessful.

McLaughlin[222] reiterated the concept originally discussed by Farabeuf[215] that it is possible to convert a simple dorsal dislocation of the metacarpophalangeal joint into a complex dislocation by attempting to reduce the deformity by traction alone. Closed reduction should be performed by first hyperextending the proximal phalanx about 90 degrees on the metacarpal and then pushing against the dorsal surface of the base of the phalanx, with the interphalangeal joints flexed. Longitudinal traction applied to the finger and attempts at pulling it back into position may possibly allow the volar plate to become entrapped in the widened joint space. A simple dislocation is easily reduced by the maneuver described, but attempts at closed reduction by any means will be unsuccessful in the complex dislocation. If the dislocation cannot be reduced, open reduction should not be delayed.

The original operative approach to this injury was described by Farabeuf[215] as a dorsal releasing incision. Kaplan[220] presented the logical reasons why a volar approach offers the surgeon more direct visual access to the injury and facilitates the release. Of extreme importance in the operation is the vulnerable location of the neurovascular bundle caused by displacement of the metacarpal head into the palm.[217] Invariably the radial digital nerve and artery in the index finger (and the ulnar bundle in the small finger) are tented very tightly and superficially over the prominent metacarpal head and lie immediately beneath the skin (Fig. 6-62). An overly aggressive transverse skin incision can easily injure the neurovascular bundle. The single most important element preventing reduction is interposition of the volar plate within the joint space[212,214,217,228,230] (Fig. 6-63), and it must be extricated surgically.

It remains a moot and frequently argued point, whether or not a true complex dislocation can be reduced by closed manipulation. Our operative experience has led us to believe that it is not possible, but the issue is difficult to resolve, since the mere fact of a successful reduction eliminates the opportunity to look and see if the volar plate was in fact entrapped.

Postoperative Care

If care is taken in removing the volar plate from the joint, it is usually intact with a firm insertion remaining into the base of the proximal phalanx. The joint is invariably stable after reduction, a fact easily confirmed at the operating table by passively moving the joint through a full range of motion. For this reason, we feel that it is neither necessary nor desirable to immobilize the digit postoperatively. Some authors prefer to splint the finger for 3 weeks, but we believe that this is more likely to result in prolonged or even permanent stiffness than if the joint is allowed active motion from the outset.[222] A soft dressing is usually sufficient protection postoperatively, but if the surgeon is concerned about possible instability in hyperextension, a dorsal extension block splint can be used, which allows full active range of flexion but protects against hyperextension.

A simple metacarpophalangeal dislocation treated by closed reduction can either be splinted for 3 weeks or allowed early active motion with buddy taping. We prefer the latter, but even if the finger is splinted, residual stiffness is not as likely as it is following the complex dislocation.

Complications

The treatment of a late, untreated, or inadequately treated complex dislocation is considerably more complicated, and the end results are significantly compromised. Murphy and Stark[224] have reported their experience with these difficult injuries, and they note that a second, dorsal, incision is necessary to excise the shortened ulnar collateral ligament. None of their 6 patients with late complex dislocations regained normal range of motion in the finger.

CARPOMETACARPAL DISLOCATIONS (EXCLUDING THE THUMB)

Dislocations of the carpometacarpal joints are uncommon. Table 6-1 lists a compilation of cases reported in the literature, drawn from the excellent review article by Waugh and Yancy[244] in 1948, and adding cases reported in the English literature since that time. Although the injury is probably not as rare as these figures would imply, the fact remains that it is relatively uncommon.

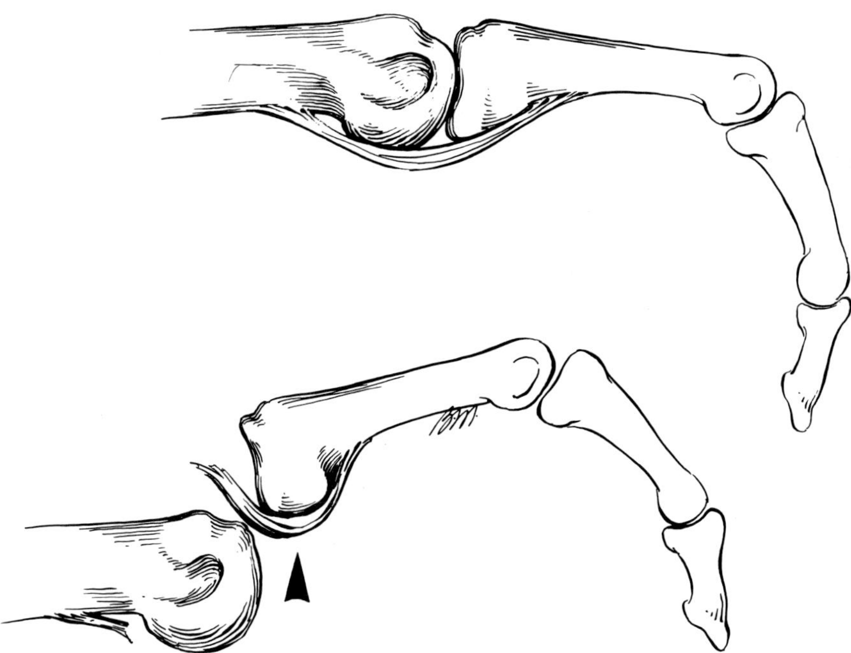

Fig. 6-63. The single most important element preventing reduction in a complex metacarpophalangeal dislocation is interposition of the volar plate within the joint space, and it must be extricated surgically.

TABLE 6-1. Carpometacarpal Dislocations Reported in the Literature (Excluding the Thumb)

	Involved Finger	Number of Reported Dislocations
Isolated	II	7
	III	3
	IV	3
	V	13
Combined	II, V	32
	III, V	4
	IV, V	13
	II, III	10
	II, III, V	4
	II, IV	3

Anatomy

The carpometacarpal joints of the palmar digits (except the fifth) are arthrodial diarthroses,[7] which means that the contiguous bone surfaces are covered with articular cartilage and that only gliding movement takes place at the joint. The bases of the metacarpals articulate with the distal row of carpal bones by an intricate, multifaceted arrangement that makes this one of the most secure articulations in the body.[239] This interlocking combination of joints is further strengthened by tough intermetacarpal and carpometacarpal ligaments, which span the joints on both volar and dorsal aspects. Additional reinforcement is provided by the insertions of the wrist flexors and extensors into the bases of the second, third, and fifth metacarpals. Essentially, no movement is possible at the third carpometacarpal joint, which functions as the stable central post of the hand as described by Flatt.[5] A very limited amount of anterior-posterior gliding is permitted at the base of the second metacarpal, considerably more in the fourth, and the most motion is present at the base of the fifth metacarpal (approximately 20 to 30 degrees). The fifth carpometacarpal joint is more mobile, because it is actually a saddle joint similar to the articulation between the thumb metacarpal and the trapezium.[7] A saddle joint is an articulation in which the opposing surfaces are reciprocally concavoconvex. The articular surface of the base of the fifth metacarpal is convex in a volar-dorsal direction and concave in a radio-ulnar direction. Motion in the joint between the fifth metacarpal and the hamate is much more restricted than at the base of the thumb, however. Flexion is limited by the hook of the hamate, and motions in all directions are restricted by the strong interosseous ligaments. Abduction is limited by the deep transverse metacarpal ligament, which tethers the neck of the metacarpal to the adjacent fourth metacarpal, and adduction is, of course, blocked by the presence of the fourth metacarpal itself.

Mechanism of Injury

Attempts have been made to reproduce carpometacarpal dislocations experimentally on cadaver hands, but usually a fracture of the metacarpal shaft resulted.[244] A precise mechanism of injury has not been clearly defined, therefore, but carpometacarpal dislocations can apparently result from both direct and indirect violence.[244] Most combined dislocations are dorsal (i.e., the bases of the metacarpals are displaced posterior to the carpus), and this probably most commonly results from a force applied to the dorsum of the hand with the wrist in acute palmar flexion. A direct force striking the hand at the level of the metacarpal bases may account for some of these injuries as well, with the resulting volar or dorsal dislocation determined by the direction of the force.

Isolated volar dislocations of the fifth metacarpal appear to represent a slightly different problem.[232,235,238] Nalebuff[241] noted that two types can occur, although both are caused by a direct blow to the ulnar border of the hand. One type displaces the base of the metacarpal radialward, tearing all of its ligament and tendon attachments. The dislocation may be extreme, with the base lying anterior to the third or fourth metacarpal. In this type, open reduction may be necessary to restore the anatomical position of the metacarpal base, although closed reduction has been successful when attempted early.[240] In the second type, the direction of displacement of the metacarpal is ulnarward. Some ligament and tendon attachments remain intact, and closed reduction can usually be achieved as with the combined carpometacarpal dislocations.

Diagnosis

The obvious clinical deformity that one might expect to see with this injury is often obscured by marked swelling of the hand. The fact that many of the carpometacarpal dislocations reported in the literature were missed on initial examination implies that the diagnosis is not always immediately obvious and that roentgenograms are necessary to identify the displacement. The standard three views of the hand, including a true lateral, will usually demonstrate the dislocation, but other views may be necessary to identify precisely which metacarpals are involved and to delineate accompanying fractures. For example, Murless[240] has stated that an isolated dislocation of the fifth carpometacarpal joint is probably always a fracture-dislocation (analagous to a Bennett's fracture dislocation in the thumb), although the fracture may be missed with routine roentgenograms. He demonstrated that an anteroposterior view (hand in supination) may reveal information not seen on the standard posteroanterior view (hand in pronation).

Dislocation of the carpometacarpal joints can occur in association with fractures of other metacarpals and they are frequently missed under such circumstances. Whenever there is a displaced or angulated fracture of the base or shaft of a metacarpal, one should be particularly careful to look for dislocation of one or more adjacent carpometacarpal joints (Fig. 6-64).

Methods of Treatment

No Treatment. There are several case reports in the literature[242,243] that state or imply that an old, unreduced carpometacarpal dislocation has no functional disability. These were cases in which the diagnosis was not made initially or in which a reduction was not maintained. The validity of these conclusions must be questioned in most reported instances because of the ex-

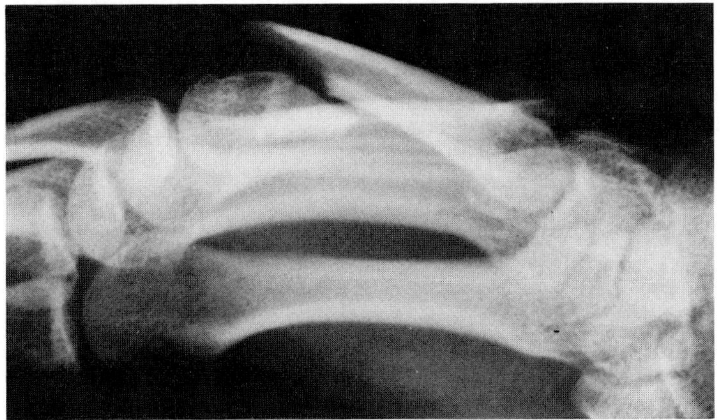

Fig. 6-64. Whenever there is a displaced or angulated fracture of the base of the shaft of the metacarpal, one should be particularly careful to look for dislocation of one or more adjacent carpometacarpal joints. In this patient, there is an angulated and shortened fracture of the fifth metacarpal and dislocation of the base of the fourth metacarpal.

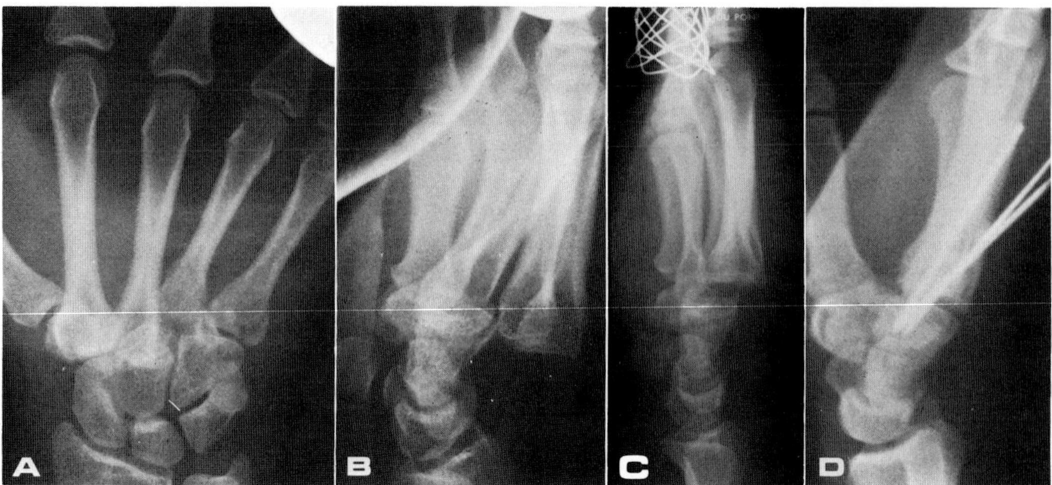

Fig. 6-65. The steps in closed reduction of a carpometacarpal dislocation: (*A*) The anteroposterior view shows proximal displacement of the bases of the second and third metacarpals. Note also the fracture of the base of the fifth metacarpal. (*B*) The lateral view dramatically demonstrates dorsal dislocation of the bases of the second and third metacarpals. (*C*) The first step in reduction is to apply a strong traction force, best accomplished by finger traps with countertraction across the upper arm. Traction brings the metacarpals out to length, but it does not necessarily reduce the dislocation. Note that there is still dorsal subluxation of the bases of the metacarpals. (*D*) Direct pressure must be applied to the bases of the metacarpals to restore their normal anatomical position. Because of the great propensity for recurrent subluxation following closed reduction alone, we believe that percutaneous pin fixation should routinely be done at the time of closed reduction.

tremely short follow-up periods. Having seen several patients with significant pain and functional disability from old, unreduced dislocations, we suspect that the long-term results from inadequate reduction are not always entirely satisfactory.

Closed Reduction and Cast Immobilization. Acceptable closed reduction is usually not difficult to achieve if the injury is recognized and treated early. A strong traction force must be applied as the first step in reduction, best accomplished by finger traps, with countertraction across the upper arm. Traction brings the metacarpals out to length, but it does not necessarily reduce the dislocation (Fig. 6-65), and direct pressure must be applied to the bases of the metacarpals to restore them to their normal positions. While reduction itself is not difficult, maintenance of that reduction is often troublesome.[234] For the usual type of dorsal dislocation, the hand should be immobilized with the wrist in extension following reduction. If this is done, however, careful roentgenographic follow-up must be done to insure maintenance of the reduction.

Closed Reduction and Percutaneous Pin Fixation. Clement[233] and Nalebuff[240] have both demonstrated that the reduction can be maintained by percutaneous fixation with Kirschner wires. As in the Wagner[178] technique of transfixing a Bennett's fracture-dislocation, the pins are passed from the metacarpal into either the base of an adjacent undislocated metacarpal or the carpus itself, or into both. The surgeon must be certain that the dislocation is completely reduced as the pins are inserted, but if this is assured and if the pins have solid purchase, this technique obviates the problem of loss of reduction during the healing phase. The wires should be left in place for at least 6 weeks, for late residual subluxation has been noted following earlier removal of the pins.

Open Reduction and Internal Fixation. Open reduction is necessary only if closed reduction fails. This is most likely to be the situation in delayed, untreated dislocations in which the correct diagnosis was not made at the time of injury. In the literature, most of the cases that require open reduction are late dislocations, and in such instances it may be necessary to reconstruct some of the ligamentous support of the carpometacarpal joint. If this is not possible, or if sufficient time has elapsed to allow the development of posttraumatic joint changes, then arthrodesis of the carpometacarpal joint may be indicated, as advocated by Watson-Jones.[116]

Authors' Preferred Method of Treatment

Early recognition and prompt reduction greatly facilitate the management of carpometacarpal dislocations. If the diagnosis is made early, we prefer to treat the dislocation by closed reduction and percutaneous pin fixation. The reduction is considerably facilitated by an initial 10-minute period of uninterrupted traction with finger traps. The bases of the metacarpals are then pressed directly into position, and while one surgeon holds the reduction, another passes two or more 0.045- or 0.0625-inch nonthreaded Kirschner wires across the carpometacarpal joint. The propensity for loss of reduction is so great that we believe percutaneous pin fixation should be done routinely at the time of closed reduction. Critical assessment of the immediate postreduction films must be made, and if residual subluxation persists, open reduction and internal fixation should be performed.

If the patient is first seen late, within a few weeks of injury, an attempt at closed reduction may be done, but it is unlikely to be successful, and open reduction is indicated.

The treatment of chronic, unreduced dislocations should be dictated by the degree of functional disability and the severity of pain. Those that are asymptomatic and cause no disability should not be treated. Those that are painful and disabling should have arthrodesis of the appropriate carpometacarpal joints.[116]

DISLOCATIONS AND LIGAMENTOUS INJURIES IN THE THUMB

Anatomy

The carpometacarpal joint of the thumb is a saddle joint, with articular surfaces that are reciprocally concavoconvex.[7] The base of the first metacarpal is convex in the radioulnar direction and concave in the dorsovolar plane. The trapezium, which forms the "saddle," is concave in the transverse plane and convex in the dorsovolar plane. The volar lip of the metacarpal base is somewhat elongated, providing added stabilization of the joint. Eaton[3] has noted that the most important soft-tissue support of the carpometacarpal joint is the deep ulnar or anterior oblique ligament, which runs from the volar beak of the metacarpal to the tubercle of the trapezium. Hyperextension of the carpometacarpal joint is limited by this ligament. Additional reinforcement is provided by a lateral ligament and the overlying insertion of the abductor pollicis longus into the dorsoradial aspect of the base of the metacarpal.

Kaplan[10] has pointed out that although these ligamentous structures are strong, they are not tight, and the contiguous surfaces of the joint are not held together firmly. This laxity of the joint capsule allows a limited amount of rotation, and Haines[253] demonstrated that the carpometacarpal ligaments act to guide the axial rotation of the metacarpal.

Lasserre, Pauzat, and Derennes[260] demonstrated how the base of the metacarpal fills the concavity of the trapezium during abduction but slides laterally in adduction. A true anteroposterior view (Robert view)[260] is necessary to show the carpometacarpal joint adequately; it is taken

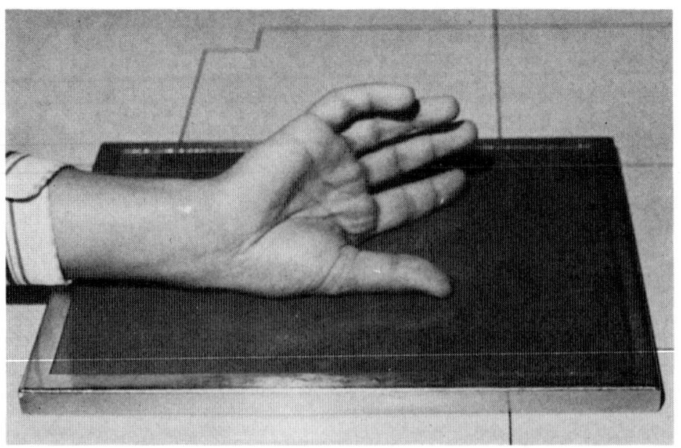

Fig. 6-66. A true anteroposterior view (Robert view) is necessary to adequately show the carpometacarpal joint of the thumb. It is taken with the hand in extreme pronation.

with the hand in maximum pronation (Fig. 6-66).

The metacarpophalangeal joint of the thumb is basically a condyloid joint, allowing flexion, extension, abduction, adduction, and possibly a very limited amount of rotation.[7] Studies of normal thumb movements have revealed that wide variations of passive motion exist. Coonrad and Goldner[249] found that flexion varied from as little as 10 degrees to as much as 100, with an average of 75 degrees. Extension ranged from 0 to 90 degrees, with an average of 20 degrees. Harris and Joseph[254] further noted that many individuals cannot passively extend the metacarpophalangeal joint even to neutral, and that limitation may be as great as 34 degrees short of full extension. In their studies, the degree of passive hyperextension possible seemed to be directly related to the shape of the metacarpal head. A "flat" metacarpal head, as seen in the lateral view, did not allow motion beyond neutral, while greater hyperextension was found in those thumbs with "round" heads.

The head of the metacarpal is also broader and more nearly quadrilateral than that of the other metacarpals, presumably a factor in providing added stability against lateral stress, although some passive lateral motion is normal. Coonrad and Goldner[249] reported that with the joint held in 15 degrees flexion, normal thumbs are capable of a range of 0 to 20 degrees of passive abduction-adduction, with an average of 10 degrees.

Like those in the fingers, the volar plate of the metacarpophalangeal joint of the thumb has two parts, a tough distal fibrocartilaginous plate firmly attached to the base of the proximal phalanx and a flexible, noncartilaginous proximal component. With flexion of the joint, the soft proximal part folds in between the fibrocartilaginous plate and the head of the metacarpal. In extension, the volar plate affords stability against hyperextension, although, as noted above, the extent of this varies considerably among individuals. Lying in the lateral margins of the volar plate are two sesamoids, which are also incorporated into the tendons of the flexor pollicis brevis (radial side) and adductor pollicis (ulnar side).

DISLOCATIONS IN THE THUMB

Metacarpophalangeal Joint

Three types of dislocations—dorsal, radial, and ulnar—can occur in the metacarpophalangeal joint of the thumb. Discussion here will be confined to the dorsal dislocation, as the latter two injuries are covered in the section on collateral ligament injuries in the thumb, which follows.

Mechanism of Injury. Dorsal dislocation of the metacarpophalangeal joint of the thumb invariably results from forcible hyperextension. In order to allow displacement of the proximal phalanx dorsally, the volar plate must be torn, usually from its

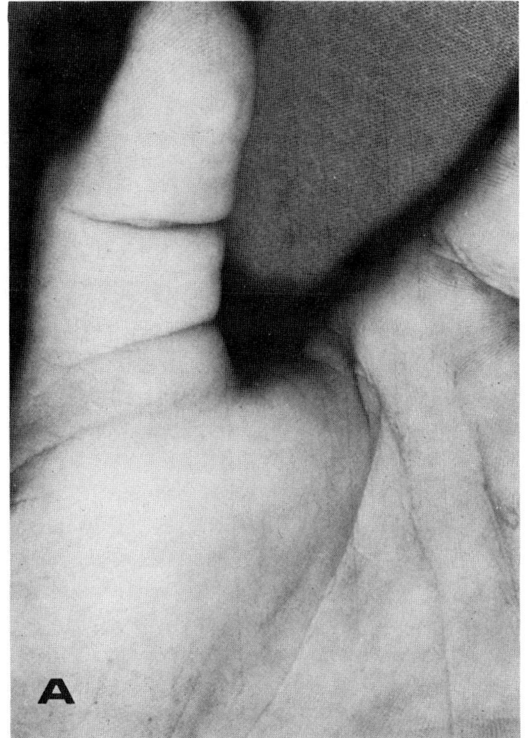

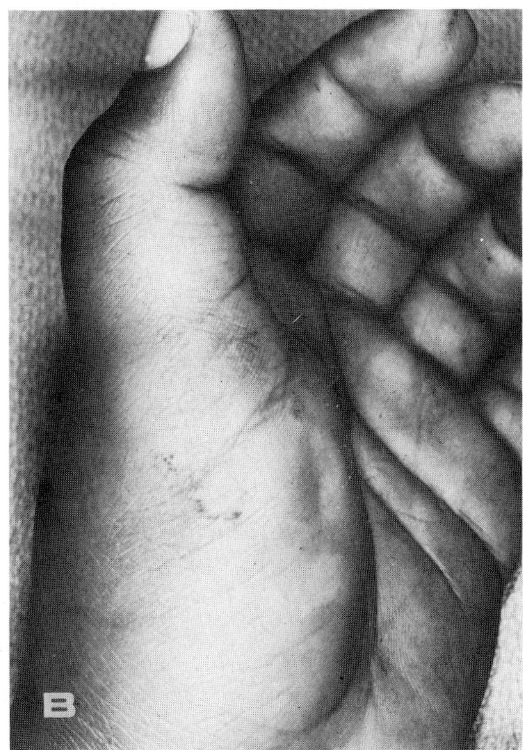

Fig. 6-67. The most important diagnostic clinical sign of a complex dislocation in the thumb is a skin dimple found on the volar aspect of the thenar eminence. (*A*) This patient had a dislocation of the metacarpophalangeal joint of the thumb, but no skin dimple was present. This was a simple dislocation which was easily reduced by closed manipulation. (*B*) This patient also had a dislocation of the metacarpophalangeal joint of the thumb, but the characteristic skin dimple was present over the thenar eminence. Closed reduction was unsuccessful, and open reduction, which revealed interposition of the volar plate in the joint, confirmed the diagnosis of the complex dislocation.

membranous attachment at the neck of the metacarpal. Usually the collateral ligaments are not torn, but instead flip up like the visor on a knight's helmet. Depending on the direction of the force, however, one or both of the collateral ligaments may be ruptured, resulting in lateral instability of the joint after reduction of the dislocation.

Occasionally the volar plate may become interposed between the base of the proximal phalanx and the head of the metacarpal, resulting in a complex, or irreducible, dislocation.

Diagnosis. The most important initial step in management of the dorsal dislocation is to differentiate between a simple and a complex dislocation. As with metacarpophalangeal dislocations in the fingers, it is usually possible to make this distinction on the basis of clinical findings rather than to arrive at such a decision after repeated unsuccessful attempts at closed reduction. The attitude of the finger offers the first clue, for in a simple dislocation the phalanx usually rests on the head of the metacarpal in nearly 90 degrees of hyperextension. In the complex dislocation, the proximal phalanx is more nearly parallel to the metacarpal, with only slight hyperextension. The most important diagnostic clinical sign of a complex dislocation is a skin dimple found on the volar aspect of the thenar eminence (Fig. 6-67). The presence of a sesamoid within the widened joint space on roentgen-

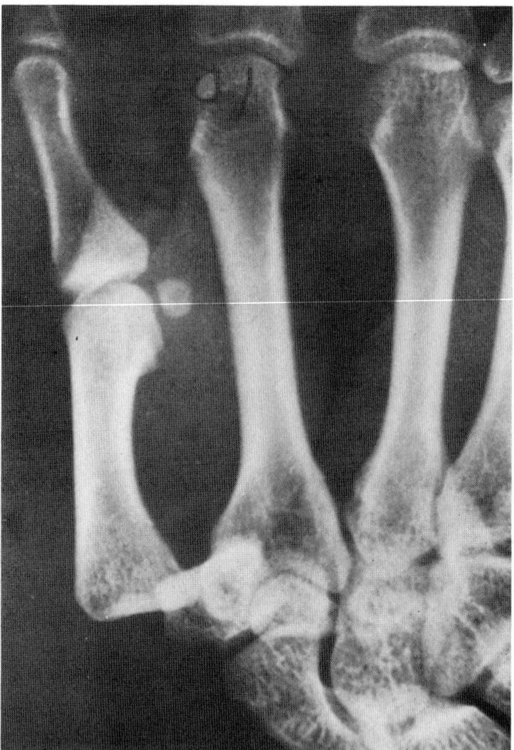

Fig. 6-68. A pure dislocation of the carpometacarpal joint of the thumb without associated fracture is an uncommon injury. Closed reduction is simple but extremely unstable.

ograms is also a pathognomonic sign of a complex dislocation.

Methods of Treatment. Simple dislocations of the metacarpophalangeal joint can be reduced easily by closed manipulation; complex dislocations cannot. Even in the presence of the pathognomonic skin dimple, however, we believe that a single attempt at closed reduction under adequate anesthesia should be made in all dorsal dislocations of this joint. McLaughlin[222] emphasized the point originally made by Farabeuf[215] that a simple dislocation can be converted into a complex dislocation by improper reduction. Closed reduction should be performed by first hyperextending the proximal phalanx as far as possible on the metacarpal and then pushing against the dorsal surface of the base of the phalanx with the interphalangeal joint in flexion. Attempting to reduce the deformity by traction and pulling the phalanx back into position may cause the volar plate to become interposed in the joint, thereby rendering it irreducible.

Following a successful closed reduction, lateral stability of the joint should be carefully tested to check the integrity of the radial and ulnar collateral ligaments. If there is evidence of complete rupture of one of the collateral ligaments, treatment should be directed toward management of this injury, as outlined in the section on injuries of the collateral ligament.

Usually the joint will be stable after closed reduction, and 3 weeks of cast immobilization will generally give an excellent result. Very few authors advocate immediate repair of the volar plate following a successful closed reduction, since satisfactory healing usually occurs with adequate immobilization. In rare cases, improper healing of the plate may result in chronic pain with either instability in hyperextension or flexion contracture from scarring, necessitating late reconstruction.

If closed manipulation of the dorsal dislocation fails, the surgeon should be prepared to follow this with an immediate open reduction. The joint is exposed through a volar approach, and the entrapped volar plate is extricated from the joint. The tendon of the flexor brevis may also be interposed, and the head of the metacarpal may be found to protrude through the bellies of the thenar intrinsic muscles. In two cases, we have found the tendon of the flexor pollicis longus wrapped around the neck of the metacarpal. Early protected motion should be instituted postoperatively, since stiffness is more common following complex dislocation than it is after a simple dislocation.

Carpometacarpal Joint

Pure dislocations of the carpometacarpal joint of the thumb are uncommon (Fig. 6-68). The mechanism of injury is usually a longitudinally directed blow along the metacarpal shaft with the carpometacarpal joint in slight flexion. Because of the strong support afforded by the anterior oblique ligament and its firm attachment to the volar beak of the base of the metacarpal, this mechanism is more likely to avulse off a fragment of the beak, resulting in the familiar Bennett's fracture-dislocation (see p. 305).

Closed reduction of the dislocation is simple but extremely unstable. Maintenance of reduction may be difficult because of the natural tendency of the base of the metacarpal to shift even in the normal thumb, compounded by the loss of ligamentous support. Immobilization with the thumb in abduction is more likely to seat the metacarpal correctly, but a true anteroposterior roentgenogram (Robert view, Fig. 6-66) is necessary to ascertain the congruity of the articular surfaces after closed reduction.

Percutaneous pin fixation of the reduced joint provides temporary stabilization during the period of immobilization, but even this may not result in healing of the ligament sufficient to prevent late subluxation and instability of the joint.[189]

Late Complications. The diagnosis may be entirely missed initially, since spontaneous reduction of the dislocation may occur at the time of injury. Such patients are particularly likely to have persistent pain secondary to residual instability. However, Eaton[189] has pointed out that chronic symptoms of instability are common, even after closed reduction, owing to inadequate healing of the important anterior oblique ligament. He and Littler have described an operation for late reconstruction of this ligament with half of the flexor carpi radialis tendon. Previous operations for late stabilization of the carpometacarpal joint were reported by Slocum,[264] Eggers,[250] and Kestler.[259] Untreated incongruity in this joint leads to early arthritic changes, however, and if damage to the joint surfaces is found at surgery, arthroplasty or arthrodesis of the joint is the preferred treatment.

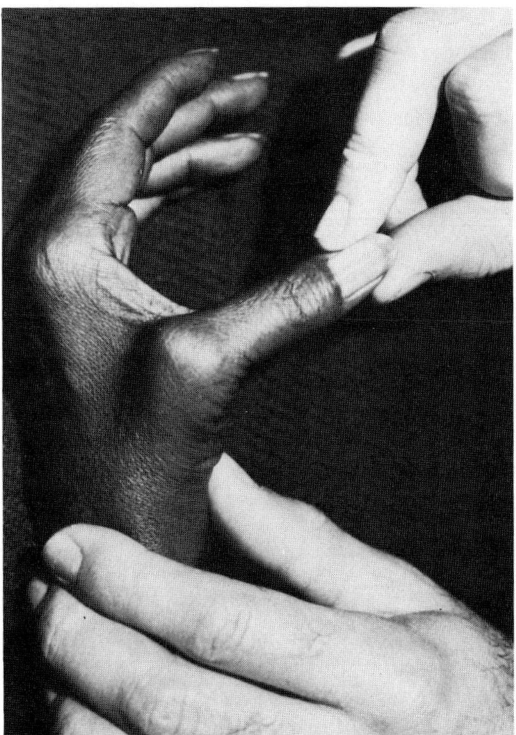

Fig. 6-69. Valgus stress applied to the metacarpophalangeal joint of the thumb in a patient with complete rupture of the ulnar collateral ligament (so-called gamekeeper's thumb).

COLLATERAL LIGAMENT INJURY OF THE METACARPOPHALANGEAL JOINT (GAMEKEEPER'S THUMB)

Mechanism of Injury

A sudden valgus stress applied to the metacarpophalangeal joint of the thumb results in partial or total disruption of the ulnar collateral ligament. Accompanying tears of the dorsal capsule and adductor aponeurosis may occur as well, but the primary injury is to the collateral ligament itself. In 1955, Campbell[248] discovered that a similar ligamentous insufficiency may develop without a specific incident of acute trauma, and he found this to be an occupational characteristic in the hands of British gamekeepers. Their customary method of killing wounded rabbits is such that lateral stress is applied to the metacarpophalangeal joint of the thumb. This does not necessarily result in an acute tearing of the ligament, but repeated maneuvers of this type may ultimately stretch the ulnar collateral ligament to the point of chronic laxity. Through common usage, the term gamekeeper's thumb has come to include any injury of the ulnar collateral ligament, whether from acute trauma or repeated stretching.

Diagnosis

Following an acute abduction injury to the metacarpophalangeal joint of the thumb, the patient presents with diffuse local swelling and pain in the region of the joint. Usually the point of maximal tenderness can be localized to the ulnar collateral ligament. Valgus stress applied to the joint is painful and may show varying degrees of lateral instability (Fig. 6-69). It is particularly important to ascertain the precise amount of instability in order to differentiate partial tears ("sprains") from complete ruptures of the ligament. Pain and resulting spasm in the adductor muscle may prevent passive movement of the joint and give a false impression of stability. Kessler[257] has therefore recommended testing after local anesthetic injection into ulnar collateral ligament if there is a question of instability.

Rupture of the radial collateral ligament can result from adduction injury, but this is decidedly less common. The clinical findings are similar to those seen in the ulnar collateral ligament tears.

Routine roentgenograms of the thumb may show no abnormality or may demonstrate a variable sized avulsion fracture at the base of the proximal phalanx (Fig. 6-70). Sutro[267] has emphasized the importance of obtaining a true anteroposterior view of the metacarpophalangeal joint, as flexion, from an oblique view, can easily be interpreted as lateral subluxation of the phalanx. If even the slightest amount of

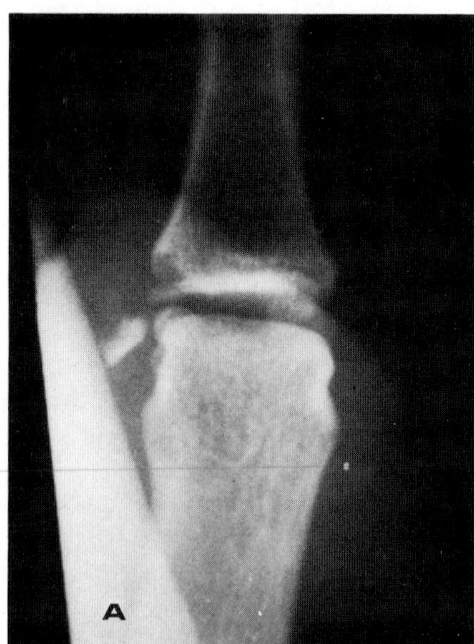

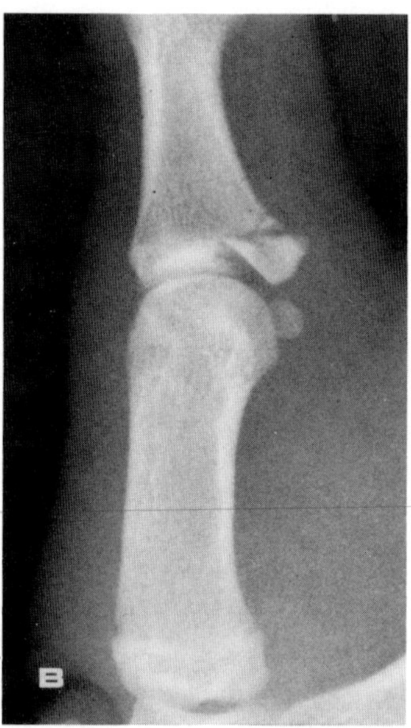

Fig. 6-70. A gamekeeper's thumb may be associated with an avulsion fracture from the base of the proximal phalanx. (*A*) This may be a very small fragment. (*B*) It may be a large fragment involving one-third or more of the articular surface. Either type, if displaced, requires open reduction. (*A* from Green, D. P.: Amer. Family Physician, 7:118, 1973)

instability is found on clinical examination, stress films should be taken to distinguish between partial and complete tears (Fig. 6-71). Again, local or regional block anesthesia will insure greater validity of the films. Since there may normally be some laxity to lateral stress in the metacarpophalangeal joint, comparison views of the opposite thumb must be taken.

Methods of Treatment

Acute Injuries. There is general agreement that partial tears ("sprains") of the ulnar collateral ligament can be satisfactorily managed by nonoperative methods. For all but the most minimal sprains, plaster immobilization is the treatment of choice. A snug fitting spica extending from the tip of the thumb to just below the elbow should be worn for 3 to 6 weeks, depending on the degree of severity (see p. 312). Care must be taken to position the metacarpophalangeal joint in optimal position for healing (i.e., in slight flexion), with mild varus angulation to relax tension on the ligament. Hyperextension of the joint must be avoided.

There is some disagreement about the proper treatment of acute complete ruptures of the ligament. In 1962, Stener[265] published an important article offering strong support for the advocates of open repair of the ligament. He reported that frequently the ruptured end of the ligament may become displaced and folded back upon itself beneath the proximal edge of the adductor aponeurosis (Fig. 6-72). Of 39 consecutive cases of total rupture of the ligament operated on by Stener himself, 25 demonstrated this interposition of the aponeurosis between the ligament and its attachment to the phalanx. Other authors have noted wide gaps at the site of ligament rupture at the time of operative repair.

Coonrad and Goldner[249] do not support the concept of surgical repair as the initial primary treatment of choice. They favor cast immobilization because their results indicated that primary repair does not necessarily offer a better result than delayed repair.

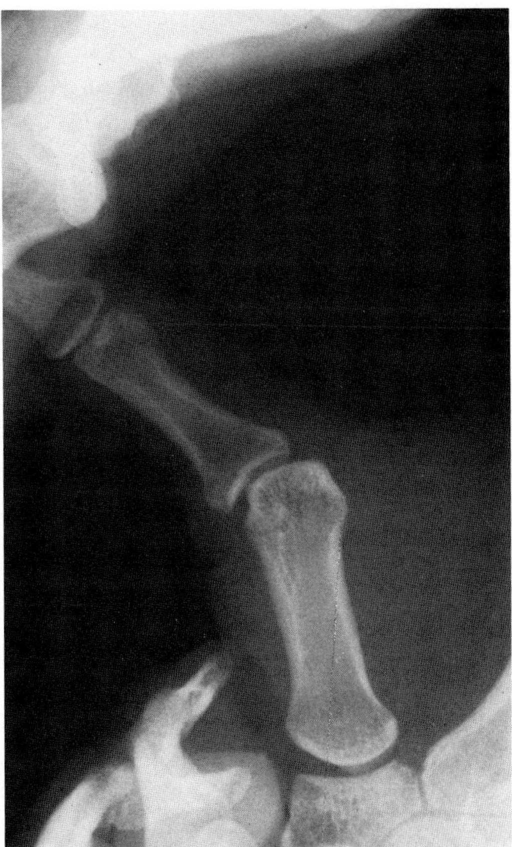

Fig. 6-71. Routine roentgenograms of the thumb in a patient with a suspected gamekeeper's thumb may show no abnormality. If the slightest amount of instability is found on clinical examination, stress films should be taken to distinguish between a partial and a complete tear. This patient has a complete tear.

While it is certainly true that some patients with complete ruptures can and do achieve excellent results with cast immobilization, we believe that the results are too unpredictable to warrant this as the treatment of choice. Supported by Stener's impressive figures explaining why some of these ruptures are destined to heal improperly or not at all, it is our belief now that all complete ruptures of the ligament should be treated by early operative repair. Since we adopted a policy of primary repair for all acute complete ulnar collateral ligament injuries, we have found interposition of the aponeurosis in more than half of our cases. Operative treatment is not warranted, however, unless the preoperative diagnosis of total rupture is confirmed by the presence of a displaced avulsion fracture or by unequivocally positive stress films.

Those injuries in which the ligament has torn loose from its distal attachment to the base of the proximal fragment, with or without a small avulsion chip fracture, are best treated with a pull-out wire technique.[251] If the fragment is larger, internal fixation with small Kirschner wires is preferable[251] (Fig. 6-73). Those less common injuries in which the ligament is torn through its substance can be easily approximated with direct suture if they are treated within the first few days after injury. Postoperative cast immobilization for 4 to 6 weeks is necessary.

Late Injuries. A more difficult management problem is the patient who presents with an ulnar collateral ligament injury several weeks old or more. The usual complaint is weakness in pinch because of the instability, and pain may be a significant feature as well. Chronic swelling and local tenderness on the ulnar side of the joint is often noted, due to callus formation at the site of healing in the attenuated ligament.[262]

If the ligament cannot be repaired, the treatment alternatives are reconstruction of the ligament or arthrodesis of the joint. If there is posttraumatic arthrosis, all agree that fusion is the treatment of choice. No form of soft-tissue reconstruction, no matter how stable it makes the joint, is likely to

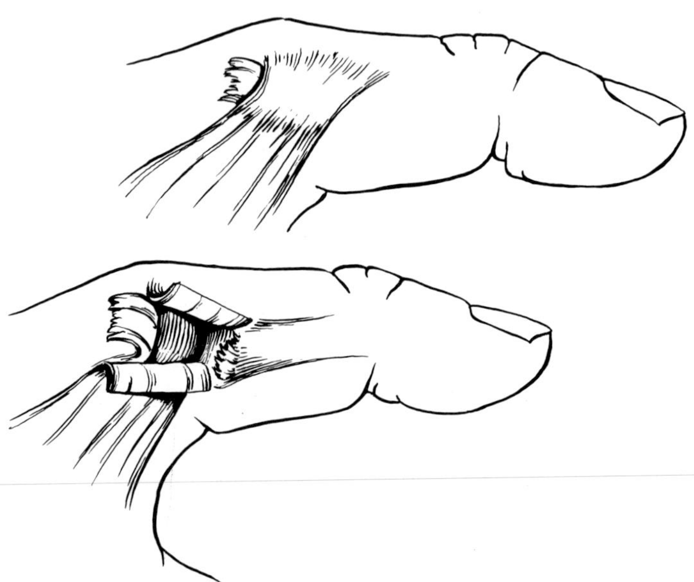

Fig. 6-72. Stener has described how the ruptured end of the ulnar collateral ligament may become displaced and folded back upon itself beneath the proximal edge of the adductor aponeurosis. Because of this frequent finding, many authors favor operative repair of complete rupture of the ulnar collateral ligament. (Redrawn from Stener, B.: J. Bone Joint Surg., *44B*:870, 1962)

relieve the patient's pain if significant damage has already developed in the articular surface.

In the absence of arthrosis, ligament reconstruction can be undertaken with a variety of procedures previously described in the literature. Alldred[246] and others have reported the use of free tendon or fascia lata grafts to reconstruct the ligament itself. This operation is technically difficult, and often stability is regained at the expense of joint motion. Substitution of an adjacent tendon for the ligament has been used by two authors. Strandell[266] reported two cases in which he substituted the extensor pollicis brevis, and the abductor pollicis longus was used by Frykman and Johansson[252] in one case.

Recently, Neviaser, Wilson, and Lievano[263] described an operation in which the tendon of the adductor pollicis is advanced into the base of the proximal phalanx after the scarred residual of the collateral ligament is reefed. Although we have had no experience with this operation, their report of good results in 6 of 8 patients in whom the operation was performed suggests that this may be a reasonably predictable operative solution for a difficult problem.

The choice between ligament reconstruction and arthrodesis demands mature judgment and careful consideration of several factors. The age of the patient, his occupational need for motion or stability of the thumb, and the amount of motion of which the opposite thumb is capable, all must be taken into account.

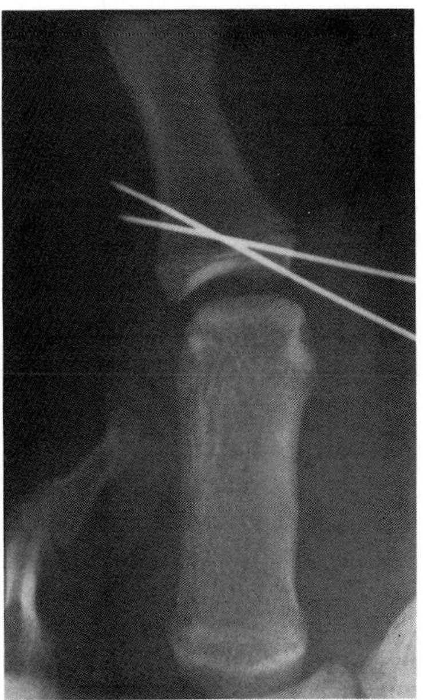

Fig. 6-73. A large, displaced fragment avulsed by the ulnar collateral ligament is best treated by open reduction and internal fixation with small, smooth Kirschner wires. Smaller fragments are sometimes more readily fixed with a pull-out wire.

REFERENCES

Anatomy

1. Allen, E. V.: Thromboangiitis obliterans: methods of diagnosis of chronic occlusive arterial lesions distal to the wrist with illustrative cases. Amer. J. Med. Sci., *178*: 237-244, 1929.
2. Cleland, J.: On the cutaneous ligaments of the phalanges. J. Anat. Physiol., *12*: 526, 1878.
3. Eaton, R. G.: Joint Injuries of the Hand. Springfield, Charles C Thomas, 1971.
4. Eyler, D. L., and Markee, J. E.: The anatomy and function of the intrinsic musculature of the fingers. J. Bone Joint Surg., *36A*:1-9; 18-20, 1954.
5. Flatt, A. E.: The Care of Minor Hand Injuries. St. Louis, C. V. Mosby, 1959.
6. Gad, P.: The anatomy of the volar part of the capsules of the finger joints. J. Bone Joint Surg., *49B*:362-367, 1967.
7. Goss, C. M.: Gray's Anatomy. ed. 26. Philadelphia, Lea & Febiger, 1954.
8. Grayson, J.: The cutaneous ligaments of the digits. J. Anat., *75*:164-165, 1941.
9. Haines, R. W.: The extensor apparatus of the finger. J. Anat., *85*:251-259, 1951.
10. Kaplan, E. B.: Functional and Surgical Anatomy of the Hand. ed. 2. Philadelphia, J. B. Lippincott, 1965.
11. Kuczynski, K.: The proximal interphalangeal joint: anatomy and causes of stiffness in the fingers. J. Bone Joint Surg., *50B*:656-663, 1968.

12. Landsmeer, J. M. F.: Anatomical and functional investigations of the human finger, and its functional significance. Acta Anat. *24*[Suppl.]:1-69, 1955.
13. Milford, L. W.: Retaining Ligaments of the Digits of the Hand: Gross and Microscopic Anatomic Study. Philadelphia, W. B. Saunders, 1968.
14. Smith, R. J.: Non-ischemic contractures of the intrinsic muscles of the hand. J. Bone Joint Surg., *53A*:1313-1331, 1971.
15. Tubiana, R., and Valentin, P.: The anatomy of the extensor apparatus of the fingers. Surg. Clin. North Amer., *44*:897-918, 1964.

Fractures (Excluding the Thumb)

16. Berkman, E. F., and Miles, G. H.: Internal fixation of metacarpal fractures exclusive of the thumb. J. Bone Joint Surg., *25*:816-821, 1943.
17. Blazina, M. E., and Lance, C.: Rupture of the flexor digitorum profundus tendon in student athletics. J. Amer. Coll. Health Assoc., *14*:248-249, 1966.
18. Bloem, J. J. A. M.: The treatment and prognosis of uncomplicated dislocated fractures of the metacarpals and phalanges. Arch. Chir. Neerl., *23*:55-65, 1971.
19. Böhler, L.: The Treatment of Fractures. ed. 5. New York, Grune & Stratton, 1956.
20. Borden, J.: Complications of fractures and ligamentous injuries of the hand. Orthop. Rev., *1*:29-38, 1972.
21. Borgeskov, S.: Conservative therapy for fractures of the phalanges and metacarpals. Acta Chir. Scand., *133*:123-130, 1967.
22. Bosworth, D. M.: Internal splinting of fractures of the fifth metacarpal. J. Bone Joint Surg., *19*:826-827, 1937.
23. Boyes, J. H.: Bunnell's Surgery of the Hand. ed. 5. Philadelphia, J. B. Lippincott, 1970.
24. ———: Bunnell's Surgery of the Hand. ed. 4. Philadelphia, J. B. Lippincott, 1964.
25. ———: Bunnell's Surgery of the Hand. ed. 3. Philadelphia, J. B. Lippincott, 1956.
26. Boyes, J. H., Wilson, J. N., and Smith, J. W.: Flexor-tendon ruptures in the forearm and hand. J. Bone Joint Surg., *42A*:637-646, 1960.
27. Brown, H.: Closed crush injuries of the hand and forearm. Orthop. Clin. North Amer., *1*:253-259, 1970.
28. Bunnell, S.: Surgery of the Hand. Philadelphia, J. B. Lippincott, 1944.
29. Burkhalter, W. E., Butler, B., Metz, W., and Omer, G.: Experiences with delayed primary closure of war wounds of the hand in Viet Nam. J. Bone Joint Surg., *50A*:945-954, 1968.
30. Burnham, P. J.: Physiological treatment for fractures of the metacarpals and phalanges. J.A.M.A., *169*:663-666, 1959.
31. Burton, R. I., and Eaton, R. G.: Common hand injuries in the athlete. Orthop. Clin. North Amer., *4*:809-838, 1973.
32. Butt, W. D.: Rigid wire fixation of fractures of the hand. Henry Ford Hosp. Bull., *4*:134-143, 1956.
33. ———: Fractures of the hand: I. Description. Can. Med. Assoc. J., *86*:731-735, 1962.
34. ———: Fractures of the hand: II. Statistical review. Can. Med. Assoc. J., *86*:775-779, 1962.
35. ———: Fractures of the hand: III. Treatment and results. Can. Med. Assoc. J., *86*:815-822, 1962.
36. Carr, R. W.: A finger caliper for reduction of phalangeal and metacarpal fractures by skeletal traction. South. Med. J., *32*:543-546, 1939.
37. Carroll, R. E., and Match, R. M.: Avulsion of the flexor profundus tendon insertion. J. Trauma, *10*:1109-1118, 1970.
38. Clifford, R. H.: Intramedullary wire fixation of hand fractures. Plast. Reconstr. Surg., *11*:366-371, 1953.
39. Clinkscales, G. S., Jr.: Complications in the management of fractures in hand injuries. South. Med. J., *63*:704-707, 1970.
40. Conwell, H. E., and Reynolds, F. C.: Key and Conwell's Management of Fractures, Dislocations, and Sprains. ed. 7. St. Louis, C. V. Mosby, 1961.
41. Coonrad, R. W., and Pohlman, M. H.: Impacted fractures in the proximal portion of the proximal phalanx of the finger. J. Bone Joint Surg., *51A*:1291-1296, 1969.
42. Cotton, F. J.: Dislocations and Joint Fractures. ed. 2. Philadelphia, W. B. Saunders, 1924.
43. Curry, G. J.: Treatment of finger fractures, simple and compound. Amer. J. Surg., *71*:80-83, 1946.
44. Dobyns, J. H.: Articular fractures of the hand [abstr.]. *In* Proc. Amer. Soc. Surg. Hand. J. Bone Joint Surg., *48*A:610, 1966.

45. Eichenholtz, S. N.: Fractures of the neck of the fifth metacarpal bone—is overtreatment justified? J.A.M.A., *178*:151-152, 1961.
46. Emmett, J. E., and Breck, L. W.: A review and analysis of 11,000 fractures seen in a private practice of orthopaedic surgery 1937-56. J. Bone Joint Surg., *40A*:1169-1175, 1958.
47. Goldberg, D.: Metacarpal fractures. A new instrument for the maintenance of position after reduction. Amer. J. Surg., *72*:758-766, 1946.
48. Green, D. P.: Commonly missed injuries in the hand. Amer. Fam. Physician, *7*: 111-119, 1973.
49. Green, D. P., and Anderson, J. R.: Closed reduction and percutaneous pin fixation of fracture phalanges. J. Bone Joint Surg., *55A*:1651-1654, 1973.
50. Gunter, E. S.: Traumatic avulsion of the insertion of flexor digitorum profundus. Aust. N. Z. J. Surg., *30*:1-8, 1960.
51. Haggart, G. E.: Fractures of the metacarpal, metatarsal bones, and phalanges treated by skeletal traction. Surg. Clin. North Amer., *14*:1203-1210, 1934.
52. Howard, L. D., Jr.: Fractures of the small bones of the hand. Plast. Reconstr. Surg., *29*:334-335, 1962.
53. ———: The problem of metacarpal fractures of the hand due to war wounds. *In* Instructional Course Lectures, The American Academy of Orthopaedic Surgeons, *2*:196-201. Ann Arbor, J. W. Edwards, 1944.
54. Hunter, J. M., and Cowen, N. J.: Fifth metacarpal fractures in a compensation clinic population. J. Bone Joint Surg., *52A*:1159-1165, 1970.
55. Jahss, S. A.: Fractures of the proximal phalanges: alignment and immobilization. J. Bone Joint Surg., *18*:726-731, 1936.
56. ———: Fractures of the metacarpals: a new method of reduction and immobilization. J. Bone Joint Surg., *20*:178-186, 1938.
57. James, J. I. P.: Fractures of the proximal and middle phalanges of the fingers. Acta Orthop. Scand., *32*:401-412, 1962.
58. ———: Common, simple errors in the management of hand injuries. Proc. R. Soc. Med., *63*:69-71, 1970.
59. James, J. I. P., and Wright, T. A.: Fractures of metacarpals and proximal and middle phalanges of the finger. *In* Proc. Br. Orthop. Assoc. J. Bone Joint Surg., *48B*:181-182, 1966.
60. Kaplan, L.: The treatment of fractures and dislocations of the hand and fingers. Surg. Clin. North Amer., *20*:1695-1720, 1940.
61. Karbelnig, M. J.: Fracture of the metacarpal shaft: a method of treatment. Calif. Med., *98*:269-270, 1963.
62. Key, J. A., and Conwell, H. E.: The Management of Fractures, Dislocation, and Sprains. ed. 5. St. Louis, C. V. Mosby, 1951.
63. Kilbourne, B. C.: Management of complicated hand fractures. Surg. Clin. North Amer., *48*:201-213, Feb., 1968.
64. Kilbourne, B. C., and Paul, E. G.: The use of small bone screws in the treatment of metacarpal, metatarsal, and phalangeal fractures. J. Bone Joint Surg., *40A*:375-383, 1958.
65. Koch, S. L.: Disabilities of hand resulting from loss of joint function. J.A.M.A., *104*: 30-35, 1935.
66. Lamphier, T. A.: Improper reduction of fractures of the proximal phalanges of fingers. Amer. J. Surg., *94*:926-930, 1957.
67. Lee, M. L. H.: Intra-articular and periarticular fractures of the phalanges. J. Bone Joint Surg., *45B*:103-109, 1963.
68. Lipscomb, P. R.: Management of fractures of the hand. Amer. Surg., *29*:277-282, 1963.
69. London, P. S.: Sprains and fractures involving the interphalangeal joints. Hand, *3*:155-158, 1971.
70. Lord, R. E.: Intramedullary fixation of metacarpal fractures. J.A.M.A., *164*:1746-1749, 1957.
71. Magnuson, P. B.: Fractures of metacarpals and phalanges. J.A.M.A., *91*:1339-1340, 1928.
72. ———: Fractures. Philadelphia, J. B. Lippincott, 1942.
73. Mansoor, I. A.: Fractures of the proximal phalanx of fingers: a method of reduction. J. Bone Joint Surg., *51A*:196-198, 1969.
74. McLaughlin, H. L.: Trauma. Philadelphia, W. B. Saunders, 1960.
75. McMaster, P. E.: Tendon and muscle ruptures: clinical and experimental studies on the causes and location of subcutaneous ruptures. J. Bone Joint Surg., *15*:705-722, 1933.
76. McNealy, R. W., and Lichtenstein, M. E.: Fractures of the metacarpals and the phalanges. Surg. Gynecol. Obstet., *60*:758-761, 1932.

77. ———: Fractures of the metacarpals and phalanges. Western J. Surg. Obstet. Gynecol., *43*:156-161, 1935.
78. ———: Fractures of the bones of the hand. Amer. J. Surg., *50*:563-570, 1940.
79. Meltzer, H.: Wire extension treatment of fractures of fingers and metacarpal bones. Surg. Gynecol. Obstet., *55*:87-89, 1932.
80. Milford, L.: The Hand. *In* Crenshaw, A. H. (ed.): Campbell's Operative Orthopaedics. ed. 5. St. Louis, C. V. Mosby, 1971.
81. Moberg, E.: The use of traction treatment for fractures of phalanges and metacarpals. Acta Chir. Scand., *99*:341-352, 1950.
82. ———: Emergency Surgery of the Hand. Edinburgh, E. & S. Livingstone, 1968.
83. Mock, H. E., and Ellis, J. D.: The treatment of fractures of the fingers and metacarpals with a description of the authors' finger caliper. Surg. Gynecol. Obstet., *45*:551-556, 1927.
84. Moore, D. C.: Regional Block. ed. 4. Springfield. Charles C Thomas, 1967.
85. Morton, H. S.: Fractures of the wrist and hand. Can. Med. Assoc. J., *51*:430-434, 1944.
86. Murray, C. R.: Fractures of the bones of the hand. New York State J. Med., *36*: 1749-1761, 1936.
87. Nemethi, C. E.: Phalangeal fractures treated by open reduction and Kirschner-wire fixation. Indust. Med. and Surg., *23*:148-150, 1954.
88. Nichols, H. M.: Manual of Hand Injuries. ed. 2. Chicago, The Year Book Publishers, 1960.
89. ———: Repair of extensor tendon insertion in the fingers. J. Bone Joint Surg., *33A*:836-841, 1951.
90. Norman, H. R. C.: Fractures of the metacarpals treated by a new method. Can. Med. Assoc. J., *49*:173-175, 1943.
91. Owen, H. R.: Fractures of the bones of the hand. Surg. Gynecol. Obstet., *66*: 500-505, 1938.
92. Peacock, E. E.: Management of conditions of the hand requiring immobilization. Surg. Clin. North Amer., *33*:1297-1309, 1953.
93. Pieron, A. P.: Correction of rotational malunion of a phalanx by metacarpal osteotomy. J. Bone Joint Surg., *54B*:516-519, 1972.
94. Posch, J. L., Walker, P. J., and Miller, H.: Treatment of ruptured tendons of the hand and wrist. Amer. J. Surg., *91*: 669-681, 1956.
95. Pratt, D. R.: Exposing fractures of the proximal phalanx of the finger longitudinally through the dorsal extensor apparatus. Clin. Orthop., *15*:22-26, 1959.
96. Quigley, T. B., and Urist, M. R.: Interphalangeal joints: a method of digital skeletal traction which permits active motion. Amer. J. Surg., *73*:175-183, 1947.
97. Rider, D. L.: Fractures of the metacarpals, metatarsals, and phalanges. Amer. J. Surg., *38*:549-559.
98. Riordan, D. C.: Fractures about the hand. South. Med. J., *50*:637-640, 1957.
99. Roberts, N.: Fractures of the phalanges of the hand and metacarpals. Proc. R. Soc. Med., *31*:793-798, 1938.
100. Ruedi, T. P., Burri, C., and Pfeiffer, K. M.: Stable internal fixation of fractures of the hand. J. Trauma, *11*:381-389, 1971.
101. Rush, L. V., and Rush, H. L.: Evolution of medullary fixation of fractures by the longitudinal pin. Amer. J. Surg., *78*:324-333, 1949.
102. Saypool, G. M., and Slattery, L. R.: Observations on displaced fractures of the hand. Surg. Gynecol. Obstet., *79*:522-525, 1944.
103. Schlein, A. P., and Nathan, F. F.: A dual finger fracture. Hand, *4*:171-172, 1972.
104. Schulze, H. A.: An improved skin-traction technique for the fingers. J. Bone Joint Surg., *29*:222-224, 1947.
105. Scobie, W. H.: Crush fracture of sesamoid bone of thumb. Br. Med. J., *2*:912, 1941.
106. Scudder, C. L.: The Treatment of Fractures. Philadelphia, W. B. Saunders, 1926.
107. Simonetta, C.: The use of "A.O." plates in the hand. Hand, *2*:43-45, 1970.
108. Smith, C. H.: Compound fracture of the fingers. Ann. Surg., *119*:266-273, 1944.
109. Smith, F. L., and Rider, D. L.: A study of the healing of one hundred consecutive phalangeal fractures. J. Bone Joint Surg., *17*:91-109, 1935.
110. Speed, K.: A textbook of fractures and dislocations. Philadelphia, Lea & Febiger, 1942.
111. Stark, H. H.: Troublesome fractures and dislocations of the hand. Instructional Course Lectures, AAOS, *19*:130-149, 1970.
112. Sutro, C. J.: Fracture of metacarpal bones and proximal manual phalanges: treat-

ment with emphasis on the prevention of rational deformities. Amer. J. Surg., *81*:327-332, 1951.

113. Swanson, A. B.: Fractures involving the digits of the hand. Orthop. Clin. North Amer., *1*:261-274, Nov., 1970.
114. Vom Saal, F. H.: Intramedullary fixation in fractures of the hand and fingers. J. Bone Joint Surg., *35A*:5-16, 1953.
115. Watson-Jones, R.: Fractures and Joint Injuries. ed. 3. Edinburgh, E. & S. Livingstone, 1943.
116. ———: Fractures and Joint Injuries. ed. 4. Edinburgh, E. & S. Livingstone, 1956.
117. Waugh, R. L., and Ferrazzano, G. P.: Fractures of the metacarpals exclusive of the thumb. A new method of treatment. Amer. J. Surg., *59*:186-194, 1943.
118. Weckesser, E. C.: Rotational osteotomy of the metacarpal for overlapping fingers. J. Bone Joint Surg., *47A*:751-756, 1965.
119. Wise, R. A.: An unusual fracture of the terminal phalanx of the finger. J. Bone Joint Surg., *21*:467-469, 1939.
120. Wright, T. A.: Early mobilization in fractures of the metacarpals. Can. J. Surg., *11*:491-498, 1968.

Mallet Finger and Boutonniere

121. Abouna, J. M., and Brown, H.: The treatment of mallet finger. Br. J. Surg., *55*: 653-667, 1968.
122. Backdahl, M.: Ruptures of the extensor aponeurosis at the distal digital joints. Acta Chir. Scand., *111*:151-157, 1956.
123. Brooks, D.: Splint for mallet fingers. Br. Med. J., *2*:1238, 1964.
124. Casscells, S. W., and Strange, T. B.: Intramedullary wire fixation of mallet-fingers. J. Bone Joint Surg., *39A*:521-526, 1957.
125. ———: Intramedullary wire fixation of mallet-finger (follow-up note). J. Bone Joint Surg., *51A*:1018-1019, 1969.
126. Elliott, R. A.: Injuries to the extensor mechanism of the hand. Orthop. Clin. North Amer., *1*:335-354, 1970.
127. Flinchum, D.: Mallet finger. J. Med. Assoc. Ga., *48*:601-603, 1959.
128. Fowler, F. D.: New splint for treatment of mallet finger. J.A.M.A., *170*:945, 1959.
129. Harris, C., Jr.: The Fowler operation for mallet finger. *In* Proc. Amer. Soc. Surg. Hand. J. Bone Joint Surg., *48A*:613, 1966.
130. Hillman, F. E.: New technique for treatment of mallet fingers and fractures of distal phalanx. J.A.M.A., *161*:1135-1138, 1956.
131. Howie, H.: The treatment of mallet finger: a modified plaster technique. New Zealand Med. J., *46*:513, 1947.
132. Kaplan, E. B.: Mallet or baseball finger. Surgery, *7*:784-791, 1940.
133. ———: Anatomy, injuries, and treatment of the extensor apparatus of the hand and the digits. Clin. Orthop., *13*:24-41, 1959.
134. Lewin, P.: A simple splint for baseball finger. J.A.M.A., *85*:1059, 1925.
135. Mason, M. L.: Mallet finger. Lancet, *266*: 1220, 1954.
136. Mason, M. L.: Rupture of the tendons of the hand. Surg. Gynecol. Obstet., *50*: 611-624, 1930.
137. Matev, I.: The boutonniere deformity, Hand, *1*:90-95, 1969.
138. McCue, F. C., and Abbott, J. L.: The treatment of mallet finger and boutonniere deformities. Virginia Med. Monthly, *94*:623-628, 1967.
139. Pratt, D. R.: Internal splint for closed and open treatment of injuries of the extensor tendon at the distal joint of the finger. J. Bone Joint Surg., *34A*:785-788, 1952.
140. Ramsey, R. A.: Mallet finger. Lancet, *2*:1244, 1968.
141. Ratliff, A. H. C.: Mallet finger: a review of forty-five cases. Manch. Med. Gaz., *26*:4, 1947.
142. Robb, W. A. T.: The results of treatment of mallet finger. J. Bone Joint Surg., *41B*: 546-549, 1959.
143. Roemer, F. J.: Hyperextension injuries to the finger joints. Amer. J. Surg., *80*:295-302, 1950.
144. Rosenzweig, N.: Management of the mallet finger. South African Med. J., *24*:831-832, 1950.
145. Smillie, I. S.: Mallet finger. Br. J. Surg., *24*:439-445, 1937.
146. Souter, W. A.: The boutonniere deformity. J. Bone Joint Surg., *49B*:710-721, 1967.
147. Spigelman, L.: New splint for management of mallet finger. J.A.M.A., *153*: 1362, 1953.
148. Stack, H. G.: Mallet finger. Hand, *1*:83-89, 1969.
149. Stark, H. H., Boyes, J. H., and Wilson, J. N.: Mallet finger. J. Bone Joint Surg., *44A*:1061-1068, 1962.
150. Stewart, I. M.: Boutonniere finger. Clin. Orthop., *23*:220-226, 1962.

151. Van Demark, R. E.: A simple method of treatment for recent mallet finger. Milit. Surg., *107*:385-386, 1950.
152. Williams, E. G.: Treatment of mallet finger. Can. Med. Assoc. J., *57*:582, 1947.

Fractures of the Thumb Metacarpal

153. Badger, F. C.: Internal fixation in the treatment of Bennett's fractures. J. Bone Joint Surg., *38B*:771, 1956.
154. Bennett, E. H.: On fracture of the metacarpal bone of the thumb. Br. Med. J., *2*:12-13, 1886.
155. ———: Fractures of the metacarpal bones. Dublin J. Med. Sci., *73*:72-75, 1882.
156. Billing, L., and Gedda, K.-O.: Roentgen examination of Bennett's fracture. Acta Radiol., *38*:471-476, 1952.
157. Blum, L.: The treatment of Bennett's fracture-dislocation of the first metacarpal bone. J. Bone Joint Surg., *23*:578-580, 1941.
158. Charnley, J.: The Closed Treatment of Common Fractures. Edinburgh, E. & S. Livingstone, 1961.
159. Cotton, F. J.: Dislocations and Joint Fractures. Philadelphia, W. B. Saunders, 1910.
160. Ellis, V. H.: A method of treating Bennett's fracture. Proc. R. Soc. Med., *39*:21, 1946.
161. Gedda, K.-O.: Studies on Bennett's fracture: anatomy, roentgenology, and therapy. Acta Chir. Scand. (Suppl. 193), 1954.
162. Gibson, A., and James, E. S.: Fractures of the first metacarpal bone. Can. Med. Assoc. J., *43*:153-155, 1940.
163. Goldberg, D.: Thumb fractures and dislocation, a new method of treatment. Am. J. Surg., *81*:227-231, 1951.
164. Green, D. P., and O'Brien, E. T.: Fractures of the thumb metacarpal. South. Med. J., *65*:807-814, 1972.
165. Griffiths, J. C.: Fractures at the base of the first metacarpal bone. J. Bone Joint Surg., *46B*:712-729, 1964.
166. ———: Bennett's fracture in childhood. Br. J. Clin. Pract., *20*:582-583, 1966.
167. Johnson, E. C.: Fracture of the base of the thumb: a new method of fixation. J.A.M.A., *126*:27-28, 1944.
168. Macey, M. B., and Murray, R. A.: Fractures about the base of the first metacarpal with special reference to Bennett's fracture. South. Med. J., *42*:931-935, 1949.
169. McNealy, R. W., and Lichtenstein, M. E.: Bennett's fracture and other fractures of the first metacarpal. Surg. Gynecol. Obstet., *56*:197-201, 1933.
170. Pollen, A. G.: The conservative treatment of Bennett's fracture-subluxation of the thumb metacarpal. J. Bone Joint Surg., *50B*:91-101, 1968.
171. Roberts, J. B., and Kelly, J. A.: Treatise on Fractures. Philadelphia, J. B. Lippincott, 1916.
172. Robinson, S.: The Bennett fracture of the first metacarpal bone: diagnosis and treatment. Boston Med. and Surg. J., *158*:275, 1908.
173. Rolando, S.: Fracture de la base du premier metacarpien: et principalement sur une variete non encore decrite. Presse Med., *33*:303, 1910.
174. Ross, J. W., and Sinclair, A. B.: The treatment of Bennett's fracture with the stader splint. J. Can. Med. Serv., *3*:507-511, 1946.
175. Spangberg, O., and Thoren, L.: Bennett's fracture: a method of treatment with oblique traction. J. Bone Joint Surg., *45B*:732-739, 1963.
176. Thoren, L.: A new method of extension treatment in Bennett's fracture. Acta Chir. Scand., *110*:485-493, 1956.
177. ———: Basal fractures of the first metacarpal bone—a method of treatment by extension. Acta Orthop. Scand., *27*:40-48, 1957.
178. Wagner, C. J.: Method of treatment of Bennett's fracture dislocation. Amer. J. Surg., *80*:230-231, 1950.
179. Wiggins, H. E., Bundens, W. D., Jr., and Park, B. J.: A method of treatment of fracture-dislocations of the first metacarpal bone. J. Bone Joint Surg., *36A*:810-819, 1954.

Interphalangeal Joints (Excluding the Thumb)

180. Adams, J. P.: Correction of chronic dorsal subluxation of the proximal interphalangeal joint by means of a criss-cross volar graft. J. Bone Joint Surg., *41A*:111-115, 1959.
181. Aufranc, O. E., Jones, W. N., and Bierbaum, B. E.: Fracture dislocation of the proximal interphalangeal joint of the finger. J.A.M.A., *204*:815-819, 1968.
182. Bate, J. T.: An operation for the correction of locking of the proximal interphalangeal joint of finger in hyperextension. J. Bone Joint Surg., *27*:142-144, 1945.

183. Boyes, J. H.: Bunnell's Surgery of the Hand. ed. 5. Philadelphia, J. B. Lippincott, 1970.
184. ———: Bunnell's Surgery of the Hand. ed. 4. Philadelphia, J. B. Lippincott, 1964.
185. ———: Bunnell's Surgery of the Hand. ed. 3. Philadelphia, J. B. Lippincott, 1956.
186. Coonrad, R. W.: *In* Discussion of Athletic Injuries of the Proximal Interphalangeal Joint Requiring Surgical Treatment. J. Bone Joint Surg., *52A*:956, 1970.
187. Curtis, R. M.: Joints of the hand. *In* Flynn, J. D. (ed.), Hand Surgery. Baltimore, Williams & Wilkins, 1966.
188. Curtis, R. M.: Treatment of the injuries of the proximal interphalangeal joints of fingers. Curr. Pract. Orthop. Surg., *2*:125-135, 1964.
188. ———: Treatment of the injuries of the proximal interphalangeal joints of fingers. Curr. Pract. Orthop. Surg., *2*:125-135, 1964.
189. Eaton, R. G.: Joint Injuries of the Hand. Springfield, Charles C Thomas, 1971.
190. Flatt, A. E.: Athletic injuries of the Hand. J. La. State Med. Assoc., *119*:425-431, 1967.
191. Furlong, R.: Injuries of the Hand. Boston, Little, Brown, 1957.
192. Johnson, F. G., and Greene, M. H.: Another cause of irreducible dislocation of the proximal interphalangeal joint of a finger. J. Bone Joint Surg., *48A*:542-544, 1966.
193. Kaplan, E. B.: Extension deformities of the proximal interphalangeal joints of the fingers: anatomical study. J. Bone Joint Surg., *18*:781, 1936.
194. Kleinert, H. E., and Kasdan, M. L.: Reconstruction of chronically subluxated proximal interphalangeal finger joint. J. Bone Joint Surg., *47A*:958-964, 1965.
195. London, P. S.: Sprains and fractures involving the interphalangeal joints. Hand, *3*:155-158, 1971.
196. McCue, F. C., Honner, R., Johnson, M. C., Jr., and Gieck, J. H.: Athletic injuries of the proximal interphalangeal joint requiring surgical treatment. J. Bone Joint Surg., *52A*:937-956, 1970.
197. McElfresh, E., Dobyns, J. H., and O'Brien, E. T.: Management of fracture-dislocation of the proximal interphalangeal joints by extension-block splinting. J. Bone Joint Surg., *54A*:1705-1711, 1972.
198. Milford, L.: The Hand. *In* Crenshaw, A. H. (ed.): Campbell's Operative Orthopaedics. ed. 5. St. Louis, C. V. Mosby, 1971.
199. Moberg, E.: Fractures and ligamentous injuries of the thumb and fingers. Surg. Clin. North Amer., *40*:297-309, April, 1960.
200. Neviaser, R. J., and Wilson, J. N.: Interposition of the extensor tendon resulting in persistent subluxation of the proximal interphalangeal joint of the finger. Clin. Orthop., *83*:118-120, 1972.
201. Portis, R. B.: Hyperextensibility of the proximal interphalangeal joint of the finger following trauma. J. Bone Joint Surg., *36A*:1141-1146, 1954.
202. Redler, I., and Williams, J. T.: Rupture of a collateral ligament of the proximal interphalangeal joint of the fingers. J. Bone Joint Surg., *49A*:322-326, 1967.
203. Robertson, R. C., Cawley, J. J., and Faris, A. M.: Treatment of fracture-dislocation of the interphalangeal joints of the hand. J. Bone Joint Surg., *28*:68-70, 1946.
204. Schulze, H. A.: Treatment of fracture-dislocations of the proximal interphalangeal joints of the fingers. Milit. Surg., *99*:190-191, 1946.
205. Spinner, M., and Choi, B. Y.: Anterior dislocation of the proximal interphalangeal joint. J. Bone Joint Surg., *52A*:1329-1336, 1970.
206. Spray, P.: Finger fracture-dislocation proximal at the interphalangeal joint. J. Tenn. Med. Assoc., *59*:765-766, 1966.
207. Trojan, E.: Fracture dislocation of the bases of the proximal and middle phalanges of the fingers. Hand, *4*:60-61, 1972.
208. Wiley, A. M.: Instability of the proximal interphalangeal joint following dislocation and fracture dislocation: surgical repair. Hand, *2*:185-191, 1970.
209. Wilson, J. N., and Rowland, S. A.: Fracture-dislocation of the proximal interphalangeal joint of the finger. J. Bone Joint Surg., *48A*:493-502, 1966.

Metacarpophalangeal Joints (Excluding the Thumb)

210. Alldred, A.: A locked index finger. J. Bone Joint Surg., *36B*:102-103, 1954.
211. Baldwin, L. W., Miller, D. L., Lockhart, L. D., and Evans, E. B.: Metacarpophalangeal-joint dislocations of the fingers. J. Bone Joint Surg., *49A*:1587-1589, 1967.

212. Barash, H. L.: An unusual case of dorsal dislocation of the metacarpophalangeal joint of the index finger. Clin. Orthop., *83*:121-122, 1972.
213. Barnard, H. L.: Dorsal dislocation of the first phalanx of the little finger; reduction by Farabeuf's dorsal incision. Lancet, *1*:88-90, 1901.
214. Burman, M.: Irreducible hyperextension dislocation of the metacarpophalangeal joint of a finger. Bull. Hosp. Joint Dis., *14*:290-291, 1953.
215. Farabeuf, L. H. F.: De la luxation du ponce en arriere. Bull. Soc. Chir. *11*:21-62, 1876.
216. Flatt, A. E.: Fracture-dislocation of an index metacarpophalangeal joint and an ulnar deviating force in the flexor tendons. J. Bone Joint Surg., *48A*:100-104, 1966.
217. Green, D. P., and Terry, G. C.: Complex dislocation of the metacarpophalangeal joint: correlative pathological anatomy. J. Bone Joint Surg., *55A*:1480-1486, 1973.
218. Gustilo, R. B.: Dislocation of the metacarpophalangeal joint of the index finger. Minn. Med., *49*:1119-1121, 1966.
219. Hunt, J. C., Watts, H. B., and Glasgow, J. D.: Dorsal dislocation of the metacarpophalangeal joint of the index finger with particular reference to open dislocation. J. Bone Joint Surg., *49A*:1572-1578, 1967.
220. Kaplan, E. B.: Dorsal dislocation of the metacarpophalangeal joint of the index finger. J. Bone Joint Surg., *39A*:1081-1086, 1957.
221. Le Clerc, R.: Luxations de l'index sur son metacarpien. Rev. d'Orthop., *2*:227-242, 1911.
222. McLaughlin, H. L.: Complex "locked" dislocation of the metacarpophalangeal joints. J. Trauma, *5*:683-688, 1965.
223. Milch, H.: Subluxation of the index metacarpophalangeal joint: case report. J. Bone Joint Surg., *47A*:522-523; 585, 1965.
224. Murphy, A. F., and Stark, H. H.: Closed dislocation of the metacarpophalangeal joint of the index finger. J. Bone Joint Surg., *49A*:1579-1586, 1967.
225. Nutter, P. D.: Interposition of sesamoids in metacarpophalangeal dislocations. J. Bone Joint Surg., *22*:730-734, 1940.
226. Ridge, E. M.: Dorsal dislocation of the first phalanx of the little finger. Lancet, *1*:781, 1901.
227. Robins, R. H. C.: Injuries of the metacarpophalangeal joints. Hand, *3*:159-163, 1971.
228. Speed, K.: Textbook of fractures and dislocations. ed. 4. Philadelphia, Lea & Febiger, 1942.
229. Sweterlitsch, P. R., Torg, J. S., and Pollack, H.: Entrapment of a sesamoid in the index metacarpophalangeal joint: report of two cases. J. Bone Joint Surg., *51A*:995-998, 1969.
230. Von Raffler, W.: Irreducible dislocation of the metacarpophalangeal joint of the finger. Clin. Orthop., *35*:171-173, 1964.
231. Wilhelmy, J., and Hay, R. L.: Dual dislocation of metacarpophalangeal joints. Hand, *4*:168-170, 1972.

Carpometacarpal Joints (Excluding the Thumb)

232. Buzby, B. F.: Palmar carpo-metacarpal dislocation of the fifth metacarpal. Ann. Surg., *100*:555-558, 1934.
233. Clement, B. L.: Fracture-dislocation of the base of the fifth metacarpal: a case report. J. Bone Joint Surg., *27*:498-499, 1945.
234. Hsu, J. D., and Curtis, R. M.: Carpometacarpal dislocations on the ulnar side of the hand. J. Bone Joint Surg., *52A*: 927-930, 1970.
235. Ker, H. R.: Dislocation of the fifth carpometacarpal joint. J. Bone Joint Surg., *37B*:254-256, 1955.
236. Lyman, C. B.: Backward dislocation of the second carpo-metacarpal articulation. Ann. Surg., *43*:905-906, 1906.
237. McLean, E. H.: Carpometacarpal Dislocation. J.A.M.A., *79*:299-300, 1922.
238. McWhorter, G. L.: Isolated and complete dislocation of the fifth carpometacarpal joint: open operation. Surg. Clin. Chicago, *2*:793-796, 1918.
239. Metz, W. R.: Multiple carpo-metacarpal dislocations. New Orleans Med. Surg. J., *79*:327-330, 1926.
240. Murless, B. C.: Fracture-dislocation of the base of the fifth metacarpal bone. Br. J. Surg., *31*:402-404, 1943.
241. Nalebuff, E. A.: Isolated anterior carpometacarpal dislocation of the fifth finger: classification and case report. J. Trauma, *8*:1119-1123, 1968.
242. Roberts, N., and Holland, C. T.: Isolated dislocation of the base of the fifth metacarpal. Br. J. Surg., *23*:567-571, 1936.
243. Shorbe, H. B.: Carpometacarpal dislocations. J. Bone Joint Surg., *20*:454-457, 1938.

244. Waugh, R. L., and Yancey, A. G.: Carpometacarpal dislocations. J. Bone Joint Surg., *30A*:397-404, 1948.
245. Whitson, R. O.: Carpometacarpal dislocation: a case report. Clin. Orthop., *6*: 189-195, 1955.

Dislocations and Ligamentous Injuries in the Thumb

246. Alldred, A. J.: Rupture of the collateral ligament of the metacarpo-phalangeal joint of the thumb. J. Bone Joint Surg., *37B*:443-445, 1955.
247. Bailey, R. A. J.: Some closed injuries of the metacarpo-phalangeal joint of the thumb. J. Bone Joint Surg., *45B*:428-429, 1963.
248. Campbell, C. S.: Gamekeeper's thumb. J. Bone Joint Surg., *37B*:148-149, 1955.
249. Coonrad, R. W., and Goldner, J. L.: A study of the pathological findings and treatment in soft-tissue injury of the thumb metacarpophalangeal joint. J. Bone Joint Surg., *50A*:439-451, 1968.
250. Eggers, G. W. N.: Chronic dislocation of the base of the metacarpal of the thumb. J. Bone Joint Surg., *27*:500-501, 1945.
251. Frank, W. E., and Dobyns, J.: Surgical pathology of collateral ligamentous injuries of the thumb. Clin. Orthop., *83*: 102-114, 1972.
252. Frykman, G., and Johansson, O.: Surgical repair of rupture of the ulnar collateral ligament of the metacarpo-phalangeal joint of the thumb. Acta Chir. Scand., *112*:58-64, 1956.
253. Haines, R. W.: The mechanism of rotation at the first carpo-metacarpal joint. J. Anat., *78*:44-46, 1944.
254. Harris, H., and Joseph, J.: Variation in extension of the metacarpo-phalangeal and interphalangeal joints of the thumb. J. Bone Joint Surg., *31B*:547-559, 1949.
255. Joseph, J.: Further studies of the metacarpo-phalangeal and interphalangeal joints of the thumb. J. Anat., *85*:221-229, 1951.
256. Kaplan, E. B.: The pathology and treatment of radial subluxation of the thumb with ulnar displacement of the head of the first metacarpal. J. Bone Joint Surg., *43A*:541-546, 1961.
257. Kessler, I.: Complete avulsion of the ulnar collateral ligament of the metacarpophalangeal joint of the thumb. Clin. Orthop., *29*:196-200, 1961.
258. Kessler, I., and Heller, J.: Complete avulsion of the ligamentous apparatus of the metacarpophalangeal joint of the thumb. Surg. Gynecol. Obstet., *116*:95-98, 1963.
259. Kestler, O. C.: Recurrent dislocation of the first carpometacarpal joint repaired by functional tenodesis. J. Bone Joint Surg., *28A*:858-861, 1946.
260. Lasserre, C., Pauzat, D., and Derennes, R.: Osteoarthritis of the trapezio-metacarpal joint. J. Bone Joint Surg., *31B*: 534-536, 1949.
261. Milch, H.: Recurrent dislocation of thumb. Capsulorrhaphy. Am. J. Surg., *6*:237-239, 1929.
262. Moberg, E., and Stener, B.: Injuries to the ligaments of the thumb and fingers. Diagnosis, treatment, and prognosis. Acta Chir. Scand., *106*:166-186, 1953.
263. Neviaser, R. J., Wilson, J. N., and Lievano, A.: Rupture of the ulnar collateral ligament of the thumb (gamekeeper's thumb): correction by dynamic repair. J. Bone Joint Surg., *53A*:1357-1364, 1971.
264. Slocum, D. B.: Stabilization of the articulation of the greater multangular and the first metacarpal. J. Bone Joint Surg., *25A*:626-630, 1943.
265. Stener, B.: Displacement of the ruptured ulnar collateral ligament of the metacarpo-phalangeal joint of the thumb. J. Bone Joint Surg., *44B*:869-879, 1962.
266. Strandell, G.: Total rupture of the ulnar collateral ligament of the metacarpophalangeal joint of the thumb. Acta Chir. Scand., *111*:72-80, 1959.
267. Sutro, C. J.: Pollex valgus (a bunion-like deformity of the thumb corrected by surgical intervention). Bull. Hosp. Joint Dis., *18*:135-139, 1957.
268. Zilberman, Z., Rotschild, E., and Krauss, L.: Rupture of the ulnar collateral ligament of the thumb. J. Trauma, *5*:477-481, 1965.

7 Fractures and Dislocations of the Wrist

James H. Dobyns, M.D.
Ronald L. Linscheid, M.D.

The wrist joint, situated between the forearm and the hand, includes the articular and metaphyseal portions of the distal radius and ulna. The word wrist is derived from *wraestan* meaning "to twist." The wrist is the terminal joint in the system of levers and articulations that constitute the upper extremity. By virtue of its unique structure, the wrist provides flexion and extension in the sagittal plane and abduction and adduction in the frontal plane. These functions are augmented by the axial rotations, pronation, and supination in the coronal plane that are afforded by the two-bone configuration of the forearm, which provides a stable yet highly movable universal joint. This useful anatomical arrangement apparently developed as a consequence of evolution in the anthropoid line to provide efficient arboreal progression by brachiation. With the advent of bipedal locomotion, the upper extremity was freed to be used for various tasks.

Consequences of the more unstable bipedal posture and the multitude of uses to which the upper extremity is put provide the bases for numerous injuries. The type of injury that occurs depends on many factors, including the forces exerted, the energy absorbed, the geometric configuration of the articular segments, the strength and disposition of supporting ligaments and muscles, the rigidity of the osseous structures, the position of the hand and wrist at impact, and the length of exposure to the injuring force.

Undoubtedly, the ancients were aware of wrist problems, but not much is written until the beginning of the 19th century. At that time, as reflected in the writings of the continental physicians,[75,76,87,184] the general belief was that most injuries in this area were dislocations of the wrist. It remained for Abraham Colles[54] of Dublin to make the important differentiation, in 1814, between dislocations and the much more common fracture that now bears his name. In France, the same distinction had been made, in 1783, by Pouteau,[220] but the distinction was not clearly established either in Great Britain or on the continent until presented vigorously and ably by Dupuytren[87] in 1820. The pendulum then swung the other way, to the opinion that dislocations of the wrist did not occur. However, the advent of the roentgenograph demonstrated that fractures and dislocations could and did take place in the carpus. Although roentgenographic interpretation was difficult, certain patterns of deformity were recognized by the early 20th century as being dislocations or fracture-dislocations in the carpus. A remarkably complete discussion of these injuries was given in various papers and finally in book form by E. Destot.[77]

Perhaps because of the frequent mistake of calling a fracture of the carpal scaphoid a sprain, and thereby missing the diagnosis until an inappropriate time, the literature has continued up until the present time to deny the significance or even the presence of sprains. Only now does current medical literature begin to suggest that there is a high incidence of sprains of the wrist. Many sprains are of immediate significance and most are of eventual importance in creating disability. While work is still being done on understanding the various types of wrist sprains and the resulting secondary collapse deformities and degenerative phenomena, we have come full cycle from a period when all wrist injuries were considered dislocations through a period when none were considered dislocations. We now have a spectrum of injuries whose frequency pattern is almost established and whose causes and mechanisms are partially understood,[14,36,37,63,101,114,154,155,176,232,236,271,274,281,288,289,292] though considerable work is still being done.[134,295]

The most common mode of injury to the wrist is a fall on the outstretched hand. The energy absorbed is a function of the body weight and the distance through which the body falls. The energy is distributed through the soft tissues, bones, and articulations.[45,105] If the force at the wrist is attenuated by the coordinated absorption of energy by the proximal musculotendinous units, as in the athlete who "knows how to fall," no injury occurs. For the elderly woman with significantly decreased structural strength of the radius due to osteoporosis, diminished muscle strength, and poor neuromuscular coordination, a fall on the outstretched hand is likely to produce a fracture, usually through the cancellous bone of the metaphysis of the distal radius. In an actively growing youngster a similar fall on the outstretched hand usually produces an injury to the weakest structural component of the wrist for that age group; that is, the zone of provisional calcification of the epiphyseal plate. A more forceful fall suffered by an energetic young person engaged in athletics or vigorous work results commonly in a fracture of the scaphoid bone. The scaphoid is particularly at risk because of its unique loading characteristics secondary to an unusual contour, a link position between the proximal and distal carpal rows and stout ligamentous support.

In falls on the dorsiflexed wrist, the osseous components as well as the ligaments are subjected to differing stresses, depending on the point of application of the force. Thus, impact on the heel of the hand is likely to produce radial fractures, whereas impact on the distal palm is likely to produce scaphoid fracture or carpal dislocation. Even more discrete localization to the thenar or hypothenar region imparts rotation and additional shearing and torsional stresses to the forearm on the fixed hand. Excursion exceeding the normal limits of ligamentous lengths results in ligamentous rupture or bone yielding, with the amount of disruption dependent on the energy of the particular injury.[107,134,295]

SURGICAL ANATOMY

General Anatomy

The wrist, that area defined by Kaplan[142] as extending from the carpometacarpal joints to the distal border of the pronator quadratus proximally, can be considered a constricted area of controlled access. Most soft-tissue structures that pass the wrist are rather rigidly compartmentalized, and all are close to some bone or joint. This suggests that damage to these structures or compromise of their function might be common, and this is true. All the extensor tendons lie in compartments dorsally (usually six in number). In this area, only the brachioradialis tendon is not in a compartment, but throughout its wrist course, this tendon is attached to bone of the radial styloid and distal metaphysis. On the palmar side of the wrist, all the flexor tendons to the digits plus the median nerve lie in the carpal tunnel, while the ulnar nerve and vessels lie in the adjacent Guyon's canal. Both the flexor carpi radialis, radially, and

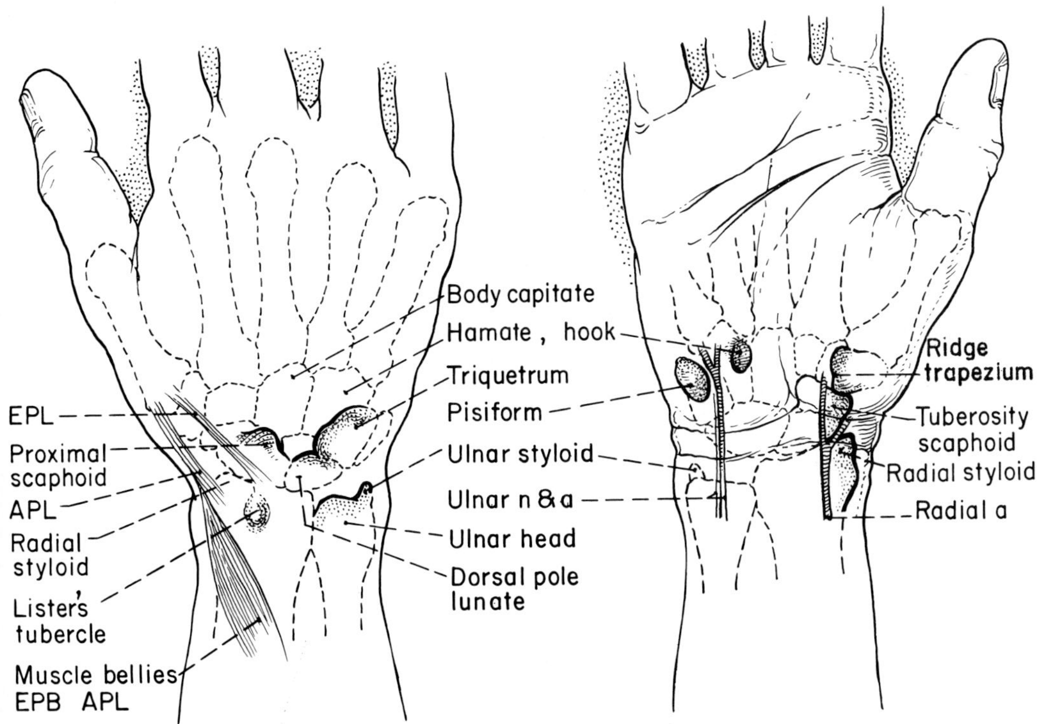

Fig. 7-1. Topographical anatomy of the right hand. Bony prominences, readily palpated at the wrist, may be used to locate most major structures, either by palpation or stereotactic approximation. Various movements of the wrist increase the accessibility of certain bony prominences, for example, the dorsal pole of the scaphoid and lunate, the tuberosity of the scaphoid, the body of the scaphoid in the snuffbox, the hamate, the triquetrum, and the pisiform. The ulnar styloid occurs in various positions, depending on rotation of the wrist. It is at the ulnopalmar position on full pronation and the dorsoradial position on full supination.

the flexor carpi ulnaris, ulnarly, have their own compartments as they pass to their metacarpal base insertions. Only the palmaris longus tendon has no deep canal, though it has a compartment between the layers of fascia. The disciplined courses allotted to structures as they pass the wrist are demonstrated by the positioning of the tendons. The digital flexors and extensors, which contribute little to wrist and hand deviation, are grouped centrally, whereas the motor muscles of the wrist are grouped peripherally so as to be most effective in wrist positioning. The disposition of structures in the carpal tunnel implies that tearing of the palmar wrist capsule or periosteum might endanger one of the deep tendons. This is true. Knowledge of the anatomy of the wrist with its eight carpal bones, five metacarpal bases, distal radius and ulna, and the associated ligamentous connections is important. Excellent detailed accounts of the anatomy can be found in other sources.[99,142,286]

Topographical Anatomy

For the clinician, certain features are particularly important (Fig. 7-1). The overall topology of the wrist area is well known, and individual variations in a given wrist generally can be easily assessed by comparing it with the opposite wrist. Every bone, most of the arteries, and many of the tendons and nerves can be palpated in the normal wrist. The most important topographical landmarks are the radial styloid,

Lister's tubercle, and the head and styloid of the ulna. The position of the ulnar styloid and head varies with rotation of the forearm. The styloid is prominent at the ulnar side of the wrist with the forearm in the mid-position. It moves to the ulnar-palmar aspect of the wrist (pointing toward the pisiform) in pronation and moves dorsally in supination. The extensor carpi ulnaris maintains a constant adjacent dorsal relationship to the styloid. The head is palpable dorsally in pronation and palmarly in supination.

An elliptical bony prominence at the base of the thenar muscles, representing a combination of the greater trapezial ridge and the scaphoid tuberosity, is the most obvious bony landmark on the radial-palmar side of the wrist. This prominence lies at the intersection of the flexor carpi radialis tendon and the distal wrist crease. Deep to this crease lie the distal scaphoid, the head of the capitate, the body of the triquetrum, and the pisiform bones. On the ulnar-palmar side of the wrist, the most obvious bony landmarks are the pisiform, lying at the junction of the flexor carpi ulnaris tendon and the distal wrist crease, and the hook of the hamate, lying somewhat more deeply just distal and slightly radial to the pisiform.

These bony landmarks indicate the attachment boundaries of the transverse carpal ligament, which contains the contents of the carpal tunnel. The area just proximal to this, lying between or just proximal to the two wrist flexion creases, will contain the abnormal prominences of bony elements displaced toward the palmar surface in perilunar dislocations. Between the creases, such a prominence would be the lunate centrally, perhaps with part or all of either scaphoid or triquetrum accompanying it. More proximally, the ulnar head at the ulnar side or the distal radius at the radial side may be prominent. Dorsally, the abnormal bony prominences most often encountered are the distal radius, as in Colles' fracture, and the proximal row of the carpus thrust posteriorly by the dorsal tilt of the deformed radial articular surface. The distal ulna may be displaced dorsally or merely relatively elongated in comparison to the shortened radius. Infrequently, it may be displaced palmarward instead.

With the forearm bones intact, the landmarks previously discussed serve as excellent guides to common pathological carpal changes. Just distal to the radial styloid, for instance, in the anatomic snuffbox, the waist of the scaphoid can be palpated. Just distal to Lister's tubercle, the scapholunate junction is palpable and is prominent when the wrist is in palmar flexion. Just distal to the ulnar head and radial to its styloid lie the lunate-triquetral junction and the triquetral-hamate joint. All of these areas are common sites of wrist injury. Within the opened carpal tunnel, the palmar projections previously mentioned, which provide attachments for the transverse carpal ligaments, are easily palpable at the sides. Along the deep or dorsal surface of the carpal tunnel, many bony surfaces can be felt, but the most prominent are the palmar lip of the lunate and, just proximal to that, the palmar lip of the radius. Either or both may be unusually prominent as a result of old trauma.

The tendons most easily felt dorsally are those of the first, second, third, and sixth compartments, though any of the extensor tendons can be felt by precise palpation while they are acting. The abductor pollicis longus and extensor pollicis brevis can be felt together and separately at the radial boundary of the snuffbox, and the extensor pollicis longus ridges at the ulnar border of the snuffbox. Almost underneath the extensor pollicis longus at the base of the second metacarpal, the extensor carpi radialis longus can be palpated, and just ulnarly, the extensor carpi radialis brevis can be palpated. Just distal to the ulnar head and directly across it in supination, the extensor carpi ulnaris tendon is easily found. Readily palpated, on the flexor surface, are the radially located flexor carpi radialis tendon, running next to the scaphoid tuberosity; the ulnar flexor carpi ulnaris tendon, running to the pisiform; and the centrally located palmaris longus (when present).

Pulses are usually easy to locate. The more common ones are the radial artery pulse, just radial to the flexor carpi radialis at the wrist, and the ulnar artery pulse, just radial to the flexor carpi ulnaris. The continuation of the radial artery through the snuffbox and dorsally into the first web space, as well as the thenar branch, is frequently palpable. Normal nerves are more difficult to palpate, but the dorsal cutaneous branches of both the radial and ulnar nerves usually can be located just proximal and dorsal to the radial styloid and ulnar head, respectively.

Bones and Joints

The wrist is composed of the distal metaphyseal portions of the radius and ulna, three functional units of the carpus, and the investing soft tissues (Fig. 7-2).

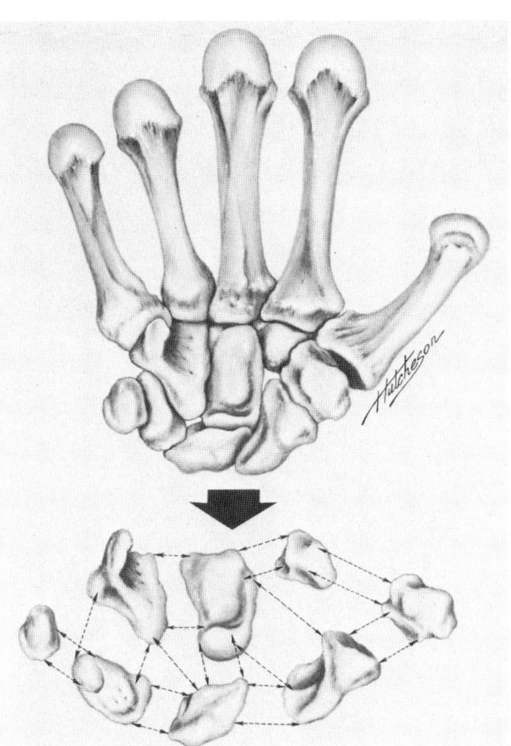

Fig. 7-2. Exploded view of carpal bones. Ligaments are attached to roughened areas on the palmar horn of the lunate, the palmar surface of the triquetrum, and the neck of the capitate in two arcades of fibers that join in the pisotriquetral area. Additional strong ligamentous attachments are noted on the tuberosity of the scaphoid, the trapezium, the trapezoid, and the carpometacarpal joints. The proximal carpal row consists of the lunate and triquetrum. The distal carpal row consists of the trapezoid, hamate, and capitate. Two carpal rows are joined by the scaphoid. This acts to coordinate movement between the two carpal rows and, with the trapezium, provides a firm base for the thumb axis. The scaphoid position, between the carpal rows, makes it uniquely susceptible to injury. (Modified from Taleisnik, J., and Kelly, P. J.: J. Bone Joint Surg., *48A*:1125-1137, 1966)

The distal radius provides a large articular surface for the proximal carpal row as a result of metaphyseal flaring (Fig. 7-3). The articular surface is biconcave, with an inclination of the articular facets that averages 12 degrees in the palmar direction and 14 degrees tangential to the lunate fossa in the ulnar direction from the longitudinal axis of the radius. The articular surface is divided into facets for the scaphoid and lunate bones. Another concave articular surface, the ulnar or sigmoid notch of the radius, accepts the convex distal articular surface of the ulna. The ulnar head is an expanded area of the distal end of the ulna, with an approximately circular cross section. This contour allows rotation of the distal radius around it, through an arc of approximately 160 degrees, thus providing the distal joint for axial rotation of the forearm in pronation and supination. The distal articular surface of the ulna is covered by the triangular fibrocartilage. This fibrocartilage attaches to the distal margin of the sigmoid notch of the radius and to the radial base of the ulnar styloid. The triangular fibrocartilage blends distally into the ulnar collateral ligament and peripherally into the distal radioulnar ligaments and dorsal and palmar radiocarpal ligaments. The cartilage is thinnest near the

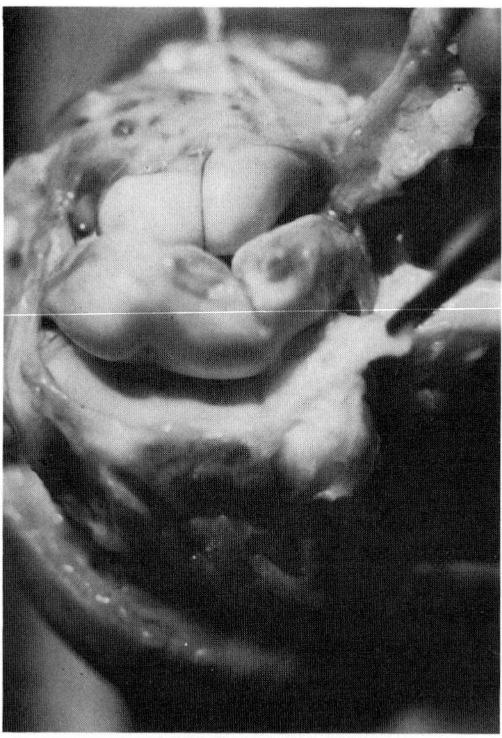

Fig. 7-3. Intraarticular anatomy of the wrist joint. The proximal carpal row is at the center of the figure; the scaphoid is on the left; lunate, in the middle; and triquetrum, on the right. Note the darker areas for ligamentous attachment of the radiotriquetral ligament on these three bones and from the radial styloid. The radial collateral ligament is at the far left. The radial articular surface consists of two fossae for articulation of the scaphoid and lunate. The triangular fibrocartilage is grasped by a clamp. It is attached to the ulnar border of the radial articular surface and is invested by the dorsal radioulnar ligament. Its attachment to the ulnar styloid is not visualized. Its prestyloid recess is seen between the triquetrum and the clamp. The proximal carpal row is connected by interosseous membranes. The articular surface of the capitate and hamate is seen at the top of the figure, and the triquetral surface of the hamate to the right.

radial attachment, where it may be fenestrated, allowing continuity between the distal radioulnar joint and the radiocarpal joint. The space between the distal ulna and the triangular fibrocartilage is the recessus sacciformis. This space allows the movement of pronation and supination around the distal ulna while maintaining the integrity of the radiocarpal articular surface. With evolutionary regression of the ulnar styloid, whose tip may be vestigially covered with cartilage, the meniscus of the ulnar-triquetral joint has joined the triangular fibrocartilage.[161,162] A residual prestyloid recess in the meniscal portion may lead to a joint space around the styloid process. In some cases, the styloid still articulates with the triquetrum. Proximally, this triangular disk holds and controls the relative motion of the radius around the distal ulna. The dorsal and palmar distal radioulnar ligaments are fibrous investments that supplement the stability of the distal radioulnar joint and are intimately attached at the periphery of the triangular fibrocartilage. The dorsal and palmar ligaments are tightened, respectively, during pronation and supination. The stability of the distal radioulnar joint also depends on the depth of the ulnar notch of the radius and the integrity of the extensor carpi ulnaris tendon held in the notch of the ulna adjacent to the ulnar styloid by its fibrous sheath.[256]

The carpal bones may be grouped into the proximal row of the lunate and triquetrum, along with the articulation of the latter to the pisiform bone; the distal carpal row of trapezoid, capitate, and hamate bones; and the scaphoid and trapezium. The trapezium provides a carpal base for the independent motion of the thumb. The scaphoid, lying between the two carpal rows, aids in structural support of the intercarpal row.

The proximal carpal row of lunate and triquetrum and the proximal segment of the scaphoid are closely bound together by the interosseous membranes, which separate the radiocarpal joint from the intercarpal joint (Fig. 7-4). The lunate has a convex curvature proximally and a concave curvature distally, where it articulates with the capitate. The radius of curvature of the distal articulation is approximately half that of the proximal. The triquetral bone articulates with the lunate, hamate, and pisiform bones, as well as with the triangular fibrocartilage. It has a trochoid distal surface that articulates with the similar though opposite curvature of the hamate. The pisiform bone articulates with the triquetrum on its palmar articular surface, which is inclined approximately 20 degrees to the long axis of the forearm. As the wrist is dorsiflexed, the pisiform slides distal- and palmarward, thus increasing the moment arm of the flexor carpi ulnaris with increasing dorsiflexion. The pisohamate ligament connects the pisiform to the hook of the hamate distally. The pisotriquetral joint may communicate with the radiocarpal joint proximally.

The distal carpal row is composed of the trapezoid, capitate, and hamate bones. The capitate is the largest carpal bone and, with the trapezoid, supports the second and third metacarpal bases. The rigidity of these metacarpals is due to the tight fit of the V-shaped trapezoid into the base of the second metacarpal, a flat capitate articular surface, and strong ligamentous investments. The hamate supports the base of the mobile fourth and fifth metacarpals.

The radial strut of the wrist is composed of the scaphoid, which bridges the proximal and distal carpal rows, and the trapezium. The scaphoid lies at an angle of approximately 47 degrees to the long axis of the forearm, being inclined distally and palmarly, where it articulates with the trapezium and trapezoid (see Fig. 7-31A). The latter arrangement allows for an independently mobile, opposable thumb. The bridging effect of the scaphoid supports the carpal rows.

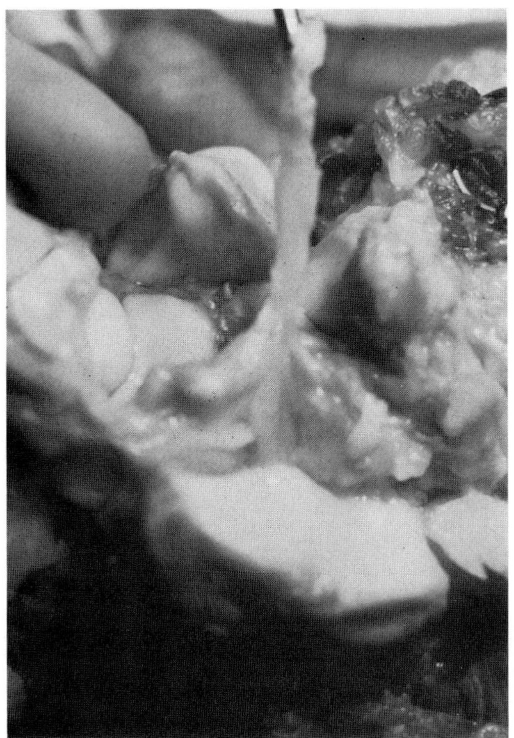

Fig. 7-4. Scapholunate interosseous ligament. The interosseous ligament has been dissected from its dorsal attachment to the rim of the radius, then distally to the dorsal scapholunate junction, where it was dissected from between these bones and is seen as it courses through the palmar radiocarpal ligament to the volar lip of the radius. It is closely enmeshed by more superficial arcades of fibers. This ligament is responsible for maintaining scapholunate stability and assuring the proper sequence of kinematic configurations of the proximal row. This ligament was described by Testut and Kuenz. On the right, triangular fibrocartilage has been partially cut away, exposing the distal radioulnar joint. The continuation of the lunotriquetral ligament is partially seen on the palmar radiocarpal ligament and is also important in providing proximal row stability.

Ligaments

The fibrous capsule of the wrist joint is interlaced by strengthening ligaments (Fig. 7-5).[156,285] Probably as a result of the plantigrade and brachiate activities of our remote ancestors, the palmar ligamentous apparatus of the wrist is much stronger than the dorsal.

The arcades of fibers of the palmar radiocarpal ligament are more prominent from the intraarticular aspect of the joint. The thickest ligaments extend from a roughened

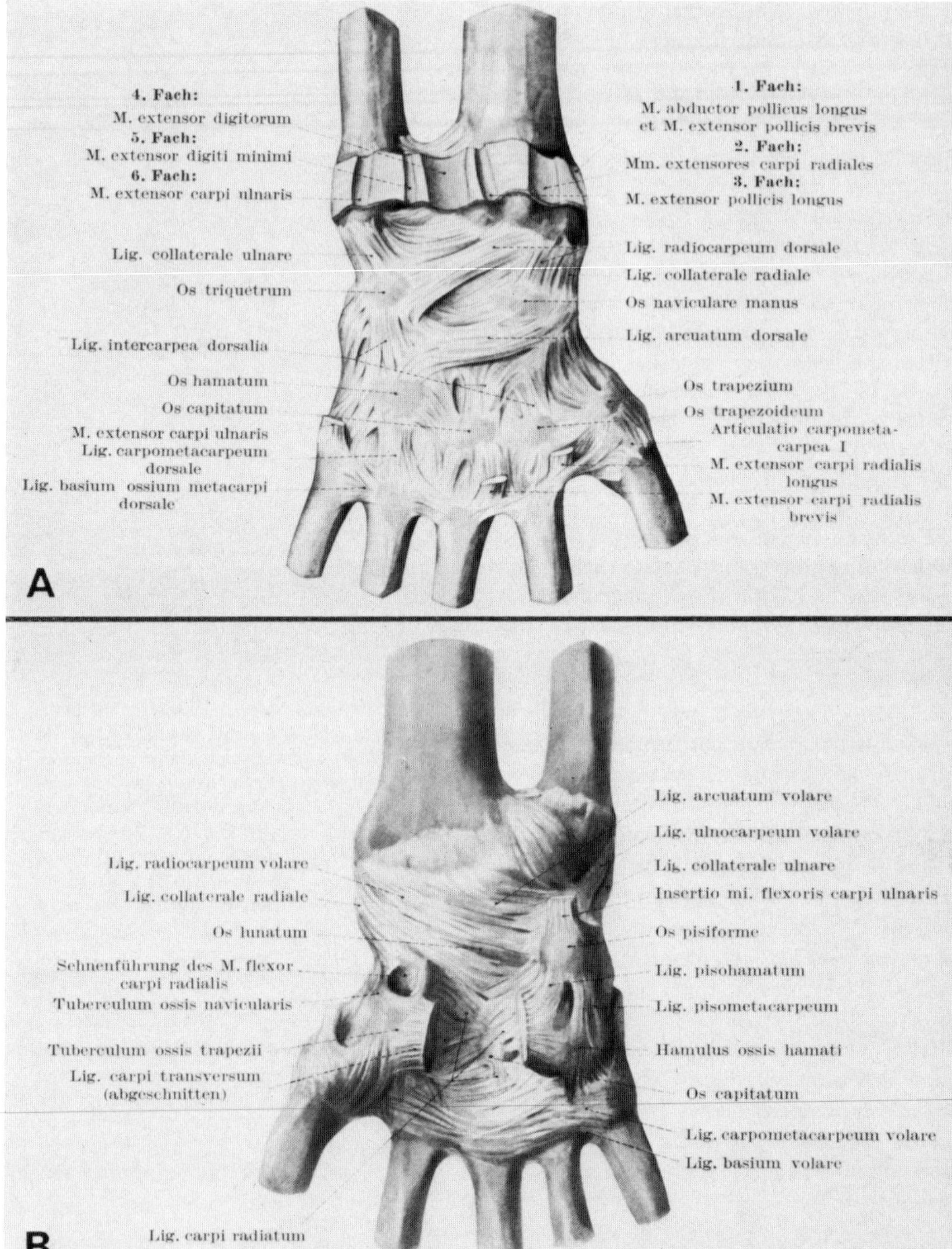

Fig. 7-5. (*A*) Dorsal ligaments of the wrist. A double arcade structure that arches from the distal radius to the proximal and distal carpal rows and then back into the ulnar carpal ligament is illustrated. Oblique disposition of the fibers acts to restrain ulnar translation of the carpus down the inclined plane of the radial articular surface. An arcade structure permits a wide range of motions in two planes while constraining abnormal motion. A thin, weak area is located over the proximal pole of the scaphoid in a site

area on the radial-palmar aspect of the radial styloid to the palmar pole of the lunate, then across to the palmar ridge of the triquetrum and to the pisotriquetral ligament. A second strong arcade of fibers extends from the radius to the palmar body of the capitate, then arches across the palmar aspect of the hamate to the pisotriquetral ligament. An area of weakness lies between these arcades just distal to the palmar surface of the lunate and just proximal to the strong ligamentous attachments to the body of the capitate. This area of weaker fibers is largest when the wrist is in extreme dorsiflexion and is hidden by overlap of the two arcuate systems when the wrist is in palmar flexion. It is through this area that a rent forms during the usual dislocations and fracture-dislocations of the wrist. It is through this interval that the lunate is displaced into the carpal canal.

The dorsal ligaments describe an arcade from the dorsal aspect of the radial styloid to the base of the ulnar styloid. The strongest portion of the dorsal ligament extends from the radial styloid to the dorsal pole of the lunate and triquetrum. At this area, it is heavily reinforced by axially directed fibers from the ulnar prominence of the radius and the fibrous investments of the third and fourth dorsal tendinous compartments. This arcade then blends into the ulnar collateral ligament and pisotriquetral ligament. The capsule is thinnest over the dorsal pole of the scaphoid. A second strong arcade of fibers extends from the dorsal ridge of the scaphoid and scaphoid tuberosity ulnarly to the trapezoid-capitate-hamate and the dorsal aspects of the carpometacarpal joints.

The radial collateral ligament resembles a hammock, with strong fibers running from the styloid to the scaphoid tuberosity and trapezium palmarly and from the styloid to the scaphoid body and trapezium dorsally. In addition, strong fascial fibers crisscross the area from the sheaths of the flexor carpi radialis and the first extensor compartments. The disposition of the fibers seems appropriate to an area that needs to resist some adduction stress but more commonly is subject to excesses of either dorsiflexion or palmar flexion stress.

The ulnar collateral ligament extends from a broad expanse of the ulnar head and the base of the ulnar styloid to a roughened area on the ulnar aspect of the triquetrum and the pisotriquetral ligament. This band of fibers is much more prominent palmarly when the wrist is in full pronation and is drawn out into a more dorsal-ulnar position with the wrist in supination.

The various bones of the proximal row, the distal row, and the metacarpal row are bound to each other by short, interosseous ligaments that pass from bone to bone. A more interesting variety of connecting interosseous ligament is represented by the

---

commonly replaced by dorsal ganglia. Triquetral attachments are strong and insert over a wide area of bone. (*B*) Palmar wrist ligaments. The proximal arcade of fibers inserting on the palmar pole of the lunate and triquetrum is extremely strong. The weak area between the radiolunotriquetral ligament and the radiocapitate ligament is much more pronounced on dorsiflexion of the wrist and represents an area that gives way during perilunar dislocations. The section of the radial collateral ligament that extends to the scaphoid tuberosity is also strong. The ulnar aspect of the wrist is well supported by the ulnar collateral, pisohamate, and pisotriquetral ligaments. During pronation, the ulnar collateral ligament is twisted so that support of distal radioulnar joint palmarly is increased. The transverse carpal ligament, which is shown cut away, further strengthens the proximal carpal arch. Dynamic functions of radiocarpal ligaments in constraining carpal motions are best understood in a fresh anatomic specimen, as the wrist is moved through a wide range of motions. (von Lanz, T., and Wachsmuth, W.: Praktische Anatomie: Ein Lehr- und Hilfsbuch der Anatomischen Grundlagen Ärztlichen Handelns. ed. 2. vol. 1. Berlin, Springer-Verlag, 1959)

scapholunate ligament and triquetrolunate ligament. These are strong and resist the distraction imposed by the distal carpal row during axial loading and rotatory motion. The proximal surface is covered with a thin layer of articular cartilage, such that it is frequently difficult to identify the interosseous ligament at the time of exposure. Both ligaments have palmar and dorsal connections to the respective radial lip and follow the proximal convex outline of the respective intercarpal joint (ligament of Testut and Kuenz[142]; Fig. 7-4). These interosseous ligaments of the proximal carpal row are intimately associated with the radiocarpal ligaments. The disposition of these ligaments and their strengths are of considerable importance in the kinematics of the joint and the mechanisms of injury.

Neurovascular Supply

The nerve and blood supplies of the wrist come from the regional nerves and vessels. These include the ulnar nerve main trunk, running deep to the flexor carpi ulnaris tendon and into Guyon's canal; the main trunk median nerve, running between the flexor carpi radialis and the palmaris longus into the carpal tunnel; the anterior interosseous branch of the median nerve, lying on the interosseous membrane between the ulna and the radius; the posterior interosseous branch of the radial nerve, lying on the posterior surface of

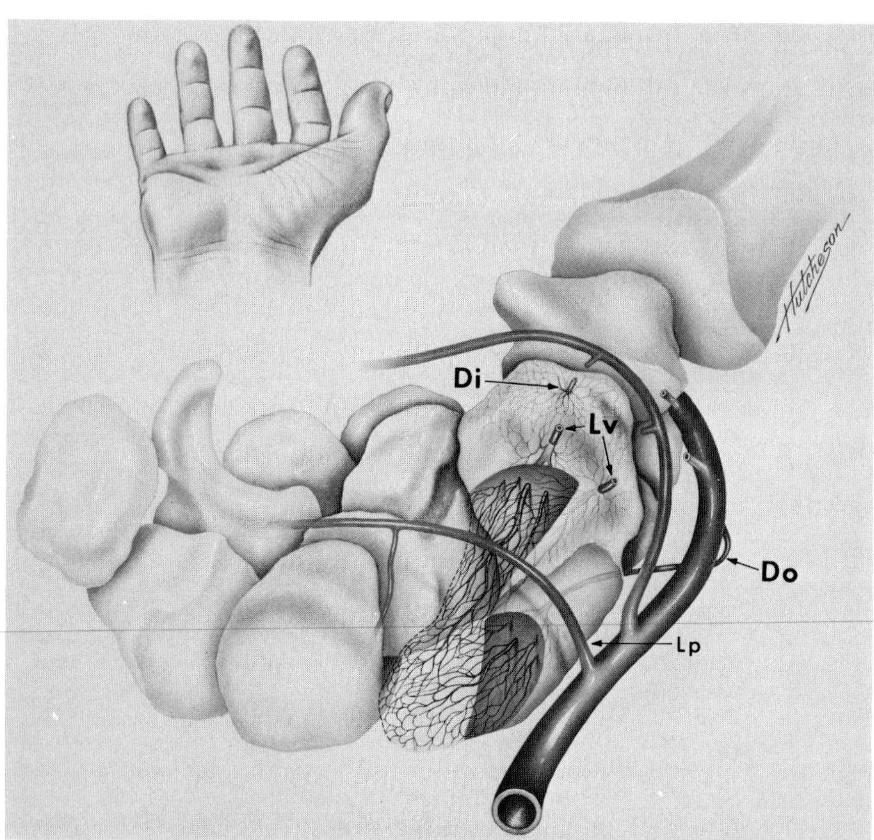

Fig. 7-6. Ideal representation of extraosseous and intraosseous blood supply of the scaphoid. *Lv*, laterovolar vessels; *Do*, dorsal vessels; *Di*, distal vessels; and *Lp*, lateral palmar vessels. (Taleisnik, J., and Kelly, P. J.: J. Bone Joint Surg., *48A*:1125-1137, 1966)

the radioulnar interosseous membrane; the superficial sensory branch of the radial nerve, emerging dorsally from underneath the brachioradialis tendon about 5 cm. proximal to the radial styloid; and the dorsal cutaneous branch of the ulnar nerve, which branches from the main ulnar trunk and lies subcutaneously across the ulnar aspect of the ulna at a point about 5 cm. proximal to the ulnar styloid. The palmar cutaneous branch of the median nerve arises from its main trunk, about 4 cm. proximal to the wrist crease. These subsidiary branches of the median, ulnar, and radial nerves are readily damaged by lacerations and incisions. They are easily visualized and should be protected. The potential for a neuralgic pain syndrome is common to all of them.

Circulation is obtained through the radial and ulnar arteries and the anterior and posterior interosseous arteries. Several of these arteries usually join to form a dorsal carpal arch. The usual concern for circulation in the wrist area is with the maintenance of adequate blood supply to the carpal scaphoid and the carpal lunate (Fig. 7-6), both of which are likely to undergo ischemic changes after trauma. Well conceived studies[157,270] of the circulation to both bones have confirmed the earlier supposition made by observation of the vascular foramina: that most of the blood supply of each bone enters the bone in its distal half.[208] There is no interval by which the scaphoid can be approached without endangering some of the three branches that constantly, but in different proportions, supply its circulation. However, the branches usually can be identified and protected, particularly in the snuffbox area. When, in addition, the radial styloid is removed, most of the scaphoid is exposed through this gap, and there are no vessels directly in the way. The lunate blood supply is constantly endangered by the usual dorsal approaches to the carpus, but the blood supply that reaches it through the palmar radiocarpal ligament is generally sufficient. Furthermore, this ligament is seldom endangered either during trauma or by surgical approaches, since the openings made by either trauma or surgery in the palmar capsule are usually just distal to the lunate.

MECHANISMS OF INJURY

Probably 90 per cent or more of injuries to the wrist area are due to stress applied when the wrist is dorsiflexed. In dorsiflexion, compression and shear stresses are concentrated along the dorsum, and tension stresses are concentrated along the palmar aspect. There are a few instances of injury sustained when the wrist is in palmar flexion, with a reversal of stresses just mentioned. These stresses cause the more uncommon types of injury, such as some of the Smith-type fractures of the distal radius and the palmar perilunate dislocation of the carpus. The amount of radial and ulnar deviation and the degree of supination and pronation are undoubtedly factors in the types of injury produced.[271] Some of these modifications of the basic positions have been investigated, but a detailed and exact delineation of all these factors has not been made. However, most investigators agree that, in the typical dorsiflexion injury, the distal radius yields with a lower level of force and a lower angle of dorsiflexion than when carpal injuries are involved.[107,134] Recent experience in our own biomechanical laboratory suggests that the classic waist fracture of the carpal scaphoid is incurred in a position of about 97 degrees dorsiflexion and 7 to 10 degrees of radial deviation.[295] The more common injuries, such as the Colles-type fracture, fractures of the carpal scaphoid, and the various dislocations and fracture-dislocations around the lunate, are failures in tension of bone or ligament, or both.

Kinematics

Wrist motions are complex because of the unusual geometric conglomerate of ball-and-socket with gliding types of joints restrained by an intricate ligamentous apparatus.[99,137,143,176,304] The wrist may move in either a dorsal-palmar plane or a radio-ulnar plane to allow circumduction, but its natural motion is a composite of these, with the preferred arc being from extension and radial deviation to flexion and ulnar deviation.

Dorsiflexion of the wrist averages 70 degrees, and palmar flexion of the wrist averages 75 degrees. This pronounced angular excursion of the wrist allows the linear excursion of the finger tendons to be greatly augmented. This range of motion is achieved by concurrent and synchronous motion at both the radiocarpal and intercarpal joints (Fig. 7-7). Each joint accounts for about half of the angular motion of the wrist. The proximal carpal row, as exemplified by the lunate, is an intercalated articular segment and has no direct tendinous support to guide its motion. Therefore, its synchronous motion with the distal row during flexion and extension depends on the geometry and the ligamentous support afforded to the joint. As will be seen later, when the support is interrupted, the intercalated segment tends to undergo a zig-zag collapse under compressive stress. The scaphoid, lying in the sagittal plane obliquely between the apparent centers of rotation of the proximal and distal carpal rows, acts as a stabilizing crank to prevent this collapse. The integrity of the scaphoid bone, the scapholunate ligament, the radioscaphoid ligament, and the radiocapitate ligaments is essential for this stability.

In the frontal plane, radial abduction is

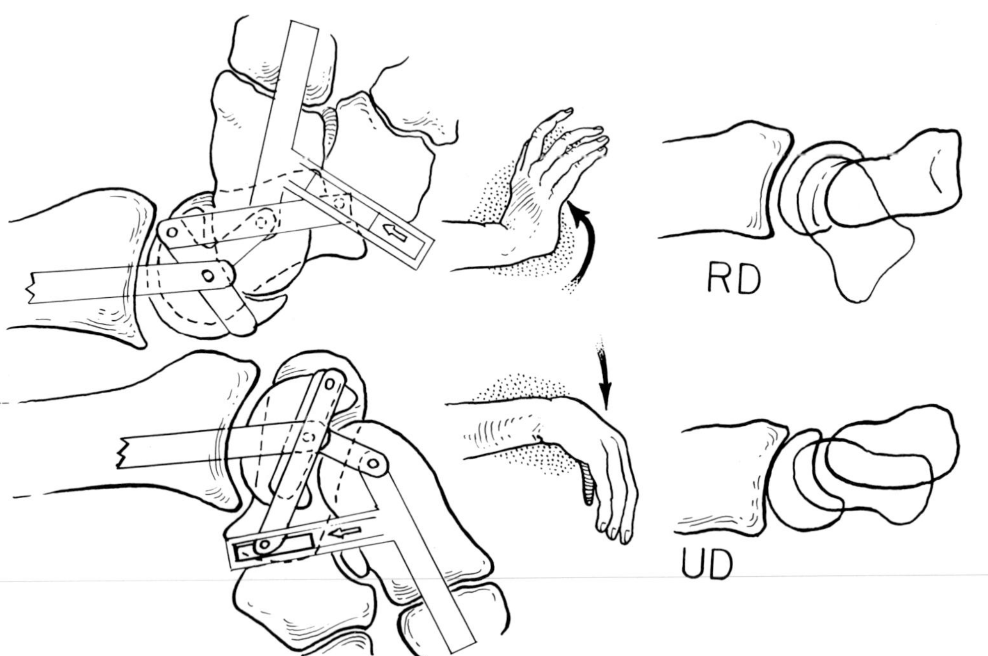

Fig. 7-7. Scaphoid link mechanism in flexion-extenison movements. During flexion and extension, nearly equal angular displacement occurs at the radiocarpal and intercarpal joints. This motion is stabilized by the scaphoid bone, which acts as a connecting rod across the two carpal rows. It also acts as a stop mechanism to prevent hyperflexion motions. Without this oblique linkage between the two carpal rows, a zig-zag collapse tends to occur. A similar mechanical linkage is known as a slider crank mechanism. Conjunct dorsiflexion of the proximal row on ulnar deviation (*UD*) and palmar flexion on radial deviation (*RD*) are shown on the right. (Modified from Linscheid, R. L., Dobyns, J. H., Beabout, J. W., and Bryan, R. S.: J. Bone Joint Surg., *54A*:1612-1632, 1972)

possible to approximately 15 to 25 degrees, and ulnar abduction to 30 to 60 degrees. This motion occurs at both the radiocarpal joint and the intercarpal joints, the respective amounts varying among persons (Figs. 7-7, 7-8). In order to achieve this motion, the proximal carpal row undergoes adjunct dorsiflexion during ulnar deviation and palmar flexion during radial deviation. Thus, there is reciprocal motion of the proximal and distal carpal rows in the sagittal plane. This is probably produced by the pressure

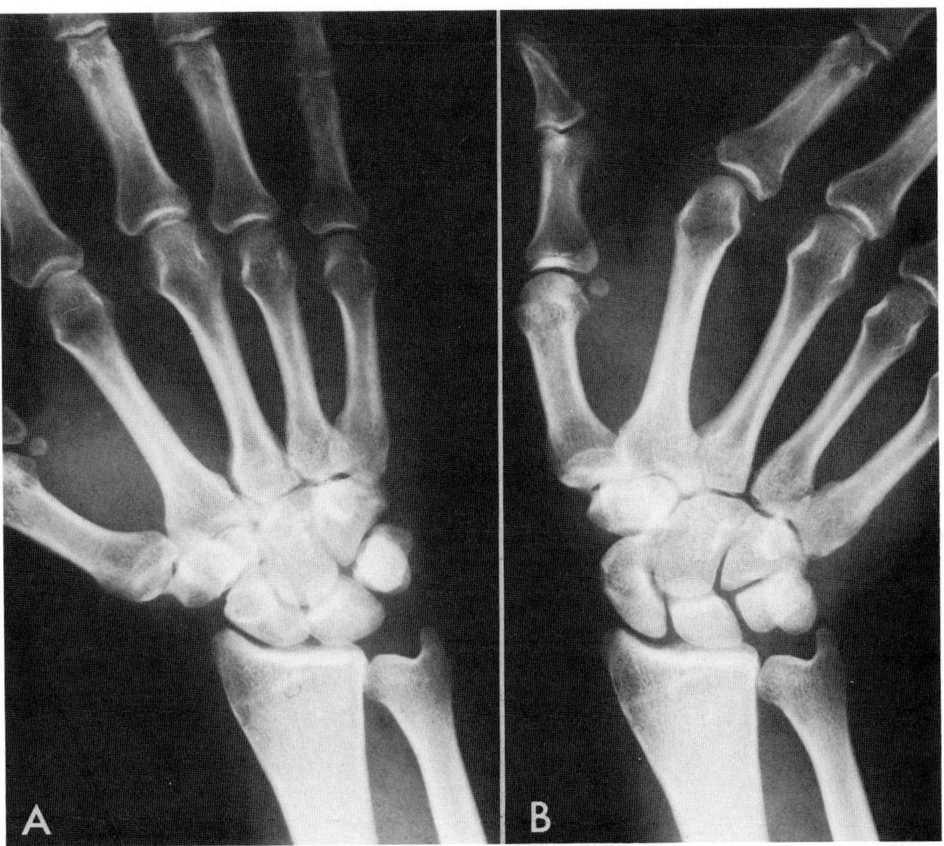

Fig. 7-8. Roentgenographic variation in carpal configuration of the right hand during radial and ulnar deviation. (*A*) In full radial deviation the scaphoid appears foreshortened, owing to palmar flexion. The scaphoid tuberosity produces a ring sign adjacent to the radial styloid. The lunate appears triangular in shape, owing to superimposition of the dorsal pole over the capitate, as the lunate is relatively palmar flexed along with the scaphoid. (*B*) In ulnar deviation, the scaphoid appears in longitudinal silhouette. As it is dorsiflexed, it skids distally on the radius. The ring sign of the tuberosity is absent. The lunate has translated completely onto the radial articular surface, and its silhouette is now more nearly trapezoidal in shape, owing to the palmar horn of lunate being superimposed beneath the capitate, because of its relative dorsiflexion. Intercarpal joint motion consists of the capitate and hamate swinging on the concavity of the distal articular surface of the proximal row. Conjunct motion of the proximal row with radial and ulnar deviation is caused by variation in contact points in the intercarpal joint. Changing contact points from palmar to dorsal along the trochoidal surfaces of triquetrohamate articulation and the ball in socket surfaces of the capitolunate articulations induces this shift.

of the capitate as it moves on the concave distal articular surface of the lunate and the varying contact area between the trochoidal surfaces of the hamate and triquetrum. This movement of the capitate is a combination of rotation and gliding along an oblique course. The arc of motion is influenced by the radiocarpal extensors pulling in a dorsoradial direction during radial deviation and by the ulnocarpal flexors pulling in a palmar-ulnar direction during ulnar deviation. During radial deviation, the scaphoid must flex palmarward in order to avoid impinging against the radial styloid. This composite motion is complex, varying from a screw-like motion ulnarly to a slider-crank motion radially. The variable joint contact area afforded by the irregular geometry of the proximal and distal rows and the differential tensions on the various components of the dorsal and volar radiocarpal ligaments are important in constraining the movement patterns. The carpal joint motions probably are slightly altered by the position of pronation and supination in the wrist.

In addition to their roles in wrist motion, several of the carpal bones are involved in important hand relationships and motions. The arches of the hand, which contribute strength, functional positioning, and structural protection, are both transverse and longitudinal.[103] The apex of the transverse arch is in the carpus itself, but the arch continues into the proximal metacarpus and is dynamically present even at the distal metacarpal level. The longitudinal arch is composed of the carpus, particularly the capitate and the metacarpal rays of the index and long fingers. Stability at this site is most important, and motion between the capitate and the metacarpus is very limited. However, the border digits are mobile, particularly the thumb. The scaphoid must participate in its action and does so through intermediary joints with the trapezium and trapezoid bones. The hamate has no intermediary joints but permits 15 to 30 degrees of motion of the fourth and fifth metacarpals, which is sufficient to permit the ulnar border digits to descend and the distal transverse arch to be restored. The mobility and power of the thumb are such that compression stresses across the thumb axis joints are probably greater and more continuous than in any other area of the carpus.

FRACTURES OF THE DISTAL RADIUS

FRACTURE OF THE DISTAL RADIUS WITH POSTERIOR DISPLACEMENT (COLLES' FRACTURE)

Rarely, this injury is called Pouteau's[220] fracture. Nevertheless, of all the eponymous fractures, probably none is so well associated with a man's name as is that of the distal radius with Abraham Colles.[54] His description has not been improved in 160 years:

> This fracture takes place at about an inch and a half above the carpal extremity of the radius, and exhibits the following appearances.
>
> The posterior surface of the limb presents a considerable deformity; for a depression is seen in the fore-arm, about an inch and a half above the end of this bone, while a considerable swelling occupies the wrist and metacarpus. Indeed, the carpus and base of the metacarpus appear to be thrown backward so much, as on first view to excite a suspicion that the carpus has been dislocated forward.
>
> On viewing the anterior surface of the limb, we observe a considerable fulness, as if caused by the flexor tendons being thrown forwards. This fulness extends upwards to about one-third of the length of the fore-arm, and terminates below at the upper edge of the annular ligament of the wrist. The extremity of the ulna is seen projecting towards the palm and inner edge of the limb; the degree, however, in which this projection takes place, is different in different instances.
>
> If the surgeon proceed to investigate the nature of this injury, he will find that the end of the ulna admits of being readily moved backwards and forwards.
>
> If the surgeon lock his hand in that of the patient's, and make extension, even with a moderate force, he restores the limb to its natural

form, but the distortion of the limb instantly returns on the extension being removed. Should the facility with which a moderate extension restores the limb to its form, induce the practitioner to treat this as a case of sprain, he will find, after a lapse of time sufficient for the removal of similar swellings, the deformity undiminished. Or, should he mistake the case for a dislocation of the wrist, and attempt to retain the parts *in situ* by tight bandages and splints, the pain caused by the pressure on the back of the wrist will force him to unbind them in a few hours; and if they be applied more loosely, he will find, at the expiration of a few weeks, that the deformity still exists in its fullest extent, and that it is now no longer to be removed by making extension of the limb. By such mistakes the patient is doomed to endure for many months considerable lameness and stiffness of the limb, accompanied by severe pains on attempting to bend the hand and fingers. One consolation only remains, that the limb will at some remote period again enjoy perfect freedom in all its motions, and be completely exempt from pain: the deformity, however, will remain undiminished through life.[54]

It is with this last sentence that we take issue, because complications that pose continuing problems occur frequently during all phases in the treatment of Colles' fractures.

Mechanisms of Injury

The fracture occurs most often from falls on the outstretched hand. The amount of force necessary experimentally to produce this fracture statically varies in the dorsiflexed wrist from 105 to 440 kg., with a mean of 195 kg. for women and 282 kg. for men. Fractures of the distal radius are produced when the dorsiflexion of the wrist varies from 40 to 90 degrees, lesser amounts of force being required at the smaller angles.[107] Although the exact mechanism of fracture is not yet clear, the generally sharp fracture on the palmar aspect of the radial metaphyseal area, compared with the dorsally comminuted fragments, suggests that the radius may first fracture in tension on its palmar surface, with the fracture propagating and compacting cancellous bone on the dorsum, which then becomes comminuted. If this hypothesis is correct, a high tensile loading of the palmar radiocarpal ligament is necessary to transmit the tensile loading to the anterior cortex.

Table 7-1. Classification of Colles' Fractures*

Fractures	Distal Ulnar Fracture Absent	Distal Ulnar Fracture Present
Extraarticular	I	II
Intraarticular involving radiocarpal joint	III	IV
Intraarticular involving distal radioulnar joint	V	VI
Intraarticular involving both radiocarpal and distal radioulnar joints	VII	VIII

*Data from Frykman, G.: Acta Orthop. Scand., *108* [Suppl.]:1-155, 1967.

Classification

Although a number of systems of classification have been advanced, that advocated by Frykman,[107] though cumbersome, seems reasonable (Table 7-1). This classification is based on the distinction between extra- and intraarticular fractures of the distal radius and on the presence of a concomitant fracture of the distal ulna. No attempt is made to ascertain the degree of comminution or initial displacement. Any classification is of limited value, unless it provides information on treatment or prognosis. With this classification, the more complex the fracture, the higher the number and the more likely the complications of fracture healing.

Signs and Symptoms

The patient complains of deformity of the wrist, with pain, swelling, and weakness. Signs include posterior angulation of the hand and carpal area, with radial deviation, supination, anterior fullness, crepitus, limitation of finger motion, and numbness. There is tenderness to palpa-

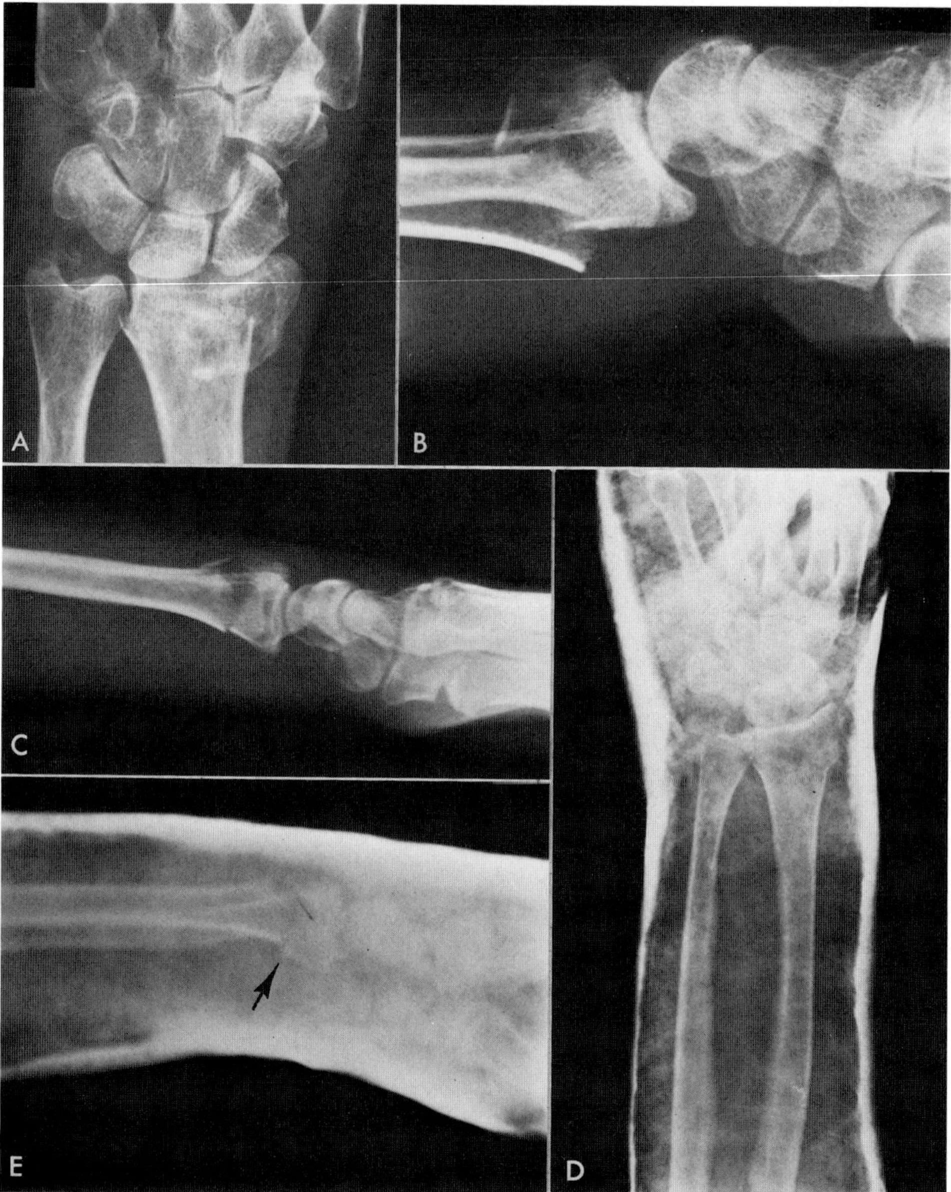

Fig. 7-9. A 54-year-old housewife fell on the palm of her left hand after slipping on ice, suffering a Type VI Colles' fracture. (*A, B*) The fracture line enters the distal radioulnar joint. There is a small avulsion fracture of the ulnar styloid, dorsal angulation of 25 degrees, radial shortening, and dorsal displacement. (*C*) Dorsal angulation was corrected with traction in Chinese fingertraps. There is a sharp fracture line on the palmar aspect. The distal fragment lacks approximately 1 mm. of complete reduction. There is a comminuted fracture surface dorsally, with evidence of compaction of cancellous bone. (*D*) Postreduction films after a circular plaster cast was applied above elbow, with forearm in slight supination, show correction of radial length and radial angulation. (*E*) The lateral view shows that the volar cortex was overcorrected slightly (*arrow*), thus locking its position. Angulation of the articular surface approaches normal palmar flexion of 10 to 15 degrees. The cast is well molded about the forearm, and three-point fixation has been achieved. The cast was split along its ulnar margin to accommodate

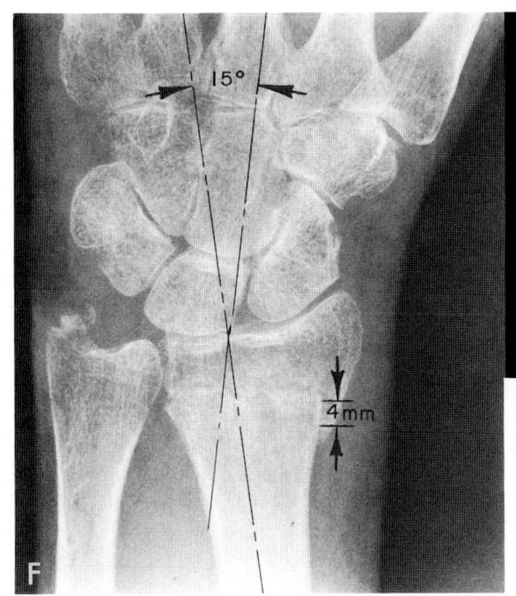

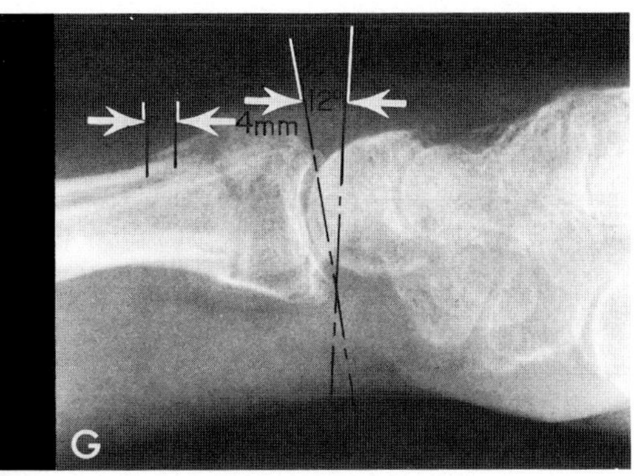

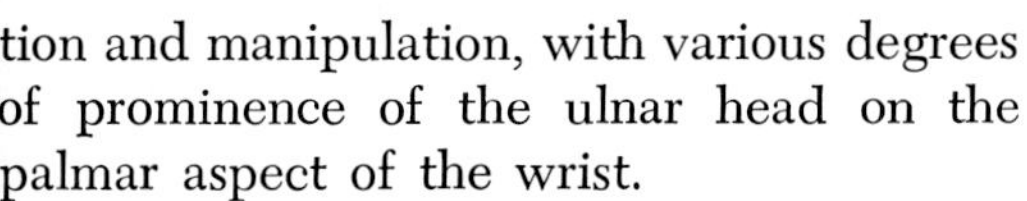

tion and manipulation, with various degrees of prominence of the ulnar head on the palmar aspect of the wrist.

Roentgenographic Findings

The findings in two views are usually typical, although they may vary considerably in degree of displacement and comminution (Figs. 7-9–7-15). Anteroposterior views of the wrist show a comminuted fracture through the metaphyseal area of the distal radius. The fracture line may enter into the distal radioulnar joint or emerge proximal to it. An additional fracture line extending into the radial articular surface or a comminuted fracture line with displacement of part of the articular surface may be noted. The distal fracture fragment may be displaced minimally or dramatically, and there are varying amounts of radial angulation and radial shortening. The ulnar styloid is fractured through the base in approximately 60 per cent of patients, and occasionally the ulnar neck is fractured.[107]

Because of the superimposition of the radius on the ulna, the lateral views require careful examination to obtain the fine details. Dorsal displacement of the distal fragments with a sharp fracture through the palmar surface is noted. Dorsal displacement varies. Generally, there is comminution of the dorsal cortex with compaction of the cancellous bone. Subluxation of the distal radioulnar joint may be apparent on a lateral view, particularly if the superimposed triquetral shadow no longer lies in line with the distal ulna. The distal articular surface of the radius, which normally has a palmar inclination of 5 to 15 degrees, may have variable degrees of dorsal inclination from fracture deformity.

The roentgenograms should be carefully reviewed to exclude carpal fractures, and roentgenograms of the elbow should be taken if there is severe displacement in the distal radial fracture or tenderness about the elbow, which suggests a concomitant elbow fracture.

---

swelling. (*F*, *G*) Six weeks after, fracture shows settling in cast. Radial angulation of 12 degrees, radial shortening of 4 mm., and loss of normal palmar flexed position of the articular surface to a neutral position have occurred in cast. The ulnar styloid appears to be uniting. Nevertheless, this is considered a good result. Six months after fracture, there was full range of motion of the fingers, but dorsiflexion was limited to 50 degrees. The woman had slight residual discomfort on supination and active use of the hand.

Treatment

The classic method of treatment includes closed reduction and plaster-of-paris splint or cast support (Fig. 7-9).[46,183,218] The method of reduction by hyperextension and disimpaction has lost favor. Reduction now is performed by applying traction through the grasped injured hand and countertraction to the humerus, with the elbow flexed.[35,40,41] After disimpaction of the fracture, which may be aided by dorsal angulation when tension is maintained, the fracture is reduced by palmar displacement of the distal fragment, mild palmar flexion, and ulnar deviation. Extreme flexion or pronation of the wrist[60] at the completion of reduction is contraindicated because of the frequent complication of median nerve compression and the difficulty in maintaining digital function.[179] Pronation of the distal fragment on the proximal fragment is important in reduction. Some authors advocate immobilization of the forearm in pronation,[40,41,59,189] and some advocate supination.[95,237] Generally, the forearm in the midposition or slight supination is favored, because this tends to open the interosseous space between the radius and the ulna and to decrease the tension of the brachioradialis. The wrist is placed in slight flexion and ulnar deviation.[43,61,69,109,219]

Extension of the plaster splint about the elbow as "sugar tongs" or the application of a long-arm cast with the elbow in flexion is frequently advocated.[84,239]

Roentgenograms should be obtained immediately on reduction and also after application of the cast or splint. Satisfactory reduction is not obtained until the dorsal displacement and supination of the distal fragment have been corrected and the angulation of the distal radial articular surface has been restored to a neutral position at least. Incomplete reduction of the palmar fracture line is the most frequent failure. If reduction is not complete, there is no fulcrum of cortical bone to maintain the radial length and to control the dorsal angulation.

Settling of the fracture after reduction should be anticipated, particularly when there is severe dorsal comminution of the fracture site.[84,109,212] Remanipulation of the fracture between 10 days and 3 weeks may be necessary if the fracture deformity has recurred. During this period of the healing process, while the fracture is "sticky," it is probably easier to hold the reduced position.[95]

General anesthesia, regional block, and local injection may be satisfactory; however, in our experience, aspiration of the fracture hematoma and injection of 5 to 20 ml. of 1- to 2 per cent local anesthesia has been less satisfactory. The decision regarding the type of anesthesia is based on such factors as the patient's general health, recent oral intake, associated injury, anesthesia risk, obesity, ecchymosis, and swelling. The better the anesthesia, the more deliberate and painstaking the surgeon can be in reduction and fixation. There is generally minimal enthusiasm for the open reduction of Colles' fractures, although extensive comminution, impacted articular fragments, median nerve entrapment, or associated injuries, particularly in the young productive patient, may on occasion suggest that some form of open reduction using pins or plates may be carried out (Fig. 7-10).[151] Percutaneous pinning may be used to fix the fragment position, maintain the length of the distal radial fragment, or maintain protracted traction (Fig. 7-15)[9,52,74,84,111,122,123,239] Three methods of pinning are available: (1) multiple fracture transfixing pins, (2) proximal and distal transverse pins held in plaster or by metal struts, and (3) a transfixing pin that supports the internal cortex of the radial styloid. Pinning should be considered only after careful skin preparation and under strict aseptic operating room conditions.

Authors' Preferred Method of Treatment. Treatment should depend on a careful evaluation of many factors. Except for moderate and severe displacements, reductions may be delayed for several hours or days if elevation and splinting with compression dressings are used. For the minimally displaced fracture, protective splinting is satisfactory. For the moderately displaced fracture with minimal comminution, we prefer regional anesthesia followed by distraction of the fracture in Chinese fingertraps. Distraction is allowed to occur over a period of 5 to 10 minutes, with 8- to 10-lb. (3.6 to 4.5 kg.) countertraction suspended over a wide, soft strap located above the elbow. This frees the surgeon's hands. Manipulation is accomplished with thumb pressure over the distal fragment

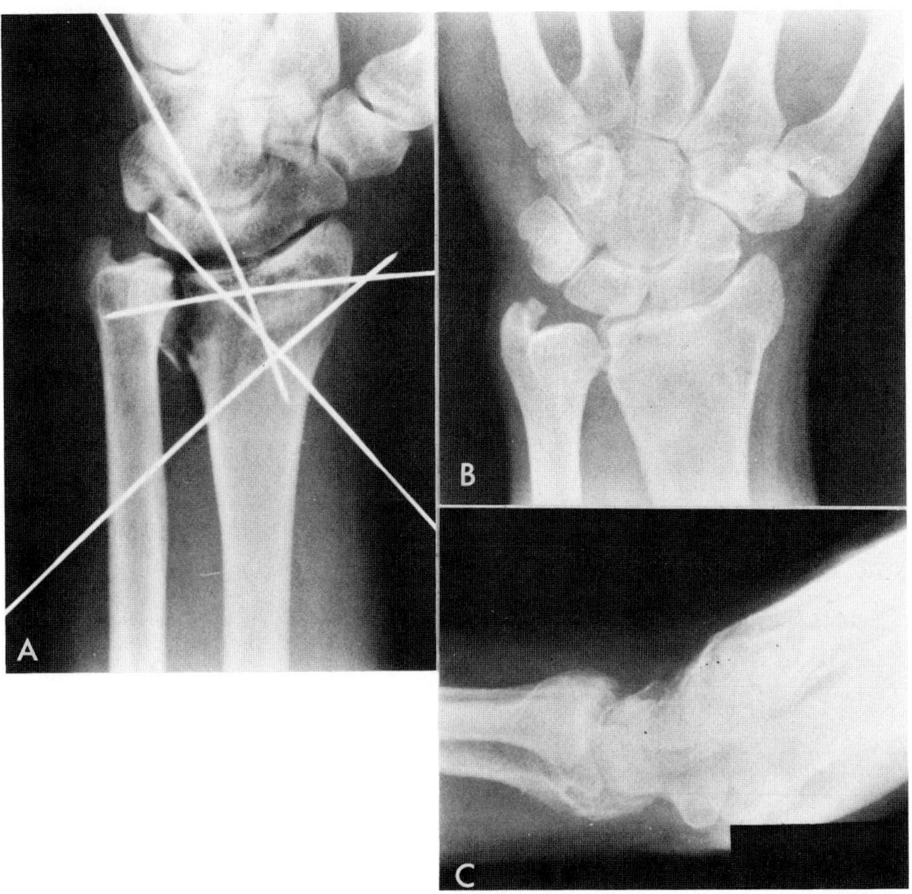

Fig. 7-10. A markedly comminuted Type VII Colles' fracture was suffered by a 36-year-old man who fell from a ladder. After closed reduction failed to improve the articular surface, open reduction was performed, and an attempt was made to hold the numerous fragments in close apposition to preserve the articular surface with multiple percutaneous pins. (*A*) The anteroposterior view shows four 0.045-inch Kirschner wires inserted at various angles to hold the fragments of the articular surface in alignment. (*B*) An anteroposterior view 1 year after injury shows good preservation of radiocarpal joint space and of radial articular surface and minimal radial shortening. There is a small ununited ulnar styloid fracture and minimal ulnar translation of the carpus on the radial articular surface. (*C*) A lateral view shows that the articular surface of the distal radius has perpendicular orientation relative to the longitudinal axis. At 1 year, there was moderate limitation of wrist motion and excellent grip strength.

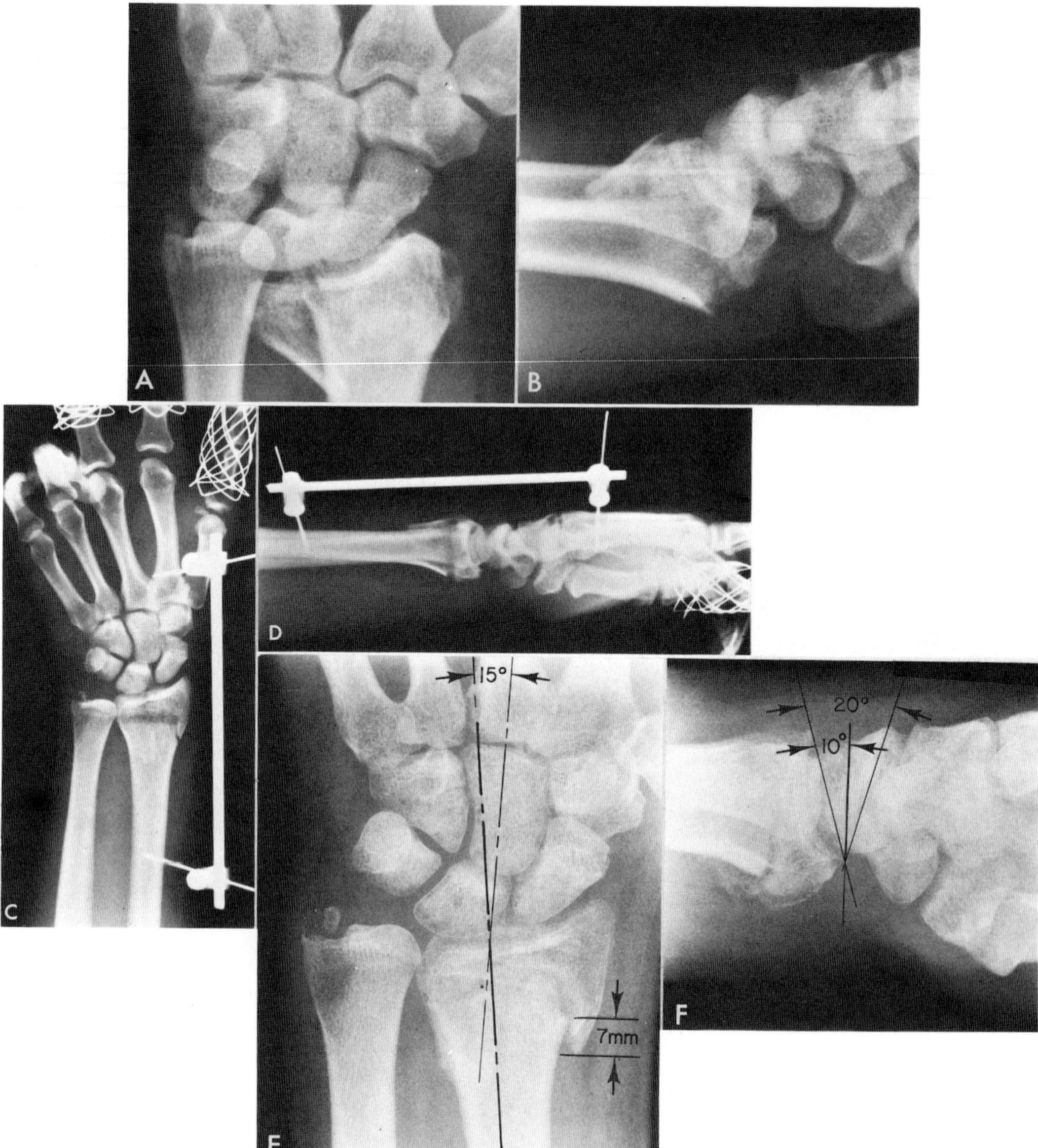

Fig. 7-11. A 41-year-old man fell backward on an icy step and suffered a comminuted distal radial fracture, Type IV. (*A, B*) Anteroposterior and lateral views show comminution of the distal radial articular surface, radial shortening, and 50 degrees dorsal angulation of the articular surface. The fracture line appears to be proximal to the radioulnar articulation. The triangular fibrocartilage probably remained intact, though avulsing ulnar styloid. (*C, D*) Correction was carried out using Chinese fingertraps and 10 lb. of traction placed on a strap over the brachium, followed by manipulation. Kirschner wires (0.045-inch) were inserted at an angle of 45 degrees to the radioulnar plane, into the base of the second metacarpal and radius, just proximal to the abductor pollicis longus. These have been connected with a baby Roger Anderson apparatus. It appears that reduction of the fracture, correction of radial angulation, and correction of radial length have been achieved. (*E, F*) Eight weeks after fracture, it is healing but there is moderate recurrence of the deformity, with loss of radial length of approximately 7 mm., recurrence of radial angulation of approximately 15 degrees, and recurrence of dorsal angulation of the fracture site of 10 degrees. The ulnar styloid fragment is slightly displaced and ununited, and there is osteoporosis of the carpus associated with immobilization. A double-pin system probably would have improved the result.

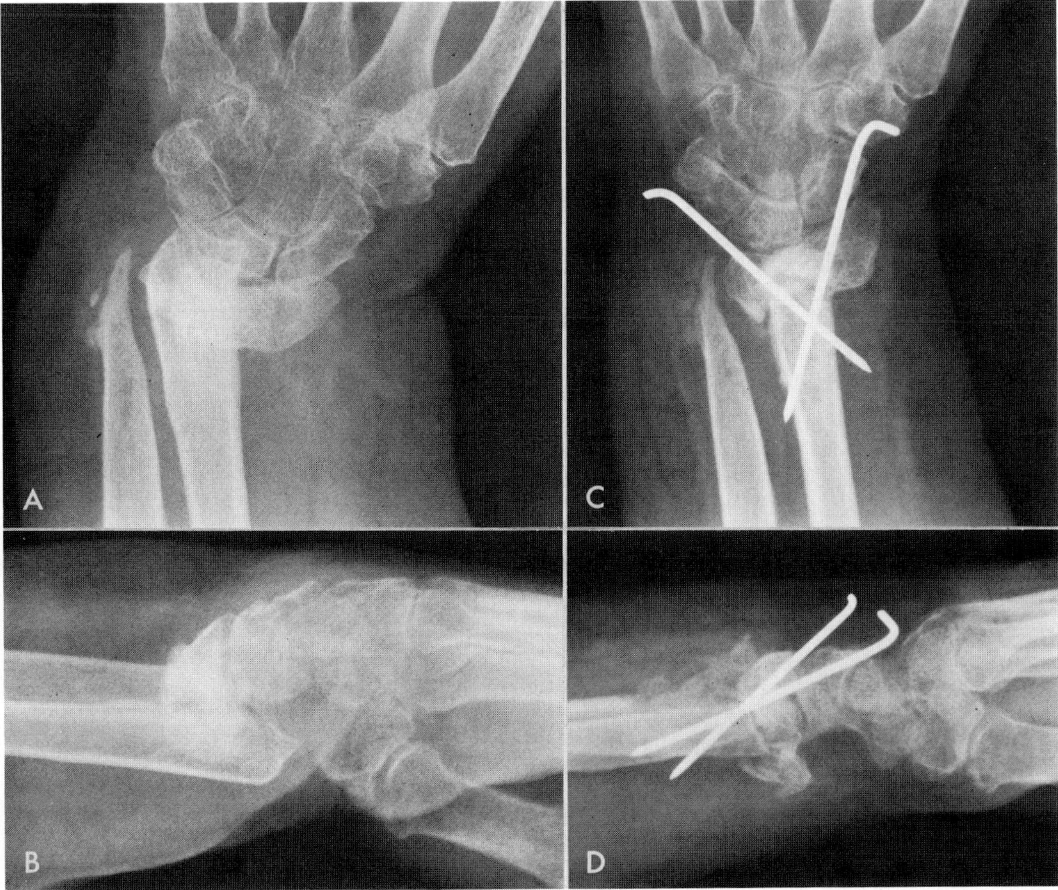

Fig. 7-12. Nonunion of Colles' fracture. (*A*) The anteroposterior view shows radial deviation and dorsal translation of the articular fragment. Previous resection of the distal ulna, with "pencilling" of the end. (*B*) The lateral view shows dorsal displacement of the ununited fragment. Darrach resection performed 6 weeks after injury may have contributed to the development of nonunion. (*C, D*) An attempt was made to stretch out the contracture by traction on external skeletal fixation pins. Anteroposterior and lateral views followed surgical replacement of the radial articular fragment and internal fixation with Kirschner wires. Late result 3 months after surgery shows early degenerative change in the radial articular surface.

and with the fingers exerting a counterforce on the palmar aspect of the proximal fragment. The distal fragment is pronated on the proximal fragment and displaced palmarward. Roentgenograms are taken in two planes, with traction still applied, to ensure that dorsal displacement has been corrected. After this, dorsal and palmar plaster splints are applied above the elbow, with the forearm in 10 to 20 degrees of supination. These splints are held in place by voluminous wrapping or completion of a circular cast. Careful molding of the plaster is important, so that three-point pressure is applied dorsally over the distal fragment and the mid-forearm and palmarly over the distal aspect of the proximal fragment. Additional molding along the index metacarpal, the radial styloid, and the ulnar neck aids immobilization. To minimize swelling after reduction, no attempt is made to obtain circumferential snug fitting of the cast. The hand is placed in 10 to 20 degrees of palmar flexion and

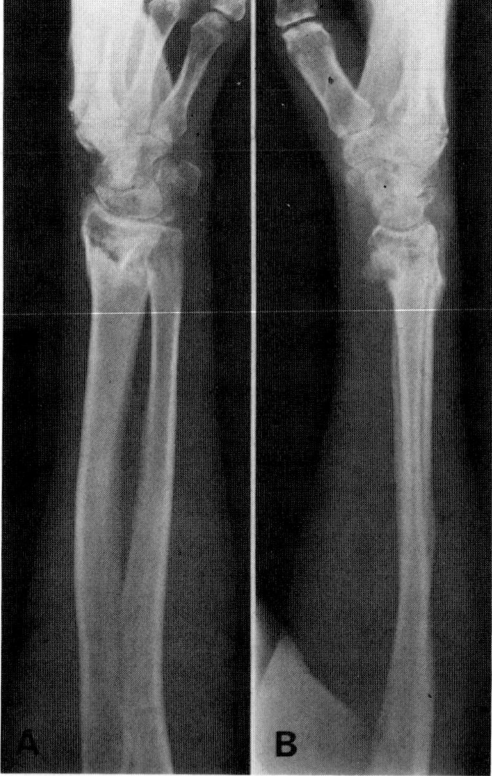

Fig. 7-13. (*A, B*) A 54-year-old man suffered a markedly displaced fracture through the distal radius. The fracture was reduced and held in plaster immobilization shortly after the accident. He had severe pain at the fracture site and complained of increasing numbness and swelling of the fingers. The cast was subsequently changed, but when seen 3 months after injury, the man had Volkmann's ischemic contracture involving the distal third of the forearm, the wrist area, and the thenar and hypothenar eminences. Extensive atrophy occurred at both eminences, where cast margins crossed muscular prominences. Three subsequent procedures were undertaken to obtain neurolysis of the median and ulnar nerves, tenolysis of flexor tendons of the fingers, and tenolysis of extensor tendons beneath the dorsal carpal ligament. Pedicle grafting for release of scars over the thenar and hypothenar eminences and capsulorrhaphies of the metacarpophalangeal joints also were necessary. Although ischemic myositis in distal radial fractures is rare, its signs and symptoms are present, as with fractures and dislocations that are more proximal. Note "Coke-bottle" appearance of the distal forearm, with atrophy of subcutaneous tissues and indentation over the thenar and hypothenar eminences, as well as the osteoporotic appearance of the carpal area. Good fracture alignment was maintained.

15 to 30 degrees of ulnar deviation. The plaster is carried out over the well-padded heads of the metacarpals dorsally to prevent occlusion of the veins and lymphatic vessels in the web spaces. The cast is trimmed just proximal to the palmar creases and about the thumb, so that full-finger flexion and full opposition are possible.

The patient is usually kept in the hospital during the first night, with the arm elevated. Instructions in exercise of the fingers and shoulder begin immediately on recovery from anesthesia.

Because of the difficulty in holding a fracture that is comminuted and unstable, we frequently employ external skeletal fixation in one of two forms. The rationale for this approach is that the unstable fracture tends to displace despite external support if the dorsal bone fragments cannot be locked into some semblance of stability. With the palmar fracture line acting as a fulcrum, the compressive force acting against the central radial articular surface due to the tension of the tendons crossing the joint has a moment arm that favors redisplacement. If a dorsally applied tensile force can be incorporated, this tendency to angular and compressive displacement will be minimized.

Accordingly, a 0.0625-inch Kirschner wire is drilled through the basilar metaphyseal areas of the second and third metacarpals and a similar pin through the radius, while the fractured extremity is hanging in the Chinese fingertraps.[30,52,185] After satisfactory reduction has been obtained, the pins are incorporated in plaster to maintain length.

A separate technique that we have employed more commonly is to insert a 0.0625-

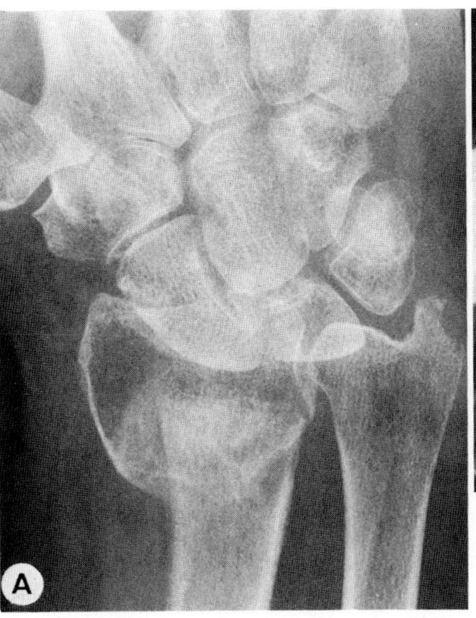

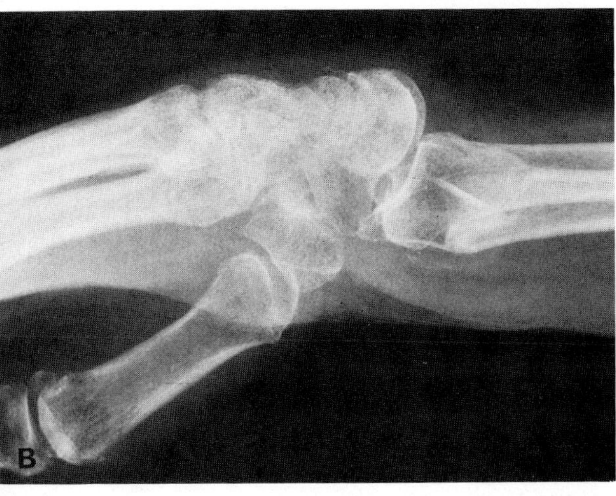

Fig. 7-14. A 40-year-old woman had malunion of a distal radial fracture. She had severe limitation of dorsiflexion. (*A*, *B*) Examination revealed radial deviation of 20 degrees, dorsal angulation of the articular surface of 35 degrees, and dorsal translation of the proximal carpal row. This subluxation occurred during her treatment period, but some instability at the time of original injury seems likely. Dorsal inclination of the articular surface provided an inclined plane on which subluxation occurred.

inch Kirschner wire from the dorsoradial aspect into the base of the second metacarpal and a wire through both cortices of the radius just proximal to the abductor pollicis longus muscle belly.[21,139] Both wires are at 45 degrees to the radioulnar plane and are parallel to each other. With the fracture in a reduced position under the image intensifier or with check roentgenograms, the two wires are connected with a ⅛-inch aluminum rod and baby Roger Anderson clamps. Occasionally, a second such system is added to the base of the third metacarpal perpendicular to the plane of the dorsum of the hand. This tensile force acting across the dorsal and radial aspects of the fracture site tends to maintain radial length and normal radial and palmar angulation of the radial articular surface. An ulnar-palmar plaster splint is then applied from the distal metacarpal crease to just proximal to the elbow over cotton cast padding, and the entire assemblage is wrapped lightly with an elastic bandage. We have been impressed with the advantages that this provides in decreasing pain and swelling, in obtaining finger and elbow motions, and in maintaining the fracture reduction. All the steps must be carried out with careful attention to details (Fig. 7-11).

Postoperative Care and Rehabilitation

Regardless of the technique of reduction, the postoperative treatment is very important. Swelling of the fingers must be minimized. The arm should be elevated above the level of the heart for 48 hours after reduction. Suspension from an overhead frame or intravenous pole is often helpful. Care must be taken that the additional support bandages are not constricting. Swelling of the fingers is pathognomonic of decreased venous and lymphatic return due to constriction. Finger exercises are important in reducing swelling and preventing finger stiffness. Wiggling the fingers is much less efficacious than full excursion

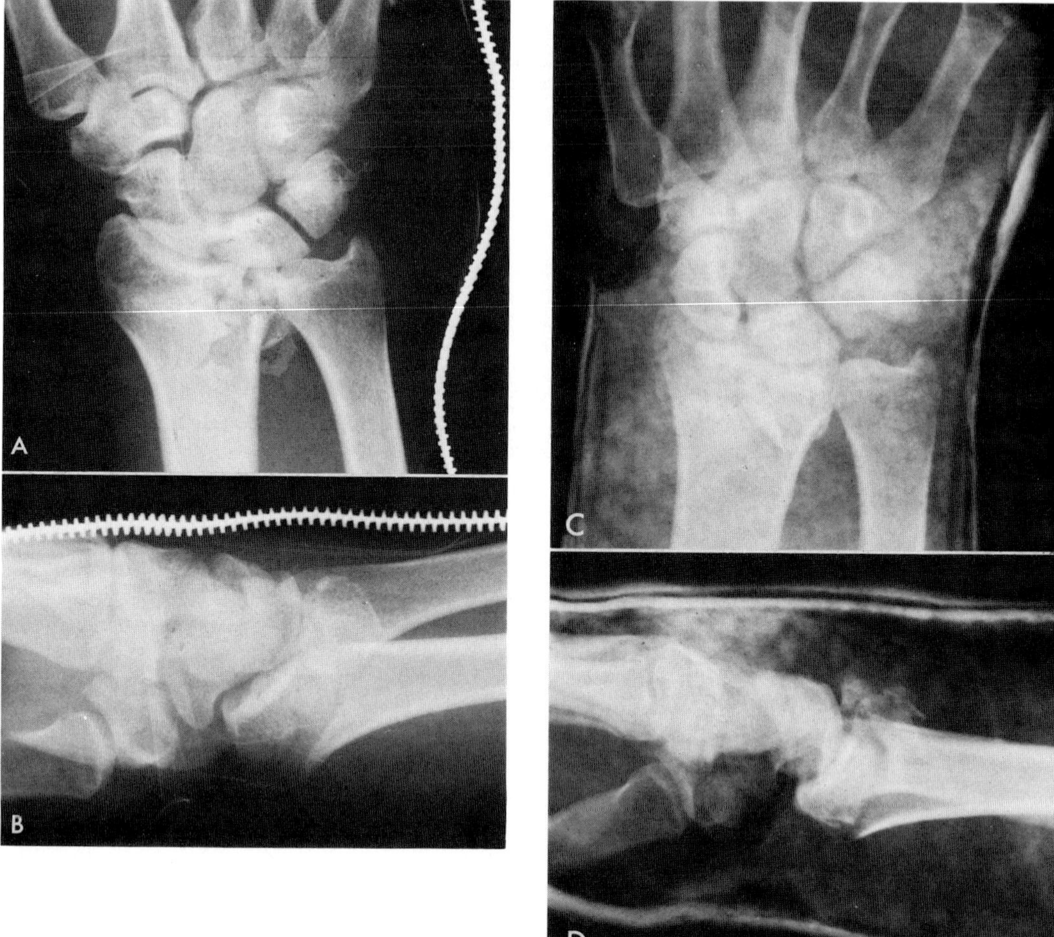

Fig. 7-15. A 25-year-old man fell from a roof, sustaining a comminuted fracture of the right distal radius. (*A, B*) Colles' fracture, Type VIII. Note comminution of the radial articular surface (particularly in the lunate fossa), dorsal angulation of the distal radial fragment, and displacement of the carpus with the dorsal rim fragment. (*C, D*) Reduction done elsewhere shows persistent dorsal angulation and displacement.

held to a count of 2 or more. The fingers should be moved from full extension to full flexion and from a claw position to an intrinsic-plus position. These should be repeated with the hand above the level of the heart not less than ten times every half hour while the patient is awake. Exercises should be maintained as long as the hand has a tendency to swell. Check roentgenograms should be taken again within 10 days, and remanipulation should be used if the fracture position is not satisfactory. It is usually necessary to rewrap splints or to reapply a plaster cast between 10 and 15 days because the swelling has decreased. Roentgenograms are taken to ensure that no change in position has occurred. The patient should be observed several times during the first 48 hours—a time when the postoperative complications are most likely to occur. The dressings or cast should be split full length if pain persists. Healing of the Colles' fracture in an area of cancellous bone is usually solid enough to re-

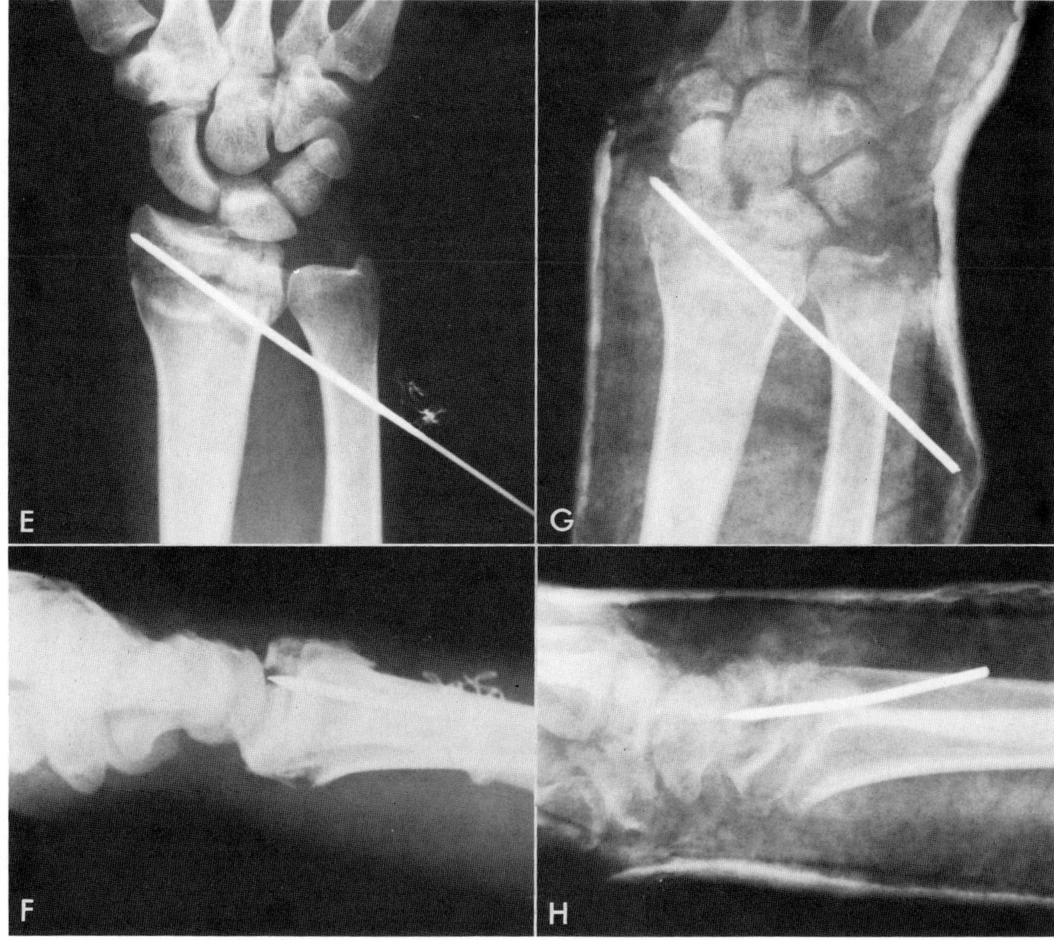

Fig. 7-15 (*Continued*) (*E, F*) Remanipulation with traction and percutaneous transulnar internal fixation (De Palma technique) was performed at 1 week. Note that the pin exits through the fracture line on the lateral view. (*G, H*) Eight weeks after fracture settling has taken place, with recurrent dorsal angulation. The patient was advised to proceed with rehabilitation procedures and return for reevaluation for possible osteotomy at 1 year.

move constant external support in 5 to 7 weeks; if the two-pin technique is used, 6 to 8 weeks is suggested.

Prognosis

Nonunion of the distal radial fracture is extremely uncommon, though various degrees of malunion are not (Fig. 7-12). The patients most at risk are elderly women,[8] who may subsequently fracture the opposite wrist, femoral neck, or intertrochanteric area. The period of disability after a Colles' fracture varies widely. In general, this depends on the severity of the complications, though the period of improvement usually lasts for more than a year.

Complications

Patient dissatisfaction is common. Complications of Colles' fractures are frequent[16,31,35,43,47,84,91,109,119,127,129,132,148,153,167,168,174,182,246,247,277,305] and are given less attention than they deserve. They may be divided into those that present within the first 2

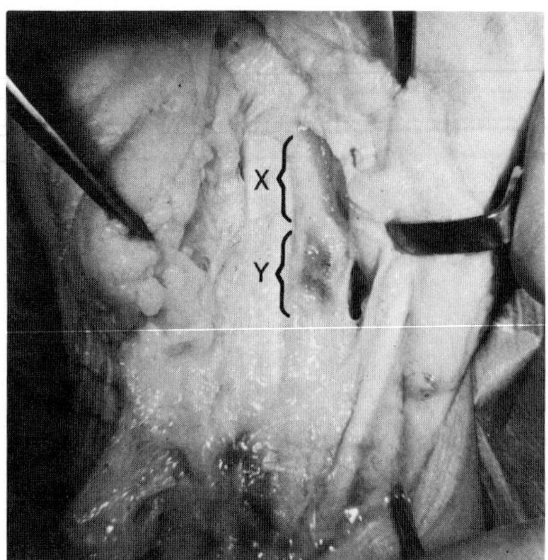

Fig. 7-16. Median nerve injury with Colles' fracture. The patient complained of acroparesthesias and pain in median distribution immediately after the fracture. Pain persisted despite reduction. Early decompression disclosed ecchymosis (*Y*) within the substance of the nerve. There was an impression (*X*) in the nerve, presumably caused by the transverse carpal ligament impinging on the nerve just distal to an ecchymotic area.

weeks of injury and those that persist after immobilization is removed. The late complications usually have their inception at the time of fracture or during the early treatment period (Figs. 7-13, 7-14).

Early adequate reduction is the most effective means of preventing complications (Fig. 7-15). To do this without running the risk of constrictive splinting, peripheral edema, and secondary arthrofibrosis is difficult. The patient who complains of moderate to severe pain after reduction often has severe median nerve compression (Fig. 7-16). This should be surgically released if it persists after cast splitting, cast removal, or secondary reduction, even if reduction is lost temporarily. The shoulder-hand syndrome, regardless of when it appears, should be treated appropriately, but is better prevented by adequate reduction,

---

Complications of Colles' Fractures

Early:

- Inadequate anesthesia
- Difficult reduction; unstable reduction maintained only by extreme position
- Depressed major articular components
- Distal radioulnar subluxation, dislocation
- Injury to proximal segments
- Median or ulnar nerve stretch, contusion, or compression
- Postreduction swelling; constrictive dressings; compartment syndromes (Fig. 7-13)
- Errors in external fixation
- Tendon damage
- Pain or dystrophy syndromes

Intermediate and Late:

- Loss of reduction and secondary deformity
  - Radial shortening, radial angulation
  - Dorsiflexion of distal segment, intercarpal collapse deformity
  - Inadequate articular reduction
  - Distal radioulnar dissociation and arthrosis
  - Interosseous membrane contracture, pronation
  - Persistent carpal translations (Fig. 7-14)
- Stiff hand; shoulder-hand syndrome; arthritic flare
- Cosmetic defect
- Weakness associated with immobilization and shortening of skeletal segments and changes in the force moment arm, particularly detrimental to efficient function of the wrist extensors
- Median nerve compression; occasionally ulnar or radial nerve compression (usually from the apparatus for the latter)
- Tendinous adhesions in the flexor compartment
- Extensor pollicis longus tendon rupture
- Radiocarpal arthrosis
- Nonunion

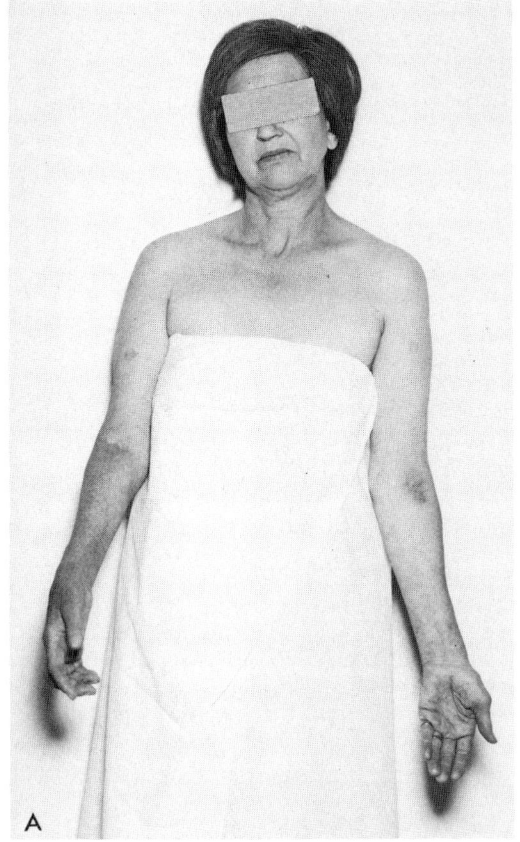

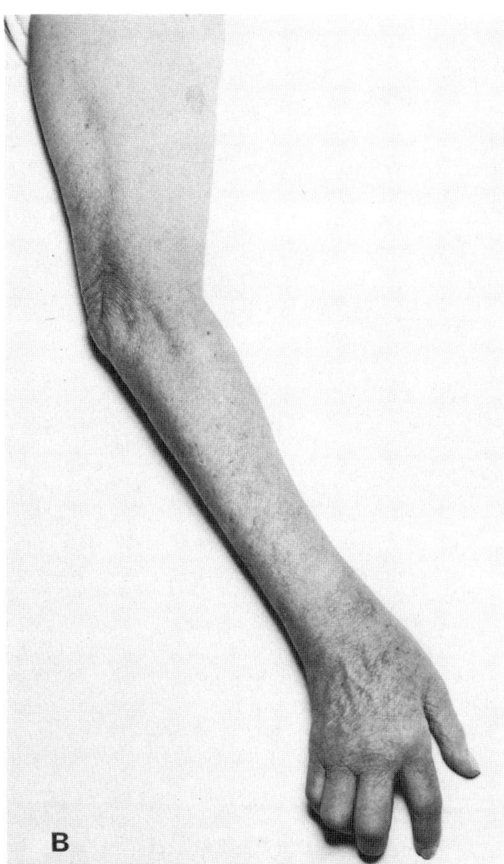

Fig. 7-17. (*A*) Shoulder-hand dystrophy after Colles' fracture. The patient holds the right arm in protective fashion with forearm supination markedly limited, the elbow moderately flexed, and the wrist and fingers flexed. Note the discouraged and depressed facial appearance. (*B*) The forearm muscles are atrophic. Skin and subcutaneous tissues about the wrist and hand are swollen. The skin of the hand and forearm has a cyanotic hue. The fingers are slightly clawed and metacarpophalangeal flexion and proximal interphalangeal extension are limited. Closely supervised therapy resulted in considerable improvement.

control of swelling, and freedom to exercise the fingers and shoulder (Fig. 7-17).[198,199]

The late complications in the distal radioulnar joint may require resection of the ulnar head (Darrach procedure) for relief (Fig. 7-18).[68,78,144,172,194-196,227] Although it is generally considered innocuous, this procedure is followed by occasional complications and is sometimes disliked by the patient because of the poor esthetic result. Resection should not be undertaken without careful evaluation and demonstration that pain or limited motion is arising from this joint. Corrective osteotomy through a healed Colles' fracture site may be useful in some patients with malunion.[38,39,126,254] A bone graft is usually necessary to maintain this position (Fig. 7-19).

Colles' fracture, because it occurs most often in osteoporotic elderly women, may be a vexing problem. Attention paid to detail in the adequacy of the reduction, the prevention of constrictive swelling, an adequate exercise program, and careful follow-up procedures prevents many complications. The esthetic awareness of a per-

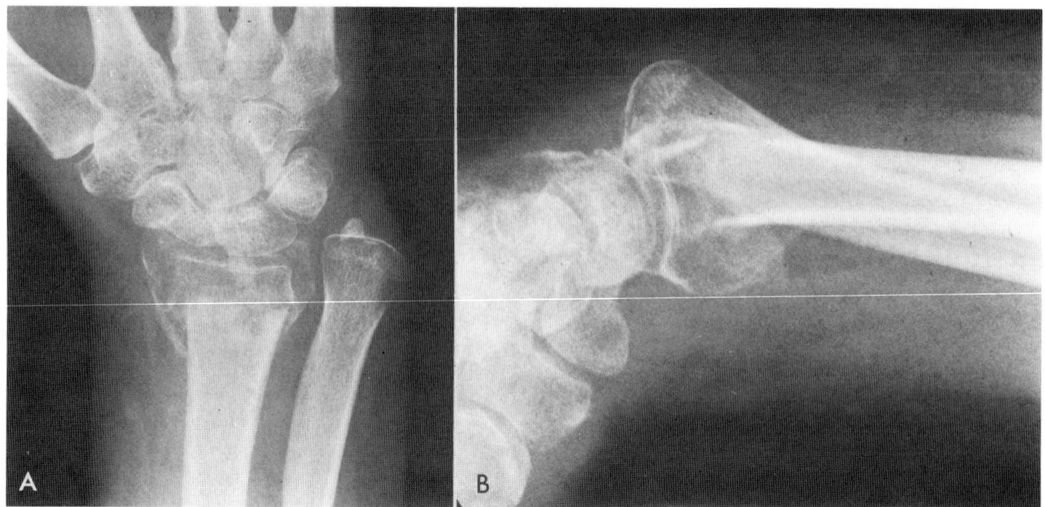

Fig. 7-18 (*A, B*) a 57-year-old school superintendent fell on ice and sustained a Colles' fracture. She was treated by cast immobilization for 6 weeks in a short-arm cast with the hand pronated and in volar flexion. When seen 9 months later, she had severely restricted motion in the wrist, stiffness of the hand, a pronation contracture of approximately 40 degrees, and a prominent distal ulna. There was also evidence of median nerve compression, with markedly decreased two-point discrimination, dryness of skin, atrophy of finger pulps in median distribution, and stiff and painful finger motion. She received some help from resection of the distal ulna and release of the transverse carpal ligament, followed by intensive rehabilitation therapy.

son of any age regarding the deformity of the distal forearm should not be underestimated.

DORSAL RIM FRACTURE

The dorsal rim fracture of the distal radius, a variant of the usual Colles' fracture and commonly known as Barton's fracture,[19,93,273] probably is produced by dorsiflexion and pronation of the distal forearm on the fixed wrist, with an intraarticular fracture line propagating to the dorsum.

The fracture is seen best on the lateral roentgenographic view, where the dorsal lip of the distal radial articular surface is displaced proximally and posteriorly and may be associated with dorsal subluxation of the carpus (Fig. 7-20).

Conservative treatment by plaster immobilization in a short-arm cast with the wrist in neutral position is usually sufficient. To prevent redisplacement, palmar flexion positioning should be avoided. If the fragment is large and there is posterior subluxation of the carpus, closed reduction by traction and manipulation is necessary. A tendency to instability or redisplacement requires percutaneous pin fixation or open reduction with a small plate or bone screws after careful replacement of the dorsal rim. Exposure of the intraarticular fracture line is warranted to ensure anatomic replacement. Healing, prognosis, and complications are similar to those for Colles' fracture.

RADIOCARPAL DISLOCATION

Radiocarpal dislocation[76] is extremely uncommon. It is often associated with a fragment of the dorsal rim and is produced by strong pronatory action of the forearm on

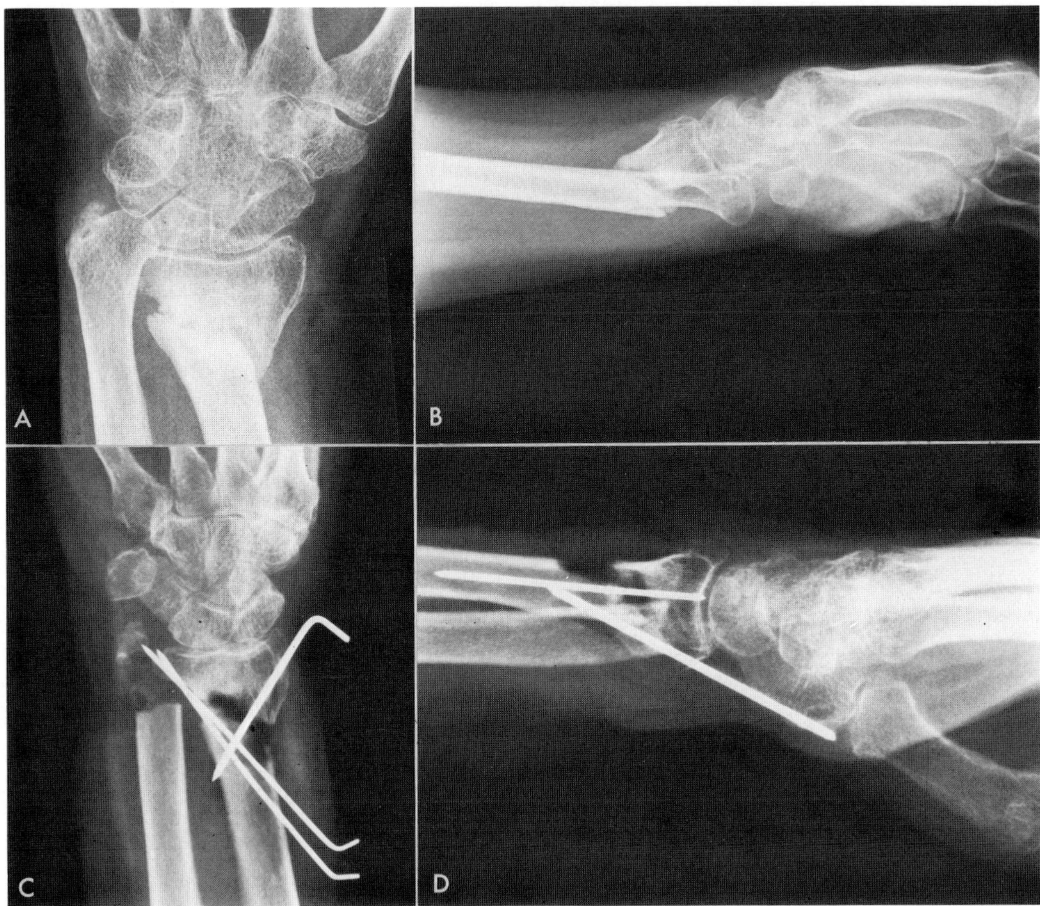

Fig. 7-19. Palmar dislocation of the distal ulna was apparent at the time a Colles' fracture was diagnosed in a 63-year-old woman. (*A, B*) Failure to reduce the radioulnar dislocation may have contributed to severe radial shortening and dorsal angulation. Persistence of pain with attempted pronation and limited flexion resulted in sufficient disability for the patient to request reconstructive measures. (*C, D*) This consisted of Darrach resection of the distal ulna and its insertion into an osteotomy site on the radius to correct dorsoradial angulation.

the fixed hand. The palmar radiocarpal ligament is always ruptured. Accessory fractures may include those of the radial and the ulnar styloids. Irreducible fracture-dislocation,[297] an extremely rare injury, occurs, with entrapment of the fragments of the dorsal rim between the proximal carpal row and the radial articular surface.

Dorsal displacement of the hand, significant prominence of the palmar aspect of the wrist, pain, tenderness, crepitus, and signs of median nerve compression are noted.

Anteroposterior roentgenograms of the wrist show a superimposition of the carpus on the distal radius with fragments of the dorsal lip of the radius. The lateral roentgenograms show complete dorsal dislocation, with the dorsal rim of the radius being carried posteriorly with the carpus (Fig.

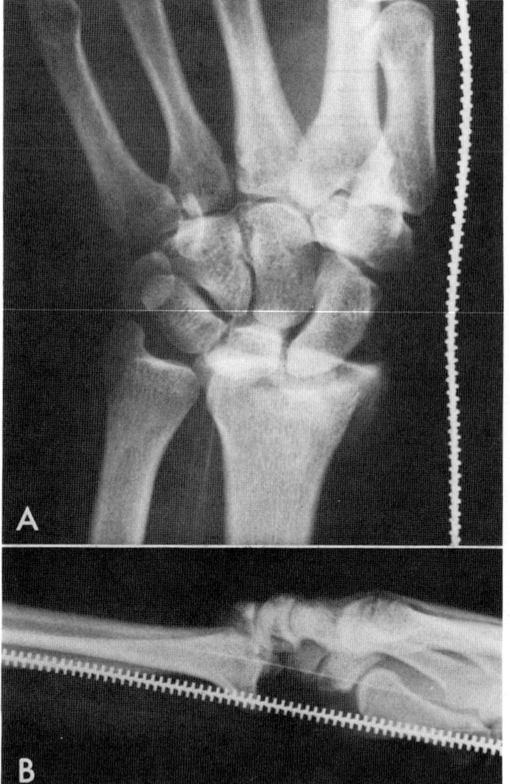

Fig. 7-20. (*A, B*) A 23-year-old surveyor fell onto his dorsiflexed left wrist sustaining a Barton's fracture, with the carpus dislocated dorsally with the dorsal rim of the radius. Closed reduction was carried out with intraarticular lidocaine anesthesia, and the wrist was immobilized in neutral position—initially with a bulky dressing stabilized with plaster splints and later with a short-arm cast in neutral position. Severe limitation of motion was noted immediately after removal of the plaster cast, but significant improvement occurred with normal use and activities during the ensuing year.

7-21). The distal radioulnar joint may or may not be dislocated. Treatment of this injury is reduction and support in a neutral wrist position.

RADIAL STYLOID FRACTURE

The radial styloid fracture is similar to the posterior marginal fracture. It was recognized commonly in the early part of the century as a result of the starting crank of an engine being suddenly reversed by a backfire. Its eponym is Hutchinson's fracture.[77,92,102]

The mechanism of injury probably is the direct transmission of force from the scaphoid against the articular surface of the radius, shearing a triangular fragment of bone transversely from the remainder of the radius. A small distally displaced radial styloid fragment suggests avulsion by the radial collateral ligament. While technologic progress has virtually eliminated the starting crank as a cause, the injury still is associated with vehicle components, such as steering wheels and handlebars.

Pain, tenderness, swelling, crepitus, and deformity of the radial styloid area are noted.

The fracture is seen best on the anteroposterior roentgenogram as a transverse one. It runs from within the scaphoid fossa laterally to the radial metaphysis. The displacement of the fragment varies but usually remains closely associated with the carpus. The fracture may be missed in the lateral view because of the superimposition of the distal radioulnar area and proximal carpal row.

If there is significant displacement, distraction and manipulation ulnarly will effect satisfactory reduction. Percutaneous fixation with Kirschner wires is helpful if the fragment is unstable. Plaster immobilization in slight ulnar deviation for 5 to 6 weeks is sufficient. If the fragment is large, fixation will be necessary to prevent collapse (Fig. 7-22).

FRACTURE OF THE DISTAL RADIUS WITH ANTERIOR DISPLACEMENT (SMITH'S FRACTURE)

Confusion persists about fractures of the distal radius with anterior displacement because of the terminology and eponyms involved in their description.[15,19,73,77,93,249] This fracture is much less common than the posteriorly displaced distal radial fracture. Failure to differentiate posterior from anterior displacement leads to misdirected treatment, with resulting deformity and functional impairment.

Mechanisms of Injury

Smith[249] reported that this fracture results from a fall on the back of the hand, thus providing a mechanism opposite that in Colles' fracture. This assumption has been challenged, and a fall with the forearm supinating on the fixed dorsiflexed hand has been suggested as a more frequent mechanism of production.[93,273] A direct blow to the dorsum of the flexed hand or knuckles, as in motorcycle crashes, may be the mechanism of injury in young adults. A clean fracture surface dorsally, with comminution of the anterior meta-

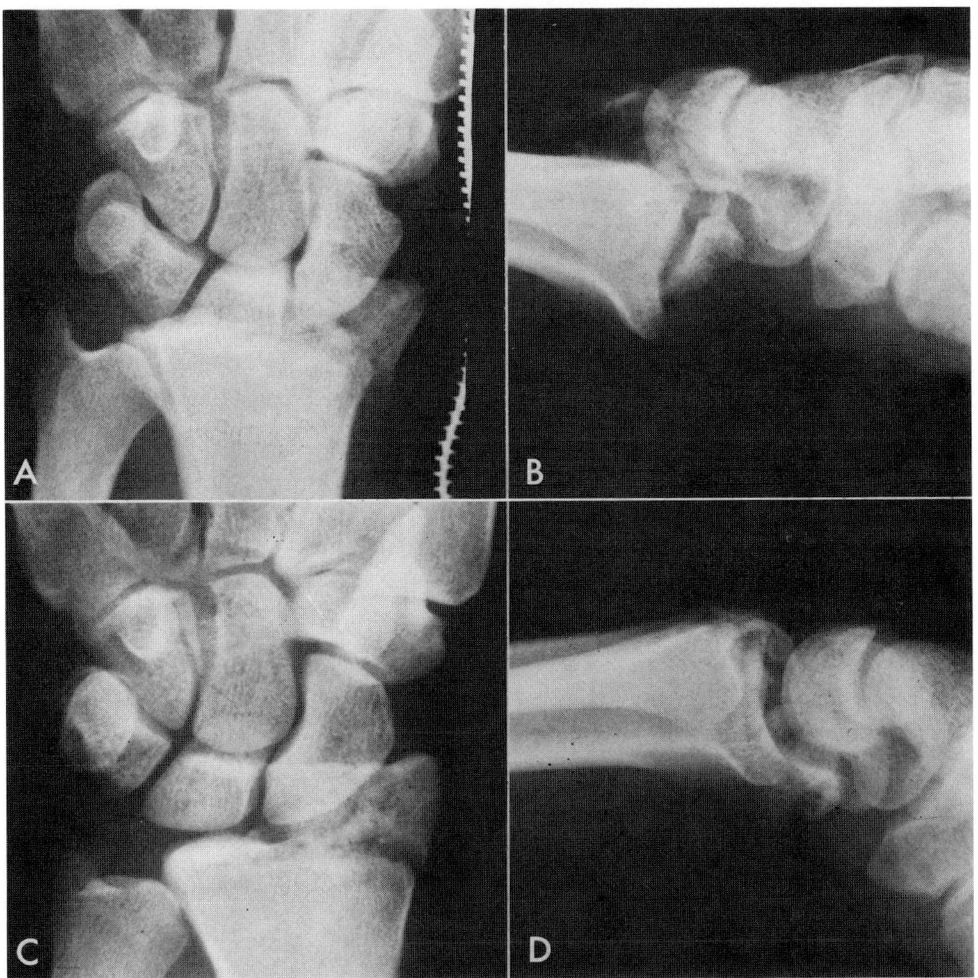

Fig. 7-21. Dorsal fracture-dislocation. A 27-year-old iron worker fell from the third floor of a building under construction, injuring both wrists. (*A, B*) At the time of injury, there was dorsal dislocation of the carpus with a thin rim of dorsal articular surface of the distal radius. There was also a radial styloid fracture with comminution of the articular surface. (*C, D*) Reduction films show disruption of the intra-articular surface. This resulted in some late discomfort and loss of motion, which prevented the patient from returning to working at heights in steel construction. Open reduction might have made a better final result.

physeal surface, suggests that compressive and rotational stresses applied to the radial articular surface through the proximal articular row initiate the fracture dorsally in tension.

Classification

Smith's fracture (Fig. 7-23) has been classified into three types by Thomas,[273] depending primarily on the obliquity of the fracture line[73,93,273]: Type 1 is a trans-

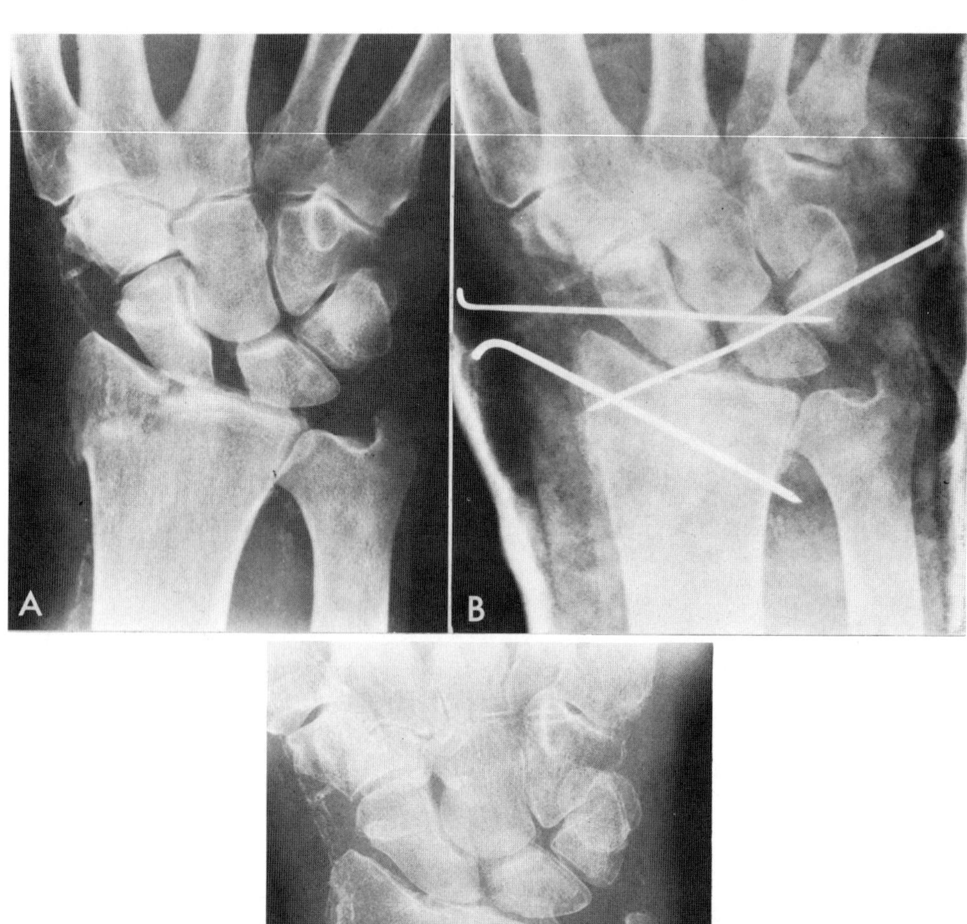

Fig. 7-22. A 77-year-old man fell from roof, suffering a radial styloid fracture of the right wrist and a depressed fracture of the zygoma and inferior orbital ridge. (*A*) The anteroposterior view shows an oblique fracture through the radial styloid, with slight ulnar tilting and proximal displacement. There is also an increased space between the scaphoid and the lunate, suggesting rupture of the scapholunate ligament. (*B*) Manipulation of the fracture was carried out under longitudinal traction. The scapholunate gap was closed and held with percutaneous Kirschner wires. Another Kirschner wire held the position of the radial styloid. (*C*) Three months after fracture, the patient had little pain or discomfort, and motion and strength were rapidly increasing.

verse fracture extending from the dorsal to the anterior cortex through the metaphysis; Type 2 is an oblique fracture from the dorsal lip to the palmar metaphysis; and Type 3 is an oblique fracture beginning in the articular surface of the distal radius and extending anteroproximally.

Signs and Symptoms

The patient complains of pain, swelling, and tenderness. The hand is anteriorly displaced in reference to the forearm, and the palmar aspect of the wrist is swollen and tense. The ulnar head is abnormally prominent dorsally. Crepitus may be less noticeable to palpation, particularly if the fracture line does not penetrate the dorsal cortex.

Roentgenographic Findings

The anteroposterior roentgenograms reveal that the carpus is proximally displaced and that the fracture line extends transversely through the distal metaphysis. Lateral views disclose anterior displacement of the fragment and palmar angulation of the radial articular surface. Type 3 fractures become evident on careful interpretation of the silhouette of the distal articular surface. The superimposition of the styloid process, distal ulna, and proximal carpal row makes interpretation difficult. The articular surface is angulated palmarward, and the carpus follows the anteriorly displaced articular surface. The ulnar styloid is usually fractured.

Fracture Eponyms

Smith[249] described the fracture in 1847, and it is most commonly associated with his name, though the term reverse Colles' fracture is also used. Barton,[19] 9 years earlier, described the intraarticular fracture, the Type 3 fracture. Because he also described the posterior fracture-dislocation, the term "reverse Barton's fracture" is used. Earlier similar descriptions were made by Lecomte (Types 1 and 2 Smith's fracture) and by Lentenneur (Type 3 Smith's fracture).[77]

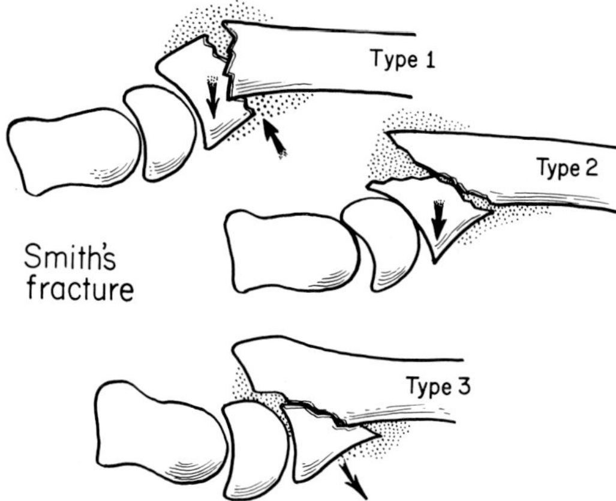

Fig. 7-23. Smith fractures. Three clinical types of anteriorly displaced distal radial fractures.[93]

Treatment

For Types 1 and 2 fractures, the initial treatment includes longitudinal distraction of the fracture and manipulation of the distal fragment by increasing the deformity and by displacing it posteriorly into position. Immobilization in a short-arm plaster cast or molded plaster splints will be sufficient when the fracture is stable, though this is seldom the case, and redisplacement is common. A long-arm cast with the forearm in supination and the wrist in slight flexion is preferred (Fig. 7-24). Dorsiflexion places the radiocarpal joint contact area volarly, thus increasing the displacement force. Fractures in which the fracture line is more oblique (Type 2) or begins intraarticularly (Type 3) tend to be unstable. Instability of the Type 3 fracture can be minimized by avoiding the dorsiflexed position after reduction.

Percutaneous 0.045-inch Kirschner wires help hold the reduction. Two or more Kirschner wires through the fragment, through the proximal cancellous bone of the shaft, and into the proximal cortex are necessary to suitably fix the fracture. Traction must be removed, while check roentgenograms are taken, to ensure that there is no displacement. In the event the frac-

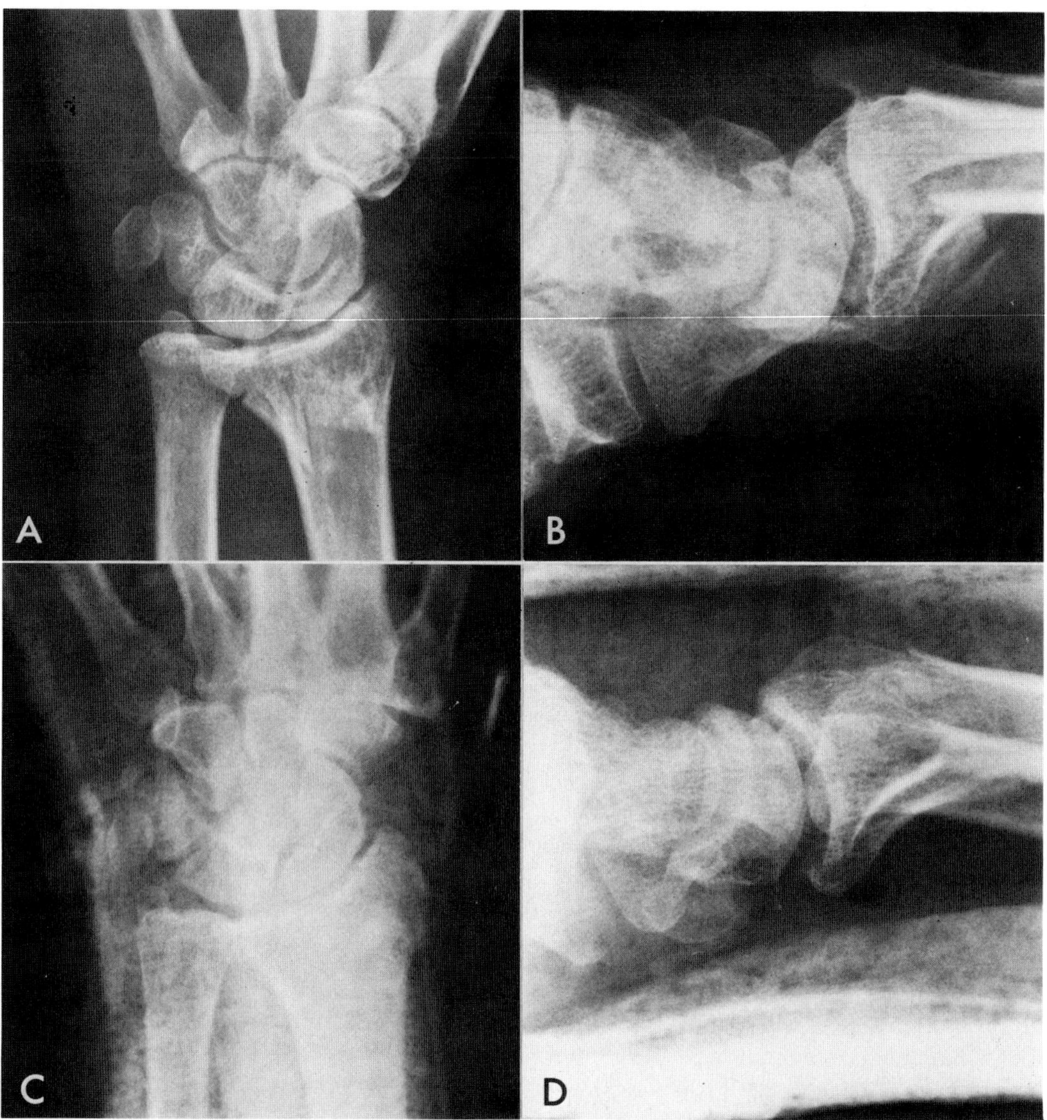

Fig. 7-24. A Type 1 Smith fracture in a 35-year-old man who fell from a stationary motorcycle. He kept a firm grip on the handlebars throughout the fall. (*A*) Comminuted distal radial fracture. (*B*) There was 40 degrees Palmar angulation of the distal fragment. (*C, D*) In the reduced position, palmar angulation of the radial articular surface is 16°. The wrist was held in neutral position.

ture cannot be readily reduced, we prefer open reduction through an anterior wrist incision, displacing the tendons of the fingers in an ulnar direction and the flexor carpi radialis and flexor pollicis longus radially. This brings into view the pronator quadratus and the palmar lip of the radius. The muscle may be partially released from its distal attachment, and the fracture fragment is visualized, replaced, and held either with Kirschner wires or a small bone plate bent to fit the curvature of the distal metaphysis. The plate is fixed with screws proximally, while the distal portion of the plate buttresses the fragment (Fig. 7-25).[73,93]

Postoperative care in a short-arm cast or

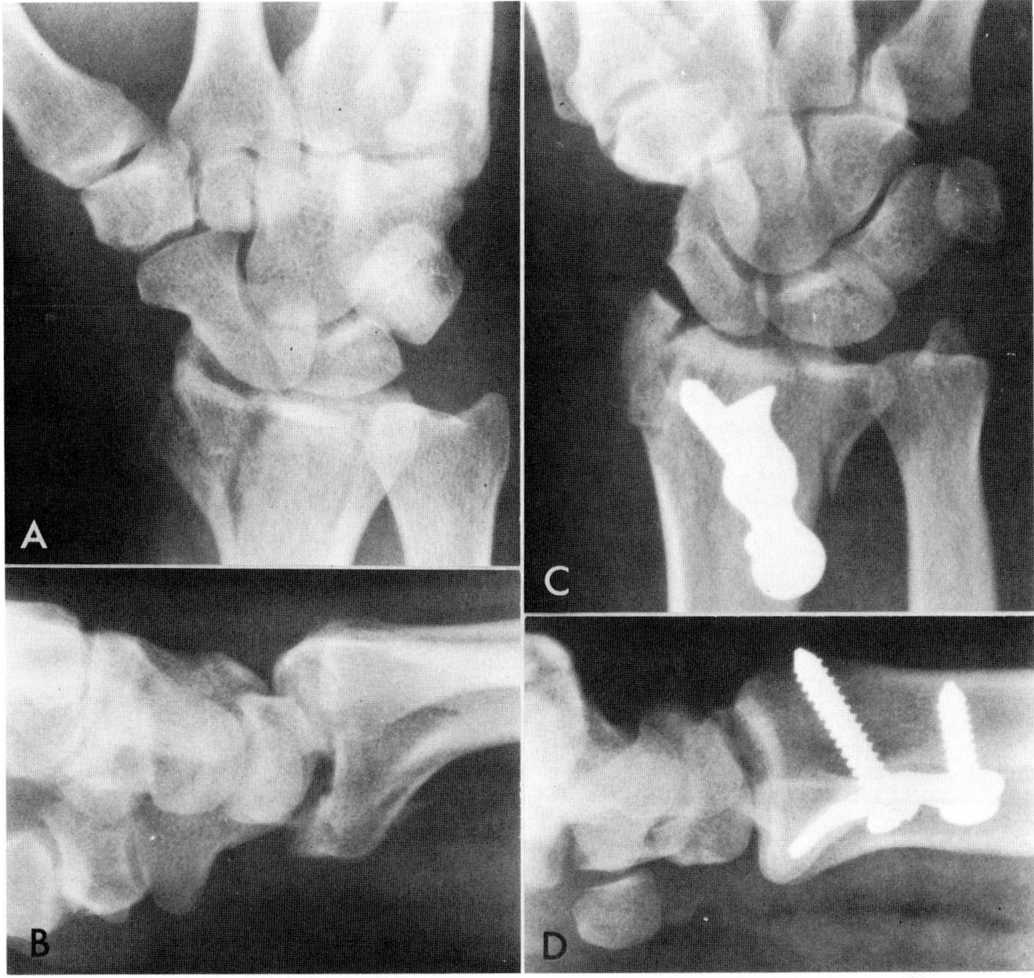

Fig. 7-25. A 51-year-old public health nurse fell backward on stairs, landing on the heel of her palm. (*A*) She sustained a comminuted fracture of the distal radius, with proximal migration of the carpus. (*B*) The palmar articular fragment was displaced palmarly and proximally. (*C, D*) Open reduction, using an Ellis buttress plate formed from a small four-hole plate, gave satisfactory reduction. At 3 months the patient returned to work. Her grip strength was 50 per cent; dorsiflexion was 40 degrees, and palmar flexion, 15 degrees. She reported little discomfort.

a plaster splint for 5 to 6 weeks is advisable. Long-arm support may be necessary.

Prognosis

With a well-reduced fracture, healing is generally completed in 5 to 6 weeks, and motion, strength, and freedom from pain should be anticipated. Incompletely reduced fractures or displaced fractures that are allowed to heal result in loss of motion, particularly in dorsiflexion, with weakness and variable amounts of discomfort on use of the wrist.

Complications

The most common problem in this fracture is misinterpretation of the roentgenograms. If this injury is considered a Colles' fracture and treated like one, the reduction is incomplete and the deformity may be

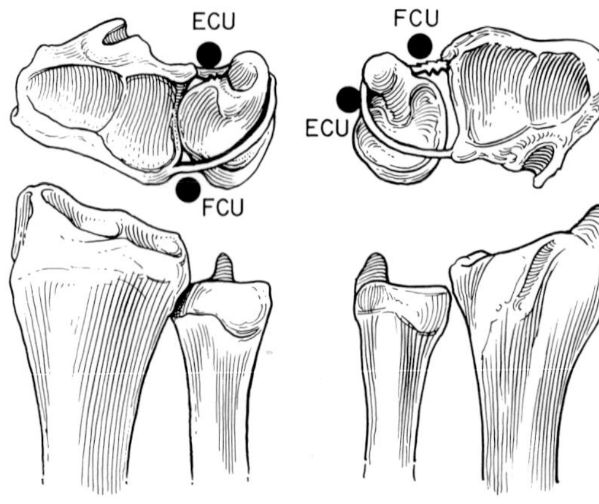

Fig. 7-26. End-on view of the distal radioulnar articulation. During pronation and supination, the ulna maintains its relative position with the radius rotating about it. The ulna performs a relative circumduction motion about the axis of rotation, but in a conical fashion; the ulna itself does not rotate, except for a few degrees of torque, which produces rotation in bone at extremes of motion (exaggerated in drawing). The extensor carpi ulnaris (*ECU*) retains its relative position in reference to the head of the ulna, but it lies in dorsoradial position in supination and a palmoulnar position in full pronation. There is a tendency for the distal radioulnar joint to dissociate at extremes of motion, but it is constrained by the dorsal and palmar radioulnar ligaments and the triangular fibrocartilage with which it is closely invested. (*FCU*, flexor carpi ulnaris)

increased, leading to loss of strength, limitation of motion, and discomfort. Further complications of the fracture are essentially the same as those seen in other fractures of the distal radius.

INJURIES OF THE DISTAL RADIOULNAR JOINT

Injuries of the distal radioulnar joint as a result of Colles', Smith's, Essex-Lopresti's, and Galeazzi's fractures are recognized as integral parts of these fractures but usually assume secondary importance to the fracture. Excision of the distal ulna as a preliminary to reducing a severely displaced Colles' fracture has been suggested.[87,292] However, isolated dislocation of the distal radioulnar joint is uncommon and frequently unrecognized so that treatment is often delayed or ignored.[7,67,124,177,233,250,283]

Ulnar styloid fractures are frequent concomitants of all the injuries discussed, and occasionally they occur independently as well. They are often assumed to be minor. Injuries of the triangular fibrocartilage[53,296] and osteochondral fractures of the convex surface of the ulnar head are difficult to diagnose and are often treated expectantly in the hopes that the symptoms will regress and disappear. However, this is far from the case, and injuries of the distal radioulnar joint frequently result in prolonged disability. The late problem is often relegated to the expediency of the Darrach resection[68,78,144,172,194-196,227] which, regardless of its reported efficacy, often leaves behind its own special problem.

An eponym formerly applied to those luxations of the distal ulna associated with fracture of the distal radius was Moore's fracture.[201]

Surgical Anatomy[142,161,162,283]

When viewed in coronal sections, the distal radioulnar joint discloses a shallow concavity on the ulnar aspect of the distal radius that slides around the nearly hemispheric circular convexity of the distal ulna during pronation and supination. The articular cartilage of the ulna continues to cover the distal face, which articulates with the basilar portion of the triangular fibrocartilage. The motion about the distal radioulnar joint is constrained by the relationship of the radius and ulna proximally, the radioulnar interosseous membrane, the triangular fibrocartilage, and the distal radioulnar ligaments. The distal ulna undergoes virtually no rotation about its long axis during pronation and supination but does describe a small arc of rotation about the distal radius (Fig. 7-26).[85] The ulnar styloid seems to change position during this motion so that it is posterior during full supination and is ulnar and anterior during full pronation. The extensor carpi ulnaris resides in a sulcus on the posterior aspect of the ulna lateral to the ulnar styloid. It is fixed in position in a fibro-osseous sheath separate from the dorsal carpal ligament.[256] Its position seems to change so that during full pronation it is an ulnar abductor of the hand. The stability of the distal radioulnar joint depends largely on the triangular fibrocartilage and the distal radioulnar ligaments into which it merges peripherally.[124,233] In addition, the depth of the ulnar notch of the radius, the extensor carpi ulnaris, and the dorsal carpal ligament add to the stability.

The triangular fibrocartilage attaches to a thin arc along the distal aspect of the ulnar notch of the radius and converges to a point of attachment on the base of the ulnar styloid process. The peripheral fibers of this ligament alternately tighten dorsally during full pronation and palmarly during full supination. They are intimately bound to the distal radioulnar ligament, which arises from the dorsal and palmar surfaces of the medial aspect of the distal radius, encompasses the articular surface of the distal ulna, and merges strongly with the transverse ligament component of the triangular fibrocartilage proximally and the meniscal portion and ulnar collateral ligament distally.[162,233] There are no strong ligamentous attachments to the ulnar styloid, except at the base. The pronator quadratus is the strongest pronator of the forearm. It lies on the distal 4 to 6 cm. of both bones.

Mechanisms of Injury

Isolated subluxations or dislocations of the distal radioulnar joint occur from falls, twisting injuries, or lifting heavy loads suddenly with the wrist outstretched. Dorsal subluxation or dislocation of the ulna occurs with the hand in the pronated position or with hyperpronation stresses. In the anatomic specimen during full pronation, the ulnar collateral ligament strongly supports the anterior distal radioulnar ligament. In addition, the dorsal fibers of the triangular fibrocartilage are taut. Together this system produces a dorsal subluxation force during pronation.

In contrast, during full supination, the ulnar collateral ligament is in a dorsal position and the anterior fibers of the triangular fibrocartilage are taut, inducing a palmar distraction of the distal ulna tangential to the ulnar notch of the radius. The anterior radioulnar ligament and the anterior capsule are stretched. This stretching sets the stage for rupture and attenuation of the ligaments as continued supination occurs against the fixed hand. Although there is some controversy concerning the relative importance of the distal radioulnar ligaments and the triangular fibrocartilage, these probably are parts of the same structure, and the distal ulna probably cannot be dislocated completely without rupture of the triangular fibrocartilage or fracture of the ulnar styloid process.

Ulnar styloid avulsions are produced by forces applied to the styloid base through the triangular fibrocartilage or the ulnar collateral ligaments. Forced radial deviation, dorsiflexion, or rotatory stresses are all capable of inducing this injury. Tears of the triangular fibrocartilage are produced by similar forces.

Classification

Because the radius rotates about the distal ulna, it is anatomically correct to speak of a dislocation of the radius on the ulna. However, convention and the appearance of the wrist lead to the continued use of the terms dorsal- and palmar ulnar dislocations. The triangular fibrocartilage can be torn from its radial attachment or at its center, or it may have transverse or lingular tears.

Signs and Symptoms

Pain and deformity are immediately apparent after a fall or twisting injury of the wrist. Dorsal subluxation results in prominence of the distal ulna with painful and limited supination. Palmar dislocation results in a wrist that is narrower in its anteroposterior diameter. There is a fullness on the ulnar-palmar aspect of the wrist, and pronation is markedly limited. With ulnar styloid fracture, tenderness and instability of the ulnar head are noted. Tears of the cartilage and chondral injuries may be associated with crepitus and pain at a specific position of wrist rotation.

Roentgenographic Findings

Dorsal subluxation is difficult to detect because a true lateral view may not be possible.[124] The appearance of the ulnar head dorsally above the radius, particularly if the triquetrum is not directly in line with the ulna, is helpful in diagnosis. Positioning the lateral view under the image intensifier may be useful.

Palmar dislocation is easier to recognize. The anteroposterior view reveals that the ulnar head lies partially superimposed on the radial metaphysis, the forearm is narrowed, and the ulnar styloid may be fractured. The lateral view shows the ulna displaced beneath the radial metaphysis. The styloid fracture may be confused with an accessory bone at the tip of the styloid known as the lunula or os triangulare.

Arthrograms of the wrist may be helpful in diagnosing fibrocartilage tears.[145,225,296] The test is performed with a needle introduced into the radiocarpal joint, either beneath the radial styloid or in the sulcus between the second and third dorsal compartments. Approximately 1 to 2 ml. of lidocaine, followed by 2 to 4 ml. of water-soluble radiopaque dye, are injected. Dye flowing into the distal radioulnar joint or into apparent rents within the substance of the triangular fibrocartilage may be helpful in diagnosis (Fig. 7-27). However, one must be cognizant of the prestyloid recess (see p. 350), which is a normal structure, and of the fact that dye in this region does not indicate a tear. Arthrograms of the

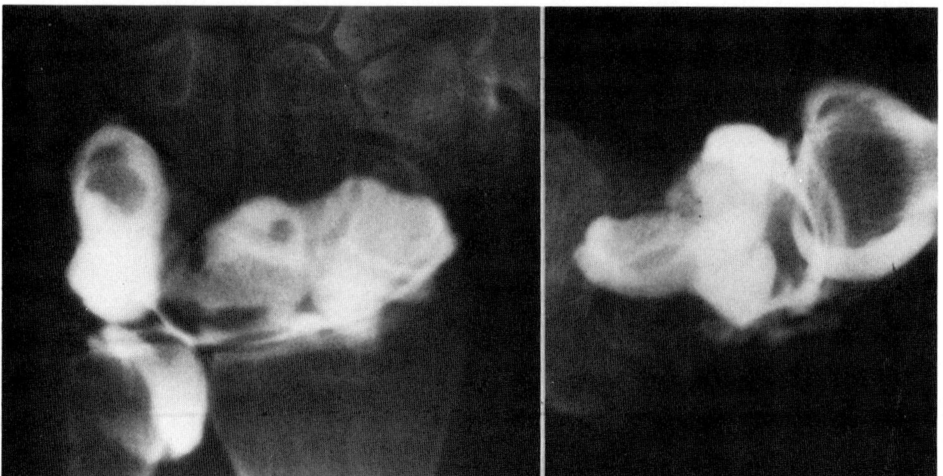

Fig. 7-27. Arthrogram of the wrist. Two milliliters of 60 per cent Renografin have filled the radiocarpal joint and (through a perforation of triangular fibrocartilage) the distal radioulnar joint as well. Sacculus recessiformis is that space filled with dye located between the triangular fibrocartilage and the head of the ulna. Dye has filled the pisotriquetral joint, giving better detail of the pisotriquetral area. Perforations of the triangular fibrocartilage are found more commonly with increasing age but are seldom clinically significant unless associated with a distinct tear in the triangular fibrocartilage. Dye is also seen to fill the center of the recess on the palmar aspect of the radius adjacent to the radial scapholunate ligament. No significant prestyloid recess is noted.

wrist are difficult to evaluate, and there may be both underdiagnosis and overdiagnosis.

Treatment

Dorsal subluxation (Fig. 7-28), when seen in the acute stage, should be managed by reducing the ulnar head, rotating the forearm into full supination, and applying an above-elbow cast with the elbow flexed to 90 degrees and the ulnar head held in reduction for 6 weeks by careful molding of the cast about the wrist. If dorsal subluxation is present 2 weeks or longer, laxity of the distal radioulnar joint with recurring subluxation in pronation is likely. This may require ligamentous reconstruction.[67,124,233,283]

Palmar dislocation (Fig. 7-29) is often locked and is painful to reduce without adequate anesthesia. Direct pressure on the ulnar head prominence anteriorly, with counterpressure over the radial metaphysis, allows reduction if the dislocation is seen early. Hypersupination may be necessary to unlock the ulnar head. The forearm should be held in pronation. The deformity is unlikely to recur once it is reduced. The ulnar styloid may be fractured and displaced. The deformity, if seen after 10 days to 2 weeks, may require open reduction.[67,124,233,283]

Frequently, an ulnar styloid fracture (Fig. 7-30) is considered to be of minor importance, especially when the fracture is associated with the more serious fractures of the distal radius. Failure of union may lead to instability of the distal radioulnar joint, inasmuch as the triangular fibrocartilage and distal ulnar collateral ligament lose their attachments on the distal ulna. This increased instability may lead to weak-

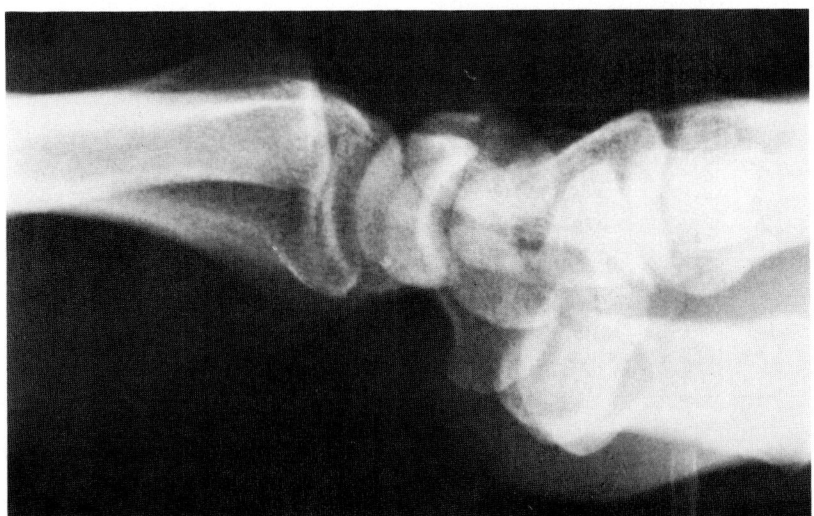

Fig. 7-28. A 32-year-old surgical resident attempted to hold heavy fiberboard in his outstretched arm through a basement window. He felt sudden pain and deformity in the left wrist. Examination 3 days later disclosed a prominent ulnar head and increased laxity of the distal radioulnar joint. There was tenderness on manipulation and discomfort on attempted supination; a click occurred before full supination could be obtained. The distal ulna was in dorsal subluxation in relation to the radius. A true lateral view was obtained under the image intensifier. Note that the distal ulna is displaced somewhat dorsally from the triquetrum. Five weeks of immobilization in a well molded above-elbow plaster cast, with the wrist supinated and the ulnar head molded anteriorly, resulted in satisfactory recovery.

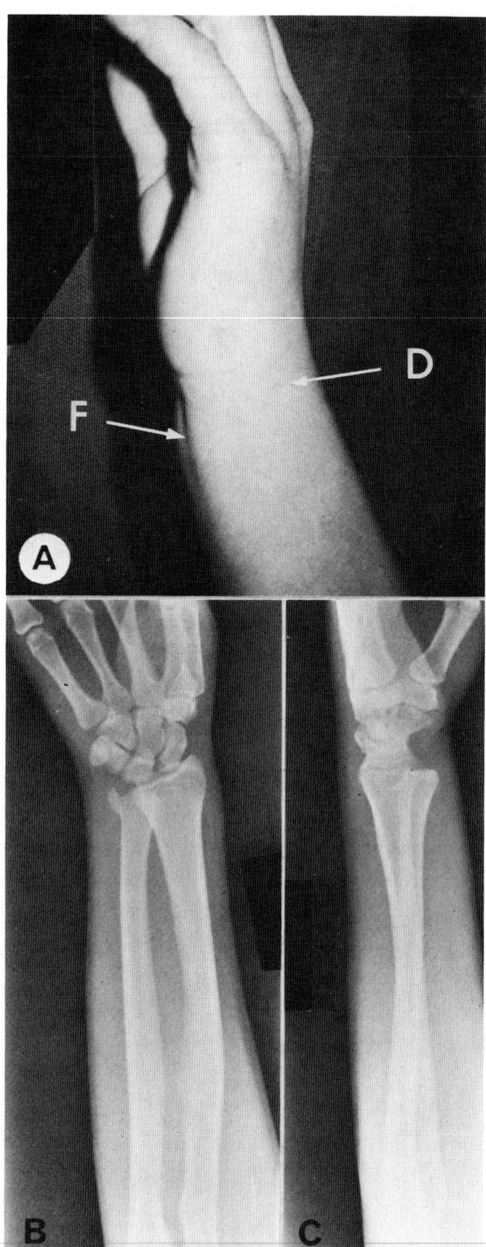

Fig. 7-29. A 24-year-old laborer fell backward onto his supinated left hand. He noted immediate pain and was referred because of persistent deformity of the wrist 1 month after injury. (*A*) At examination there was fullness (*F*) on the ulnar side and depression (*D*) over the dorso-ulnar aspect of the wrist. There was inability to supinate the left hand to neutral position. (*B*) An anteroposterior view shows superimposition of the radius on the ulnar head, fracture of the ulnar styloid, and narrowing of the interosseous space. (*C*) A lateral view shows the ulnar head to be displaced and locked under the radius. Open reduction was necessary to unlock the distal ulna. Triangular fibrocartilage was replaced over the end of the ulna, and the ulnar styloid was held by a Kirschner wire. Three months after injury, he had nearly a full range of pronation and supination and normal strength in the left wrist.

ness and discomfort and predispose to future injuries with lesser stresses. If the ulnar styloid is not significantly displaced, support of the wrist in a gauntlet cast, with the wrist in slight ulnar deviation and neutral position, relaxes its ligamentous attachments and allows it to seek the proximal fragment. With immobilization, healing is usually complete in 5 to 6 weeks. If displaced, the triangular fibrocartilage may be sutured back to the base of the ulnar styloid.

If a tear in the fibrocartilage is suspected, 4 to 6 weeks of immobilization should be undertaken before arthrography and exploration are considered. Removal of the cartilage is indicated on the basis of severity of the symptoms. Resection of the distal ulna (Darrach resection) may be a last resort if painful arthrosis of the distal radioulnar joint persists.[68,78,144,172,194-196,227]

Prognosis

Dorsal subluxations of the distal ulna are likely to recur, particularly if treatment is delayed or inadequate. Palmar dislocations are unlikely to recur if they are adequately reduced, although an unreduced dislocation results in severe limitation of pronation. Union in styloid fractures may be delayed if they remain displaced. Triangular fibrocartilage injuries often improve with time.

Complications

Osteochondral fractures of the radioulnar and ulnocarpal articulation, tears of the triangular fibrocartilage, unrecognized proximal forearm injuries, ulnar nerve irritations in Guyon's canal, and late distal radioulnar laxity may coexist to complicate each other and the physician's treatment.[106] Unrecognized dorsal subluxation fixed in position during a treatment period for a month or longer will become irreducible and may limit forearm motion unless corrected by reconstructive surgery.

CARPAL INJURIES

Classification

Fractures and dislocations of the carpal bones and joints are said to constitute approximately 6 per cent of all fractures and dislocations, but this figure is probably too small, because many subtle problems have not been identified in previous surveys.[24,57,255,292] Table 7-2 compares the distribution of diagnoses in a fairly equal group of patients surveyed at the Böhler Clinic by Schnek[24,241] and at the Mayo Clinic by the present authors. With some regrouping of the Schnek categories to fit those used in our review, there is a close correspondence between the numbers and types of injuries. The largest discrepancy is in the identification of the subluxation type of posttraumatic carpal instability,[165] a diagnosis not recognized at the time of Schnek's study.[241]

A breakdown of the various traumatic entities in the carpus according to their relative incidences includes (1) carpal scaphoid fractures, (2) dorsal chip fractures, (3) posttraumatic carpal instability,

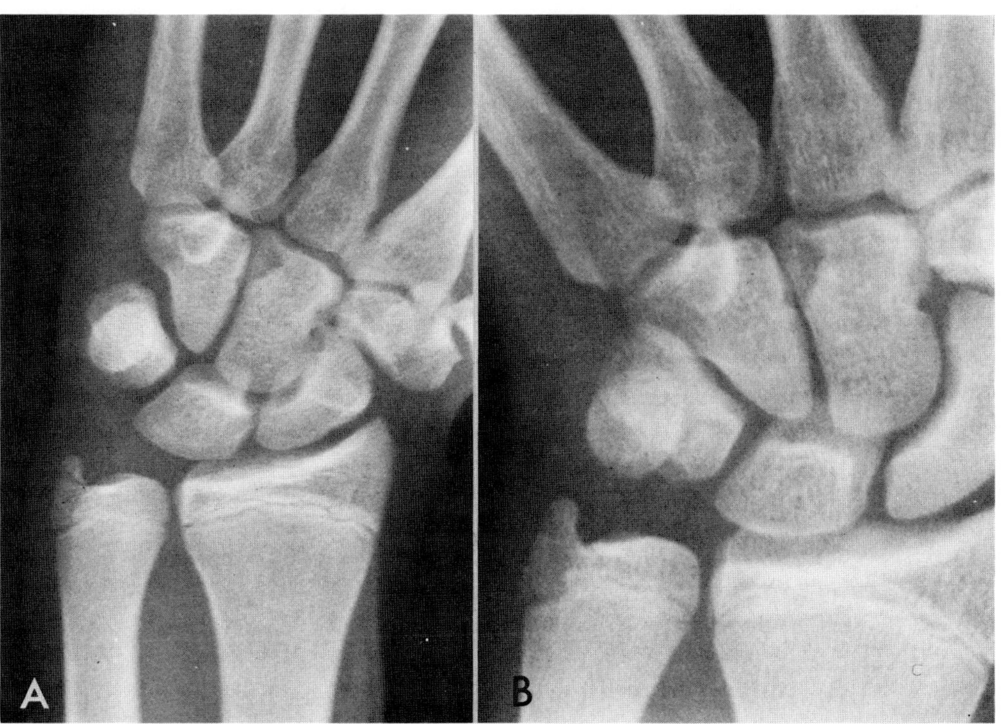

Fig. 7-30. Isolated fracture of the ulnar styloid. A 16-year-old gymnast felt sharp pain in his left wrist with the hands in marked radial deviation during practice on still rings. (*A*) A transverse fracture through the ulnar styloid, with slight displacement during radial deviation. (*B*) The fracture was well reduced with ulnar deviation. It healed with 4 weeks of immobilization, and the patient returned to gymnastics.

Table 7-2. Comparison of the Incidences of Various Carpal Injuries

Type	Böhler Clinic (6 yr.)		Mayo Clinic (10 yr.)	
Scaphoid fractures	234		367	
New		154		215
Old		80		152
Dorsal chip fractures	59		36	
Dislocations and fracture-dislocations	59		25	
Transscaphoid perilunar		17		9
Perilunar or lunate		25		7
Others		17		9
Subluxations and collapse deformities			57	
Dorsiflexion instability (new)				13
Dorsiflexion instability (old)				35
Palmar flexion instability (new)				7
Palmar flexion instability (old)				2
Lunate fractures (including Kienböck's)	23		15	
Triquetral fractures	18		7	
Trapezium fractures	13		5	
Pisiform fractures	13		4	
Hamate fractures	2		3	
Capitate fractures	6		2	
Trapezoid fractures	1		2	
Total	428		523	

with dislocations and without dislocations, (4) carpal lunate fractures, and (5) all other carpal fractures.

Fractures of the carpal scaphoid probably constitute 60 to 70 per cent of all diagnosed carpal injuries.[24,57,255,292] The combination of dislocations and subluxations or collapse deformities probably accounts for another 10 per cent of carpal injuries, dorsal chip fractures for another 10 per cent, carpal lunate fractures for about 3 per cent, and all other carpal fractures for about 7 per cent of the total.[82]

Signs and Symptoms

The most constant and dependable sign of carpal injury is well-localized tenderness. Fractures of the carpal scaphoid, for instance, are most tender to pressure in the anatomic snuffbox. Scapholunate and carpal lunate injuries cause tenderness just distal to Lister's tubercle. Triquetral and triquetrohamate injuries result in tenderness over the dorsal margin of the appropriate bone, usually a fingerbreadth distal to the ulnar head. Similar findings are noted with fractures of the pisiform, hook of the hamate, trapezium, and capitate. Other clinical findings are highly variable and depend on the extent of carpal disruption. There may be swelling that is severe and generalized or discrete and barely detectable. Changes of shape, attributable to swelling, internal realignment of the bony architecture, or both, may occur. A specific diagnosis is difficult to make from changes in shape, contour, or swelling, although such changes may be suggestive. Central, dorsal swelling over the proximal carpal row, extending into the forearm proximally and the metacarpals distally, is suggestive of a chip fracture. A marked prominence of the entire carpus dorsally is suggestive of a perilunate dislocation. Compressive stresses

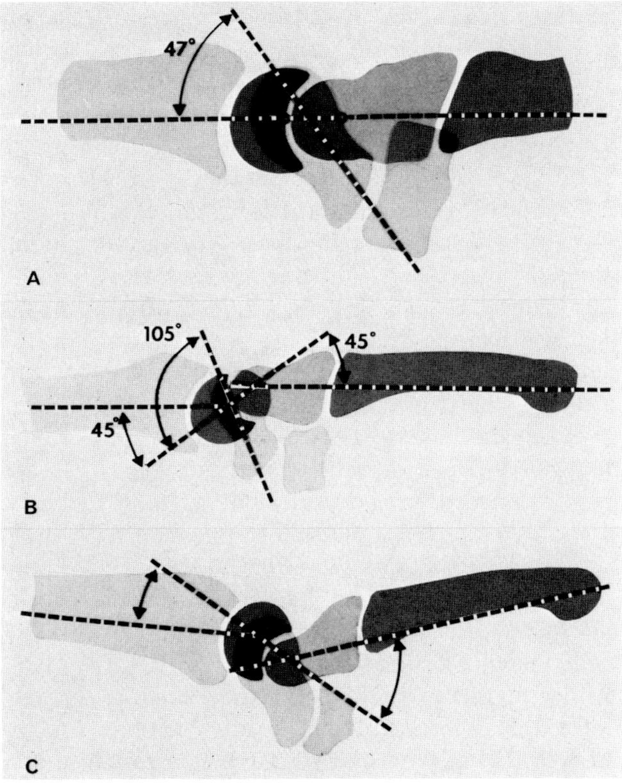

Fig. 7-31. Drawings depict the axes of the carpal bones in lateral view. (*A*) In neutral position, the axes of the radius, lunate, and capitate are colinear. The scaphoid lies at an average of 47 degrees to the longitudinal axis of the lunate, with a range of 30 to 70 degrees. (*B*) Dorsiflexed, intercalated segment instability (dorsiflexion instability) is obtained when the capitolunate angle is greater than 20 degrees and the scapholunate angle is greater than 70 degrees. (*C*) Palmar flexed, intercalated instability pattern (palmar flexion instability) presents the opposite pattern: the scapholunate angle is decreased to an average of 35 degrees. (Linscheid, R. L., Dobyns, J. H., Beabout, J. W., and Bryan, R. S.: J. Bone Joint Surg., *54A*:1612-1632, 1972)

applied actively or passively produce pain at the site of damage. Other contributory diagnostic signs include those of difficulties with tendon function and those of neural or vascular compromise.

General Roentgenographic Findings

Roentgenographic findings are the chief determinant for the specific diagnosis of wrist area fractures and dislocations, even though valuable information is available from the history and clinical examination. The two most important views are the anteroposterior and the lateral, each taken in an exact neutral position. To these two views, we often add four more and consider the entire group of six as a motion study of the wrist. The added four are anteroposterior views in maximal radial deviation and maximal ulnar deviation and lateral views in maximal flexion and maximal extension. These six views are adequate in more than 90 per cent of cases in diagnosing fractures and dislocations in this area. The shifting of the carpal bones in the various positions changes the overlap pattern sufficiently that most fracture lines can be seen readily on one or more of the views.

In addition, the more subtle changes in the normal relationships of the carpal bones usually can be visualized and measured in one or more of the views. The important angular relationships are probably best visualized in the lateral views. In the normal wrist in neutral position, the longitudinal axes of the long finger metacarpal, the capitate, the lunate, and the radius all fall on the same line—a line drawn through the center of the head of the third metacarpal, the center of the head of the capitate, the midpoints of the convex proximal and the concave distal joint surfaces of the lunate, and the midpoint of the distal articular surface of the radius. The longitudinal axis of the scaphoid is drawn through the midpoints of its proximal and distal poles. Use of these axes makes it possible to measure angles that define the positions of the carpal bones. For instance, the scapholunate angle formed by the intersection of the longitudinal axes of the scaphoid and the lunate averages 47 degrees and ranges from 30 to 60 degrees in normal wrists (Fig. 7-31A). An angle greater than 70 degrees suggests instability, and one greater than 80 degrees is almost certain proof of carpal instability of the dorsiflexion type. A capitolunate angle of more than 20 degrees is also strongly suggestive of carpal instability.

When the lunate lies palmar to the capitate but is flexed dorsally, the collapse pattern is referred to as dorsiflexion instability, and this pattern is much more common in posttraumatic situations (Fig. 7-31B). If the lunate lies dorsal to the capitate and is flexed palmarward, the collapse pattern is called palmar flexion instability (Fig. 7-31C). Either of these instability patterns may be associated with scapholunate dissociations as well, though there are instances in each category in which scapholunate dissociation cannot be demonstrated, at least by standard roentgenograms.

In addition to these angular changes, scapholunate dissociation is marked by more dramatic changes on the anteroposterior view. The normal roentgenogram shows a fairly constant space between the various carpal bones, which is maintained throughout the range of motion. For instance, the joint width between the scaphoid and the lunate is normally 1 to 2 mm., no matter where the measurement is taken or what position the wrist is in during the measurement. However, with scapholunate dissociation, an increasing gap appears, which may in time be wide enough to accept proximal migration of the entire capitate head. A spread of more than 3 mm. is considered abnormal (see Figs. 7-41A, 7-42G, 7-47F, and 7-50A, B). In addition, the scaphoid flexes palmarward; this gives the scaphoid less of an elongated profile on the anteroposterior view and projects the cortical waist of the scaphoid as an overlapping ring of bone, inside the scaphoid projection, similar to the projection of the hook of the hamate. The lunate also moves into one or the other of the two collapse positions, and this can also be noted on the anteroposterior view by the increasing overlap of the capitate silhouette by a lunate horn. Another associated deformity which may be seen with either dorsiflexion or palmar flexion instability is that of ulnar translocation of the carpus.[165]

Many special views and techniques have been described and are used occasionally for further clarification of wrist injuries. These include motion studies under the image intensifier,[12] cinefluoroscopy,[12] arthrography,[145,225] special oblique projections,[175,217] carpal tunnel,[121,302] and carpal bridge views,[159] and special techniques such as tomography, with or without grid cassettes,[187] and electronic detail enhancement.[230] The ancillary roentgenographic methods used most commonly by the authors are the carpal tunnel view, arthrography, and compression views.

The carpal tunnel view is especially valuable for showing changes in the depth of the tunnel, deformities of the palmar projecting pillars, such as the hook of the hamate (see Fig. 7-62), and calcific deposits in the region of the carpal ligaments and the two wrist flexors.[42,217] Arthrography has not been sufficiently exploited in the wrist. This procedure can show communications (congenital, traumatic, or attritional) between the major synovial-lined compartments—the distal radioulnar joint, the radiocarpal joint (which usually includes the pisotriquetral joint), the midcarpal joint (which includes most of the carpometacarpal joints), and the thumb carpometacarpal joint. Not only are communications between the various compartments revealed but the appearance of the radiopaque dye may indicate the condition of the synovium, and even chondral defects occasionally may be suggested by lines of double density. Communication between the normal synovial cavities and the cystic masses frequently seen about the wrist also may be evident, whether these masses are common ganglia or proliferating synovial herniations. Fracture lines of the carpal bones are usually transverse. Active 'fist' compression by the patient while neutral anteroposterior and neutral lateral wrist roentgenograms are being made often shows a scapholunate gap or an increased scapholunate angle that standard roentgenograms may miss.

Roentgenographic findings about the wrist that may be confusing during the search for trauma stigmata are accessory ossification centers,[44,51,89,211,215,216,293] congenital absences, fusions, or deformities,[49,89,125,138,216,293,300] periarticular calcareous deposits,[42,217] cystic deformities,[141,159,231] and tumors.[2,66] In the past, osteochondroses[278] were said to occur in the carpus, and Kienböck's disease[147] for the carpal lunate and Preiser's disease[221,222] of the carpal scaphoid were names given to the better known conditions. Most of these instances, perhaps all, are in our opinion associated with trauma residua.

There are about 16 secondary ossification centers reported as possibilities in the carpal region. The ones most commonly seen are the lunula (also called os triangulare and many other names), lying between the ulnar styloid and the triquetrum, and one or the other of two associated with the distal scaphoid, the os radiale externum, or the os centrale carpi. Most cases shown in various texts or articles as bipartite carpal scaphoids with a separation at the wrist level are, in fact, old fractures, even when they are bilateral.[97,216,244,293] Degenerative changes around accessory carpal bones are unusual, but such changes around the so-called bipartite navicular are common. Congenital changes in the wrist are fairly common and may be represented by absences, deformities, or coalitions. The most common absences are those in the thumb axis, with a portion of or all of the scaphoid, trapezoid, and trapezium missing. Carpal coalitions are rare, but the most common is that of the lunate with the triquetrum. Wedge-shaped deformities of carpal bones are the rule in the various achondroplasias and dyschondroplasias and are common in growth or developmental disturbances involving the hand.[149,150] Except for the deposit of calcium frequently seen in the musculotendinous cuff at the shoulder, such deposits are most commonly found about the wrist and hand. They may be found on dorsal, palmar, or lateral surfaces and may be deep or superficial. However, the deposits are usually extraarticular and look like calcific deposits rather than bone.[42,217] Cystic changes in the carpal area are frequently associated with swelling, erosions, generalized radiolucency, and other signs of inflammatory disease, usually rheumatoid arthritis.[13,55,136] They also may be associated with sclerosis, spurring, deformity, and other signs of degenerative disease. Discretely outlined cysts in either single or multiple carpal bones without associated findings are occasionally seen. These may be the residua of old trauma. They are frequently empty cysts, with or without cyst walls or intraosseous ganglia and are not, in themselves, associated with recent injury and are seldom symptomatic.[141,159,231] Degenerative disease frequently results from old injuries and may be aggravated by recent trauma, but the narrowed joint spaces and the sclerosis, exostosis formation, and deformity are usually unmistakable. However, intraarticular calcification or even ossification may accompany degenerative or posttraumatic joint disease and mimic a fracture fragment.[149,150] Chondrocalcinosis[149,150] may be a cause of intraarticular calcification with associated calcification of the triangular fibrocartilage. Other confusing roentgenographic findings are noted in synovial chondromatosis, which may show scattered areas of calcification, intraosseous tumors such as osteoid osteoma with its osteoblastic reaction, and tumors that appear to be cystic, such as enchondromata and giant cell tumor.[2,135,278] Seldom is there real confusion between these and traumatic changes, however, if the appropriate diagnosis is considered.

Fracture Eponyms

Fortunately, fractures of the wrist have never been cursed with any eponyms that have persisted (although a transscaphoid perilunar fracture-dislocation is still sometimes referred to as de Quervain's fracture[75,266]). In Desault's text[76] in 1805, the classic deformities, though recognized, were usually called dislocations of one sort or another. However, less than 50 years later, Dupuytren[87] could say that he had never seen a dislocation of the wrist. He ascribed all deformities in the area to fractures of the distal radius or ulna. By the early 20th century, just another 50 years later, most of the traumatic entities that we know today were being diagnosed correctly because roentgenograms had made it much easier to differentiate among them. However, no eponyms became permanently attached to injuries in this area, except for those of the distal radius.

SCAPHOID INJURIES

The scaphoid is an irregular bone linking and forming the radial part of both the proximal and distal carpal rows.[142] It lies obliquely at about 45 degrees to the longitudinal axis of the two rows. Approximately two-thirds of its external surface is occupied by four surfaces that articulate with five bones. The largest articular surface is proximal and is convex in two planes to permit articulation with the radius. A concave ulnar articular area is for capitate motion. Distally, a bi-articular surface composed of the trapezium and trapezoid presents to the scaphoid. The last of the four surfaces is relatively small and permits a limited range of motion between the proximal pole and the lunate. A roughened ridge lying between these articular surfaces runs obliquely across the dorsal scaphoid for the insertion of the dorsal radiocarpal ligament, with multiple foramina for the entrance of the blood supply. A central indentation, known as the waist, has no ligamentous attachments, though a strong band of the palmar radiocarpal ligament passes by on its way to the capitate. The ligamentous insertion into the tuberosity is thick, and there are vascular foramina throughout this nonarticular surface.[285,286] In addition to its link function, wherein it helps to push or pull the proximal carpal row into position during various wrist motions, the scaphoid also responds directly to the compressive stresses that pass through the capitate and the separate compression stresses that are mediated by the thumb axis. Since the scaphoid crosses two carpal rows, it is also the principal bony block to continued excessive dorsiflexion stresses and eventually comes to lie between the radial lip dorsally and a fascicle of the palmar radiocarpal ligament which is under high-tension loading palmarly. This combination produces the susceptibility of the carpal scaphoid to fracture, the most common significant injury of the carpal bones. Nevertheless, the bone is well adapted to its role, as demonstrated by the experimental findings that compression loads that can fracture it are well above those required to fracture the distal radius.[134,295]

Classification

Since fracture of the scaphoid is common, it has been classified in many ways,[22,25,178,181,190,191,235,263] usually by anatomic location (Fig. 7-32). Almost everyone differentiates between proximal-third and middle-third fractures, although some disagree about whether to classify all fractures of the distal third as one entity or as distal-third fractures and tuberosity fractures. The clinical basis for differentiating among these four types is the variation in average healing time, which may be as short as 4 weeks for the tuberosity fracture and 20 weeks or longer for the proximal pole fracture. Associated with these differing healing times is the problem of diminished blood supply at the proximal levels.[169,173,270,286] This is not a problem for the tuberosity fracture and is rarely one for the distal-third fracture; but it is a problem for approximately 30 per cent of middle-third fractures and approaches 100 per cent in fractures of the proximal fifth of the scaphoid. Additional methods of classification are based on the direction of the fracture line, as stability is correlated with obliquity.[22,235,282]

Dislocations of the scaphoid have not been classified, but differing types have been described, varying from the so-called rotary subluxation to complete dislocation (reducible or irreducible) to the completely displaced scaphoid with loss of all ligamentous attachment.[11,14,28,34,36,37,56,63,80,94,101,114,152,164,165,236,259,271,272,274,281,290,292,301] All forms of the reduced dislocated scaphoid tend to be unstable, usually adopting a more vertical posture with the distal end facing palmarward and the proximal end dorsally and radially with some displacement away from the lunate. This is the position of rotary subluxation and is the position adopted in dorsiflexion instability. Our discussion of the treatment of this condition is included under the discussion of dorsiflexion instability collapse with associated scapholunate dissociation.

Signs and Symptoms

The general signs and symptoms of injury to the scaphoid are as discussed previously for the carpal area. However, there may be palpable abnormalities if a portion or all of the scaphoid is displaced significantly. Such displacements are rare, especially palmarward. The most common displacements are palpable just distal to the radial styloid and may represent distal fragments.

Roentgenographic Findings

As noted previously, the six motion study views show most scaphoid fractures and usually any associated instability. The signs of instability are (1) displacement of one of the fracture fragments (see Fig. 7-41), (2) motion between the fracture fragments, and (3) presence of one of the carpal collapse patterns (see Fig. 7-39). If doubt still remains, and it is important to know immediately if the fracture is present, anteroposterior tomograms, giant views, or special scaphoid views can be helpful.[146,163,234,235]

The most common carpal fracture is the transverse fracture of the middle third of the scaphoid, though fracture lines of the proximal third, distal third, and tuberosity also are seen. One of the chief difficulties in evaluating scaphoid fractures is estimating the age of the fracture. Signs that the fracture is old are (1) a space between the fragments similar in appearance and width to the other carpal spaces, (2) subspace sclerosis similar to, or even more marked than, the subchondral sclerosis elsewhere in the carpus, (3) surrounding degenerative changes, and (4) variations in the gap between the two fragments during the motion studies. Cystic changes at the fracture line and minor degrees of sclerosis have been said to indicate old fractures, but this appearance can be simulated immediately after a fresh fracture by rotation and overlap of the fracture surfaces. Large cystic

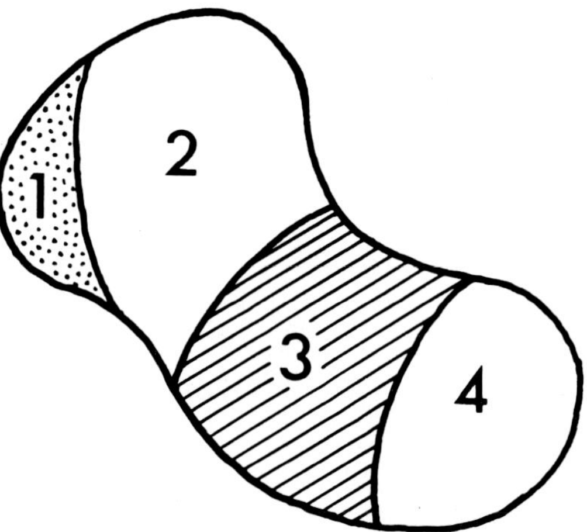

Fig. 7-32. The usual four sites of fracture of scaphoid are (*1*) the capsular attachment of the scaphoid tuberosity; (*2*) through the distal third of the scaphoid; (*3*) through the waist (by far the most common fracture); and (*4*) through the proximal pole. Prognosis for healing is distinctly affected by the site and obliquity of the fracture.

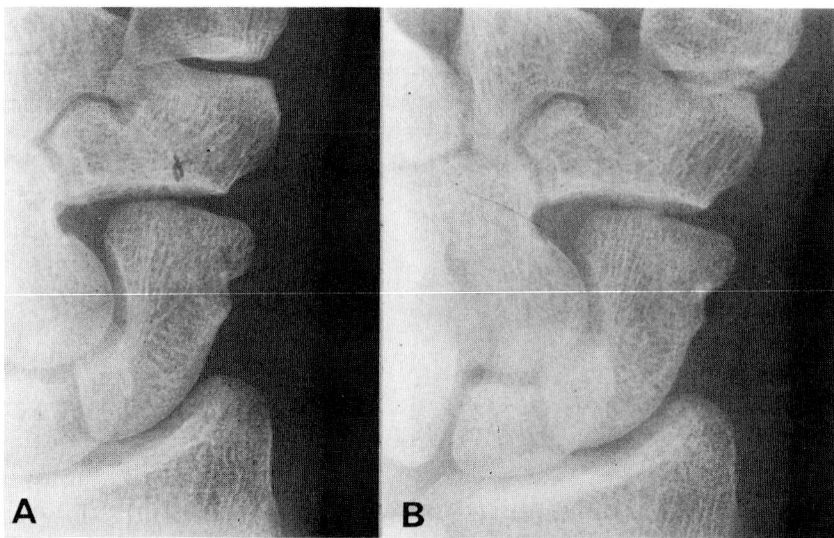

Fig. 7-33. Fracture of the tuberosity of the scaphoid. A 21-year-old man injured his left wrist in a fall from a motorcycle. (*A*) The fracture line went through the tuberosity and entered the scaphotrapezial joint. (*B*) Healing was uneventful in a plaster gauntlet cast. The patient returned to full activities after cast removal at 4½ weeks.

cavities probably indicate a fracture that is not fresh, but unless combined with one of the four points previously mentioned, this finding does not confirm an established pseudarthrosis.

Another significant problem with the roentgenographic diagnosis of scaphoid fractures is the occasional lack of sufficient fracture line distinction to make the diagnosis. This problem can be a feature of

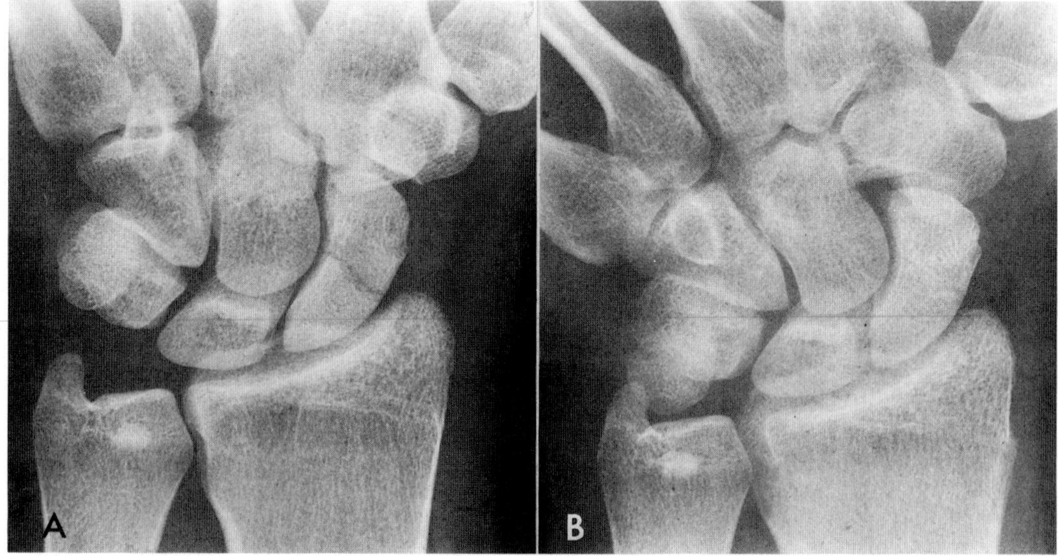

Fig. 7-34. A 24-year-old salesman incurred a transverse waist fracture of the left scaphoid while playing baseball. (*A*) The fracture line was more apparent at 2 weeks. Cast immobilization continued to 6 weeks, and a removable splint was worn for an additional 4 weeks. (*B*) The fracture line is still apparent, but it was healing well at 3 months.

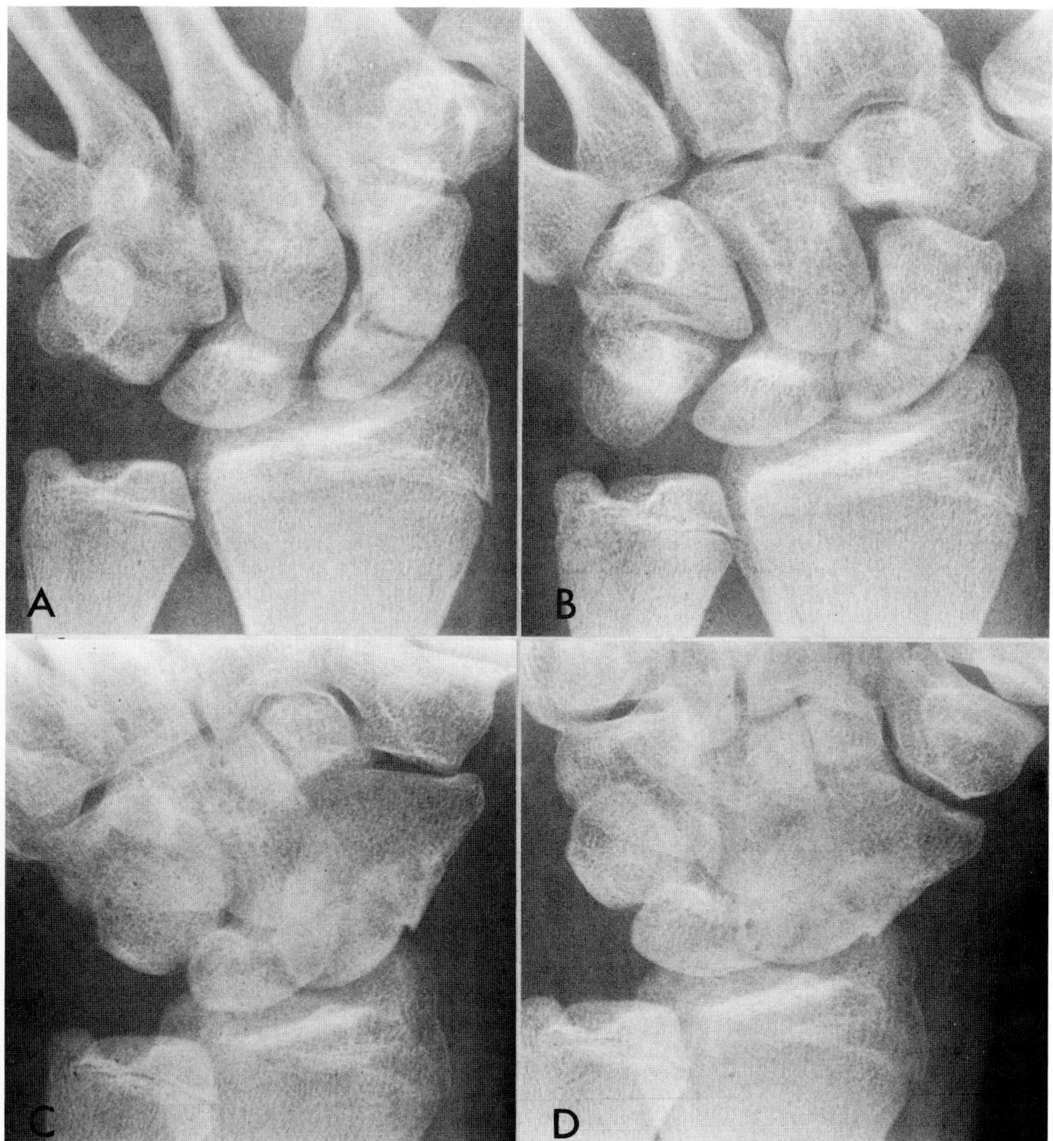

Fig. 7-35. A 16-year-old high school football player sprained his left wrist 4 months earlier. Roentgenograms were "negative." The patient noted increasing pain and crepitus 1 month prior to consultation. (*A*) Appearance of transverse fracture at the junction of the middle and proximal thirds 4 months after sprain. There is 1 mm. of ulnar displacement of the proximal fragment, and osteolysis at fracture line. (*B*) Six weeks after immobilization in a long-arm cast with neutral forearm position, 20 degrees of dorsiflexion, and neutral position of the thumb. Early trabeculation is visible across the fracture line. A short-arm cast that extended to the interphalangeal joint of the thumb was applied. (*C*) Fourteen weeks from beginning immobilization, trabeculation across fracture line is complete with slight persistent localized osteoporotic appearance. The patient was allowed to begin football practice in a protective isoprene splint. (*D*) Healing was complete after 5 months of immobilization (9 months after fracture). There is a slight step off of the articular surface.

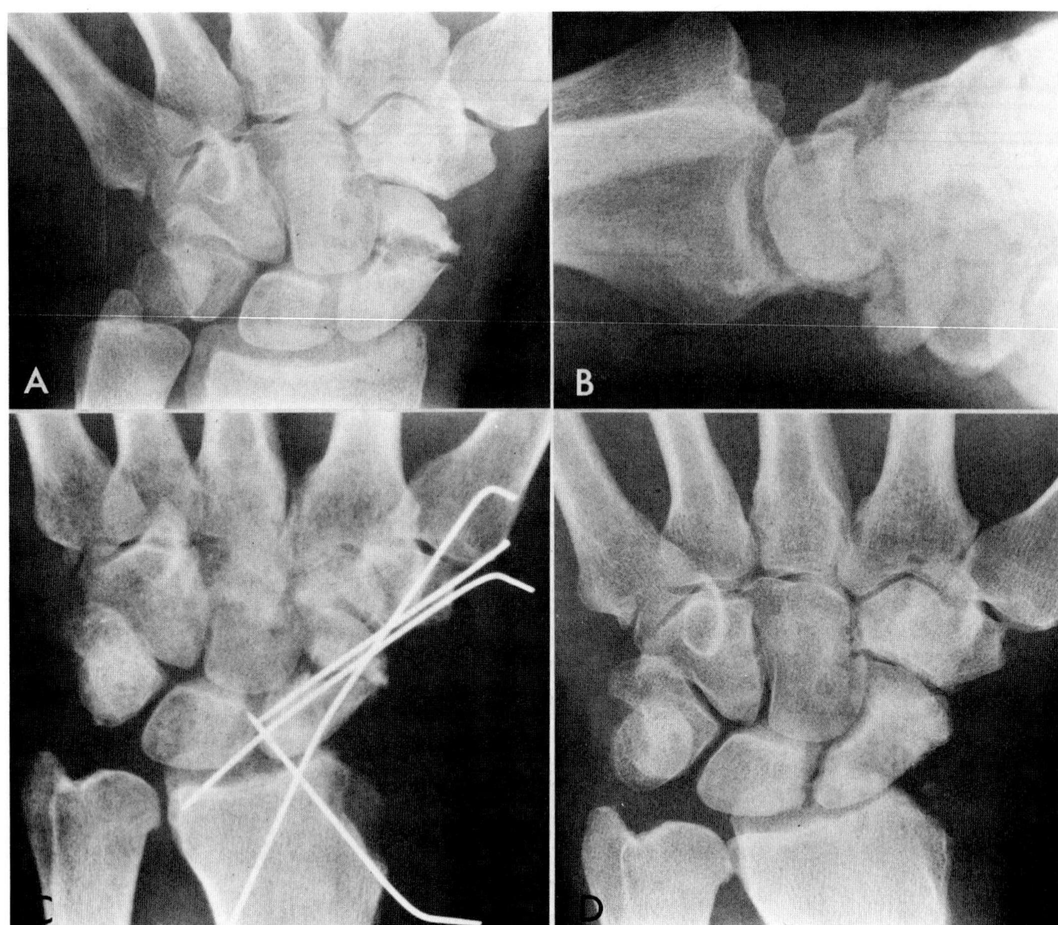

Fig. 7-36. (*A*) A 44-year-old farmer with a 9-month nonunion of the scaphoid of the nondominant left hand. (*B*) A true lateral view confirmed the clinical impression of dorsal subluxation of the distal ulna. This caused only minor discomfort, and no treatment was recommended. (*C*) Bone grafting, using the radial styloid as the donor site, and cross-fixation of the scaphoid and radioscaphoid joints with Kirschner wires were carried out, in an attempt to hasten rehabilitation. Long-arm cast immobilization was continued for 6 weeks. Then Kirschner wires were removed and a short-arm cast was employed for another 10 weeks. (*D*) One year later, union was complete. Grip strength and range of motion were near normal. Note the mild degenerative changes.

fracture of other carpals as well. Some of the special roentgenographic views previously discussed occasionally clarify the situation.[282,292]

Alternate Methods of Treatment

Closed methods of treatment are used for most of these injuries[24,29,104,207,224] (Figs. 7-33, 7-34), though the popularity of operative methods has slowly increased for some of the more difficult problems.[110,178,188,202,282,292] The major problem with the scaphoid fracture has been the inability to recognize the fracture early. This problem has led to the clinical aphorism that all patients with an appropriate stress or injury to the wrist and tenderness in the region of the scaphoid should be treated as if they had a fracture until a fracture has been disproved by negative roentgenograms at 2 and 4 weeks. We

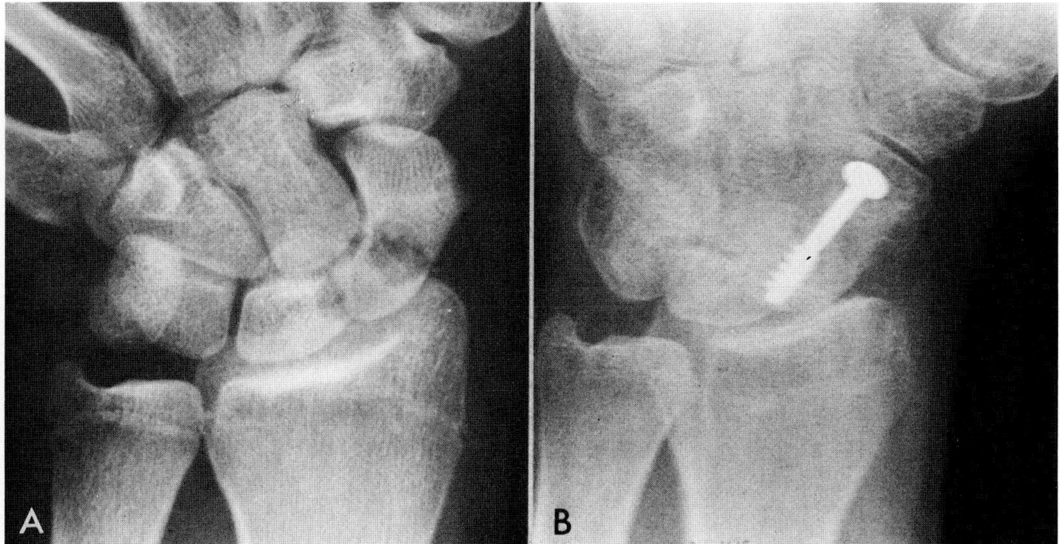

Fig. 7-37. A 19-year-old student fractured the left scaphoid in a sandlot wrestling match. Immobilization was initiated 4 months later and continued 4 more months, at which time the patient was lost to follow-up. (*A*) He returned with reinjury and delayed union at 18 months. Note the large cyst in the scaphoid, with a transverse waist fracture. (*B*) Open reduction, radial styloidectomy, and bone grafting were carried out. Fixation was accomplished with a corticocancellous bone screw, 24 mm. long. Further immobilization for 4 months was followed by gradual return to activity and nearly full range of painless motion.

see no reason to challenge this tenet and, in fact, would add to it that two other exceedingly common wrist injuries occur in the same area and may be equally difficult to see on the original roentgenogram. These are the scapholunate tears and the lunate fractures. Once a fractured scaphoid has been diagnosed, the principal treatment has been support of the wrist and thumb and inhibition of overall hand function. These recommendations were codified by Böhler,[24] who recommended a gauntlet-type short-arm cast from the proximal forearm to the midpalmar crease, with the proximal phalanx of the thumb included.[116,251-253] Modifications of this basic cast have included less support, even leaving the thumb entirely unsupported,[108] or supporting only to the thumb metacarpophalangeal joint.[57,235] Advocates of more support have recommended (1) inclusion to the thumbnail or tip,[263] (2) including thumb and index and long fingers,[72] (3) including all digits,[228] (4) carrying the proximal support above the elbow sufficient to inhibit supination and pronation,[282] and (5) carrying the proximal support far enough above the elbow to inhibit elbow motion as well.[32,118]

Some have advocated surgical measures, usually a direct attack on the fracture itself with pin or screw fixation.[178,191] Such treatment is particularly recommended when the scaphoid fracture remains displaced. Closed percutaneous Kirschner wire fixation plus plaster support also has been used.[72] At least one group has suggested Z-lengthening of the flexor carpi radialis tendon as an adjunct to external support.[238] There is a consensus that fresh fractures identified early and treated uninterruptedly with any of the standard techniques will heal in at least 90 per cent of the instances, with roentgenographic evidence of beginning consolidation at about 6 weeks.[170,192,235,282]

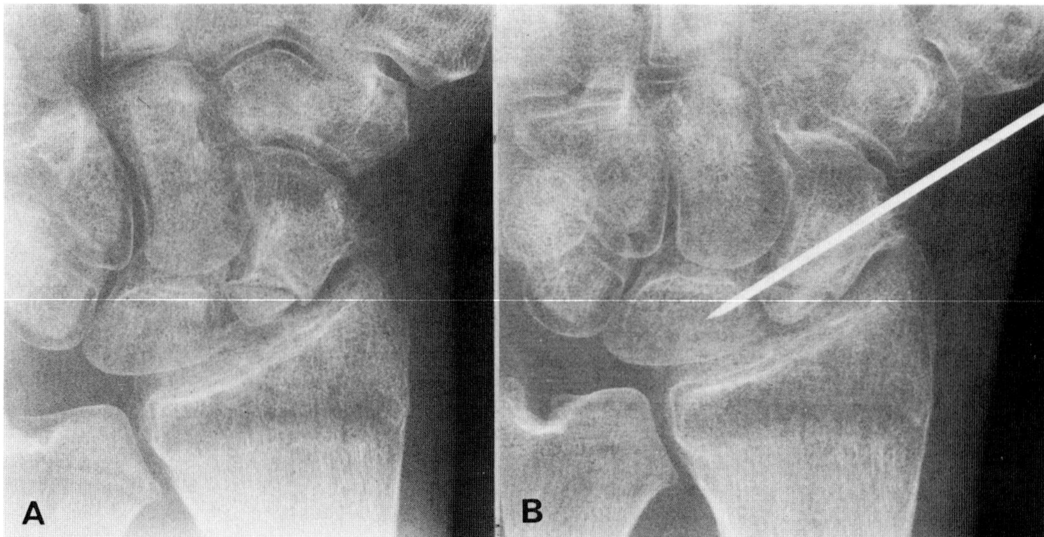

Fig. 7-38. This patient fell with a motorcycle, injuring his left wrist. Roentgenograms revealed a fracture through the proximal pole of the scaphoid. He was treated with short-arm-cast immobilization for 4 months. (*A*) There were no signs of union, and there was a persistent fracture line. Because of the position of the fracture, it was believed that union would be hastened by bone grafting. (*B*) A Matti-Russe technique was carried out through a palmar approach, packing the proximal pole and a trough in the body of the scaphoid with cancellous bone and fixing the scaphoid with a percutaneous Kirschner wire. The result was satisfactory at 6 months. Osteonecrosis of the proximal fragment is occasionally a sequela of both proximal pole fracture and osteosynthetic intervention.

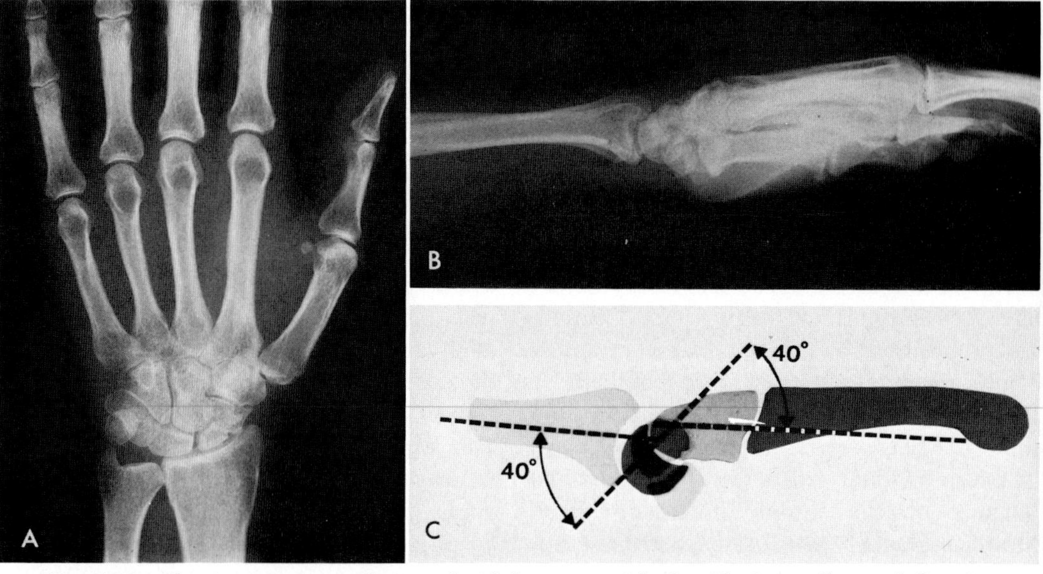

Fig. 7-39. Classic nonunion of a scaphoid fracture with dorsiflexion collapse deformity of the intercarpal joint. (*A*) The anteroposterior view shows an ununited fracture of the scaphoid. Note the palmar horn of the lunate superimposed distally on the capitate neck. (*B*) The lateral view shows dorsiflexion of the lunate interposed between the radius and capitate. (*C*) The drawing shows the dorsiflexed intercalated lunate as a result of loss of scaphoid stability. The authors have been impressed with the frequency of this condition in nonunions. (Linscheid, R. L., Dobyns, J. H., Beabout, J. W., and Bryan, R. S.: J. Bone Joint Surg., *54A*:1612-1632, 1972)

Delayed unions of the scaphoid (Fig. 7-35), which are those fractures showing absorption at the fracture line, moderately advanced cystic changes, and perhaps some sclerosis, are treated by most authors in the same way as are acute fractures,[191,253,263,291] though some prefer to treat them as established nonunions.[110,181,188,202,235] With proper selection, union is usual, though the time involved is highly variable and may be more than 1 year.

The treatment of established nonunion of the scaphoid can be divided into the following categories: supportive measures, osteosynthesis or attempts to obtain union (Figs. 7-36 to 7-38), arthroplasty techniques, and arthrodesis techniques. The factors to be evaluated in making a choice usually are age, health, and functional needs of the patient, age of the nonunion, the functional capacity of the wrist at the time of evaluation, the circulatory status and deformity of the fragments (Fig. 7-40), and the degree of degenerative arthritis present locally or regionally. When the fragments and the local and regional joints are in good condition, and the patient is healthy and young, the decision is almost always in favor of an attempt to regain union. When the patient is middle-aged or older and the wrist is functionally adequate or almost so, measures such as part-time support, intermittent analgesic medication, or occasional steroid injection are usually elected. When wrist difficulty is increasing, and the condition of fracture fragments or regional joints suggests that continued joint pain is likely, one of the arthroplasty or arthrodesis techniques is frequently employed.

Union may be attempted by internal fixation, bone grafting, or both. Popular devices for internal fixation are Kirschner wires and small corticocancellous bone screws (Fig. 7-37).[110,181,235] Popular methods of bone grafting include the use of a bone peg inserted through a drill hole across the fracture line[18,48,192,203-205,263,287] and the use of a prepared bed from surface to interior of the scaphoid and crossing the fracture line.[186,235,279,282] This bed is then filled with cancellous autograft material, with the possible addition of a corticocancellous plug (Figs. 7-36, 7-38). Multiple drilling of both fracture fragments is seldom used any more.[240]

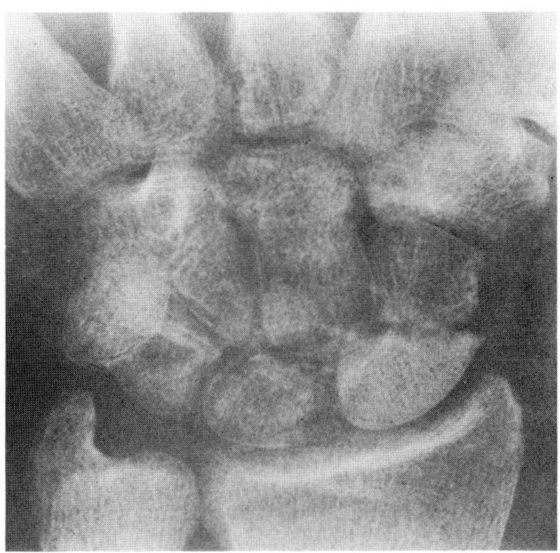

Fig. 7-40. A transverse waist fracture of the scaphoid with significantly increased density of the proximal fragment, suggesting vascular compromise. Immobilization continued for 6 months, with satisfactory union, movement, and function at 8 months.

The preferred approaches are either on the palmar surface of the wrist[235,282] between the flexor carpi radialis tendon and the radial artery or dorsoradially in the snuffbox area.[18,110,181,188,192,202-205,235,263,287] In the latter approach, removal of the radial styloid is optional. Two advantages are claimed for the palmar approach. One is that the blood supply to the scaphoid is protected better. This is not necessarily so, since the lateral volar artery to the scaphoid is endangered in this approach (Fig. 7-6). It nearly always contributes significantly to the scaphoid circulation and may contribute most of the circulation to the proximal two-thirds.[270] The other advantage claimed is that bone grafting from this approach can better restore the scaphoid to its normal contour, since it tends to collapse on the palmar surface and angulate and open on the dorsal surface after fracture and absorption.[101]

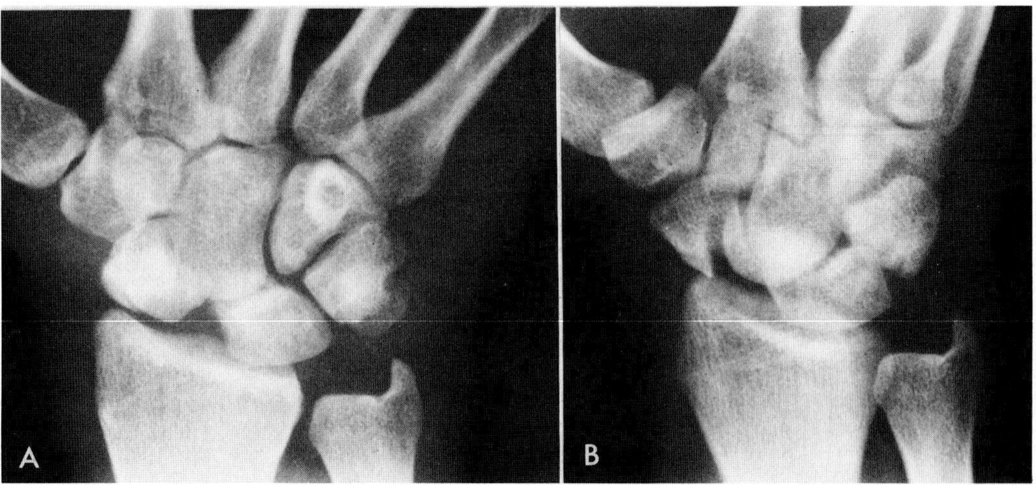

Fig. 7-41. A 21-year-old foreman fell from a horse 3 months before coming for treatment. The dorsal pole of the scaphoid is prominent and tender. (*A*) The anteroposterior view shows a scapholunate gap and a narrow end on the silhouette of the scaphoid. (*B*) The oblique view shows a possible scaphoid fracture with dorsal displacement of the proximal pole. Rupture of the scapholunate interosseous ligament was required to assume this position. The patient deferred treatment.

The proponents of the snuffbox approach claim other advantages. The bone graft can be obtained easily from the radial styloid at the time of approach, and if the styloid is removed in the approach,[18] a much better view of the scaphoid is obtained than from any other approach. The transstyloid interval is removed from the scaphoid arterial supply, and these branches can be seen distally and easily protected.

The treatment elected for patients whose wrist joint condition is not considered sufficiently normal to proceed with fracture union attempts is related to age and functional requirements of the wrist. Fusion techniques are often elected if the patient is young, if the other hand and wrist are normal, and if much stressful activity is required. Various methods described include fusion of the radius to one or more of the proximal carpal row, midcarpal fusions, fusion of the radius to the distal carpal elements, and fusion of the radius across the carpus to the bases of the second and third metacarpals. The only joints always left free unless some special problem exists are the thumb axis joints (scaphotrapezial and trapeziometacarpal), the distal radioulnar joint, the ulnocarpal joint, and the carpometacarpal joints of the fourth and fifth digits.

Arthroplasty techniques are more likely to be selected for older patients or those with less likelihood of persistent, unrelenting wrist stress. The simplest of these techniques and the one most consistently given favorable reports in the literature is excision of the radial styloid.[248] This is applicable only when most of the symptomatic, degenerative joint changes lie between the radial styloid and the distal half of the scaphoid. With scaphoid nonunion, the pattern of wrist motion changes and some shortening of the scaphoid occurs.[24,29,138,255,292] Both tend to bring about greater contact between the distal scaphoid fragment and the radial styloid, with resulting severe degenerative changes between these two. Another simple method designed to cope with the problem of the associated degenerative changes between the two fragments is the placement of a soft-tissue flap between the two scaphoid fragments.[5,23,213] This, in fact, can be done more easily by combining the flap placement with excision of the radial styloid.[71] Excision of part or all of the scaphoid also has been described, though collapse and degenerative changes are inevitable sequelae.[70,90,287] Often no replacement is used, because the natural scar formation probably will fill the defect; however, soft-tissue flaps and various implants,[4,6,158] including molded Silastic ones, have been used.[267,268]

Indications for Operative Treatment. Although some have disagreed, the consensus in the literature is that operative treatment has no place in the management of the acute fracture of the scaphoid, except for the displaced fracture that cannot be reduced with closed manipulation (Fig. 7-41). At the delayed union stage, opinion still is sharply divided as to the need for operative treatment; some authors believe that all or almost all of these fractures will unite with continued conservative measures. For those who believe differently, the most popular current method is that of internal fixation with a corticocancellous bone screw. For the definite pseudarthrosis, treatment varies from supportive measures only, to attempts at regaining union, to reconstructive measures, the selection depending on the individual case.

Authors' Preferred Method of Treatment. Although we often differ in our preferred treatments with regard to fractures of the scaphoid, we both believe that many fractures of the scaphoid are stable—even to the extent of having an intact cartilage shell around the osseous fracture—and that some fractures of the scaphoid are subtly unstable, though not grossly displaced. Such instability may be detected by slight angulation and malrotation at the fracture site or by evidence of dorsiflexion collapse instability. Observation of carpal motion under the image intensifier or by cinefluoroscopy has been suggested. Usually, our attempt to determine instability stops with the six motion study views. We also believe that distal fractures heal better than proximal ones, that transverse fractures heal better than oblique ones, and that all compressive stresses across the wrist can and do cause slight increments of scaphoid motion. In fact, one of us (J. H. D.) has been so impressed with the easy mobility of the carpal fragments, as noted at more than 100 operative procedures for scaphoid nonunion, that he automatically assumes scaphoid instability and places the carpus as near complete rest as is possible with closed methods. This technique is that of applying a long-arm plaster cast with all digits included to just past the fingertips and thumb tip. This is usually not applied until near the end of the first week, to permit initial swelling to subside, and is maintained for 6 weeks. The other author (R. L. L.) uses a thumb-spica-type long-arm cast that stops distally at the thumb interphalangeal joint. We treat all fractures in this manner except those that fulfill the criteria for nonunion (as given previously) and those with displacement that will not reduce manually or with traction. This latter group constitutes a rare but definite indication for open reduction and internal fixation in our opinion. This treatment is followed by the same external support regimen just described.

We both proceed similarly after the initial 6 weeks. Clinical and roentgenographic checks at 6 weeks determine whether the wrist should be returned to plaster or whether an orthoplast support thumb-spica splint may be used instead. Frequently the plaster cast can be removed safely after 6 weeks and usually after 3 months. If cast treatment is to be continued, the cast may be a long-arm or a short-arm one, depending on the healing progress as interpreted from the roentgenogram. The next checkpoint is usually 4 to 6 weeks later. Reinjury is fairly common, however, and a protective support is usually recommended for a month after the more formal support period is over. We both treat fractures that would be considered delayed unions similarly for about 6 weeks. If there is some evidence of healing or even of increased vascularization, such as enlarged cyst formation, we continue treatment for another 6 weeks. Otherwise, we discontinue casting for a week or two so that the patient can regain mobility and strength, and we recommend operative treatment.

When operative treatment is elected for such a delayed union in a young person, one of us (R. L. L.) prefers the Matti-Russe procedure[186,235,282] accomplished via the palmar approach; the other (J. H. D.) uses the snuffbox approach, inserts a corticocancellous bone screw, and places a few cancellous chips across the fracture line but deep to the articular margins. In generalized carpal instability or definite pseudarthrosis, this latter approach is modified by removing the styloid, preparing a trench across the fracture line laterally, and packing it with cancellous and corticocancellous strips. After this, multiple Kirschner wires are used to fix the relationship of the adjoining carpal bones and of the carpus to the radius. This technique, while somewhat worrisome with regard to possible additional damage to articular surfaces, has been almost completely successful in obtaining scaphoid union, though there have been a few infections.

Avascular changes do not alter our approach except in the occasional instance of a very small, ischemic, proximal fragment. We prefer to do nothing with these, but we do occasionally excise them and fill the defect with some interposition material.

For scaphoid nonunion with significant degenerative changes, there are many individual variations. If most of the pain arises from impingement of the scaphoid fragment and the radial styloid, radial styloidectomy (with or without a soft-tissue flap between the scaphoid fragments) is a worthwhile procedure. If more than this is involved, the selection process becomes complex and is beyond the scope of this chapter, though it has been discussed in general terms in the indications for operative treatment.

TRAUMATIC CARPAL INSTABILITY (INCLUDING PERILUNAR AND LUNATE DISLOCATIONS)

Another common group of injuries includes those bone and ligamentous injuries associated with carpal instability.[101,114,165] The term *traumatic* refers to both early and late cases but primarily early cases. It is used to differentiate carpal instability due to trauma from similar problems arising from rheumatoid arthritis and other causes. The surgical anatomy, mechanism of injury, classification, signs and symptoms, and some of the roentgenographic findings have been discussed. The more forceful injuries associated with dislocations or fracture-dislocations are well known by their bizarre roentgenographic appearance, the frequent difficulty in obtaining and maintaining satisfactory reduction, and the frequent complications, both early and late.[36,37,274] These are so commonly the result of palmar tension and dorsal compression stresses that the few injuries from opposite stresses will not be discussed. The stresses involved are forceful. Thus, even the exceedingly strong support ligaments of the palmar aspect of the carpus are torn to permit the dislocations and fracture-dislocations, and they do not repair easily after reduction. It is no wonder, then, that recurrent dislocation or at least subluxation is the rule rather than the exception after these injuries.[242]

Those familiar with most literature about wrist injuries will note the conspicuous absence of a separate section on dislocations and fracture-dislocations of the wrist or a lengthy dissertation on the perilunate dislocation versus lunate dislocation controversy. It is our opinion that the dislocations, fracture-dislocations, and those collapse deformities secondary to less severe ligament injuries (sprains) have similar mechanisms, similar tendencies to deform, and require similar treatment techniques. We, therefore, include them in one group called traumatic instability. We believe that the lunate and the proximal scaphoid are the most protected of the carpal bones and that "yielding" takes place around them, leading to the common perilunate or transscaphoid perilunate dislocation. Nevertheless, lunate dislocations certainly occur, whether primarily or secondarily to the above. In almost all instances of lunate malposition, the palmar radiolunate ligament remains intact, and the management techniques described later by the authors are appropriate. In the few instances when the lunate is dislocated to the extent of being totally stripped of its soft-tissue attachments, a decision must be made to replace a completely avascular bone or excise it. Compared to this critical decision, the other issues in the lunate versus perilunate dislocation theories are relatively trivial.

The more subtle subluxations or carpal instability collapse deformities have been mentioned by many authors, including Destot[77] and Watson-Jones,[292] but the true incidence of these injuries has not been recognized, the two basic collapse patterns[165] have not been emphasized, and a subsidiary phenomenon of scapholunate dissociation has been over emphasized.[14,63,274,281] An early paper by Gilford *et al.*[114] set the stage by comparing the wrist joint to a link system and noting that a link could collapse in two different ways under compression and was stable only in tension. The struggle to properly equate this concept with the clinical presentation is still under way. We believe that this type of injury is extremely common and that it is misdiagnosed as a simple sprain in much the same way that a fracture of the scaphoid is frequently misdiagnosed as a sprain. These injuries constitute a sprain—but not a simple one—and the residua are bothersome and may be crippling. Little attention has been paid to the treatment of this condition in prior literature unless the symptoms are severe, in which case the usual reconstruction methods of arthroplasty or arthrodesis were invoked.

Roentgenographic Findings

Dislocations and fracture-dislocations of the carpus often are thought to be diagnostic puzzles, but this need not be so.[149,150,303] Almost every carpal bone has been described as being individually dislocated, and there are also instances in which most or all of the carpal bones are grossly distorted. Nevertheless, the great majority of fracture-dislocations of the carpus are of the perilunate type. Anteroposterior views show soft-tissue swelling, shortening of the wrist, and a considerable increase in the overlap pattern. Lateral views show the capitate absent from the lunate cup. The lunate itself may be still aligned with the radius, palmarly displaced, or (rarely) even dorsally displaced. Fracture lines may be evident in one or more of the carpal bones and even through one or both styloids of the forearm component. The usual associated fractures are transscaphoid, transcapitate, transtriquetral, or combinations of these.[29,77,255,292,298] Often the best view for determining the number of fractures and the position of the various fragments is obtained when the carpus is distracted after anesthesia is induced prior to reduction attempts. Occasionally, a fragment or an entire bone is displaced so far from its normal habitat that it must be assumed to have lost all of its ligamentous and circulatory attachments.[98,117,261,292] The lunate is the usual bone around which the remainder of the carpus dislocates, but another common combination is the lunate and the proximal half of the scaphoid. The lunate dislocation is thought to be a variant of the perilunate dislocation. Any combination of the bones of the proximal row remaining together while the others separate from them is possible. Radiocarpal, midcarpal, and carpometacarpal dislocations are seen but are rare (Figs. 7-42 to 7-45).[29,77,255,294]

On the roentgenogram, a generalized or patchy radiopacity of certain bones may be detected after various dislocations about

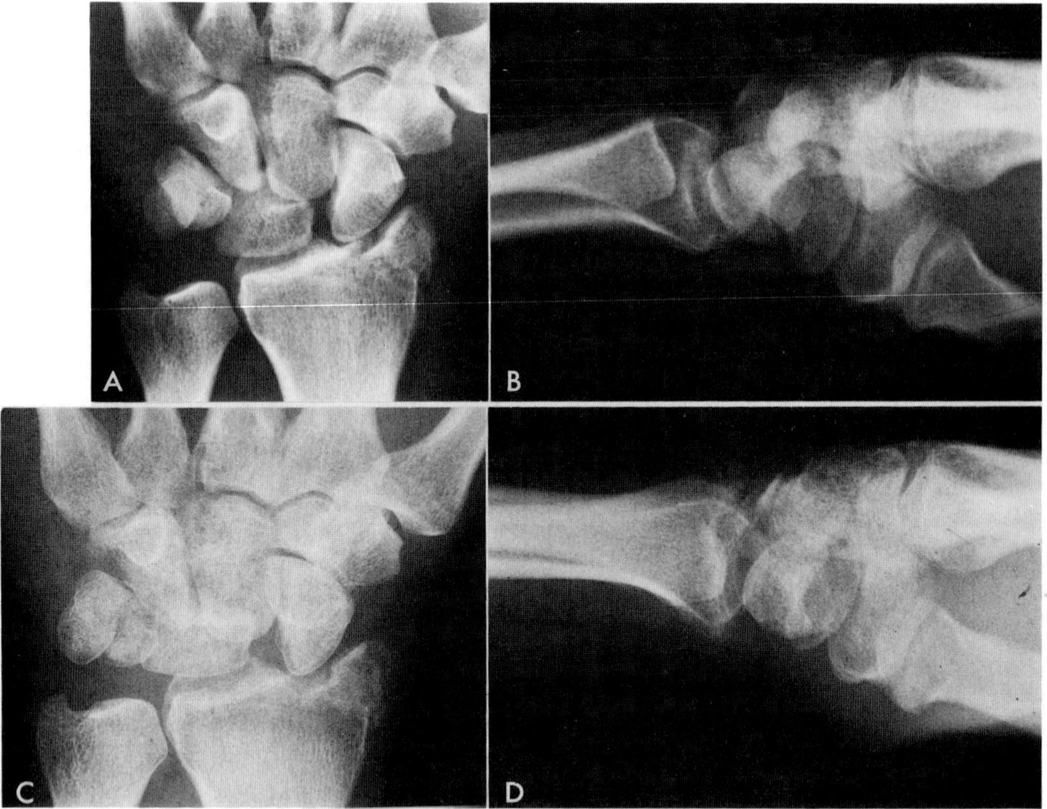

Fig. 7-42. A transstyloid perilunar dislocation in a 39-year-old man who was seen in the emergency room immediately after he fell while running. (*A, B*) A radial styloid fracture was seen, but the perilunar dislocation was missed on the lateral view. He was treated with 8 weeks of immobilization for his radial styloid fracture before the dislocation was noted. (*C, D*) Appearance of the dislocation 6 weeks after fracture, with further subluxation of scaphoid and radial styloid fracture.

the wrist. Most commonly involved are the carpal lunate or the scaphoid, or both, or the lunate plus the proximal half of the scaphoid. These changes indicate decreased circulation.[149,290] However, in these instances, deformity rarely occurs, and revascularization usually takes place when the treatment is appropriate. Similar changes can be seen in any of the carpal bones, with or without accompanying dislocation, but are rare except in fractures of the proximal articular end of the capitate.[1,261] This small, proximal fragment is usually rotated 90 to 180 degrees and is completely deprived of its blood supply. If replaced, the fragment undergoes circulatory changes as described.

Treatment

There have been varied recommendations for the treatment of dislocations and fracture-dislocations of the wrist, although the trend toward operative reduction and internal fixation, if a completely satisfactory reduction cannot be obtained by closed methods, is increasing.[37,81,274,298] The associated displaced fractures, such as the transscaphoid fracture or the capitate head fracture, should be anatomically replaced and internally fixed. However, the more subtle manifestations of instability, such as the dorsiflexion collapse pattern and the associated scapholunate dissociation, have not received much attention. A few scattered reports

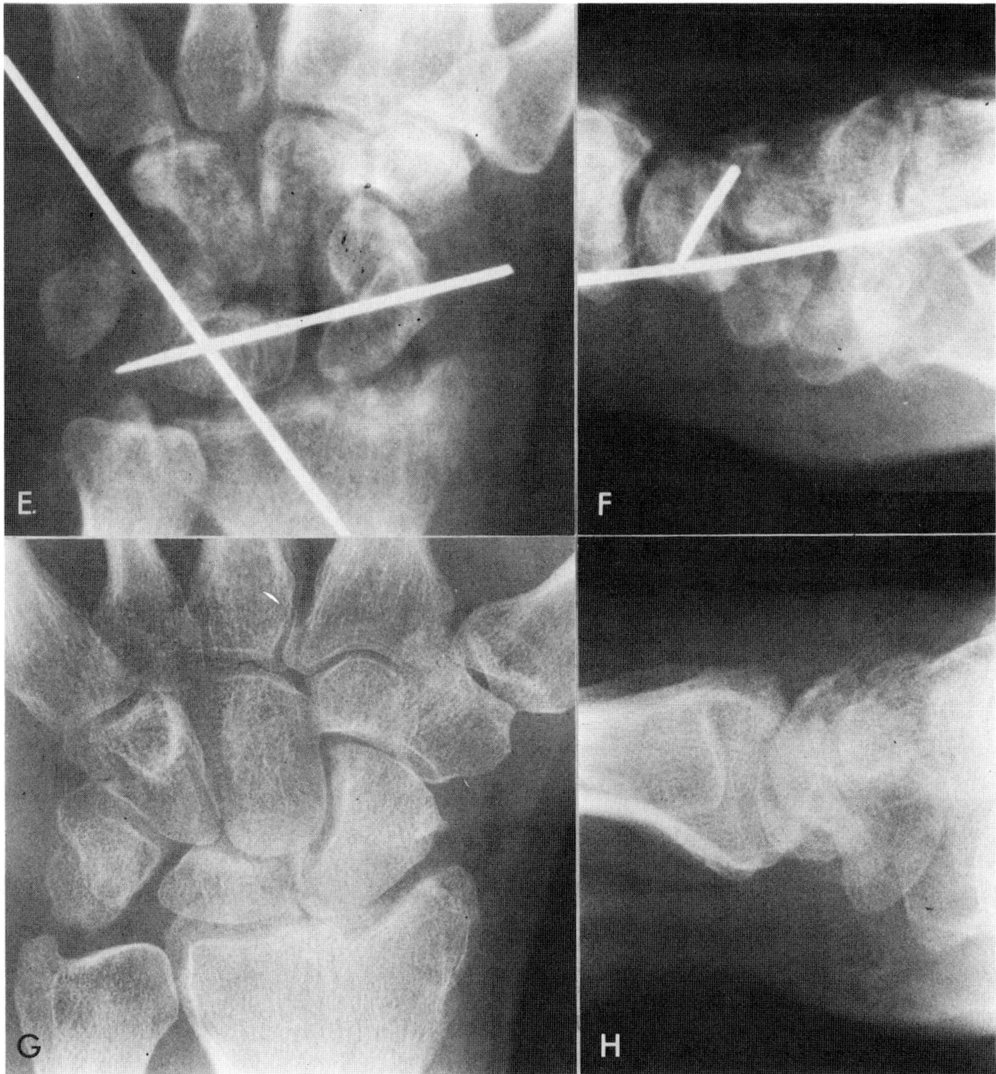

Fig. 7-42. (*Continued*) (*E, F*) At open reduction and internal fixation, considerable difficulty in reduction was noted because of extensive fibrotic reaction in the capsule. Note incomplete reduction of the intercarpal joint. (*G, H*) Five months after reduction there was resultant incongruity in the radial articular surface, persistent dorsal subluxation of the distal carpal row, and a moderate scapholunate dissociation pattern. Clinically, dorsiflexion was 30 degrees; palmar flexion, 15 degrees; and grip strength, 30 lb. on the left and 100 lb. on the right.

have mentioned an occasional need for open reduction.[94,130,165] For the most part, the condition is ignored or treated by various supportive measures until reconstruction is needed.

For the overt dislocations and fracture-dislocations, most authors recommend closed reduction techniques initially, and traction has been the common ingredient of the suggested maneuvers.[24,57,232,255,292] Both palmar flexion and dorsiflexion, or each alternately, plus direct pressure over the displaced bony prominences, have been suggested. Our observations at surgery in-

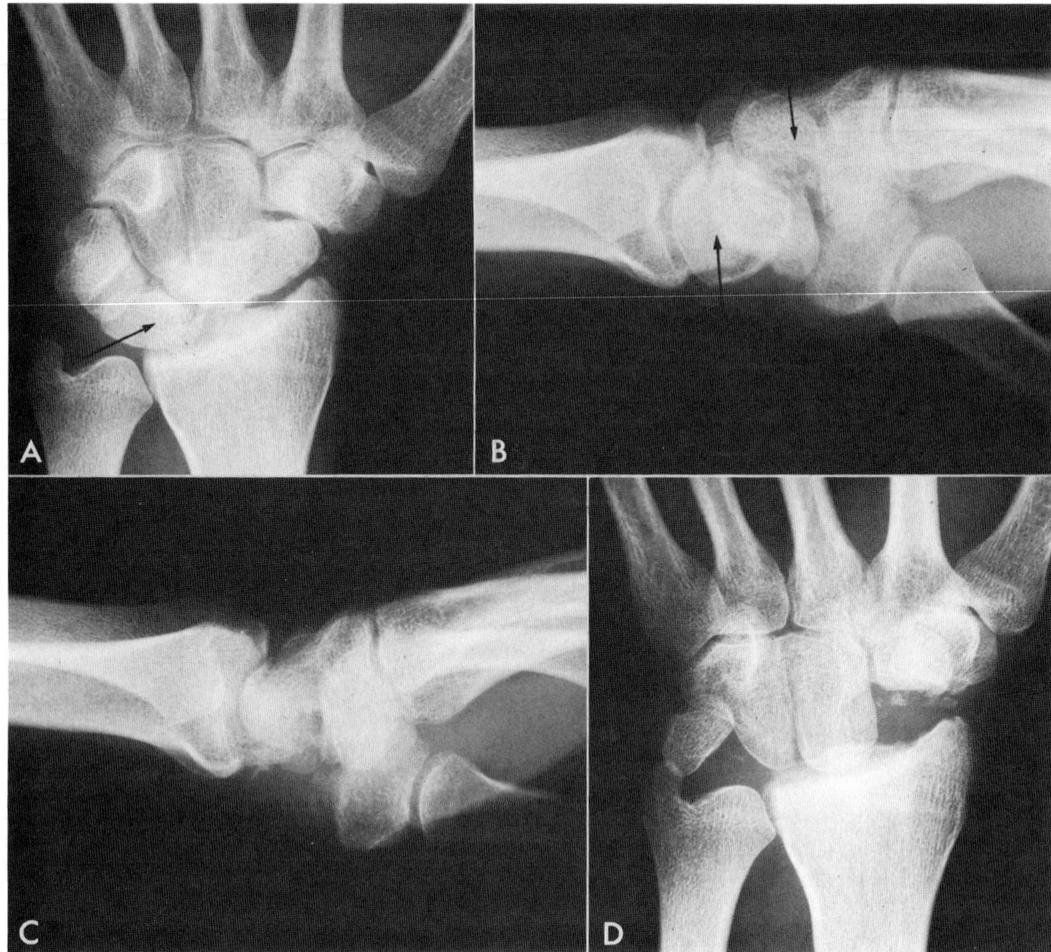

Fig. 7-43. A 24-year-old physical education instructor fell from a horse 1 year prior to our review. The original films were interpreted as negative. He had persistent pain and disability from the time of his original injury. (*A, B*) Perilunar dislocation. The scaphoid has been displaced so that it is lying beneath the distal carpal row and on the distal concave surface of the lunate. Arrows indicate fracture into the lunate. (*C, D*) Proximal row carpectomy resulted in considerable alleviation of pain. Range of motion: dorsiflexion, 35 degrees; palmar flexion, 25 degrees. The patient resumed calesthenics, gymnastics, and weight lifting.

dicate that a strong, distracting force, followed by dorsally directed pressure on the palmar dislocated lunate plus pressure directed palmarward on the dorsally dislocated carpus, is the key maneuver. Unfortunately, some of these grossly deformed wrists are not seen until late. Closed reduction after 3 weeks is usually not practical. In such instances, recommended treatment has varied from open reduction to excision of the more displaced carpal bones to proximal row excision.[36,62,90,140,180,257,292] Similarly varied recommendations have been made for fractures that are treated early but in which there is recurrent subluxation during the postreduction stage.

Authors' Preferred Method of Treatment (Operative Indications Included). In theory, we credit a closed reduction that was absolutely anatomic and remained so as a satisfactory method of treatment. In practice, this can rarely be done, although some reductions remain near normal and function satisfactorily over an extended period (Fig. 7-46). If closed reduction is not possible with reasonable force, open reduction is indicated. If closed reduction is possible, the wrist should be supported in a splint and compression dressing in the neutral position. If, during the next few days, there is redislocation, rotary subluxation of the scaphoid, development of a scapholunate gap, or other signs of dorsiflexion instability, these, too, are considered as indications for

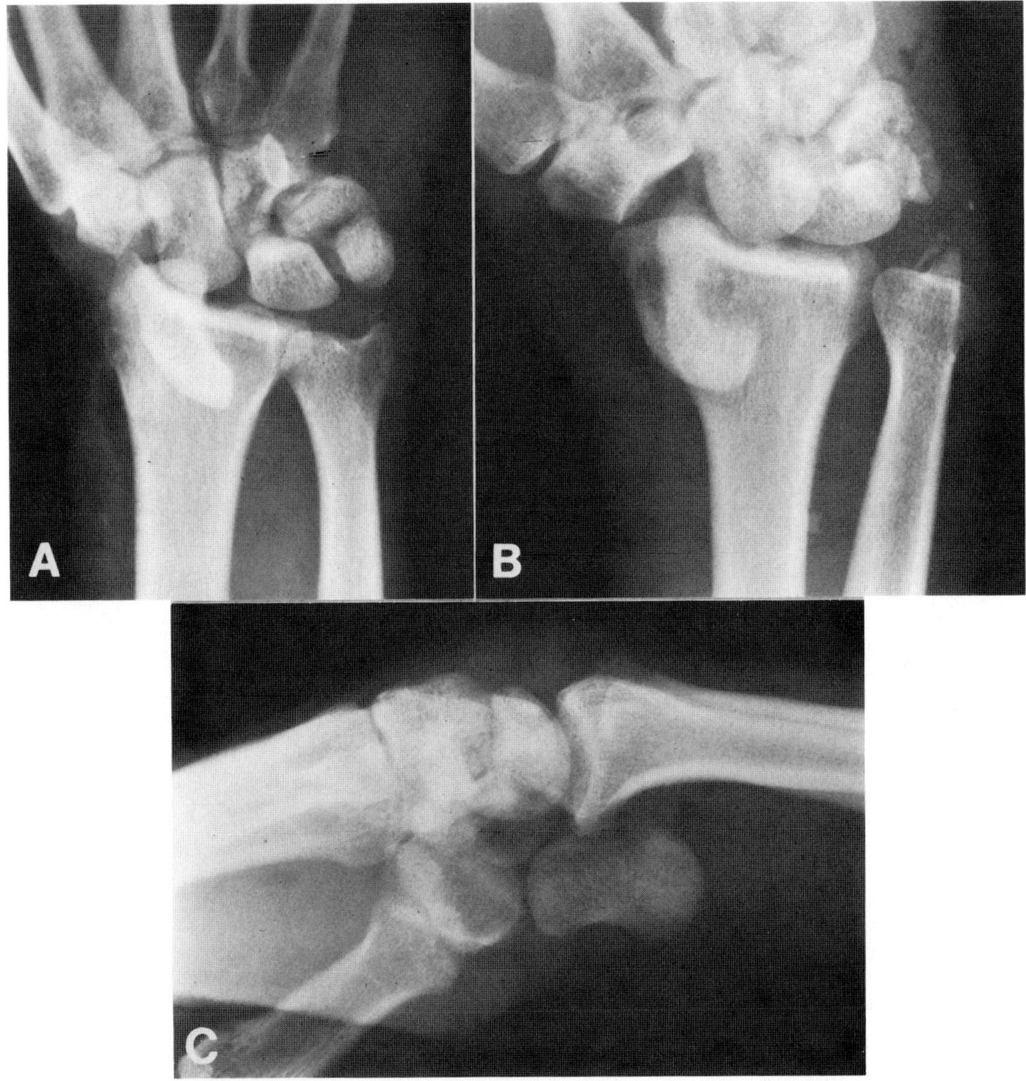

Fig. 7-44. Open dislocation of the scaphoid with intercarpal subluxation and triquetral fractures. A 30-year-old farmer had his right hand caught in the cinching bar of a hay baler. (*A*) There is palmar dislocation of the scaphoid. There are intraarticular and subcutaneous air spaces. Additional fractures of the triquetrum and ulnar styloid and subluxation of the intercarpal joint are noted. (*B*) Oblique view. (*C*) Lateral view. Treatment consisted of open reduction, delayed primary closure, and 6 weeks' immobilization. Secondary stiffness persisted despite dynamic splinting and active assisted exercises.

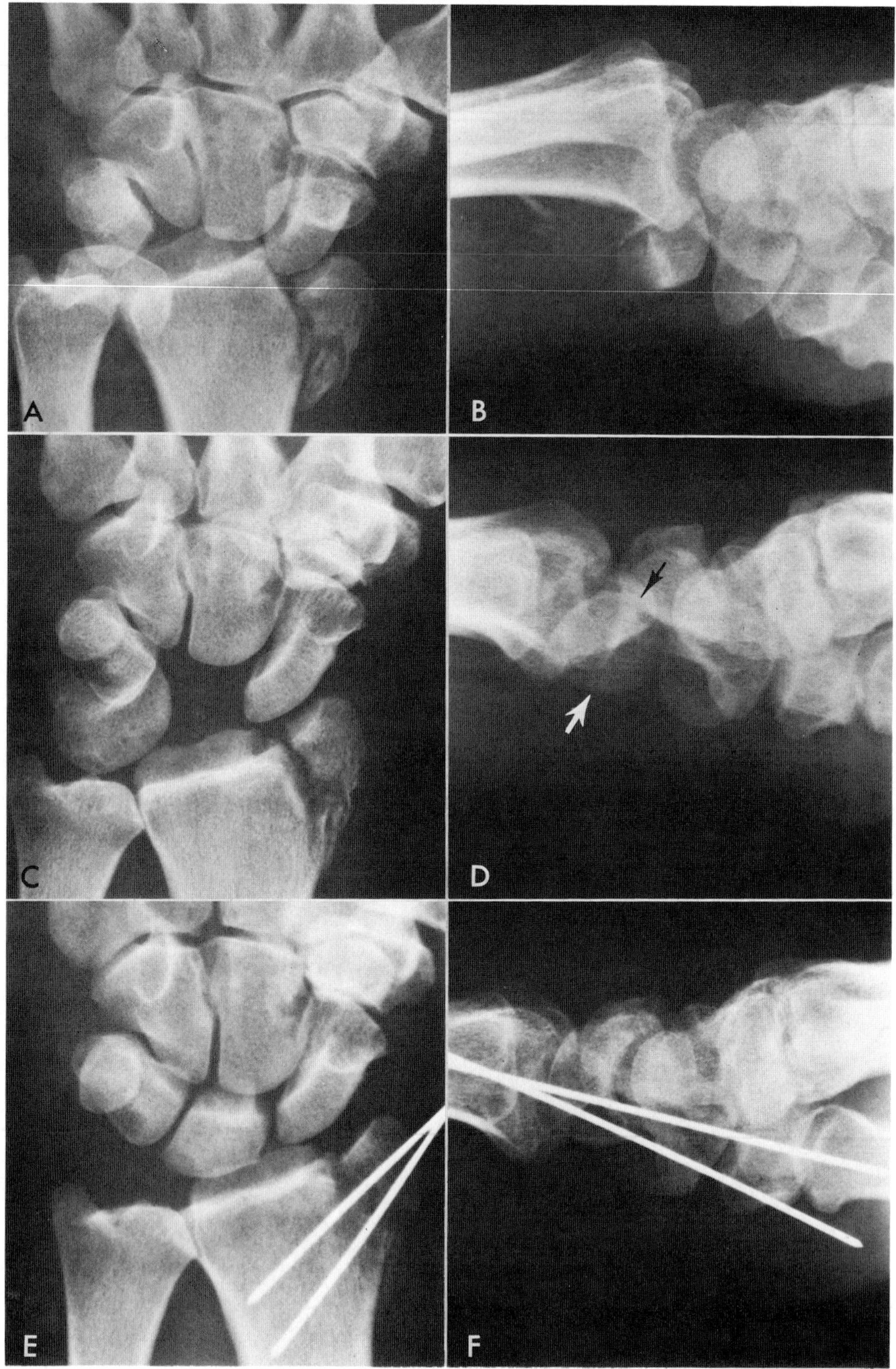

Fig. 7-45. (*See opposite.*)

open reduction (Fig. 7-47). Preferably, open reduction for these injuries should include both dorsal and palmar approaches, with the palmar approach including a carpal tunnel release. A rent is found across the palmar carpal capsule just distal to the palmar horn of the lunate. If, in fact, reduction has not already been achieved when this approach is made, the lunate usually is situated in the central part of the rent, with the distal articular surface facing toward the flexor tendons. This rent traverses the part of the ligament system that stabilizes the distal carpus so that the capitate and all bones still connected to it easily move into dorsal subluxation. We believe, therefore, that this rent should be repaired, even to the extent of utilizing local fascial flaps or tendon graft material if the edges cannot be brought together satisfactorily. Another advantage of the palmar approach is that it assists greatly in obtaining and maintaining proper reduction. The lunate, once reduced, still tends to slide under the capitate and to dorsiflex. Pushing directly dorsalward on the lunate from the palmar incision and pushing the capitate palmarward with an impactor permits a good alignment, though a surprising amount of force is required. This alignment will not remain, however, unless it is fixed by passing a Kirschner wire through the radial styloid, across the lunate, and into either the capitate or the hamate. With this portion of the instability fixed, the scaphoid can be reduced to the lunate by lifting the thumb and the distal scaphoid dorsally and pushing the proximal pole of the scaphoid palmarward. Reducing the scaphoid, fixing it in position with a Kirschner wire that traverses the radial styloid, scaphoid, and capitate, and closing the dorsal capsule may be sufficient.

However, we prefer reconstruction of a scapholunate ligament prior to this step. This should be done before scaphoid reduction, because it entails drilling a hole and passing a tendon graft from the dorsal pole of the scaphoid to the scapholunate surface of the scaphoid and then from the opposing surface of the lunate dorsally and ulnarward, the graft emerging dorsally at the proximal pole of the lunate. This tendon graft is then passed dorsally back across the scapholunate interval, tightened after reduction and fixation are achieved, and then sutured to itself. If the tendon graft is long enough, it is then directed ulnarward again and sutured to the dorsal capsular insertions into the triquetrum.

Modifications of the basic perilunar dislocation require some modification in the management program. If there is a fracture of the scaphoid, it, too, is reduced and fixed (Fig. 7-48). The scapholunate ligament is probably intact but not necessarily so. Both may break. If the capitate is fractured (Fig. 7-49) the articular fragment is usually displaced, rotated, and without soft-tissue attachments. Nevertheless, this fragment will survive and revascularize and should be replaced anatomically and fixed in position. Similarly, other fractures associated with the basic dislocations may be treated as required. One must, of course, avoid compromising the only remaining blood supply

---

Fig. 7-45. Transstyloid perilunar dislocation with dislocation of the lunate in a 71-year-old contractor involved in an automobile accident. Enucleation of the left eye also occurred. (*A*) Transstyloid perilunar dislocation. (*B*) The lateral view shows the lunate dislocation. Note that the lunate is in 90-degree ulnar rotation. The radiolunate ligament remains intact. (*C, D*) With 16 lb. traction, closed reduction was attempted. The lunate was manipulated by pressure from the palmar aspect of the wrist. Note the failure of the lunate to replace and persistent transverse displacement (*arrows*). (*E, F*) The second manipulation satisfactorily reduced the lunate. Percutaneous Kirschner wires were used to hold the radius. At 4 months, grip strength was 30 per cent of normal and motion was moderately restricted.

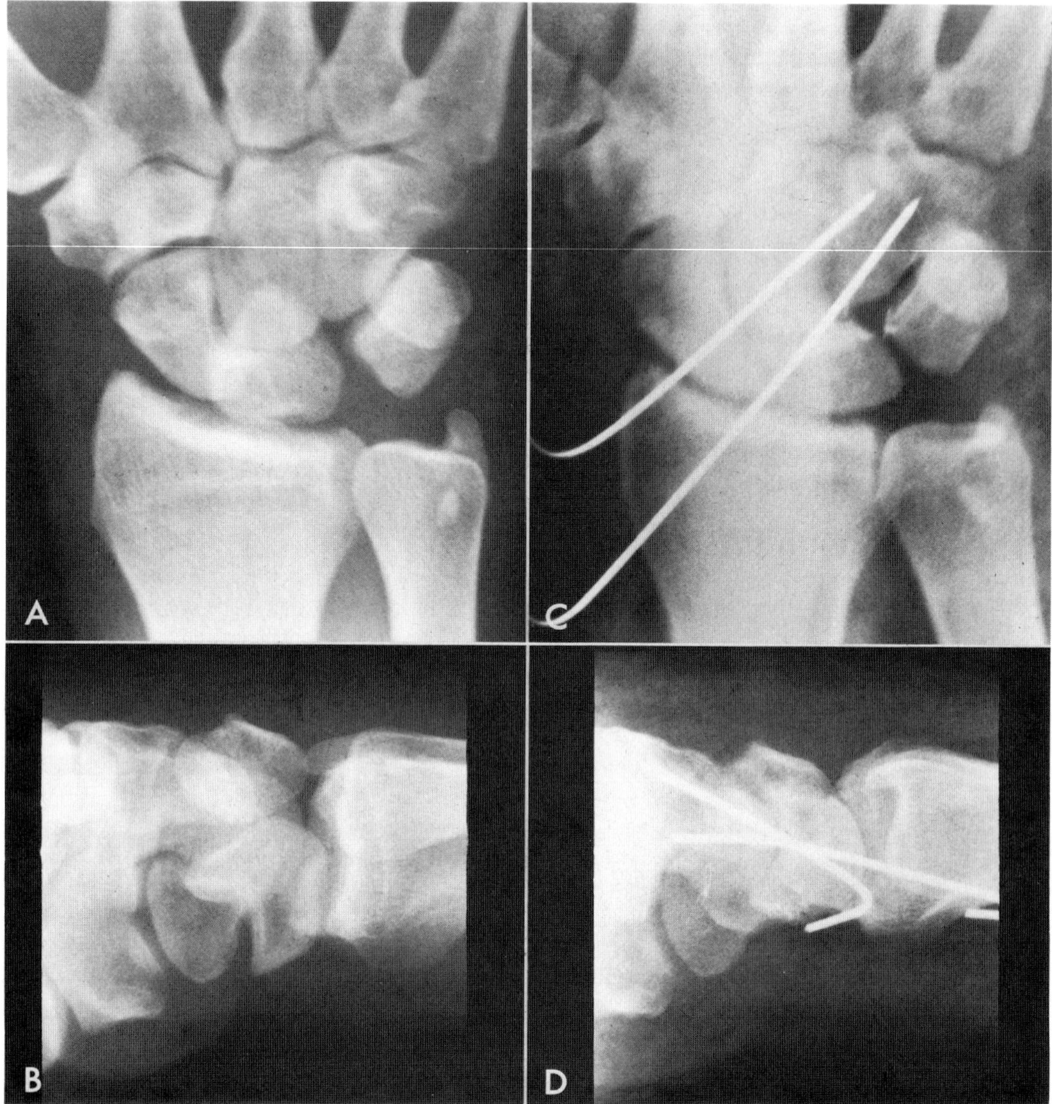

Fig. 7-46. Perilunar dislocation in a 41-year-old man who injured his wrist 3 weeks earlier when he was thrown from a horse. (*A*) Dislocation could be easily missed on the anteroposterior view. Note the triangular profile of the lunate. (*B*) The carpus is dorsally displaced in relation to the radius and the ulna. The lunate is flexed palmarward 30 degrees and is lying beneath the head of the capitate. (*C, D*) After closed reduction, the lunate and scaphoid were carefully positioned and fixed with percutaneous Kirschner wires to ensure that late subluxations through the carpus would not occur. Kirschner wires were removed at 5 weeks, and gradually increased active, passive, and active assisted exercises were begun. Five weeks later, the range of wrist motion was 50 per cent of normal and grip was 25 per cent of normal.

to the carpal lunate, that which enters it through the intact portion of the palmar radiocarpal ligament. However, there is seldom any need to enter the wrist through this area, since the rent is already present and lies well distal to the strategic area. Even so, ischemic changes in the carpal lunate and half of the scaphoid do occur if the common transscaphoid perilunate dislocation is present. However, revascularization usually takes place in time, and deformity is seldom noted. Furthermore, fracture healing seems unimpaired, except that it takes longer.

The wrist sprain injuries are usually due to much less stress and, therefore, frequently do not have the transverse palmar capsular rent. Nevertheless, the same carpal instability pattern may appear either immediately or gradually, and residua that vary from mild wrist lameness to severe incapacity may result. Our experience in treating absolutely fresh carpal collapse instability has been limited, but we have alerted ourselves and our associates to detect this early stage. The results of early treatment of the acute collapse deformities by splint and cast support are not known as yet, though a few such patients have been treated. Patients who have this condition for 6 weeks or longer are best treated as those with dislocations and fracture-dislocations of the carpus, unless there are significant degenerative changes or near-normal strength and endurance in spite of the instability. Degenerative changes may be aggravated by such treatment.

Patients with near normal function may elect, like similar patients with scaphoid nonunion, to continue without further treatment. Because a palmar capsular rent is seldom present in this condition, a dorsal approach with reduction, fixation, and ligamentous reconstruction is usually sufficient. However, there are two basic types of collapse deformity, and the type of ligament reconstruction differs. The dorsiflexion instability injuries (Fig. 7-50) have deformity similar to the residua of the dislocations and are currently being treated by similar methods. Reduction, with normal neutral alignment of the carpals, is fixed by Kirschner wires. A ligamentous support is fashioned to restore scapholunate integrity, and an attempt is made to tether the proximal row so that it cannot slip so easily into the palmar displacement—dorsiflexion pattern. This may be accomplished by free tendon graft, but currently it is accomplished by using a tendon end obtained by splitting half of the distal tendon of the extensor carpi radialis longus. This tendon is left attached distally but is passed through the radial capsule, then through the scaphoid and across the scapholunate interval. It is passed around itself and then directed ulnarward to the radiocarpal ligament insertions into the triquetrum, where it is sutured.

Palmar flexion instability (Fig. 7-51) is treated similarly, except that the tethering tendon is run proximally to the region of Lister's tubercle. If there is no scapholunate dissociation and, therefore, no complete loss of scapholunate ligament integrity, the tethering segment of tendon may be all that is necessary. In a few of these cases, there is also extensive ulnar translocation (Fig. 7-52). In these instances, those portions of the radiocarpal ligament between the radial styloid and the lunate and the capitate should be reconstructed either dorsally or palmarward.[79,131]

DORSAL CHIP FRACTURES OF THE CARPAL BONES

With current diagnostic sophistication, dorsal chip fractures are the second most common carpal bone injury, though we believe that traumatic carpal instabilities may yet prove to be more common. We include all fractures of this group in one category, even though they may be from differing bones, since they occur frequently, are mostly due to dorsal shear stresses, and are relatively easy to manage. Most often the chip fractures are from the

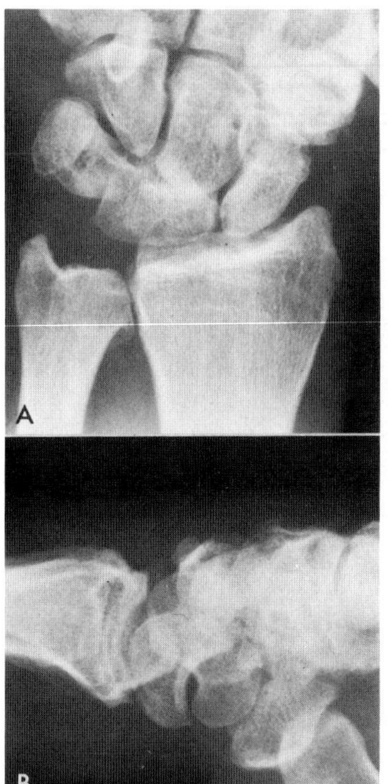

Fig. 7-47. A 47-year-old farmer was injured in fall from tractor. He continued to work despite increasing pain and numbness in his fingers. He was referred approximately 48 hours after injury because of pronounced median nerve paresthesias. (*A, B*) Perilunar dislocation was noted. He was taken to surgery for decompression of median nerve. (*C*) At surgery, with the flexor tendons and median nerve (*continued on facing page*)

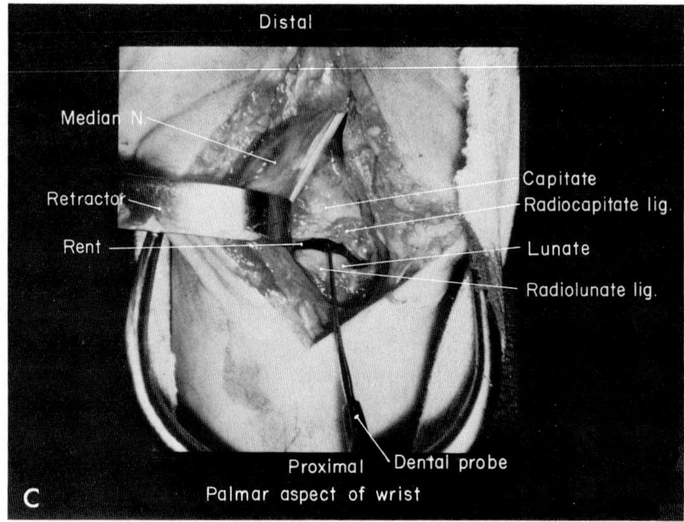

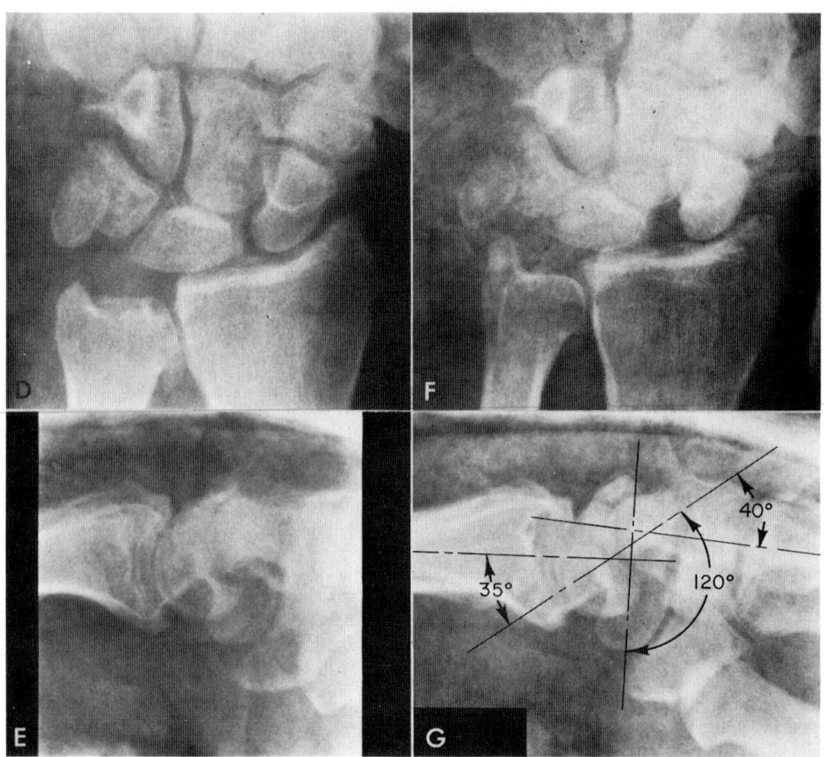

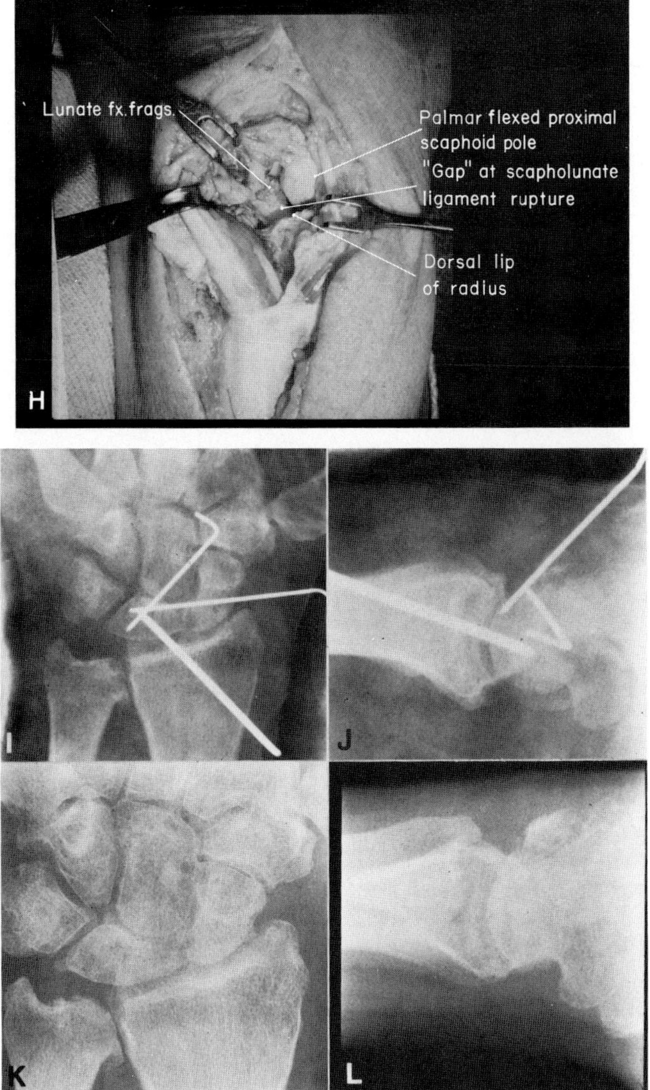

Fig. 7-47. (*Continued*) (*C*) displaced ulnarly by retractor, a large rent was shown between radiolunate and radiocapitate ligaments. This defect occurs in a weak space between two ligaments at the time of perilunar dislocation.

(*D, E*) The patient was immobilized with plaster splints after reduction and repair of rent, with satisfactory roentgenographic reduction. When seen for reexamination 18 days later, however, there was an obvious instability pattern in wrist. (*F, G*) This consisted of dorsiflexion of the lunate, dorsal subluxation of the capitate, and scapholunate dissociation. (***H***) The dorsal aspect of the wrist at the time of open reduction. The proximal pole of the scaphoid shows an area of cartilaginous loss. There is a chip fracture of the dorsal aspect of the lunate. A bone fragment and the radiocarpal ligament are retracted dorsoulnarly. There is a gap between the scaphoid and lunate. The lunate has slid palmarward and is dorsiflexed. (*I, J*) The wrist was flexed palmarward to reduce the lunate, and an 0.0625-inch Kirschner wire was drilled through the radial styloid to hold the reduction. The scaphoid was then reduced by direct pressure over the dorsal pole and fixed with a second transverse wire. Lunate fragments were held with a third wire. (*K, L*) Six months after injury, the wrist showed moderate residual deformity on lateral view, but the scapholunate gap had closed. The injured left dominant hand was improving, with dorsiflexion of 40 degrees palmar flexion of 40 degrees, radial deviation of 10 degrees, ulnar deviation of 20 degrees, and grip strength of 120 lb. right and 45 lb. left.

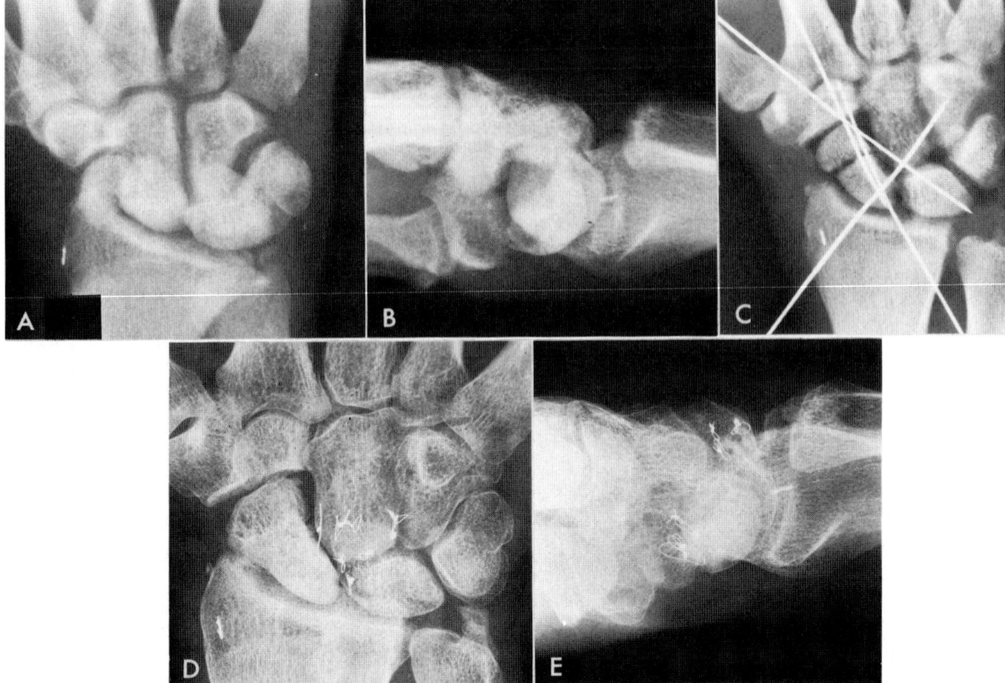

Fig. 7-48. A 19-year-old American tourist fell five floors from a Finnish hotel while sleepwalking, suffering multiple injuries, including a transscaphoid perilunar dislocation of the right wrist. (*A, B*) Although the original closed reduction was done in Europe, when the patient returned to the U.S.A. 6 weeks after injury, dislocation had recurred. (*C*) Open reduction and internal fixation with percutaneous Kirschner wires was carried out. (*D, E*) Anteroposterior and lateral views taken 1 year from time of original open reduction, with repair of torn ligaments using fine wire sutures. Note the persistent dorsiflexed position of the lunate, consistent with dorsiflexion instability. The proximal pole of the scaphoid is radiodense. Dorsiflexion is 30 degrees; palmar flexion is 20 degrees; radial deviation is 10 degrees; ulnar deviation is 30 degrees; and grip strength is 85 per cent of normal.

triquetrum (Fig. 7-53), and the mechanisms involved are discussed further under fractures of the triquetrum.[20] However, similar fractures can and do occur at the dorsal rims of the lunate, radius, hamate, scaphoid, and other bones.

These fractures are easily seen on the lateral roentgenographic view, particularly

Fig. 7-49. A 47-year-old man fell from ladder, injuring his right wrist. (*A, B, C*) Initial roentgenograms disclosed a transscaphoid perilunar dislocation, which was reduced. Reduction films, however, showed a rotated displaced head of the capitate (*arrows*). (*D, E*) Open replacement of the free head of the capitate and fixation with Kirschner wire immobilization resulted in healing, with good alignment and position. There was moderate residual limitation of wrist motion at 5 months, but the patient, a farmer, returned to full activity. (*F, G*) Four months later, both scaphoid and capitellar fractures were satisfactorily healed, with good joint space and no evidence of avascular necrosis of the head of capitate. Three years after injury, the patient had normal strength and motion of the wrist, with return to normal activities.

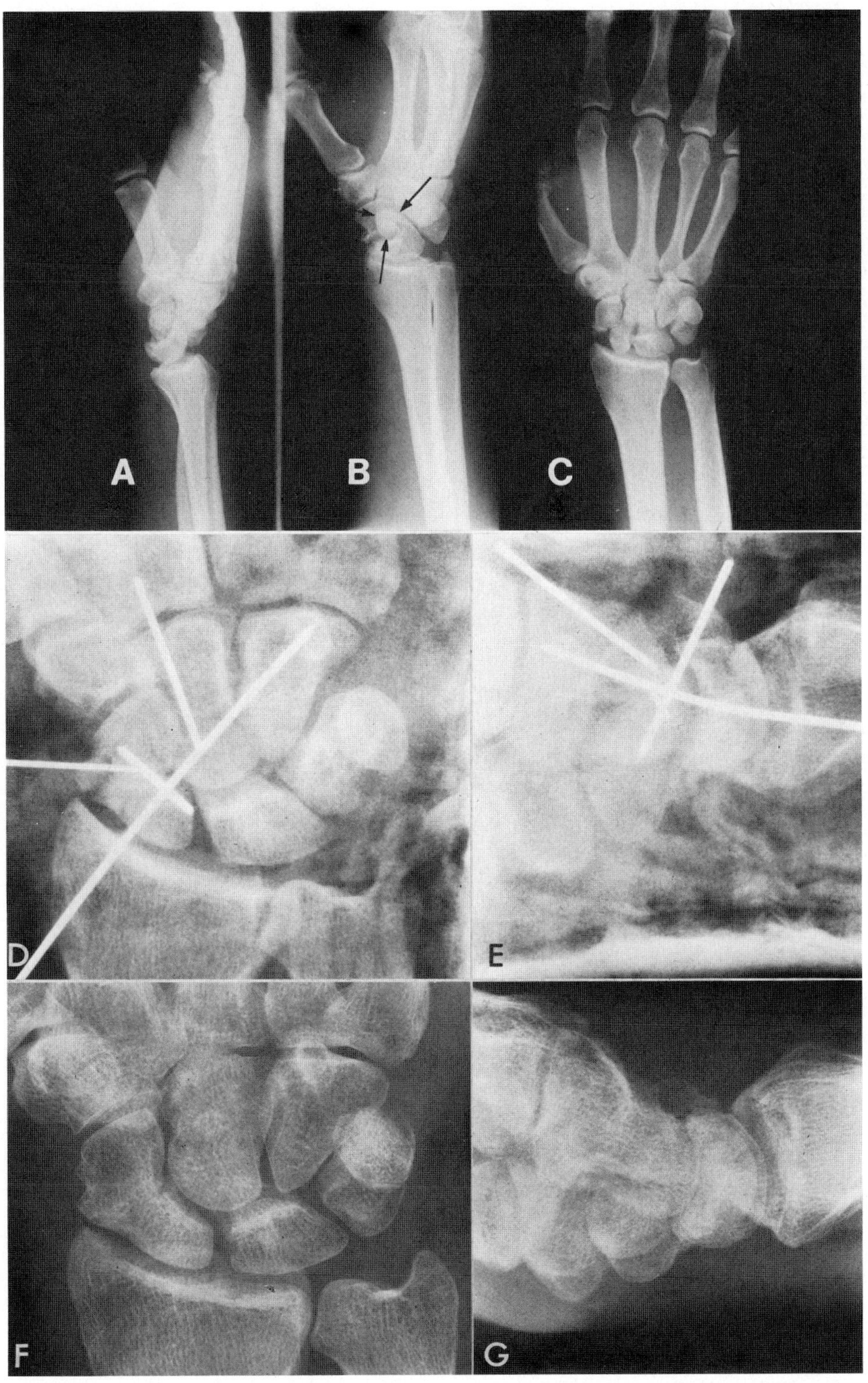

Fig. 7-49. (*See opposite.*)

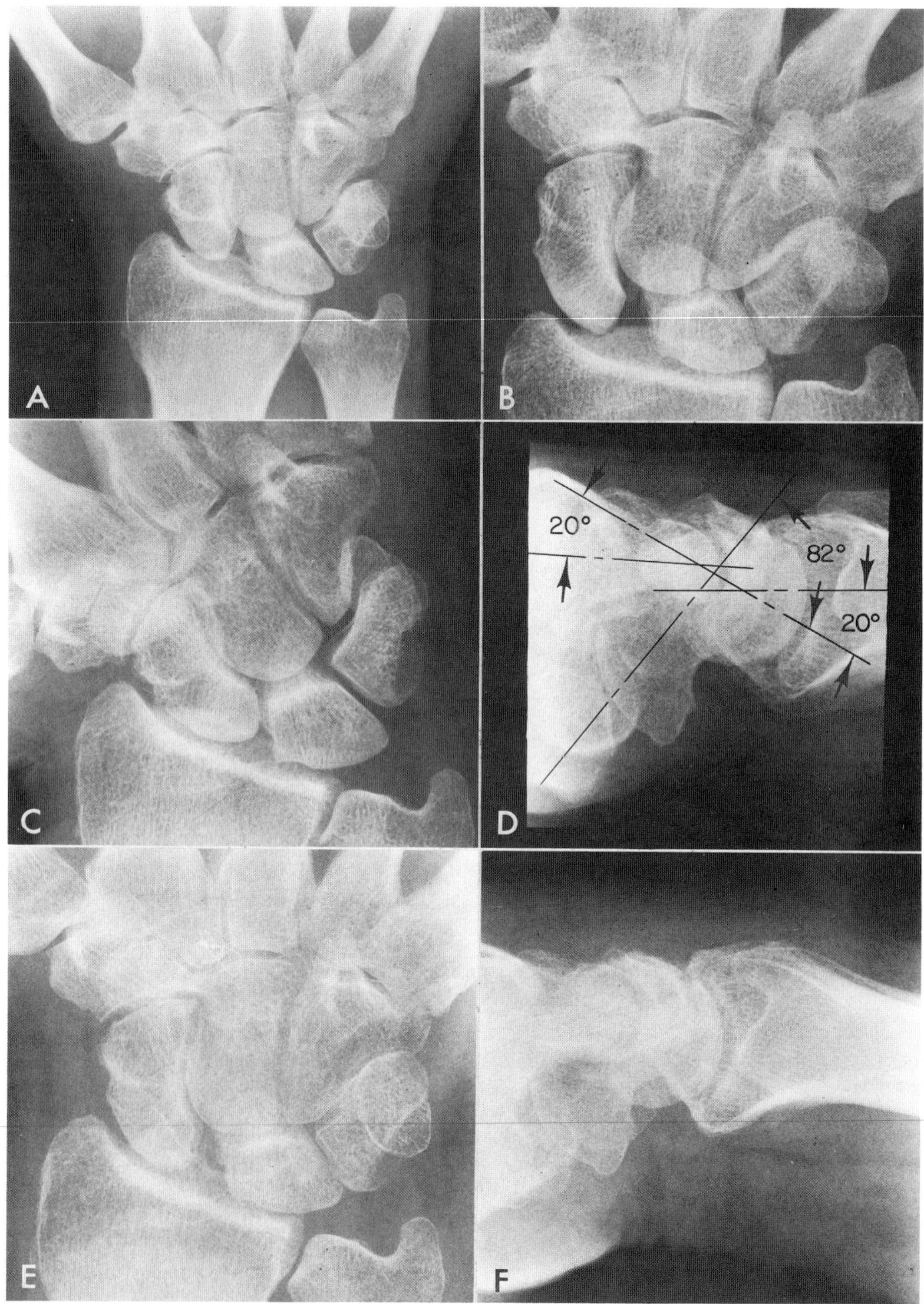

Fig. 7-50. Dorsiflexed instability pattern and scapholunate dissociation. A 49-year-old airline pilot and vigorous tennis player noted increasing discomfort in his wrist, especially when serving in tennis. There was clicking motion of the wrist between radial and ulnar deviation and prominence of the proximal pole of the scaphoid dorsoradially, with

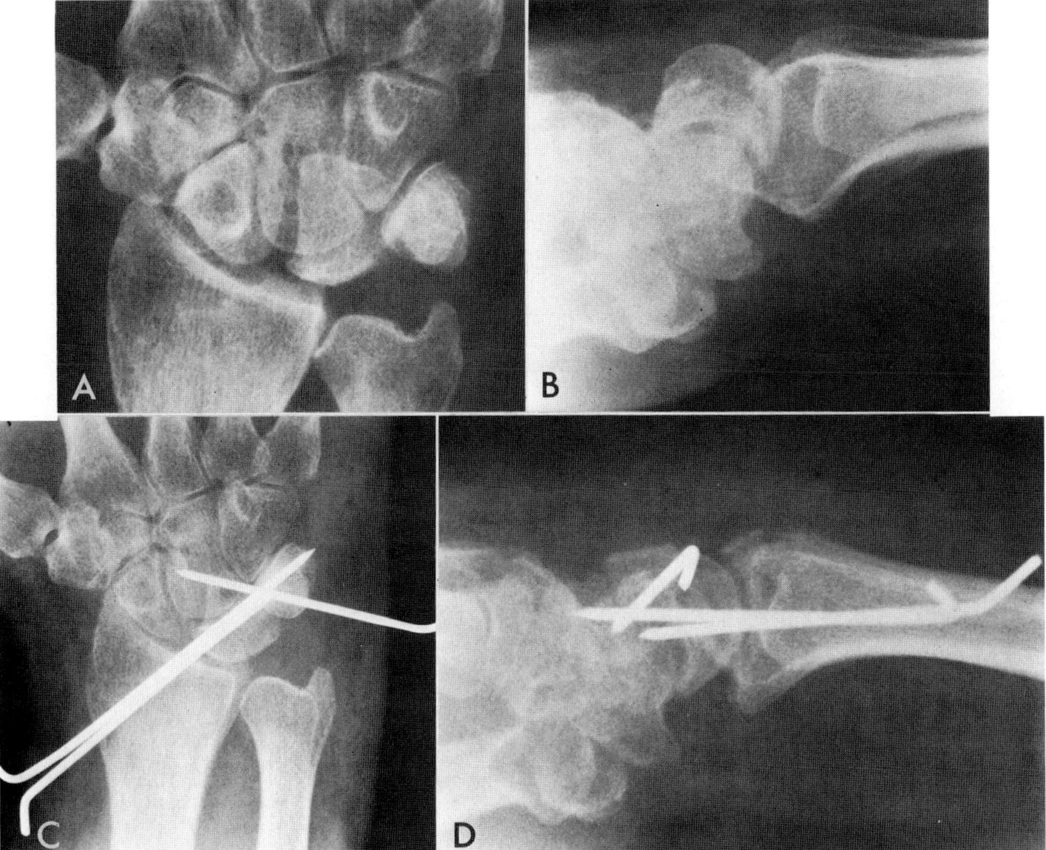

Fig. 7-51. A 54-year-old hospital administrator had a painful wrist after hyperextension of his hand in supination when he attempted to catch a man falling from a ladder. Persistent pain and a click for 9 months were followed by a sudden change in the contour of the wrist with increasing weakness and pain. (*A, B*) Palmar flexion instability of the lunate. Both the scaphoid and the lunate are in rather pronounced palmar flexion on lateral view. On anteroposterior view, the scaphoid is seen end-on; the triangular dorsal horn of the lunate is superimposed distally over the capitate. The space occupied by the proximal carpal row is narrowed. Initial roentgenograms had shown no alteration in the carpal bones, and this instability pattern developed suddenly 9 months after the initial injury. (*C, D*) An attempt was made to replace the proximal carpal row in normal position and hold it by Kirschner wires. Intercarpal lunotriquetral arthrodesis and a ligamentous tethering procedure from the dorsal pole of the lunate to the area of Lister's tubercle were performed. The patient had moderate residual deformity, better function, and less pain.

---

tenderness to palpation. (*A*) With the wrist in neutral position, slight foreshortening of the scaphoid, prominence of the ventral horn of the lunate beneath the capitate, and a scapholunate gap of 5 mm. could be missed easily. (*B*) In full ulnar deviation, the scapholunate gap is more easily visualized, and there appears to be a small osseous fragment lying between the scaphoid and the lunate. (*C*) On full radial deviation, the gap is closed. (*D*) A lateral view shows the lunate angulated dorsally, approximately 20 degrees in relation to the capitate, and a scapholunate angle of 82 degrees. (*E, F*) Four months after ligamentous reconstruction of the wrist, there is still a noticeable scapholunate gap on anteroposterior view and moderate residual dorsiflexion instability of the lunate. Symptoms associated with motions of the wrist, however, were improved after ligamentous reconstruction of the scapholunate ligament with portions of the extensor carpi radialis longus.

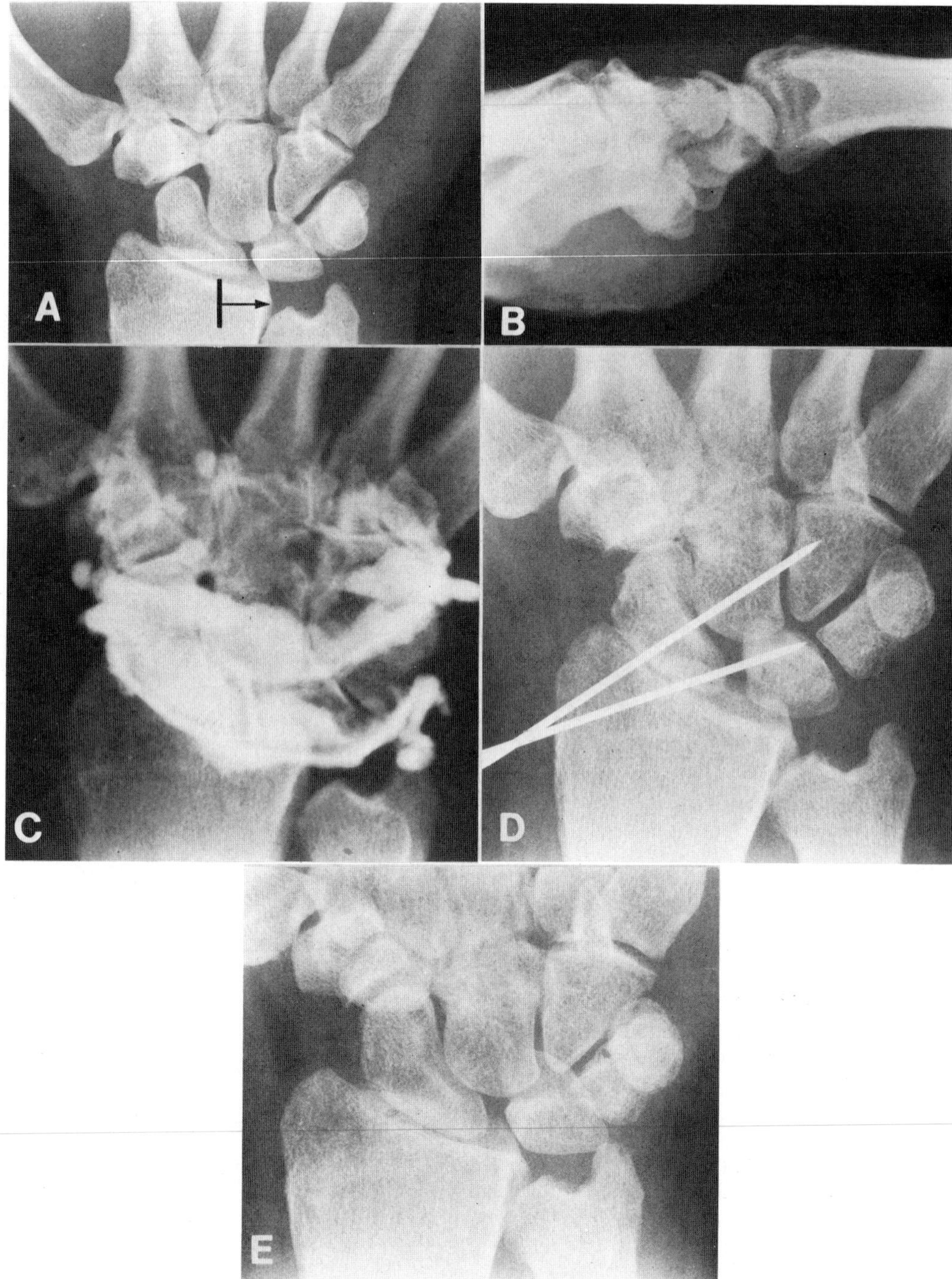

Fig. 7-52. A 40-year-old man hyperextended his right wrist in a fall. He was seen 3½ months after injury, with persistent swelling and tenderness of the wrist and 75 per cent loss of grip strength. Initial anteroposterior views (*A, B*) show ulnar translation of the carpus (*arrow*) and the lunate is not articulating with the radial surface. The scaphoid appears in longitudinal silhouette. A lateral view shows the dorsiflexed position of the

the lateral view in flexion. Exact localization is difficult on the anteroposterior view because of bone overlap. Special views may help, but are seldom warranted, since localization by clinical signs such as tenderness is usually adequate. The only problems with these injuries are to recognize that they are common, to differentiate them from the other carpal injuries, and to treat them appropriately with simple, supportive measures. This usually involves a splint-compression dressing until the swelling subsides, followed by a short-arm-wrist support cast for about 3 weeks and then the use of a removable wrist support splint for another 2 to 3 weeks, as symptoms require. Early surgery is never indicated unless there is a serious associated injury—a very common occurrence, however, as seen in the case documented in Figure 7-53. The only indication for surgery may be a late one, that is, the development of a painful impaction between the fracture area and some adjacent bony margin that can impinge during dorsiflexion (Fig. 7-54).

CARPAL LUNATE INJURY

The most common entity next to dorsal chip fracture is fracture of the body of the carpal lunate.[209,223] This, too, has received little attention in the literature until it reaches a stage recognizable as Kienböck's disease.[131,214,221,222,258] This is the most common and the most discussed posttraumatic residuum of lunate injury, but there is not general agreement that the original episode is one of fracture. At that point, many treatments have been recommended, including prolonged rest in a wrist support cast.[83,131,269] Results from this treatment have been poor, however, except in the young teen-age group. Proceeding from a premise that a minus variant[83,131,269] or short distal ulna allowed more stress loading of the lunate and therefore predisposed it to such changes, various authors have recommended and carried out lengthening of the distal ulna,[214,275] and some have even reversed the procedure and shortened the distal radius in order to equalize the level of the articular surfaces of the distal radius and ulna.[200] Reported results from these procedures have been equivocal, and neither procedure has been popular in Great Britain or the United States. Prolonged support has often been used, but the most popular treatment in the United States is surgery.

Surgical Anatomy

The lunate tends to be well protected within the lunate fossa on the distal radial articular surface. In the neutral position, approximately 70 per cent of its proximal articular surface resides on the radius; the remaining ulnar portion articulates with the triangular fibrocartilage.

---

lunate. This position suggests that both the dorsal and palmar radiolunate ligaments were attenuated. (*C*) An arthrogram of the radiocarpal joint shows dye flowing through the scapholunate joint, suggesting rupture of the scapholunate ligament. (*D, E*) Post-reduction films show the result of ligamentous reconstruction utilizing one-half the extensor carpi ulnaris interwoven through the dorsal radiocarpal ligament from the fifth metacarpal base to the radial styloid, 5 weeks after operation. (*D*) The lunate is partially restored into its position in the radiolunate sulcus. There is slight widening of the scapholunate space. (*E*) Three months after repositioning and reconstruction of ligaments, ulnar translation has recurred, and the scapholunate gap persists. Immobilization was discontinued at 2 months. The wrist felt as if it would give way after the patient returned to work. Early recognition of this deformity, followed by adequate reduction and internal fixation with ligamentous reconstruction or repair, if needed, would markedly enhance the chances of improving results in this type of injury. Both dorsal and palmar approaches to radiocarpal ligaments are necessary.

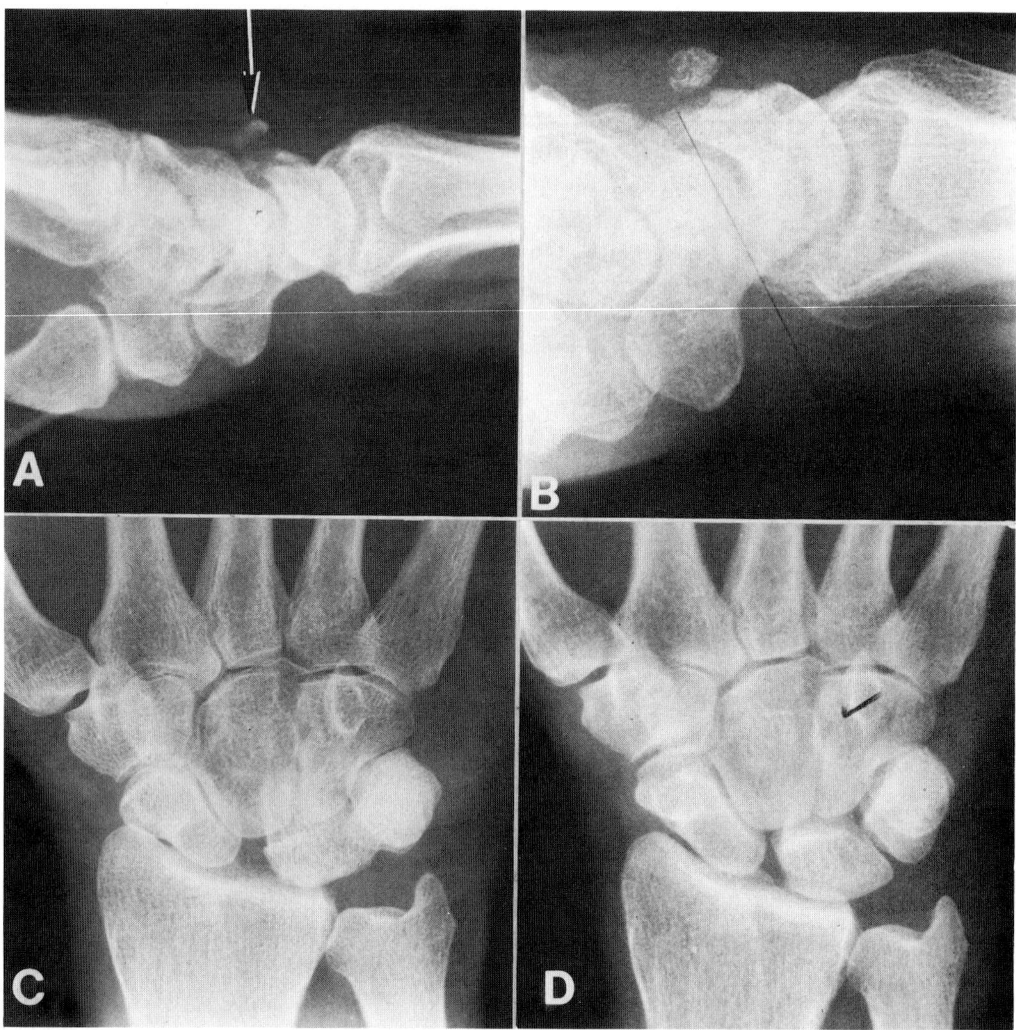

Fig. 7-53. A dorsal chip fracture of the triquetrum was sustained by a 63-year-old minister who fell on his outstretched hand. (*A*) The original lateral view shows a large chip fracture (*arrow*) off the dorsal aspect of the triquetrum. The hand was immobilized in a cast for 6 weeks. Loss of strength persisted, and pain slowly increased with use. (*B, C*) Thirty months later, volar instability pattern was present. Note the volar flexed position and dorsal translation of the lunate. (*D*) Reexamination of the original anteroposterior view discloses a scapholunate gap of 4 mm. suggesting rupture of the scapholunate ligament at the time of the original injury. Most dorsal chip fractures heal uneventfully with 6 weeks of immobilization.

The frequent development of osteonecrosis suggests that this injury is associated with injuries to its blood supply. Studies have shown that the lunate is generally well supplied both dorsally and palmarly and that osteonecrosis of the lunate is extremely uncommon even after dislocations involving the lunate.[36,236] However, an osteochondral fracture through the proximal half of the lunate deprives the proximal fragment of its blood supply.[157,258]

Mechanisms of Injury

Most of the patients have histories of trauma.[258] There is usually a dorsiflexion injury from a fall or strenuous push on the heel of the hand. The appearance of the usual fracture suggests an osteochondral shearing fracture through the proximal half of the bone. Many fractures of the body are not obvious until the later stages, though tomography does reveal some.[113] This type of fracture might well be induced by a translational force applied to the heel of the hand as the lunate is forced posteriorly against the dorsal aspect of the radial articular surface. The tendency for shearing fracture may be exaggerated by a shortened ulna. The triangular fibrocartilage, being more resilient, offers less dispersion of the force to the articular surface of the lunate. This fracture has not yet been routinely reproduced in laboratory situations.

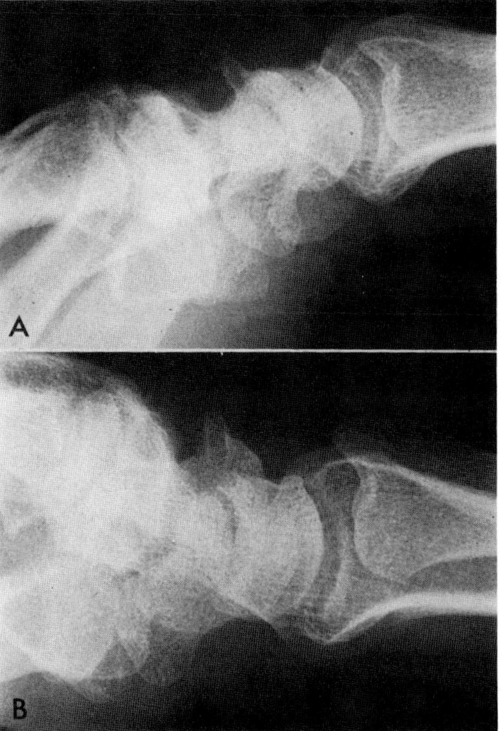

Fig. 7-54. Osteochondral exostosis of the dorsal aspect of the right triquetrum. This 44-year-old "ham boner" had injured his wrist when he dropped a tackle box on it 20 years earlier. He had incurred repeated industrial injuries since then. Despite numerous injections of hydrocortisone, he had continuing discomfort over the dorsoulnar aspect of the wrist. He had pain on dorsiflexion and ulnar deviation of the wrist. Roentgenograms showed osteochondral exostosis, considered to be an impaction injury to the dorsal rim of the triquetral bone. (*A*) On volar flexion, exostosis is clearly delineated. (*B*) On dorsiflexion, impaction between the exostosis and the hamate was noted. Removal and debridement of the triquetrohamate surface resulted in considerable improvement of symptoms.

Classification

Lunate fractures other than dorsal chip fractures may occur in any or all of the three planes with varying comminution. Transverse fractures in the dorsal-palmar coronal plane are likely to progress to lunatomalacia. Dislocation of the lunate may occur as an isolated injury, but we believe that most of such reported injuries are secondary to perilunate dislocation.

Signs and Symptoms

Symptoms are generally pain and weakness in the wrist, aggravated by motion or compression along the third digit ray. Limitation of motion and tenderness over the lunate are readily elicited.

Roentgenographic Findings

Fractures of the body of the carpal bones are relatively infrequent, compared to those of the scaphoid, but such fractures may occur in any one of the bones. The carpal lunate probably is the next most frequently affected bone. A search is made on the anteroposterior view for a thin, lucent, transverse line across the lunate (Fig. 7-55). This fracture is also difficult to visualize. If clinically suspected, it must be treated and roentgenograms taken at intervals over even longer a time than for the scaphoid fracture. Roentgenograms may be misinterpreted as normal, either because the fracture line in the lunate is not evident or because it is superimposed on the dorsal radial rim. The fracture line may be difficult to see on the lateral view because of

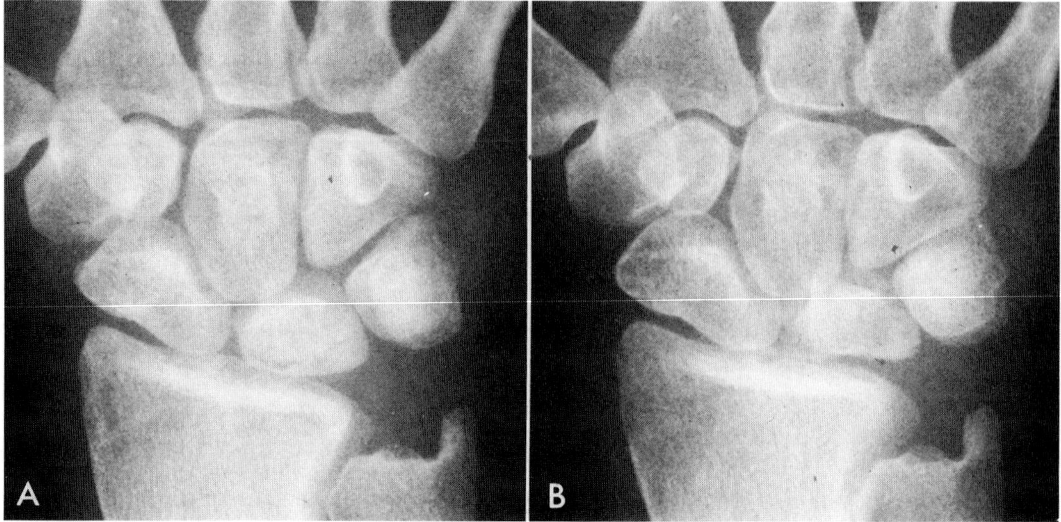

Fig. 7-55. A young mental patient injured his wrist while vigorously pushing a door. (*A*) The initial view discloses a transverse fracture of the lunate. (*B*) Three months later the proximal portion of the lunate collapsed, and the wrist was painful. This is the classic early appearance ascribed to Kienböck's disease.

the numerous superimpositions. All too frequently a carpal lunate fracture is diagnosed at the stage of osteonecrosis. In the early stages, osteonecrosis is visible as a relatively mottled radiodense shadow of the proximal lunate, when compared to the other carpal bones, which are usually more radiolucent than normal. Subsequently, deformity and collapse of the carpal lunate develop, with later fragmentation and absorption (Fig. 7-56).[258] Occasionally, healing in a deformed shape occurs.[83,258,269]

Fracture Eponyms

Osteonecrosis of the lunate (which we believe results from a fracture of the lunate) is generally known as Kienböck's disease[147] or lunatomalacia.

Treatment

For fractures of the carpal lunate body, we prefer a rest support cast, similar to that described for fractures of the scaphoid. Control of rotation helps to prevent small shearing motions in the wrist. After 6 to 8 weeks, a short-arm cast or gauntlet splint is continued for 6 weeks, until healing is well established. When there is evidence that Kienböck's disease is definitely present and progressing, treatment by excision of the carpal lunate is offered.[83] Such evidence includes relative density of the bone seen on the roentgenogram and deformity or fragmentation (or both). After excision of the lunate, we have used either no replacement[115] or soft-tissue flap replacement[206] in the past but are currently using a special model of Silastic implant[267,268] that is larger than normal in both longitudinal and vertical directions. Occasionally, we bond Silastic-Dacron fascia to both palmar and dorsal sides of the lunate implant and suture the dorsal fascia to capsular and ligamentous tissues. Other types of implants[3,166] used in the past appear to offer too much opportunity for complications.

Prognosis

The prognosis for healing of the lunate fracture, if the fracture is detected early and treated well, is excellent in patients who are less than 16 years old. In older patients, healing is frequently complicated by lunatomalacia.

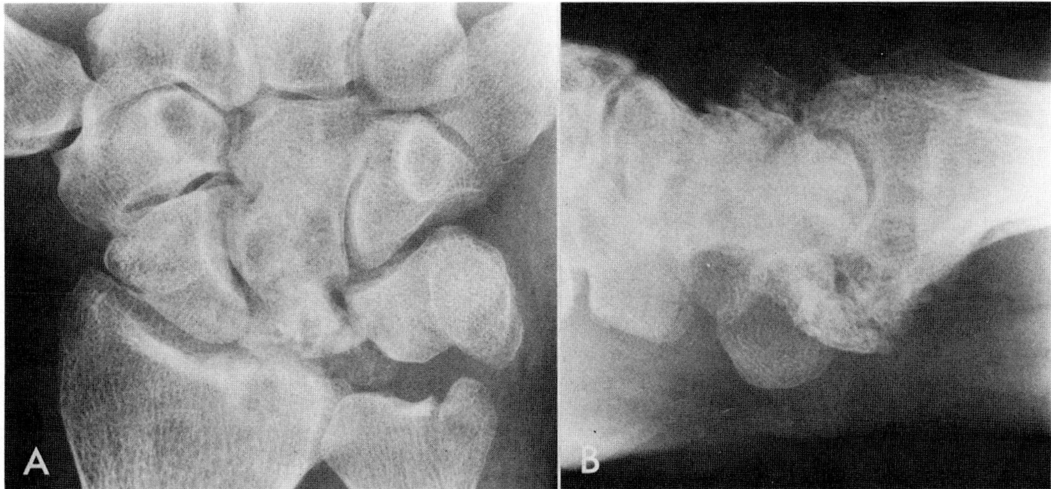

Fig. 7-56. A 43-year-old truck driver had moderate continual pain in the left wrist. There was a recent fracture of the right scaphoid and a history of injury to the left wrist 8 years earlier. (*A*, *B*) There is fragmentation of the lunate, foreshortening of the scaphoid, and cystic degeneration in the radius and capitate. Kienböck's disease secondary to lunate fracture is the probable cause. Arthrodesis was carried out.

Complications

Many lunate fractures develop progressive disorganization of the carpus, with increasing disintegration of the lunate.

INJURIES OF OTHER CARPAL BONES

Injuries to carpal bones (other than the lunate and the scaphoid and dorsal chip injuries) probably account for only 7 to 10 per cent of overall carpal injuries. Nevertheless, this is a significant group, and a brief discussion of each carpal bone is warranted. The carpal bones that are involved are, in approximate order of frequency of injury, the triquetrum, trapezium, pisiform, hamate, capitate, and trapezoid.

Surgical Anatomy

The triquetrum is located on the ulnar side of the wrist between the resilient, triangular fibrocartilage proximally and the trochoidal surface of the hamate distally. Laterally, the triquetrum articulates with the lunate to which it is approximated by an interosseous ligament, and during radial deviation, the triquetrum may articulate with the capitate. Anteriorly, there is an articulating surface for the pisiform.

The trapezium presents a saddle-shaped surface distally for articulation with the matching base of the first metacarpal. Proximally, the trapezium articulates with the distal surface of the scaphoid and ulnarly with the base of the second metacarpal and the trapezoid. On the palmar surface, there is a prominent ridge for the attachment of the transverse carpal ligament and a groove for the passage of the flexor carpi radialis to its attachment on the base of the second metacarpal.

The pisiform acts as a sesamoid bone that articulates with the palmar aspect of the triquetrum.[299] The pisiform is heavily invested proximally by the tendon of the flexor carpi ulnaris and distally by the pisohamate and pisometacarpal ligaments. Ulnarly, the pisotriquetral ligament and attachment of the dorsal carpal ligament provide a strong, fibrous investiture, and radially the proximal arcade of fibers of the radiocarpal joint is attached. During dorsiflexion, the pisiform is approximated

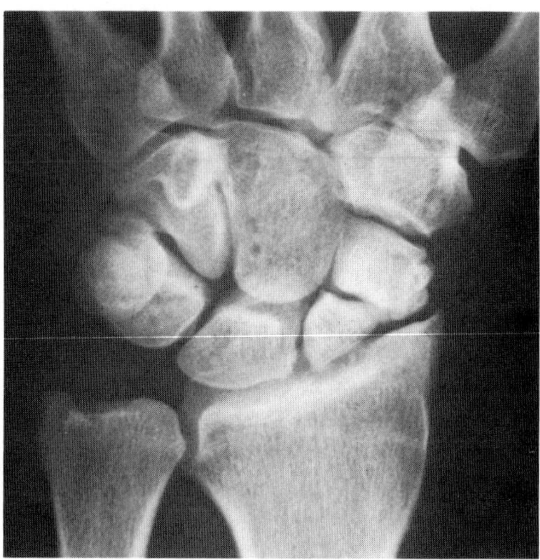

Fig. 7-57. A 36-year-old painter fell from a ladder while cleaning paint from statues of the Mayo brothers. The roentgenogram demonstrated an old ununited scaphoid fracture and a recent triquetral fracture through the body of the bone. A predisposition to triquetral injury by hyperdorsiflexion may be secondary to loss of support of the scaphoid strut.

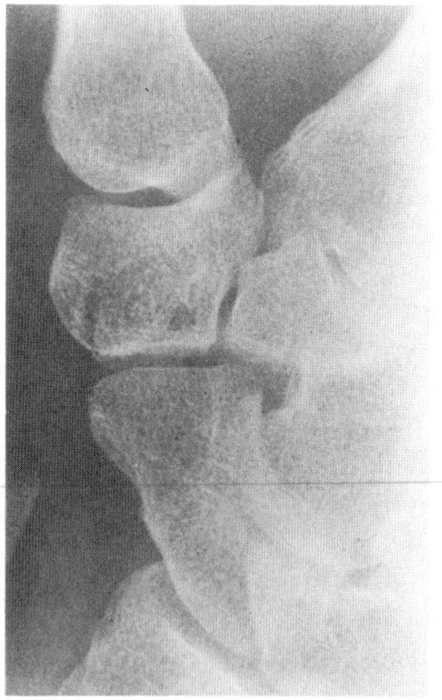

Fig. 7-58. A 47-year-old housewife fell on her right thumb on a boat deck. A roentgenogram disclosed a nondisplaced intraarticular fracture through the greater trapezial ridge. This fracture is an analog of Bennett's fracture.

to the articular surface of the triquetrum, and with increasing dorsiflexion, excursion continues distally. Owing to the inclination of the articulation, the pisiform increases its leverage as it slides distally.

The hamate articulates distally with the bases of the fourth and fifth metacarpals, which have approximately 15 and 30 degrees of flexion, respectively. The hamate articulates closely with the capitate laterally and, during full ulnar deviation, articulates with the lunate. The palmar hook is strongly attached to the pisohamular, pisometacarpal, and transverse carpal ligaments.

The capitate is the largest bone in the carpus, articulating with the hamate ulnarly, the lunate proximally, the trapezoid and scaphoid radially, and the base of the third and fourth metacarpals distally. The ligamentous support apparatus is strong. The most narrow part is the constricted waist, lying between articular expansion proximally and the even more expanded body distally.

The trapezoid is wedge-shaped distally, where it articulates with the base of the second metacarpal as a ridged, unyielding joint forming the keystone of the proximal palmar arch. The trapezoid is also strongly attached to the capitate and trapezium, and articulates proximally with the distal pole of the scaphoid, particularly during palmar flexion of the wrist.

Mechanisms of Injury

The triquetrum may be fractured transversely during a perilunar dislocation (Fig. 7-57), but it is rarely dislocated because of the strong ligamentous support dorsally, volarly, and ulnarly.[26,79,88,96] The most common fracture occurs at the dorsal lip during hyperextension and ulnar deviation, when the hamate shears the posteroradial projection. This fracture may have a second mechanism of injury in palmar and radial flexion, when the radiotriquetral ligaments avulse their triquetral attachments.

Fracture through the articular surface of

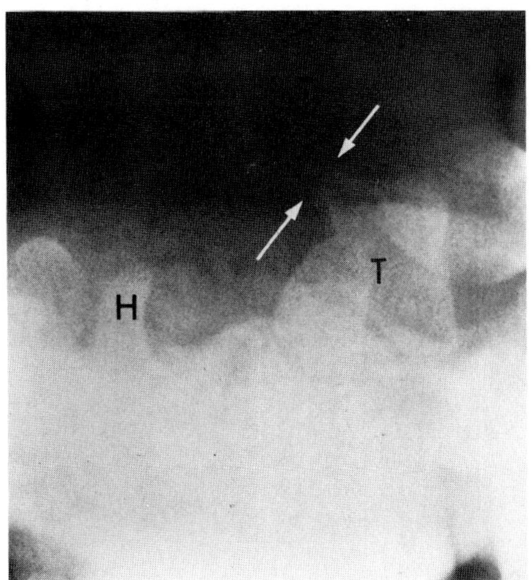

Fig. 7-59. A 30-year-old medical librarian fell against a door jam. She noted pain in the palm of her hand. Tenderness over the trapezial ridge and a carpal tunnel-view roentgenogram confirmed a fine fracture line in the ridge of the trapezium (*T*) at the insertion of the transverse carpal ligament. Hamulus of hamate (*H*).

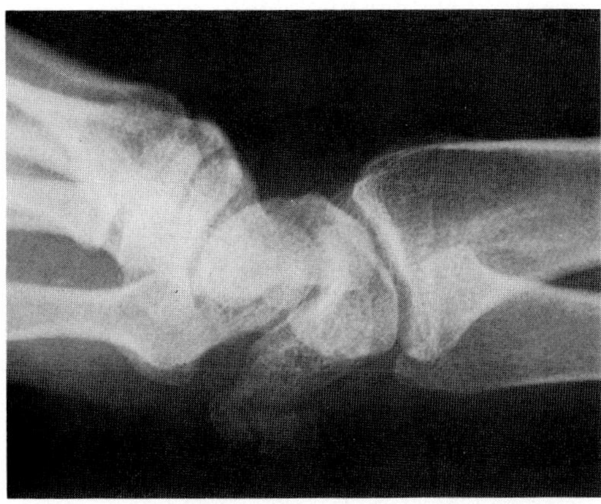

Fig. 7-60. Fracture of the left pisiform. A 32-year-old woman fell on the ulnar aspect of her left wrist. Immediate and continuing pain over the base of the hypothenar eminence and a roentgenogram taken with the wrist in 20 degrees supination demonstrated a comminuted fracture of the pisiform. Treatment consisted of 6 weeks' immobilization in a gauntlet cast with the wrist in 30 degrees flexion and slight ulnar deviation. Mild symptoms of traumatic arthrosis persisted.

the trapezium is produced by the base of the first metacarpal being driven into the articular surface of the trapezium by force on the adducted thumb (Fig. 7-58).[58] Avulsion fractures caused by the capsular ligament during forceful deviation of the thumb rarely occur. Direct injury to the heel of the hand or forceful distraction of the proximal palmar arch may result in avulsion of the ridge of the trapezium by the transverse carpal ligament (Fig. 7-59).[175] Dislocations are occasionally seen.[243,245]

The pisiform is generally injured during a fall on the dorsiflexed, outstretched hand (Fig. 7-60).[280] A direct blow, with the pisiform under tension from the flexor carpi ulnaris and held firmly against the triquetrum, leads to avulsion of its distal portion or a vertical fracture or an osteochondral fracture of the articular surface. Subluxation or dislocation may occur.[133]

The hamate may be fractured in its distal articular surface (Fig. 7-61), through the hook of the hamate (Fig. 7-62), the proxi-

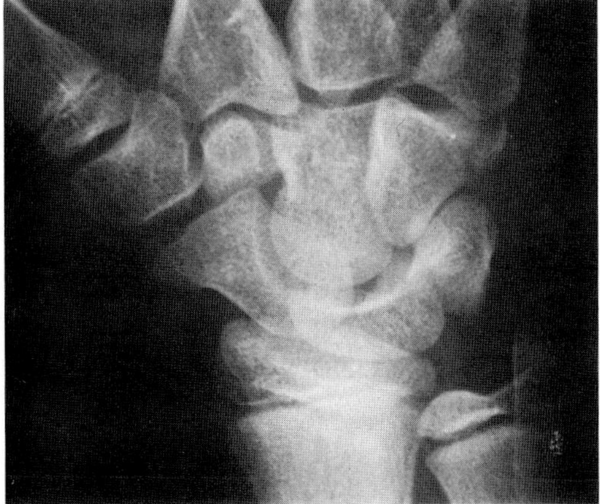

Fig. 7-61. Fracture of the metacarpal articular surface of the hamate. A 14-year-old boy fell from his bicycle, injuring his right hand. Roentgenographic examination showed an essentially undisplaced crack through the fifth metacarpal hamate articular surface. This is analogous to the mechanism that produces Bennett's fractures of the thumb.

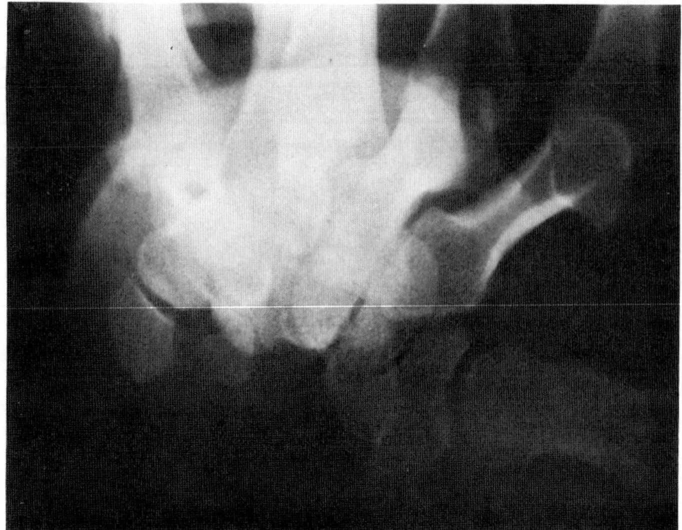

Fig. 7-62. A 47-year-old man injured his right hand in a fall. There was pronounced tenderness over the base of the hypothenar eminence. Carpal tunnel views showed displacement of the hook of the hamate. The patient was immobilized for 6 weeks, with rapid resolution of symptoms and return to normal activities.

mal pole, or the body.[27,193] The hamate also may be dislocated by direct violence.[86,112] A displaced, articular fracture of the distal portion of the hamate occurs when force is applied along the shaft of the fifth metacarpal, as from a fall or a blow on the flexed and ulnarly deviated fist. A fracture of the hook of the hamate may occur from a fall on the dorsiflexed wrist, with tension exerted through the transverse carpal ligament and pisohamate ligament.[10,276] The fracture generally occurs at the base of the hamulus, though avulsion fracture of the tip also may be seen. Osteochondral fracture of the proximal pole likely occurs from impaction injuries against the articular surface of the lunate during dorsiflexion and ulnar deviation. Osteochondral fractures of the triquetral articular surface of the hamate may occur in a similar fashion (Fig. 7-63) or from a shearing injury, such as occurs when a trapped hand is wrenched violently against a steering wheel. Fractures of the body of the hamate and dislocations of the hamate are generally caused by direct crushing injuries, such as punch-press accidents (Fig. 7-64).

Because of its protected position, the body of the capitate[1,229] is seldom fractured except by direct force or crushing blows. There is often an associated injury to the metacarpals and other carpal bones. The capitate is more susceptible to fracture through the neck of the bone, frequently associated with some type of fracture-dislocation. A fairly common variation of this is the naviculocapitate syndrome, in which the capitate and the scaphoid are fractured but no dislocation is observed.[98,261] In this situation, the capitate fragment is frequently rotated 90 to 180 degrees so that the articular surface is displaced anteriorly or is facing the fracture surface of the neck. The mechanism is impingement of the capitate against the dorsal lip of the radius during hyperdorsiflexion, though an opposite mechanism—that of a fall on the hyperflexed wrist—also has been suggested.

Injury to the trapezoid is generally associated with forces applied through the second metacarpal. Because of its shape and position, the trapezoid is rarely fractured, though axial loading of the second metacarpal can cause dorsal dislocation with rupture of the capsular ligaments. Palmar dislocation also has been reported.[65,160,236,260] Ligamentous instability produced by similar injury or osteochondral injuries to the trapezoid-second metacarpal joints also may occur.

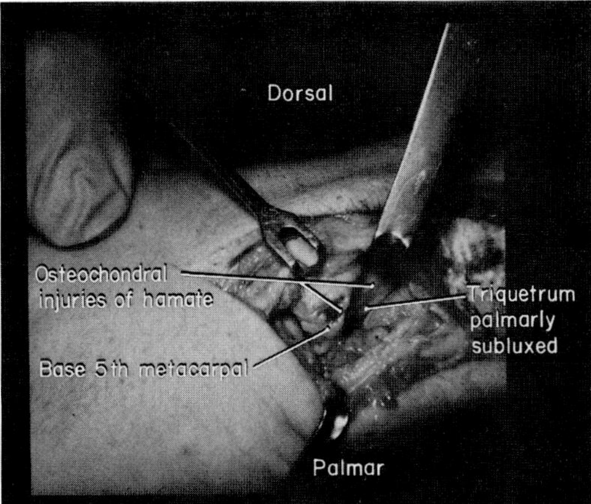

Fig. 7-63. A 22-year-old man injured his left hand in a fight. There is unusual dorsal prominence of the hamate, a palmar subluxation of the triquetrum, and drooping of the fourth and fifth metacarpals. There is an osteochondral injury of the hamate surface. Overlying ligaments show evidence of distortion.

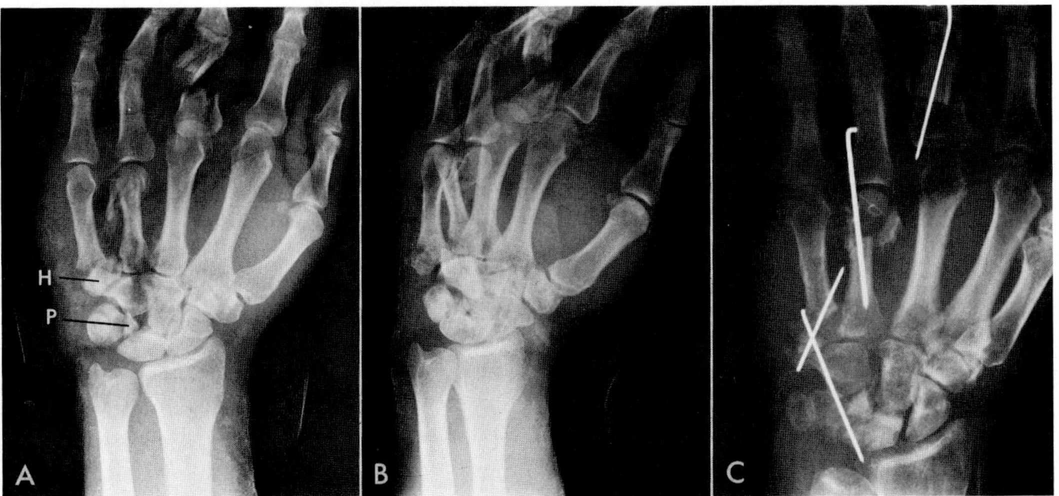

Fig. 7-64. A 47-year-old man suffered a severe crushing injury. (*A, B*) The hamate has a fractured proximal pole (*P*) and there is 90 degrees rotatory subluxation. Note the position of the hamulus (*H*). Instability produced by this type of injury results in disruption of the proximal carpal arch, with flattening of the palm or dorsal displacement of the ulnar border of the hand. In addition, there are fractures of the bases of the fourth and fifth metacarpals, the fourth metacarpal neck, and the proximal phalanx of the middle finger. Motor ulnar palsy was present. (*C*) The patient was referred 5 weeks after the original injury. Open reduction was carried out to correct angulation at the base of the fourth and fifth metacarpals. An attempt was made to correct angulation of the fourth metacarpal neck, and osteotomy was performed through the proximal phalanx of the long finger. An attempt was made to rotate the hamate back into its normal position, but complete reduction was not obtained. Late secondary neurolysis of the ulnar branch of the motor nerve resulted in return of intrinsic activity.

Roentgenographic Findings[149]

Dorsal chip fractures of the triquetrum are easily overlooked on the anteroposterior view because of the normal superimposition of the dorsal lip on the hamate. Such fractures are usually seen in one of the three lateral views of the recommended motion studies of the wrist; if not, a slightly oblique, pronated lateral view will project the triquetrum even more dorsal to the lunate. Transverse fractures of the triquetral body are usually easily identified on the anteroposterior view.

If fractures of the body of the trapezium cannot be seen on the recommended general views, an oblique view of the hand to outline the trapezium and first metacarpal base without superimposition may be useful.

Fracture of the trapezial ridge is difficult to identify without special carpal tunnel views that silhouette the ridge.[121,175,302]

If a special view for pisiform injury is required, a lateral view with the hand in 20 degrees of supination is useful, or the carpal tunnel view may be needed. If subluxation of the pisotriquetral joint is suspected, the following criteria may be necessary when the roentgenograms are made with the wrist in neutral position and the joint well visualized: (1) a joint space more than 4 mm. in width, (2) loss of parallelism of the joint surfaces greater than 20 degrees, and (3) proximal or distal overriding of the pisiform amounting to more than 15 per cent of the width of the joint surfaces.[280]

Fractures and dislocations of the hamate are usually identified on anteroposterior views, particularly with the three views available on the motion studies. A dislocation usually results in some rotation that alters the contour of the bone and the normal oval appearance of the hamulus. Fracture of the hook of the hamate is best visualized on the carpal tunnel view or on a 20-degree supination oblique view.[276] The hook of the hamate is said to ossify independently and occasionally may fail to fuse with the body of the hamate. This separate bone, known as the os hamulus proprium, could be mistaken for a fracture.[216] Chondral articular injuries are seldom visualized on roentgenograms.[64]

Fractures of the capitate usually can be identified on the standard recommended motion study views. A lucent line through the neck of the capitate may be isolated or may be combined with other fractures or fracture-dislocations. In such instances, the head of the capitate should be identified on the lateral view to determine if it has been rotated or displaced.[1,98,261]

A trapezoid injury,[65,77,160,236] frequently a dislocation or fracture-dislocation, is seen on the anteroposterior view as a loss of the normal relationship between the second metacarpal base and the trapezoid. The trapezoid may be superimposed over the trapezium, or the capitate and the second metacarpal may be proximally displaced.

Signs and Symptoms

As noted previously, the signs and symptoms of injuries to the individual carpal bones are those of any fracture or dislocation, with pain and tenderness being appropriately situated for the injury. Localized swelling or prominence and limited motion may be present, and stress of muscle tendon units inserted or supported by the injured structure causes symptoms. Briefly, a knowledge of the deep and topographical anatomy should locate the injury specifically. Neurovascular signs are unusual with these isolated carpal injuries, except for injury of the pisiform and the hook of the hamate, which may irritate the ulnar nerve and artery.

Methods of Management

All isolated injuries of the carpal bones are treated similarly. If undisplaced, most of these injuries respond to 6 weeks of support in a short-arm plaster cast. In a few instances, such as the fracture of the neck of the capitate in which there generally is instability and vascular deprivation, more complete rest of the upper limb muscles is gained by using a long-arm, full-digit cast, as recommended for scaphoid fractures.

Dislocations or displaced fractures may be treated in the same fashion. If satisfactory reduction can be obtained, this is usually accomplished in a fingertrap apparatus with countertraction on the arm and good muscle relaxation. Direct manipulative pressure may be required occasionally. If such attempts do not shortly produce a satisfactory reduction, open reduction, and possibly internal fixation with Kirschner wires, should be used. Even some fractures that are satisfactorily reduced closed may be unstable enough to require percutaneous wire fixation. Fractures at the carpometacarpal joint frequently need such fixation. Occasionally, there are other indications for open procedures, such as gross comminution involving an important joint, the trapezium, and the thumb carpometacarpal joints. Significant or persistent neuropathy, as is occasionally seen with pisiform or hamate hook fractures, may be another indication.[129]

COMPLICATIONS OF CARPAL INJURIES

Refracture

The incidence of refracture in the carpal bones is not known. However, the frequent injuries and excessive stress to this area suggest the likelihood of refracture, as does the incidence of carpal scaphoid fractures that seem to be healing at 6, 8, or even 12 weeks but are found a few years later to have nonunion. The use of a protective splint for a considerable time, even after the formal support apparatus has been removed, therefore, is recommended.

Nerve Injury

Nerve injury is relatively uncommon with carpal injuries. Almost all dislocations and fracture-dislocations of the carpus have at least transient median nerve symptoms, and many have a sufficient neuropathy to suggest a partial or total axonotmesis. Those with immediate significant signs of neuropathy are more likely to be due to direct contusion or direct stretching of the nerve. Those with slowly increasing signs during the first week are more likely to be due to an incipient carpal tunnel syndrome aggravated by the injury. Some patients have both lesions.

The other carpal injuries most frequently associated with neuropathy are the fractures of the hamate hook and the pisiform.[17,129] Both bones are juxtaposed to the ulnar nerve, and an ulnar neuropathy of variable degree is frequent. Damage to both of these nerves, or any of the other nerves in the area, is possible but infrequent—with one exception. Damage to the articular branches is probably common, but the results of this damage are unknown. Damage to or irritation of the dorsal sensory branches of the radial nerve is not uncommon but probably is due to the pressure of the support apparatus rather than to direct injury from the fracture or dislocation. Vascular injury of significant degree associated with carpal injuries is uncommon.

Nonunion

Nonunion is common throughout the carpal bones because of frequent and forceful compressive stresses crossing the area, the extreme difficulty of maintaining immobility, and the frequent difficulty in making an early diagnosis. Scaphoid nonunion is the most common, of course, but similar problems have been observed in almost every bone. Malunion and delayed union are also fairly common, for the same reasons.

Upper Limb Dystrophy

The dysfunction and dystrophy, which combine to be a common serious complication of wrist area injuries, can be introduced by a quotation from John Rhea Barton.[19]

> I do not know of any subject on which I have been more frequently consulted than on deformities, rigid joints, inflexible fingers, loss of the pronating and supinating motions and on neuralgic complaints resulting from injuries of the wrist, and of the carpal extremity of the forearm—one or more of these evils having been left, not merely as a temporary inconvenience, but as a permanent consequence.

The many upper limb disabilities that lead to upper limb dysfunction, which are referred to as the shoulder-hand syndrome, are common complications of wrist injuries, particularly those that occur more frequently in the older age group. The dramatic presentation of the causalgia type has drawn particular attention to the effect of reflex sympathetic dystrophy in such conditions.[171,197-199,262] Nevertheless, the number of cases in which this is the principal factor is relatively small. The other popular name is perhaps a better choice, since shoulder and hand are the most commonly involved, although hand involvement is more common than shoulder involvement. However, wrist involvement is exceedingly common, particularly with the group of injuries we are discussing now. In addition, we have seen many instances in which the forearm and even the elbow have been involved, regarding both pain and limitation of motion.

To cover this spectrum of disabilities, we use the term upper limb dystrophy. The common denominator of all forms of upper limb dystrophy with their gradually increasing involvement of the entire upper limb, even including the shoulder girdle and the neck, is that of dysfunction. This lack of normal function is usually precipitated by pain—local, from multiple sites throughout the limb, or even referred. However, there are other causes of functional inhibition including fear, neurosis, anxiety, and even volition. Sudeck's atrophy or osteoporosis associated with pain and dysfunction is one portion of the spectrum of upper limb dystrophies that can occur after carpal injuries, particularly injuries with median nerve irritability and sensitivity. Nevertheless, this form of upper limb dystrophy is no more common than the other types. Furthermore, the osteoporosis commonly seen after carpal injury and treatment is usually not the Sudeck type.[264,265] Treatment of upper limb dystrophy consists of identifying and coping with as many of the causes of lack of function as possible.

Ischemic Contractures

Closed compartment syndromes, both of the forearm or Volkmann type[284] and of the intrinsic compartments of the hand,[33] are not uncommon, particularly if the carpal injury is associated with a crush injury. Thus, rigid encasements must be avoided, and careful attention must be paid to all severe and increasing pains that are referred to muscle compartments. If rest, elevation, and resilient bulky dressings are unavailing, surgical decompression is the only remaining treatment of value.

Posttraumatic Changes

The usual type of stress fracture has not been noted in the carpal bones. However, osteolytic and cystic changes, secondary to episodes of single or repetitive stress, have been reported.[100,128] In addition, we have noted reactions to repetitive stress in certain athletes. In boxers, a condition similar to carpe bossu or os styloideum has been noted, with ridging and exostosis formation, plus chondral changes and even chondral fractures at the carpometacarpal joints, intercarpal joints, and the joints between the bases of the index and long finger rays. Similar chondral defects, eburnation, and ridging have been noted at areas where radius and carpus or adjacent carpal bones make contact during extreme dorsiflexion, as in gymnastics. Similar impingement syndromes, usually with considerably more exostosis formation, have been seen after trauma, such as dorsal chip fractures or Colles' fractures. Associated with these or presenting alone are other lesions that could be posttraumatic residua.[226] These include intraarticular meniscoids, osteochondral fragments, and localized areas of synovitis and ganglia.

Other Complications

Skin loss, infection, and pathological fractures are rare and do not warrant discussion. Injuries to neighboring muscles and joints are uncommon from acute carpal injuries, though the secondary arthrosis may, much later, lead to damage of the deep flexors or of the deep radial extensors. Traumatic arthritis is present to some degree in almost all carpal injuries and may be severe. The amount seems to depend on the degree of chondral surface damage. Fibrous ankylosis of the carpal joints is common and is associated with the extent of traumatic arthritis or arthrosis, the degree and persistence of hemorrhage and edema, the length of immobility, and the position during immobility. The wrist ankylosed in flexion makes satisfactory hand function impossible.

PROGNOSIS IN CARPAL INJURIES

In general, the prognosis for recovery from these injuries is excellent, provided diagnosis is made early and appropriate management is carried out swiftly. The time for recovery varies, depending on the type of injury and the treatment requirements, particularly the length of time required for support and adequate healing of all damaged tissues. With residual deformity, particularly if this involves a joint surface, recovery is practically never complete. Severe deformity, such as recurrent or persistent dislocation or a severe collapse deformity or severe chondral damage, nearly always results in disability sufficient to warrant a reconstructive procedure. These procedures range from various arthroplasties, such as bone excision with or without replacement, to various types of arthrodesis involving radius, carpus, and metacarpus. For increasing comfort and strength, most of these procedures, when properly selected, are adequate. Nevertheless, significant disability always results. Partly for this reason, the search for a total wrist arthroplasty is currently being conducted in many centers.[120,268]

POSTTREATMENT CARE AND REHABILITATION OF CARPAL INJURIES

The type of support apparatus used for each condition has been included under the individual topics. Generally, palmar surface splints combined with compression dressings are used during the immediate posttrauma period of reaction and swelling. After this, the minimal support used should be a short-arm wrist-support splint for such entities as dorsal chip fractures, and the maximal support should be a long-arm cast that includes all five digits for scaphoid fractures and other carpal body fractures. Dislocations and fracture-dislocations are treated with supports similar to those used in carpal body fractures, unless there has been associated internal fixation. Kirschner wires, when used percutaneously or for open reduction, are usually left protruding, with the external portion bent at right angles to avoid the occasional migration. These cause little trouble (less so in our experience than do buried pins) but must be monitored closely for evidence of looseness or inflammation, or both.

Generally, the inflammation is preceded by loosening of the pin. A loose pin should be removed immediately. The first sign of loosening is that the pin can be rotated with manual force alone. In most instances, even snug Kirschner wires are removed in about 6 weeks. The return of a complete range of motion, even in normal joints, can be expected to take about as long as the given joint was totally immobilized during the treatment period. The return of full comfort and full strength as judged by the return of grip power and repetitive grip endurance takes about four times as long as the time that the part is rigidly supported. Nevertheless, the permanently disabling residua associated with upper limb dystrophy almost always can be avoided by careful attention to the following: (1) instituting and maintaining shoulder-elevation exercises throughout the course of treatment,[198,199] (2) observing and halting the progression of any neurologic or circulatory deficits, (3) observing and remedying all pain and swelling,[210] (4) avoiding extreme positioning of any joint or part, (5) initiating digit exercises as soon as feasible,[199] and (6) bringing the wrist to a neutral or slightly extended position as soon as this is safe.

Shoulder exercises of the Codman type[50] are helpful and may be undertaken, particularly when some disability of the shoulder restricts elevation or makes it impossible. However, the key shoulder exercise to avoid upper limb dystrophy is that of active elevation and rotation. This should be carried out a minimum of 50 times each day if possible. Almost any digit exercise is useful, provided a full range of possible motion is carried out, with the maximal force that is comfortable. The usual wiggling and waving exercises are inadequate. To ensure that each joint has the maximal chance of being carried through its particular range of motion, we use a set of six exercises: (1) maximal extension of all digits, (2) thumb to each fingertip, (3) the grasp or "fist" exercise with all fingers flexing to the palmar crease or as near as possible to it, (4) the "claw" exercise with the metacarpophalangeal joints of the fingers kept extended but the interphalangeal joints maximally flexed, (5) the "tabletop" exercise with the metacarpophalangeal joints maximally flexed but the interphalangeal joints extended, and (6) abduction-adduction of all digits in the radioulnar plane.

With these precautions and a gradual increase of function with both time and force carefully controlled, rehabilitation is seldom a problem. Occasionally, however, special treatments may be required, including physical therapy modalities, splinting, and particularly reeducation. Inhibition of some or all of the motors that control the wrist and digits may be so ingrained a pattern that special training may be necessary. The most common instance of this is inhibition of the wrist extensors when pain is associated with wrist extension or when deformity decreases the moment-arm distance between the center of wrist motion and the wrist extensor tendon.

REFERENCES

1. Adler, J. B., and Shaftan, G. W.: Fractures of the capitate. J. Bone Joint Surg., *44A*: 1537-1547, 1962.
2. Aegerter, E., and Kirkpatrick, J. A., Jr.: Orthopedic Diseases: Physiology, Pathology, Radiology. Philadelphia, W. B. Saunders, 1958.
3. Agerholm, J. C., and Goodfellow, J. W.: Avascular necrosis of the lunate bone treated by excision and prosthetic replacement. J. Bone Joint Surg., *45B*:110-116, 1963.
4. Agerholm, J. C., and Lee, M. L. H.: The acrylic scaphoid prosthesis in the treatment of the ununited carpal scaphoid fracture. Acta Orthop. Scand., *37*:67-76, 1966.
5. Agner, O.: Treatment of ununited fractures of the carpal scaphoid by Bentzon's operation. Acta Orthop. Scand., *33*:56-65, 1963.
6. ———: Treatment of non-united navicular fractures by total excision of the bone and the insertion of acrylic prostheses. Acta Orthop. Scand., *33*:235-245, 1963.

7. Albert, S. M., Wohl, M. A., and Rechtman, A. M.: Treatment of the disrupted radio-ulnar joint. J. Bone Joint Surg., *45A*:1373-1381, 1963.
8. Alffram, P.-A., and Bauer, G. C. H.: Epidemiology of fractures of the forearm: a biomechanical investigation of bone strength. J. Bone Joint Surg., *44A*:105-114, 1962.
9. Anderson, R., and O'Neil, G.: Comminuted fractures of the distal end of the radius. Surg. Gynecol. Obstet., *78*:434-440, 1944.
10. Andress, M. R., and Peckar, V. G.: Fracture of the hook of the hamate. Brit. J. Radiol., *43*:141-143, 1970.
11. Andrews, F. T.: A dislocation of the carpal bones—the scaphoid and semilunar: report of a case. Mich. Med., *31*:269-271, 1932.
12. Arkless, R.: Cineradiography in normal and abnormal wrists. Amer. J. Roentgenol. Radium Ther. Nucl. Med., *96*:837-844, 1966.
13. ———: Rheumatoid wrists: cineradiography. Radiology, *88*:543-549, 1967.
14. Armstrong, G. W. D.: Rotational subluxation of the scaphoid. Canad. J. Surg., *11*:306-314, 1968.
15. Aufranc, O. E., Jones, W. N., and Turner, R. H.: Anterior marginal articular fracture of distal radius. J.A.M.A., *196*:788-791, 1966.
16. Bacorn, R. W., and Kurtzke, J. F.: Colles' fracture: a study of two thousand cases from the New York State Workmen's Compensation Board. J. Bone Joint Surg., *35A*:643-658, 1953.
17. Baird, D. B., and Friedenberg, Z. B.: Delayed ulnar-nerve palsy following a fracture of the hamate. J. Bone Joint Surg., *50A*:570-572, 1968.
18. Barnard, L., and Stubbins, S. G.: Styloidectomy of the radius in the surgical treatment of non-union of the carpal navicular: a preliminary report. J. Bone Joint Surg., *30A*:98-102, 1948.
19. Barton, J. R.: Views and treatment of an important injury to the wrist. Med. Examiner, *1*:365, 1838.
20. Bartone, N. F., and Grieco, R. V.: Fractures of the triquetrum. J. Bone Joint Surg., *38A*:353-356, 1956.
21. Bate, J. T.: Apparatus for use in reduction and fixation of fractures of distal radius. Clin. Orthop., *63*:190-195, 1969.
22. Baumann, J. U., and Campbell, R. D., Jr.: Significance of architectural types of fractures of the carpal scaphoid and relation to timing of treatment. J. Trauma, *2*:431-438, 1962.
23. Bentzon, P. G. K., and Randløv-Madsen, A.: On fracture of the carpal scaphoid. Acta Orthop. Scand., *16*:30-39, 1946.
24. Böhler, L.: The Treatment of Fractures. ed. 4. Baltimore, William Wood & Co., 1942.
25. Böhler, L., Trojan, E., and Jahna, H.: Behandlungsergebnisse von 734 frischen einfachen Brüchen des Kahnbeinkörpers der Hand. Weiderherstell. Chir. Traumatol, *2*:86-111, 1954.
26. Bonnin, J. G., and Greening, W. P.: Fractures of the triquetrum. Brit. J. Surg., *31*:278-283, 1944.
27. Bowen, T. L.: Injuries of the hamate bone. Hand, *5*:235-238, 1973.
28. Boyes, J. H.: Bunnell's Surgery of the Hand. ed. 4. Philadelphia, J. B. Lippincott, 1964.
29. ———: Bunnell's Surgery of the Hand. ed. 5. Philadelphia, J. B. Lippincott, 1970.
30. Brady, L. P.: Double pin fixation of severely comminuted fractures of the distal radius and ulna. South. Med. J., *56*:307-311, 1963.
31. Broder, H.: Rupture of flexor tendons, associated with a malunited Colles' fracture. J. Bone Joint Surg., *36A*:404-405, 1954.
32. Broomé, A., Grönqvist, B., and Telhag, H.: Långtidsresultat vid hög Gipsfixation av Navicularefrakturer. Lakartidningen, *65*:1950-1951, 1968.
33. Bunnell, S.: Ischaemic contracture, local, in the hand. J. Bone Joint Surg., *35A*:88-101, 1953.
34. Buzby, B. F.: Isolated radial dislocation of carpal scaphoid. Ann. Surg., *100*:553-555, 1934.
35. Caldwell, J. A.: Device for making traction on the fingers. J.A.M.A., *96*:1226, 1931.
36. Campbell, R. D., Jr., Lance, E. M., and Yeoh, C. B.: Lunate and perilunar dislocations. J. Bone Joint Surg., *46B*:55-72, 1964.
37. Campbell, R. D., Jr., Thompson, T. C., Lance, E. M., and Adler, J. B.: Indications for open reduction of lunate and perilunate dislocations of the carpal bones. J. Bone Joint Surg., *47A*:915-937, 1965.
38. Campbell, W. C.: Malunited Colles' fracture. J.A.M.A., *109*:1105-1108, 1937.
39. ———: Malunited fractures. Surg. Gynecol. Obstet., *66*:466-474, 1938.
40. Carothers, R. G., and Berning, D. D.:

Colles' fracture. Amer. J. Surg., *80*:626-628, 1950.

41. Carothers, R. G., and Boyd, F. J.: Thumb traction technic for reduction of Colles' fracture. Arch. Surg., *58*:848-852, 1949.
42. Carroll, R. E., Sinton, W., and Garcia, A.: Acute calcium deposits in the hand. J.A.M.A., *157*:422-426, 1955.
43. Cassebaum, W. H.: Colles' fracture: a study of end results. J.A.M.A., *143*:963-965, 1950.
44. Cave, E. F.: The carpus, with reference to the fractured navicular bone. Arch. Surg., *40*:54-76, 1940.
45. Chao, E. Y. S.: Principles of Biomechanics. Resident Lecture Series, Mayo Clinic, Rochester, Minnesota.
46. Charnley, J.: The Closed Treatment of Common Fractures. ed. 3. Baltimore, Williams & Wilkins, 1961.
47. Christophe, K.: Rupture of the extensor pollicis longus tendon following Colles' fracture. J. Bone Joint Surg., *35A*:1003-1005, 1953.
48. Cobey, M. C., and White, R. K.: An operation for non-union of fractures of the carpal navicular. J. Bone Joint Surg., *28*: 757-764, 1946.
49. Cockshott, W. P.: Carpal fusions. Amer. J. Roentgenol. Radium Ther. Nucl. Med., *89*:1260-1271, 1963.
50. Codman, E. A.: The Shoulder: Rupture of the Supraspinatus Tendon and Other Lesions in or About the Subacromial Bursa. Boston, Thomas Todd Company, 1934.
51. Codman, E. A., and Chase, H. M.: The diagnosis and treatment of fracture of the carpal scaphoid and dislocation of the semilunar bone: with a report of thirty cases. Ann. Surg., *41*:321-362; 863-902, 1905.
52. Cole, J. M., and Obletz, B. E.: Comminuted fractures of the distal end of the radius treated by skeletal transfixion in plaster cast: an end-result study of thirty-three cases. J. Bone Joint Surg., *48A*:931-945, 1966.
53. Coleman, H. M.: Injuries of the articular disc at the wrist. J. Bone Joint Surg., *42B*: 522-529, 1960.
54. Colles, A.: On the fracture of the carpal extremity of the radius. Edinb. Med. Surg. J., *10*:182-186, 1814.
55. Collins, L. C., Lidsky, M. D., Sharp, J. T., and Moreland, J.: Malposition of carpal bones in rheumatoid arthritis. Radiology, *103*:95-98, 1972.
56. Connell, M. C., and Dyson, R. P.: Dislocation of the carpal scaphoid: report of a case. J. Bone Joint Surg., *37B*:252-253, 1955.
57. Conwell, H. E., and Reynolds, F. C.: Key and Conwell's Management of Fractures, Dislocations, and Sprains. ed. 7. St. Louis, C. V. Mosby, 1961.
58. Cordrey, L. J., and Ferrer-Torells, M.: Management of fractures of the greater multangular: report of five cases. J. Bone Joint Surg., *42A*:1111-1118, 1960.
59. Cotton, F. J.: The pathology of fracture of the lower extremity of the radius. Ann. Surg., *32*:194-218; 388-415, 1900.
60. ———: Dislocations and Joint-Fractures. ed. 2. Philadelphia, W. B. Saunders, 1924.
61. Cozen, L.: Colles' fracture: a method of maintaining reduction. Calif. Med., *75*: 362-364, 1951.
62. Crabbe, W. A.: Excision of the proximal row of the carpus. J. Bone Joint Surg., *46B*:708-711, 1964.
63. Crittenden, J. J., Jones, D. M., and Santarelli, A. G.: Bilateral rotational dislocation of the carpal navicular: case report. Radiology, *94*:629-630, 1970.
64. Crock, H. V.: Post-traumatic erosions of articular cartilage. J. Bone Joint Surg., *46B*:530-538, 1964.
65. Curtiss, P. H., Jr.: The hunchback carpal bone. J. Bone Joint Surg., *43A*:392-394, 1961.
66. Dahlin, D. C.: Bone Tumors: General Aspects and Data on 3,987 Cases. Springfield, Illinois, Charles C Thomas, 1967.
67. Dameron, T. B., Jr.: Traumatic dislocation of the distal radio-ulnar joint. Clin. Orthop., *83*:55-63, 1972.
68. Darrach, W.: Partial excision of lower shaft of ulna for deformity following Colles' fracture. Ann. Surg., *57*:764-765, 1913.
69. ———: Fractures of the lower extremity of the radius: diagnosis and treatment. J.A.M.A., *89*:1683-1685, 1927.
70. Davidson, A. J., and Horowitz, M. T.: An evaluation of excision in the treatment of ununited fracture of the carpal scaphoid (navicular) bone. Ann. Surg., *108*:291-295, 1938.
71. Dawkins, A. L.: The fractured scaphoid: a modern view. Med. J. Austral., *1*:332-333, 1967.
72. Dehne, E., Deffer, P. A., and Feighney, R. E.: Pathomechanics of the fracture of the carpal navicular. J. Trauma, *4*:96-113, 1964.
73. De Oliveira, J. C.: Barton's fractures. J. Bone Joint Surg., *55A*:586-594, 1973.

74. DePalma, A. F.: Comminuted fractures of the distal end of the radius treated by ulnar pinning. J. Bone Joint Surg., *34A*: 651-662, 1952.
75. De Quervain, F.: Clinical surgical diagnosis for students and practitioners. ed. 4. New York, William Wood & Co., 1913.
76. Desault, P. J.: A Treatise on Fractures, Luxations, and Other Affections of the Bones. Philadelphia, Fry & Kammerer, 1805.
77. Destot, E.: Injuries of the Wrist. London, Ernest Benn, 1925.
78. Dingman, P. V. C.: Resection of the distal end of the ulna (Darrach operation): an end-result study of twenty-four cases. J. Bone Joint Surg., *34A*:893-900, 1952.
79. Dobyns, J. H., and Linscheid, R. L.: Posttraumatic instability of the wrist (instructional course). Presented at the Annual Meeting of the American Academy of Orthopaedic Surgeons, Dallas, January 19 to 24, 1974. [In press]
80. Dobyns, J. H., and Perkins, J. C.: Instability of the carpal navicular (abstr.). J. Bone Joint Surg., *49A*:1014, 1967.
81. Dobyns, J. H., and Swanson, G. E.: A 19-year-old with multiple fractures (fracture conference). Minn. Med., *56*:143-149, 1973.
82. Dobyns, J. H., Swanson, G. E., and Linscheid, R. L.: A review of incidence and management of dislocations and fracture dislocations of the carpus. Presented at the Annual Meeting of the American Academy of Orthopaedic Surgeons, Dallas, January 19 to 24, 1974.
83. Dornan, A.: The results of treatment in Kienböck's disease. J. Bone Joint Surg., *31B*:518-520, 1949.
84. Dowling, J. J., and Sawyer, B., Jr.: Comminuted Colles' fractures: evaluation of a method of treatment. J. Bone Joint Surg., *43A*:657-668, 1961.
85. Duchenne, G. B. A.: Physiology of Motion: Demonstrated by Means of Electrical Stimulation and Clinical Observation and Applied to the Study of Paralysis and Deformities. Philadelphia, W. B. Saunders, 1959.
86. Duke, R.: Dislocation of the hamate bone: report of a case. J. Bone Joint Surg., *45B*:744, 1963.
87. Dupuytren, B.: On the Injuries and Diseases of Bones. London, The Sydenham Society, 1847.
88. Durbin, F. C.: Non-union of the triquetrum: report of a case. J. Bone Joint Surg., *32B*:388, 1950.
89. Dwight, T.: A Clinical Atlas: Variations of the Bones of the Hands and Feet. Philadelphia, J. B. Lippincott, 1907.
90. Dwyer, F. C.: Excision of the carpal scaphoid for ununited fracture. J. Bone Joint Surg., *31B*:572-577, 1949.
91. Edwards, H., and Clayton, E. B.: Colles' fracture (correspondence). Brit. Med. J., *1*:523, 1929.
92. Edwards, H. C.: Mechanism and treatment of backfire fracture. J. Bone Joint Surg., *8*:701-717, 1926.
93. Ellis, J.: Smith's and Barton's fractures: a method of treatment. J. Bone Joint Surg., *47B*:724-727, 1965.
94. England, J. P. S.: Subluxation of the carpal scaphoid. Proc. Roy. Soc. Med., *63*:581-582, 1970.
95. Fahey, J. H.: Fractures and dislocations about the wrist. Surg. Clin. North Amer., Feb.:19-40, 1957.
96. Fairbank, T. J.: Chip fractures of the os triquetrum (carpal cuneiform). Brit. Med. J., *2*:310-311, 1942.
97. Faulkner, D. M.: Bipartite carpal scaphoid. J. Bone Joint Surg., *10*:284-289, 1928.
98. Fenton, R. L.: The naviculo-capitate fracture syndrome. J. Bone Joint Surg., *38A*:681-684, 1956.
99. Fick, R.: Handbuch der Anatomie und Mechanik der Gelenke: Unter Berücksichtigung der bewegenden Muskeln. I. Anatomie der Gelenke. II. Allgemeine Gelenk- und Muskelmechanik. III. Spezielle Gelenk- und Muskelmechanik. Jena, Gustav Fischer Verlag, 1904-1911.
100. Fischer, E.: Posttraumatische karpale Osteolysen nach isolierter Fraktur am distalen Radius. Fortschr. Geb. Roentgenstr. Nuklearmed. *112*:541-542, 1970.
101. Fisk, G. R.: Carpal instability and the fractured scaphoid. Ann. Roy. Coll. Surg. Engl., *46*:63-76, 1970.
102. Fitzsimons, R. A.: Colles' fracture and chauffeur's fracture. Brit. Med. J., *2*:357-360, 1938.
103. Flatt, A. E.: The Care of Minor Hand Injuries. ed. 3. St. Louis, C. V. Mosby, 1972.
104. Flynn, J. E. (ed.): Hand Surgery. Baltimore, Williams & Wilkins, 1966.
105. Frankel, V. H., and Burstein, A. H.: Orthopaedic Biomechanics. Philadelphia, Lea & Febiger, 1970.
106. Freundlich, B. D. and Spinner, M.: Nerve compression syndrome in derangements of the proximal and distal radial ulnar

joints. Bull. Hosp. Joint Dis., *29*:38-47, 1968.

107. Frykman, G.: Fracture of the distal radius including sequelae—shoulder-hand-finger syndrome, disturbance in the distal radio-ulnar joint, and impairment of nerve function: a clinical and experimental study. Acta Orthop. Scand., *108* [Suppl.]:1-155, 1967.
108. Furlong, R.: Injuries of the Hand. Boston, Little, Brown & Company, 1957.
109. Gartland, J. J., Jr., and Werley, C. W.: Evaluation of healed Colles' fractures. J. Bone Joint Surg., *33A*:895-907, 1951.
110. Gasser, H.: Delayed union and pseudarthrosis of the carpal navicular: treatment by compression-screw osteosynthesis: a preliminary report of twenty fractures. J. Bone Joint Surg., *47A*:249-266, 1965.
111. Geckeler, E. O.: Treatment of comminuted Colles' fracture. J. Int. Coll. Surg., *20*:596-601, 1953.
112. Geist, D. C.: Dislocation of the hamate bone. J. Bone Joint Surg., *21*:215-217, 1939.
113. Gentaz, R., Lespargot, J., Levame, J.-H., and Poli, J.-P.: La maladie de Kienböck approche tomographique: analyse de 5 cas. Nouv. Presse Med., *1*:1207-1210, 1972.
114. Gilford, W. W., Bolton, R. H., and Lambrinudi, C.: The mechanism of the wrist joint: with special reference to fractures of the scaphoid. Guys Hosp. Rep., *92*:52-59, 1943.
115. Gillespie, H. S.: Excision of the lunate bone in Kienböck's disease. J. Bone Joint Surg., *43B*:245-249, 1961.
116. Goldman, S., Lipscomb, P. R., and Taylor, W. F.: Immobilization for acute carpal scaphoid fractures. Surg. Gynecol. Obstet., *129*:281-284, 1969.
117. Gordon, S. L.: Scaphoid and lunate dislocation: report of a case in a patient with peripheral neuropathy. J. Bone Joint Surg., *54A*:1769-1772, 1972.
118. Grace, R. V.: Fracture of the carpal scaphoid. Ann. Surg., *89*:752-761, 1929.
119. Green, J. T., and Gay, F. H.: Colles' fracture—residual disability. Amer. J. Surg., *91*:636-642, 1956.
120. Gschwend, N., and Scheier, H.: Die GSB-Handgelenksprothese. Orthopade, *2*:46-47, 1973.
121. Hart, V. L., and Gaynor, V.: Roentgenographic study of the carpal canal. J. Bone Joint Surg., *23*:382-383, 1941.
122. Haynes, H. H.: Treating fractures by skeletal fixation of the individual bone. South. Med. J., *32*:720-723, 1939.
123. ———: Skeletal fixation of fractures. Amer. J. Surg., *59*:25-36, 1943.
124. Heiple, K. G., Freehafer, A. A., and Van't Hof, A.: Isolated traumatic dislocation of the distal end of the ulna or distal radio-ulnar joint. J. Bone Joint Surg., *44A*:1387-1394, 1962.
125. Hindenach, J. C. R.: Bilateral congenital fusion of the semilunar and cuneiform bones: report of a case. Brit. J. Surg., *35*:104-105, 1947.
126. Hobart, M. H., and Kraft, G. L.: Malunited Colles' fracture. Amer. J. Surg., *53*:55-60, 1941.
127. Hoffman, B. P.: Fractures of the distal end of the radius in the adult and in the child. Bull. Hosp. Joint Dis., *14*:114-124, 1953.
128. Horvath, S. F., Kakosy, T., and Villanyi, G.: Structural changes of carpal bones in motor saw workers. Magy Radiol., *21*: 257-266, 1969.
129. Howard, F. M.: Ulnar-nerve palsy in wrist fractures. J. Bone Joint Surg., *43A*:1197-1201, 1961.
130. Howard, F. M., Fahey, T., and Wojcik, E.: The rotating navicular—voluntary subluxation (abstr.). J. Bone Joint Surg., *55A*:877, 1973.
131. Hultén, O.: Uber anatomische Variationen der Handgelenkknocken: ein Beitrag zur Kenntnis der Genese zwei verschiedener Mondbeinveränderungen. Acta Radiol., *9*:155-168, 1928.
132. Hyman, G., and Martin, F. R. R.: Dislocation of the inferior radio-ulnar joint as a complication of fracture of the radius. Brit. J. Surg., *27*:481-491, 1940.
133. Immermann, E. W.: Dislocation of the pisiform. J. Bone Joint Surg., *30A*:489-492, 1948.
134. Iwamoto, Y., Fujiwara, A., and Liang, F.: Experimental study on the carpal navicular fracture. *In* Proceedings of the 15th Annual Meeting of the Japanese Society for Surgery of the Hand. Niigata, 1972.
135. Jaffe, H. L.: Tumors and Tumorous Conditions of the Bones and Joints. Philadelphia, Lea & Febiger, 1958.
136. ———: Metabolic, Degenerative, and Inflammatory Diseases of Bones and Joints. Philadelphia, Lea & Febiger, 1972.
137. Johnston, H. M.: Varying positions of the carpal bones in the different movements at the wrist. J. Anat. Physiol., *41*:109-122, 1907.

138. Jones, F. W.: The Principles of Anatomy as Seen in the Hand. ed. 2. Baltimore, Williams & Wilkins, 1942.
139. Jones, K. G.: Experiences with extraskeletal fixation for Colles' type fractures. Personal Communication.
140. Jorgensen, E. C.: Proximal-row carpectomy: an end-result study of twenty-two cases. J. Bone Joint Surg., *51A*:1104-1111, 1969.
141. Kambolis, C., Bullough, P. G., and Jaffe, H. L.: Ganglionic cystic defects of bone. J. Bone Joint Surg., *55A*:496-505, 1973.
142. Kaplan, E. B.: Functional and Surgical Anatomy of the Hand. ed. 2. Philadelphia, J. B. Lippincott, 1965.
143. Kauer, J. M. G.: Een analyse van de carpale flexie. Thesis, University of Leiden, 1964.
144. Kessler, I., and Hecht, O.: Present application of the Darrach procedure. Clin. Orthop., *72*:254-260, 1970.
145. Kessler, I., and Silberman, Z.: An experimental study of the radiocarpal joint by arthrography. Surg. Gynecol. Obstet., *112*:33-40, 1961.
146. Kessler, I., Silberman, Z., Heller, J., and Pupko, L.: Diagnostic considerations in fractures of the carpal scaphoid bone. Surg. Gynecol. Obstet., *110*:117-120, 1960.
147. Kienböck, R.: Uber traumatische Malazie des Mondbeins und ihre Folgezustände: Entartungsformen und Kompressionsfrakturen. Fortschr. Geb. Roentgenstr., *16*:78-103, 1910-1911.
148. Knapp, M. E.: Treatment of some complications of Colles' fracture. J.A.M.A., *148*:825-827, 1952.
149. Köhler, A., and Zimmer, E. A.: Borderlands of the Normal and Early Pathologic in Skeletal Roentgenology. [Third American edition, based on 11th German edition] New York, Grune & Stratton, 1968.
150. Kricun, M. E., and Edeiken, J.: Roentgenologic Atlas of the Hand and Wrist in Systemic Disease. Baltimore, Williams & Wilkins, 1973.
151. Kristiansen, A., and Gjersoe, E.: Colles' fracture: operative treatment, indications and results. Acta Orthop. Scand., *39*:33-46, 1968.
152. Kuth, J. R.: Isolated dislocation of the carpal navicular: a case report. J. Bone Joint Surg., *21*:479-483, 1939.
153. Kwedar, A. T., and Mitchell, C. L.: Late rupture of extensor pollicis longus tendon following Colles' fracture. J. Bone Joint Surg., *22*:429-435, 1940.
154. Landsmeer, J. M.: Studies in the anatomy of articulation. I. The equilibrium of the "intercalated" bone. Acta Morphol. Neerl. Scand., *3*:287-303, 1961.
155. ———: Les cohérences spatiales et l'equilibre spatial dans la région carpienne. Acta Anat. (Basel), 70 [Suppl. *54*]:1-84, 1968.
156. Last, R. J.: Specimens from the Hunterian collection. J. Bone Joint Surg., *33B*:114-118, 1951.
157. Lee, M. L. H.: The intraosseous arterial pattern of the carpal lunate bone and its relation to avascular necrosis. Acta Orthop. Scand., *33*:43-55, 1963.
158. Legge, R.: Vitallium prosthesis in the treatment of fracture of the carpal navicular. West. J. Surg., *59*:468-471, 1951.
159. Lentino, W., Lubetsky, H. W., Jacobson, H. G., and Poppel, M. H.: The carpal-bridge view: a position for the roentgenographic diagnosis of abnormalities in the dorsum of the wrist. J. Bone Joint Surg., *39A*:88-90, 1957.
160. Lewis, H. H.: Dislocation of the lesser multangular: report of a case. J. Bone Joint Surg., *44A*:1412-1414, 1962.
161. Lewis, O. J.: The Hominoid Wrist Joint. Amer. J. Phys. Anthropol., *30*:251-267, 1969.
162. Lewis, O. J., Hamshere, R. J., and Bucknill, T. M.: The anatomy of the wrist joint. J. Anat., *106*:539-552, 1970.
163. Lindgren, E.: Some radiological aspects on the carpal scaphoid and its fractures. Acta Chir. Scand., *98*:538-548, 1949.
164. Linscheid, R. L.: The mechanical factors affecting deformity at the wrist in rheumatoid arthritis (abstr.). J. Bone Joint Surg., *51A*:790, 1969.
165. Linscheid, R. L., Dobyns, J. H., Beabout, J. W., and Bryan, R. S.: Traumatic instability of the wrist: diagnosis, classification, and pathomechanics. J. Bone Joint Surg., *54A*:1612-1632, 1972.
166. Lippman, E. M., and McDermott, L. J.: Vitallium replacement of lunate in Kienböck's disease. Milit. Surgeon, *105*:482-484, 1949.
167. Lippmann, R. K.: Laxity of the radioulnar joint following Colles' fracture. Arch. Surg., *35*:772-786, 1937.
168. Lipschutz, B.: Late subcutaneous rupture of the tendon of the extensor pollicis longus muscle. Arch. Surg., *31*:816-822, 1935.
169. Logròscino, D., and de Marchi, E.: Vascolarizzazione e trofo-patie delle ossa

del carpo. Chir. Organi. Mov., *23*:499-524, 1938.

170. London, P. S.: The broken scaphoid bone: the case against pessimism. J. Bone Joint Surg., *43B*:237-244, 1961.
171. Lorente de Nó, R.: Analysis of the activity of the chains of internuncial neurons. J. Neurophysiol., *1*:207-244, 1938.
172. Lugnegard, H.: Resection of the head of the ulna in posttraumatic dysfunction of the distal radio-ulnar joint. Scand. J. Plast. Reconstr. Surg., *3*:65-69, 1969.
173. Lützeler, H.: Die Entstehungsursache der Pseudarthrose nach Bruch des Kahnbeins der Hand. Dtsch. Z. Chir., *235*:450-467, 1932.
174. Lynch, A. C., and Lipscomb, P. R.: The carpal tunnel syndrome and Colles' fractures. J.A.M.A., *185*:363-366, 1963.
175. McClain, E. J., and Boyes, J. H.: Missed fractures of the greater multangular. J. Bone Joint Surg., *48A*:1525-1528, 1966.
176. MacConaill, M. A.: The mechanical anatomy of the carpus and its bearings on some surgical problems. J. Anat., *75*:166-175, 1941.
177. McDougall, A., and White, J.: Subluxation of the inferior radio-ulnar joint complicating fracture of the radial head. J. Bone Joint Surg., *39B*:278-287, 1957.
178. McLaughlin, H. L.: Fracture of the carpal navicular (scaphoid) bone: some observations based on treatment by open reduction and internal fixation. J. Bone Joint Surg., *36A*:765-774, 1954.
179. ———: Trauma. Philadelphia, W. B. Saunders, 1959.
180. McLaughlin, H. L., and Baab, O. D.: Carpectomy. Surg. Clin. North Amer., *31*: 451-461, 1951.
181. McLaughlin, H. L., and Parkes, J. C., II: Fracture of the carpal navicular (scaphoid) bone: gradations in therapy based upon pathology. J. Trauma, *9*:311-318, 1969.
182. McMaster, P. E.: Late ruptures of extensor and flexor pollicis longus tendons following Colles' fracture. J. Bone Joint Surg., *14*:93-101, 1932.
183. Malgaigne, J. F.: Traité des Fractures et des Luxations. vol. 1. Paris, J. B. Baillière Tindall et Co., 1847.
184. ———: A Treatise on Fractures. Philadelphia, J. B. Lippincott, 1859.
185. Marsh, H. O., and Teal, S. W.: Treatment of comminuted fractures of the distal radius with self-contained skeletal traction. Amer. J. Surg., *124*:715-719, 1972.
186. Matti, H.: Uber die Behandlung der Navicularefrakture und der Refractura patellae durch Plombierung mit Spongiosa. Zentrabl. Chir., *64*:2353-2359, 1937.
187. Mattsson, O.: Cassette for simultaneous multiplane tomography with non-screen film. Acta Radiol. [Diag.], *6*:589-592, 1967.
188. Maudsley, R. H., and Chen, S. C.: Screw fixation in the management of the fractured carpal scaphoid. J. Bone Joint Surg., *54B*:432-441, 1972.
189. Mayer, J. H.: Colles' fracture. Brit. J. Surg., *27*:629-642, 1940.
190. Mazet, R., Jr., and Hohl, M.: Radial styloidectomy and styloidectomy plus bone graft in the treatment of old ununited carpal scaphoid fractures. Ann. Surg., *152*:296-302, 1960.
191. ———: Conservative treatment of old fractures of the carpal scaphoid. J. Trauma, *1*:115-125, 1961.
192. ———: Fractures of the carpal navicular: analysis of ninety-one cases and review of the literature. J. Bone Joint Surg., *45A*:82-112, 1963.
193. Milch, H.: Fracture of the hamate bone. J. Bone Joint Surg., *16*:459-462, 1934.
194. ———: So-called dislocation of the lower end of the ulna. Ann. Surg., *116*: 282-292, 1942.
195. ———: Colles' fracture. Bull. Hosp. Joint Dis., *11*:61-74, 1950.
196. ———: Treatment of disabilities following fracture of the lower end of the radius. Clin. Orthop., *29*:157-163, 1963.
197. Mitchell, S. W.: Injuries of Nerves and Their Consequences. Philadelphia, J. B. Lippincott, 1872.
198. Moberg, E.: The shoulder-hand-finger syndrome. Surg. Clin. North Amer., *40*: 367-373, 1960.
199. ———: Shoulder-hand-finger syndrome, reflex dystrophy, causalgia. Acta Chir. Scand., *125*:523-524, 1963.
200. ———: Discussion. J. Bone Joint Surg., *52A*:251-252, 1970.
201. Moore, E. M.: Three cases illustrating luxation of the ulna in connection with Colles' fracture. Med. Record, *17*:305-308, 1880.
202. Müller, M. E., Allgöwer, M., and Willenegger, H.: Technique of Internal Fixation of Fractures. New York, Springer-Verlag, 1965.
203. Murray, G.: Bone-graft for non-union of the carpal scaphoid. Brit. J. Surg., *22*: 63-68, 1934.

204. ———: Bone graft for non-union of the carpal scaphoid. Surg. Gynecol. Obstet., *60*:540-541, 1935.
205. ———: End results of bone-grafting for non-union of the carpal navicular. J. Bone Joint Surg., *28*:749-755, 1946.
206. Nahigian, S. H., Li, C. S., Richey, D. G., and Shaw, D. T.: The dorsal flap arthroplasty in the treatment of Kienböck's disease. J. Bone Joint Surg., *52A*:245-251, 1970.
207. Nenninger, W.: Uber die Behandlung von Kahnbeinfrakturen der Hand. Dtsch. Med. J., *6*:224-226, 1955.
208. Obletz, B. E., and Halbstein, B. M.: Non-union of fractures of the carpal navicular. J. Bone Joint Surg., *20*:424-428, 1938.
209. O'Donoghue, D. H.: Treatment of Injuries to Athletes. Philadelphia, W. B. Saunders, 1962.
210. Omer, G., and Thomas, S.: Treatment of causalgia: review of cases at Brooke General Hospital. Tex. Med., *67*:93-96, 1971.
211. O'Rahilly, R.: A survey of carpal and tarsal anomalies. J. Bone Joint Surg., *35A*:626-642, 1953.
212. Parisien, S.: Settling in Colles' fracture: a review of the literature. Bull. Hosp. Joint Dis., *34*:117-125, 1973.
213. Perey, O.: A re-examination of cases of pseudarthrosis of the navicular bone operated on according to Bentzon's technique. Acta Orthop. Scand., *23*:26-33, 1954.
214. Persson, M.: Causal treatment of lunatomalacia: further experiences of operative ulna lengthening. Acta Chir. Scand., *100*:531-544, 1950.
215. Pfitzner, W.: Beiträge zur Kenntniss des menschlichen Extremitätenskelets. VI. Die Variationen im Aufbau der Handskelets. Morphol. Arb. Jena, *4*:347-570, 1894-1895.
216. ———: Beiträge zur Kenntniss des menschlichen Extremitätenskelets. VIII. Die morphologischen Elemente des menschlichen Handskelets. Z. Morphol. Anthropol., *2*:77-157, 1900.
217. Phalen, G. S.: Calcification adjacent to the pisiform bone. J. Bone Joint Surg., *34A*:579-583, 1952.
218. Pilcher, L. S.: Fractures of the lower extremity or base of the radius. Ann. Surg., *65*:1-27, 1917.
219. Platt, H.: Colles' fracture. Brit. Med. J., *2*:288-292, 1932.
220. Pouteau, C.: Cited by Eskelund: Oeuvres Posthumes de M. Pouteau. vol. 2. Paris, P. D. Pierres, 1783.
221. Preiser, G.: Eine typische posttraumatische und zur Spontanfraktur führende Ostitis des Naviculare Carpi. Fortschr. Geb. Roentgenstr., *15*:189-197, 1910.
222. ———: Zur Frage der typischen traumatischen Ernährungsstörungen der Kurzen Hand- und Fusswurzelknochen. Fortschr. Geb. Roentgenstr., *17*:360-362, 1911.
223. Pribyl, T., Landrgot, B., and Kavan, Z.: Nase zkusenosti s lecenl′ m poraněnl′ polomesl cite′ kosti ruky. Acta Chir. Orthop. Traumatol. Cech., *34*:363-365, 1967.
224. Ralston, E. L.: Handbook of Fractures. St. Louis, C. V. Mosby, 1967.
225. Ranawat, C. S., Freiberger, R. H., Jordan, L. R., and Straub, L. R.: Arthrography in the rheumatoid wrist joint: a preliminary report. J. Bone Joint Surg., *51A*:1269-1280, 1969.
226. Redler, I.: Meniscoid of the wrist. Clin. Orthop., *88*:138-141, 1972.
227. Reeves, B.: Excision of the ulnar styloid fragment after Colles' fracture. Int. Surg., *45*:46-52, 1966.
228. Rehbein, F., and Düben, W.: Zur konservativen Behandlung des veralteten Kahnbeinbruches und der Kahnbeinpseudarthrose. Arch. Orthop. Unfallchir., *45*:67-77, 1952.
229. Reider, J. J.: Fractures of the capitate bone. US Armed Forces J., *9*:1513-1516, 1958.
230. Rittmeyer, K., and Freyschmidt, J.: Der Wert der Detailverdeutlichung bei der Beurteilung von Navikularfrakturen. Fortschr. Geb. Roentgenstr. Nuklearmed., *118*:568-573, 1973.
231. Rodholm, A. K., and Phemister, D. B.: Cyst-like lesions of carpal bones, associated with fractures, aseptic necrosis, and traumatic arthritis. J. Bone Joint Surg., *30A*:151-158, 1948.
232. Rosado, A. P.: A possible relationship of radio-carpal dislocation and dislocation of the lunate bone. J. Bone Joint Surg., *48B*:504-506, 1966.
233. Rose-Innes, A. P.: Anterior dislocation of the ulna at the inferior radio-ulnar joint: case reports, with a discussion of the anatomy of rotation of the forearm. J. Bone Joint Surg., *42B*:515-521, 1960.
234. Rothberg, A. S.: Fractures of the carpal navicular: importance of special roentgenography. J. Bone Joint Surg., *21*:1020-1022, 1939.

235. Russe, O.: Fracture of the carpal navicular: diagnosis, non-operative treatment, and operative treatment. J. Bone Joint Surg., *42A*:759-768, 1960.
236. Russell, T. B.: Inter-carpal dislocations and fracture-dislocations: a review of fifty-nine cases. J. Bone Joint Surg., *31B*: 524-531, 1949.
237. Sarmiento, A.: The brachioradialis as a deforming force in Colles' fractures. Clin. Orthop., *38*:86-92, 1965.
238. Schallmayer, J., and Hertel, E.: Zur Ruhigstellung des Handgelenkes bei der Kahnbeinfraktur. Zentralbl. Chir., *94*:89-98, 1968.
239. Scheck, M.: Long-term follow-up of treatment of comminuted fractures of the distal end of the radius by transfixation with Kirschner wires and cast. J. Bone Joint Surg., *44A*:337-351, 1962.
240. Schnek, F.: Die Behandlung der verzögerten Callusbildung des Os naviculare manus mit der Beck'schen Bohrung. Zentralbl. Chir., *57*:2600-2603, 1930.
241. ———: Die Verletzungen der Handwurzel. Ergeb. Chir. Orthop., *23*:1-109, 1930.
242. Sebald, J. R., Dobyns, J. H., and Linscheid, R. L.: The natural history of collapse deformities of the wrist. Clin. Orthop., *104*:140-148, 1974.
243. Seimon, L. P.: Compound dislocation of the trapezium: a case report. J. Bone Joint Surg., *54A*:1297-1300, 1972.
244. Sherwin, J. M., Nagel, D. A., and Southwick, W. O.: Bipartite carpal navicular and the diagnostic problem of bone partition: a case report. J. Trauma, *11*:440-443, 1971.
245. Siegel, M. W., and Hertzberg, H.: Complete dislocation of the greater multangular (trapezium): a case report. J. Bone Joint Surg., *51A*:769-772, 1969.
246. Smaill, G. B.: Long-term follow-up of Colles' fracture. J. Bone Joint Surg., *47B*: 80-85, 1965.
247. Smith, F. M.: Late rupture of extensor pollicis longus tendon following Colles' fracture. J. Bone Joint Surg., *28*:49-59, 1946.
248. Smith, L., and Friedman, B.: Treatment of ununited fracture of the carpal navicular by styloidectomy of the radius. J. Bone Joint Surg., *38A*:368-375, 1956.
249. Smith, R. W.: A Treatise on Fractures in the Vicinity of Joints, and on Certain Forms of Accidental and Congenital Dislocations. Dublin, Hodges & Smith, 1854.
250. Snook, G. A., Chrisman, O. D., Wilson, T. C., and Wietsma, R. D.: Subluxation of the distal radio-ulnar joint by hyperpronation. J. Bone Joint Surg., *51A*:1315-1323, 1969.
251. Soto-Hall, R.: Recent fractures of the carpal scaphoid. J.A.M.A., *129*:335-338, 1945.
252. Soto-Hall, R., and Haldeman, K. O.: Treatment of fractures of the carpal scaphoid. J. Bone Joint Surg., *16*:822-828, 1934.
253. ———: The conservative and operative treatment of fractures of the carpal scaphoid (navicular). J. Bone Joint Surg., *23*: 841-850, 1941.
254. Speed, J. S., and Knight, R. A.: Treatment of malunited Colles' fractures. J. Bone Joint Surg., *27*:361-367, 1945.
255. Speed, K.: Traumatic Injuries of the Carpus, Including Colles' Fracture. New York, D. Appleton & Co., 1925.
256. Spinner, M., and Kaplan, E. B.: Extensor carpi ulnaris: its relationship to the stability of the distal radio-ulnar joint. Clin. Orthop., *68*:124-129, 1970.
257. Stack, J. K.: End results of excision of the carpal bones. Arch. Surg., *57*:245-251, 1948.
258. Stahl, F.: On lunatomalacia (Kienböck's disease): a clinical and roentgenological study, especially on its pathogenesis and the late results of immobilization treatment. Acta Chir. Scand., *126* [Suppl.]: 1-133, 1947.
259. Stark, W. A.: Recurrent perilunar subluxation. Clin. Orthop., *73*:152, 1970.
260. Stein, A. H., Jr.: Dorsal dislocation of the lesser multangular bone. J. Bone Joint Surg., *53A*:377-379, 1971.
261. Stein, F., and Siegel, M. W.: Naviculocapitate fracture syndrome: a case report; new thoughts on the mechanism of injury. J. Bone Joint Surg., *51A*:391-395, 1969.
262. Steinbrocker, O., and Argyros, T. G.: The shoulder-hand syndrome: present status as a diagnostic and therapeutic entity. Med. Clin. North Amer., *42*:1533-1553, 1958.
263. Stewart, M. J.: Fractures of the carpal navicular (scaphoid): a report of 436 cases. J. Bone Joint Surg., *36A*:998-1006, 1954.
264. Sudeck, P.: Ueber die akute entzündliche Knochenatrophie. Arch. Klin. Chir., *62*: 147-156, 1900.
265. ———: Uber die akute (reflektorische) Knochenatrophie nach Entzündungen und Verletzungen an den Extremitäten und ihre klinischen Erscheinungen.

Fortschr. Geb. Roentgenstr., *5*:277-297, 1901-1902.
266. Sund, C.: Ein gleichzeitiger, beidseitiger de Quervainscher Verrenkungsbruch der Hand. Monatsschr. Unfallheilkd., *71*:114-119, 1968.
267. Swanson, A. B.: Silicone rubber implants for the replacement of the carpal scaphoid and lunate bones. Orthop. Clin. North Amer., *1*:299-309, 1970.
268. ———: Flexible implant resection arthroplasty in the hand and extremities. St. Louis, C. V. Mosby, 1973.
269. Tajima, T.: An investigation of the treatment of Kienböck's disease (abstr.). J. Bone Joint Surg., *48A*:1649, 1966.
270. Taleisnik, J., and Kelly, P. J.: The extraosseous and intraosseous blood supply of the scaphoid bone. J. Bone Joint Surg., *48A*:1125-1137, 1966.
271. Tanz, S. S.: Rotation effect in lunar and perilunar dislocations. Clin. Orthop., *57*:147-152, 1968.
272. Taylor, A. R.: Dislocation of the Scaphoid. Postgrad. Med. J., *45*:186-189, 1969.
273. Thomas, F. B.: Reduction of Smith's Fracture. J. Bone Joint Surg., *39B*:463-470, 1957.
274. Thompson, T. C., Campbell, R. D., Jr., and Arnold, W. D.: Primary and secondary dislocation of the scaphoid bone. J. Bone Joint Surg., *46B*:73-82, 1964.
275. Tillberg, B.: Kienboeck's disease treated with osteotomy to lengthen ulna. Acta Orthop. Scand., *39*:359-368, 1968.
276. Torisu, T.: Fracture of the hook of the hamate by a golfswing. Clin. Orthop., *83*:91-94, 1972.
277. Trevor, D.: Rupture of the extensor pollicis longus tendon after Colles fracture. J. Bone Joint Surg., *32B*:370-375, 1950.
278. Turek, S. L.: Orthopaedics: Principles and Their Application. ed. 2. Philadelphia, J. B. Lippincott, 1967.
279. Unger, H. S., and Stryker, W. C.: Nonunion of the carpal navicular: analysis of 42 cases treated by the Russe procedure. South Med. J., *62*:620-622, 1969.
280. Vasilas, A., Grieco, R. V., and Bartone, N. F.: Roentgen aspects of injuries to the pisiform bone and pisotriquetral joint. J. Bone Joint Surg., *42A*:1317-1328, 1960.
281. Vaughan-Jackson, O. J.: A case of recurrent subluxation of the carpal scaphoid. J. Bone Joint Surg., *31B*:532-533, 1949.
282. Verdan, C.: Fractures of the scaphoid. Surg. Clin. North Amer., *40*:461-464, 1960.
283. Vesely, D. G.: The distal radio-ulnar joint. Clin. Orthop., *51*:75-91, 1967.
284. Volkmann, R.: Die ischaemischen Muskellähmungen und Kontrakturen. Zentrabl. Chir., *8*:801-805, 1881.
285. Von Lanz, T., and Wachsmuth, W.: Praktische Anatomie: Ein Lehr- und Hilfsbuch der anatomischen Grundlagen ärztlichen Handelns. ed. 1. vol. 1. Berlin, Springer-Verlag, 1938.
286. ———: Praktische Anatomie: Ein Lehr- und Hilfsbuch der anatomischen Grundlagen ärztlichen Handelns. ed. 2. vol. 1. Berlin, Springer-Verlag, 1959.
287. Wagner, C. J.: Fractures of the carpal navicular. J. Bone Joint Surg., *34A*:774-784, 1952.
288. ———: Perilunar dislocations. J. Bone Joint Surg., *38A*:1198-1207, 1956.
289. ———: Fracture-dislocations of the wrist. Clin. Orthop., *15*:181-196, 1959.
290. Walker, G. B. W.: Dislocation of the carpal scaphoid reduced by open operation. Brit. J. Surg., *30*:380-381, 1943.
291. Watson-Jones, R.: Inadequate immobilization and non-union of fractures. Brit. Med. J., *1*:936-939, 1934.
292. ———: Fractures and Joint Injuries. ed. 4. vol. 2. Baltimore, Williams & Wilkins, 1955.
293. Waugh, R. L., and Sullivan, R. F.: Anomalies of the carpus: with particular reference to the bipartite scaphoid (navicular). J. Bone Joint Surg., *32A*:682-686, 1950.
294. Waugh, R. L., and Yancey, A. G.: Carpometacarpal dislocations: with particular reference to simultaneous dislocation of the bases of the fourth and fifth metacarpals. J. Bone Joint Surg., *30A*:397-404, 1948.
295. Weber, E. R., Chao, E. Y. S., and Linscheid, R. L.: Biomechanical Analysis of the Dorsiflexed Wrist With Emphasis on Scaphoid Waist Fracture. Read at the Annual Meeting of the Orthopaedic Research Society, Dallas, January 17, 1974.
296. Weigl, K., and Spira, E.: The triangular fibrocartilage of the wrist joint. Reconstr. Surg. Traumatol., *11*:139-153, 1969.
297. Weiss, C., Laskin, R. S., and Spinner, M.: Irreducible radiocarpal dislocation: a case report. J. Bone Joint Surg., *52A*:562-564, 1970.
298. Weseley, M. S., and Barenfeld, P. A.: Trans-scaphoid, transcapitate, transtriquetral, perilunate fracture-dislocation of

the wrist: a case report. J. Bone Joint Surg., *54A*:1073-1078, 1972.

299. Weston, W. J., and Kelsey, C. K.: Functional anatomy of the pisi-cuneiform joint. Brit. J. Radiol., *46*:692-694, 1973.
300. White, E. H.: Bilateral congenital fusion of carpal capitate and hamate. Amer. J. Roentgenol. Radium. Ther. Nucl. Med., *52*:406-407, 1944.
301. Whitefield, G. A.: Recurrent dislocation of the carpal scaphoid bone (abstr.). J. Bone Joint Surg., *44B*:963, 1962.
302. Wilson, J. N.: Profiles of the carpal canal. J. Bone Joint Surg., *36A*:127-132, 1954.
303. Wiot, J. F., and Dorst, J. P.: Less common fractures and dislocations of the wrist. Radiol. Clin. North Amer., *4*:261-276, 1966.
304. Wright, R. D.: A detailed study of movement of the wrist joint. J. Anat., *70*:137-142, 1935.
305. Zoëga, H.: Fracture of the lower end of the radius with ulnar nerve palsy. J. Bone Joint Surg., *48B*:514-516, 1966.

8 Fractures of the Shafts of the Radius and Ulna

Lewis D. Anderson, M.D.

Chapter 7 included a discussion of fractures of the distal radius and the ulna, and Chapter 9 deals with fractures of the olecranon and radial head. This chapter therefore is confined to fractures of the shaft of both bones of the forearm, single fractures of the radius, and single fractures of the ulna in adults.

I can find no eponym associated with fractures of both bones of the forearm. The fracture of the shaft of the ulna with associated dislocation of the radial head was first described by G. B. Monteggia[43,50] in 1814 and has been known as the Monteggia fracture since that time. The single bone fracture of the ulna without dislocation of the radial head is often called a "nightstick fracture," an obvious reference to one of the mechanisms of injury. The single bone fracture of the radius in the distal third associated with dislocation of the radioulnar joint has several eponyms. Galeazzi[29,50] of Italy called attention to this treacherous injury in 1934, and since then it has frequently been referred to as Galeazzi's fracture. This combination of injuries is also known as the Piedmont fracture. Hughston[32] of Columbus, Georgia, collected a series of 41 fractures treated by members of the Piedmont Orthopaedic Society and pointed out the difficulties encountered in its treatment. Hughston noted that the French referred to the fracture of the distal radius with dislocation of the ulna as a "reverse Monteggia fracture." In Memphis and among graduates of the Campbell Foundation—University of Tennessee Residency Program, one frequently hears this injury called the "fracture of necessity." The origin of this description goes back to Dr. Willis C. Campbell's early days when he emphasized that this was a fracture in which poor results could be expected with closed treatment.[61] Campbell believed that open reduction was a necessity.

SURGICAL ANATOMY

As has been pointed out in many articles and books[49,54,67] dealing with the treatment of forearm fractures, the surgical anatomy of the forearm creates problems in dealing with these fractures not found in the treatment of diaphyseal fractures of other long bones. The radius and ulna are approximately parallel, but they touch only at ends. They are bound together proximally by the capsule of the elbow joint and the annular ligament, and distally by the capsule of the wrist joint, the anterior and posterior radioulnar ligaments, and the fibrocartilaginous articular disc. The proximal and distal joints are very complex in both function and structure and are really many joints and not just two. They include the proximal and distal radioulnar joints and the ulnohumeral, radiohumeral and radiocarpal joints. The ulna is a relatively straight bone, but the radius is much more complex. In a study of 100 radii from cadavers, Sage[55] pointed out

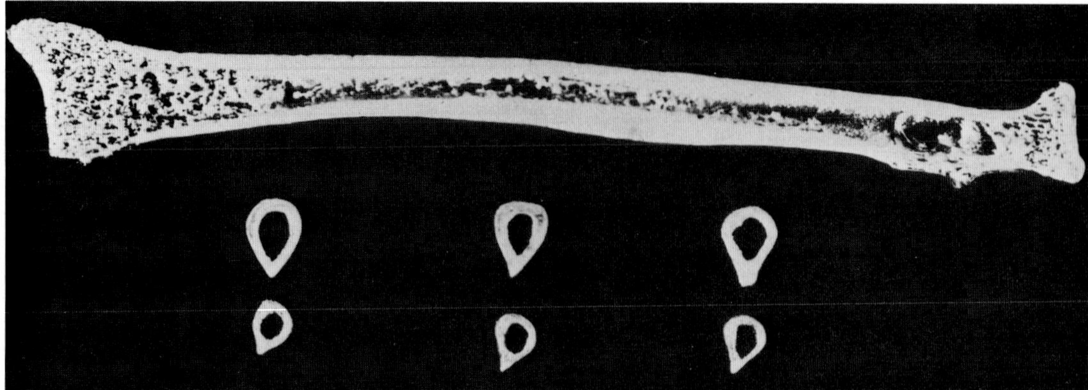

Fig. 8-1. A cross-section contour of the medullary canal of two radii at three points along the diaphysis. (Sage, F. P.: J. Bone Joint Surg., *41A*:1489-1516, 1959)

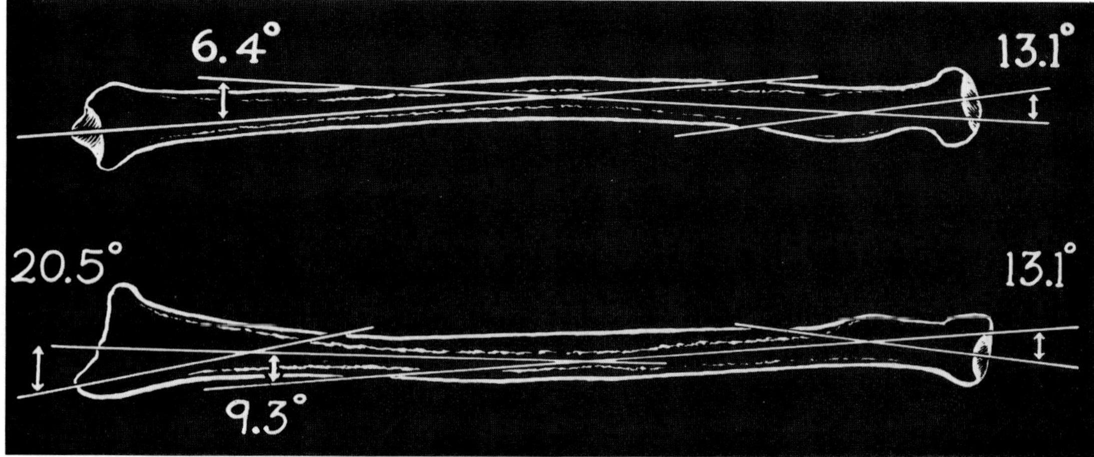

Fig. 8-2. Schematic drawings to show the two distal and two proximal angles in the longitudinal axis of the radial medullary canal. (Sage, F. P.: J. Bone Joint Surg., *41A*: 1489-1516, 1959)

the complexity of the angles and curves in this bone and the importance of maintaining them, especially the lateral bow of the radius, in achieving full pronation and supination after fracture (Figs. 8-1, 8-2).

Between the shafts of the ulna and radius is the interosseous space. The fibers of the interosseous membrane run obliquely across the interosseous space from their distal insertion on the ulna to their proximal origin on the radius. The strength of the interosseous membrane and the oblique arrangement of the fibers are what make it possible to resect the radial head when indicated and still have good function of the forearm.

Not only are the forearm bones themselves and their associated joints complex, but the muscle groups acting across the forearm cause complex deforming forces when fractures are present. The radius and ulna are joined by three muscles—the supinator, pronator teres, and pronator quadratus—which take origin on one bone and insert on the other. In addition to their named functions, when there is a fracture these muscles tend to approximate the radius and ulna and decrease the interosseous space.

As Sage[54] has pointed out, the forearm muscles which take origin on the volar side

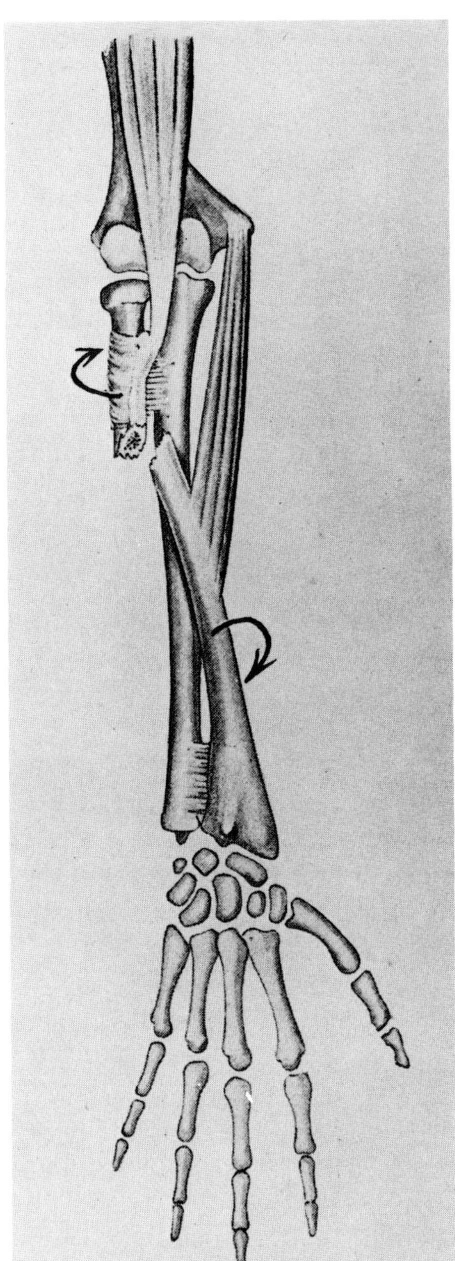

Fig. 8-3. In a fracture of the upper shaft of the radius between the insertion of the supinator and pronator teres the proximal fragment is supinated and the lower fragment pronated. (Watson-Jones, R.: Fractures and Joint Injuries. vol. 2. ed. 4. Edinburgh, E. & S. Livingstone, 1955)

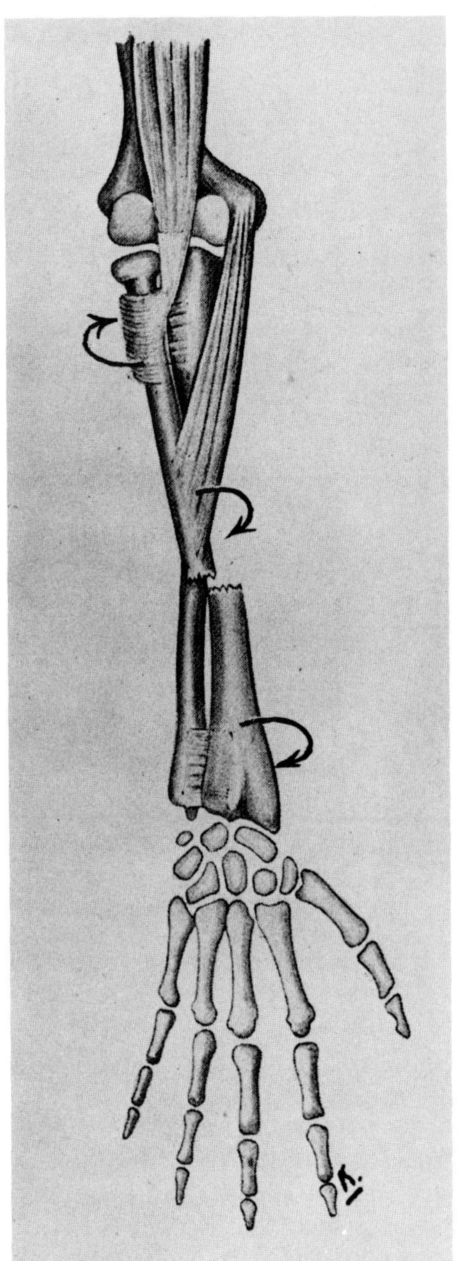

Fig. 8-4. In a fracture of the middle or lower shaft between the insertions of the pronator teres and the pronator quadratus the proximal fragment is in mid position. (Watson-Jones, R.: Fractures and Joint Injuries. vol. 2. ed. 4. Edinburgh, E. & S. Livingstone, 1955)

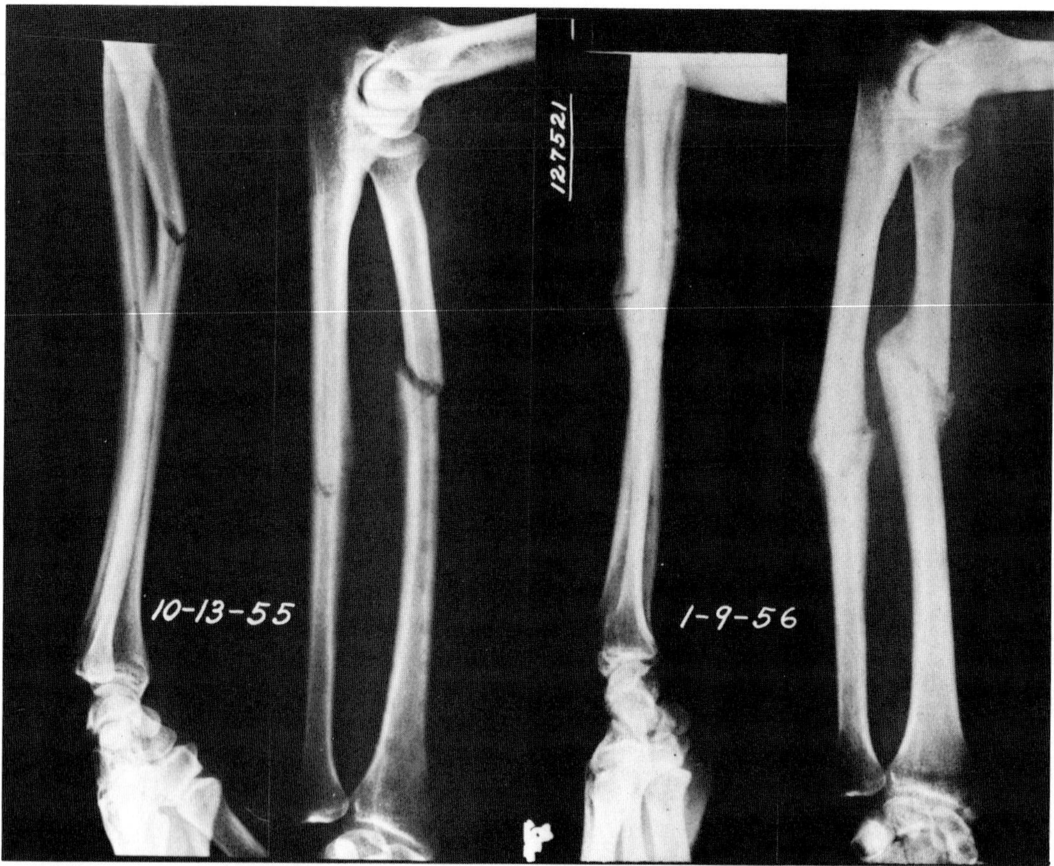

Fig. 8-5. A fracture of the proximal shaft of the radius and mid-shaft of the ulna treated by closed reduction and cast immobilization. Three months later the fracture has healed with loss of the radial bow and ulnar angulation. Pronation and supination were severely limited.

of the ulna and insert on the radial side of the wrist or hand, such as the flexor carpi radialis, tend to exert a pronating force. In a similar manner, the muscles such as the abductor pollicis longus and brevis and the extensor pollicis longus, which have their origins on the ulna and interosseous membrane on the dorsal side and are inserted on the radial side of the dorsum of the wrist, tend to exert a supinating force.

In addition to the supinator muscle itself, the biceps brachii is a powerful supinator of the radius. In fractures of the upper radius below the insertion of the supinator and above the insertion of the pronator teres there are two strong muscles that exert an unopposed force so that the proximal radial fragment comes to lie in maximum supination (Fig. 8-3). In fractures of the radius located distal to the pronator teres, the force of the supinator and biceps are somewhat neutralized. In these fractures the proximal fragment of the radius is usually in a slightly supinated or neutral position (Fig. 8-4). In closed treatment of forearm fractures therefore, the location of the fracture of the radius determines the degree of supination of the distal fragment needed to provide correct rotational alignment.

If satisfactory functional results are to be achieved in the treatment of fractures of the forearm, it is not sufficient to maintain the length of each bone. Axial and rotational alignment must be achieved as well, and the radial bow must be maintained. With the complexity of the bones and of the joints involved, and the many and varied deforming muscle forces, it is extremely difficult to obtain union with adequate restoration of the anatomy to ensure good functional results by closed treatment (Fig. 8-5). For these reasons most recent articles in the literature recommend some form of open reduction and internal fixation for displaced diaphyseal fractures of the forearm in adults.[2,3,22,54,59]

FRACTURES OF BOTH THE RADIUS AND ULNA

MECHANISM OF INJURY

The mechanisms of injury that cause fractures of the shaft of the radius and ulna are myriad. The most common by far is some form of vehicular accident. The injured person may have been driving or riding as a passenger, or he may have been a pedestrian. Motorcycle accidents have caused an increasing number of these fractures in recent years. Usually the patient does not know exactly what happened because of the sudden nature of the accident. Probably most of these vehicular accidents result in some type of direct blow to the forearm.

Automobile accidents are not the only source of direct blow injuries. For orthopaedists working in city and county hospitals, fights in which one of the adversaries is struck on the forearm with a stick is a frequent history. Not only do Monteggia and nightstick fractures result from this kind of blow but fractures of both bones as well. The person throws his forearm up to protect his head and the forearm is the recipient of the violence.

Pathological fractures of the forearm bones are not common. If they are excluded, most of the remainder of shaft fractures of the forearm bones result from some type of fall. The fall is usually worse than the minor fall required to cause a Colles' fracture. Most forearm shaft fractures resulting from falls occur in athletics or in falls from heights such as ladders or roofs.

CLASSIFICATION

Fractures of both bones of the forearm are usually classified according to the level of the fracture, the degree of displacement and angulation, the presence or absence of comminution, and whether they are open or closed. Each of these factors may have some bearing on the type of treatment to be selected and the ultimate prognosis.

SIGNS AND SYMPTOMS

Undisplaced diaphyseal fractures of the shafts of both bones of the forearm in adults are rare. An injury of sufficient force to break both the radius and ulna is almost always sufficient to cause displacement. Because shaft fractures of both the radius and ulna are usually displaced, the signs and symptoms usually make the diagnosis obvious. They include pain, deformity, and loss of function of the forearm and hand. Palpation along the subcutaneous border of the ulna usually elicits tenderness at the level of the fracture. Some degree of swelling is almost always present and is usually related to both the force causing the injury and the time since injury. The examiner should not attempt to elicit crepitus, because this may cause additional soft-tissue damage. However, it is usually noted as the forearm is aligned for splinting.

The examination should include a careful neurological evaluation of the motor and sensory functions of the radial, median, and ulnar nerves. Neurological deficits are not common in closed fractures of the shafts of the radius and ulna, but they do occur. Open fractures, especially those caused by gunshot wounds, frequently have associated nerve and major blood vessel involvement, and this must be carefully evaluated. In open fractures it is a mistake to probe the wound in the emergency room to determine the degree of soft-tissue injury. This may carry contamination deeper into the wound and increase the risk of infection. The soft-

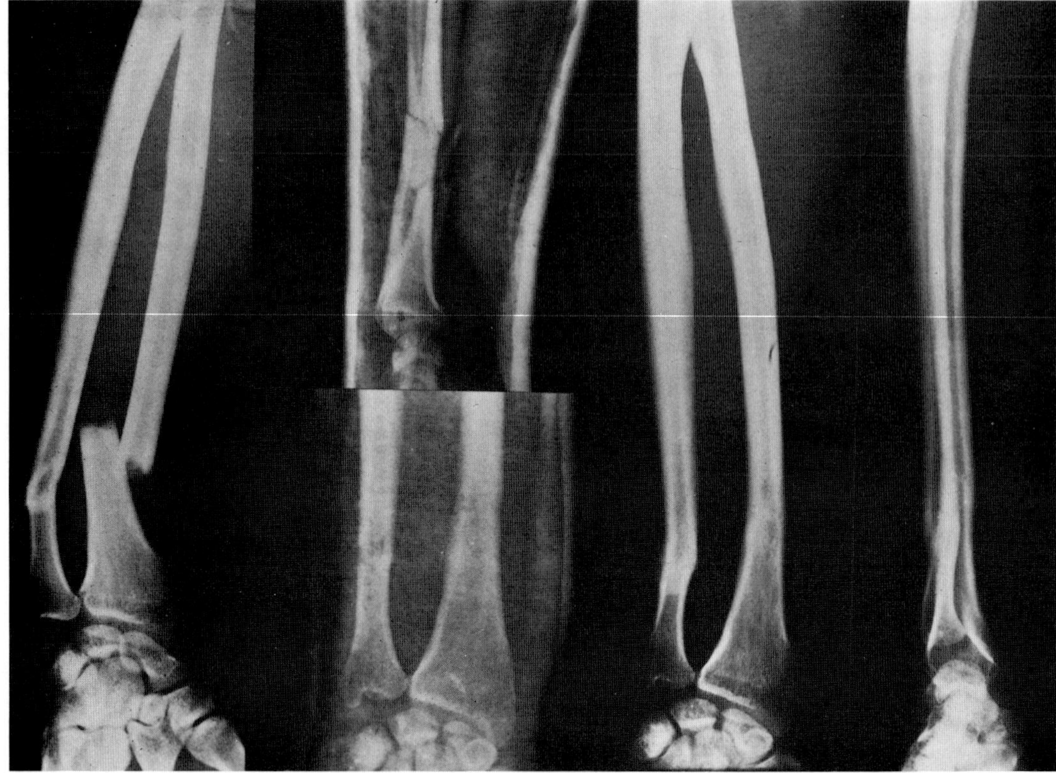

Fig. 8-6. Satisfactory closed reduction and cast fixation in fractures of the distal third of the radius and ulna. The fractures united with only mild narrowing of the interosseous space. (Sage, F. P.: Fractures of the shaft of the radius and ulna in the adult. *In* Adams, J. P., (ed.): Current Practice in Orthopaedic Surgery. vol. 1. St. Louis, C. V. Mosby, 1963)

tissue damage can be evaluated much better and more safely at the time of formal debridement in the operating room.

ROENTGENOGRAPHIC FINDINGS

Just as the clinical signs and symptoms are usually obvious in shaft fractures of both bones of the forearm, so are the roentgenographic signs. The degree of offset and angulation should be noted, as well as the amount of shortening, angulation, and comminution. Occasionally one of the fractures may be segmental. Care must be taken to include the elbow and wrist joints in the films to ascertain if there is an associated dislocation or articular fracture.

The nutrient foramen of the radius sometimes is quite prominent in the anteroposterior roentgenograms and can be confused with an undisplaced fracture by one not familiar with its location and appearance. It is located at about the junction of the proximal and middle thirds of the radius and enters obliquely from distal to proximal. Because it is not usually visualized on the lateral or oblique views anyone who knows what it looks like should not be confused.

METHODS OF TREATMENT

Undisplaced Fractures

Undisplaced fractures of the shafts of *both* the radius and ulna in adults are rare. It hardly seems justified to perform open reduction and internal fixation for a true undisplaced fracture as the initial treatment. It should be immobilized in a well molded long-arm cast in neutral pronation-supination with the elbow flexed 90 degrees. An initially undisplaced fracture of this sort can become displaced while immobilized in plaster. For this reason roentgenograms should be made in both the anteroposterior and lateral planes at weekly intervals for the first several weeks to be sure displacement does not occur. If it does, the treatment is then the same as for those fractures that are displaced when first seen.

Displaced Fractures

The treatment for displaced fractures of the shafts of the radius and ulna is difficult. The choices available include closed treatment, on the one hand, and open reduction and some form of internal fixation on the other.

Closed Reduction and External Fixation

The results of closed treatment in most series[32,46] have proved unsatisfactory in a high percentage of cases. For the reasons outlined in the discussion of surgical anatomy, it is difficult to reduce and maintain satisfactory position of the fragments. Knight and Purvis[35] analyzed 100 adults with shaft fractures of both bones of the forearm treated at the Campbell Clinic, of which approximately half had been treated by closed methods. Of those treated closed, 71 per cent had unsatisfactory results, and the incidence of nonunion and malunion was high. In our hands closed reduction has been more successful for fractures of both the radius and ulna when the fractures are located in the distal third of the bones (Fig. 8-6). If closed treatment is undertaken, the patient must be warned that the treatment may have to be changed to an open method at any time in order to assure solid union in an acceptable position.

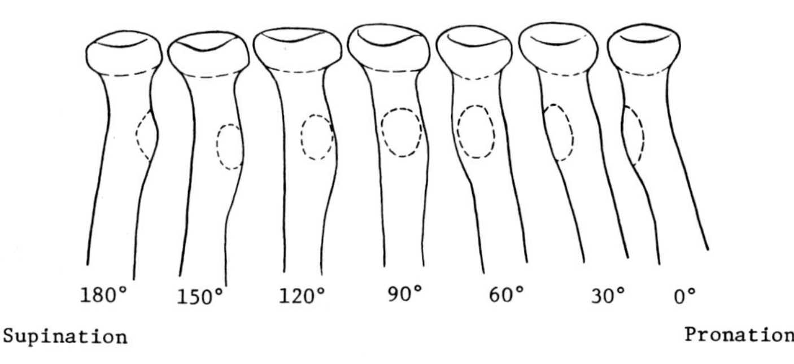

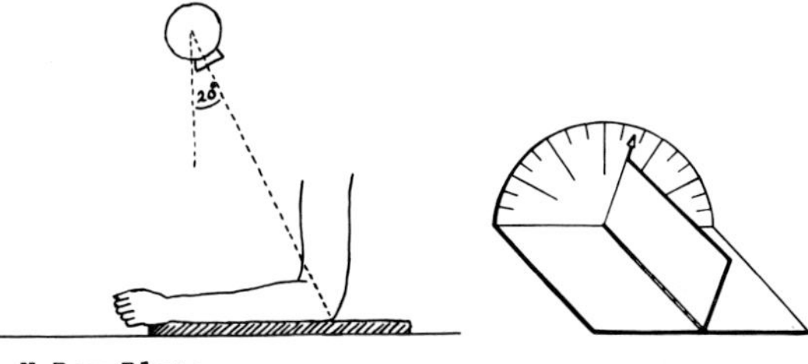

Fig. 8-7. Method of taking "tuberosity view." The position of the humeral condyles should be equal distance from the x-ray film. The appearance of the bicipital tuberosity of the radius is shown at the top in different degrees of pronation and supination. The protractor for measuring rotation is shown at the bottom right. The hand is laid against the vertical plate, and the degree of rotation is read from the calibrated scale. (Evans, E. M.: J. Bone Joint Surg., 27:373-379, 1945)

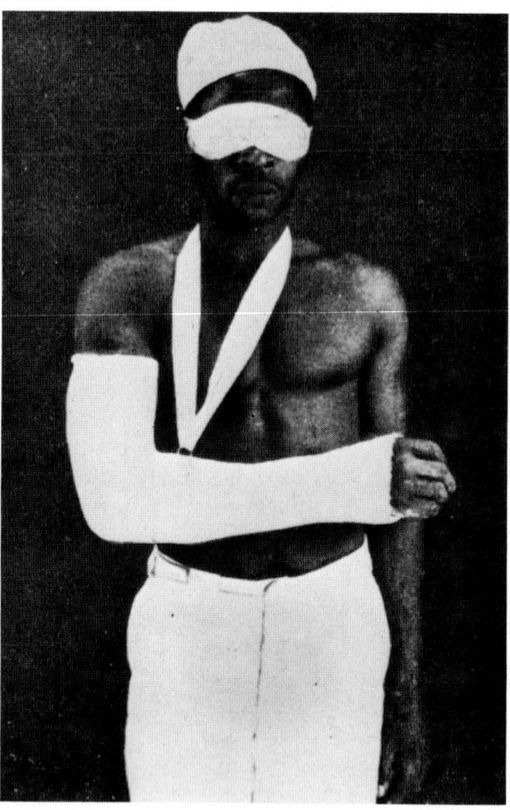

Fig. 8-8. The proper method of suspending a cast by a sling so that the ulnar border of the cast is kept snugly against the forearm to prevent ulnar angulation. (Knight, R. A., and Purvis, G. D.: J. Bone Joint Surg., *31A*:755-764, 1949)

As was pointed out earlier, if good results are to be obtained not only must longitudinal alignment be correct but also rotational alignment. The rotational alignment is difficult to determine in the ordinary anteroposterior and lateral roentgenograms. The view of the tuberosity recommended by Evans[28] is often helpful (Fig. 8-7). Because the surgeon has no control over the proximal radial fragment with closed methods, he must bring the distal radial fragment into correct relationship with the proximal one. Ascertaining the rotation of the proximal fragment from the tuberosity view prior to reduction gives some idea of how much pronation or supination of the distal fragment is needed. The tuberosity view is made with the x-ray tube tilted 20 degrees toward the olecranon with both humeral condyles and the subcutaneous border of the ulna flat on the cassette. The roentgenogram can then be compared with a diagram showing the prominence of the tubercle in various degrees of pronation or supination. As an alternative, a film of the opposite elbow can be made in a given degree of rotation for comparison.

As a practical matter, I rarely attempt closed treatment for displaced fractures of both bones of the forearm in adults, unless some other condition of the patient prohibits surgery. The results are too uncertain and the period of immobilization too long.

Technique of Closed Reduction. Good relaxation of the muscles is mandatory for closed reduction, and general anesthesia is usually best. When the patient is anesthetized, a tuberosity view is obtained if that has not already been done. Finger traps or clove hitches of gauze are then placed on the thumb, index, and middle finger to suspend the extremity from an overhead frame or intravenous stand with muslin so that the elbow is flexed 90 degrees. Another strip of muslin is used to make a loop over the distal arm about 3 inches above the elbow. This is tied at a convenient height from the floor so that the surgeon's foot can be placed in it for countertraction. The loop over the distal humerus is padded to prevent excessive pressure. Traction and countertraction are applied while the ulna is palpated, and an attempt is made to reduce it. The radius usually cannot be palpated in the proximal half because of the swelling and overlying muscles. The forearm is placed in the appropriate amount of supination as determined by the tuberosity view. When the fractures seem reduced and the alignment of the forearm appears good, a layer of padding is applied from the midpalmar crease to above the elbow with an extra layer over the bony prominences. A sugar tong splint is then applied and molded well as it sets. Anteroposterior and lateral views are taken to determine if the reduction is proper. Anything less than near anatomical reduction should not be accepted. If the reduction is not acceptable, the sugar tong is removed and the fractures are remanipulated. Once reduction is acceptable, the muslin loop is removed from the upper arm and the sugar tong is converted into a well molded, full, long-arm circular cast while the extremity is still suspended. As the cast hardens, the plaster is flattened in the area posterior to the distal humerus to prevent the cast from slipping distally.

The completed cast should extend from the midpalmar crease and metacarpal necks to the axilla. The suspension is removed and a final set of films is made. A wire or plaster loop is then incorporated on the radial side of the forearm proximal to the level of the fractures. Suspending this loop in the cast from the patient's neck with a sling helps prevent angulation of the fractures by keeping the cast snugged up against the ulna (Fig. 8-8).[46] The loop should never be placed distal to the fracture, for this increases the chance of angulation (Fig. 8-9).

After Care. The circulation and function of the hand must be observed carefully until the swelling begins to decrease. During this period the arm should be suspended from an overhead frame with the fingers uppermost. Active flexion and extension of the fingers should be carried out at frequent intervals to help reduce edema. If at any time the circulation appears in jeopardy, the cast should be cut completely down to the skin from hand to axilla on two sides. A loss of reduction is not nearly so bad as gangrene or ischemic contracture.

Roentgenograms in two planes should be made at weekly intervals through the cast for the first month and every 2 weeks thereafter until union is solid. Each new set of films should be compared to the *original films of the reduction that were accepted.* A common error is to compare the most recent films with the films from the previous visit. If this is done a gradual loss of reduction goes undetected until it is too late.

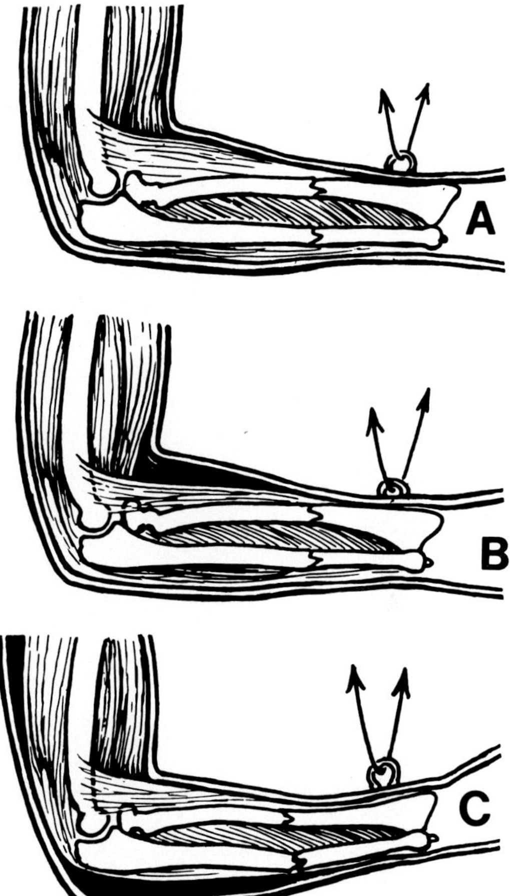

Fig. 8-9. Angulation of the radius and ulna during the period of cast immobilization is illustrated. (*A*) Immediately after reduction the cast fits snugly. (*B*) Atrophy of forearm muscles has taken place with consequent loosening of the cast in the upper half of the forearm. (*C*) Cast has sagged while still holding distal fragment firmly, thus causing angulation of radius and ulna. (Knight, R. A., and Purvis, G. D.: J. Bone Joint Surg., *31A*:755-764, 1949)

The cast should be changed at intervals of 4 to 6 weeks. Each new cast must be applied as carefully as the first one. These fractures can angulate even after some callus is present. There is no margin for error due to a sloppily applied cast.

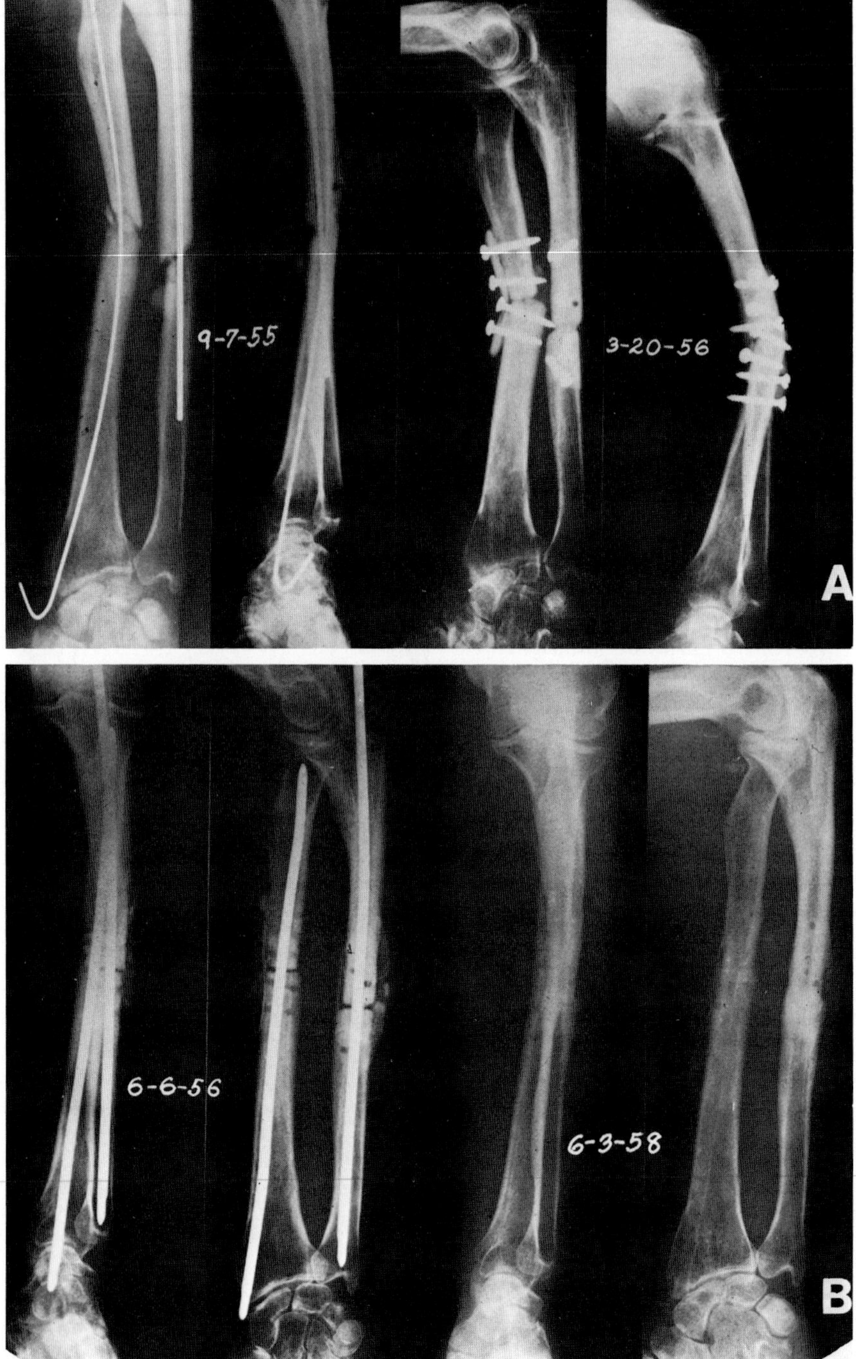

Fig. 8-10. (*A*) Failure of union in a fracture of both bones of the forearm resulted from inadequate fixation with Kirschner wires as medullary nails. A second procedure using cortical onlay bone grafts also resulted in failure. (*B*) Eleven months after injury rigid medullary fixation was achieved with Sage triangular nails. Two years later the nails have been removed. Union is good. (Sage, F. P.: J. Bone Joint Surg., *41A*:1489-1516, 1959)

Open Reduction and Internal Fixation

Over the years many methods of open reduction and internal fixation have been advocated. Open reduction without internal fixation has all the disadvantages of both open and closed treatment and has no place in the modern treatment of fractures of the shaft of the radius and ulna in adults.

In the early 1900's Lane[6,40,41] of London and Lambotte[6,38,39] of Belgium reported the use of plates on diaphyseal fractures. However, metal reaction led to frequent failures until modern metals for implantation were introduced in 1937 after the work of Venable and Stuck[66] on electrolysis. Campbell[16] used autogenous tibial grafts fixed to the radius and ulna with bone pegs or screws for acute fractures as well as nonunion. Some of these were successful, but unless external immobilization was very prolonged the grafts often developed fatigue fractures before they were revascularized.[35]

Fixation with Medullary Nails. After medullary nailing became popular for fractures of the femur in the late 1940's, various devices for medullary fixation of the radius and ulna were used. In 1957 Smith and Sage[58] reported a series of 555 fractures collected from all over the country in which some form of medullary fixation had been carried out. The devices included Rush pins, Kirschner wires, Steinmann pins, Lottes nails, and Küntscher V-nails. The results were discouraging (Fig. 8-10). Nonunion resulted in over 20 per cent of the fractures, and malunion and poor function were frequent in those that did unite. The radial bow was not maintained, and the use of a round pin in a round medullary canal could not control rotation of the fragments (Fig. 8-11). Caden[15] reported a nonunion rate of 16.6 per cent in forearm fractures treated with Rush pins.

In 1959 Sage[55] published his study of the anatomy of the radius and introduced Sage triangular forearm medullary nails. The nails for the ulna are straight and are inserted in a retrograde manner. The nail for the radius is bent to aid in maintaining the radial bow (Fig. 8-12). It is introduced from the radial styloid and driven proximally (Fig. 8-13). The ulnar nail is relatively easy to insert, but the technique for inserting the radial nail is more difficult and exacting. Sage reported good results with his nails (Fig. 8-14). Nonunion resulted in only 6.2 per cent; delayed union, in 4.9 per cent. Other triangular or rectangular nails for the forearm bones were introduced by Ritchie[52] and Street.[62] These also grip the

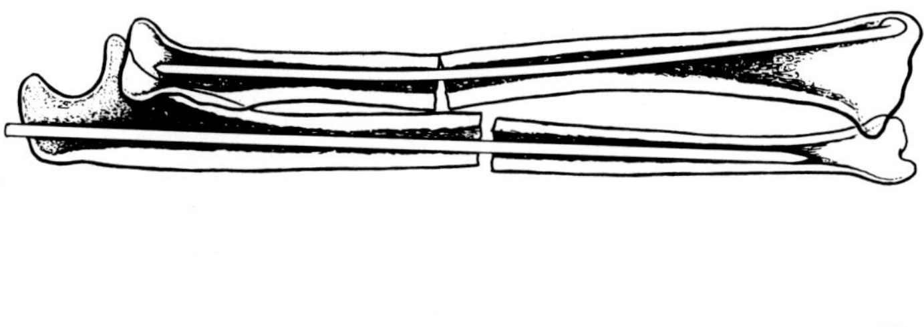

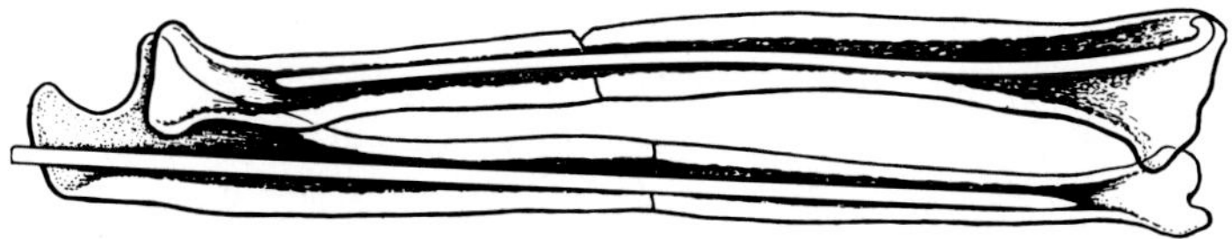

Fig. 8-11. When medullary pins are used in both bones, fixation of the radius must be sufficiently stable to prevent collapse of the radial arch; otherwise, there will be a relative elongation of the radius with distraction of the ulnar fracture, and nonunion may result in either or both bones. (Smith, H., and Sage, F. P.: J. Bone Joint Surg., 39A:91-98, 1957)

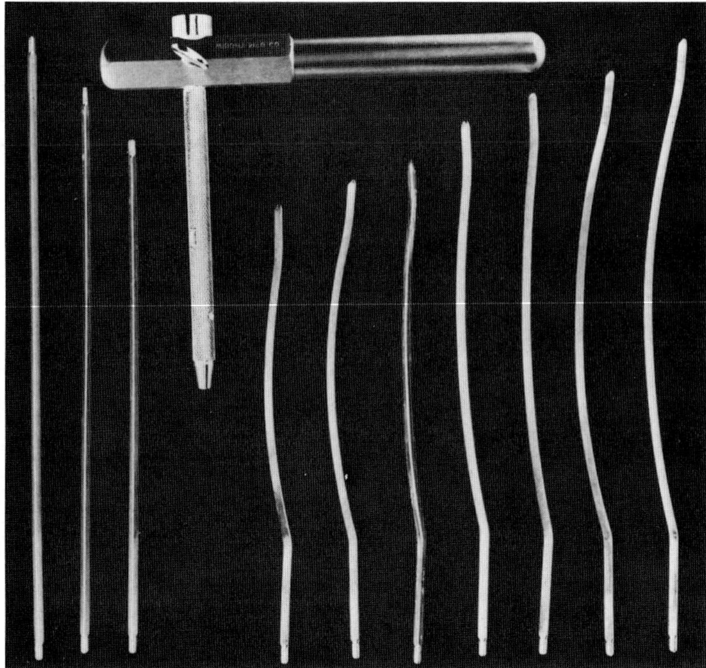

Fig. 8-12. The Sage driver-extractor and full complement of Sage nails for the radius and ulna. (Sage, F. P.: J. Bone Joint Surg., *41A*:1489-1516, 1959)

cortex well and control rotation but do not preserve the radial bow as well as the Sage nail.

Sage nails are not recommended for fractures of the distal third of the radius after the medullary canal has begun to enlarge (Fig. 8-15). Also, one should not attempt to use them if the medullary canal is less than 3 mm. in diameter. When his nails are used, Sage[54] recommends routine autogenous iliac bone grafting.

Technique for Sage Forearm Nails. The technique for fixation of fractures of the shaft of the radius and ulna with Sage[55] nails is described elsewhere and will not be reported here. It should be emphasized that a complete set of nails must be available, including both the 4-mm. and 5-mm. diameters in all lengths, along with the driver-extractor.

Fixation with Plates and Screws. Even after better metals became available, many of the early plates used for fractures of the radius and ulna were of poor design. Failures were frequent because adequate fixation was not achieved (Fig. 8-16). For a time the use of plates and screws for the internal fixation of diaphyseal fractures in general fell into disfavor. Many surgeons treating fractures thought that fixation with a plate and screws held the fracture distracted and caused delayed union and nonunion. This belief was still common in the early 1960's.

Plate-and-screw fixation slowly began regaining favor after Eggers[23-26] introduced the slotted plate (or contact splint, as he preferred to call it). The plate was designed with slots rather than round holes so that, theoretically, the longitudinal muscle pull acting across the fracture would keep the bones in contact and promote union. Whether this actually happens is debatable. After the first few days, fibrous tissue and callus probably grow into the slots, so that sliding is no longer possible. In any case, the Eggers' plate was a much stronger plate than those used previously, and it provided better fixation. Jinkins, Lockhart, and Eggers[34] reported a series of 165 forearm

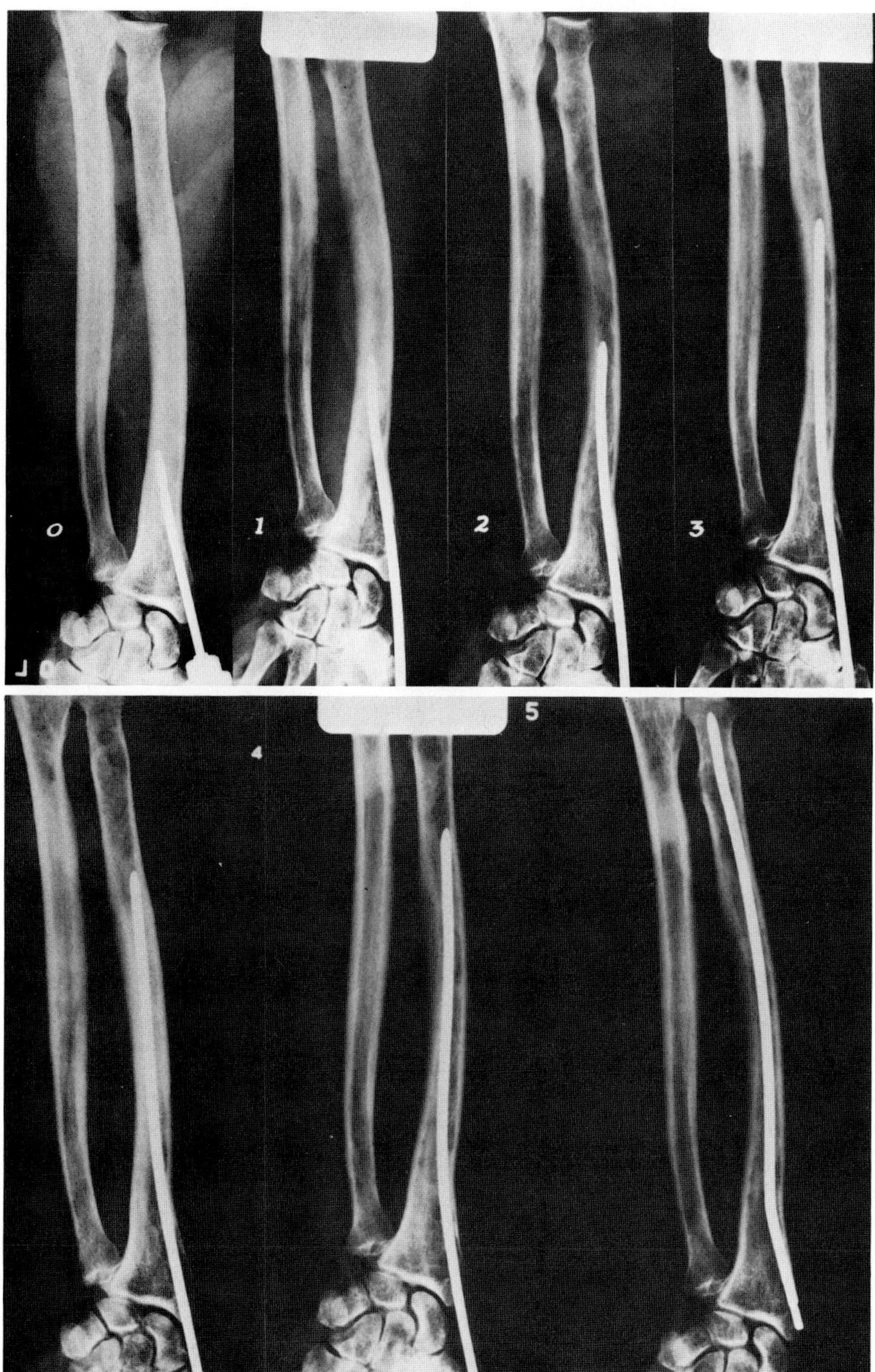

Fig. 8-13. A Sage radial nail is being driven up the radius of an amputated specimen. The nail must bend as it traverses the canal and then finally spring back to its original shape. (Sage, F. P.: J. Bone Joint Surg., *41A*:1489-1516, 1959)

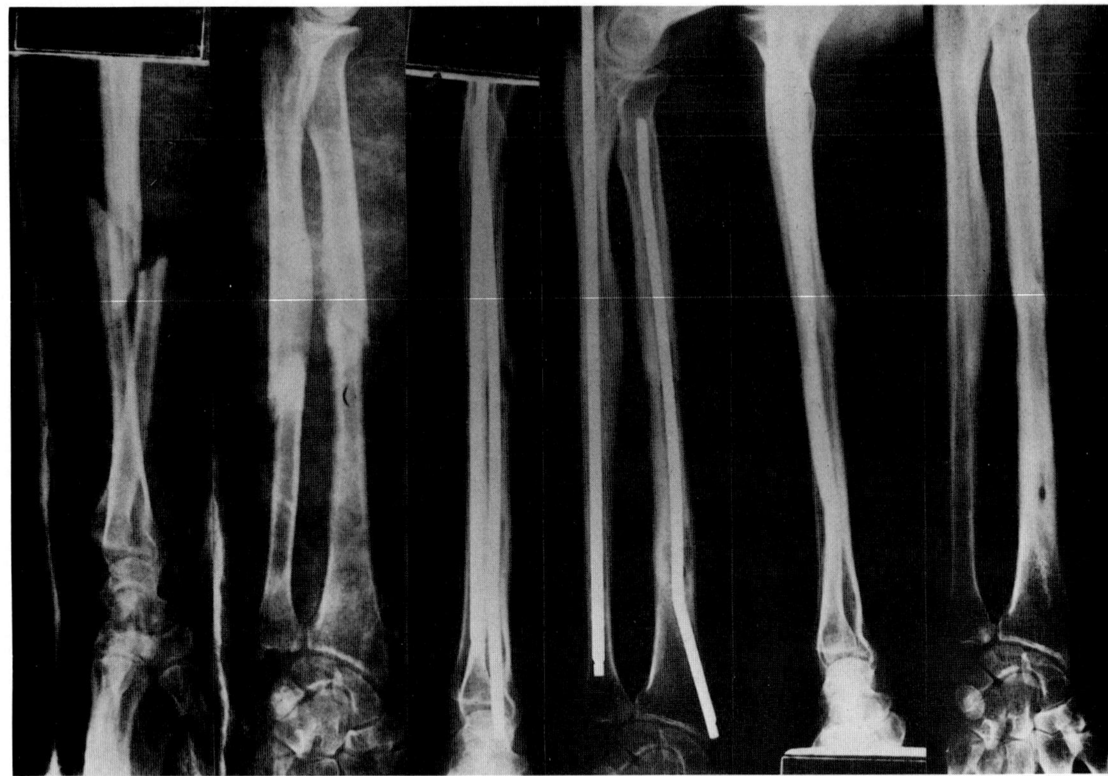

Fig. 8-14. Infection occurred in this radius 6 weeks after nailing. It was felt to be metastatic from an open draining wound of the knee present at the time of nailing. Fortunately the infection was controlled, and union was secured approximately 5 months after nailing. (Sage, F. P.: J. Bone Joint Surg., *41A*:1489-1516, 1959)

fractures in 1960 in which 145 slotted plates and 20 medullary nails had been used. The overall nonunion rate was only 4.2 per cent. They concluded that the results were best when a slotted plate was used for the ulna and either a slotted plate or a Rush pin for the radius.

As well as I can determine, the idea of using plates through which active compression could be applied began with Danis[21] of Belgium. He published a book in 1949 in which the use of such plates was described. Danis called attention to the fact that diaphyseal fractures treated with these plates healed with very little peripheral callus, a phenomenon that he referred to as primary fracture healing. The plate used by Danis had a coapting screw at one end through which compression was applied.

Venable[65] described a similar plate in 1951. Boreau and Hermann[7] introduced a plate with two parts in which a cylindrical bolt forced the fragments together. Bagby[5] modified a Collison plate with oval holes. Compression was achieved by eccentric placement of the screws.

In about 1958, Müller, Allgower, and Willenegger developed what is now known as the ASIF compression plate (Fig. 8-17). The technique for using this plate and other recommended techniques of the Association for the Study of Internal Fixation were published in 1965.[44] The plate is a modification of the plate of Danis but is much stronger, so more compression can be obtained. Müller visited the Campbell Clinic about 1959 and introduced the technique of compression plating to us. We first used

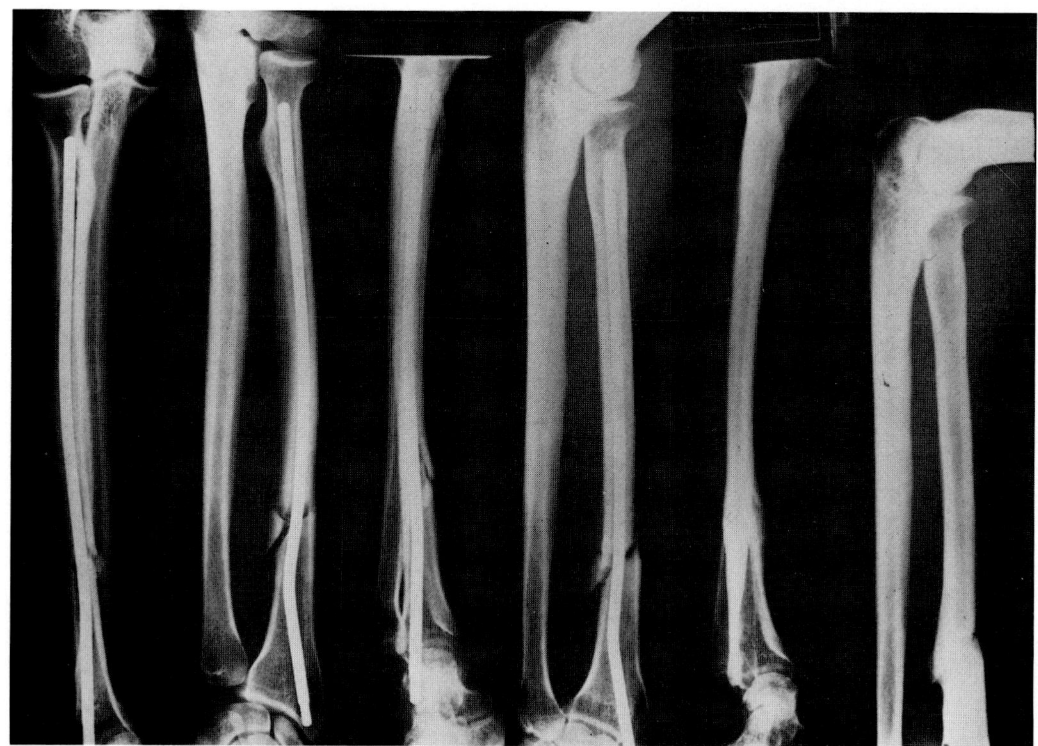

Fig. 8-15. A Sage radial nail was inserted in a fracture that we would now consider too far distal for this form of treatment. Note that telescoping of the nail occurred, resulting in radial shortening and subluxation of the distal radioulnar joint. (Sage, F. P.: J. Bone Joint Surg., *41A*:1489-1516, 1959)

compression plates in experimental fractures of the femur in dogs (Fig. 8-18).[1] Finding the results to be excellent, we began using the plates in diaphyseal fractures of the radius and ulna in adults in 1960. In the experimental fractures we found that when rigid fixation was achieved with these plates, resorption of bone at the fracture ends was not seen roentgenographically. Resorption was seen in roentgenograms only when infection was present or if the screws had loosened. It appeared that the resorption seen with earlier, less rigid plate fixation and "holding the fracture distracted" was a function of poor fixation with inadequate plates and screws.

In January of 1972 we reported our clinical experience with the ASIF compression plate for forearm fractures over the 10-year period from 1960 to 1970 at the meeting of the American Academy of Orthopaedic Surgeons in Washington, D. C.[3] During this time a total of 258 adults with displaced fractures of the radius and ulna were treated with compression plate fixation. Fourteen of these patients were lost to follow-up before the outcome was known. The remaining 244 were followed an average of 13.2 months. One hundred twelve had fractures of both bones of the forearm; 82 had single fractures of the radius, and 50 had single fractures of the ulna. All 132 patients with single-bone fractures of the radius or ulna were treated with compression plates. Of the 112 patients with both bones fractured 86 had both fractures fixed with compression plates (Fig. 8-19). Of the remainder, 25 had the fracture of the radius fixed with a compression plate and the ulna fixed with some other device (usually a

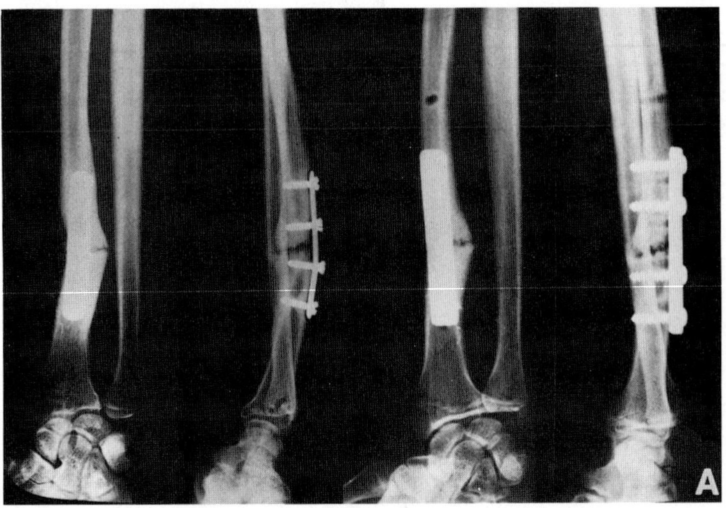

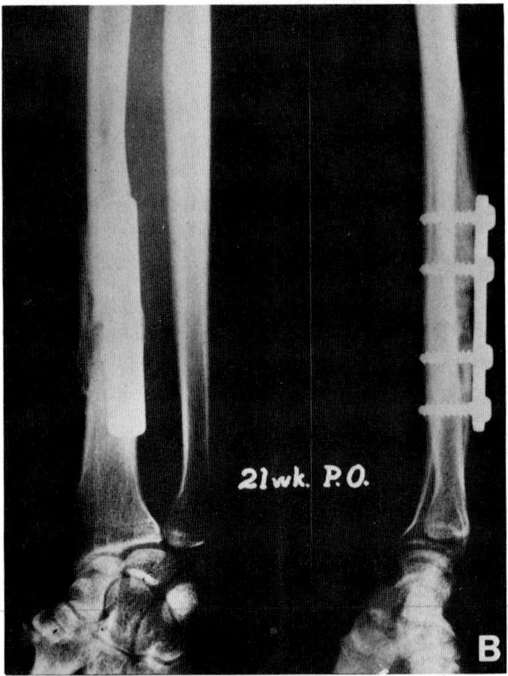

Fig. 8-16. (*A*) An inadequate plate used to treat a fracture of the junction of the middle and distal thirds of the radius. The screws loosened and nonunion resulted. The inadequate plate was removed and a compression plate was applied. Note the hole for the compression device. (*B*) Twenty-one weeks after compression plating and bone grafting good union is present.

Sage triangular nail). In one other patient the ulna was fixed with a compression plate and the radius with a Sage nail. Thus 137 fractures of the ulna and 193 fractures of the radius were treated by this method—a total of 330 forearm bones.

Twenty-eight patients (11.4 per cent) had open fractures, and 216 patients had closed fractures (88.6 per cent). It has been our policy to delay internal fixation in most open fractures until we are sure infection is not present. The period of delay in these 28 patients ranged from 1 to 3 weeks. The average time of delay was 10.6 days.

When we began using the ASIF compression plates we decided on a policy of using autogenous iliac bone grafts if one third or more of the circumference of the bone was comminuted. Also, in both-bone fractures, if one bone was grafted because of comminution, the other bone was also grafted regardless of its comminution. Following this policy 63 of the 244 patients (25.9 per cent) had bone grafts applied.

The overall results are shown in Table 8-1 for fractures of the ulna and in Table 8-2 for fractures of the radius in terms of union and nonunion of the fractures. The nonunion rate for the ulna was 3.7 per cent and for the radius it was 2.1 per cent. The percentage of fractures that united com-

Table 8-1. Results of Compression Plate Fixation for Fractures of the Ulna

	Frac-tures	Union	Non-union	Rate of Union
Ulna Only	50	48	2	96 %
Ulna and Radius	87	84	3	96.5%
Total	137	132	5	96.3%

Table 8-2. Results of Compression Plate Fixation for Fractures of the Radius

	Frac-tures	Union	Non-union	Rate of Union
Radius Only	82	80	2	97.5%
Radius and Ulna	111	109	2	98.2%
Total	193	189	4	97.9%

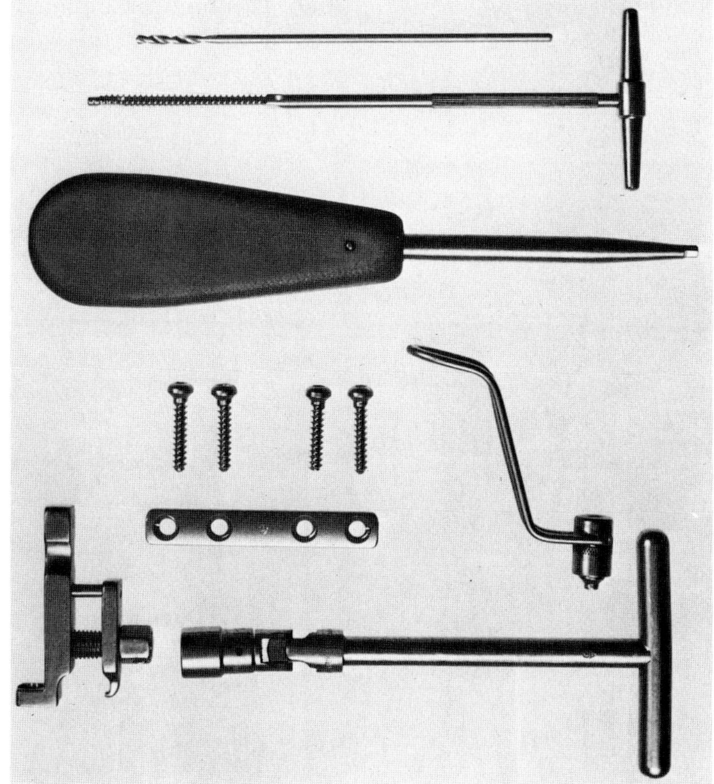

Fig. 8-17. The ASIF (AO) compression instruments. The four-hole plate designed for the human forearm is of heavy construction. The screws have small cores with large threads and are not self-tapping. The drill bit shown at the top has the same diameter as the core of the screws. The tap seen just below the drill bit is used to cut threads in the bone exactly matching those of the screws. The drill guide seen to the right of the screws is used to center the drill exactly so that the heads of the screws countersink accurately into the plate. The compression device is shown at the bottom left, and the wrench for tightening this device is at the lower right. (Anderson, L. D.: J. Bone Joint Surg., *47A*:191, 1965)

pares favorably with other reports in the literature.

The functional results were also very good. In 223 patients where sufficient information was available to determine the degree of function restored, 131 were considered excellent, 69 satisfactory, and 16 fair. Seven patients who required additional operations because their fractures failed to unite were considered failures.

There were 28 patients with 38 open fractures in whom internal fixation was delayed. None developed infection. Ninety fractures in 63 patients received bone grafts. The proportion who developed nonunion when bone grafts were used was almost identical to that when grafts were not used (Table 8-3). This fact can be interpreted in different ways. One could conclude the bone

Table 8-3. Results of Compression Plate Fixation with ($\bar{c}$) and without ($\bar{s}$) Bone Grafting

	Fractures	Union	Nonunion	Rate of Union
Radius $\bar{s}$ Graft	149	146	3	97.3%
Radius $\bar{c}$ Graft	44	43	1	97.8%
Ulna $\bar{s}$ Graft	91	87	4	95.6%
Ulna $\bar{c}$ Graft	46	45	1	97.8%
Total	330	321	9	97.3%

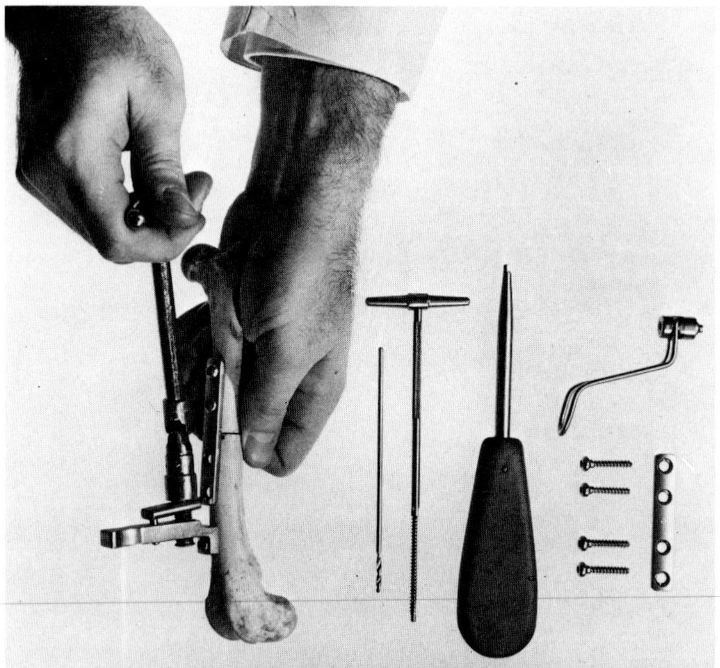

Fig. 8-18. The ASIF (AO) compression instruments and technique of application. The fracture is reduced and the plate fixed to the upper fragment with two screws. The compression device is hooked into the opposite end of the plate and fixed to the lower fragment with a screw. By tightening the compression device, the fragments are impacted. A screw is then placed into the second hole from the bottom, the compression device removed, and the final screw placed in the bottom hole. (Anderson, L. D.: J. Bone Joint Surg., *47A*:191, 1965)

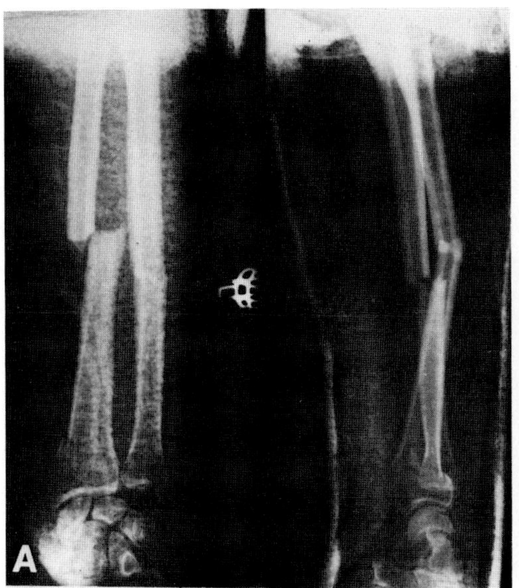

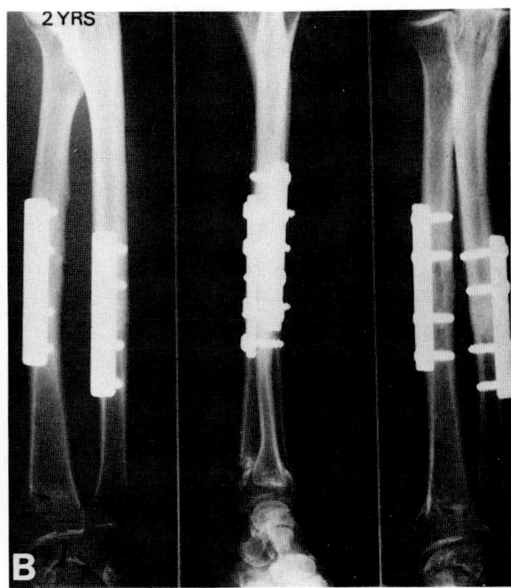

Fig. 8-19. (*A*) A fracture of the radius and ulna in the middle third temporarily immobilized in a cast prior to surgery. Note that there is also a fracture of the distal radius. (*B*) Two years after open reduction and internal fixation with compression plates the radial bow is well maintained and the fractures show good union. The fracture of the distal radius was treated by cast immobilization for 6 weeks.

grafting did not promote union. However, since grafts were used in the more comminuted fractures, a more reasonable conclusion seems to be that by using bone grafts the results in these comminuted fractures can be improved to equal the results of fractures that have no significant comminution. Obviously this is not proved; to do so one would have to treat a series of patients without any bone grafts and then determine whether the rate of nonunion was correlated to the degree of comminution.

The complications in our series of fractures treated with compression plates included nine cases of nonunion (2.7 per cent) and four of delayed union (1.2 per cent) in 330 fractures. Seven of the 244 patients developed significant infection (2.9 per cent; Fig. 8-20). Four of these infections cleared with antibiotic therapy and caused no further difficulty. The other three failed to unite, and subsequent operations were required. Almost all of the nonunions and delayed unions appeared to have been caused by infection or errors in technique (Fig. 8-21).

Two other complications that we have seen with compression plates have been refracture (if the plate is removed too early) and fracture at the end of the plate from additional trauma. The plate provides very rigid fixation, and the normal stresses acting over the bone beneath the plate are reduced. If the plate is removed early, minor trauma may cause a refracture at or near the site of the original fracture (Fig. 8-22). We do not advocate routine removal of plates. The two indications for removal, in our experience, are: (1) a prominent plate lying subcutaneously that causes the patient discomfort and (2) the intention of the patient to return to contact sports. Even in these situations, we try to leave the plate in for at least 18 months.

After the plate is removed, the extremity should be protected for about 6 weeks with a right-angle splint with Velcro straps. Since adopting this practice we have had no further difficulty with refracture. There were five such refractures early in the series, when the plates were removed after only a few months. Three fractures developed at the end of the plate through the area occupied by the screw most distal to the original fracture. In all of these there was additional trauma which was rather violent; the forearms were all struck by a baseball bat or similar club. All were minimally displaced and healed with simple immobilization.

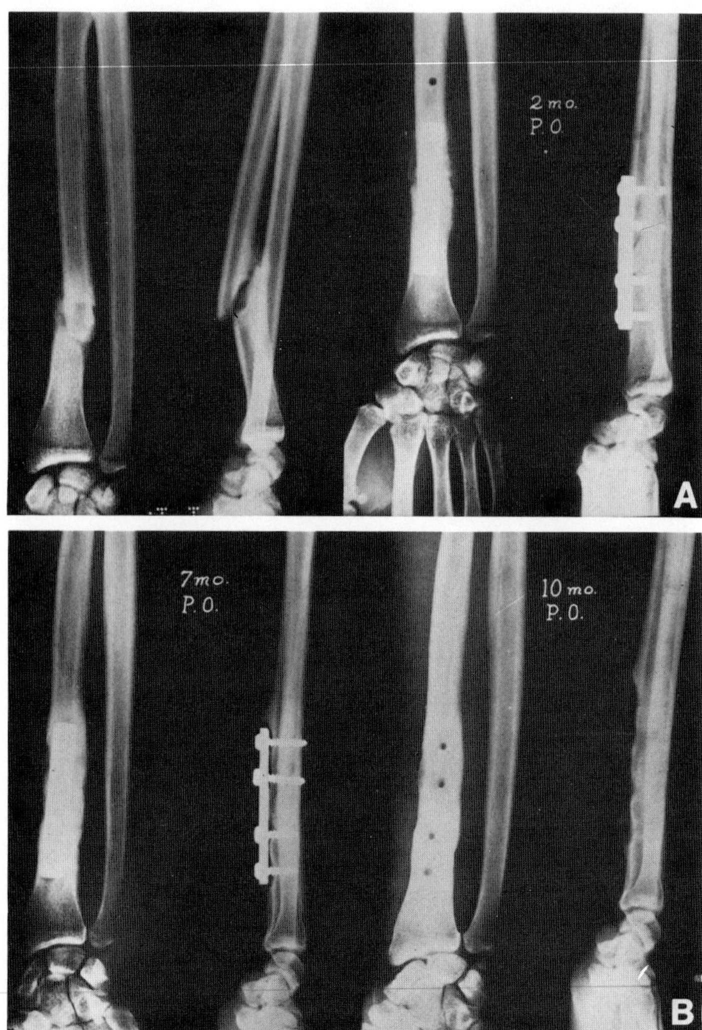

Fig. 8-20. (*A*) A 20-year-old male with an untreated fracture of the junction of the middle and distal thirds of the radius incurred 6 weeks earlier. He was treated with a compression plate applied to the volar surface of the radius. (*B*) The patient was lost to follow-up but returned at 7 months, at which time he had developed drainage secondary to a *Staphylococcus aureus* infection. Note the periosteal reaction present at the proximal end of the plate and the resorption about the screws in the distal end. The infection resolved when the plate was removed and irrigation-suction treatment was carried out.

Recently Naiman *et al.*[45] and Dodge and Cody[22] have reported series of diaphyseal fractures of the radius and ulna treated by compression plates. In Naiman's series, all 30 fractures united. Dodge and Cody encountered no nonunion in their 78 patients in whom compression plates were used. However, there were 10 infections; the incidence was 3 per cent in closed fractures and 36 per cent in open fractures.

Technique of Compression Plating. The technique of compression plating of forearm fractures is discussed in detail in other texts[2,44] and will not be repeated here. However, a few important points will be emphasized.

Most of the failures in our series and other reported series of fractures of the forearm treated with compression plates have been due to errors in technique or to infection. Before compression plating is undertaken, the surgeon must be thoroughly familiar with the technique and, ideally, should have practiced it in the laboratory. A complete set of equipment must be available, and rigid aseptic technique must be enforced in the operating room.

When the fracture of the radius is located in the distal half of the bone, the plate should be placed on the volar surface.[8,30] The bone is flatter, and the plate fits better. For fractures of the proximal half of the radius, the fracture should be approached through a dorsal Thompson[8,63] approach; the plate should be placed on the dorsal surface of the bone. There is less hazard to the deep branch of the radial nerve through this approach than through an anterior one. In very high fractures the nerve can be exposed and retracted. For fractures involving the middle third of the radius, either approach is satisfactory. The compression device should be placed at the end of the plate nearest the middle of the bone where the cortex is thicker and better compression can be obtained.

For fractures of the ulna, the plate may be placed on either the volar or dorsal surface. The surface to be used is determined by which surface the plate fits better and the location of comminuted fragments. If there is a butterfly fragment, it is reduced as accurately as possible and the plate is placed over it to hold it in place.

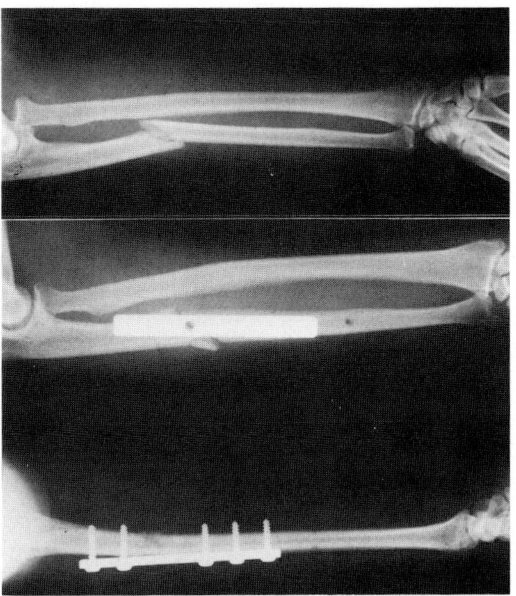

Fig. 8-21. A Monteggia fracture treated by closed reduction of the radial head and compression plate fixation of the ulna. In the bottom films the screws have loosened in the proximal fragment and fixation has been lost. There was an error in technique in that the plate was not centered accurately over the fracture. Nonunion resulted and a second operation was required.

The periosteum should not be stripped to expose the bone. Less damage is done if the muscle is dissected free from the periosteum with scissors and the plate is placed on top of the periosteum.

The ideal length for the plate varies with the amount of comminution and the configuration of the fracture. Four-hole plates are adequate only if the fracture is transverse and not comminuted. In all other fractures of the forearm bones, a five- or six-hole plate should be used. It is important to center the plate over the fracture so that no screw will be closer than 1 cm. to the fracture line. If screws are placed closer than this, a crack may develop between the screw and the fracture as compression is applied, and fixation will be lost (Fig. 8-21). It is better to select a longer plate and leave one or two holes empty than to have screws too close to the fracture.

Three self-retaining Lane or similar bone-holding forceps are needed for the application of compression plates. After the fracture is reduced and any comminuted fragments are fitted into place, a Lane bone-holding forceps is placed at each end of the plate to secure it temporarily to the bone. The third Lane forceps is placed directly over the fracture at right angles to the other two. Its purpose is to lock comminuted fragments into place and to prevent shortening of oblique fractures as compression is applied.

The compression device should be fixed to the bone directly in line with the plate. If it is fixed at an angle, tightening the device will produce angulation rather than compression.

We use autogenous iliac bone grafts if a significant degree of comminution is present. Significant comminution is arbitrarily defined as comminution that involves one third or more of the circumference of the bone.

Finally, it is of utmost importance to close only the subcutaneous tissue and skin. The deep fascia of the forearm is very dense. If it is sutured tightly, edema and hemorrhage may cause increased pressure in the forearm compartments and may lead to a Volkmann's contracture. Obviously, leaving the deep fascia unsutured is important not only with compression plating. It is equally important when other forms of internal fixation are used. A closed drainage system should be used to decrease the

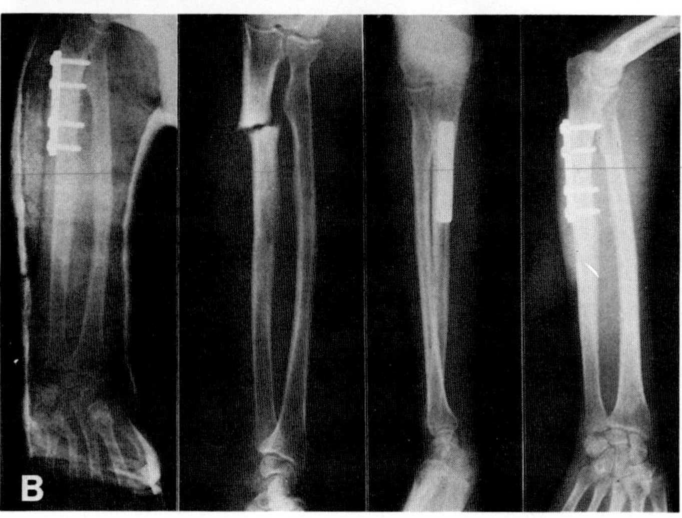

Fig. 8-22. (*A*) A Monteggia fracture treated by closed reduction of the radial head and compression plate fixation of the ulna. (*B*) The extremity was immobilized in a cast for 6 weeks to allow soft-tissue healing about the radial head (*first frame*). At 6 months the plate was removed, and the extremity was not protected. Refracture occurred a month later with minor trauma (*second frame*). A second plate was then applied. Union occurred in 8 weeks with a good functional result (*third and fourth frames*). (Courtesy L. D. Anderson and T. D. Sisk)

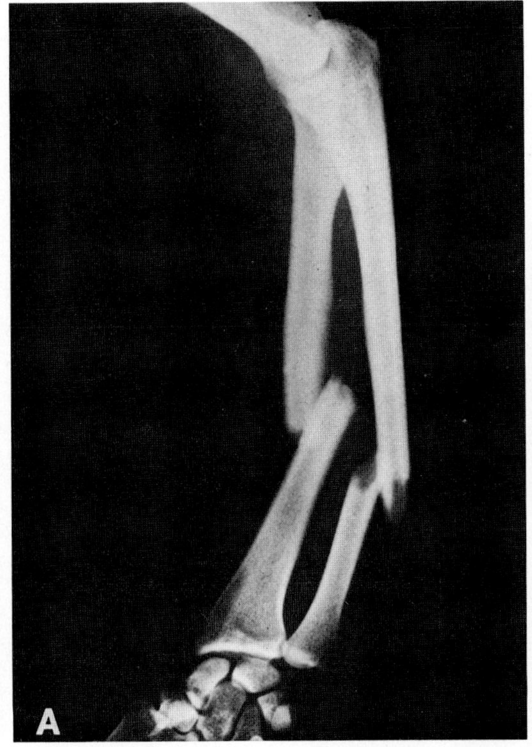

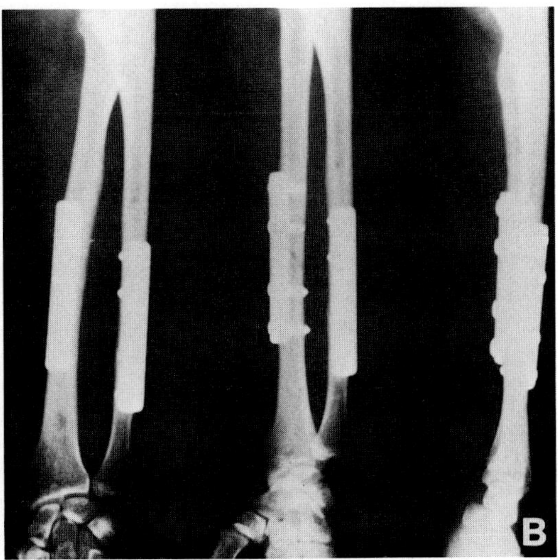

Fig. 8-23. (*A*) A closed fracture of the shaft of the radius and ulna in a cooperative patient. (*B*) Six months after open reduction and compression plate fixation. No external fixation was necessary. Motion was begun early, and functional recovery was complete. Four-hole plates were used but owing to the obliquity of the fractures, five-hole plates would have been better. (Anderson, L. D.: Fractures. *In* Crenshaw, A. H., (ed.): Campbell's Operative Orthopaedics. ed. 5. vol. 1. St. Louis, C. V. Mosby, 1971)

hematoma and resultant swelling. It is removed after 48 hours.

After Care. The postoperative care after compression plate fixation is tailored to each patient. If the patient is reliable and can be counted on to follow instructions, if the fracture is without significant comminution, and if good compression has been achieved, no external fixation is necessary (Fig. 8-23). A pressure dressing is applied, and the forearm is elevated from an overhead frame until the swelling begins to subside. As soon as the patient has recovered from the anesthetic, gentle active exercises are begun for the elbow, wrist, and hand. By the end of 10 days, such patients have usually regained most of their normal range of motion.

Another category includes the group where the fracture is not comminuted and good compression has been obtained but the patient's reliability is questionable. One approach is to leave the extremity free of a cast so that exercises can be carried out while the patient is in the hospital under observation. At about 10 to 12 days the sutures are removed and a long-arm cast is applied prior to discharge. The cast is worn until the fracture appears united by roentgenograms, usually after about 6 weeks. Because most of the motion has been regained prior to cast immobilization, these patients obtain good function rapidly once they are out of the cast.

If the fracture is comminuted or if good compression has not been obtained, a posterior plaster splint should be applied when the operation is completed. This is changed

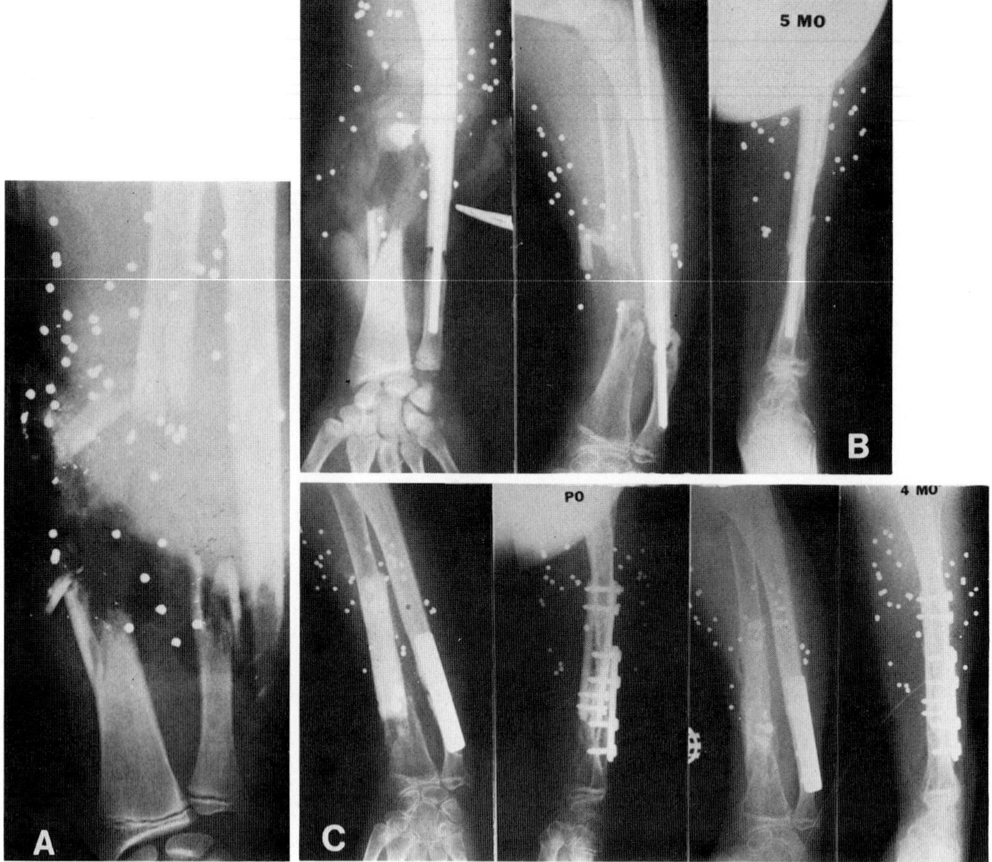

Fig. 8-24. (*A*) Open fractures of the radius and ulna in a teenage boy secondary to a shotgun wound from very close range. Note the loss of bone from the radius. (*B*) Following irrigation and debridement, temporary fixation of the ulna was secured with a Sage nail to provide enough stability for dressing of the wound and skin grafting (*first frame*). At 5 months coverage was complete and he was free of infection. There is a nonunion of the ulna as well as a large bony defect in the radius. (*C*) Fixation of the ulna was accomplished with a compression plate, and dual onlay autogenous cortical grafts from the tibia were used to bridge the defect in the radius (*first and second frames*). At 4 months the grafts have consolidated, and both bones have united.

to a long-arm cast when the sutures are removed and the patient is ready for discharge. The cast is continued until there is roentgenographic evidence of healing or until consolidation of bone grafts is noted.

Open Fractures of the Radius and Ulna

The ratio of open (compound) fractures to closed fractures is higher for the forearm bones than for any other bone except the tibia.[11] The fact that the ulna has a subcutaneous border throughout its length is the probable reason.

Compound fractures of both bones of the forearm are best divided into two groups. The first group is, fortunately, by far the more common. In this type the open wound is minor; frequently there is only a small wound where a sharp spike of bone has compounded from within to without. In these fractures the wounds should be debrided and closed. With the patient under anesthesia with good relaxation, an attempt should be made to "hook" at least one of the fractures to prevent excessive shortening. A long-arm cast is applied following the technique described for closed treatment of fractures of both bones of the forearm. When the compounding wound is healed at 10 to 21 days, one can carry out open reduction and internal fixation more safely. As previously discussed, in our series of forearm fractures treated with compression plates none of the 28 patients with 38 compound fractures developed infection when this policy of delaying open reduction was followed.

The second type of compound fracture of the forearm bones involves a major loss of soft tissue or bone. Close-range shotgun or high-velocity rifle wounds are examples (Fig. 8-24). Fortunately, in peace time they are not common. In these severe injuries some form of internal fixation must be used so that the soft tissue can be treated and coverage achieved with skin grafts or pedicle flaps, as appropriate.

Initially, only the minimal amount of metal needed to stabilize the forearm for dressings and skin grafting should be used. There is no need to internally fix both bones. Medullary nails are better for this purpose than plates and screws. If an infection should develop, screws may pull loose and fixation will be lost. A Sage nail or similar device inserted in the ulna is usually adequate for the immediate purpose. Reconstruction of the radius is left until a later date after there is good soft-tissue coverage. Rarely, there may be a significant loss of bone from the ulna but not from the radius. In this case, the radius is fixed with a medullary nail, and the ulna is left for reconstruction later.

As in all compound fractures, copious irrigation and meticulous debridement of the wound are extremely important. Antibiotics should be started intravenously in the emergency room and continued during and after surgery. Tetanus prophylaxis should be provided (see Chap. 4).

AUTHOR'S PREFERRED METHOD OF TREATMENT

For most displaced fractures of the radius and ulna in adults I prefer ASIF compression plate fixation. Closed treatment of these fractures generally yields a high incidence of poor results. On the other hand, the results of compression plate fixation in my experience over a 13-year period have been excellent. The incidence of nonunion has been low (less than 3 per cent) and the functional results have been excellent in most cases. I cannot overemphasize the importance of meticulous attention to the "details of operative technique." The need for strict asepsis in the operating room is absolute. Errors in technique and infection are the principal causes of failure. The time of external immobilization with this method is usually less than with other forms of internal fixation, and in appropriate cases I frequently use no cast at all.

For segmental fractures of the radius I have used one plate on the dorsal surface for the proximal fracture and one on the volar surface for the distal fracture. I have found it difficult to ream and insert Sage nails in segmental fractures of the radius. However, they are easier to use for the ulna, and I generally prefer the Sage nail for segmental fractures of this bone.

Moderate degrees of comminution can generally be handled with compression plates, but where there is extensive comminution I prefer a Sage nail for both the radius and ulna. The comminuted fragments are held in place with circumferential wires, and the fractures are grafted with autogenous iliac bone grafts.

I do not like to carry out primary internal fixation in compound fractures of the shafts of the radius and ulna except in patients with major soft-tissue loss as outlined above. In most instances, when the wound is relatively small and not too contaminated I irrigate, debride, and close it and use antibiotics liberally before, during, and after surgery. I then immobilize the extremity in a cast and perform internal fixation as a secondary procedure when the wound is healed.

PROGNOSIS

The prognosis for adults with fractures of the radius and ulna depends on many factors. Was the fracture compound, and if so, how extensive was the damage, and how great was the contamination? Was the fracture displaced or undisplaced, and was there comminution? The surgeon has no control over these and many other factors; they are decided at the time of injury. To be sure, the prognosis related to these may be affected by the surgeon's actions and decisions, including early and appropriate treatment.

There are other factors over which the surgeon has more direct control. These include the choice of the treatment method (open versus closed), the timing of internal fixation as related to compound fractures, and attention to details of technique and the prevention of infection.

The prognosis for displaced fractures of the radius and ulna in adults treated by closed reduction is generally considered poor in an unacceptably high percentage of patients. For such fractures treated by open reduction and rigid internal fixation, the prognosis for developing union of the fractures is in the range of 95 per cent. Sage[55] reported union of 93.8 per cent of the fractures in his series treated with triangular medullary nails and in our series[3] of forearm fractures treated with compression plates 97.3 per cent of the fractures united. Approximately 90 per cent had satisfactory or excellent function and 10 per cent had unsatisfactory or poor function after the first operation. Other recent articles concerning forearm fractures treated with compression plates report similar results.[22,45]

In a group of forearm shaft fractures treated primarily with slotted plates by Jinkins, Lockhart, and Eggers,[34] 95.8 per cent united. Caden[15] reports a union rate of 92.5 per cent with slotted plates. Other surgeons report similar results with good rigid fixation both with plates and with medullary nails.[14,52] The important feature common to all these reports where over 90 per cent of the fractures united was the rigidity of fixation. If medullary nails are used they must control rotation of the fragments and be sturdy enough to resist angulatory forces. If plates and screws are used, they must be long enough and strong enough to resist loosening and breakage of the fixation. In our experience, the results can be as good for open fractures where the wound is relatively minor if open reduction and internal fixation is delayed from 7 to 21 days.

The prognosis for union and good function is much poorer if round medullary nails or inadequate plates are used. Small forearm plates have been reported to lead to nonunion in 20 per cent of forearm fractures,[35] and round medullary pins or nails in 14 to 16 per cent.[15,58] Kirschner wire fixation was reported by Smith and Sage[58] to produce nonunion in 38 per cent of forearm fractures.

For open fractures of the shaft of the radius and ulna with major skin and soft-tissue loss, the prognosis must be more guarded. In these cases, several operative procedures are necessary, including the initial debridement and stabilization, skin grafting or pedicle flap applications, late reconstruction of the bones, and, frequently, the transfer of tendons. If infection develops, sequestrectomy and institution of irrigation-suction may be necessary. Usually, enough function can be preserved to make all this worthwhile, but the result is generally far from normal. Occasionally, infection and fibrosis of the soft tissues may necessitate an amputation.

COMPLICATIONS

Nonunion and Malunion

Nonunion of fractures of the shafts of the radius and ulna is most often seen where infection is present, when fixation after open reduction is inadequate, and when adequate reduction was not achieved and maintained following closed treatment. Accurate open reduction and rigid internal fixation will prevent most of these complications. The treatment of nonunion is discussed in Chapter 2.

Infection

In spite of all attempts to prevent infection, a proportion of compound fractures and closed fractures treated by open reduction inevitably become infected. With good technique and operating facilities, this group should be small. If infection develops, the wound should be cultured, the sensitivity of the organism should be determined, and appropriate antibiotic therapy should be begun. Superficial infections will frequently respond to this treatment alone. If the infection appears deep, the wound should be opened to provide drainage, and if the arm is not already immobilized in a cast, one should be applied. External support will rest the extremity and decrease the chance of the infection causing loss of fixation. If internal fixation is in place and the fixation has not loosened, it should not be abandoned; a fairly high percentage of fractures that have been fixed internally will unite in spite of infection if the extremity is held in a cast. After the fracture has healed the metal can be removed. The residual infection is treated by irrigation-suction (Fig. 8-20).

We probably should consider treating infections following open reduction and internal fixation more vigorously soon after they develop than we have in the past. We have had little experience with early debridement and irrigation-suction in these cases. The results of such management have been good in acute hematogenous osteomyelitis and might have a place here.

In late infections, where fixation has already been lost and nonunion has developed, the metal should be removed along with any sequestra, and irrigation-suction should be instituted. After the infection has cleared up, the extremity is maintained in a cast or leather lacer brace. When the extremity has been free of infection for 6 months, reconstructive procedures can be undertaken with less danger of flaring up the old infection. Appropriate antibiotics should be given before, during, and after the reconstructive surgery.

Nerve Injury

Nerve injuries associated with fractures of both bones of the forearm are uncommon in closed fractures or those with minor compounding wounds. They are most common in the major compound wounds with extensive soft-tissue loss, such as shotgun injuries. In such an injury, if one of the major nerves is found not to be functioning it should be explored at the time of debridement to determine whether it is intact or divided. If it is divided, the ends should be tagged with wire sutures for repair at a later time.

Vascular Injury

The collateral circulation of the forearm is good, and if either the radial or ulnar artery is functioning, the hand and forearm are usually not in jeopardy. When either vessel is patent the other can be simply ligated. It is rare to have both vessels lacerated, except in compound fractures where a traumatic near-amputation has occurred. Here the damage to nerves, tendons, and bone is usually so severe that amputation may be necessary.

Compartment Syndrome

Little has been written about compartment syndromes in the forearm. Compartment syndromes in fact do occur in the forearm both following initial injury and after surgery. If these syndromes are not recognized early and if the pressure is not relieved, the end result is similar to that in Volkmann's ischemic contracture. Either the anterior or posterior compartment of the forearm or both may be involved.

Just as in the leg, it is possible to have a palpable forearm pulse despite an increase in pressure in the forearm compartments sufficient to obliterate the capillary circula-

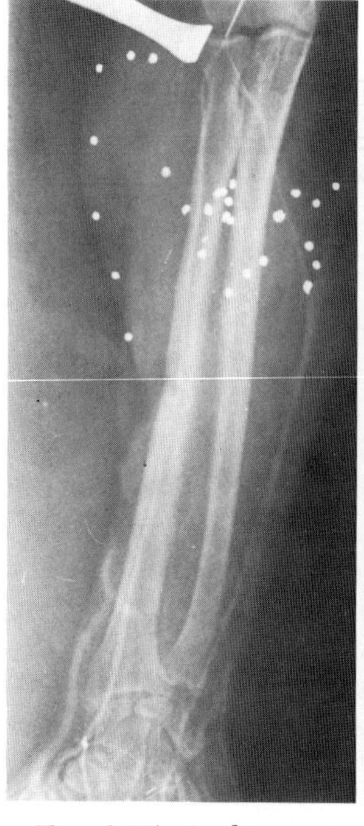
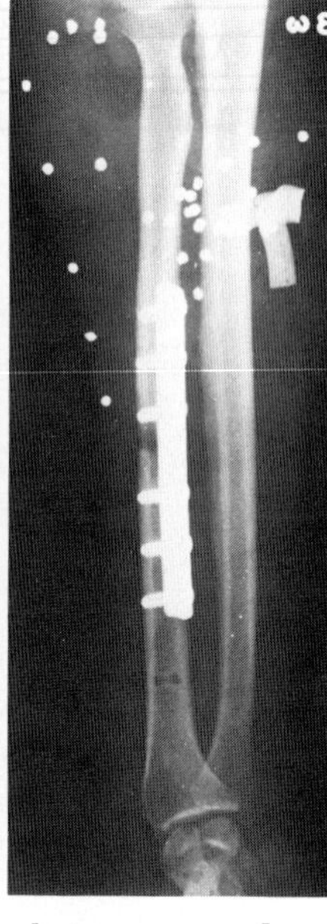

Fig. 8-25. A close-range shotgun wound resulted in a fracture of the radius in the middle third and a closed compartment syndrome. Weak pulses were present at the wrist, but there was decreased sensation in the hand, decreased function of the forearm muscles, and deep boring pain. The arteriogram showed filling of both the radial and ulnar arteries (*first frame*). An immediate anterior and posterior fasciotomy achieved almost immediate return of sensation and motor function. After achieving skin coverage the fracture of the radius was treated with a compression plate 5 weeks later.

tion to the muscles and nerves. This may confuse the picture and delay diagnosis and treatment. In such cases there is decreased sensation in the fingers, little or no function in the forearm muscles, and a deep boring pain in the forearm out of proportion to what one would expect (Fig. 8-25). The treatment is early and wide fasciotomy from the elbow to the wrist. At the time of operation the muscles bulge into the wound. The incision should be allowed to separate, and skin grafts may be applied either then or later.

Closed compartment syndromes that follow surgery on the forearm are usually due to faulty hemostasis and closure of the deep fascia. They can be avoided by releasing the tourniquet prior to wound closure, to make sure hemostasis is adequate, and by closing only the subcutaneous tissue and skin. I know of three patients who developed closed compartment syndromes after open reduction and internal fixation of forearm fractures. In all three the deep fascia had been closed. None was recognized early, and all ended in ischemic contracture. This complication is avoidable.

Synostosis

Synostosis of the radius and ulna following fracture is relatively uncommon. In our series of forearm fractures treated with compression plates there were 112 patients with fractures of both the radius and ulna, and only three developed a complete synostosis.[3] All three had badly displaced and comminuted fractures with the fracture in both bones at the same level.

Patients who develop a synostosis frequently give a history of a crushing injury. If a synostosis develops and the position of the forearm is relatively functional, it is usually best to do nothing. If the position of the forearm is poor, osteotomy to place the hand in a more functional position should be considered. A few cases of successful resection of synostoses have been reported, but usually the heterotopic bone reforms, and the synostosis recurs.

FRACTURE OF THE ULNA ALONE (Nightstick Fracture)

UNDISPLACED FRACTURES

Undisplaced or minimally displaced fractures of the shaft of the ulna are fairly common. Most occur as the result of a direct blow. Those in the distal half of the bone usually unite in good position if they are immobilized in a long-arm cast. The usual time required for union is about 3 months. Loss of position is more common in the proximal half of the bone where the cast does not provide such good fixation because the forearm is fleshier. If roentgenograms of these fractures through the cast reveal loss of position, open reduction and internal fixation should be done.

DISPLACED FRACTURES

Displaced fractures of the ulna alone do occur without fracture of the radius or dislocation of the radial head, but if there is much displacement, there is usually some associated injury. One must be sure that the elbow and wrist are well visualized in the roentgenograms, so that these injuries are not missed. In solitary fractures of the ulna, open reduction and internal fixation should be carried out if there is any significant displacement. For most fractures of the ulna, I prefer a five- or six-hole compression plate. In fractures of the middle or distal third of the ulna, triangular nails work well and may be better than plates if there is extensive comminution over a long area or if the fracture is segmental. These severely comminuted fractures should be bone grafted. In the proximal third of the ulna, the medullary canal is large, and a nail will not provide rigid fixation. Compression plate fixation is better at this level (Fig. 8-26).

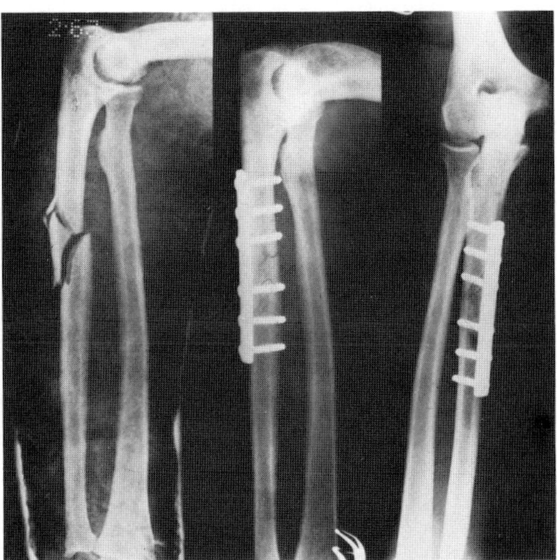

Fig. 8-26. A closed comminuted fracture of the ulna with a large butterfly fragment (*first frame*). Rigid fixation was achieved with a six-hole compression plate and screws. The butterfly fragment was anatomically reduced and held beneath the plate. Films made in the operating room show the fracture line to be barely visible (*second and third frames*).

MONTEGGIA'S FRACTURE

Monteggia[43,50] of Milan published his classic description of the fracture that is associated with his name in 1814. Strictly speaking, a Monteggia fracture is a fracture of the proximal third of the ulna with an anterior dislocation of the radial head (Fig. 8-27). As pointed out by Bado[4] and Boyd and Boals,[10] this strict definition accounts for only 60 per cent of ulnar fractures with associated dislocation of the radiohumeral articulation. Bado[4] coined the term "Monteggia lesion" to include the entire spectrum of these injuries. He classified these injuries as follows and gave these percentages for each type:

Type I (60 per cent of cases) Anterior dislocation of the radial head. Fracture of the ulnar diaphysis at any level with anterior angulation.

Type II (15 per cent of cases) Posterior or posterolateral dislocation of the radial head. Fracture of the ulna diaphysis with posterior angulation.

Type III (20 per cent of cases) Lateral or anterolateral dislocation of the radial head. Fracture of the ulnar metaphysis.

Type IV (5 per cent or less of cases) Anterior dislocation of the radial head. Fracture of the proximal third of the radius. Fracture of the ulna at the same level.

Other authors classify these injuries somewhat differently, but it seems clear that the fracture of the proximal third of the ulna with anterior dislocation of the radial head is the most common (Type I). In the report of Speed and Boyd[60] in 1940, 83.3 per cent of the radial head dislocations were anterior, 10 per cent posterior, and 6.7 per cent were lateral. Thus, in their series, Bado's Type I lesion was by far the most common,

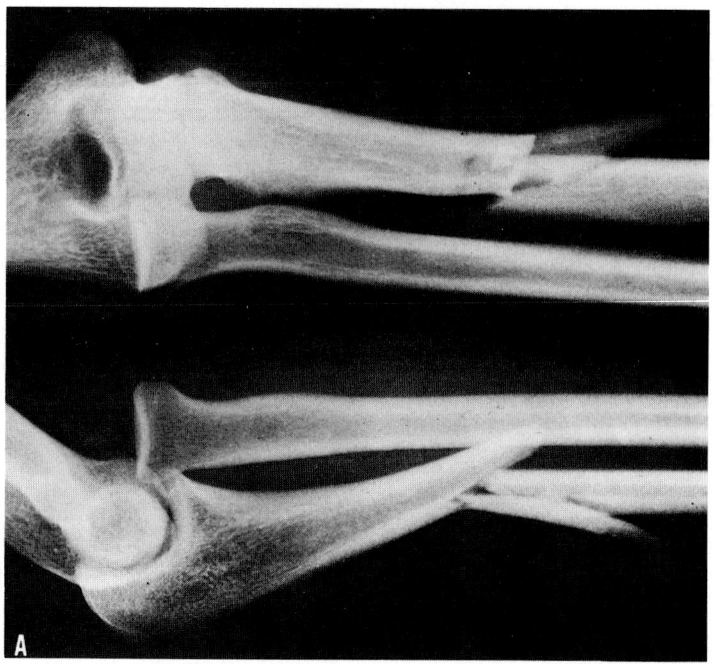

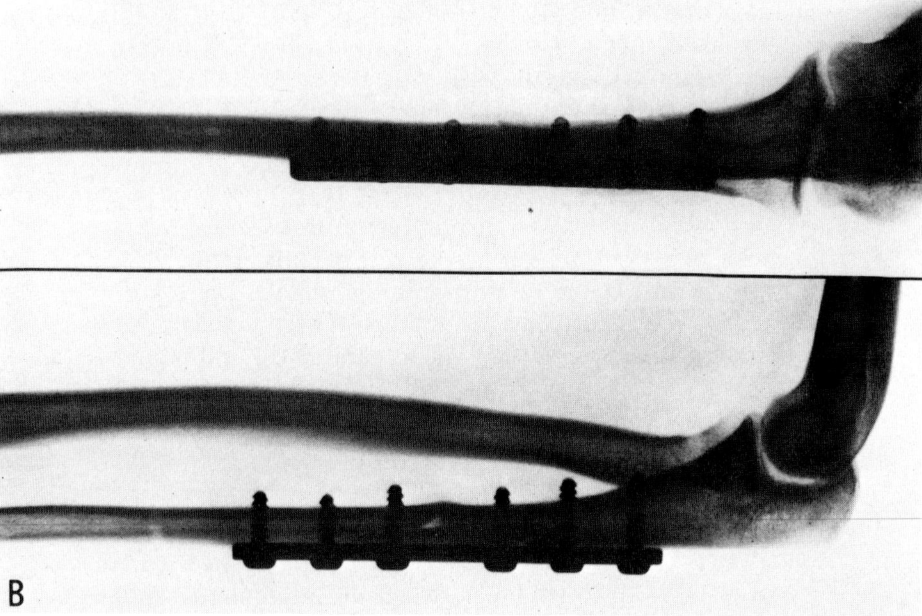

Fig. 8-27. (*A*) Preoperative roentgenograms of an acute Monteggia lesion in an adult. Note the comminution of the ulna. (*B*) Roentgenograms 3 months postoperatively (Boyd, H. B., and Boals, J. C.: Clin. Orthop., *66*:94-100, 1969)

but the Type II lesion was more frequently seen than the Type III.

Mechanism of Injury

There has been a great deal of discussion in the literature about the mechanism of injury in Monteggia lesions. The mechanism obviously must vary depending on the type of lesion. The greatest discussion has been whether the true Type I Monteggia fracture is caused by forced pronation of the forearm or by a direct blow over the posterior aspect of the ulna, as when it is struck by a club. Evans[27] was able to reproduce the Monteggia fracture in cadaveric specimens. He placed the humerus in a vise and applied strong pronation to the forearm with a wrench. The shaft of the ulna fractured, and the radial head dislocated anteriorly. Bado[4] agreed with Evans and pointed out that in lateral roentgenograms of the elbow in Type I lesions, the bicipital tuberosity is located posteriorly, indicating full pronation. Evans pointed out that in falls, the hand and forearm are usually in full pronation. With the hand planted on the ground, the added weight of the body causes an external rotatory force on the extremity which has the effect of producing greater pronation. Evans also cited the lack of hematoma and contusion over the fractured ulna as further evidence that the Monteggia Type I fracture is caused by forced pronation in a fall.

On the other hand, I have seen a number of patients with Type I lesions who gave no history of a fall but had a definite history of having been struck over the ulna with a baseball bat or similar object. This group of patients did have contusion and hematoma over the ulna, and it seems clear that a direct blow to the ulna was the cause of their injury. Probably the truth is that the Type I Monteggia lesion can be produced either by a fall with forced pronation or by a direct blow over the posterior ulna.

In 1951 Penrose[47] described the mechanism of injury for the Type II Monteggia lesion as a variation of posterior dislocation of the elbow. In these Type II lesions the ligamentous attachments of the proximal ulna are stronger than the ulna itself. Thus the radial head dislocates posteriorly, but the humeroulnar joint remains intact, and the ulna fractures.

Bado[4] states that the mechanism of injury in the Type III Monteggia lesion is a direct blow over the inner aspect of the elbow and that this type occurs only in children. However, I can recall at least one such lesion in an adult. Bado does not describe the mechanism of injury in the Type IV Monteggia lesion other than to note that it is a Type I lesion with associated fracture of the radial shaft. Possibly a second blow over the radial side of the forearm after the radial head has already dislocated accounts for this injury.

Signs and Symptoms

The signs and symptoms in Monteggia lesions vary with the type. In Type I lesions the radial head can be palpated in the antecubital fossa, and there is shortening of the forearm with anterior angulation of the fractured ulna. In Type II lesions the radial head can be palpated posterior to the distal humerus, and there is posterior angulation of the ulna. The radial head can be felt laterally in the Type III lesions, and there is lateral angulation of the ulnar metaphysis. In the Type IV lesions the radial head is located anteriorly, and there is tenderness and deformity of the radial and ulnar shafts at the level of fractures.

In all four types of Monteggia lesions there is marked pain and tenderness about the elbow. The patient resists any attempts to move the elbow in flexion-extension and pronation-supination as it is painful.

Paralysis of the deep branch of the radial nerve is the most common associated neurological lesion. Boyd and Boals[10] reported five such cases in their series of 159 patients treated at the Campbell Clinic. These authors noted that spontaneous recovery is the usual course and that exploration of the nerve is not indicated.

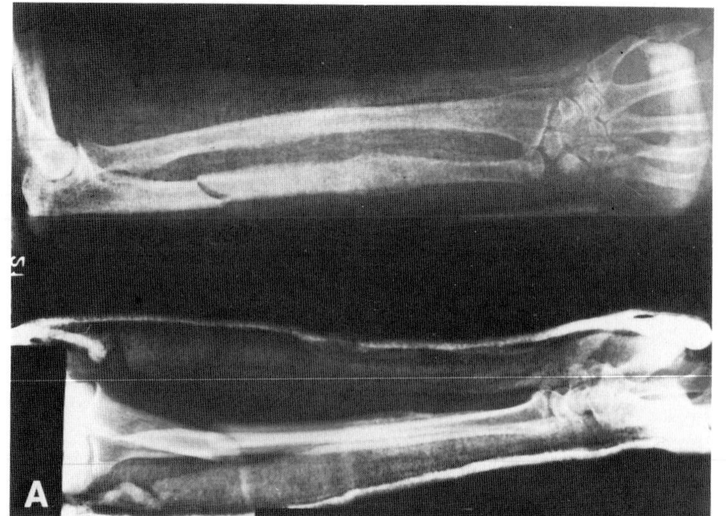

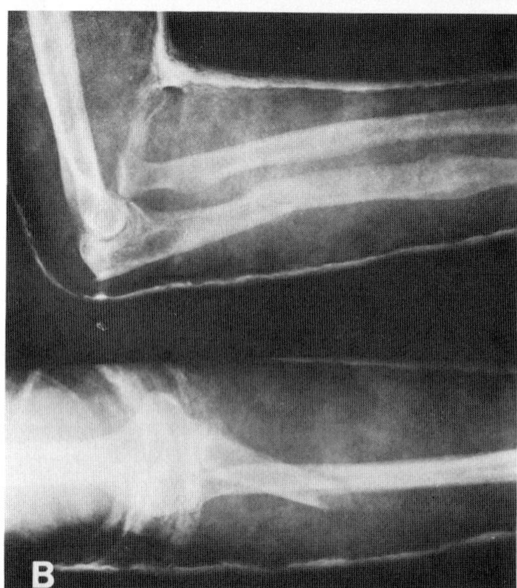

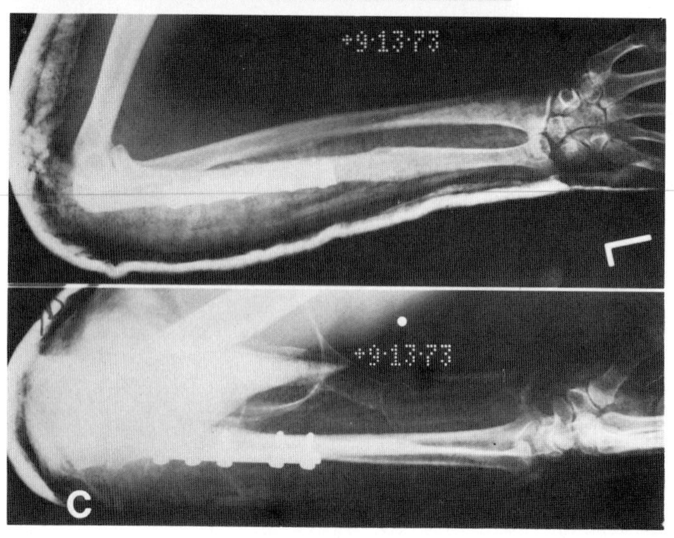

Fig. 8-28. (*A*) Films following application of a long-arm cast for what was felt to be a minimally displaced fracture of the ulna. (*B*) Films made 1 week later show dislocation of the radial head and increased angulation of the fracture of the ulna. Careful questioning at that time revealed that the patient probably had reduced her own dislocation of the radial head initially. (*C*) Postoperative films showing a five-hole compression plate applied to the ulna and the elbow maintained 20 degrees above a right angle in a posterior plaster splint.

Roentgenographic Findings

It would seem that the Monteggia lesions would be obvious in roentgenograms, but this is not always so. In the 62 patients reported by Speed and Boyd[60] in 1940, 52 per cent of the patient's lesions were not detected until over 4 weeks after injury. By the 1965 report of Boyd and Boals,[10] which added 97 additional patients to the series, the proportion of patients with old lesions had decreased to 24 per cent. They concluded that physicians in recent years are doing a better job of recognizing Monteggia fractures. However, it appears we still have some way to go.

The fracture of the ulna is usually obvious and difficult to miss. In the 97 patients reported by Boyd and Boals, the fracture was located in the region of the olecranon or metaphysis in 19, in the proximal third in 69, the middle third in eight, and in the distal third in only one. There were 12 patients with associated radial head fractures. Six of the 97 patients had Bado Type IV lesions with an associated fracture of the shaft of the radius.

There are probably several reasons why the dislocation of the radial head is missed so often. First, the roentgenograms may not include the elbow. Second, the x-ray tube may not be centered over the elbow, so that even though the elbow is included in the film, the dislocation may not be obvious. Third, the physician who first sees the patient may be unfamiliar with the lesion and may not realize that dislocation of the radial head is present. He may unknowingly reduce the dislocation when he aligns the arm to splint it. If such a patient arrives elsewhere for definitive care without the initial roentgenograms, the new films may appear to be a fracture of the ulna with minimal displacement. A fourth reason for missing the dislocation of the radial head was pointed out by an incident that happened recently on my service at the City of Memphis Hospital. A patient arrived in the emergency room with pain in the forearm after a fall (Fig. 8-28). She came directly without having been referred by another physician. Her roentgenograms showed a minimally displaced fracture of the proximal third of the ulna, and the radial head was in normal position. The arm was placed in a long-arm cast with the elbow at 90 degrees, and the patient was told to visit the Fracture Clinic 1 week later. At that time, check roentgenograms through the cast revealed displacement of the fractured ulna and anterior dislocation of the radial head (Fig. 8-28). Upon more careful questioning at that time, the patient related that the extremity had been so painful after her fall that she had pulled on the arm vigorously and felt a snap in her elbow. After this the pain was much less severe. Apparently she had reduced her own dislocation and fracture prior to arriving in the emergency room. A more detailed history and careful examination of the lateral elbow for tenderness might have led to the proper diagnosis initially. Fortunately the diagnosis was picked up after 1 week, the dislocated radial head was reduced, and the ulna was fixed with a compression plate (Fig. 8-28). The final result was excellent, but if the patient had not returned early for check-up roentgenograms the outcome might not have been a happy one.

There are several lessons to be learned from this case. The Monteggia fracture remains a treacherous one, just as Monteggia himself pointed out in 1814.

Methods of Treatment

There is general agreement that closed treatment is satisfactory in children[4,10] for most Monteggia fractures, but there is a great deal of controversy as to how these fractures should be treated in adults.

Monteggia[43,50] used closed reduction in his two cases and found it unsatisfactory. The dislocation recurred. Watson-Jones[68] reported that the incidence of myositis ossificans was increased by open reduction of the radial head and reported poor results in 32 of 34 patients initially treated by other

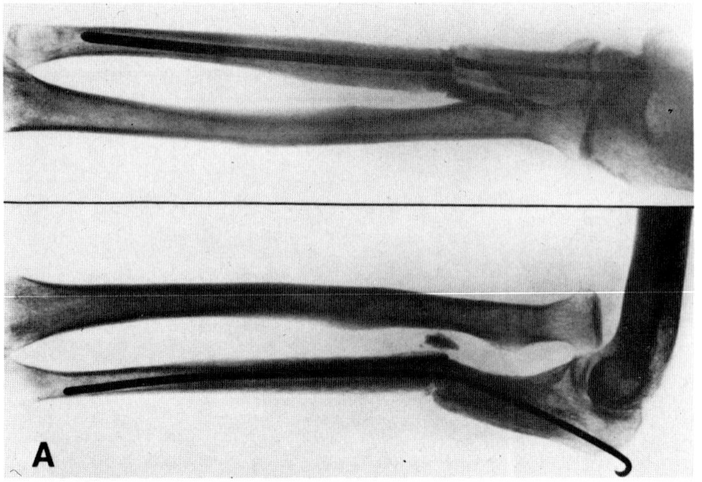

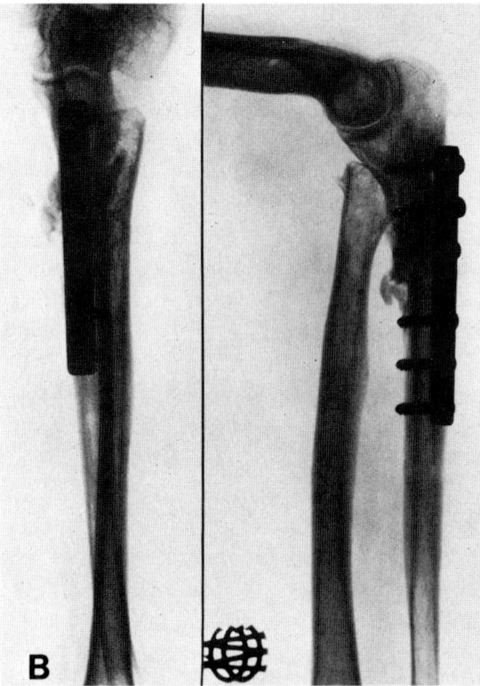

Fig. 8-29. (*A*) Nonunion with recurrence of the dislocation of the radial head 4 months after inadequate internal fixation. (*B*) Same patient 4 months after compression plate fixation, bone grafting, and resection of the head of the radius. (Boyd, H. B., and Boals, J. C.: Clin. Orthop., *66*: 94-100, 1969)

surgeons. Bado[4] along with Evans[27] emphasized the importance of reducing the dislocation by supination and maintaining the forearm in that position for 6 to 8 weeks. Bado maintained that conservative treatment is always best for fresh cases of dislocated radial head and usually is best for the fractured ulna.

In their 1940 article, Speed and Boyd[60] found closed treatment unsatisfactory in most acute Monteggia fractures in adults. At that time they advocated open reduction and internal fixation of the ulna with a Vitallium plate along with reconstruction of the annular ligament with a fascial loop. At that time the authors thought the fascial loop repair gave added stability and helped prevent redislocation of the radial head. With the relatively inadequate devices available for fixation of the ulnar fracture at that time, the fascial repair may have been helpful.

In the more recent report of 1969, Boyd and Boals[10] recommended rigid internal fixation of the fractured ulna with a compression plate or medullary nail. However, they then stated that open reduction of the dislocated radial head was not indicated unless closed reduction failed. When there is a significant fracture of the head of the radius, Boyd and Boals recommend resec-

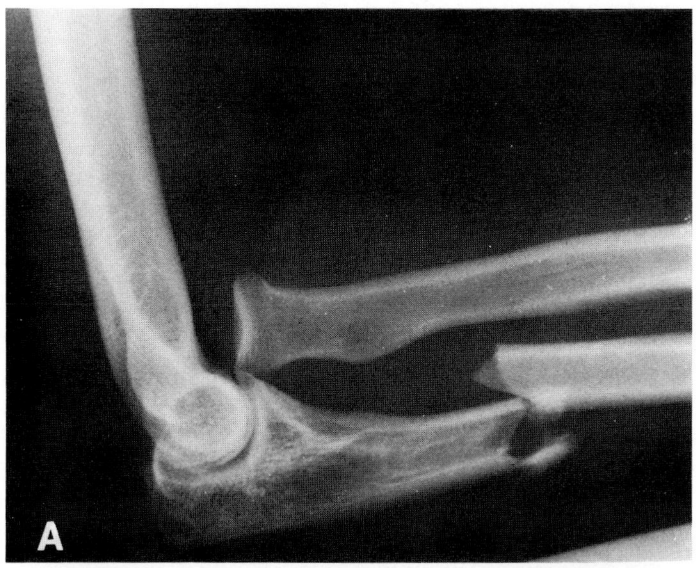

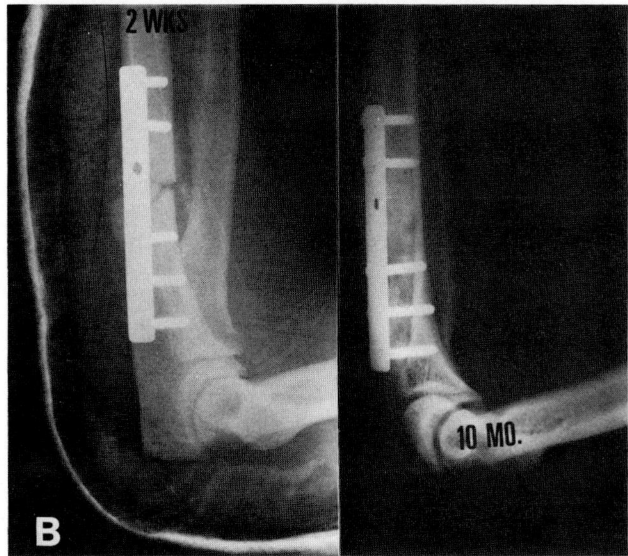

Fig. 8-30. (*A*) A Monteggia fracture in which the intact annular ligament held the radial head dislocated. (*B*) Two weeks after surgery in which the annular ligament was incised, the radial head is reduced, and the fracture of the ulna is fixed with a compression plate. Iliac grafts were applied because of comminution (*first frame*). Ten months after surgery, function is full except for 10 degrees loss of extension (*second frame*). (Anderson, L. D.: Fractures. *In* Crenshaw, A. H., (ed.): Campbell's Operative Orthopaedics. ed. 5. vol. 1. St. Louis, C. V. Mosby, 1971)

tion of the radial head at the same time the ulna is internally fixed. Their results were excellent to good in 77 per cent of the acute fractures.

Untreated or inadequately treated Monteggia fractures that are not seen until 4 to 6 weeks or more after injury present many problems (Fig. 8-29). Usually the ulna has angulated, and the radial head is either unreduced or has dislocated again. Malunion or nonunion of the ulna may be present.

If the patient presents with malunion of the ulna with only a few degrees of angulation and subluxation of the head of the radius, it is best to accept the mild malunion and resect only the head of the radius. If the malunion has occurred with moderate or severe angulation, osteotomy and rigid internal fixation of the ulna along with resection of the radial head is usually indicated.

When there is nonunion of the ulna and subluxation or dislocation of the radial head, realignment of the nonunion, rigid internal fixation, and bone grafting of the ulna should be done. The radial head should usually be resected, except in the rare case where subluxation is insignificant.

Author's Preferred Method of Treatment

I believe that the most important factors in achieving good results in adults with Monteggia lesions are (1) early accurate diagnosis, (2) rigid internal fixation of the fractured ulna, (3) complete reduction of the dislocated radial head, (4) cast immobilization in the appropriate position (depending on the type of Monteggia lesion) for a period of about 6 weeks, and (5) early open reduction and internal fixation of the fractured radial shaft in Bado's Type IV lesions.

The importance of early diagnosis is apparent. If the dislocation is not recognized, the treatment will be inappropriate. Generally I prefer compression plate fixation for the fractured ulna. Most of these fractures are in the proximal third of the ulna. A medullary nail in this location may not fill the medullary canal and thus provide less than rigid fixation. For very comminuted fractures in the middle third of the ulna, a triangular medullary nail may be better, but these are not common. Whenever significant comminution is present, I apply autogenous iliac grafts about the fracture.

When the radial head can be reduced completely by closed means it is unnecessary to perform open reduction. Open reduction of the radial head is indicated only when an infolded portion of the annular ligament prevents complete reduction or when the radial head is telescoped proximally through an intact annular ligament and hung behind the lateral epicondyle (Fig. 8-30). In the former, the infolded part of the ligament should be removed from the joint to permit reduction of the radial head. In the latter, the ligament must be incised so that the head of the radius can be removed from behind the lateral epicondyle and returned to its proper position. In both, the ligament is repaired after the radial head is reduced. Fascial reconstruction of the annular ligament is very rarely indicated in acute cases of Monteggia fractures. When open reduction of the radial head is required, I prefer the approach recommended by Boyd[8,9] which utilizes one incision to expose both the fracture and the dislocation.

In the Type IV Monteggia lesions, early open reduction and internal fixation of both the fractures of the shaft of the radius and ulna is important. The dislocation can usually be treated closed with postoperative immobilization, as outlined above.

After Care

The position in which the elbow and forearm are placed after surgery is of utmost importance. I think that in the Type I, II, and IV lesions the elbow should be held in about 110 degrees of flexion. With rigid fixation of the ulna, I have never seen the radial head redislocate if the elbow is held in this position for 6 weeks after surgery. Supination is probably important when closed treatment is used, but forced supination is unnecessary with good fixation of the ulna if the elbow is maintained in 110 degrees of flexion. The Type II lesions with posterior dislocation of the radial head should be maintained in about 70 degrees of elbow flexion for 6 weeks.

Following surgery, roentgenograms of the forearm and elbow should be made at 2 weeks and again at 6 weeks. After 6 weeks with the elbow immobilized in plaster as outlined above, the cast is removed and active exercises are instituted. Passive stretching exercises are contraindicated. Improvement in elbow function generally continues over several months.

Complications

Many of the complications of Monteggia lesions are the same as those for other fractures of the shafts of the forearm bones. These include infection and nonunion. Redislocation or subluxation of the head of the radius and loss of reduction of the fracture of the ulna are almost always the result of inadequate internal fixation of the fractured ulna or improper positioning of the elbow during the postoperative period. Paralysis of the deep branch of the radial nerve is not uncommon, but function nearly always returns with time, and exploration of the nerve is not indicated.

Prognosis

The prognosis for regaining satisfactory or even excellent function following most Monteggia fractures is good, provided the diagnosis is made early and treatment is adequate. In the series reported by Boyd and Boals[10] in 1969, 77 per cent of the results were good or excellent. Twenty-three per cent were fair or poor. This series included all patients treated from 1940 until 1967, and a number of the fair and poor results were from the earlier years, when methods for fixation of the ulnar fracture were not as good as they are now. With rigid fixation of the ulna the percentage of good and excellent results should be higher, except when infection develops or when there is major soft-tissue damage from compound wounds.

FRACTURE OF THE RADIUS ALONE

Fractures of the shaft of the radius alone are divided into two distinct groups: (1) the fractures in the proximal two-thirds of the bone and (2) those that are located at the junction of the middle and distal thirds.

FRACTURES OF THE PROXIMAL RADIUS

Fractures of the upper two-thirds of the radial shaft alone are not common in adults. The radial shaft in the proximal two-thirds is relatively well padded by the forearm muscles. Most injuries severe enough to fracture the radius at this level will also fracture the ulna. Also, the anatomic position of the radius in most positions of function makes it less likely than the ulna to receive a direct blow.

The rare undisplaced fracture of the shaft of the radius in the proximal two-thirds should be immobilized in a long-arm cast with the forearm in mild or full supination, depending on whether the fracture is located above or below the insertion of the pronator teres. The reasons for placing the forearm in supination are outlined under the sections of this chapter dealing with surgical anatomy and fractures of both the radius and ulna.

Even undisplaced fractures can become displaced. Frequent roentgenograms must be made during the first few weeks, and the cast must be maintained until healing has occurred.

Displaced fractures of the proximal one-fifth of the radius are probably best treated closed with the forearm in full supination. These fractures are too high for good fixation with a plate and screws, and the proximal fragment is to short for a medullary nail to control rotation. If they are completely displaced and cannot be reduced, axial alignment can be achieved and maintained

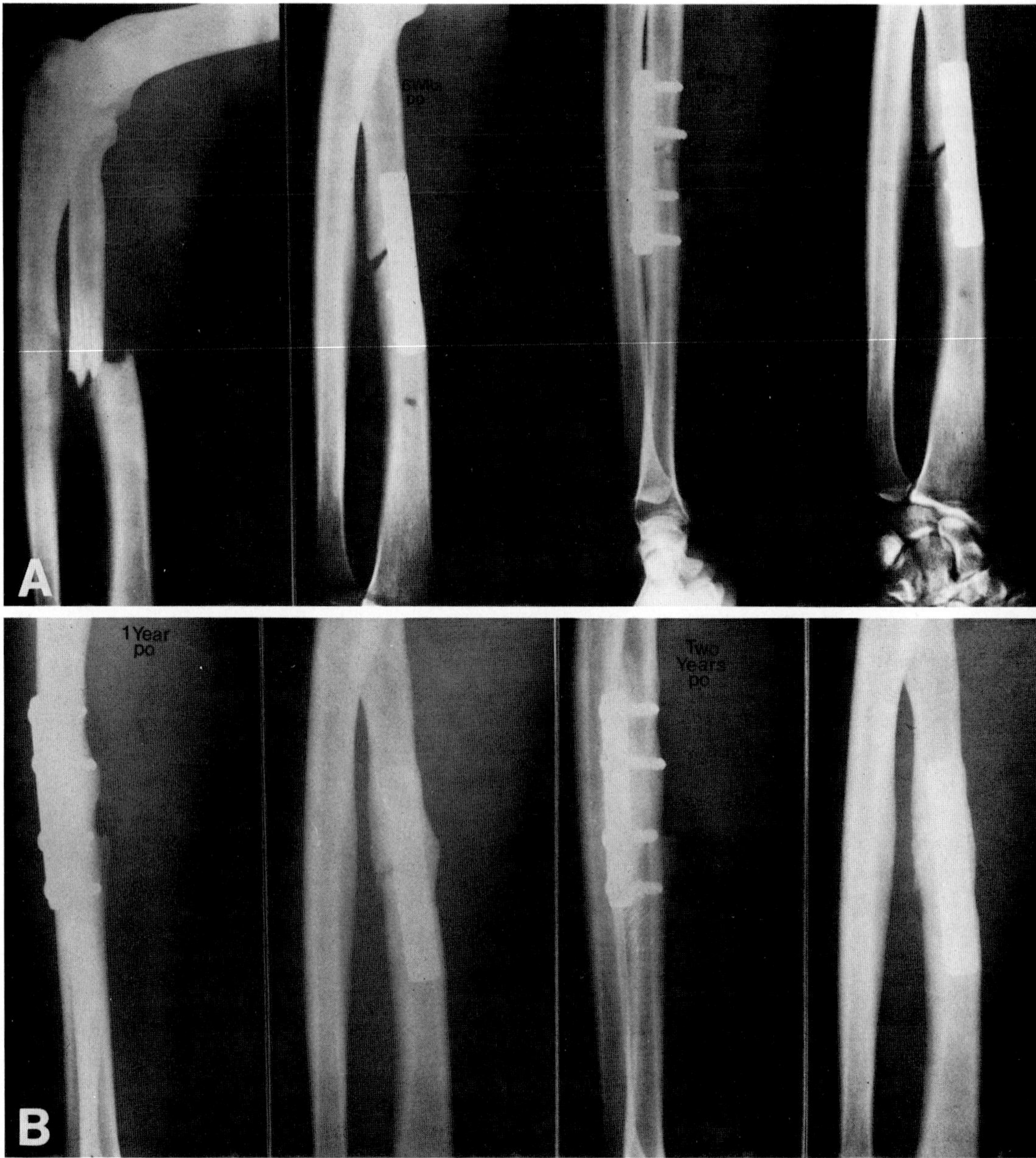

Fig. 8-31. (*A*) A fracture of the shaft of the radius at the junction of the proximal and middle thirds with intact ulna. Open reduction and internal fixation with a four-hole compression plate was carried out. Note that the plate was placed on the dorsal aspect of the radius. At 6 months, a portion of the fracture line is still visible. A five-hole plate would have been better, and bone grafts should have been applied. (*B*) Films at 1 year and 2 years showing good union. He had a full range of motion.

with a medullary nail, and rotational alignment, with a cast holding the forearm in full supination.

Except for the very high proximal one-fifth fractures, displaced fractures of the radius in the upper two-thirds can be treated with plate-and-screw fixation or with an adequate medullary nail as outlined under the section in this chapter on fractures of both the radius and ulna. I usually prefer a compression plate, because it is easier for me and the results have been good (Fig. 8-31). On the other hand, I have no quarrel with using a medullary nail, provided it controls rotation and maintains the radial bow. The after treatment is the same as for fractures of both bones of the forearm treated by open reduction and internal fixation.

FRACTURES OF THE DISTAL SHAFT (GALEAZZI'S FRACTURE)

The solitary fracture of the radius at the junction of the middle and distal thirds has several eponyms. The French, at least as early as 1929, referred to this lesion as a reverse Monteggia fracture.[64] Galeazzi[29,50] described the fracture in 1934 and called attention to the associated dislocation or subluxation of the distal radioulnar joint. He pointed out that subluxation of this joint may be present initially or may occur gradually during treatment. Galeazzi advocated treating the fracture by strong traction through the thumb. Campbell[61] is said to have called this lesion "the fracture of necessity" by which he meant that open reduction and internal fixation was necessary if a good result was to be obtained.

Probably the best description of the fracture of the distal shaft of the radius associated with dislocation of the distal radioulnar joint is that published by Hughston[32] in 1957. He collected 41 cases from members of the Piedmont Orthopaedic Club and called attention to the frequent mistakes in management. His criteria for a satisfactory result were very strict. They included union with perfect alignment, no loss of length, no subluxation of the distal radioulnar joint, and full pronation and supination. Of the 38 fractures treated initially by closed reduction and immobilization, Hughston found that 35 (92 percent) resulted in failure. Only three had a satisfactory result.

As pointed out by Hughston, there are four major deforming factors that cause loss of reduction. (1) Gravity acting through the weight of the hand, even in a cast, tends to cause subluxation of the distal radioulnar joint and dorsal angulation of the fractured radius. (2) The insertion of the pronator quadratus on the volar surface of the distal fragment rotates it towards the ulna and pulls it in a proximal and volar direction. (3) The brachioradialis tends to use the distal radioulnar joint as a pivot point upon which to rotate the distal fragment of the radius and at the same time causes shortening. (4) The abductors and extensors of the thumb cause shortening and relaxation of the radial collateral ligament so that one is not able to keep the soft-tissue bridge on stretch, even though the wrist is placed in ulnar deviation.

Mechanism of Injury

The two principal causes of the Galeazzi fracture are direct blows on the dorsilateral side of the wrist and falls. According to Galeazzi,[29,50] this lesion is approximately three times as common as is the Monteggia fracture.

Signs and Symptoms

The signs and symptoms vary with the severity of injury and the degree of displacement. In undisplaced or relatively undisplaced fractures the only deformity may be swelling and tenderness about the fracture. If the displacement is greater, there will be shortening of the radius and posterolateral angulation. Subluxation or dislocation will be evident in the distal radioulnar joint with prominence of the head of the ulna and tenderness over the joint. Most of these are closed fractures. In compound ones, the wound is usually a small puncture wound from within where the distal end of the proximal fragment has protruded through the skin. Nerve and vascular damage are rare.

Roentgenographic Findings

The fracture at the junction of the middle and distal thirds of the radius usually has a transverse or short oblique configuration (Fig. 8-32). Most do not have significant comminution. If there is much displacement of the fractured radius, the distal radioulnar joint will be dislocated. On the anteroposterior film the radius appears relatively shortened, with an increase in the space be-

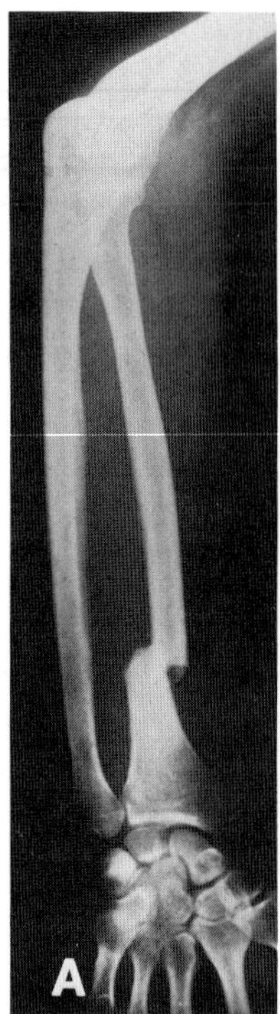

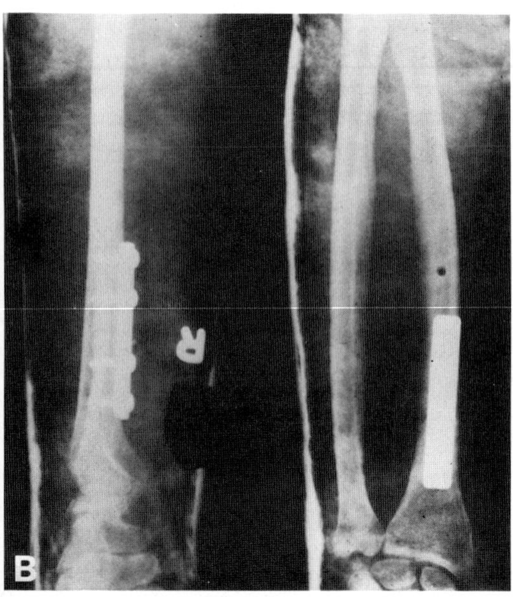

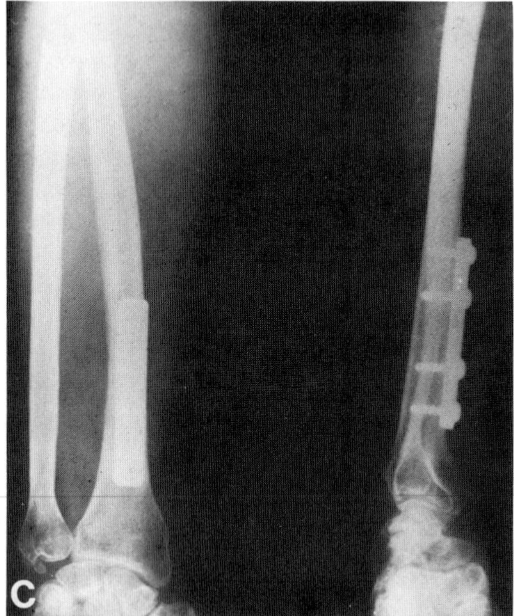

Fig. 8-32. (*A*) A Galeazzi fracture of the distal radial shaft with dislocation of the radioulnar joint. (*B*) Successful internal fixation using a four-hole compression plate. Note that the plate was applied on the volar surface of the radius where the bone is flatter. Compression was applied proximally. (*C*) One year later union is complete and function is normal.

tween the distal radius and ulna where they articulate. In the lateral view, the fractured radius is usually angulated dorsally and the head of the ulna is prominent dorsally. The injury to the radioulnar joint may be purely ligamentous, or the ligament may remain intact and the ulnar styloid may be avulsed.

Methods of Treatment

From the introductory discussion, it should be apparent that the results of closed treatment are poor. The deforming forces are so great that even if the fracture is undisplaced initially or if good position is obtained by closed reduction, displacement in a cast is the rule rather than the exception (Fig. 8-33). In order to obtain good pronation and supination and avoid derangement and arthritic changes in the distal radioulnar joint, the fracture must unite in anatomic position. For these reasons, open reduction and internal fixation is almost always the preferred form of treatment.

Medullary nails do not provide satisfactory fixation for these fractures (Fig. 8-15). The medullary canal at the level of the frac-

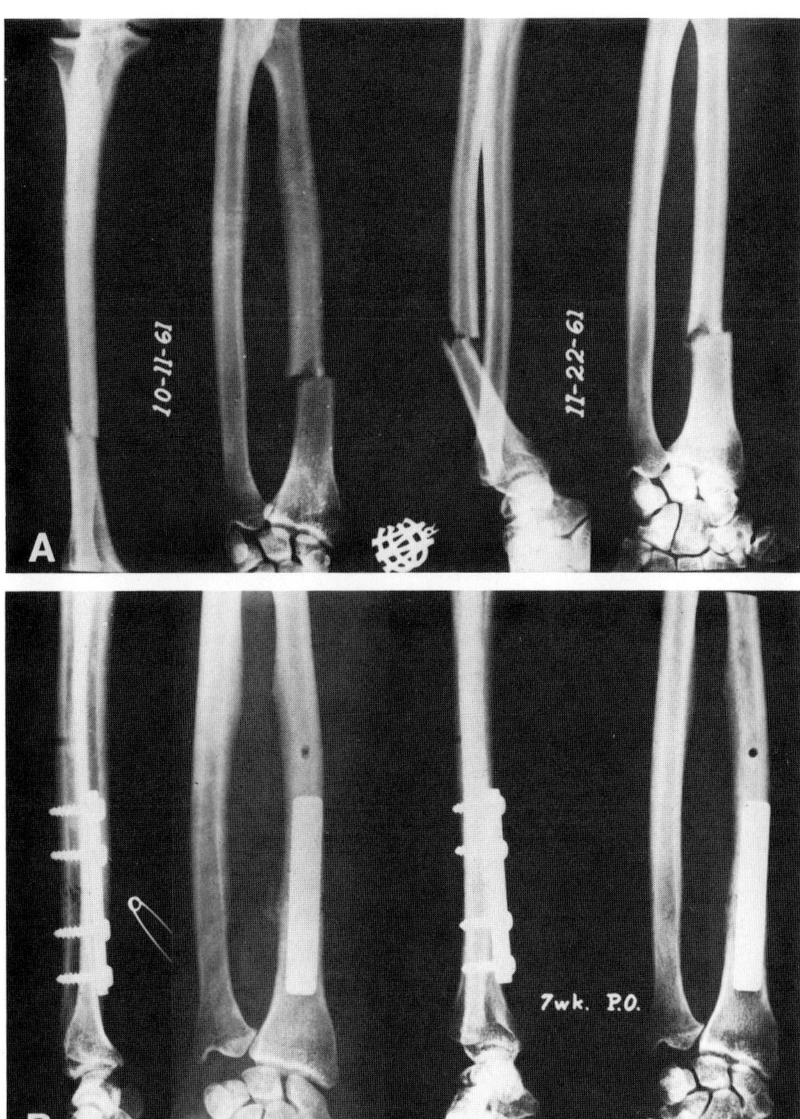

Fig. 8-33. (*A*) Solitary fracture of the distal third of the radial shaft with minimal displacement (*first and second frames*). After 6 weeks immobilization (by the family physician) and a long-arm cast, the fracture has angulated dorsally and the distal radioulnar joint is seen to be dislocated (*third and fourth frames*). (*B*) Immediate post-operative films showing the fracture fixed with a four-hole compression plate applied to the volar surface of the radius (*first and second frames*). Seven weeks later the fracture has united (*third and fourth frames*). (Anderson, L. D.: Fractures. *In* Crenshaw, A. H., (ed.): Campbell's Operative Orthopaedics. ed. 5. vol. 1. St. Louis, C. V. Mosby, 1971)

ture is large and continues to enlarge distally. The nail does not prevent medial offset of the distal fragment and shortening of the radius. Also, the medullary canal of the distal fragment is too large for the nail to control rotation.

Small plates and screws also do not provide fixation adequate to resist the deforming forces. The plates may bend or the screws pull loose and cause loss of position with malunion or nonunion. Plate-and-screw fixation is by far the best, but if good results are to be expected the plate must be long enough and the screws must obtain good purchase in both cortices.

Author's Preferred Method of Treatment

I prefer to treat fractures of the junction of the middle and distal thirds of the radius with ASIF compression plates. I have now used this method of fixation since 1960, and the results have been excellent. The details of technique are reported elsewhere[2,44] but a few points about this particular fracture should be emphasized.

At the level of this fracture I prefer the anterior approach of Henry.[8,30] The volar surface of the radius is flat and provides a better bed for the plate.

Using a hand table and tourniquet control, a 5- or 6-inch longitudinal incision is made, centered over the fracture in the plane between the flexor carpiradialis and brachioradialis muscles. The radial artery and veins are identified and retracted laterally along with the brachioradialis tendon and the superficial radial nerve. All other structures are retracted medially. The fracture is almost always located just above the proximal border of the pronator quadratus. Using scissors and extraperiosteal dissection, the insertion of the pronator quadratus is freed from the radius and reflected ulnarward. The volar surface of the proximal fragment is then exposed extraperiosteally for a distance long enough to allow placement of the plate and compression device. Using self-retaining Lane bone-holding forceps, the fracture is reduced anatomically. Usually there is little or no comminution, but if there is, the surgeon should try to fit each fragment anatomically into place. The appropriate length plate is selected, depending on the obliquity of the fracture and degree of comminution. In pure transverse fractures a 4-hole plate is adequate, but if there is any comminution or obliquity a 5- or 6-hole plate is necessary. The plate is centered accurately so that at least two screws can be placed in both the proximal and distal fragments with no screw closer than 1 cm. to the fracture, even if this means leaving a hole in the plate empty.

The plate is clamped to the proximal and distal fragments with two self-retaining Lane forceps parallel to the plate. A third Lane forceps is placed at right angles to the first two and clamped in place to prevent angulation and shortening when compression is applied. The screws are inserted into the distal fragment first. Cancellous screws with large threads are used if the standard cortical screws do not seat with adequate fixation. The bone proximal to the plate is drilled and tapped for the compression device and compression is applied in the usual way.

At this point roentgenograms are made in anteroposterior and lateral planes to be sure the relationship at the distal radioulnar joint is exactly right. If it is, the screws are inserted in the proximal fragment.

If done properly, strong compression can usually be applied to these fractures without disturbing the distal relationship of the radius to the ulna. Occasionally, however, the fracture may be so comminuted or oblique that the radius shortens when compression is applied and the distal relationship is disturbed. If the films made after compression is applied but before screws are inserted in the proximal fragment show radial shortening, the compression is released and the compression device is removed. The fracture is then reduced again, making sure the radius is out to full length, confirmed with additional roentgenograms. The screws are then inserted in the proximal fragment without compression. If there is significant comminution (there usually is if compression cannot be applied without causing the radius to shorten) autogenous iliac bone grafts are added.

The pronator quadratus is allowed to fall back in position over the plate and is tacked back to the soft tissues on the lateral side of the radius. The fascia should *not* be closed for the reasons discussed on page 462. The subcutaneous tissue and skin are closed and a well molded sugar tong splint is applied. Final films are made after the cast is in place to confirm that the distal radioulnar joint is reduced anatomically.

After Care

After 2 weeks the sutures are removed and a new sugar tong is applied. Check films are made. The splint is left in place for a total of 5 or 6 weeks to allow healing of the soft tissues. Then active exercises of the elbow, wrist, and forearm are begun, with emphasis on regaining pronation and supination. Because the plate is well covered with soft tissue, it is seldom necessary to remove it, except in young athletes. If it is removed, the precautions noted on page 463 to prevent refracture should be followed.

Prognosis

Some of the older articles emphasize the poor prognosis for regaining good function after the Galeazzi fracture.[32,68] However, these articles were published before rigid fixation with compression plates was available. The points of Campbell and Hughston are well made. Closed treatment gives poor results, as does inadequate internal fixation. The reduction of both the radial fracture and the distal radioulnar joint must be anatomical, and the fixation must be rigid. Since we began using compression plates for this fracture in 1960, the results have been excellent.

Complications

The complications of the Galeazzi fracture are those incident to all forearm fractures—nonunion, malunion, infection. The most common complication is angulation of the fracture and subluxation or dislocation of the distal radioulnar joint. In patients with acute fractures, these complications are largely avoidable with skillful surgical technique and rigid fixation.

In patients presenting for treatment late (after 6 weeks) with nonunion and malposition, it is usually best to realign the radius and bone graft it. If there has been much resorption of bone at the fracture, a full-thickness iliac graft from the crest can often be used to regain radial length, restore the distal radioulnar relationship, and obtain reasonably good function. Even if the distal ulna must be resected, it is better to allow the nonunion to heal before doing so. Resecting the distal ulna at the same time that you plate and bone graft the radius is asking for trouble. Even though the distal relationship may not be satisfactory, the ulna relieves some of the deforming forces on the radius. If it is resected at the same time, the added stress may cause the screws to pull out of the osteoporotic bone. I know of two patients in whom this complication occurred.

In patients with mild to moderate degrees of malunion of the radius, pronation and supination will be limited and painful. In these, the distal 2 cm. of the ulna should be resected, but only after the radius is solidly united. When the distal ulna is resected it should be done subperiostally, and care should be taken to reconstruct the lateral collateral ligament.

REFERENCES

1. Anderson, L. D.: Compression plate fixation and the effect of different types of internal fixation on fracture healing. J. Bone Joint Surg., *47A*:191-208, 1965.
2. ———: Fractures. *In* Crenshaw, A. H., (ed.): Campbell's Operative Orthopaedics. vol. 1. ed. 5. St. Louis, C. V. Mosby, 1971.
3. Anderson, L. D., Sisk, T. D., Park, W. I., and Tooms, R. E.: Compression plate fixation in acute diaphyseal fractures of the radius and ulna. *In* Proceedings American

Academy of Orthopaedic Surgeons. J. Bone Joint Surg., *54A*:1332-1333, 1972.
4. Bado, J. L.: The Monteggia lesion. Clin. Orthop., *50*:71-76, 1967.
5. Bagby, G. W.: The effect of compression on the rate of healing using a special plate. Am. J. Surg., *95*:761-771, 1958.
6. Bick, E. M.: Source Book of Orthopaedics. ed. 2. Baltimore, Williams & Wilkins, 1948.
7. Boreau, J., and Hermann, P.: Plague d'Osteosynthese permettant l'Impaction des Fragments. Presse Med., *1*:356, 1952.
8. Boyd, H. B.: Surgical approaches. *In* Crenshaw, A. H., (ed.): Campbell's Operative Orthopaedics. vol. 1. ed. 5. St. Louis, C. V. Mosby, 1971.
9. ———: Surgical exposure of the ulna and proximal third of the radius through one incision. Surg., Gynecol., and Obstet., *71*: 86-88, 1940.
10. Boyd, H. B., and Boals, J. C.: The Monteggia lesion. A review of 159 cases. Clin. Orthop., *66*:94-100, 1969.
11. Boyd, H. B., Lipinski, S. W., and Wiley, J. H.: Observations on non-union of the shafts of the long bones, with a statistical analysis of 842 patients. J. Bone Joint Surg., *43A*:159-167, 1961.
12. Bradford, C. H., Adams, R. W., and Kilfoyle, R. M.: Fractures of both bones of the forearm in adults. Surg., Gynecol., and Obstet., *96*:240-244, 1953.
13. Brav, E. A.: Further evaluation of the use of intramedullary nailing in the treatment of gunshot fractures of the extremities. J. Bone Joint Surg., *39A*:513-520, 1957.
14. Burwell, H. N., and Charnley, A. D.: Treatment of forearm fractures in adults with particular reference to plate fixation. J. Bone Joint Surg., *46B*:404-424, 1964.
15. Caden, J. G.: Internal fixation of fractures of the forearm. J. Bone Joint Surg., *43A*: 1115-1121, 1961.
16. Campbell, W. C., and Boyd, H. B.: Fixation of onlay bone grafts by means of Vitallium screws in the treatment of unusual fractures. Am. J. Surg., *51*:748-756, 1941.
17. Cave, E. F.: Fractures and Other Injuries. Chicago, Year Book Medical Publishers, 1958.
18. Charnley, J.: The Closed Treatment of Common Fractures. ed. 3. Baltimore, Williams & Wilkins, 1961.
19. Compere, E. L., Banks, S. W., and Compere, C. L.: Pictorial Handbook of Fracture Treatment. ed. 3. Chicago, Year Book Medical Publishers, 1952.
20. Conwell, H. E., and Reynolds, F. C.: Management of Fractures, Dislocations, and Sprains. ed. 7. St. Louis, C. V. Mosby, 1961.
21. Danis: Les Coopteurs and les Coopteurs: Uncles Theoric et Practique de l'Osteosynthese. Paris, Masson & Cie, 1949.
22. Dodge, H. S., and Cody, G. W.: Treatment of fractures of the radius and ulna with compression plates: a retrospective study of one hundred eight patients. J. Bone Joint Surg., *54A*:1167-1176, 1972.
23. Eggers, G. W. N.: Internal contact splint. J. Bone Joint Surg., *30A*:40-51, 1948.
24. ———: The internal fixation of fractures of the shafts of long bones. *In* Carter, B. N. (ed.): Monographs on Surgery. Baltimore, Williams & Wilkins, 1952.
25. Eggers, G. W. N., Ainsworth, W. H., Shindler, T. O., and Pomerat, C. M.: Clinical significance of contact-compression factor in bone surgery. Arch. Surg., *62*:467-474, 1951.
26. Eggers, G. W. N., Shindler, T. O., and Pomerat, C. M.: The influence of the contact-compression factor on osteogenesis in surgical fractures. J. Bone Joint Surg., *31A*: 693-716, 1949.
27. Evans, E. M.: Pronation injuries of forearm with special reference to anterior Monteggia fracture. J. Bone Joint Surg., *31B*: 578-588, 1949.
28. ———: Rotational deformity in the treatment of fractures of both bones of the forearm. J. Bone Joint Surg., *27*:373-379, 1945.
29. Galeazzi, R.: Arch. Orthop. Unfallchir., *35*:557-562, 1934.
30. Henry, A. K.: Extensile Exposure. ed. 2. Baltimore, Williams & Wilkins, 1957.
31. Hicks, J. H.: Fracture Forearm Treatment by Rigid Fixation. J. Bone Joint Surg., *43B*: 680-687, 1961.
32. Hughston, J. C.: Fracture of the distal radial shaft. Mistakes in management. J. Bone Joint Surg., *39A*:249-264, 1957.
33. Hutzchenreuter, P., Perren, S. M., and Steinemann, S.: Some effects of rigidity of internal fixation on the healing pattern of osteotomies. Injury, *1*:77-81, 1969.
34. Jinkins, W. J., Lockhart, L. D., and Eggers, G. W. N.: Fractures the forearm in adults. Southern Med. J., *53*:669-679, 1960.
35. Knight, R. A., and Purvis, G. D.: Fractures of both bones of the forearm in adults. J. Bone Joint Surg., *31A*:755-764, 1949.

36. Lam, S. J. S.: Delayed internal fixation for fractures of the radial shaft. Guy's Hosp. Rep., *114*:391-400, 1965.
37. ———: The place of delayed internal fixation in the treatment of fractures of the long bones. J. Bone Joint Surg., *46B*:393-397, 1964.
38. Lambotte, A.: Chirurgie Operatoire des Fractures. Paris, Masson & Cie, 1913.
39. ———: L'intervention Operatoire dans les Fractures Recentes et Anciennes Envisagee Particulierement au Point de vue de l'osteosynthese avec la Description des Plusiers Techniques nouvelles. Paris, A. Maloine, 1907.
40. Lane, W. A.: Operative Treatment of Fractures. London, 1905.
41. ———: Treatment of simple fractures by operation. Lancet, *1*:1489-1493, 1900.
42. Marek, F. M.: Axial fixation of forearm fractures. J. Bone Joint Surg., *43A*:1099-1114, 1961.
43. Monteggia, G. B.: Instituzioni Chirurgiche. vol. 5. Milan, Maspero, 1814.
44. Müller, M. E., Allgower, M., and Willenegger, H.: Technique of Internal Fixation of Fractures. New York, Springer-Verlag, 1965.
45. Naiman, P. T., Schein, A. J., and Seiffert, R. S.: Use of ASIF compression plates in selected shaft fractures of the upper extremity. Clin. Orthop., *71*:208-217, 1970.
46. Patrick, J.: A study of supination and pronation, with especial reference to the treatment of forearm fractures. J. Bone Joint Surg., *28*:737-748, 1946.
47. Penrose, J. H.: The Monteggia fracture with posterior dislocation of radial head. J. Bone Joint Surg., *33B*:65-73, 1951.
48. Perren, S. M., Allgower, M., Russenberger, M., Mathys, R., Schenk, R., Willenegger, H., and Müller, M. E.: The reaction of cortical bone to compression. Acta Orthop. Scandinavica, [Suppl.]:125, 1969.
49. Ralston, E. L.: Handbook of Fractures. St. Louis, C. V. Mosby, 1967.
50. Rang, M.: Anthology of Orthopaedics. Edinburgh, E. & S. Livingstone, 1968.
51. Reckling, F. W., and Cordell, L. D.: Unstable fracture-dislocations of the forearm. The Monteggia and Galeazzi lesions. Arch. Surg., *96*:999-1007, 1968.
52. Ritchie, S. J., Richardson, J. P., and Thompson, M. S.: Rigid medullary fixation of forearm fractures. Southern Med. J., *51*: 852-856, 1958.
53. Rush, L. V.: Atlas of Rush Pin Technics. Mississippi Doctor, *31*:book section, Aug. 1953; March 1954.
54. Sage, F. P.: Fractures of the shaft of the radius and ulna in the adult. *In* Adams, J. P., (ed.): Current Practice in Orthopaedic Surgery. vol. 1. St. Louis, C. V. Mosby, 1963.
55. Sage, F. P.: Medullary fixation of fractures of the forearm. A study of the medullary canal of the radius and a report of fifty fractures of the radius treated with a prebent triangular nail. J. Bone Joint Surg., *41A*:1489-1516, 1959.
56. Sargent, J. P., and Teipner, W. A.: Treatment of forearm shaft fractures by double-plating. A preliminary report. J. Bone Joint Surg., *47A*:1475-1490, 1965.
57. Smith, F. M.: Monteggia fractures; analysis of 25 consecutive fresh injuries. Surg., Gynecol., and Obstet., *85*:630-640, 1947.
58. Smith, H., and Sage, F. P.: Medullary fixation of forearm fractures. J. Bone Joint Surg., *39A*:91-98, 1957.
59. Smith, J. E. M.: Internal fixation in the treatment of fractures of the shaft of the radius and ulna in adults. J. Bone Joint Surg., *41B*:122-131, 1959.
60. Speed, J. S., and Boyd, H. B.: Treatment of fractures of the ulna with dislocation of head of radius (Monteggia fracture). J.A.M.A., *115*:1699-1704, 1940.
61. Stewart, M. J.: Personal communication. Dec., 1973.
62. Street, D. M.: Spectator Letter. 1955.
63. Thompson, J. E.: Anatomical methods of approach in operations on the long bones of the extremities. Ann. Surg., *68*:309-329, 1918.
64. Valande, M.: Luxation en Arriere du Cubitus avec Fracture de la diaphyse radiale. Bull. et Mem. de la Soc. Nat. de Chir., *55*: 435-437, 1929.
65. Venable, C. S.: An impacting bone plate to attain close apposition. Ann. Surg., *133*: 808-812, 1951.
66. Venable, C. S., Stuck, W. G., and Beach, A.: The effects on bone of the presence of metals; based upon electrolysis; an experimental study. Ann. Surg., *105*:917-938, 1937.
67. Watson-Jones, R.: Fractures and joint injuries. vol. 1. ed. 4. Edinburgh, E. & S. Livingstone, 1952.
68. ———: Fractures and Joint Injuries. vol. 2. ed. 4. Edinburgh, E. & S. Livingstone, 1955.

9 Fractures and Dislocations of the Elbow

Richard H. Eppright, M.D.
Kaye E. Wilkins, M.D.

Trauma about the elbow joint is often poorly tolerated by adults. Fortunately, fractures near the elbow account for only about 6 per cent of all fractures treated.[62,311] The injury may present as a fracture, a dislocation, or a profound injury of soft tissue. Often it is a difficult and challenging combination of these. In order to achieve the best possible result, it is important to be accurate and decisive in the initial evaluation and management. The surgeon must promptly differentiate those injuries that respond best to surgical intervention from those that lend themselves better to nonoperative treatment. It is inappropriate to institute closed treatment routinely for all elbow injuries and to rely upon open reduction and internal fixation only as a late secondary procedure. There are many injuries of the elbow in which prompt operative intervention is the treatment of choice.

Because of the anatomical structure of the bones that comprise the joint, very few elbow fractures are instrinsically stable. The muscles that attach to the bony prominences about the elbow joint may produce persistent displacement of the fracture fragments. Closed methods of treatment often require extremes of positioning to achieve an adequate reduction. Maintaining such a position in the adult patient until the fracture becomes stable can result in residual stiffness and significant elbow disability.

Many of the operative procedures for reassembling a shattered elbow are technically difficult. They may require extensive soft-tissue dissection to achieve a good anatomical reduction. This surgical insult superimposed upon already severely traumatized soft tissue may lead to further postoperative adhesions. Thus surgery, performed improperly or done where not indicated, may result in disability as great as that resulting from a nonoperative method.

It is therefore mandatory for the responsible surgeon to have a thorough knowledge of the anatomy and potential complications, both early and late. He must be very familiar with the various methods of management of these complicated fractures.

ANATOMY

The humerus, radius, and ulna come together at the elbow to form a complex called the cubital articulation[109] (Fig. 9-1). The elbow joint is composed of three articulations: humeroradial, humeroulnar, and radioulnar, all within a continuous synovial cavity. Magnuson[174] viewed the ulna as a distal extension of the arm and the radius as a proximal extension of the hand. Most of the strength and stability of the elbow lies in the articulation of the ulna with the humerus; the radius facilitates the dextrous motions of the hand. This is an important concept, because residual deformities of the

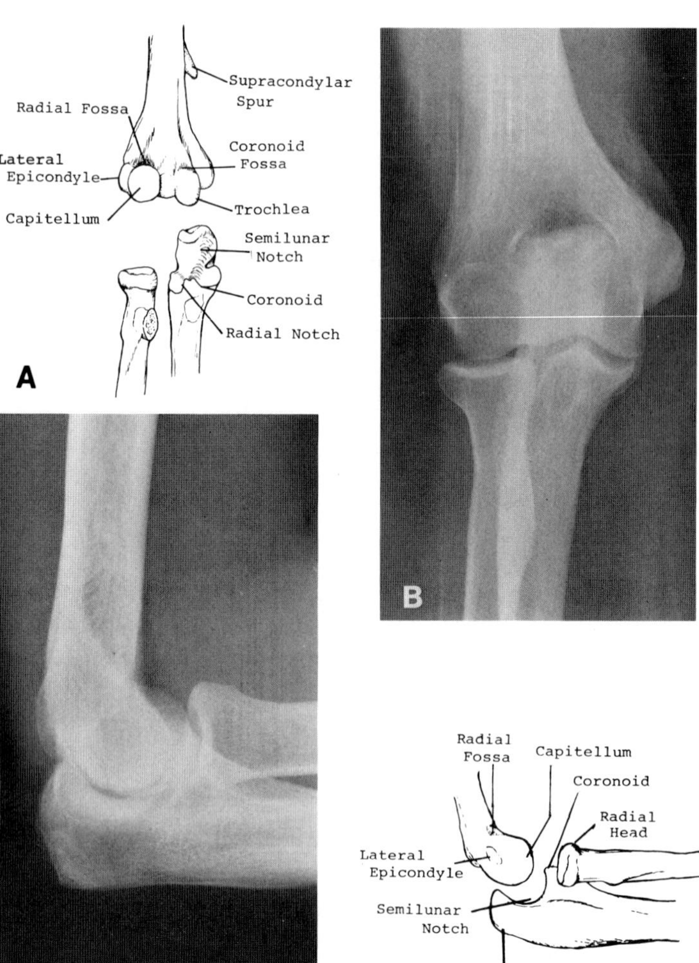

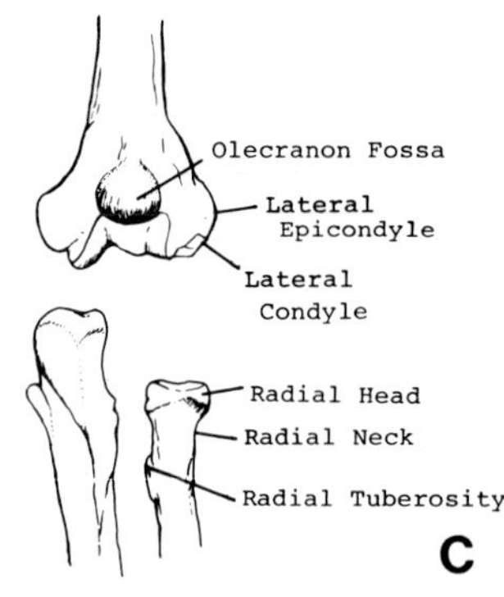

Fig. 9-1. Normal anatomy. (*A*) The normal bony landmarks on the anterior aspect of the radius, ulna, and humerus at the elbow joint. The supracondylar spur is seen in only about 1 per cent of normal individuals. (*B*) The same bony landmarks as seen on the anteroposterior roentgenogram of a normal elbow. (*C*) The normal landmarks on the lateral aspect of the bones comprising the elbow. (*D*) A lateral roentgenogram of the normal elbow shows the landmarks demonstrated in 1C. (*E*) The normal bony landmarks as seen on the posterior aspect of the elbow.

radius with the humerus or the proximal ulna lead to loss of manual dexterity. Residual deformities of the humeroulnar joint can lead to loss of strength, stability, or flexion—an extension motion of the elbow joint.

When the elbow is extended, the forearm forms a valgus angulation with the arm. Supination of the forearm makes this angulation more apparent. When the arm is hanging at the side of the body, this angulation positions the hand a convenient distance away from the thigh, thus facilitating its carrying function.[275] This carrying angle is normally 5 to 20 degrees (average 15 degrees) in adults.[174,254]

General anatomical descriptions are presented in the following sections. Additional anatomical details relating specifically to particular injuries are presented in the discussions of those injuries.

TOPOGRAPHICAL ANATOMY

Several bony landmarks of the elbow can be palpated readily. In full extension both epicondyles and the olecranon process lie in the same horizontal plane on the posterior aspect of the elbow. When the elbow is flexed 90 degrees these points form a nearly equilateral triangle in a plane parallel to the posterior surface of the humerus.[13] In flexion, a fourth bony prominence, the outer border of the capitellum, becomes more evident on the lateral aspect of the humerus. It lies distal and anterior to the lateral epicondyle and should not be confused with it. Just distal to the capitellum the radial head can be palpated; it is most easily found by passively rotating the forearm. A familiarity with the bony prominences of the elbow and their relationships to one another greatly assists the surgeon in perceiving subtle abnormalities in the examination of the injured elbow.

When the elbow is flexed, the anconeous muscle lies just distal and posterior to the radiohumeral joint in a triangular area outlined by the radial head, the lateral epicondyle, and the tip of the olecranon. The main portion of the radial collateral ligament extends anteriorly and distally, leaving only the fibrous capsule of the elbow joint underlying this rather small, thin muscle. Any distension of the joint with fluid can best be detected here, and this is the preferred site for aspiration of the joint.

THE BONES

Lower End of the Humerus

The distal aspect of the humerus divides into medial and lateral columns (Fig. 9-2). Each of these columns is roughly triangular and is bounded on its outer border by a supracondylar ridge. The divergence of these two columns increases the diameter of the distal humerus in the medial-lateral plane. From a structural and functional standpoint, the distal humerus is divided into separate medial and lateral components, called condyles, each containing an articulating portion and a nonarticulating portion. Included in the nonarticulating

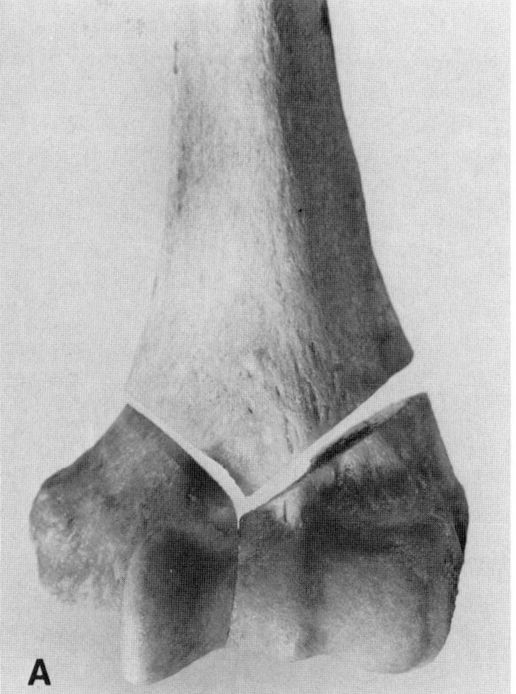

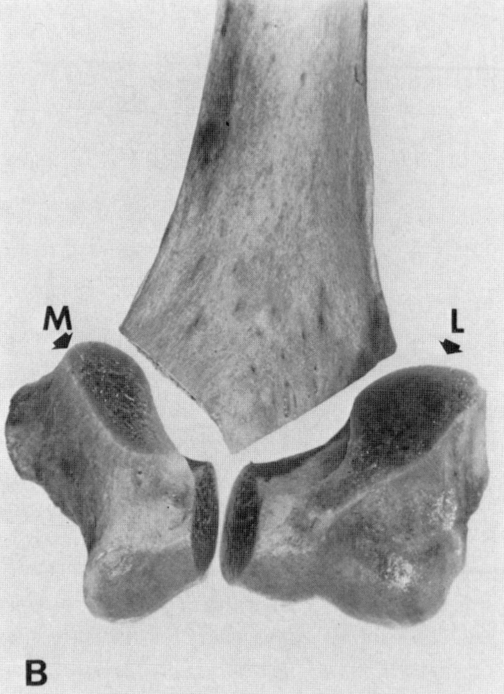

Fig. 9-2. Internal structure of the distal humerus. (*A*) Photograph of the anterior surface of a normal distal humerus with cuts through the medial and lateral supracondylar columns. (*B*) Rotation of the medial (M) and lateral (L) supracondylar columns demonstrates their internal structure. The diameter of the medial column (M) is smaller than the lateral (L).

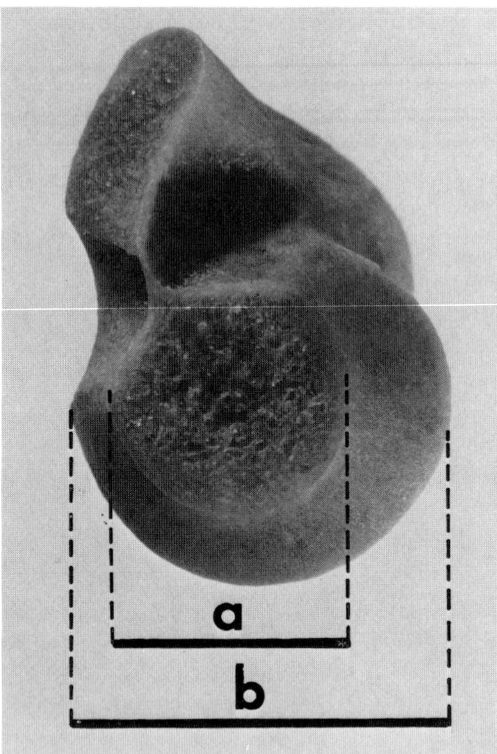

Fig. 9-3. Cross-section of the medial condyle through the trochlear groove of the medial condyle. The diameter of the bony portion of the center of the groove (*a*) is slightly over one-half that of the medial trochlear ridge (*b*).

portions are the epicondyles, which are the terminal points of the supracondylar ridges. The lateral epicondyle contains a roughened anterolateral surface from which the superficial forearm extensor muscles arise. The medial epicondyle is larger than its lateral counterpart and serves as the origin of the forearm flexor muscles. The posterior distal portion of the medial epicondyle is smooth and is in contact with the ulnar nerve as it crosses the elbow joint. When a condyle loses continuity from its supporting column, as in a fracture, displacement can occur, because there are no muscles attached to the condyles to oppose those attached to the epicondyles.

The articulating surface of the lateral condyle is hemispherical and projects anteriorly; it is called the capitellum (capitulum), or "little head." The capitellum is much smaller than the trochlea, and its convex surface articulates with the reciprocally concave head of the radius. These surfaces are in contact throughout only a small portion of the full range of elbow motion.

The articular surface of the medial condyle, the trochlea, is more cylindrical, or spool-like. It has very prominent medial and lateral ridges, which Milch believed are very important in maintaining medial and lateral stability of the elbow.[189] Between these ridges is a central groove that articulates with the greater sigmoid (semilunar) notch of the proximal ulna. The diameter of the trochlea at this groove is approximately half that of the medial ridge (Fig. 9-3), and the groove occupies nearly the entire circumference of the trochlea. It originates anteriorly in the coronoid fossa and terminates posteriorly in the olecranon fossa. On the posterior surface of the trochlea the groove is directed slightly laterally. It is this obliquity of the trochlear groove that produces the valgus carrying angle of the forearm when the elbow is extended. Between the lateral ridge of the trochlea and the hemispherical surface of the capitellum, a sulcus separates the medial and lateral condyles. This capitulotrochlear sulcus articulates with the peripheral ridge of the radial head.

Proximal to the condyles on the anterior surface of the humerus lie the coronoid and radial fossae. They receive the coronoid process and radial head, respectively, when the elbow is flexed. Posteriorly, the olecranon fossa is a deep hollow for the reception of the olecranon, making it possible for the elbow to go into full extension. The bone that separates these anterior and posterior fossae is extremely thin, usually translucent, and occasionally even absent. The presence of any extraneous material in the olecranon fossa, such as fracture fragments or an internal fixation device, necessarily impedes full extension of the elbow (see Fig. 9-13).

The articular cartilage surfaces of the capitellum and trochlea project downward and forward from the end of the humerus at an angle of approximately 45 degrees.[64] The centers of the arcs of rotation of the articular surfaces of each condyle lie on the same horizonal line through the distal humerus. Thus, malalignment of the relationship of one condyle to the other changes their arcs of rotation, limiting flexion and extension[172] (Fig. 9-4).

A bony spine, called the supracondylar process, occasionally projects downward from the anteriomedial surface of the humerus (Fig. 9-5). It arises approximately 5 cm. superior to the medial epicondyle, and it is attached to the medial epicondyle by a fibrous band. The process, the shaft of the humerus, and the fibrous band form a foramen through which the median nerve and the brachial artery pass. The spur gives origin to a part of the pronator teres muscle and may receive a lower portion of the insertion of the coracobrachialis muscle.

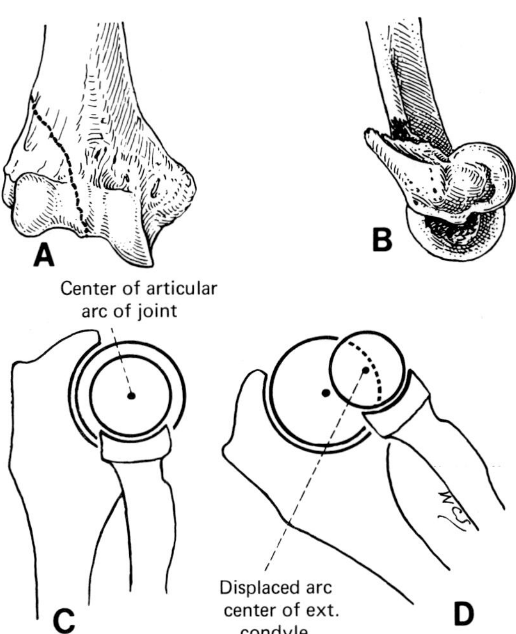

Fig. 9-4. Effects of condylar malalignment. The centers of the articular arc of the separate condyles are located on the same horizontal line through the distal humerus (*A*, *C*). When there is malalignment of one condyle with another (*B*, *D*), flexion and extension of the elbow are blocked. (Magnuson, P. B., and Stack, J. K.: Fractures. ed. 5. Philadelphia, J. B. Lippincott, 1949)

Upper End of the Radius

The proximal end of the radius (see Fig. 9-1) consists of the disc-shaped head, the neck, and the radial tuberosity; the head and part of the neck lie within the joint. The shallow concavity of the radial head articulates with the convex surface of the capitellum, and the border of the radial head articulates with the lateral side of the coronoid process in the lesser sigmoid (radial) notch. The tuberosity, which is extraarticular, has a rough posterior portion for the insertion of the tendon of the biceps, and a smooth anterior surface over which lies a bursa that separates the tuberosity from the tendon.

Upper End of the Ulna

The proximal end of the ulna (see Fig. 9-1) consists of the olecranon and coronoid processes, which together form the greater sigmoid (semilunar) notch, although their articular surfaces may not always be continuous.[282] The articulation of this notch with the trochlea of the humerus provides inherent bony stability to the hinge joint of the elbow. It is notable that both the medial and lateral collateral ligaments attach to the proximal portion of the ulna.

The triceps inserts by a broad tendinous expansion into the olecranon posteriorly, and on the anterior surface, the brachialis muscle inserts into the distal (nonarticular) side of the coronoid process and the tuberosity of the ulna, which lies at the base of the coronoid process.

The head of the radius rests within the lesser sigmoid (radial) notch on the lateral side of the coronoid process. The orbicular (annular) ligament consists of bands of strong fibers, which are intimately and inseparably connected with—but somewhat thicker than—the capsule of the elbow

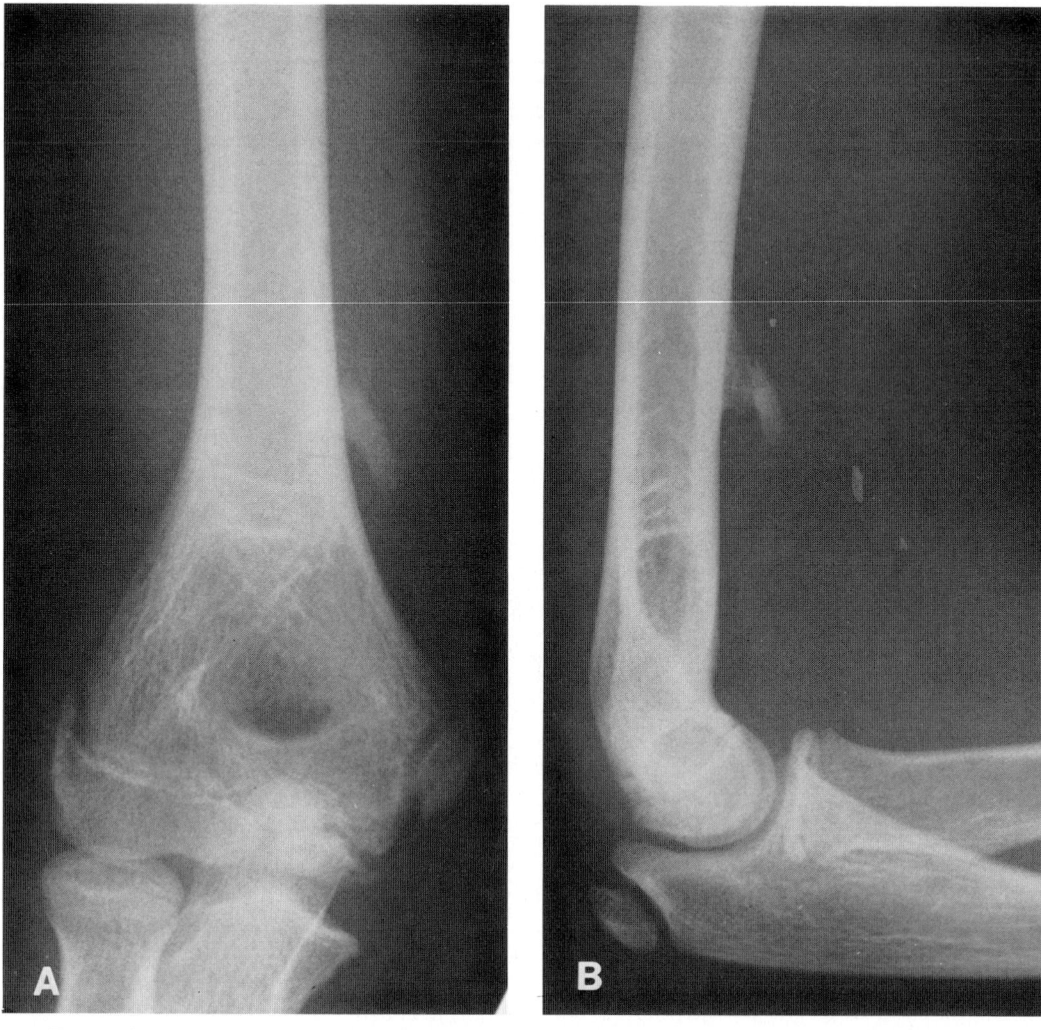

Fig. 9-5. Anteroposterior (*A*) and lateral (*B*) views of a distal humerus which has a supracondylar process.

joint. The ligament encircles the head of the radius, retaining it within the radial notch but allowing it enough freedom to rotate easily.

THE JOINT

Collateral Ligaments

The collateral ligaments of the elbow supplement the natural stability of the elbow joint. The fan-shaped radial collateral ligament originates from the lateral epicondyle and inserts into the orbicular (annular) ligament of the radius. Some of the posterior fibers go to the ulna just proximal to the posterior origin of the orbicular ligament. The thicker and stronger ulnar collateral ligament consists of two portions, both arising from the medial epicondyle. The anterior portion attaches to a tubercle (sublime tubercle) on the medial surface of the coronoid. The posterior portion attaches to the medial surface of the olecranon process. The humeral attachment of the ulnar collateral ligament is eccentrically placed, so that the posterior fibers are taut in flexion and the anterior fibers are taut in extension.[111]

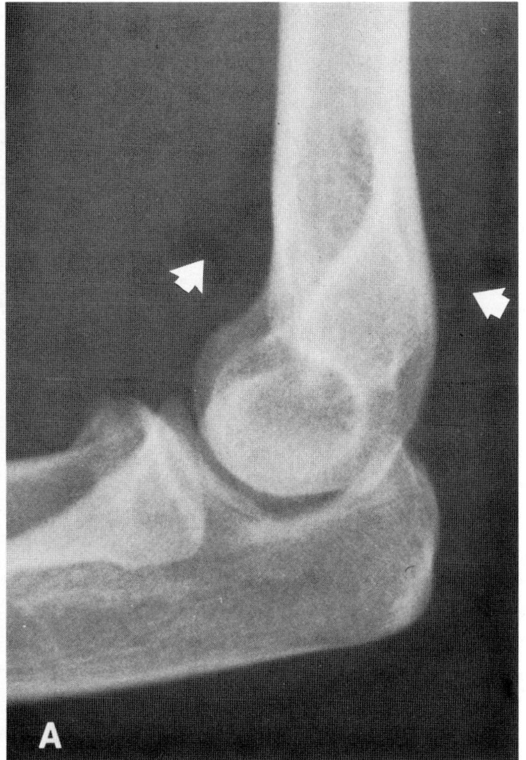

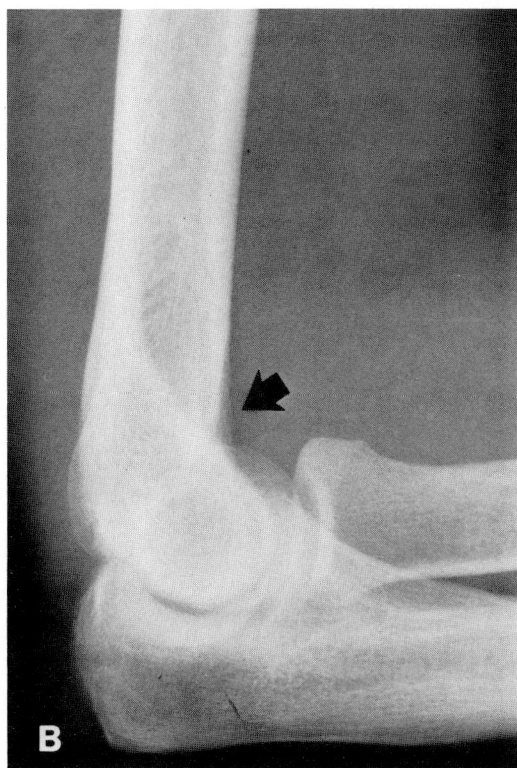

Fig. 9-6. Fat pad sign. (*A*) A lateral view of the elbow joint shows a joint effusion secondary to a minimally displaced fracture of the radial head. There is anterior and superior displacement of the anterior fat pad in the presence of an effusion (*anterior arrow*), and the posterior fat pad is very prominent as well (*posterior arrow*). (*B*) Lateral roentgenogram of a normal elbow for comparison. The anterior fat pad is barely visualized (*arrow*); the posterior fat pad is not seen.

Joint Capsule

Grant[111] described two separate capsules of the elbow joint. There is an outer fibrous layer that extends from the upper margins of the coronoid and radial fossa anteriorly. It does not quite reach the top of the posterior aspect of the olecranon fossa. Distally, it attaches to the margins of the trochlear notch of the ulna and to the annular ligament. The inner synovial capsule arises farther distally in the respective humeral fossae. It also bulges from beneath the distal free margin of the annular ligament. This loose sac-like protrusion surrounds the neck of the radius, permitting free rotation. Between the synovial and fibrous capsules in the coronoid and olecranon fossa are fat pads (Haversian glands). Normally, the posterior fat pad lies wholly within the depression of the olecranon fossa.

ROENTGENOGRAPHIC ANATOMY

Fat Pad Sign

Precise interpretation of roentgenograms in a patient with an injured elbow may be difficult. Minimally displaced fractures may be poorly visualized on the initial anteroposterior and lateral views, and oblique views of the elbow may uncover a fracture line not seen on these routine views. The presence of the so-called fat pad sign should alert the physician to the likelihood of an occult, usually intraarticular, fracture (Fig. 9-6A). This roentgenographic sign is an area of radiolucency posterior to the distal humerus in the lateral view. Since the posterior fat pad lies deep within the olecranon fossa, it is not visible on the lateral roentgenogram of a normal elbow. Distension of the joint capsule by effusion or hemarthrosis displaces it from beneath the cover of the overlying bone, producing a radiolucency posterior to the humerus.[159,202] Since the coronoid fossa is shallower, a portion of the anterior fat pad may be seen in the normal elbow (Fig. 9-6B), but distension of the joint capsule causes the fat pad to become more anteriorly and superiorly displaced.

FRACTURES OF THE DISTAL HUMERUS

SUPRACONDYLAR FRACTURES

Fractures through the supracondylar area are extraarticular. They involve a fracture through the medial and lateral columns of the distal humerus and the thin piece of bone that separates the coronoid and olecranon fossae. When the distal fragment is displaced posterior to the shaft of the humerus, it is considered an extension type of supracondylar fracture (Fig. 9-7A). When the distal fragment is displaced anteriorly, the fracture is a flexion type (Fig. 9-7B). Roberts and Kelly[229] cited Kocher as originally describing four types of supracondylar fractures: extension, flexion, abduction, and adduction. Since the last two types occur with the elbow in extension, they will be considered as variants of the extension type.

Classification of Distal Humerus Fractures Based on Involved Structures

- Supracondylar fractures
  - Extension type
  - Flexion type
- Transcondylar fractures
- Intercondylar (dicondylar **T** or **Y**) fractures
- Fractures of the condyles
  - Lateral (external)
  - Medial (internal)
- Fractures of the articular surface only
  - Capitellum
  - Trochlea
- Fractures of the epicondyles
  - Lateral
  - Medial
- Fractures of the supracondylar process

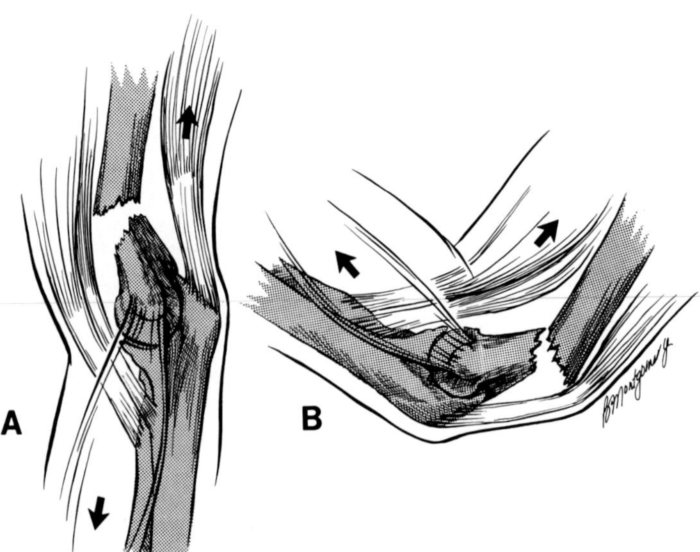

Fig. 9-7. (*A*) Extension type, lateral view of a supracondylar fracture. The obliquity of the fracture line from anterior distal to posterior proximal is demonstrated. The fragment is pulled posteriorly and proximally by the action of the triceps. The forearm muscles flex the distal fragment at the elbow. (*B*) In a flexion-type supracondylar fracture, the distal fragment lies anterior to the proximal humeral portion. The obliquity of the fracture is opposite that from the extension type.

Extension-Type Supracondylar Fractures

Extension-type fractures are usually caused by a fall on the outstretched hand with the elbow in extension. Roberts and Kelly[229] stated that in children the anterior capsule and collateral ligaments are usually stronger than bone. Thus, in the younger age group, when the elbow is locked in extension, the anterior capsule and anterior portion of the collateral ligaments become taut, concentrating all the force in the supracondylar region. Since the bone is the weaker area, supracondylar fractures are more common in children. This was confirmed in Speed's[266] series where 60 per cent of these fractures occurred before the age of 15. Høyer[132] found it to be rare after the age of 20.

Mechanism of Injury

In the adult, the mechanism that produces the extension-type fracture is not entirely clear. In Kocher's original classification of supracondylar fractures the abduction and adduction fractures were thought to be due to pure abduction and adduction forces while the elbow was in extension.[229] While in some cases hyperextension may be a mechanism, there are authors who cite direct violence to the elbow as a cause.[229,266] Speed[226] pointed out that burglars were especially prone to this injury because of injuries sustained to the distal humerus when jumping from a window or from the sharp blow of a policeman's hickory club on the elbow. (After the injury the resultant deformity of the elbow inhibited the burglar's ability to use a gun.)

In the lateral view, the fracture usually extends obliquely upward from the anterior distal aspect to posterior proximal aspect (Fig. 9-7A). In the extension type, the distal fragment is displaced posteriorly and proximally by the force of the initial injury and of the triceps acting on the proximal ulna. The distal fragment is also usually flexed at the elbow because of the pull of the origins of the forearm muscles on the epicondyles. The sharp fractured end of the proximal fragment projects forward into the antecubital fossa, where it may contuse or even impale the brachial artery or median nerve. Even if the artery escapes direct injury, massive swelling of the elbow secondary to the frequently severe associated soft-tissue injury often results. Neurovascular complications are an ever-present threat in the management of these difficult injuries.

Signs and Symptoms

The findings in an extension-type supracondylar fracture vary with both the degree of swelling and the displacement of the fracture. When one sees an injury of this nature early, there is little swelling about the elbow, which makes it possible to palpate the bony landmarks. More commonly, however, the patient is seen only after considerable swelling has developed, when the landmarks are not palpable. With posterior displacement of the distal fragment this fracture may easily be confused with a posterior dislocation. Malgaigne's early emphasis on differentiating it from a dislocation[85] led to the association of the fracture with his name (Malgaigne fracture).[115] In a supracondylar fracture the three bony landmarks, the medial and lateral epicondyles and the olecranon, maintain their normal spatial relationships. The plane of the equidistant triangle that these points form now lies farther back and not necessarily parallel to the long axis of the humerus. In a posterior dislocation of the elbow the relationship of these three points is disrupted. The tip of the olecranon is posterior to the two epicondyles.

While Dupuytren[85] pointed out that another pathognomonic sign of this fracture was crepitus, no attempt should be made to elicit it. Uncontrolled manipulation could cause neurovascular damage. The extension-type supracondylar fracture frequently is associated with intense pain and is usually grossly unstable.

Roentgenographic Findings

The roentgenographic findings depend upon the degree of displacement. On the anteroposterior view, the fracture line is usually transverse in the minimal or undisplaced fracture, lying just proximal to the articular capsule. In moderately displaced fractures the distal fragment can lie either medially or laterally in relation to the humeral shaft. In those cases with marked displacement there may be either axial rotation of the fragment or angulation in the medial-lateral plane as well. In the lateral roentgenogram, if the fracture is undisplaced there may be only a positive fat sign (see p. 493). In those minimally displaced, there may be only a decrease in the angulation of the articular surface with the long axis of the humerus. With marked displacement, the distal fragment is displaced posteriorly and proximally.

Methods of Treatment

The course of treatment of extension-type supracondylar fractures is influenced greatly by the associated soft-tissue injuries (especially neurovascular). In all cases, prompt reduction of the fracture is desirable, but impairment of circulation constitutes an absolute surgical emergency.

Nonoperative Treatment. *Closed reduction* is usually attempted first. This relieves tension on the vital neurovascular structures anterior to the elbow joint. First, however, the surgeon must thoroughly examine the roentgenograms and plan his manipulative maneuvers carefully. He must determine the degree of displacement of the distal fragment, noting especially the extent of abduction, adduction, medial or lateral displacement, and rotation. Reduction of those markedly displaced fractures requires an anesthetic that can give both adequate relaxation and pain relief. This requires, at the minimum, a proximal regional block of the entire extremity or preferably, if the condition of the patient permits, a general anesthetic. An assistant is necessary to apply countertraction, by grasping the upper arm. He must also hold the proximal fragment steady while the surgeon manipulates the distal portion. This is usually best performed by applying traction at the wrist with one hand and guiding the distal fragment during manipulation with the other hand. The proximal pull of the triceps and biceps must first be overcome by longitudinal traction with the elbow *extended.* Smith[254] cautioned against flexion before reduction is obtained, as this may impinge the anteriorly placed neurovascular structures between the sharp ends of the fracture fragments. Once length has been regained, the elbow may be hyperextended slightly, if extreme care is taken not to overstretch the anterior structures. This tends to unlock the fracture fragments. Once the fragments are free, forward pressure is applied to the distal fragment, and backward pressure is applied to the proximal one. At the same time medial or lateral angulation can be corrected. With the fracture fragments now in their proper relationship the elbow can be flexed gradually. This usually locks the fracture fragment securely in place. The degree of flexion obtainable is usually limited by the amount of swelling about the elbow. The arm must be immobilized in sufficient flexion to maintain fracture reduction. Too much flexion does not permit adequate venous return and may even cause occlusion of the brachial artery. The elbow may be flexed just to the point where the radial pulse disappears, and then it should be extended 5 to 10 degrees to accommodate additional swelling. The arm is immobilized in this position with a posterior plaster-of-paris splint. Patients who have displaced fractures or considerable swelling must be hospitalized after reduction. This allows close observation for the development of any delayed vascular complications.

The decision as to whether to immobilize the forearm in supination or in pronation is somewhat controversial. Smith[254] pointed out that during reduction the hand must be supinated and directed toward the anterior portion of the shoulder. This helps to obtain adequate rotary alignment. In the past, various authors[266,229] had maintained this position of supination with flexion (the so-called natural splint technique) after reduction had been obtained. Others have placed no special emphasis on the position of the forearm,[64,144,240,254,275,301] DePalma recommends that the forearm be in neutral position.[76] Some of the more recent thinking is that the position of the forearm does influence the position of the distal fragment. This is very important because it is angulation of the distal fragment that is responsible for the cubitus valgus or varus deformities.[150,175,256] Böhler[32] felt very strongly that the forearm should be in pronation to prevent the more common varus angulation. On the basis of his cadaver- and clinical studies he felt that the varus angulation of the distant fragment resulted from the unopposed pull on the fragment by the pronators of the forearm. Placing the forearm in pronation relaxes these muscles. In full pronation, the rotation of the radius has been exhausted, thus all the forces directed to the forearm are transmitted via the ulna to the humerus. Full pronation tenses the medial collateral ligament, correcting the varus angulation of the distal fragment. Salter,[237] treating this fracture in children, determines the intact periosteum by the location of the distal fragment in the medial-lateral plane. He then uses this intact periosteum as a hinge to secure the fragments in place. If there is medial displacement (intact medial periosteum), he recommends that the forearm be pronated. If there is lateral displacement (intact lateral periosteum), the forearm is supinated. While the periosteum of adults is not as strong as that of children, these general principles can be useful. D'Ambrosia[71] also confirmed with cadaver studies (on the basis of ligament tension) that these fractures were more stable in pronation.

In extension-type fractures with minimal or moderate displacement the principles are essentially the same as for the severely displaced fractures. In many of these there is only loss of the normal condylar angulation. If only less than 20 degrees of the condyle-shaft angulation is lost, the position can be accepted.[254] This may result in some decrease of flexion but the patient should be able to reach his mouth with his hand. In fractures where the angulation loss is greater than 20 degrees, manipulation should be performed.

In those cases where there is considerable swelling and reduction is difficult, the extremity can be placed in Dunlop's[82] side arm traction or overhead olecranon pin traction[254,256] until the swelling subsides and a reduction can be attempted with greater ease.

Care After Reduction. Roentgenograms must be taken immediately after reduction. They should be repeated on about the third and seventh days, because occasionally loss of reduction occurs. Special attention needs to be given to the recognition of varus or valgus angulation of the distal fragments. This can be visualized on a tangential view of the distal humerus through the flexed elbow. The alignment of the distal articular surface with the long axis of the humerus is then measured and compared with a similar film of the opposite humerus.

Postoperative immobilization is accomplished by the use of a posterior plaster slab in the proper amount of flexion. This can be suspended by a collar and cuff arrangement or a sling. A posterior slab probably should be used even in undisplaced fractures, instead of a collar and cuff alone. This provides protection for the tender injured elbow. Circular plaster casts should never be used as the initial method of immobilization. The period of immobilization after reduction lasts from 4 to 6 weeks. Periodic active motion out of the protective splint may be initiated as soon as the fracture is clinically stable. Active motion is facilitated by the application of heat. Passive stretching exercises should *never* be attempted.

Overhead Olecranon Traction. In a number of fractures skeletal pin traction through the olecranon may be the treatment of choice. Smith[254] listed four types of severe supracondylar fractures for which Kirschner-wire traction is indicated: (1) when it is impossible to reduce the fracture by other closed methods; (2) when it is possible to reduce the fracture, but impossible to maintain the reduction by flexion without compromising the circulation; (3) when swelling is excessive, circulatory impairment is present, or Volkmann's ischaemia already threatens; and (4) when associated lesions are present such as compounding of the fracture, additional fractures in the same extremity, or paralysis of a nerve.

The main advantage of this method is that skeletal traction is easier to apply and adjust than skin traction. Also, the arm is suspended overhead, facilitating control of edema. Motion of the elbow can be started early; flexion is aided by gravity. Dressing changes are easily accomplished.[254] Lyman Smith[256] feels that angulation of the distal fragment can be better controlled as well. Conn and Wade[62] warned against some of the problems encountered with skeletal pin traction. Too early discontinuance of the traction can result in a loss of reduction with poor results. They also described two cases with pin tract infection. The infection cleared readily, but there was marked residual limitation of motion. Another disadvantage of this method is that it does necessitate a lengthy period of hospitalization.

Operative Methods. Two operative techniques are available to the surgeon in the treatment of extension-type fractures. One is fixation of the distal fragment with percutaneous Kirschner wires after reduction has been obtained by closed methods. The second is primary open reduction and internal fixation.

Percutaneous Pin Fixation. Miller[191] first described percutaneous pinning of intercondylar fractures of the distal humerus in 1939. By directing the wires in a different direction, Swenson[280] adapted its use for supracondylar fractures in children. While most of the use of this technique is applied to supracondylar fractures in children and adolescents, it has been extended to use in adults.[140] This technique finds application in those fractures that are unstable except in extreme flexion. Stabilization of the fracture by this technique allows the arm to be immobilized in much less flexion, in some cases 90 degrees or less. Another indication for this technique is the presence of a fracture of the forearm in the same extremity.[11] In the adult, Kirschner wires may not be strong enough to provide rigid fixation, and small Steinmann pins may be necessary instead. Pin fixation must not be done, of course, unless an adequate reduction can be accomplished. The technique relies heavily upon the surgeon's ability to palpate the bone landmarks. Since both of these may be difficult or even impossible in the severely swollen elbow, a preliminary period of traction may be necessary to allow the swelling to subside. Power equipment for insertion of the pins greatly facilitates the procedure.

In the original descriptions[140,280] the wires were passed medially and laterally through the epicondyles and continued proximally up the respective supracondylar columns. This technique entails some risk to the ulnar nerve during placing of the medial pin. In an effort to avoid this risk Fowles *et al.*[102] used two pins laterally. One is passed laterally through the lateral epicondyle in the usual manner. A second pin traverses the joint just lateral to the olecranon in the region of the capitulotrochlear sulcus. This pin continues in an axial direction up the humeral shaft. Childress[56] has employed a single pin through the olecranon crossing the joint and continuing up the shaft of the humerus.

Open Reduction and Internal Fixation. Primary open reduction is indicated in those fractures where there is inability to obtain a satisfactory closed reduction or where there is a vascular injury. In those cases where reduction cannot be obtained, muscle, especially the brachialis, may be interposed between the fracture fragments. In rare instances the proximal humeral fragment may be buttoned-holed through the brachialis. Attempts at longitudinal traction only tighten the muscle around the protruding fragment. In those with vascular injury where arterial repair is necessary, the fracture must be stabilized as well. Access to both the antecubital fossa and the distal humerus can be accomplished by the surgical approach of Fiolle and Delmas as described by Henry.[124] After the underlying pathology is corrected, a reduction is obtained by direct visualization. Stabilization is then achieved with percutaneous pinning by one of the techniques described previously.

Flexion-Type Supracondylar Fractures

This type of injury is quite rare.[64] In Smith's[254] series it occurred in less than 2 per cent of supracondylar fractures. It is generally agreed that this fracture is caused by a force directed against the posterior aspect of the flexed elbow.[32,226,229,254] This results in anterior displacement of the distal fragment with the elbow joint (Fig. 9-7B). The posterior periosteum is torn, but the anterior periosteum may remain attached, having separated only from the anterior surface of the proximal fragment. Because direct violence is usual in this injury, the fracture is often open, with the sharp proximal fragment piercing the triceps tendon and skin.[32] Vascular injuries are rare.

Signs and Symptoms

As in the extension-type fracture, the relationship between the epicondyles and the ulna remains the same, but the plane of their triangle is shifted anterior to the shaft of the humerus. The elbow is flexed, with resistance encountered on attempts at extension.[66] There is an absence of the normal prominence of the posterior aspect of the elbow.

Roentgenographic Findings

The obliquity of the fracture through the supracondylar region on the lateral roentgenogram is from proximal anterior to distal posterior (opposite that seen in the extension type). The distal fragment lies anterior to the humerus and is flexed at the elbow. The fracture line, as a rule, is transverse on the anteroposterior projection.

Methods of Treatment

Nonoperative Treatment. Closed reduction is usually obtained by first applying traction with the forearm flexed. Applying traction with the forearm in extension before reduction is obtained increases the pull of the forearm muscles on the condyles, increasing the flexion of this fragment at the elbow joint. This inhibits reduction and can injure the anterior structures. As the traction is maintained, the distal humeral fragment is pushed posteriorly into position by pressure on its anterior aspect and counterpressure posteriorly on the proximal fragment. Once the fracture is reduced, the fracture fragments can be locked into place by extension of the elbow.

Opinions vary as to the best method of immobilization after reduction.[64,76,301] If the anterior periosteum is intact, it can be used as a hinge to hold the distal fragment in place while pressure is applied to the anterior portion of the distal fragment in a posterior direction. This can be achieved by extension of the elbow with the posterior force being applied to the distal fragment through the anterior capsule and collateral ligaments. The usual obliquity of the fracture line also helps to buttress the posteriorly applied force on the distal fragment. A second method of holding the distal fragment posteriorly is to direct an axial force down the ulna through the coronoid process to the trochlea of the humerus. This can be obtained by flexing the elbow 90 degrees or more and forcing the forearm posteriorly. The posterior axial force can then be applied by molding over the palm with the wrist dorsiflexed and the forearm pronated or over the dorsum of the flexed wrist and hand with the forearm supinated. Counterpressure is maintained by molding proximally over the posterior aspect of the humerus. Even though the fracture is stable

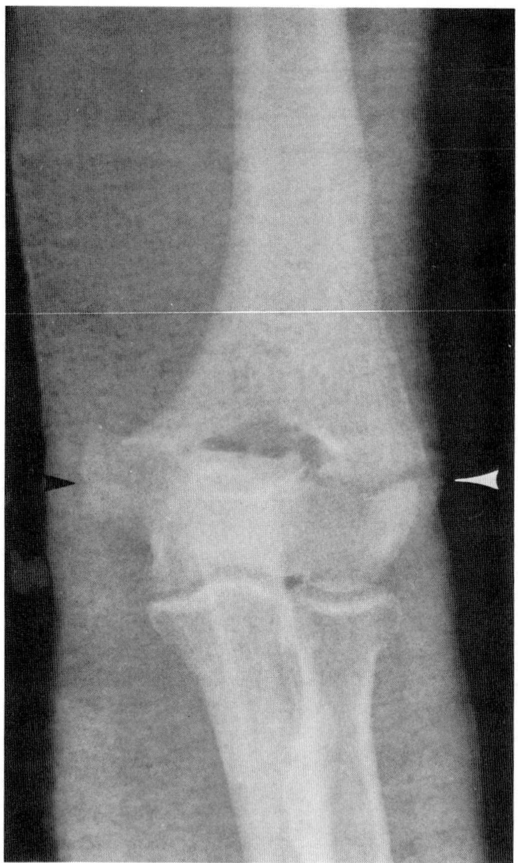

Fig. 9-8. An anteroposterior roentgenogram of a transcondylar fracture demonstrates a transverse fracture line through the distal humerus. The fracture line extends from the medial epicondyle through the coronoid and olecranon fossae to the lateral epicondyle (*arrows*).

in extension, we are opposed to immobilizing the arm in this position, for fear of not being able to regain flexion of the elbow after the fracture heals.

Operative Treatment. For those fractures that cannot be held by closed methods except by extremes of extension, percutaneous pin fixation may be indicated. After the reduction has been accomplished the pinning should be performed with the elbow flexed. When the elbow is in extension the bony landmarks may be obscured, making pin placement difficult. Also, flexing the elbow after it has been stabilized in extension can result in a loss of reduction.

Because of the rarity of vascular injury in this type of fracture the main reason for primary open reduction would be failure to achieve a closed reduction because of interposed muscle. In this instance the direct posterior approach of Campbell[47] to the distal humerus provides the best access to the fracture.

TRANSCONDYLAR (DICONDYLAR) FRACTURES

There is some controversy as to whether the transcondylar fracture should be classified as a separate entity. While most of the earlier fracture texts distinguished it as a separate fracture,[32,64,76,229,240,266,301,309] others did not.[66,115,254] Smith[254] classified transcondylar and supracondylar fractures as a single entity. He felt that for practical purposes the treatment, prognosis, and complications are essentially identical with those of a supracondylar fracture.

We suggest that those fractures that pass through both condyles and are within the joint capsule be classified as transcondylar fractures (Fig. 9-8). There appear to be two types, extension and flexion, based on the position of the elbow when fractured. Kocher, Ashurst, and Chutro are credited with distinguishing the extension type from supracondylar fractures.[64,229] In the extension variety the fracture line is characteristically crescent-shaped or transverse, passing just proximal to the articular surface of the condyles. It also enters the coronoid and olecranon fossae. This fracture occurs just proximal to the old epiphyseal line. Many of these are undisplaced. The mechanisms of injury and principles of treatment that apply to extension supracondylar fractures are basically the same in this fracture. There are some differences that merit discussion, however. First, this type of injury is more common in elderly persons with fragile osteoporotic bone. Secondly, since this fracture lies within the joint cavity, excessive callus production can result in residual loss of motion. This is especially true if callus develops in the olecranon or coronoid fossae.[64,301,309]

A second type of transcondylar fracture is recognized as being caused by trauma to the elbow in flexion. This is the so-called Posadas fracture[229,240,266] (Fig. 9-9). The condylar fragment is carried forward, and there is a posterior dislocation of the radius and ulna. The coronoid process appears to become wedged between the anteriorly displaced dicondylar fragment and the proximal supracondylar portion of the shaft. There is no record of the method of treatment of this fracture, but it appears that closed reduction may be difficult. Scudder[240] described how, with improper treatment, the ulna subsequently can develop a pseudarthrosis with the distal portion of the humerus (i.e., a type of traumatic arthroplasty).

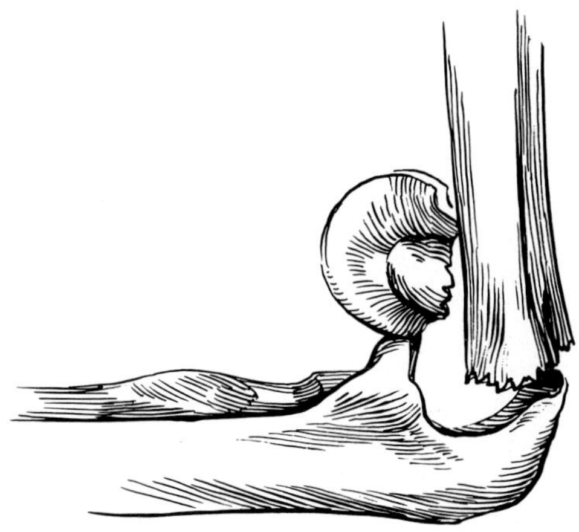

Fig. 9-9. Posada's fracture is a flexion type of transcondylar fracture in which the condylar fragment is flexed anteriorly. The ulna is dislocated posteriorly with the coronoid process wedged between the condyles and the humeral shaft.

INTERCONDYLAR T- OR Y-FRACTURES

Intercondylar fractures are some of the most complicated and difficult fractures of the distal humerus to treat. The fracture consists of a vertical component through the articular surface, most commonly through the trochlear sulcus into the humeral fossae. From this area there is either a single transverse or two diverging oblique fractures through the supracondylar humeral columns. This **Y**- or **T**-shaped fracture produces varying degrees of separation of the condyles from each other and from the main humeral fragment. The significance of the presence of condylar separation in determining prognosis was not appreciated by the early authors until Pierre Desault's classical description of this injury in the very early 1800's.[77] He emphasized the necessity of reestablishing condylar alignment.

This type of injury is rare, fortunately. Because of its rarity, however, very few surgeons are able to gain much experience in treating it. Two large series from the fracture service of the Massachusetts General Hospital averaged only three or four per year.[227,311] It is usually seen in adults in later life[64,76,301,309]; the average age was 54 in Miller's series[192] and 44 at the Mayo Clinic.[30]

Mechanism of Injury

The splitting of the condyles appears to be created by the wedgelike action of the proximal ulnar articular surface against the trochlea of the humerus. This has been seen to occur in flexion and in extension.[76,138,311] In flexion, the force is usually directed against the posterior portion of the elbow. The fracture can be produced by relatively minor trauma such as a simple fall. In this situation one would suspect that the condyles are prestressed by the contraction of the forearm muscles in the individual's attempt to break his fall. This prestressing of the condyles enables them to be separated with much less force. In many instances, however, the forces applied to the posterior flexed elbow are violent, as seen in motor vehicle injuries. In the flexion type of fracture the condyles are usually found anterior to the humeral shaft. In the extension type of injury the ulna is directed anteriorly against the posterior aspect of the

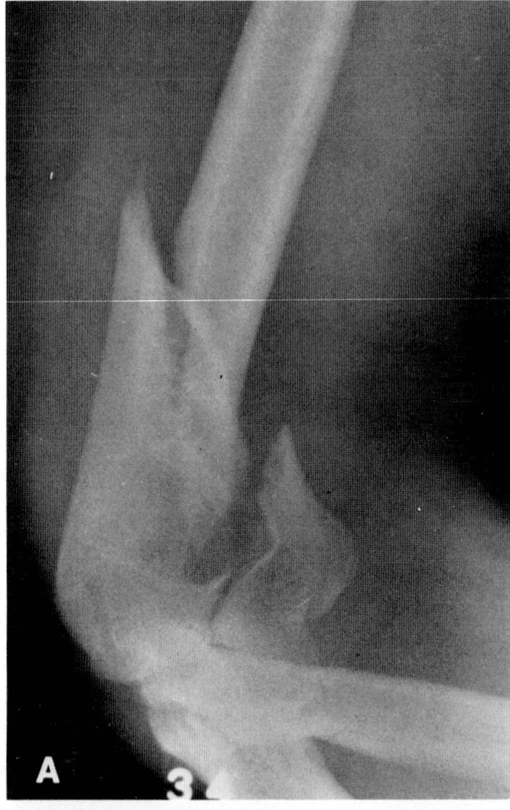

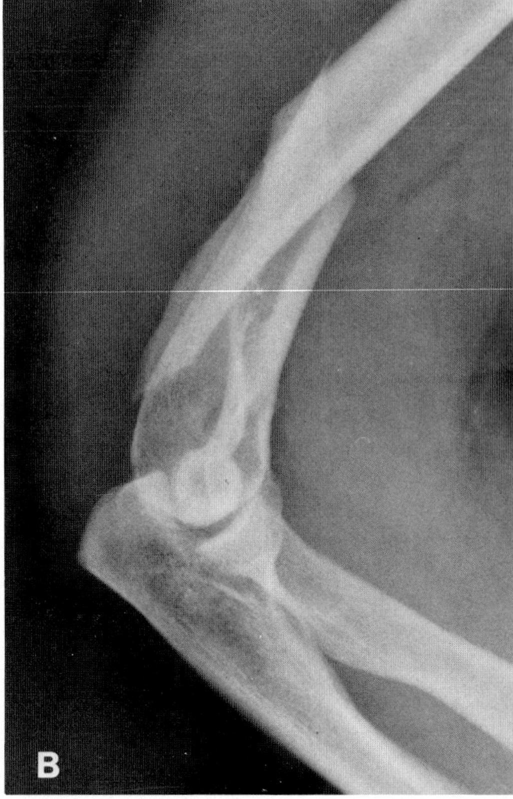

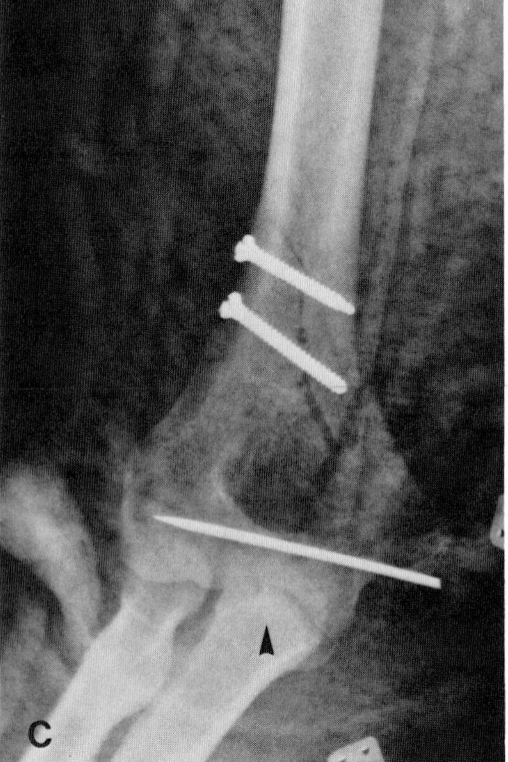

Fig. 9-10. (*A*) Oblique view of an intercondylar **Y**-Fracture, Type II, showing the vertical fracture line through the trochlear groove. This fracture joins oblique fractures through the medial and lateral supracondylar columns. There is little separation of the condyles. (*B*) A lateral view of the same fracture shows that the condylar fragments are displaced anteriorly. (*C*) The same fracture after open reduction and internal fixation. The **Y** configuration of the fracture lines is better visualized after reduction. The articular surface of the trochlea has been restored (*arrow*).

trochlea separating the condyles at the same time as the supracondylar portion is fractured. Another mechanism is that proposed by Wilson and Cochrane,[309] who felt the separation of the condyles in this type of fracture may be created by the splitting effect of the humeral shaft as it is forced distally. In the extension type of injuries the condyles are usually found to lie behind the humeral shaft. Whatever the mechanism, there is usually considerable associated soft-tissue injury. Some may have open lacerations extending into the fracture site. Comminution of the bony fragments is not unusual. Because of loss of bony continuity the fracture fragments are displaced by unopposed muscle action. In those with severe displacement the origins of the forearm muscles pull the epicondyles distally, rotating the condyles so that their articular surfaces face a more proximal direction. This converts the trochlear sulcus into a narrow inverted **V**, making it no longer congruous with the articular surface of the ulna (Fig. 9-10). The action of the biceps anteriorly and the triceps posteriorly pull the articular surface of the ulna proximally. In an opposing fashion the humeral shaft is forced distally between the rotated condyles.

Signs and Symptoms

Little can be added to points in diagnosis as outlined by Desault[77] in his original description of this injury.

> If the fingers, placed before or behind, press on the limb in the direction of the longitudinal fracture, the two condyles will be separated from each other, the one yielding in an outward, and the other in an inward direction, leaving a fissure or opening between them. The part at the same time expands in breadth. The forearm is almost constantly in a state of pronation. When we take hold of one of the condyles in each hand, and endeavour to make them move in opposite directions, they can be brought alternately forward or backward, and if their surfaces touch, a manifest crepitation is heard.

The key to distinguishing an intercondylar **T**- or **Y**-fracture from others is determining the presence of separation of the condyles from each other and from the humeral shaft. With proximal migration of the ulna the arm appears shortened. It is also widened by concomitant condylar separation. The independent mobility of the condyles can be determined by pressing the condyles between the index finger and the thumb. There is crepitus when the condyles are pressed together. Since they are still under the influence of the forearm muscles the condyles tend to spring back into displacement when the pressure is released. Both the pressure and its release are a source of pain to the patient. The relationship of the epicondyles with the tip of the olecranon process has been disrupted. In those fractures with an extensive degree of displacement there is usually gross instability in all directions.

Roentgenographic Findings

In those fractures with considerable displacement of the fragments the diagnosis is easy. Because of considerable comminution of the fracture fragments, it may be difficult to determine the origin of many of the small fragments. In those that are undisplaced or minimally displaced the surgeon must look carefully for the presence of a vertical intercondylar fracture to distinguish this from a simple supracondylar fracture.

Classification

Riseborough and Radin[227] have devised a very useful classification of this type of fracture, based upon its roentgenographic appearance. This classification provides some guide to management and prognosis. They have defined four types:

I. Undisplaced fracture between the capitellum and trochlea
II. Separation of the capitellum and trochlea without appreciable rotation of the fragments in the frontal plane (Fig. 9-10)
III. Separation of the fragments with rotary deformity (Fig. 9-11)
IV. Severe comminution of the articular surface with wide separation of the humeral condyles (Fig. 9-12)

Methods of Treatment

Selection of the proper treatment for intercondylar fractures requires the utmost in judgment and discretion. Each case must be individualized. In the young adult it is important to obtain as near an anatomical reduction of the articular surface as possible. In the older adult with an excessively comminuted fracture motion is more desirable, and the congruity of the articular surface is not as important.

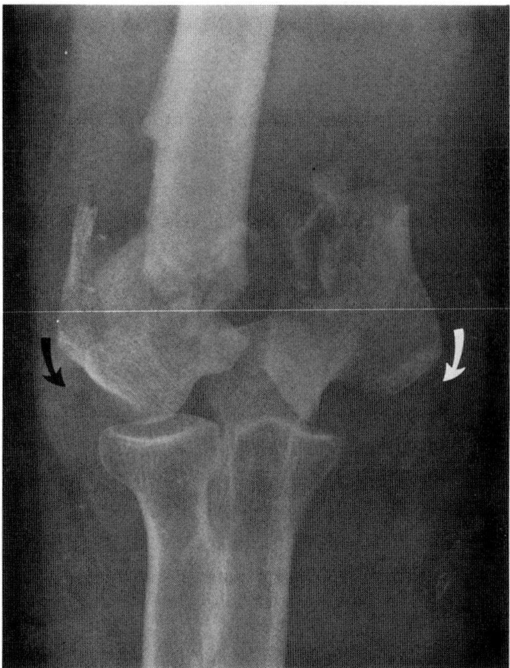

Fig. 9-11. In this intercondylar **T**-Fracture, Type III, there is comminution of the supracondylar area, but the articular surfaces of the separate condyles are intact. The distal portion of the humeral shaft fragment is advanced toward the ulna by the action of the triceps and biceps muscles. The condyles are rotated distally by the origins of the muscles of the forearm (*arrows*).

The final roentgenographic appearance does not always coincide with the functional result. Those with excellent function of the elbow may demonstrate a very distorted roentgenographic appearance. The opposite is also true. On the final roentgenogram there may be nearly perfect anatomical restoration but very poor functional capacity, usually due to joint stiffness. Because of this, one may need to compromise appearance, both clinically and roentgenographically, for function.[254]

Initially, many types of closed techniques were utilized. The goal of these early surgeons was to place the elbow in the maximum flexion allowable at the time of fracture. The basis of this was twofold. First, extension is easier to obtain than flexion because of the assistance of gravity. Secondly, should ankylosis or restrictive motion of the elbow develop, the upper extremity is in a better functional position in flexion. In recent years, with refinement of surgical technique, there has been an emphasis on reconstructing the distal humerus by operative intervention. Once rigid fixation has been established early motion and rehabilitation can be initiated. There still remain, however, those intercondylar fractures of the humerus for which there is no optimum treatment.

In order to gain a better understanding of the problems in the treatment of these fractures it is important to review the various methods of treatment, both operative and nonoperative, which have been proposed. From this, some specific guidelines to aid the reader in his approach to this difficult problem can be appreciated.

Nonoperative Treatment. All of the nonoperative methods attempt to maintain the alignment of the fragments, especially the two condylar fragments. Some of these allow early motion; others do not. The nonoperative methods can be divided into three main categories: (1) cast or posterior slab immobilization; (2) traction; and (3) the "bag of bones" technique.

Cast or posterior slab immobilization is usually preceded by manipulation of the fracture. Bicondylar pressure is applied while the fracture is being reduced. After reduction, the arm is placed at 90 degrees in either a long-arm cast or a posterior plaster slab. The bicondylar pressure is applied by molding the cast well over the condyles or using a posterior splint and applying well-padded secondary splints medially and laterally.[66] As the swelling subsides, the bandage holding the side pads is tightened. Total immobilization may be useful only in those fractures with little or no displacement. In the comminuted fractures it combines two major disadvantages: (1) poor maintenance of fracture alignment and (2) lack of early motion.

Traction is a popular technique among

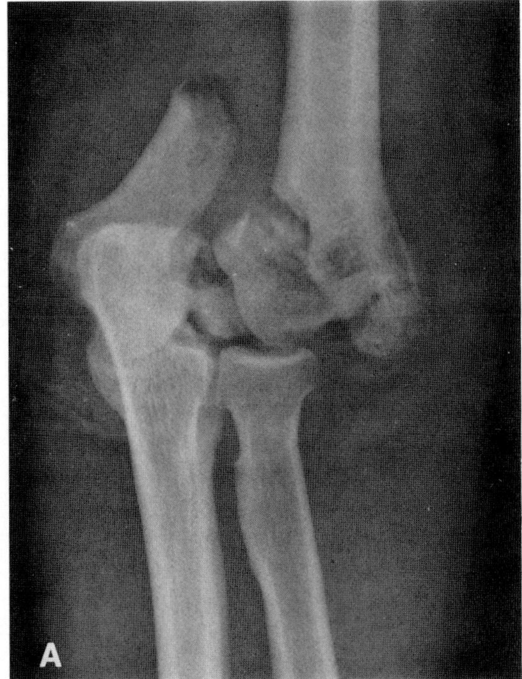

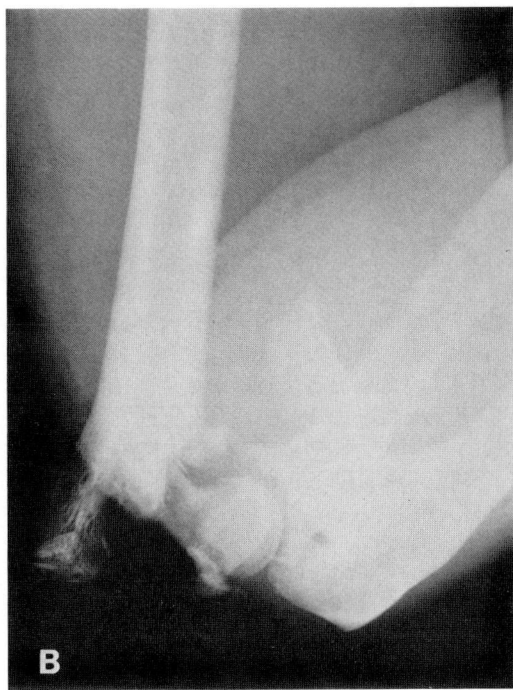

Fig. 9-12. (*A*) An anteroposterior roentgenogram of an open intercondylar fracture, Type IV, shows marked comminution of the lateral condylar fragment. (*B*) In a lateral roentgenogram of the same fracture, a portion of the proximal humeral fragment is seen protruding through the soft tissues to the exterior.

the proponents of nonoperative treatment.[64,76,127,144,174,211,223,227,284] While many of these authors would use traction for all types of displaced intercondylar fractures, there appear to be two specific conditions in which it should be used. First is the Riseborough and Radin Type IV fracture, in which there is severe comminution of the condyles and of the articular surface. The goal in this type of fracture is to obtain as good alignment as possible and go for early motion. The second instance is the fracture with a large open wound or a markedly contaminated wound in which the chances of infection would be increased with internal fixation. Many of the advantages and disadvantages of using traction with supracondylar fractures apply in this type of fracture as well (see p. 498).

Traction is especially useful for maintaining the condylar fragments at the proper length in relationship to the humeral shaft. It is also easy to initiate elbow motion at the same time reduction is being maintained. With loss of intercondylar continuity the force upon the condyles transmitted via the collateral ligaments is unopposed. Thus traction tends to increase the rotation of the condyles, especially if it is skeletal traction where all the force originates at the proximal ulna. An attempt to maintain better intercondylar contact has resulted in numerous modifications of the basic traction principle. Patterson[211] used a well molded long-arm cast with the ulnar pin incorporated in the cast. This technique does not provide the advantage of early motion. Two other means of maintaining condylar control include: the use of ice tongs applied directly to the condylar fragments[223] and closed reduction with primary percutaneous pinning of the two condylar fragments.[76]

Because skeletal traction adds the danger

of infection with resultant stiffness, other surgeons felt skin traction if properly applied could be as useful.[127,309] With skin traction, lateral compression over the condyles can be applied simultaneously using well padded lateral splints[64] or the Magnuson felt cuff.[174] Skin traction has its limitation—no more than 5 to 7 pounds may be used. In addition, if there is considerable swelling, the skin may not tolerate the adhesive tapes under traction. Skin traction is best utilized as side-arm traction; olecranon pin traction can be used either as side-arm or overhead traction.

In an attempt to maintain traction yet allow the patient mobility, many ambulatory techniques were tried. These included the Robert Jones- and modified Thomas arm splints.[223,309] The Michael Hoke plaster traction technique has also been adapted for this type of fracture.[289] These methods have not gained much acceptance. They are cumbersome for the patient and most do not allow elbow motion.

"Bag of Bones" Technique. Eastwood,[86] who popularized this method in England during the 1930's, credited Hugh Owen Thomas as being its originator. It involves simply placing the arm in a collar and cuff initially, in as much flexion as possible. The elbow is left hanging free, which is an important point. The effect of gravity on the dependent elbow is thought to enable the fracture fragments to settle into a more natural alignment. Some attempt at initial reduction is made, but the permanent success of this maneuver is questionable. Hand and finger motion are started immediately. Pendulum shoulder motion begins at about 7 to 10 days. As the swelling and pain subside, the patient is allowed gradually to actively extend the elbow. In a recent series reported by Brown,[37] his patients achieved an average of 70 degrees of elbow motion. One author[290] had modified this method by the application of a large padded wooden carpenter's clamp to the condyles, suspending it from the neck. The clamp was tightened as the swelling subsided. In addition to some inherent dangers, patients might not accept this modification.

Watson-Jones[301] noted that many of the patients treated with this method had residual loss of extension from excessive anterior tilting of the condyles. Evans felt that while many of his patients treated in this manner had a satisfactory range of motion, there were a significant number who complained of weakness and instability in the elbow.[93] The "bag of bones" technique appears to be suitable for the elderly patient in whom early ambulation is desired. It does require a good deal of patient motivation and cooperation to achieve a satisfactory result.

Operative Methods. The operative techniques can also be categorized into four basic methods: (1) pins in plaster; (2) open reduction and internal fixation; (3) arthroplasty; and (4) prosthetic (distal humerus) replacement.

Pins in plaster was originally called blind nailing by Miller.[191] He initially placed the upper extremity in traction with a Kirschner wire in the olecranon. The condyles were then manually reduced and transfixed percutaneously with a second Kirschner wire. A third wire was likewise passed percutaneously through the proximal fragment. While the fracture was maintained in traction a long-arm cast was applied, incorporating all three wires. Böhler[31] appears to be one of the few other surgeons to have utilized this technique. While this method may facilitate maintaining alignment, it contains no provision for elbow motion. The presence of at least two pins penetrating into the fracture site greatly enhances the chances of infection and its resultant disability.

Open Reduction and Internal Fixation. In performing open reduction and internal fixation the surgeon usually has one of two possible goals in mind. He can perform limited surgery on the condyles, attempting to reestablish primarily only the articular surface. This method is usually followed by postoperative traction. His second alternative can be to achieve total anatomical restoration of the distal humerus. This, of course, requires more surgical exposure. The fixation obtained should be rigid enough to allow early motion.

The best candidate for open reduction

and internal fixation is the younger patient with three or four large fragments. Elderly patients, those in poor physical condition, and those with contaminated open wounds are not candidates for this method.[11,254]

The posterior approach to the distal humerus and elbow appears to be the one most widely accepted by the proponents of open reduction and internal fixation.[30,47,155,192,194,262,291] Originally described by Campbell,[47] it involves reflecting distally an inverted V-shaped portion of the triceps aponeurosis. Van Gorder[291] believed this incision has four major advantages:

> (1) It affords a more adequate exposure of the broken parts; (2) it allows more freedom in the use and selection of metal fixation; (3) it involves dissection of soft parts that contain no large vessels or important nerve structures (the ulnar nerve having been previously identified and gently retracted); and (4) it is the only approach that gives a clear view of the involved articular surfaces and joint line.

Its one disadvantage is that it affords poor visualization of the anterior surface of the joint.

The transolecranon approach popularized by Cassebaum has also gained wide acceptance.[50,51,138,192,194] It provides much better visualization of the total articular surface, especially anteriorly. While this approach involves less muscle dissection, thus lessening the chances of postoperative fibrosis, it does add another fracture, which requires fixation. In addition, it provides less exposure of the supracondylar area than the posterior approach.

Because poor exposure makes extensive soft-tissue dissection necessary, the medial-lateral approaches have few advocates.[93] Kelly and Taylor[143] reported a series that used the anterior approach of Henry. Their results were equal to other open methods. They believe it may have an advantage where there are associated neurovascular injuries.

Before undertaking surgical reconstruction of these fractures the surgeon needs to review some anatomical points regarding the distal humerus. First, in obtaining transcondylar fixation it must be remembered that the diameter of the trochlear sulcus is much smaller (approximately one-half) than that of the medial trochlear ridge and the lateral condyle (see Fig. 9-3). Thus the transfixation device must be centered exactly or it may enter the articular surface. Secondly, in reattachment of the condyles to the humeral shaft the placement of the screws must be within the centers of the supracondylar columns (see Fig. 9-2B). Inaccurate placement may impinge on the olecranon fossa with resultant limitation of motion (Fig. 9-13).

Each of the fractures has its own pattern. The surgeon must have at his disposal a variety of instruments and fixation devices. While no standard surgical technique can be cited the surgeon will do well to follow some of the basic principles outlined by those who have had considerable experience with these fractures.[11,38,50,51,156,227,262] These merit summarizing at this point:

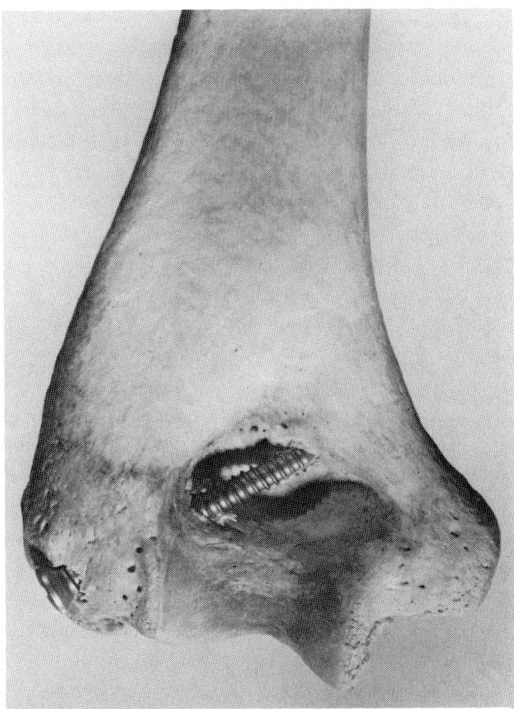

Fig. 9-13. Improper placement of a screw into the lateral supracondylar column can result in its entering the olecranon fossa. This produces a block to extension of the elbow.

The order of reduction is important. The condyles should be attached together first.

The articular surface of the condyles must be accurately reduced. Loss of articular surface can be accepted; incongruity cannot.

In reestablishing condylar shaft fixation, the epitrochlear ridges, which are often separate fragments, serve as essential buttresses to the condyles. Their continuity with the humeral metaphysis must be reestablished before the condyles can be stabilized to the shaft.

For fixation of the condyles to the shaft there is little purchase achieved from the central cancellous bone of the supracondylar columns. The proximally directed screws need to engage the opposite cortex of the humeral shaft.

In general, screws are the more desirable fixation devices. Kirschner wires do not provide sufficient stability for reattaching the condyles to the shaft. Plates require more soft-tissue dissection.

The distal humeral fossae need to be kept clear of fixation devices.

The proper anterior angulation of the condyles with the shaft needs to be maintained. Significant alteration in the normal anterior angulation (45 degrees) can result in loss of elbow motion.

Prophylactic removal of a portion of the tip of the olecranon process at the time of surgery may help to assure adequate extension postoperatively, should the olecranon fossa become filled with callus or fibrous tissue.

Arthroplasty. To the surprise of some of the earlier surgeons[115,275] wide debridement of those fractures with open wounds, including removal of the condylar fragments, often resulted in an elbow with acceptable function. Thus, primary arthroplasty at the time of injury has become a mode of treatment in fractures with severe comminution.[127,301] Others, however, strongly condemn this method as a primary procedure.[156,262,311] They feel it leads to too much weakness and instability. Since the outcome of the most severely comminuted fracture may be surprising, it would appear that arthroplasty should be a delayed procedure.

Prosthetic Replacement. There are several reports of the prosthetic replacement of the distal humerus in the literature using various materials such as Vitallium.[24,83,171,186,292] Most of these have been secondary procedures for poor results after healing of the fracture has occurred. In two instances[171,292] the insertion of the prosthesis was the primary treatment for comminuted fractures. The long-term results have not been reported. The indications for this mode of treatment are a long way from being clearly established.

Authors' Preferred Method of Treatment

We have found the classification of Riseborough and Radin useful for evaluating these fractures. Because each fracture is different we do not have one standard method of treatment. For Type I undisplaced fractures, we usually employ simple posterior splint for immobilization. These fractures are usually stable, and active motion can be initiated after about 2 to 3 weeks of immobilization. In approaching Type II and III fractures, the age of the patient and the size and type of the fragments are considered. If there are large fragments and the patient is young, we prefer to use open reduction with internal fixation. This allows the most rapid return of function. Our feeling is that the posterior approach to the elbow provides the best exposure for this fracture. If there is moderate comminution of the distal humerus but two or three large condylar fragments, we attempt to fix them and follow this with olecranon pin traction. In those with severe comminution (Type IV) we use traction exclusively. An attempt to improve the position of the fragments is made by initial manipulation. It is important to make some differentiation between extension and flexion injuries. This can be accomplished by combining the history with the roentgenographic appearance. Those with the condyles lying anterior to the shaft are considered flexion injuries and are manipulated in flexion. Those with the condyles lying posterior to the shaft are manipulated initially in extension and then brought into flexion.

Patients with open wounds and those who are poor surgical risks are treated in traction; the one exception being those with Type I injuries, which can be treated in a posterior slab. We do not believe that age alone is necessarily a contraindication to surgery.

Postoperative Care and Rehabilitation

The primary goal here is to provide enough stabilization to facilitate early motion. Some type of motion needs to be started as soon as the wound has begun to heal or when the swelling has been reduced. The motion must be active. Passive stretching only delays rehabilitation and is to be condemned.

Complications

While neurovascular injuries are common in fractures of the distal humerus there appear to be no specific neurovascular injuries associated with this fracture. The general principles of management of neurovascular injuries associated with fractures are discussed elsewhere in this text (see p. 534). Union usually occurs between the condylar fragments without difficulty. Nonunion of the supracondylar portion does occur occasionally. Avascular necrosis of the bony fragments is extremely rare.[30] Apart from these initial complications the major problems associated with this fracture lie in the residual disability resulting from loss of elbow function. Knight[156] lists four major causes of elbow disability after this fracture: (1) limitation of motion, (2) deformity, (3) pain, and (4) weakness and instability.

Limitation of motion may be due to a bony block, obliteration of the humeral fossae, or periarticular fibrosis. Deformity results from persistent contracture or bone angulation. Pain, fortunately, is rarely a problem. Weakness and instability may be due to altered joint mechanics or secondary muscle atrophy.

FRACTURES OF THE HUMERAL CONDYLES

Anatomy and Classification

There appears to be some confusion regarding the nomenclature of the various anatomical structures of the distal humerus. Some standard anatomy texts[13,109,111] do not differentiate between medial and lateral condyles as separate entities. Gray's Anatomy[109] describes the distal end of the humerus as being basically *a condyle* with articular and nonarticular surfaces. The articular portion is divided into two areas, the capitulum and the trochlea. (We use the term capitellum instead of capitulum as it is more commonly used in the orthopaedic literature. In our discussion we hope to demonstrate that the terms capitellum and lateral condyle are not synonymous. The same is true for the terms trochlea and medial condyle.)

In the discussion of fractures, separation of the distal humerus into medial and lateral condyles is widely accepted. The capitulotrochlear sulcus is the terminal dividing point for these condyles. Each of the condyles contains an articular and a nonarticular portion. The epicondyle is considered part of the nonarticular portion. The articulating portion of the lateral condyle is called the capitellum (capitulu rotuli humeri, eminentia capitata). The articular surface of the medial condyle is called the trochlea. It must be appreciated at this point that fractures of the condyles do not always follow these anatomic boundaries. For example, in a fracture of the lateral condyle or capitellum a portion of the trochlea is often involved.

During growth there are four separate ossification centers in the distal humerus.[109] The ossification center in the lateral condyle appears during the first year. It forms the bulk of the lateral condyle and a portion of the bone underlying the lateral aspect of the trochlea. The ossification of the medial condyle does not appear until the ninth or tenth year. The epicondyles also have separate ossification centers. The lateral epicondyle center appears at about 12 years only to fuse 1 or 2 years later with the main lateral condylar centers. The center for the medial epicondyle appears at about 4 to 6 years. Fusion with the main condylar segment does not occur until about the 20th year. In rare instances fusion never occurs.[115] These separate ossification centers have considerable significance in the discussion of fractures of the distal humerus in children. In adults, however, there does not appear to be any residuum in the trabecular pattern within the distal humerus from these separate ossification centers (Fig. 9-14). Thus it would appear that in adults, fractures of the distal humerus are dependent upon the external contour of the bone and the forces applied rather than upon intrinsic weakness.

Distinction between the condyles and their various portions is important in the diagnosis and treatment of these fractures. We shall stipulate that the fracture of the condyle includes separation of both the articular and nonarticular portions, including the epicondyle (Fig. 9-15A). There can be isolated fractures of either the articular portion (Fig. 9-15B) or the epicondylar portion of the condyle. In this instance the remainder of the condyle is still attached to the shaft and to the opposite condyle.

This distinction has practical significance, and some generalities can be made. Fracture of the articular portion alone results in loss of motion, but stability of the elbow by and large remains. The fracture fragment is not influenced by muscle forces. There is minimal swelling, because the hematoma is usually restricted by the joint capsule. Fracture of the epicondyles in adults results in local tenderness. There may be some instability. The fracture fragment can also be displaced by muscle forces. Fracture of the entire condyle results in both restriction of motion and instability. There is usually considerable swelling. Fracture of the articular surface alone may be treated by simple excision of the fragment. Fracture of the condyle requires anatomic reduction to restore free motion and fixation to assure stability.

Mechanism of Injury

A number of external forces act upon the distal humerus. Avulsion forces are usually applied via tension on the collateral ligaments. The tension forces on these collateral ligaments can be increased by leverage through the forearm with the elbow in extension. Abduction or adduction of the ex-

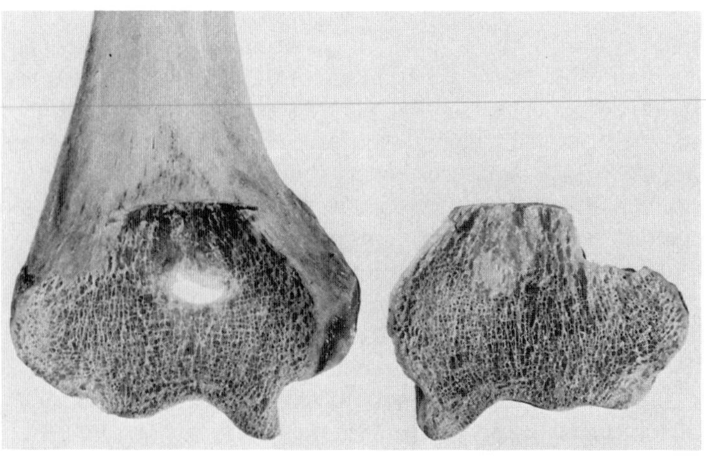

Fig. 9-14. The trabecular pattern of the distal humerus shows no residua of the old ossification centers.

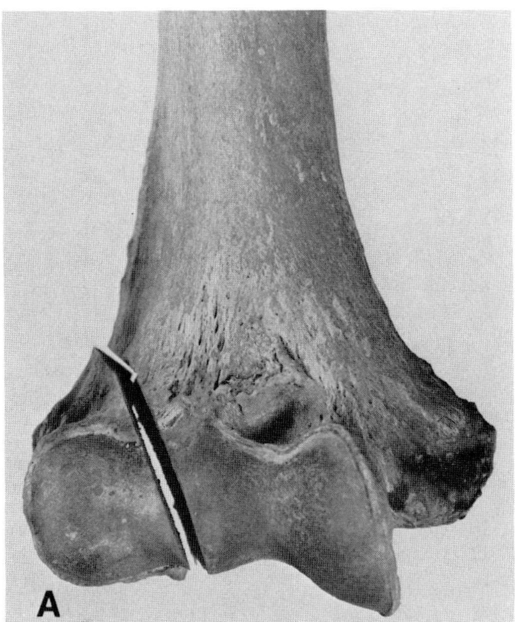

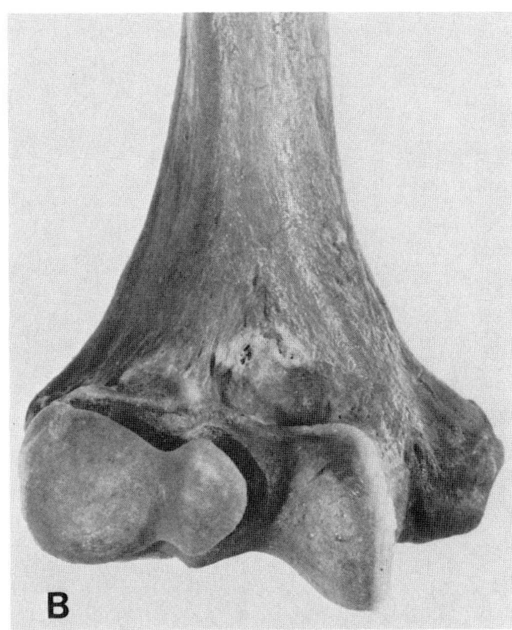

Fig. 9-15. (*A*) Demonstration of a fracture pattern as seen in a true lateral condyle fracture. Articular and nonarticular portions are present in the fragment. (*B*) A fracture limited to the articular surface. This large anterior fragment, which includes a small portion of the trochlea, is typical of a Type I fracture of the capitellum.

tended forearm concentrates these forces to one side of the distal humerus. In addition, compressive forces can be applied to the articular surface. These forces may be indirect, being transmitted axially via the radius or ulna from forces applied to the distal portion of the extremity. There are specific areas of the articular surface where greater concentration of force can occur (e.g., by the wedge-shaped articular portion of the ulna against the groove of the trochlea or by the rim of the radial head in the capitulotrochlear sulcus). Abduction or adduction of the forearm in extension can further concentrate the force in a given area. Direct forces can be applied to the elbow as well. This usually occurs on the posterior aspect of the flexed elbow. In this position the lateral condyle is more exposed on the lateral side, while medially the epicondyle is more vulnerable to injury from a direct force. Forces applied directly to the posterior border of the proximal ulna are concentrated in the trochlear groove. If applied centrally, both condyles may be wedged apart, producing an intercondylar fracture. If the force is applied eccentrically, fracture of an isolated condyle is produced. Rarely are the forces applied during an injury pure. They are often mixed, resulting in a variety of fracture patterns.

Milch[190] pointed out that the lateral trochlear ridge is a very important structure in stability of the elbow after fracture of a single condyle. He divided fractures of the condyles into two classes, based upon the preservation or loss of the integrity of this ridge (Fig. 9-16). Type I fractures are simple fractures. In this type of fracture the lateral trochlear ridge remains with the intact condyle. Thus the medial-lateral stability of the elbow is maintained. This medial-lateral stability refers to the medial-lateral translocation of the ulna with respect to the distal humerus. Valgus or varus instability can be present, however, with a

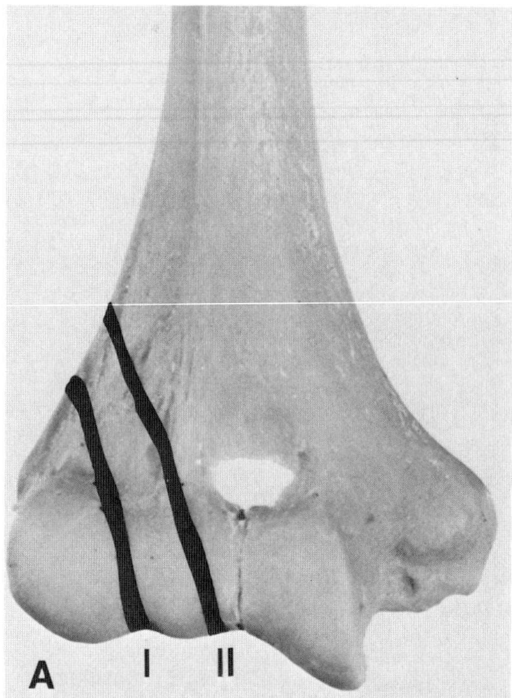

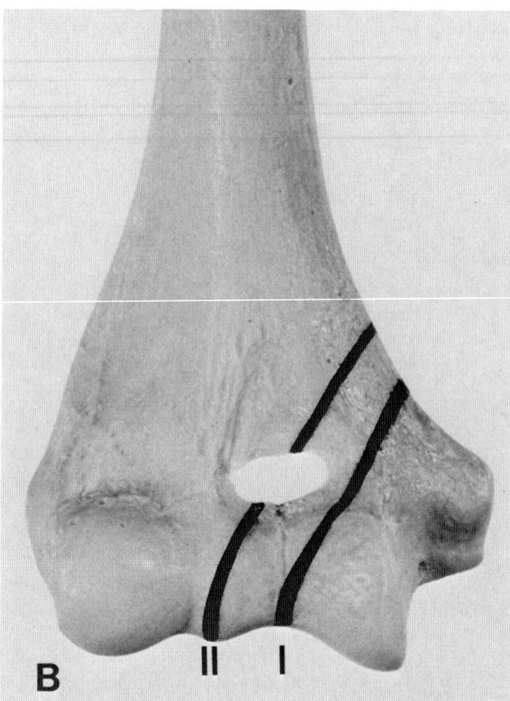

Fig. 9-16. Classification of condylar fractures according to Milch.[189] Location of the common fracture lines seen in Type I and Type II fractures of the lateral (*A*) and medial (*B*) condyle.

Type I fracture. Displacement of the fractured condyle can be proximal or distal, depending upon the type of injury involved. In the Type II fracture the lateral trochlear ridge is a part of the fractured condyle. This allows the radius and ulna to translocate in a medial-lateral direction with respect to the long axis of the humerus, thus the Type II fracture is called a fracture-dislocation. This classification has therapeutic application. Some Type I fractures can be treated by closed methods. All Type II fractures require open reduction and internal fixation.

Incidence

Fractures of the humeral condyles or their components are uncommon in adults.[32,62,115] In Knight's series,[155] fractures of a single condyle accounted for only about 5 per cent of the fractures of the distal humerus in adults. Fracture of the lateral condyle is more common than fracture of the medial condyle.[64,254]

Fractures of the Lateral Condyle

Signs and Symptoms

Fracture of the lateral condyle is recognized by the presence of independent motion of the lateral condyle from the medial condyle and humeral shaft. The condyle may be proximal or distal to the main portion of the humerus, depending on the type of force that created the fracture. As the arm hangs at the side, there may be a loss of the carrying angle.[262] Crepitus usually is present. Radial rotation may accentuate the crepitus.[115] While intercondylar distance may be widened, the arm does not appear shortened as in intercondylar fractures.

Roentgenographic Findings

The fracture line extends obliquely from

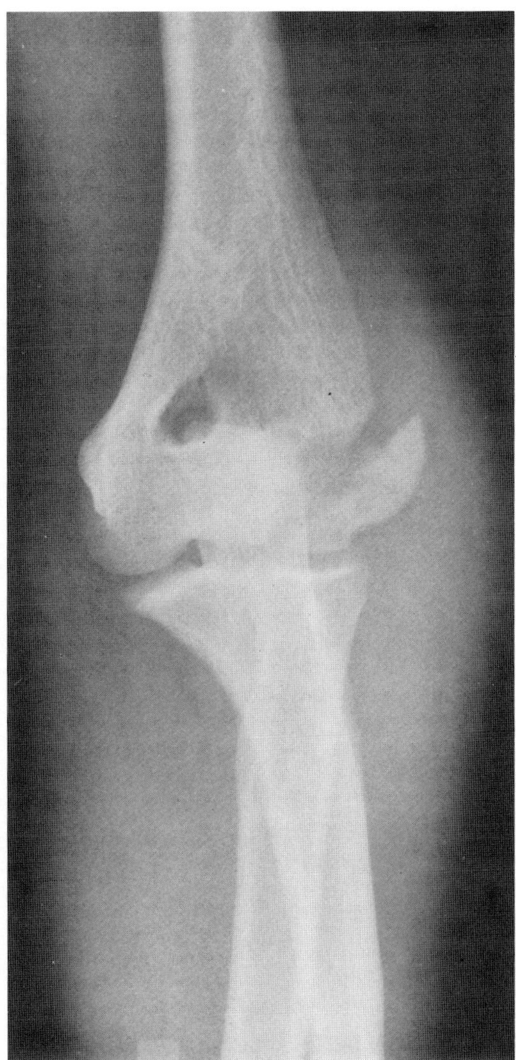

Fig. 9-17. This Type I fracture of the lateral condyle involves both the articular surface of the capitellum and the nonarticular surface, including the lateral epicondyle. The distal portion of the fracture line emerges just lateral to the capitulotrochlear sulcus.

either the capitulotrochlear sulcus or the lateral border of the trochlear groove up to the supracondylar ridge (Figs. 9-15A; 9-17). Depending upon the type of fracture, there may be lateral translocation of the ulna with respect to the shaft of the humerus. Complete rotation of the fragment by the extensor muscle origin, while common in children, is rare in adults. Lateral condylar fractures must be differentiated from fractures of the capitellum (see p. 515). A fracture of the condyle has both articular and nonarticular components. A fracture of the capitellum involves only the articular surface and its supporting bone (Figs. 9-15B; 9-18).

Methods of Treatment

Nonoperative. Many lateral condyle fractures are undisplaced or only minimally displaced. These usually can be treated by simple immobilization until stable. Conwell and Reynolds[64] described reduction of the fracture with the elbow extended. With the forearm supinated and extended, manual pressure is applied directly over the fragment for a reduction. Adduction of the fore-

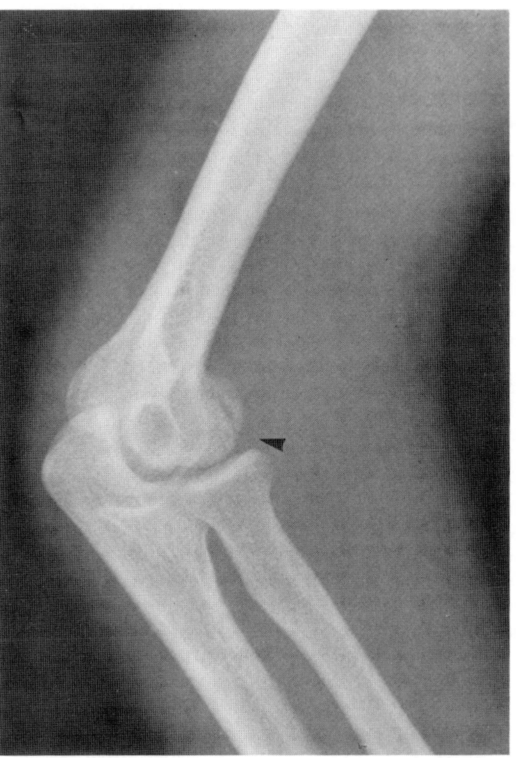

Fig. 9-18. Oblique view of the elbow with a Type II fracture of the capitellum demonstrating the small fragment involving the anterior surface of the capitellum (*arrow*).

arm opens up the lateral aspect of the joint to facilitate the reduction. The supinated forearm is then gradually flexed at the elbow. A long-arm plaster is applied with lateral molding. There is some question as to which position provides maximum stability after reduction. Based on the precedents set by R. Jones, H. L. Smith, and F. B. Lund, Cotton[66] believed that the best stability was achieved by the splinting effect of the triceps tendon in acute flexion. Milch was of the opinion that these are more stable in extension.[190] In extension the olecranon is locked into its opposing fossa of the humerus, which affords medial-lateral stability. While this position may be tolerated for a brief period of time by a child, it can result in considerable disability in an adult. We prefer to immobilize these in flexion with the forearm supinated and the wrist dorsiflexed slightly to relieve some of the muscle forces on the fragment.

Operative. The goals of operative intervention appear to be twofold. First, condylar alignment must be reestablished so that the axes of rotation of the condyles are the same (see Fig. 9-4). Secondly, in the Type II fracture the integrity of the lateral trochlear wall must be reestablished. Surgery is best performed as soon after the injury as possible. Either the posterior or lateral approach may be used. Fixation is usually achieved with screws. Smith[254] recommended repairing the medial collateral ligament, if it is torn, through a separate medial approach.

Complications and Prognosis

The outcome depends upon the degree of comminution of the condyle. Rigid fixation allowing early motion usually improves the final result. If the fracture is a Type I and improperly reduced, cubitus valgus can result. If it is a Type II fracture, cubitus valgus plus lateral transposition of the forearm occurs. This results in a greater deformity because the prominence of the medial epicondyle is accentuated.[190]

Fractures of the Medial Condyle

The medial condyle is fractured less often than the lateral one, probably because direct blows to the medial side of the elbow more often fracture the prominent medial epicondyle than the deeper medial condyle. Generally the fracture originates at the depth of the trochlear groove and ascends obliquely to end at the supracondylar ridge (Type I; Fig. 9-16B). If the primary wedging force on the articular surface is applied by the rim of the head of the radius, then the fracture may originate in the capitulotrochlear sulcus, producing a Type II injury (Fig. 9-16B). Because it usually involves the trochlear groove, there may be more disability associated with fracture of this condyle.

Signs and Symptoms

Motion of the entire condyle occurs when the medial epicondyle is manipulated. If the radial head is displaced medially with the ulnar and medial condyle fragment, there may be an apparent increased prominence of the lateral condyle and capitellum. Extension of the elbow tends to produce motion of the fragment, due to increased tension on the origin of the forearm flexor muscles.

Methods of Treatment

Nonoperative. In undisplaced fractures, satisfactory treatment can be achieved with a posterior splint. The elbow is flexed and the forearm is pronated with some wrist flexion to relax the muscles that originate on the medial epicondyle.[64,254] Roentgenograms must be taken at frequent intervals to be sure that late displacement of the fragment does not occur.

Operative. While many of the displaced fractures can be reduced closed, it is virtually impossible to maintain a reduction that will prevent a step-off in the articular surface. We prefer anatomical restoration of the articular surface by open reduction and internal fixation. In approaching the fragment, the ulnar nerve must be carefully exposed and protected. Conwell and Reynolds[64] recommended anterior transposition if the ulnar groove is involved in the fracture or if there is injury to the nerve. Firm fixation may be difficult to obtain. The medial supracondylar column is long and narrow (see Fig. 9-2B). Placement of screws up this column or through the narrow central portion of the trochlear groove (see Fig. 9-3) may be difficult. Also it is more difficult to obtain initial purchase of the screws on the pointed medial epicondyle than on the flattened surface of the lateral condyle. If the fixation is not solid after operation, the extremity should be immobilized as with closed reduction (i.e., with the elbow and wrist flexed and the forearm pronated).

Prognosis and Complications

Because of involvement of the trochlear groove there is more chance for residual incongruity. This increases the incidence of posttraumatic arthritis. Malunion with the fragment displaced proximally can result in cubitus varus.

One interesting complication was reported by Roaf,[228] who described a case where the median nerve had become trapped between the fracture fragments. With healing, two foramina were created through which the median nerve passed. With time and continued motion of the elbow the nerve became frayed at the distal foramen. Total disruption of the nerve resulted.

FRACTURES OF THE ARTICULAR SURFACE OF THE DISTAL HUMERUS

Compressive wedging or shear forces are usually involved in the production of fractures of the articular surfaces. Because there are no soft-tissue attachments, avulsion forces do not play a role in the production of these fractures. The initial displacement is produced by the causative force. Further displacement can occur, however, because the fragment has no soft-tissue attachments and lies freely within the joint cavity. The fragment involves primarily the articular cartilage. In some cases large amounts of subchondral bone are attached. Often there may be more than one articular surface involved. We will discuss the various types of articular fractures based on the primary area of involvement.

Fractures of the Capitellum

While the first case was described by Hahn in 1853,[162,165] Kocher is credited with calling attention to this fracture in his classic monograph "Fractura Rotuli Humeri."[64,162,165,181] Thus, fractures of the capitellum are often called *Kocher fractures.*[238] Fractures of the capitellum are rare. The incidence of this fracture in the numerous series reported[42,62,88,232,310] varies from 0.5 to 1 per cent of all the elbow injuries seen.

Both Kocher and Lorenz recognized two separate types of fractures of the capitellum.[100,162] Type I or the Hahn-Steinthal type involves a large part of the osseous portion of the capitellum. The Type II or Kocher-Lorenz type involves articular cartilage with very little bone attached (Fig. 9-18). Wilson[310] described a third type in which the articular surface is driven proximally and impacted into the osseous portion.

Emphasis needs to be placed again on the differentiation between fractures of the capitellum and lateral condyle (see p. 510). A fracture of the capitellum involves only the articular portion of the condyle. A fracture of the lateral condyle involves the capitellum plus the nonarticular portion, which often includes the epicondyle.

Mechanism of Injury

Milch[188] believed that the location of the fragment gives a clue to the position of the elbow when injured. If the elbow is in extension, the anterior surface of the capitellum is sheared off and the fragment is displaced anteriorly. Injury with the elbow flexed results in the fragment lying in the posterior aspect of the joint. Kocher originally felt that in the Type I the anterior capsule avulsed the fragment when the elbow was forced into hyperextension.[101,162] There are no recent adherents to this mechanism. Because the lateral surface of the capitellum is exposed when the elbow is in a position of semiflexion and semipronation, some authors feel that Type I injuries can result from a direct blow to this area.[101,162]

In some instances, especially in the Type I fracture, a portion of the lateral trochlear ridge may be included (see Fig. 9-15B). Robertson and Bogart reported a fracture "*en masse*" of both articular surfaces.[232] This type of fracture may be confused with the Posada type of transcondylar fracture (see Fig. 9-9). The latter type of fracture extends through both condyles to their posterior borders, while the fracture *en masse* involves only articular surfaces.

Signs and Symptoms

There is a fair amount of consistency in the reported clinical findings. Since most of the acute symptoms are due to the distension of the joint with blood, there may be a silent interval between the time of injury and the development of symptoms.[225] Anterior displacement of the fragment results in its impingement in the radial or coronoid fossa, producing a bony block. With posteriorly placed fragments there is no bony block, only pain with flexion as the fragment is forced against the capsule.[162] Crepitus may be present. Often the fragment can be palpated anterior to the radial head when the elbow is extended. Since the external bony landmarks maintain their normal relationship, the clinical findings often do not correlate with the acute disability displayed with fracture of the capitellum.[181] While the presence of fractures of both the radial head and the capitellum is rare, it does occur. Milch[188] emphasized that the presence of dual tenderness on the lateral side of the elbow may be an important sign of the existence of fractures in both areas.

Roentgenographic Findings

Lindem[165] pointed out that the roentgenographic signs are best appreciated on the lateral view (Fig. 9-18). The fragment most commonly lies anterior and proximal to the main portion of the capitellum. The articular surface usually faces anteriorly. There may be a lack of the normal cortical margin in the area of the defect on the surface of the capitellum. If seen later there may be union of the fragment with the humerus in the area of the radial fossa. Often the fragment is not well visualized on the anteroposterior view. The rare instances of dual fractures of both the radial head and the capitellum must always be kept in mind. In all fractures of the capitellum the radial head must be carefully evaluated, clinically and roentgenographically. This is especially important where closed reduction is to be utilized, using pressure from the radial head to secure the fragment. The opposite is also true. That is, in evaluation of an isolated radial head fracture, the capitellum should be checked carefully for the presence of a fracture as well. In Milch's[188] experience, fracture fragments from a comminuted radial head are rarely displaced in a proximal direction. Thus, if a large fragment is seen in the joint anterior and proximal to the radial head, it should be suspected to have originated from the capitellum rather than from the comminuted radial head (Fig. 9-19).

Methods of Treatment

Nonoperative. The Type I injury is the one most amenable to closed reduction. Reduction must be very accurate, because the smallest amount of displacement can restrict motion of the radiohumeral joint. Most surgeons prefer to manipulate the fracture with the elbow extended.[32,64,76,225,232] Traction is applied to the forearm with the

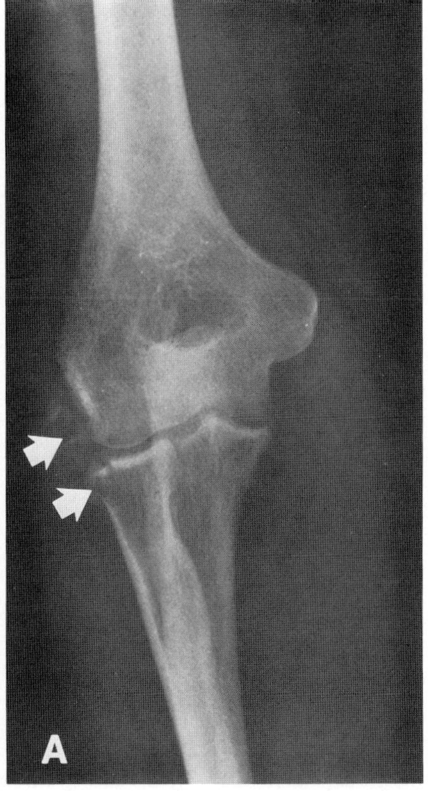

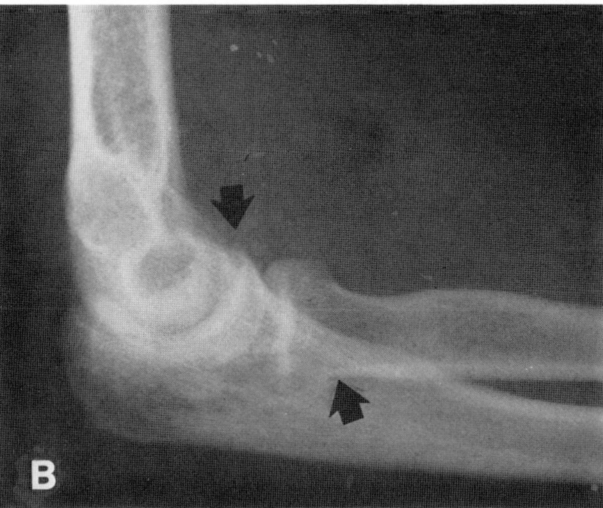

Fig. 9-19. Concomitant fractures of the capitellum and the radial head. This injury, sustained by a direct blow, shows fractures of both the capitellum and radial head (*arrows*): (*A*) anteroposterior and (*B*) lateral roentgenograms. The fragments from the capitellum (*upper arrow*) characteristically lie in the anterior aspect of the joint proximal to the radial head.

elbow extended. Pressure is then placed directly over the fracture fragment to effect reduction. Placing a varus stress on the forearm opens the lateral side of the elbow and facilitates replacement of the fracture fragment. Once reduction is accomplished it is maintained by holding the elbow flexed. The fragment is held in place by the head of the radius. Pronation of the forearm seems to secure the radial fixation of the fragment. The ability of the radius to hold the fragment in place has been confirmed at the time of open reduction by Rhoden and Darrach.[73,225]

Operative. Simple excision of the small fragments is the usual means of treating the Type II fracture. In the Type I fracture where an inadequate closed reduction was obtained or where there is marked comminution of the fragment, surgical intervention must be performed. Keon-Cohen[144] has found that once an open reduction is obtained, the fragment may be stable and can, thus, be held in place with the opposing radial head similar to a closed reduction. Others[41,155,262] fix the fragment with a screw. The screw is usually inserted from the posterior aspect of the condyle. The tip engages the bony portion of the fragment securing it to the condyle. The articular cartilage is therefore not penetrated. If the fragment is comminuted, then excision may be the better treatment.

The real problem in management arises where there are multiple large fragments, often involving both articular surfaces. Smith[254] believed that these should always be removed. The lateral instability that is present has not lead to ulnar nerve problems or disability, in his opinion. Attempting to replace the fragment necessitates immobilization, which can lead to residual disability. Excision allows early motion with less morbidity. Anderson[11] used the epicondyles as the point for deciding on retention or excision of the fragments. If resection proximal to the condyles is required, an attempt should be made to reestablish the contour of the distal humerus. If all the resection can be performed distal to the epicondyles, then excision of the fragments is the procedure of choice. In those cases where wide excision of the fragments would be necessary, he recommends a primary hemiarthroplasty.

We feel that early motion is essential to the rehabilitation of articular injuries. If the fragment is large enough to allow firm fixation and early motion, then it should be replaced. If it is comminuted, the fragments should be excised.

The significance of avascularity of the fragment is unclear. Speed[262] and Anderson[11] have not found it to be a problem. Smith felt, however, that it is and can lead to delayed traumatic arthritis.[254] This was his rationale for removing even a large single fragment.

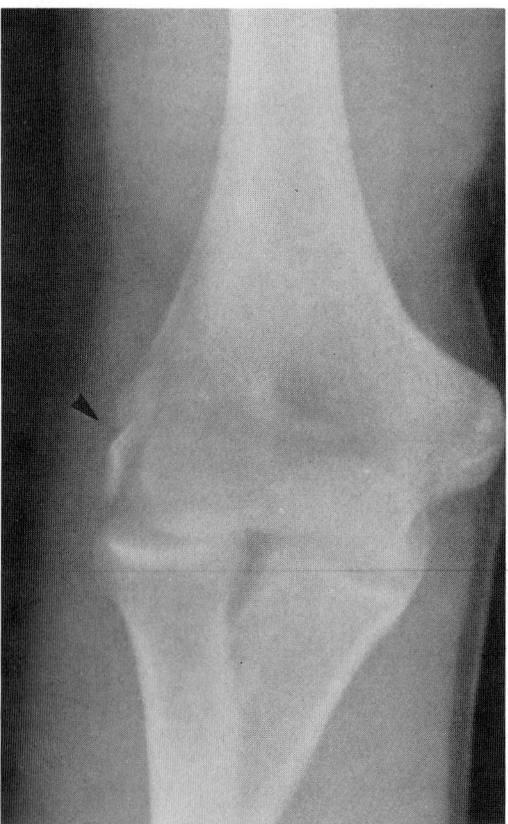

Fig. 9-20. Fracture of the lateral epicondyle (*arrow*) with a small portion of the capitellum as well.

Fractures of the Trochlea

Isolated fractures of the trochlea are extremely rare. Stimson[275] credits the original description to Laugier in 1853. Hence the term, Laugier's fracture. Very few authors report having seen it as an isolated fracture.[88,115,229,254,275]

The very structure of the trochlea probably contributes to the rarity of its existence as an isolated injury. The capitellum is subject to shear and compressive forces from the head of the radius. It can also be fractured by a direct blow. The trochlea, on the other hand, is deep within the elbow joint and thus protected from direct injury. The transmitted force of the ulna against the trochlea tends to produce more of a wedging action than a tangential shearing force.

In making the clinical diagnosis the signs of effusion, pain, restriction of motion, and crepitus indicative of an intraarticular fracture are usually present. The one specific finding that would lead the surgeon to suspect a fracture of the trochlea would be a fragment lying on the medial side of the joint just distal to the medial epicondyle.

The fracture may extend from the trochlea into the distal portion of the epicondyle.[254] Large fragments may be replaced. The smaller fragments are better excised.

FRACTURES OF THE EPICONDYLES

Each of the epicondyles has its own separate ossification center. This has special significance in children, because with tension on the collateral ligaments the point of weakness is at the epiphyseal growth plate rather than the ligaments. Thus fractures of the epicondyles in children are usually epiphyseal separations most often caused by avulsion. As primary isolated fractures in adults they are uncommon.

Fractures of the Lateral Epicondyle

Fracture of the lateral epicondyle is extremely rare (Fig. 9-20). In fact, many authors have doubted that it even exists as an isolated fracture in adults.[66A,115,275,301] The ossification center of the lateral epicondyle is small and appears about the twelfth year. After it fuses with the main portion of the lateral condyle at puberty, avulsion fractures are even rarer. The lateral epicondyle is almost level with the flattened outer surface of the lateral condyle. Thus it has only minimal exposure to a direct blow. The treatment involves simple immobilization until the pain subsides, then early motion, similar to an undisplaced lateral condyle (see p. 513).

Fractures of the Medial Epicondyle

Fracture of the medial epicondyle or epitrochlea (Figs. 9-21; 9-22) is more common than fracture of the lateral epicondyle. Its existence as a separate entity has been known since Granger reported on ten cases in 1818.[115,275] Fusion of the ossification center of the medial epicondyle with the distal humerus does not occur until about the 20th year.[109] In some adults fusion may never occur.[115]

Mechanism of Injury

In the child and adolescent this fragment is commonly avulsed from the humerus during a posterior dislocation of the elbow. In many of these fractures associated with dislocations (see p. 532), the epicondylar fragment may be carried into the joint and remain lodged there when the elbow is reduced (Fig. 9-22). The ulnar nerve can also become trapped with this fragment. After the age of twenty it rarely occurs as a single fracture or associated with a dislocation. In Smith's[254] series of medial epicondyle fractures, only six of 143 were found in adults. There is no residua of the old epiphyseal plate after fusion with the main osseous portion of the distal humerus occurs (Fig. 9-14). Fractures in the adult are not necessarily limited to the area originating from the medial epicondylar ossification center. They can extend into part of the main medial condylar mass as well. These isolated fractures in the adult are most commonly caused by a direct blow to the epicondyle. Its prominence on the medial aspect of the elbow makes it especially vulnerable to this type of force.

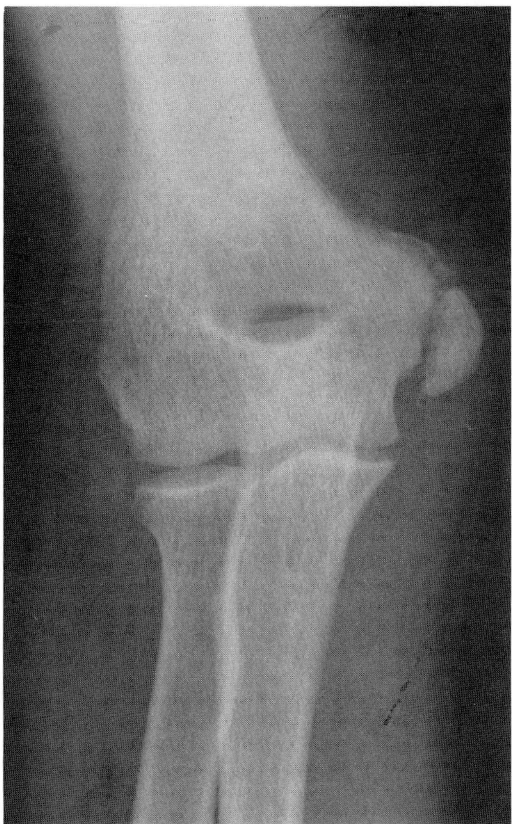

Fig. 9-21. This fracture of the medial epicondyle is relatively undisplaced. There is evidence of periosteal new bone formation proximally along the supracondylar ridge.

Signs and Symptoms

In displaced fractures the fragment is usually pulled anterior and distal by the forearm flexor muscles. Local tenderness and crepitus over the medial epicondyle are characteristic. Active flexion of the elbow and wrist along with pronation of the

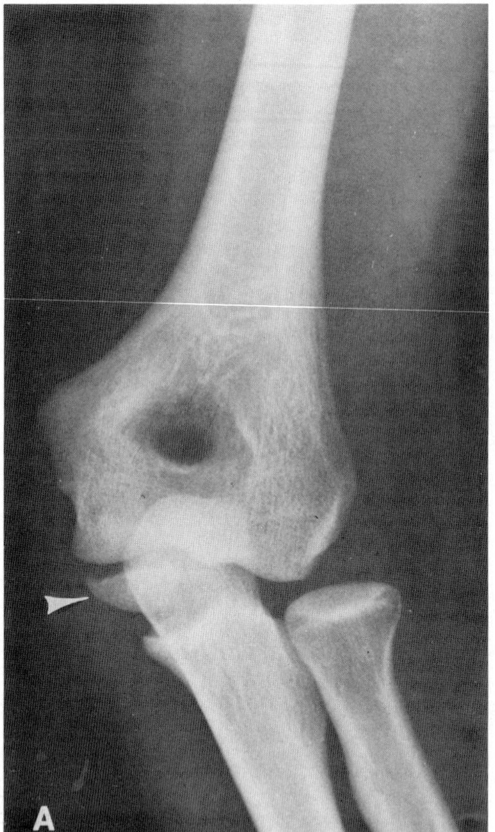

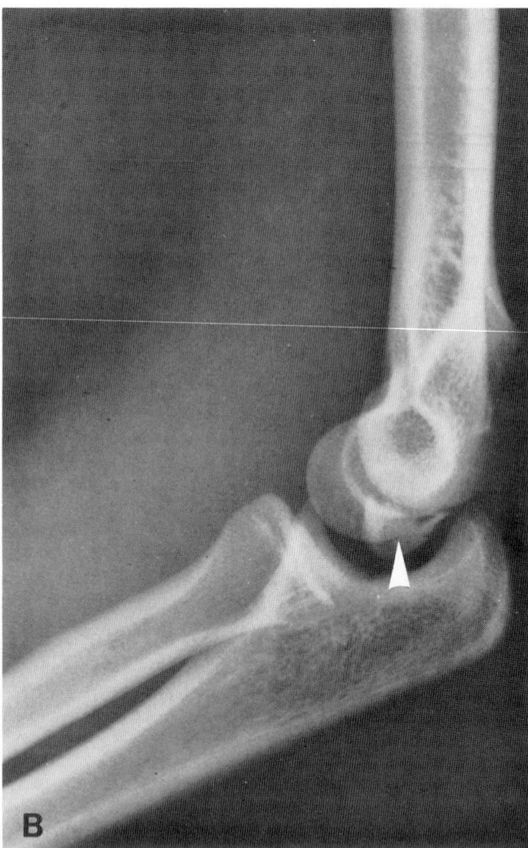

Fig. 9-22. Avulsion of the medial epicondyle with displacement into the joint. (*A*) The epicondyle (*arrow*) is lodged between the medial articular surface of the trochlea and ulna, inhibiting reduction. (*B*) Lateral view of the same patient demonstrating intraarticular location of the medial epicondyle (*arrow*).

forearm may accentuate the local tenderness. Because of its proximity to the epicondyle the function of the ulnar nerve must be evaluated carefully.

Roentgenographic Findings

There may be a tendency to confuse the normal radiolucent epiphyseal growth plate with an acute fracture of the epicondyle in the adolescent patient. Comparison views of the opposite elbow may be helpful. In those cases where the epicondylar fragment has been avulsed during a posterior lateral dislocation its presence within the joint must be ruled out. A roentgenographic clue to its lodgement within the joint was demonstrated by Patrick.[210] With simple avulsion of the epicondyle the fragment never migrates distally as far as the joint level. Thus if the fragment is seen lying at the level of the joint, its intraarticular incarceration must be ruled out (Fig. 9-22).

Methods of Treatment

General agreement exists as to the proper method of treatment of either the minimally displaced fractures or those which are lodged within the joint.[11,64,76,144,254] In the minimally displaced fracture the generally accepted method of treatment is short-term immobilization (7 to 10 days) with the elbow and wrist flexed and the forearm pronated. Likewise, those fragments lying within the joint that cannot be extracted by the closed methods advocated by Patrick[210] (see p. 532) must be removed operatively.

It is on the subject of moderately- to severely displaced fragments that difference of opinion exists. Three methods of treatment are available to the surgeon: (1) manipulation and short-term immobilization; (2) open reduction with internal fixation; and (3) excision of the fragment.

Smith[254] advocated nonoperative treatment with early motion in nearly all cases. In his extensive review of patients with this injury he was unable to confirm the presence of any of the previously described disabilities resulting from persistent displacement of the fragment.[251] None of those with fibrous union had pain or disability. Distal displacement of the epicondyle did not result in weakness of the wrist flexors. Only one of 116 cases in his series treated by nonoperative means had any delayed ulnar nerve problems. It was his conclusion that the end results with either bony- or fibrous union were the same.

Proponents of operation cite the presence of ulnar nerve symptoms as an indication for either reattachment or excision of the fragment.[11,144,155] Anderson[11] uses displacement greater than 1 cm. as another indication for internal fixation.

Authors' Preferred Method of Treatment. We feel that early resumption of motion is essential to recovery of elbow function. Thus these fractures are treated by manipulation and immobilization with the forearm pronated and the elbow and wrist flexed in a posterior slab for 10 to 14 days. Active motion is then allowed. Should the displaced fragment be unsightly or painful, or if ulnar nerve problems develop, the fragment can be excised later with a minimal operative morbidity. Treatment of the entrapped fragment is discussed under dislocation of the elbow.

FRACTURES OF THE SUPRACONDYLAR PROCESS

Fracture of this uncommon process is of clinical significance and bears discussion. The incidence of this process is very low, ranging from 0.6 to 2.7 per cent.[79] Because of its long, thin structure and muscle attachments it is easily fractured. This fracture can become troublesome by virtue of its proximity to the median nerve and brachial artery. One should always suspect its presence in the patient with median nerve dysfunction distal to the elbow.

Treatment of fractures of the supracondylar process varies.[79,160,169] Many heal spontaneously and become asymptomatic. In the ones that remain painful or produce median nerve dysfunction surgical excision is indicated.[79,169] Kolb is more cautious in recommending surgical resection.[160] He reported one case of myositis ossificans after removal of the fractured process.

DISLOCATIONS OF THE ELBOW

During the course of human activities, the elbow is frequently placed under loads and in positions that overtax its inherent mechanical stability. A sudden force applied to the arm can transcend the normal range of motion of the elbow and cause a dislocation. The only joints more often affected by dislocation are the shoulder and finger joints. While the incidence of dislocation of the elbow decreases as the development of the coronoid and olecranon processes becomes complete, it is still a relatively common injury in the adult. As with other dislocations, elbow dislocations need to be reduced as rapidly as possible after injury, not only to relieve pain, but also to avoid excessive swelling, adverse circulatory changes, and additional articular cartilage damage.

CLASSIFICATION

The standard method of classifying elbow dislocations is to describe how the radius and ulna are displaced in relationship to the distal humerus. During the very early 1800's most authors recognized only the four types of elbow dislocation that involved the radius and ulna as a unit. In addition, they also described isolated dislocations of the radial head.[77] As more cases

Table 9-1. Classification of Adult Elbow Dislocations

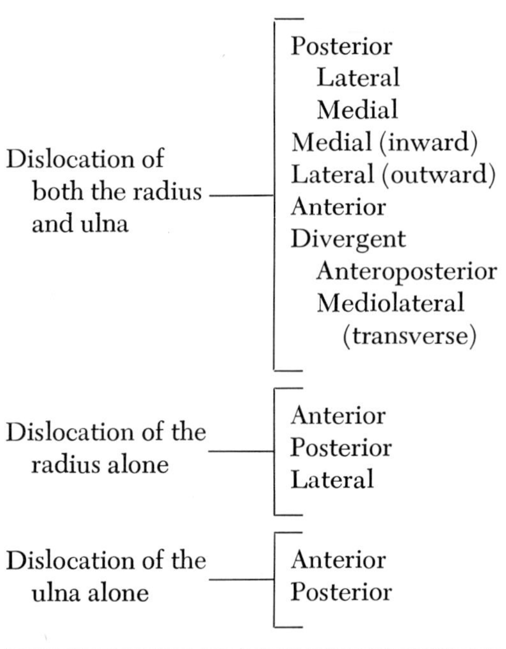

Dislocation of both the radius and ulna	Posterior Lateral Medial Medial (inward) Lateral (outward) Anterior Divergent Anteroposterior Mediolateral (transverse)
Dislocation of the radius alone	Anterior Posterior Lateral
Dislocation of the ulna alone	Anterior Posterior

(Adapted from Stimson, L. A.: A Treatise on Fractures. Philadelphia, Henry C. Lea's Son and Co., 1890.)

were reported in the medical literature some of the more rare forms of elbow dislocation became recognized. By the later part of the 1800's Hamilton[115] and Stimson[275] had developed similar classifications for elbow dislocations. Their classification has become well established, as evidenced by its use in most of the recent textbooks that deal with elbow injuries.[64,66,76,254,266] We have modified Stimson's original classification[275] (in Table 9-1) to include only the pure primary dislocations occurring in the adult's elbow. Dislocation of the radius and ulna associated with fractures of the olecranon is discussed in the section on olecranon fractures (see p. 536). Dislocation of the radial head associated with the Monteggia fracture-dislocation is discussed in Chapter 8. We will consider unreduced and recurrent dislocations as secondary conditions arising from the primary dislocation.

Posterior or posterolateral dislocations account for 80 to 90 per cent of elbow dislocations in most series.[153,166] The incidence of the other types of dislocations varies, with only sporadic cases being reported. Kini[153] reported a few lateral and no medial or anterior dislocations in 38 cases. Roberts,[231] reviewing 60 cases, had no medial or anterior dislocations but two lateral ones. Linscheid and Wheeler,[166] in their 110 cases, reported 86 posterior or posterolateral, two lateral, two anterior, and four medial dislocations. Anterior dislocations boast a more extensive literature by virtue of their rarity; 33 had been reported up to 1972, as noted by Oury, Roe, and Laning.[208] Divergent and isolated radial and ulnar dislocations are very rare.

PRIMARY ELBOW DISLOCATIONS

Posterior Dislocation of the Elbow

Mechanism of Injury

The mechanism of injury of a posterior dislocation is usually a fall on the outstretched hand with the arm in extension and abduction. The olecranon process levers in the olecranon fossa, and the shape of the trochlea may supply a cam action causing lateral rotation. The coronoid process slips posteriorly and comes to lie in the olecranon fossa or is jammed into the distal end of the humerus (Figs. 9-23; 9-24). As this happens, the distal humerus drives through the anterior joint capsule and tears the brachialis muscle. There is injury to both collateral ligaments and the joint capsule, and stripping of the periosteum and triceps mechanism posteriorly. The final position depends on the amount and direction of force. Smith[254] pointed out that searching for specific mechanisms of injury is useless, because a plan of reduction is based on roentgenograms and clinical findings and is not accomplished simply by reversing the mechanism of injury. The salient feature is a realization of the extensive disruption of soft tissue and its potential for complications.

Signs and Symptoms

Clinical diagnosis can be made easily if the injury is seen early, but it may be impossible after swelling obscures soft-tissue

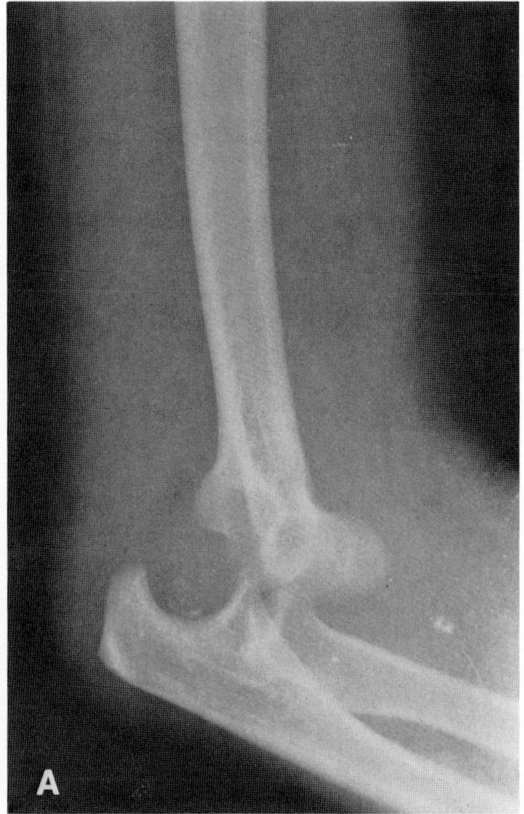

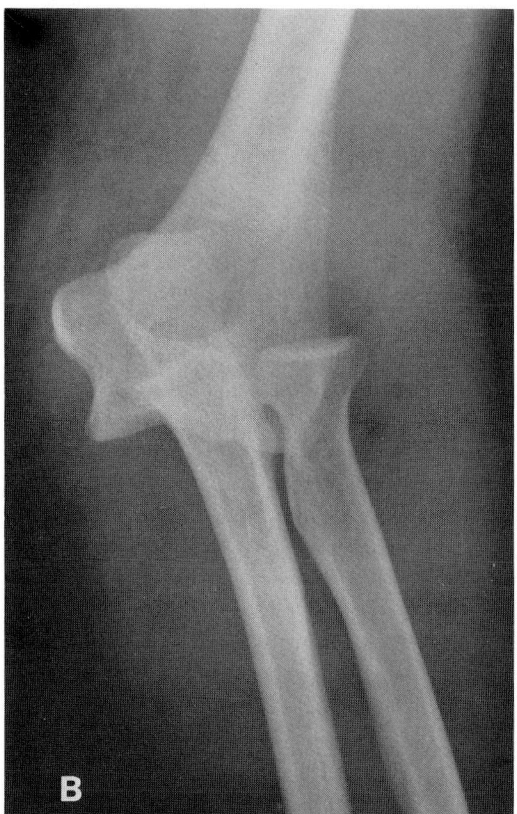

Fig. 9-23. (*A*) A posterior dislocation of the elbow. Note that the coronoid process is adjacent to the olecranon fossa. (*B*) In the anteroposterior view, note the slight lateral displacement of the radius and ulna.

configuration and bony landmarks. The appearance is relatively typical, with the extremity held in mild flexion—usually about 45 degrees. The forearm appears shortened, and the olecranon is prominent posteriorly. The antecubital fossa is full, because of the distal humerus. On the posterior aspect of the elbow the olecranon process tents the skin. Just proximal to this, the skin appears "sucked in" between the edges of the triceps tendon. Palpation reveals disturbance of the triangular relationship of the olecranon and epicondyles posteriorly. The concavity of the radial head may be palpated posteriorly, especially if the dislocation is posterolateral.

Roentgenographic Findings

Roentgenographic examination is imperative to confirm the clinical diagnosis and rule out associated fractures. Additional views other than routine anteroposterior and lateral may be required because of the unusual attitude of the arm.

Methods of Treatment

The initial step in management is careful assessment and accurate recording of the vascular and neurologic status of the extremity. This information may indicate the urgency of reduction as well as the possible need for open treatment if the neurovascular status is compromised following reduction. Armed with roentgenographic and neurovascular assessment, reduction can be accomplished by closed means in virtually all instances of pure dislocation. Several methods of reduction are reported in the literature. Early writers suggested extension, mild gentle hyperextension (to disengage the coronoid process), longitudinal traction, and then flexion. Loomis[167] con-

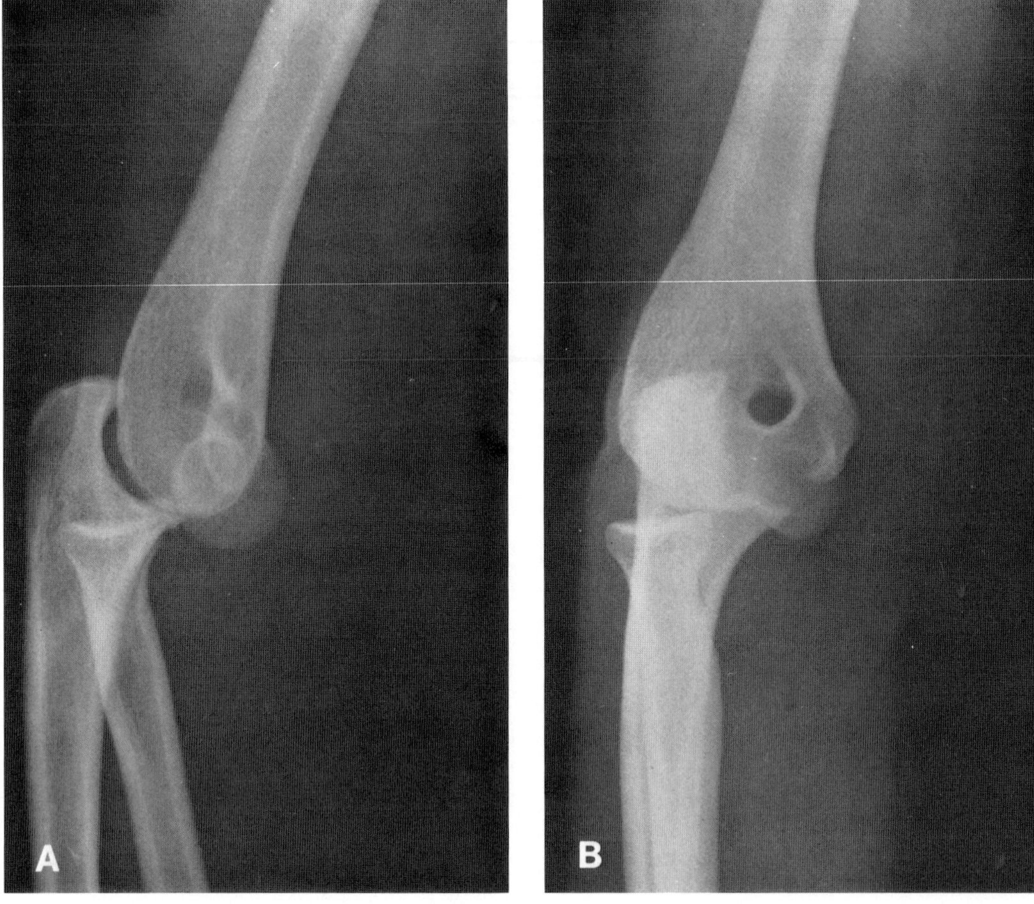

Fig. 9-24. A posterior dislocation of the elbow in which the coronoid is impaled into the trochlea; (*A*) lateral and (*B*) anteroposterior views.

demned extension and especially hyperextension because of increased trauma to the brachialis muscle, which he believed enhanced the likelihood of myositis ossificans. He recommended reduction in flexion, distal traction to the forearm, and application of posterior pressure to the anterior humerus. Starkloff[269] suggested having the patient lie supine on the table with the arm hanging over the side, then applying traction by a weight hung from a gauze bandage on the wrist. After 15 to 20 minutes, gentle traction and forward pressure were applied to the olecranon, effecting reduction. Cherry[55] described an elaborate system of muslin bandages to apply traction in four directions when an assistant was not available. Cotton[67] described a method of reduction for posterior dislocation in which he used the knee as a fulcrum and countertraction against the anterior aspect of the distal arm.

Reduction is generally easily accomplished, especially if done as soon as an accurate diagnosis is made and prior to the appearance of muscle spasm and swelling. The simplest method involves countertraction on the humerus by an assistant while the surgeon applies distal traction by gripping the wrist and the proximal forearm. Medial or lateral displacement is corrected first, and then distal traction is continued as the elbow is flexed. Downward pressure by the surgeon on the proximal forearm to disengage the coronoid out of the olecranon fossa, or a push posteriorly on the distal humerus by an assistant may be helpful as the elbow is brought into flexion. Hyperextension should be avoided.

As the reduction occurs, an audible and palpable "clunk" can usually be appreciated by the surgeon. An important part of the reduction maneuver is to flex and extend the elbow through a full range of motion immediately after reduction. This is necessary to insure that reduction has actually occurred, that the joint is stable, and that there is no mechanical block to motion within the joint (see Entrapped Medial Epicondyle, p. 532).

Complete muscle relaxation is imperative to achieve an atraumatic reduction. Whether this is accomplished by general anesthesia, regional block, or heavy sedation is a matter of judgment on the part of the surgeon. No anesthesia may be required if the diagnosis is made and gentle reduction attempted within a few minutes of injury. An example of this is on the athletic field. Even if the diagnosis is made and the reduction performed by an experienced surgeon, roentgenographic examination must be obtained following reduction. More commonly, the patient is first seen only after muscle spasm and swelling have already begun to develop, and some form of analgesia or anesthesia is mandatory. There should be no hesitation about using regional or general anesthesia, especially when spasm, swelling, and apprehension are significant.

Repeated forceful attempts at reduction are contraindicated, and if several gentle attempts at reduction under adequate anesthesia fail, open reduction is indicated. This is rarely necessary in pure dislocations. In Linscheid and Wheeler's[166] series of 110 dislocations, open reduction was required only 12 times, and in every instance this was to treat an associated fracture.

Care After Reduction

After a satisfactory seating of the reduced dislocation has occurred, the arm is extended to determine the stability of the elbow. The position at which a redislocation is likely to occur should be noted. If the reduction is stable, active motion of the elbow is instituted as pain and swelling subside. Failure to observe and carry out this step can frequently result in a permanent flexion contracture of the elbow. In cases of demonstrable instability of the elbow, longer periods of immobilization are required.

After a satisfactory reduction has been obtained clinically, anterior and lateral roentgenograms are obtained to document the adequacy of reduction and to recognize fractures not apparent prior to reduction or those caused by the manipulation itself.

If the patient is not hospitalized, strict warnings should be given to those responsible for the patient to observe the circulatory and neurological status of the extremity. The extremity is elevated above chest level, and ice packs are applied.

A long-arm plaster splint is the usual method of holding the reduction. The position of immobilization generally is flexion as far as the swelling and circulatory status allow. Most authors suggest at least 90 degrees—more if possible.

The duration of immobilization depends primarily on the stability of the elbow after reduction. In general, the sooner active motion can be started, the more favorable the result. In uncomplicated, stable dislocations, we prefer to remove the splint in 3 to 4 days for gentle active motion several times a day. At 10 to 14 days the splint is discarded, and a sling or collar and cuff is substituted rather than allowing the arm to hang free. Gentle active motion and application of heat are continued at this point. There is no place for passive motion or any form of manipulation; forceful treatment may lead to loss of motion and even bone ankylosis. This regimen must be altered if there is severe soft-tissue damage, gross instability, or an associated fracture. In such cases, immobilization must be longer, but

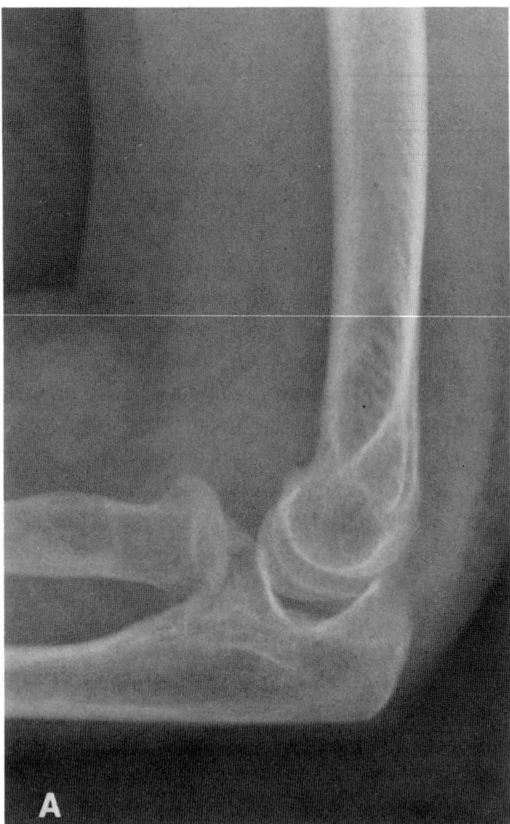

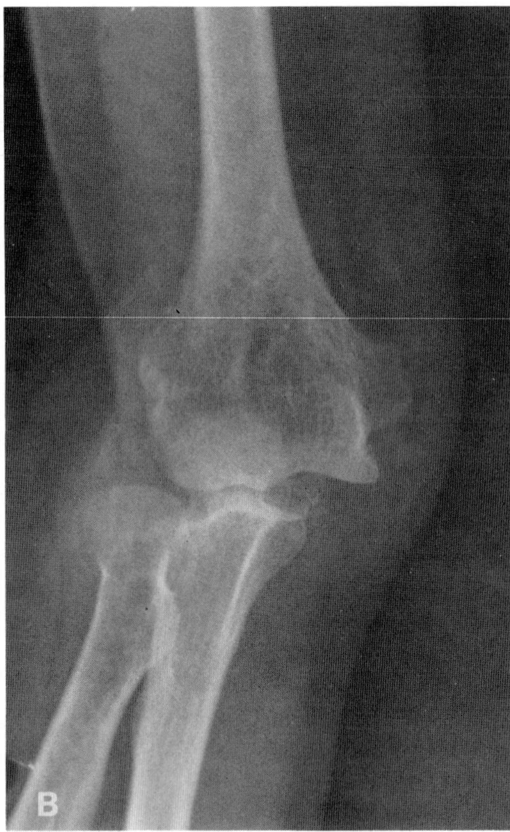

Fig. 9-25. (*A*) Lateral view of a lateral dislocation of the elbow. The semilunar notch appears to be articulating with the distal humerus. There is no anterior or posterior displacement of the proximal ulna. (*B*) The anteroposterior view shows the proximal radius and ulna to have shifted laterally as a unit. The semilunar notch of the ulna is articulating in the capitulotrochlear sulcus. This may allow some limited flexion and extension.

under no circumstances should it exceed 3 to 4 weeks, as permanent flexion contracture may result.

Medial and Lateral Dislocations of the Elbow

Diagnosis

Medial or lateral dislocations present with a widened appearance of the elbow and normal relative lengths of the arm and forearm. On roentgenograms, a pure medial or lateral dislocation shows the greater sigmoid notch of the ulna in the plane of the distal humerus on the lateral view (Fig. 9-25).

In a pure lateral dislocation the greater sigmoid notch may articulate in the capitulotrochlear sulcus (Fig. 9-25), allowing some degree of flexion and extension. This motion may lead the unsuspecting surgeon astray in diagnosing the dislocation on the clinical findings, especially if there is considerable swelling.

Methods of Treatment

Medial and lateral dislocations are reduced by countertraction on the arm, distal traction on the forearm in mild extension, and then straight medial or lateral pressure. Care should be taken to avoid converting this type into a posterior dislocation, causing further soft-tissue damage. The medial dislocation is usually a subluxation rather than a complete dislocation, and soft-tissue damage is not as extensive as in the more severe lateral dislocation. The forearm bones generally dislocate together, as they are firmly bound by the interosseous membrane and the annular ligament.

Anterior Dislocation of the Elbow

This injury has been the subject of extensive literature, perhaps because of its rarity. Cohn,[59] in an excellent review of the literature in 1922, found 23 cases and credits Everts (1787) with the original description. This case also represented the first open elbow dislocation and the first associated with brachial artery laceration.

The mechanism of injury is a blow to the flexed elbow that drives the olecranon forward.

Diagnosis

The arm appears shortened; the forearm, lengthened and supinated; and the elbow is usually in full extension. The olecranon fossa and the trochlea will be palpable posteriorly. Tenting of the biceps tendon and brachialis muscle is prominent anteriorly.

Roentgenograms show the olecranon impinging on the anterior aspect of the distal humerus.

Methods of Treatment

Reduction is obtained in partial extension with distal traction and backward pressure on the forearm; it is usually achieved with ease.

This is a severe injury associated with extensive stripping of the soft tissue and is more likely to be open or to cause vascular damage than is the posterior dislocation. It may be frequently associated with complete avulsion of the triceps mechanism.

Oury, Roe, and Laning[208] reported the first case of bilateral anterior dislocation and reviewed the literature, finding 33 cases. Their patient had excellent results. They stated that complications were unusual, and when present involved the brachial artery or ulnar nerve.

Divergent Dislocation of the Elbow

In this rare type of dislocation the radius and ulna dislocate in diverging directions. Two types are seen: anteroposterior and mediolateral (transverse).

The more common anteroposterior type was first described by M. Bulley in 1841.[115,275] It involves a posterior dislocation of the ulna with the coronoid process lodged in the olecranon fossa. The radial head is dislocated anteriorly into the coronoid fossa. In cadaver studies it was demonstrated that this dislocation could be produced by forced pronation of the forearm after the medial collateral ligament had been cut. Thus, with the forearm in forced pronation and extended, the humerus is forced distally, diverging the radius and ulna.[275] It can be appreciated that, in addition to rupture of the orbicular and collateral ligaments, the interosseous membrane is also torn. Clinically, this type of dislocation resembles a posterior dislocation, except that the radial head is palpable in the antecubital fossa. Reduction is accomplished first by reduction of the ulna in a manner similar to reduction of a posterior dislocation (see p. 523). As the ulnar dislocation is being reduced, simultaneous pressure is applied directly over the radial head to reduce it as well. Smith[254] warned that maintenance of reduction of the radial head may be difficult and may require operative intervention. Most authors recommend that following this injury the elbow be immobilized in flexion with the forearm supinated.[64,66,254]

The mediolateral (transverse) type is considered by many to be so rare as to be listed as a surgical curiosity.[66,254] In Warmont's description of Guersant's original case in 1854, the distal humerus was found to be wedged between the radius laterally and the ulna medially.[115,275] This lesion should be easily recognized clinically. The elbow appears markedly widened. The articular surface of the trochlea can be palpated readily on the posterior surface of the elbow. Conwell and Reynolds[64] recommended reducing the second type by applying traction with the elbow in extension while pressing the proximal radius and ulna together.

Dislocation of the Radial Head Alone

Isolated radial head dislocation without an associated fracture of the ulna in an adult is exceedingly rare (Fig. 9-26). It has been reported in children,[199,293] but none of the extensive reviews of consecutive elbow injuries in adults[62,310] had an isolated radial head dislocation that was not associated with a fracture of the ulna. In his classic textbook on the elbow, Smith[254] noted that the injury is extremely rare, and that most dislocations of the radius occur in conjunction with a fracture of the ulna (Monteggia's fracture-dislocation).

Mechanism of Injury

Speed[266] noted that a dislocation of the radius can occur without an associated fracture. He postulated the mechanism of injury to be a fall on the pronated forearm with the elbow flexed by muscle contraction, resulting in hyperextension of the head of the radius by lever action. Evans[92] postulated on theoretical grounds that forced pronation of the forearm could cause an anterior dislocation of the head of the radius without fracture of the ulna. He did not present any cases but instead demonstrated the anterior Monteggia fracture-dislocation, which is a far more common injury.

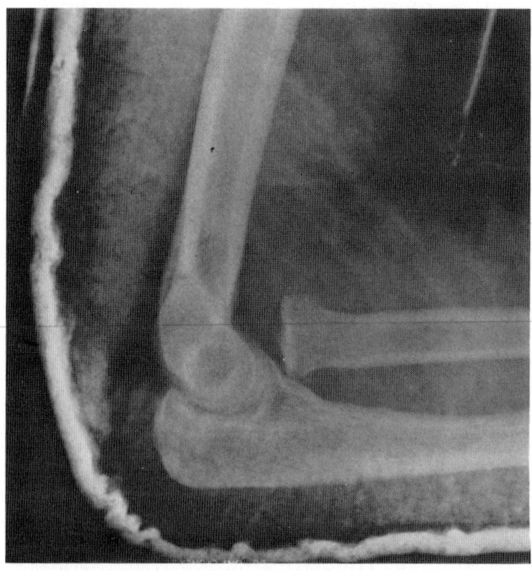

Fig. 9-26. Anterior dislocation of the radial head. Note that the axis of the radial head passes superior to the capitellum. In all dislocations of the radial head, one must look for a concomitant fracture of the ulna.

Methods of Treatment

Although some textbooks[64,266] described the injury and its treatment (agreeing that it is extremely rare), case reports in the literature are difficult to find. Wiley[305,306] reported on five anterior and five lateral dislocations of the head of the radius that occurred as isolated injuries, three caused by automobile accidents and seven by trivial injury. All were reduced under general anesthesia by gently supinating the forearm while extending the elbow. Results were not discussed, but presumably all were stable after closed reduction, as only one required Kirschner wire fixation from the capitellum to the radial head. Other authors[254,266] although they do not cite cases, suggest that the reduction may be unstable and that if open reduction is done, reconstruction of the annular ligament may be necessary.

The rarity of isolated dislocation of the radial head, if in fact it does occur in adults, should prompt the examiner to search diligently for an associated fracture of the ulna before making this diagnosis. Radial head dislocation in association with a fracture of the ulna (Monteggia's fracture-dislocation) is discussed in Chapter 8.

Dislocation of the Ulna Alone

Isolated dislocation of the ulna can occur in either an anterior or posterior direction. Stimson[275] described how the ulna can dislocate while the radius remains in position.

The radial head serves as the pivot. The medial collateral ligament is torn, while the lateral collateral and orbicular ligaments remain intact. The mechanism requires a combination of both angular and axial divergence of the forearm with the humerus. In normal supination with the proximal ulna secure, only the distal forearm can rotate with the radius. In this injury, proximal fixation of the ulna is lost, allowing the whole forearm, including the proximal ulna, to rotate with the radius. With adduction and posterior rotation of the forearm, the coronoid process becomes displaced posterior to the trochlea. Patients with this injury hold their elbows extended. The forearm loses its normal carrying angle and appears to be in varus. Reduction is achieved by applying traction in extension to the supinated forearm. The addition of a valgus force to the forearm facilitates the reduction.[64,66,254]

The anterior dislocation is much more rare. In this type the ulna rotates anteriorly, and the forearm is abducted. Again the radius remains as a fixed pivot. The olecranon is carried forward and becomes locked into the coronoid fossa. Patients with this injury are said to keep the elbow flexed.[275] There is also an increase in the carrying angle. Reduction is achieved by direct pressure applied in a posterior direction over the proximal ulna while the forearm is adducted and pronated.

UNREDUCED DISLOCATION OF THE ELBOW

While unreduced dislocations of the elbow are uncommon because of the wider availability of medical care, they are still seen occasionally. They may be the result of poor initial treatment or the fault of the patient in not seeking medical attention. If the patient is seen within a week, a closed reduction can usually be achieved under general anesthesia with total muscle relaxation. Even during this period, however, the danger of fracture is present, and the manipulation must be done with extreme care and gentleness. If there has been a delay of 7 to 21 days, the reduction is more likely to be successful if a preliminary period of traction is used. Allende and Freytes[9] reported on the treatment of 35 cases of old unreduced dislocations, and they noted that satisfactory reduction by closed means cannot be accomplished after 21 days, even after preliminary traction.

Open reduction of the dislocation may be successful up to 2 months after injury. Speed[68,261] has described in detail the extensive operation required to accomplish this. After 6 months in the unreduced position (and possibly as early as 2 months) changes in the articular surfaces are so great that Callahan[44] concluded that open reduction is not warranted. The choices for these very late dislocations are resection arthroplasty, arthrodesis, and now, possibly, total joint replacement.

RECURRENT DISLOCATION OF THE ELBOW

Recurrent dislocation of the elbow is rare as a complication of acute dislocation and is usually of the posterior type. The cause for the recurrent dislocation varies, but one or more of the following abnormalities may be present: (1) a residual defect in the articular surface of the trochlea; (2) attenuation of the collateral ligaments; (3) failure of union of the coronoid; or (4) stripping of the capsule anteriorly. Some patients may have a congenitally shallow semilunar notch that predisposes to dislocation. In others that were not properly splinted, recurrent trauma may be a cause. If sufficient follow-up roentgenograms were not obtained following the original reduction, subtle subluxation may not have been recognized. If a large fragment of the coronoid did not unite, a shallow semilunar notch might result. The radial head may slide off the capitellum if the capsule and posterolateral ligaments have not healed properly.

The precise defect that permits the recurrent dislocation to occur may not be evident initially by the usual clinical examination. An arthrogram can be helpful in establishing the cause of recurrent disloca-

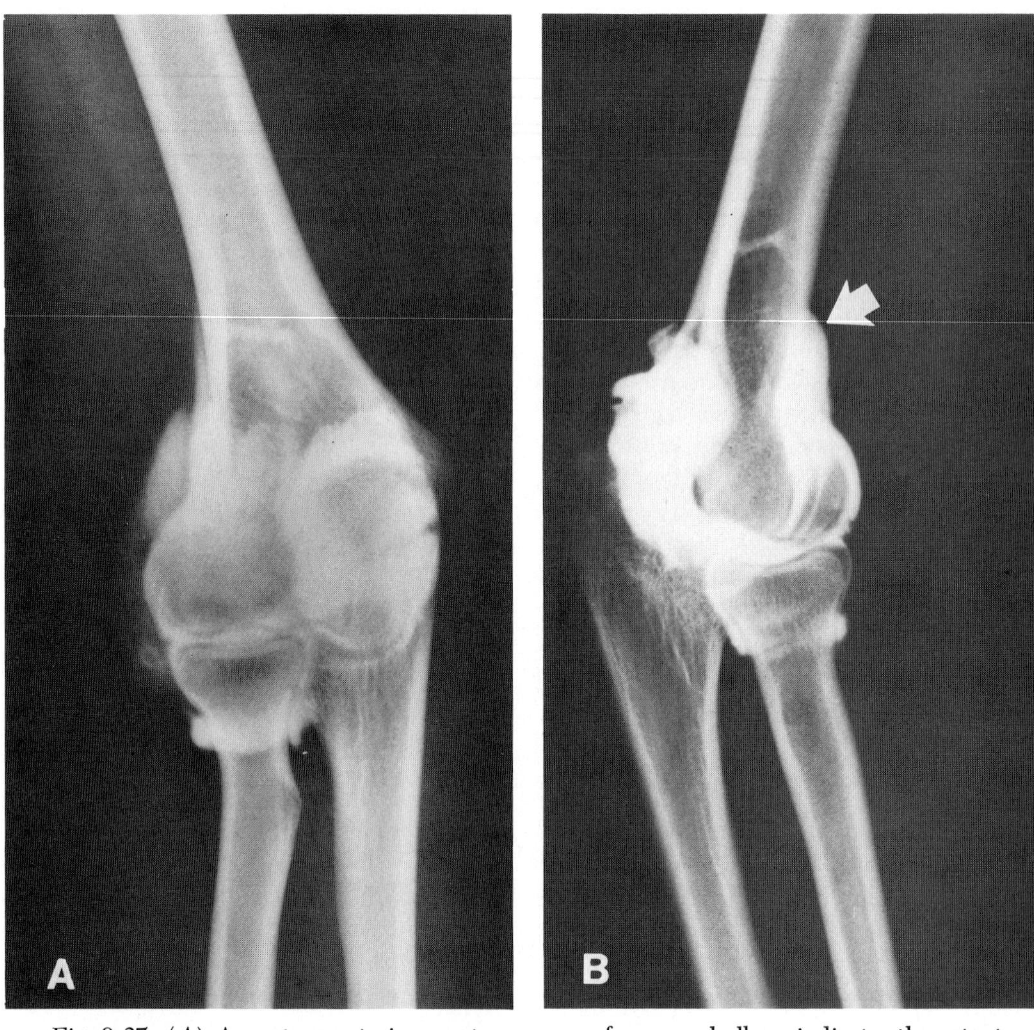

Fig. 9-27. (*A*) An anteroposterior roentgenogram of a normal elbow indicates the extent of the capsule as demonstrated by an arthrogram. (*B*) On the lateral view, note the superior extension of the joint capsule (*arrow*).

tion if the defect is in soft tissue or cartilage, instead of in bone (Figs. 9-27; 9-28).

As outlined in Campbell's Operative Orthopaedics,[68] the various surgical procedures described for treatment of recurrent elbow dislocations can be divided into: (1) a bone block in the area of the coronoid process[185]; (2) transfer of the biceps tendon insertion into the coronoid process[152,224]; (3) threading portions of the biceps and triceps tendons through the distal humerus[142]; and (4) reconstruction of the posterolateral ligamentous and capsular structures of the elbow.[206] The reader is referred to Campbell's text for the details of these operative procedures.

ASSOCIATED FRACTURES

The relative incidence of associated fracture in previous reports of elbow dislocations ranges from 12 per cent in Kini's series[153] to 38 per cent in Linscheid and Wheeler's series,[166] and 62 per cent in Roberts' series.[231] Roberts, reviewing 23 associated fractures, noted eight of the me-

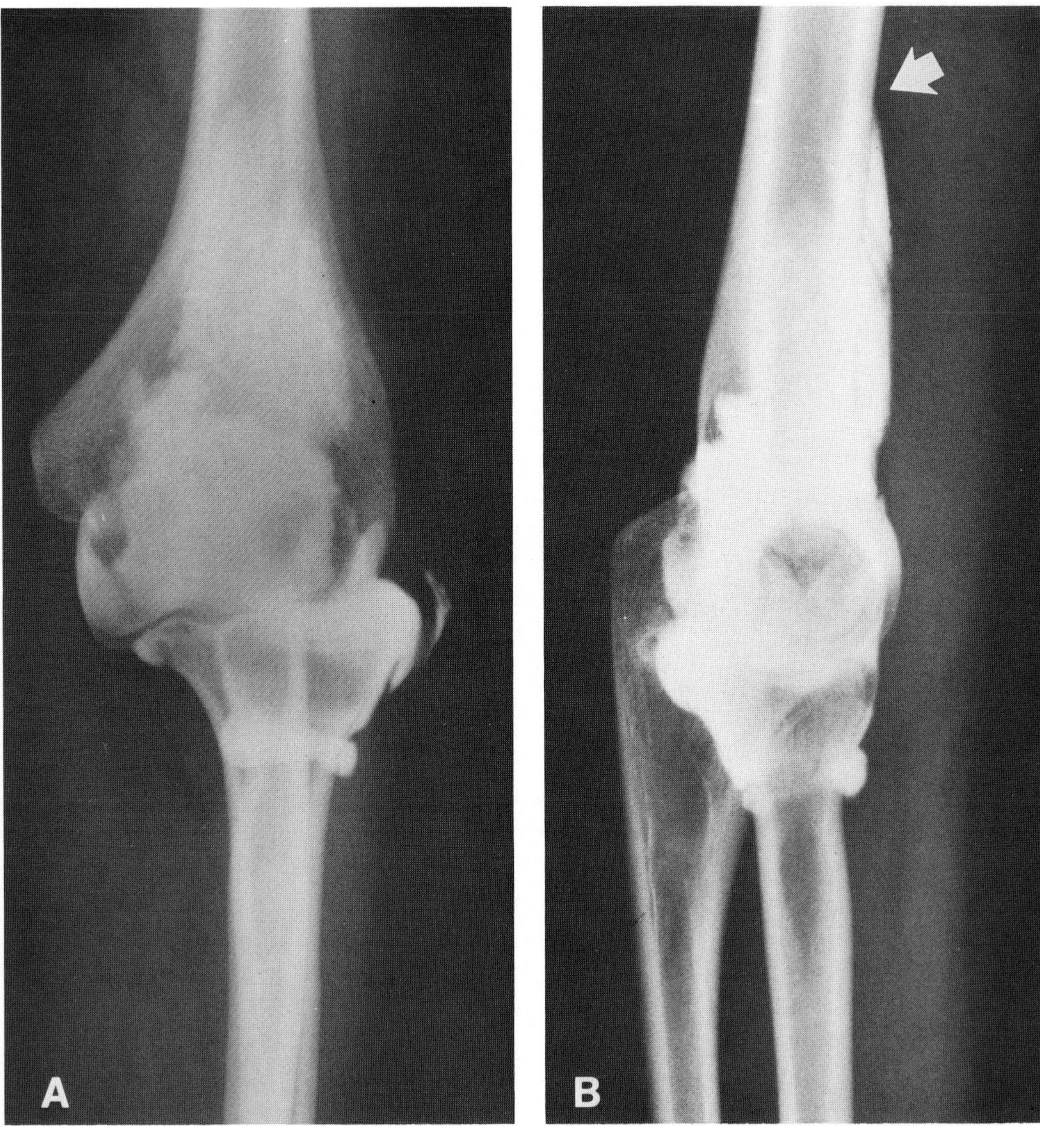

Fig. 9-28. (*A*) An arthrogram shows the superior excursion of the dye in a recurrent dislocating elbow. (*B*) Lateral view: the dye extends considerably higher than normal (*arrow*).

dial epicondyle, all in patients under 14 years of age, and 15 involving the articular portion of the joint. Of the intraarticular fractures, eight were avulsion fractures of the coronoid process, and the others involved the lateral condyle, radial head, or capitellum. Linscheid and Wheeler, in a review of 42 associated fractures, had five medial epicondyle epiphyseal injuries, all in patients less than 16 years of age, five radial head fractures, and two radial neck fractures. The most common fracture was avulsion of ligamentous or capsular attachments at the medial or lateral epicondyles and the coronoid process.

Fracture-dislocation of the elbow (fracture of the olecranon and anterior dislocation of the radial head; Fig. 9-29) is considered by the authors to be distinctly different from a pure dislocation, and is discussed in the section on fractures of the olecranon.

Entrapped Medial Epicondyle

A common pitfall for the unwary in the management of posterior dislocation of the elbow is failure to recognize an associated fracture of the medial epicondyle which becomes trapped within the joint after reduction. Immediately after a closed reduction, the elbow should be taken through a full range of motion. If smooth, unrestricted motion is not possible, or if there appears to be any type of mechanical block to motion, entrapment of the medial epicondyle should immediately be suspected as the culprit. If roentgenograms reveal the avulsed fragment to lie at the level of the joint, it should be assumed that the fragment lies *within* the joint[210] (Fig. 9-22). Comparison views of the opposite elbow are helpful in making this diagnosis.

Although it is decidedly more common in children and rare in adults,[219] the possibility of this complication must be borne in mind with every posterior dislocation that is treated. Failure to recognize this complication and to remove the fragment will rapidly lead to severe destruction of the articular cartilage.

Extrication of the entrapped epicondyle can occasionally be effected by manipulation, either by valgus stress of the forearm accompanied by supination and extension of the wrist and fingers to pull on the flexor muscles, or by adduction of the elbow associated with flexion and extension movements of the elbow to express the epicondyle from the joint.[210]

Patrick[210] described a method of attempting to extricate the entrapped epicondyle by simultaneous valgus stress on the elbow and faradic stimulation of the flexor-pronator group of muscles. Usually, however, arthrotomy is necessary to remove the bone, which may then be secured to its normal bed with Steinmann pins. Alternatively, the bone can be excised and the common flexor origin reattached directly to bone.

Fractures of the Coronoid Process

While this fracture can occur as an isolated injury, it is most often associated with posterior dislocation of the elbow. The fracture is due to avulsion by the brachialis muscle when the elbow is hyperextended. Conwell and Reynolds[64] treated a patient in whom this occurred when the elbow was momentarily subluxated in the hyperextended position. In this type, the fracture line is usually oblique, with the distal portion of the process tilted anteriorly. In those associated with posterior dislocation the coronoid process is usually more comminuted.[266] In coronoid process fractures a portion of the tip, which is intraarticular, may become loose within the joint.

Since wide displacement of a large fragment may lead to recurrent dislocation, many authors recommend that these be immobilized in as acute flexion as is obtainable.[64,66,254,266] The period of immobilization should be 3 to 4 weeks which is longer than for the routine dislocations. Operative intervention appears to be limited to those fractures that interfere with joint motion. This can occur if the fragment is intraarticular or if it unites proximally and forms a significant bony block to flexion. Because of the increased incidence of myositis ossificans with this injury, surgery should be performed at the time of injury or at a much later date when the danger of this complication is lessened.

COMPLICATIONS

Heterotopic Bone Formation

Ligament Calcification. Calcification in the elbow ligaments and capsule is common. The stimulus is ligament avulsion from bone and periosteal stripping, both of which are stimuli for new bone formation. When calcification is confined to the capsule or ligaments, there is usually no loss of function, but stiffness may be a complaint. Once formed, ligamentous new bone does not resorb.

Myositis Ossificans. Myositis ossificans refers to a heterotopic bone formation that can follow local trauma; it generally occurs in, or adjacent to, muscles, and near bone. One of the most characteristic locations for the development of myositis is around the elbow, where it virtually always is associated with an extensively damaged brachialis muscle. Loomis[167] presented an excellent review of the subject in 1944, documenting the fact that the brachialis muscle is largely fleshy at the point where it is torn by the protruding distal humerus. He urged 3 weeks of immobilization to prevent this complication.

Factors that have been implicated as favoring the development of myositis include: (1) delay in treatment, with resultant excessive force necessary to effect reduction; (2) extensive soft-tissue damage in association with the original injury or resulting from repeated or forceful attempts at reduction; (3) too brief a period of immobilization; (4) passive stretching in an attempt to regain motion; and (5) surgical intervention delayed several days after the injury. In Kini's[153] series of 38 dislocations from India, 14 developed myositis; all had been treated by primitive bone setters, and many of the above mentioned factors were noted to have occurred. Mohan[193] reported 200 cases of myositis about the elbow and noted that nearly all cases had a history of massage as part of the treatment. In Thompson and Garcia's series,[287] over half of the patients with myositis had received passive stretching in the postreduction period. In 24 of their 41 patients, the original injury was a dislocation associated with a fracture, but 11 were simple dislocations. Fortunately, this dreaded complication has become less frequent with a better understanding of the factors involved and more appropriate treatment. In the recent series of Roberts[231] and Linscheid and Wheeler[166] the incidence of myositis was one in 60 and four in 110, respectively.

Although the incidence is now relatively low, the surgeon should maintain a high index of suspicion, particularly when dealing with dislocations of the elbow associated with fractures. Clinical clues include prolonged tenderness around the elbow, undue difficulty in regaining motion, and excessive pain with motion.[64] Thompson and Garcia[287] noted that myositis will be apparent roentgenographically within 3 to 4 weeks after the initial injury.

There does not appear to be a successful method of halting the progression of myositis once it has begun to develop. Although Bush and McClain[41] reported gratifying results with the local injection of tetracaine and steroids, this treatment has not been universally successful. The generally accepted method of managing myositis is to cease all active motion and immobilize the elbow in a position of function (usually about 45 degrees in an adult) until all local tenderness has subsided and there is roentgenographic evidence that the heterotopic bone has matured. Attempts at early operative excision, before the process has become fully mature and quiescent, are definitely contraindicated.

Late excision of the bony block or bridge can be performed if necessary. Mohan[193] reported surgical excision in 90 patients with myositis who had limited motion. The operative procedure must be well planned and carried out in an atraumatic manner to ensure success.

Irreducibility

Irreducibility of an acute pure dislocation (i.e., without fracture) is rare. Pawlowski, Palumbo, and Callahan[212] reported a case of irreducible posterolateral dislocation in which the annular ligament and collateral ligaments had bowstrung proximally and inferiorly to the head, which was in subluxation. Also, part of the radial collateral ligament and anterior capsule were torn and were interposed between the coronoid process of the ulna and the posterior inferior trochlear-capitellar junction. They referred to a previous case in which the radial head had buttonholed through the posterior lateral capsule. Most irreducible elbow dislocations are associated with a major fracture.

Nerve Injury

Cotton,[67] in 1929, was the first to describe the association of ulnar nerve injury with elbow dislocation, and reported 10 cases, all in children who had associated fractures of the medial epicondyle. Roberts[231] reported one stretching injury of the ulnar nerve out of 60 fracture-dislocations, and it resolved. Linscheid and Wheeler[166] noted involvement of the ulnar nerve in 16 of their 110 cases, seven resolved in 24 hours; only one resulted in permanent ulnar nerve palsy.

Mannerfelt,[176] in 1968, reported a case of median nerve entrapment in a posterior dislocation and listed two others. The incidence of median nerve injury has been low in all of the large series of elbow dislocations cited previously. There is no report in the recent literature of radial nerve injury in association with pure dislocations, although it was mentioned by Cherry[55] in 1948.

The prognosis for return in most of these injuries is generally good, and operative intervention is not indicated unless actual interposition or entrapment of the nerve (a very rare situation) is suspected on the basis of a block to passive motion of the joint following reduction.

Vascular Injury

Disruption of the brachial artery is an unusual complication of pure elbow dislocations, but it can occur. Kerin[145] reviewed elbow dislocations in association with vascular disruption and cited Everts' case (of 1787) as the first dislocation associated with brachial artery disruption. He credited Sherrill[244] with describing the first closed dislocation of the elbow complicated by vascular disruption. In 1940 Jackson[134] reported the first simple anterior dislocation with rupture of the brachial artery; he achieved an excellent result with a primary vein graft. Linscheid and Wheeler[166] reported a 4 per cent incidence of vascular complication in their series. Two had loss of radial pulse that returned following reduction, and six others required exploration. Roberts[231] had no vascular complications in 60 injuries, of which 37 were pure dislocations.

Early recognition of vascular injury is imperative; otherwise irreversible ischemia develops. The absence of radial pulses may be the first indication of circulatory deficiency, but this is not always serious if the capillary filling is brisk and if the fingers are pink and warm. If the fingers are cyanotic or pale, cold, and swollen, with no radial pulse, an emergency does exist. The outlook is even more grim if paresthesias are present in the hand. Prompt action is required, and reduction of the dislocation is the immediate treatment indicated. If vascular compromise is recognized only after reduction, the cast or any encircling bandage should be removed and the amount of flexion at the elbow should be decreased.

Fortunately, carrying out these measures usually permits the radial pulse to return, with resultant improvement in the circulation of the hand and fingers. In the event that the circulatory status is still deficient, one should proceed immediately to obtain an arteriogram. If this is not feasible, surgical exploration of the artery must be undertaken, preferably in conjunction with a vascular surgeon, if available.

PROGNOSIS

In spite of the great amount of soft-tissue damage that is incurred with dislocation of the elbow, results are good or excellent in 75 to 80 per cent of cases. The most common problem is some loss of extension, but the patient generally has a good functional result and does not notice disability until the loss of extension exceeds 30 degrees. Results are poor, of course, with more severe initial injuries associated with the complications noted above.

FRACTURES OF THE OLECRANON

ANATOMY

The olecranon process is a large curved eminence comprising the proximal and posterior portions of the ulna. It lies in a subcutaneous position which makes it especially vulnerable to direct trauma. Together with the proximal portion of the coronoid process, the olecranon forms the greater sigmoid (semilunar) notch of the ulna, a deep depression which serves as the articulation with the trochlea of the humerus. This articulation with the trochlea allows motion only in the anteroposterior plane and thereby provides stability to the elbow joint. It is because of this unique relationship that all fractures of the olecranon are intraarticular fractures that disrupt the stability of the elbow joint.

The ossification center for the olecranon appears at age 10 years and is generally fused to the proximal ulna by the age of 16. There are reports of persistent epiphyseal plates in adults; these are usually bilateral and tend to occur in families.[204] This is not to be confused with patellae cubiti, which is a true accessory ossicle located in the triceps tendon at its insertion into the olecranon.[158] Both of these entities may be confused with a fracture, especially when there has been local trauma to the olecranon. They are often bilateral, and comparison films of the uninjured elbow help differentiate them from fractures.

Posteriorly, the triceps tendon covers the joint capsule before it inserts into the olecranon. The fascia overlying the triceps muscle spreads out medially and laterally like the retinacula of the quadriceps in the knee. These expansions and the triceps aponeurosis insert into the deep fascia of the forearm and to the periosteum of the olecranon and proximal ulna. The integrity of these expansions and extensive insertions of the triceps mechanism is a critical factor in deciding upon appropriate treatment for fractures of the olecranon. If these structures are torn, the fracture will be displaced; if they remain intact, displacement is usually minimal.

On the posterior medial aspect of the elbow the ulnar nerve passes behind the medial epicondyle to enter the volar surface of the forearm beneath the two heads of the flexor carpi ulnaris. This relationship must be remembered when a surgical procedure is performed on the olecranon.

MECHANISM OF INJURY

Fractures of the olecranon occur in response to two main types of injury. Direct violence, such as a fall on the point of the elbow or a direct blow to the olecranon, often results in a comminuted fracture. Indirect violence, such as a fall on the outstretched hand with the elbow in flexion, accompanied by a strong contraction of the triceps, can result in a transverse or oblique fracture through the olecranon.

The transverse or oblique fracture enters the semilunar notch, and the amount of separation of the fragments is influenced by the pull of the triceps muscle. Limited separation of these fragments may be due to the presence of an intact triceps aponeurosis and periosteum of the olecranon, which, in addition to the lateral ligaments and capsule of the elbow joint, resist displacement of the fracture.[254]

In cases of extreme violence to the elbow, the proximal olecranon fragment often displaces posteriorly, while the distal ulnar fragment, together with the head of the radius, may displace anterior to the humerus, resulting in the so-called fracture-dislocation of the elbow. Because of the accompanying anterior soft-tissue damage required to produce this situation, the fracture-dislocation is a far more serious injury than the isolated olecranon fracture, and persistent or recurrent deformity is likely to occur if the olecranon is not stabilized adequately.

SIGNS AND SYMPTOMS

Because all fractures of the olecranon process have some intraarticular component, there is generally a hemorrhagic effusion of the elbow joint. This results in swelling and pain over the olecranon. There may also be a palpable sulcus at the fracture site, accompanied by a painful and limited range of motion.

Inability to actively extend the elbow against gravity is the most important sign to be elicited; it indicates discontinuity of the triceps mechanism. The presence or absence of this sign often determines the plan of treatment of these fractures.

A careful neurological evaluation should be carried out, as ulnar nerve injuries may accompany fractures of the olecranon, especially in the extensively comminuted fracture that results from direct trauma.[254]

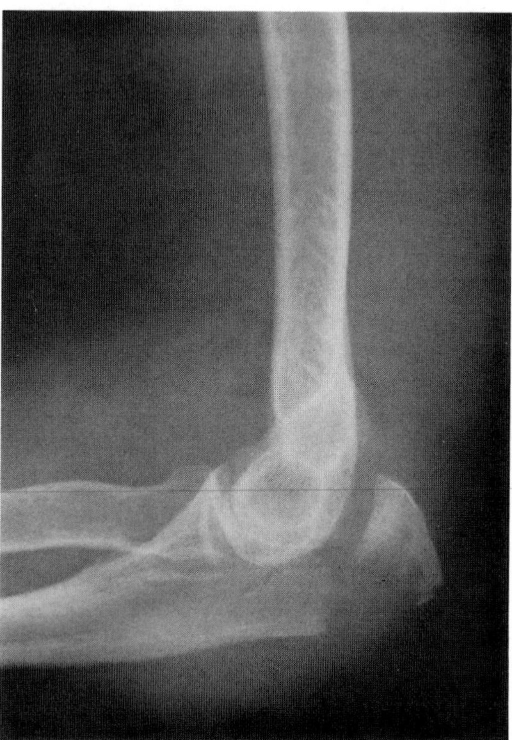

Fig. 9-29. A fracture of the olecranon. Note the comminution and disruption of the articular surface; a *true* lateral view is necessary to visualize this adequately.

ROENTGENOGRAPHIC FINDINGS

Probably the most common pitfall in the initial evaluation of a fracture of the olecranon is failure to insist upon a *true* lateral view of the elbow (Fig. 9-29). The slightly oblique view, which is frequently obtained in the emergency room, is inadequate to identify precisely the extent of the fracture, the degree of comminution, the amount of disruption of the articular surface in the semilunar notch, and any displacement of the radial head, if present. An anteroposterior view is also important to delineate a fracture line in the sagittal plane.

CLASSIFICATION

No generally accepted classification of olecranon fracture has been presented in the orthopaedic literature. A simple classification of olecranon fractures modified from that of Colton[61] is offered here to serve as a basis for selection of appropriate treatment:

- I. Undisplaced fractures
- II. Displaced fractures
  - A. Avulsion fractures
  - B. Oblique and transverse fractures
  - C. Comminuted fractures
  - D. Fracture-dislocations

As mentioned earlier, the inability to extend the elbow against gravity indicates a disruption of the triceps mechanism, which in turn results in a displaced fracture. In general, undisplaced fractures can be managed by nonoperative means; displaced fractures usually require open reduction and internal fixation.

In order to be considered undisplaced, a fracture of the olecranon must meet the following criteria: (1) displacement of less than 2 mm.[90]; (2) no increase in this minimal degree of separation with flexion of the elbow to 90 degrees; and (3) the patient's ability to actively extend the elbow against gravity.

Displaced fractures include all those that do not meet the above criteria, and they may be further subdivided as follows:

Avulsion Fractures

A transverse fracture line separates a small proximal fragment of the olecranon process from the rest of the ulna. This fracture is most common in elderly patients.

Oblique and Transverse Fractures

The fracture line runs obliquely, starting near the deepest part of the semilunar notch and running dorsally and distally to emerge on the subcutaneous crest of the proximal part of the ulna. This fracture may be a single oblique line, or it may have an element of comminution caused by a fracture in the sagittal plane or a central area of depression of the articular surface.

Comminuted Fractures

This group includes all of the severely comminuted fractures of the olecranon, which usually result from direct trauma to the posterior aspect of the elbow. There are multiple fracture planes, often with severe crushing of many of the fragments. There may be associated fractures of the distal end of the humerus, the shafts of the forearm bones, or the head of the radius.

Fracture-Dislocation

The olecranon fracture is at or very near the level of the tip of the coronoid process, so that a plane of instability is located through the fracture site and the radiohumeral joint as well, resulting in an anterior dislocation of the ulna and the radius (Fig. 9-30). This fracture is usually secondary to a severe injury, such as a blow to the posterior aspect of the elbow.

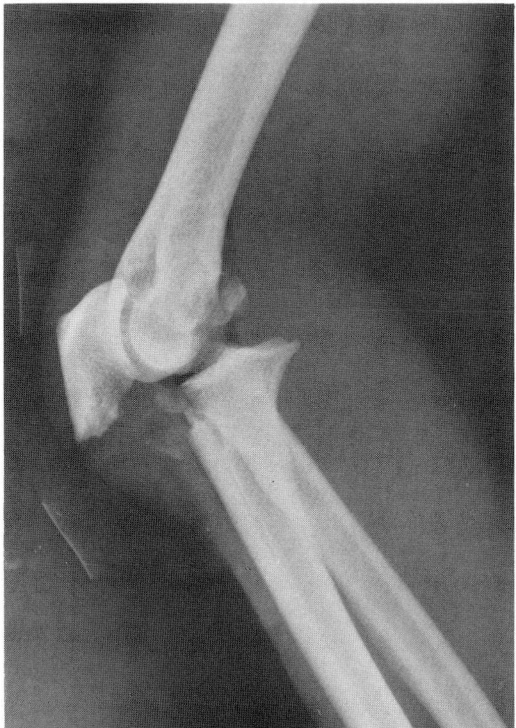

Fig. 9-30. A fracture-dislocation of the elbow (fracture of the olecranon and anterior dislocation of the radius and ulna).

METHODS OF TREATMENT

Historical Methods

The treatment of fractures of the olecranon has run the gamut from early range of motion of the elbow without regard for the fracture[89] to precise and open anatomical reduction of the fracture site.

Olecranon fractures are mentioned only occasionally in the very early treatises on fracture treatment. Prior to the era of aseptic surgery, these fractures were splinted in full extension for 4 to 6 weeks.[130] This usually resulted in a stiff elbow with loss of flexion and was the prime reason that early practitioners slowly began to use the position of mid-flexion. This frequently led to nonunion of the olecranon because of separation of fracture fragments, resulting in decreased power of the triceps mechanism. It was this dilemma of nonunion versus stiffness that led Lister in 1884 to choose the fracture of the olecranon to be the first fracture treated by open reduction and internal fixation using his method of antisepsis.[130] Lister provided fixation of the fragment with a wire loop. This method of treatment was modified somewhat as the wire was placed in the form of a ring by Berger in 1902,[28] and was later adopted by Böhler in 1929.[31] Modifications of this technique are now in current use, and it was the forerunner of the tension band wiring technique advocated by the AO group.[194]

In 1894, Sachs[89] reported excellent results with rapid restoration of function by dispensing with any form of splinting, allowing the arm to hang in extension, and instituting early massage. At the end of a 2-week period, active movements were started; Sachs reported that full function returned in 6 weeks. It must be remembered that this article was written before the discovery of roentgenography and that most of these cases undoubtedly represented fibrous union with resultant decrease of strength of the olecranon.

Daland,[70] in 1933, presented the first substantial series of olecranon fractures, in which he delineated the signs and symptoms and first recognized the need for accurate reduction of any displaced fracture. In the following year Rombold[234] was the first to publish a description of the use of the fascial strip suture to repair displaced olecranon fractures.

Excision of the proximal fragment and repair of the triceps tendon for a fractured olecranon was first suggested by Fiolle[98] in 1918. Dunn,[84] in 1939, described several cases using this technique; excellent results were reported. Excision of the proximal fragment and triceps repair was popularized in the United States by McKeever and Buck[183] in a classic article in 1947. Their indications for this method of treatment were: (1) old ununited fractures of the olecranon; (2) extensively comminuted fractures of the olecranon; (3) fractures of the olecranon in elderly people; and (4) any fracture of the olecranon that does not involve the trochlear notch. They were the first to investigate and substantiate the idea that instability of the elbow joint does not result as long as the coronoid process and the distal surface of the semilunar notch of the ulna remain intact. They stated that as much as 80 per cent of the olecranon can be removed without danger of producing instability of the elbow joint.

Fixation of displaced olecranon fractures by the use of an intramedullary screw was introduced by W. Russell MacAusland in 1942.[170] Since that time several different types of screws for intramedullary fixation have been proposed.

Watson-Jones[301] believed that reduction by closed manipulation could often be achieved in full extension of the elbow with firm pressure over the fragment. He felt that conservative treatment was only justified if the position was accurate. Immobilization was continued for 5 weeks. He noted also that full flexion would be delayed for a year and frequently required gentle manipulation at intervals for its complete return.

Current Methods

Undisplaced fractures as defined above are best treated by immobilization in a long-arm cast with the elbow in 45 to 90 degrees of flexion for a short period of time. The elbow should not be placed in full extension for immobilization because of the likelihood of stiffness and because, in general, if a fracture is not stable in partial flexion, it will not be stable in full extension.

A follow-up roentgenogram should be obtained within 5 to 7 days after cast application, to make certain that displacement has not occurred. Bony union is usually not complete for 6 to 8 weeks, but generally there is adequate stability at 3 weeks to remove the cast and allow protected range of motion exercises, avoiding flexion past 90 degrees until bone healing is complete roentgenographically.

In elderly patients, the period of immobilization should be even shorter than 3 weeks. In these patients, a sling can be used for a few days until the patient is comfortable enough to begin active range of motion of the elbow.

Displaced Fractures. Open reduction and

internal fixation or primary excision have generally become accepted as the treatments of choice for displaced fractures of the olecranon. The disadvantages of nonoperative treatment are the following: (1) Failure to reduce the fracture may allow it to heal in an elongated position by means of a fibrous union; this shortens the distance between the origin and insertion of the triceps muscle, which effectively decreases its power of extension. (2) Articular incongruity secondary to inadequate reduction can lead to posttraumatic arthrosis.[90] (3) A displaced olecranon fragment can cause a block to full extension of the elbow joint.[254] (4) Immobilization in full extension for a period of time sufficient to allow bone healing frequently results in failure to regain flexion of the elbow.

With the above considerations in mind, the aims of treatment of displaced fractures of the olecranon are: (1) to maintain power of extension of the elbow; (2) to avoid incongruity of the articular surface; (3) to restore stability of the elbow; and (4) to prevent stiffness of the joint. In order to achieve this final—and perhaps most important—goal, any mode of internal fixation selected should, ideally, allow the patient to resume protected range of motion reasonably soon after open reduction.

Internal Suture. Approximation of the fragments has been attempted with a variety of materials, including fascia, wire, catgut, and nonabsorbable sutures. In general, these do not provide true internal fixation which is rigid enough to allow early motion, and their use is not recommended (Figs. 9-31B; 9-32).

Intramedullary Fixation. Many different types of intramedullary devices have also been used, including Rush rods, cancellous (wood) screws, large threaded Steinmann pins, and several types of screws designed especially for olecranon fractures.[117] A Rush rod does not provide adequate purchase on the proximal fragment, and most screws have the disadvantage that the cancellous bone of the olecranon does not allow an adequate hold in the distal fragment.[156] The Leinbach screw, which is long enough to gain adequate purchase in the distal fragment, has been known to break at the shank-screw junction (Fig. 9-33). There-

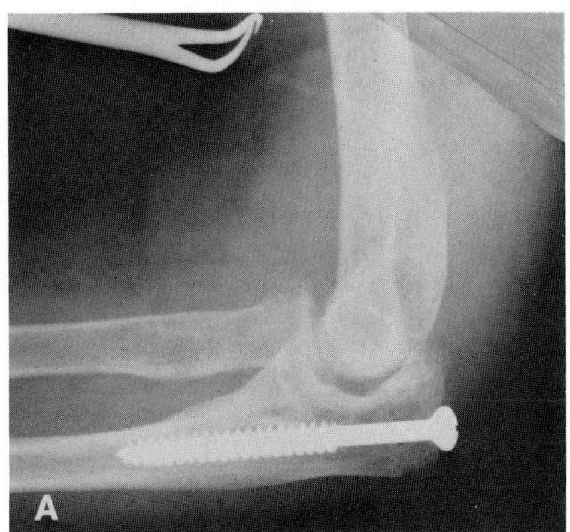

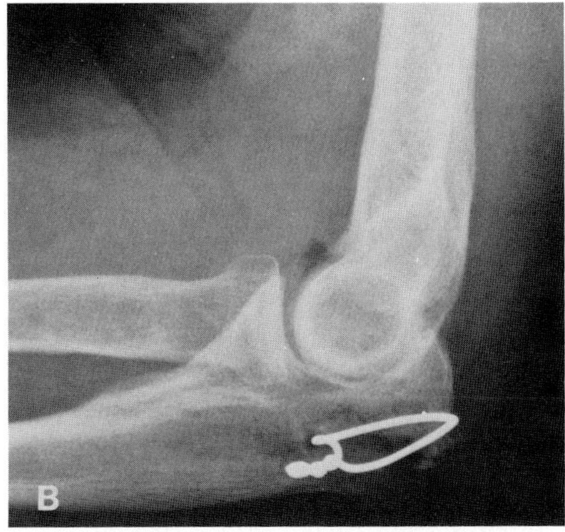

Fig. 9-31. (*A*) Wood screw fixation of an olecranon fracture. There is reasonably good purchase on the cortices of the ulna by the wide threads, although there is a slight step-off in the articular surface. (*B*) Unfortunately, the screw split the proximal fragment, causing poor fixation. The screw was removed and a cerclage wire loop was substituted. This is not a tension band wire.

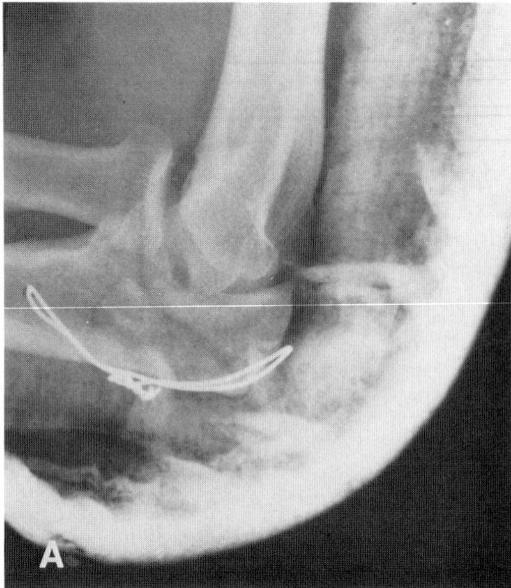

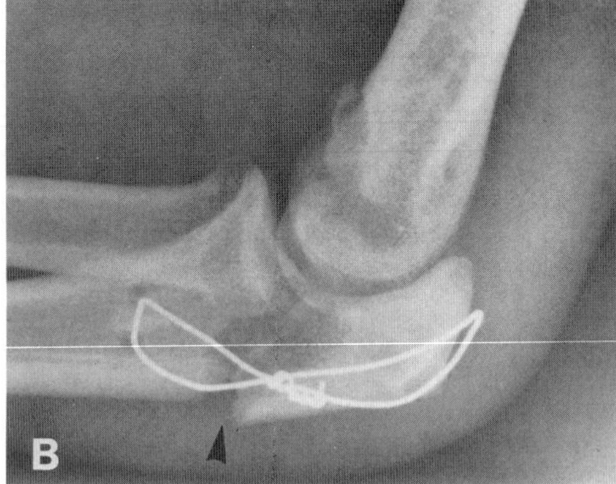

Fig. 9-32. (*A*) Good approximation of a large olecranon fragment by means of a figure-of-eight wire. (*B*) Two months later there is considerable displacement at the fracture site (*arrow*), indicating inadequate fixation by the wire.

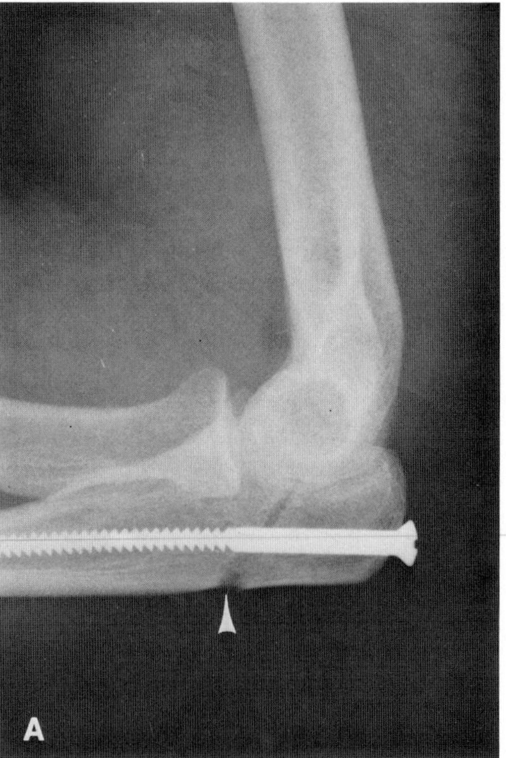

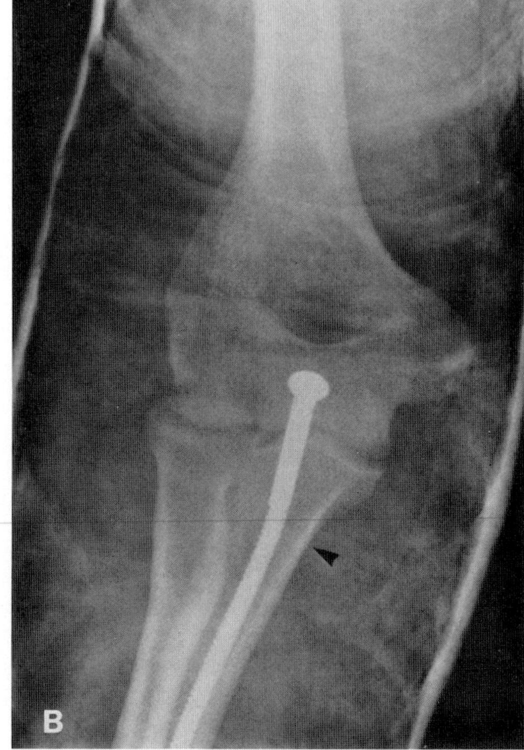

Fig. 9-33. (*A*) An olecranon fracture transfixed with a Leinbach screw. Note the close proximity of the fracture site and the junction of the thread and shank of the screw (*arrow*). (*B*) The anteroposterior view shows angulation of the threaded portion of the screw in the medullary canal (*arrow*).

fore, if an intramedullary screw is used, it must be of sufficient length to reach the diaphyseal area of the ulna, where the canal is small enough to allow contact of the screw threads with the cortices, and it must be sufficiently strong to resist breaking.

Bicortical Screw Fixation. In 1969, Taylor and Scham[282] described a modified method of screw fixation for fractures of the olecranon. They advocated its use particularly in transverse and oblique fractures, which occur most frequently at or near the junction of the olecranon and the coronoid processes. Their method utilizes a posteromedial surgical approach, which allows direct visualization not only of the fracture site but of the coronoid process as well. A cortical bone screw is passed from the posterior tip of the olecranon obliquely to engage the anterior cortex of the coronoid process near the sublime tubercle (Fig. 9-34). The strong internal fixation achieved with this method allows active range of motion by the patient within 10 to 14 days after operation.

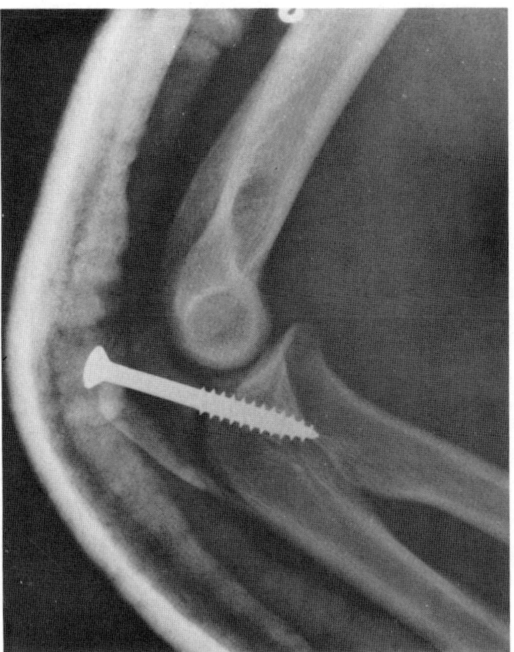

Fig. 9-34. Bicortical fixation of an olecranon fracture. Note that in this case the threads of the screw cross the fracture site, which is undesirable unless the proximal fragment is overdrilled to give a lag effect.

Tension band wiring is a method of internal fixation developed by the AO group[194]; it differs significantly in technique and principle from conventional cerclage wiring. Primarily indicated in the treatment of avulsion fractures, the basic principle is to counteract the tensile forces that act across the fracture site and convert them into compressive forces. In order to accomplish this, the wire is passed in figure-of-eight fashion around the insertion of the triceps tendon and then distally beyond the fracture site into a transverse drill hole on the posterior (subcutaneous) border of the olecranon. Improved alignment and greater stability can be provided by introducing two parallel Kirschner wires across the fracture site before applying the tension band. It might seem that this posterior position of the wire would tend to cause the fracture site to gape open at the articular surface in the semilunar notch. At the time of operation, this may in fact occur, but the counterpressure of the trochlea under tension by the triceps muscle causes a compression force across the fracture site sufficiently strong to allow immediate active range of motion. The reader is referred to the AO manual for more precise details regarding the technique of tension band wiring.[194]

Excision of the proximal fragment(s) has been advocated for both early and late treatment of fractures of the olecranon.[4,84,182,299] Over the past 20 years W. R. MacAusland, Jr.[173] has studied fractures of the olecranon extensively, with particular attention to excising the proximal fragments. On the basis of these studies, he has laid down the following guidelines regarding excision of the olecranon:

1. The entire olecranon process can be excised so long as the coronoid and anterior soft tissues are intact.

2. The triceps tendon should be securely reattached to the distal fragment with nonabsorbable sutures; wire is not recom-

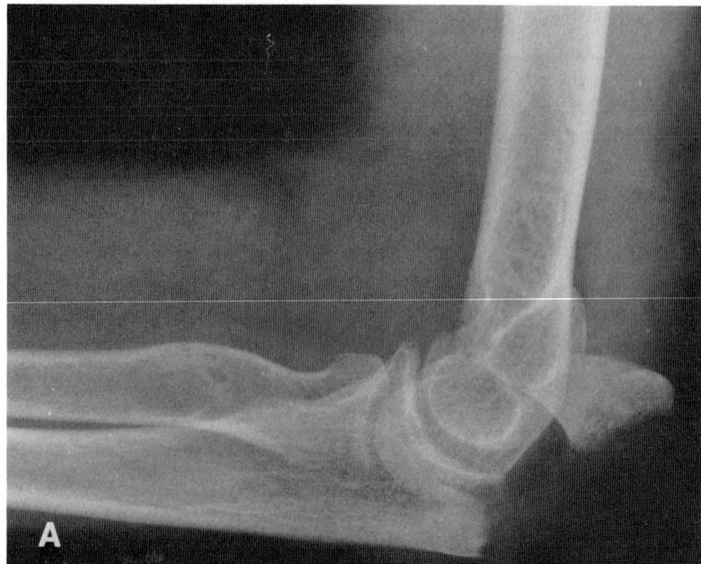

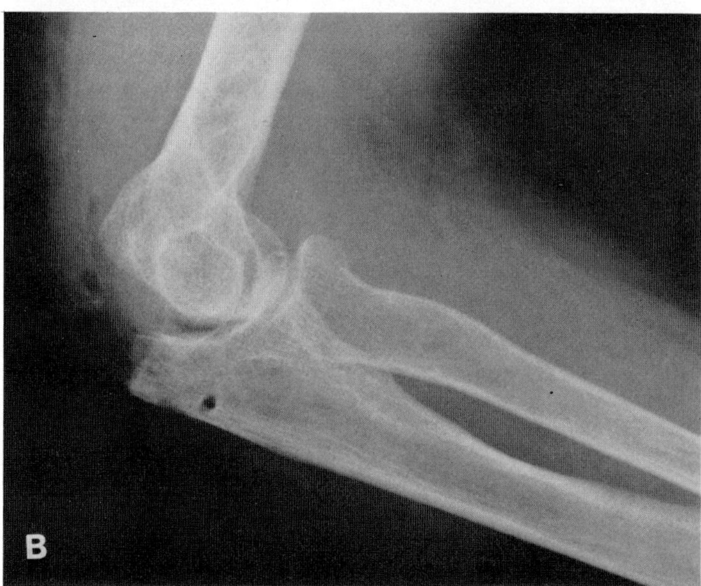

Fig. 9-35. A fracture of the olecranon with rotation of the proximal fragment. (*A*) A lateral view shows wide retraction of the proximal fragment with the elbow in flexion. (*B*) This patient was treated by primary resection of the olecranon fragment and reattachment of the triceps tendon.

mended, as motion of the elbow will cause it to break.

3. Active motion is allowed immediately after operation, but acute flexion is not permitted for several weeks.

4. A particularly important point is that excision is indicated only for *isolated* fractures of the olecranon. If there is evidence of damage to the anterior structures of the elbow (i.e., if there is anterior dislocation of the radial head and shaft of the ulna—fracture-dislocation of the elbow), primary excision is definitely contraindicated.

MacAusland[173] further points out that occasionally during the course of attempted internal fixation, comminution of the olecranon proves to be more extensive than was initially anticipated, and the surgeon's inability to achieve rigid internal fixation becomes apparent. In such cases, he believes that it is better to admit defeat, as it were, and do a primary excision of the olecranon rather than to persist with a technique which is likely to be unsatisfactory.

Authors' Preferred Method of Treatment

Undisplaced Fractures. We prefer to treat undisplaced fractures of the olecranon with a short period of immobilization followed by early protected range of motion (see p. 538).

Avulsion Fractures. Generally, the proximal fragment is rather small, and these fractures can be treated adequately either by excision of the fragment and repair of the triceps tendon (Fig. 9-35) or by tension band wiring. Both techniques allow early active range of motion, which is particularly desirable, because most of these fractures occur in older patients.

Transverse Fractures. If the surgeon has in his armamentarium a large threaded wood screw of sufficient length to obtain solid purchase on the cortices of the ulnar shaft, this will provide solid internal fixation and allow reasonably early range of motion. Tension band wiring is also applicable to these fractures.[194]

Oblique fractures lend themselves particularly well to bicortical screw fixation.[282] Intramedullary fixation is equally satisfactory if the proper screw is used. Tension band wiring, if used, should be supplemented with a bicortical screw. The surgeon should use the technique with which he is most familiar.

Comminuted Fractures. Isolated comminuted fractures (i.e., those without dislocation of the ulna and radial head and without disruption of the anterior soft tissues) are best treated by excision of the olecranon and secure reattachment of the triceps tendon with nonabsorbable suture to allow early active motion.

Fracture-Dislocations. These injuries present a challenging therapeutic problem because of the severe combination of bone- and soft-tissue damage. As noted above, primary excision is contraindicated in fracture-dislocation, as this eliminates any chance of providing stability of the elbow. Open reduction and internal fixation with some form of intramedullary device[236] may be the only feasible method of achieving any semblance of stability, but if the fracture is complicated by a severely contaminated open wound, which is frequently the case, it may be necessary to avoid the use of internal fixation and attempt to hold the reduction in plaster alone. Late excision of the olecranon can be considered after healing of the anterior soft-tissue structures is complete.

COMPLICATIONS

Complications of olecranon fractures are mainly decreased range of motion, degenerative arthritis, and nonunion. It is hoped that decreased range of motion can be limited by firm internal fixation and early range of motion of the joint. Eriksson *et al.*[90] reported that up to 50 per cent of patients have limited range of motion of the elbow following olecranon fractures, generally with loss of extension. However, the limitation was not great, and only 3 per cent were aware of it.

Development of posttraumatic arthritis in the elbow is not as common (or perhaps not as noticeable) as in a weight-bearing joint. However, this does not obviate the need for an anatomical reduction of a fracture in this area. In the event that reduction to less than 2 mm. offset cannot be obtained, the possibility of an arthritis developing later is significant.

Nonunion of the olecranon has been reported to occur in 5 per cent of olecranon fractures.[90] The treatment of a nonunion should be suited to the patient. In a young active patient the pseudarthrosis may be taken down and the fracture site reapproximated and held with a tension band wire or a suitable intramedullary device. Due to the fact that the majority of the bone is cancellous, bone grafting is seldom needed. Excision of the proximal portion of the pseudarthrosis and repair of the triceps tendon is also an acceptable method of management, especially in older patients.

Injury to the ulnar nerve, generally in the form of numbness or paresthesias in the ulnar distribution, has been reported in 10 per cent of patients.[90] These symptoms usually clear spontaneously and require no definitive treatment.

FRACTURES OF THE HEAD OF THE RADIUS

Fracture of the radial head is a common injury in the adult, and its management has long been a controversial subject. Disagreement has centered around four main points: (1) the indications for nonoperative and operative treatment; (2) the period of immobilization; (3) the need for aspiration of the elbow joint; and (4) the timing of radial head excision, if this is done.

ANATOMY

The anatomy of the proximal radioulnar joint is discussed on p. 487, but several points merit reemphasis. As Mason and Shutkin[178] noted, the elbow is a unique joint with a bicondylar configuration. Mason[179] noted that the radial head is intraarticular, and that the capitellum and the radial head are reciprocally curved. However, actual contact of these two opposing joint surfaces takes place only when the elbow is flexed 135 degrees and the radius is in the midprone position. Full rotation of the head of the radius in the lesser sigmoid notch requires accurate anatomical positioning and configuration of the head, as complete articular contact is maintained throughout the full range of elbow motion and forearm rotation. Mason believed that the key clinical application of these anatomical observations was that if more than one fourth of the radial head was damaged, it necessarily interfered with rotation of the forearm.

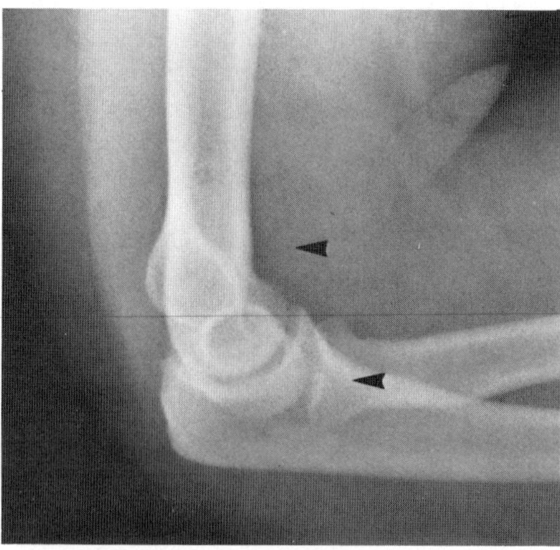

Fig. 9-36. A Type I (undisplaced) chisel fracture of the radial head (*lower arrow*). Note the elevation of the anterior fat pad (*upper arrow*), indicating hemarthrosis. The posterior fat pad is quite small, but present.

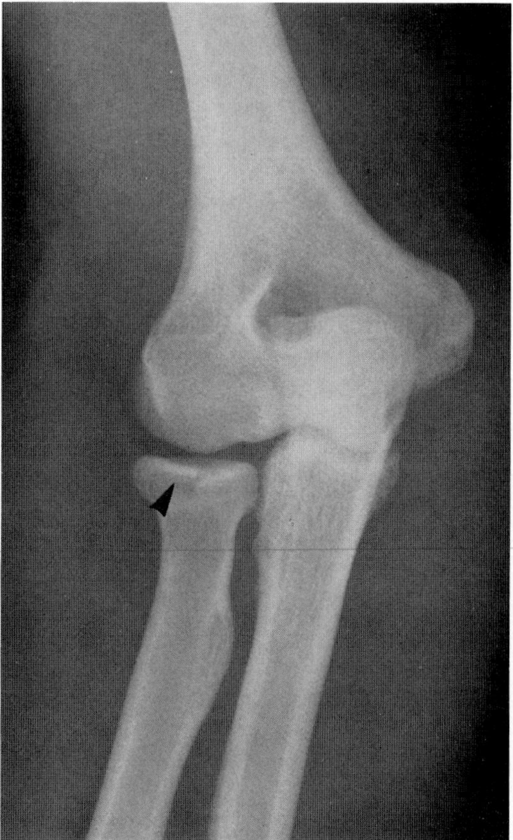

Fig. 9-37. A minimally displaced central depression fracture of the radial head (*arrow*).

MECHANISM OF INJURY

Most fractures of the radial head are caused by indirect trauma (e.g., a fall on the outstretched hand, with longitudinal thrust of the radius against the capitellum resulting in damage to the articular surface of the radius; a depression of part of the head [chisel fracture]; or an angulated fracture of the head or neck). If the injuring force is more violent, dislocation of the elbow joint may occur, and the radial head may be fractured on impact with the capitellum as it displaces posteriorly. This injury involves considerably more soft-tissue damage than an isolated radial head fracture, a factor which has significant therapeutic and prognostic implications that will be discussed later.

Direct trauma can also be a cause, and Radin and Riseborough[221] reported that, in their series, indirect and direct injuries were equally responsible for fractures of the radial head.

CLASSIFICATION

Most authors have used the classification proposed by Mason in 1954[179]:

Type I Undisplaced fractures (Figs. 9-36; 9-37)

Type II Marginal fractures with displacement (including impaction, depression, and angulation; Fig. 9-38)

Type III Comminuted fractures involving the entire head (Figs. 9-39; 9-40)

In 1949, Gaston, Smith, and Baab[104] were apparently the first to point out the different implications of fractures of the radial head associated with posterior dislocation of the elbow. These injuries are associated with considerably more soft-tissue injury, specifically, tearing of the anterior capsule of the joint and the brachialis muscle. These authors noted a significantly higher incidence of complications, especially myositis ossificans, following this injury than with isolated fractures of the radial head. Thompson and Garcia[187] in 1967 reported a series that substantiated this earlier observation. It would therefore seem important to separate these fractures when considering the treatment and prognosis of radial head fractures. Thus, we would include a final category in the classification:

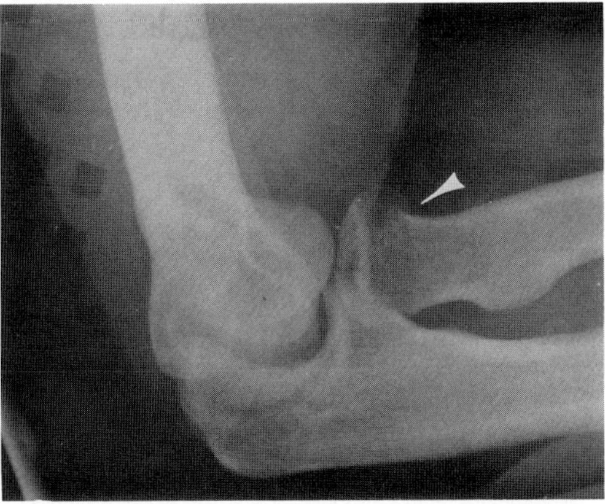

Fig. 9-38. A Type II (displaced) fracture of the radial head (*arrow*) involving more than 50 per cent of the articular surface.

Type IV Fracture of the radial head in association with a dislocation of the elbow

DIAGNOSIS

Isolated fractures of the radial head often do not produce dramatic physical findings. Although pain over the lateral side of the elbow may be severe, frequently there is minimal swelling, and the diagnosis is made by determining well-localized tenderness directly over the radial head. Passive rotation of the forearm by the examiner, especially supination, is usually painful. Occasionally, crepitus can be palpated over the radial head or elicited with motion. Active range of motion is usually limited by pain. If the fracture is in association with a dislocation of the elbow, the physical abnormalities are, of course, more striking.

Not infrequently, an undisplaced fracture of the radial head is very difficult to see on the initial anteroposterior and lateral roentgenographs. Almost invariably, however, a

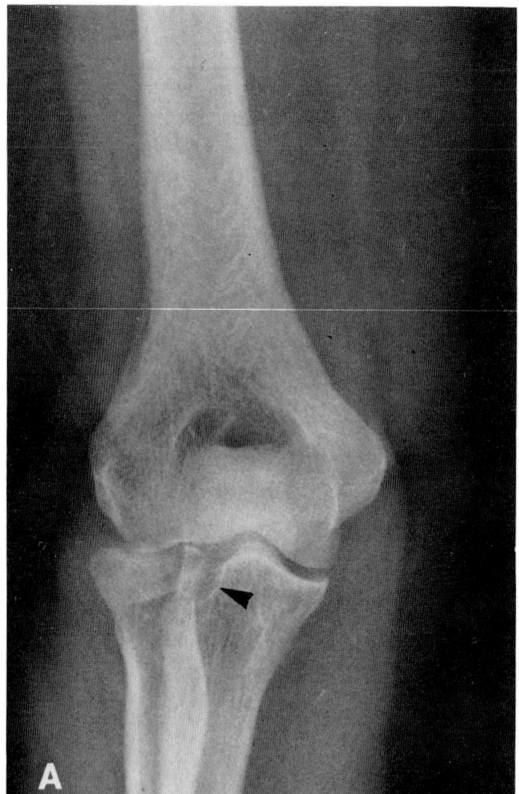

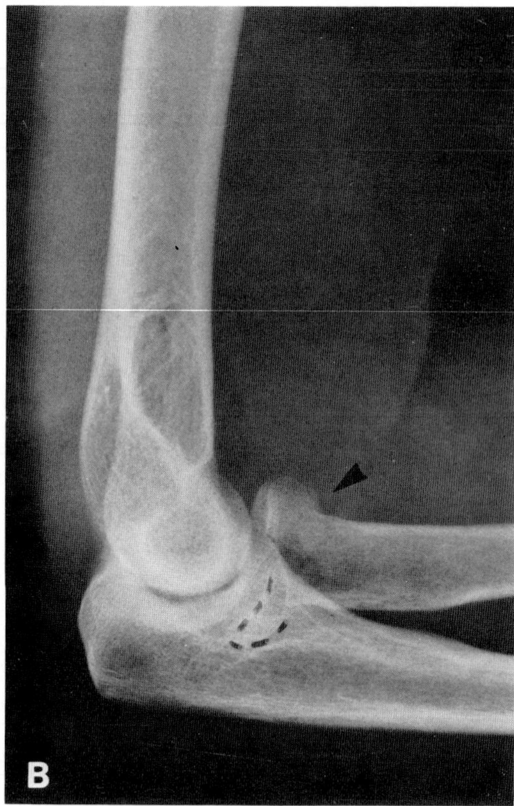

Fig. 9-39. (*A*) A Type III (comminuted) fracture of the radial head (*arrow*). (*B*) A lateral view of the same fracture (*arrow*), showing marked displacement not appreciated on the anteroposterior view.

positive fat pad sign is present (see Fig. 9-6 and p. 493), suggesting the likelihood of an intraarticular fracture, the most common type in the elbow being the radial head fracture. Physical findings localized to the radial head, as described above, plus the presence of a fat pad sign are virtually pathognomonic of a radial head fracture, and additional oblique views of the elbow usually delineate the fracture line.

In the evaluation of all radial head fractures, the capitellum should also be carefully scrutinized for the presence of a fracture. Fracture fragments from a comminuted radial head rarely are displaced proximally.[188] The presence of fracture fragments lying free within the joint proximal to the radial head should alert the surgeon to the presence of an associated fracture of the capitellum (see Fig. 9-19).

METHODS OF TREATMENT

Type I

There is essentially universal agreement that undisplaced fractures of the radial head can be treated by nonoperative means. Controversy arises, however, as to when motion should be begun, ranging from the first 24 hours[3,104,178,184,198,218] to as long as 3 weeks in a long-arm splint or cast, with all variations in between. McLaughlin[184] was particularly strong in advocating early motion, stating that immobilization was unnecessary and harmful. Neuwirth, in 1942,[198] and Mason and Shutkin in 1943[178] were among the first to advocate early mobilization of an undisplaced radial head fracture. The latter authors offered as the rationale for this method that the small fragments in a radial head fracture are uncontrollable

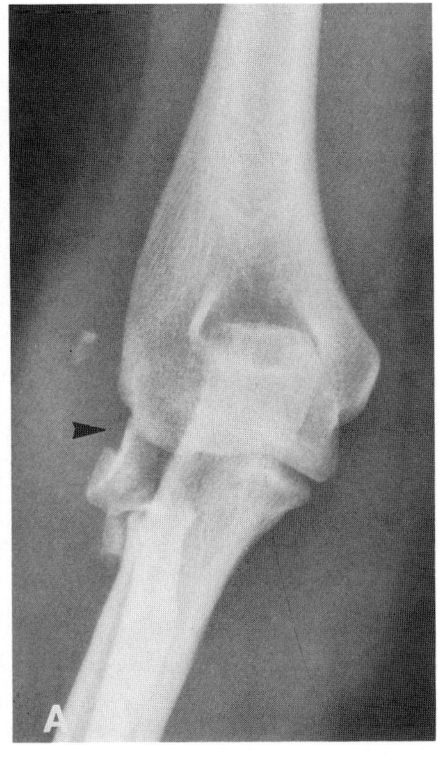

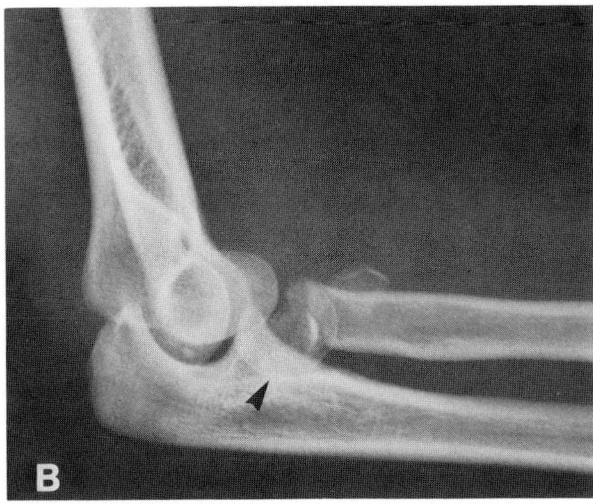

Fig. 9-40. (*A*) A markedly comminuted and displaced fracture of the radial head (*arrow*) and neck. (*B*) A lateral view shows the fracture of the radial neck and rotation of the radial head (*arrow*).

by cast immobilization, and they are thereby more likely to be molded back into better alignment (or kept in normal alignment if undisplaced) through motion than by immobilizing the elbow. Most authors have noted that displacement of the fracture is not likely to take place with early motion, but Radin and Riseborough[221] reported that 10 of their 30 patients with undisplaced fractures treated by early motion had some loss of position of the fragments. We believe that early motion is desirable in undisplaced fractures of the radial head, beginning within 24 to 48 hours after injury, as pain subsides.

Aspiration of the elbow joint has been advocated by many[104,135,184,215,216,218,220,298] for the initial management of the patient with a radial head fracture, noting also that relief of pain allows the patient to begin active range of motion much sooner and much more easily. One has only to observe the rather dramatic relief of pain in a patient after a tense hemarthrosis has been aspirated to appreciate the value of this therapeutic maneuver. Pinder[216] reported a series in which he treated alternate patients with Type I and II fractures with and without aspiration, noting better results in the Type II fractures treated with aspiration. Even if aspiration does not affect the end result, as Radin and Riseborough[221] have suggested, the immediate benefit to the patient in the emergency room is definitely worthwhile.

The timing of the aspiration is debated by many. Some authors[135,220] say that it should be deferred for at least 24 hours, until active bleeding has subsided; others, including these authors, believe that its benefit to the patient by immediate relief of pain on the day of injury merits its use when the patient is first seen.

The technique of aspiration of the elbow joint is quite simple, but it must be done under strict aseptic conditions. Three easily palpable landmarks on the lateral aspect of the elbow (the radial head, the lateral epicondyle, and the tip of the olecranon) form a triangle directly overlying the joint, with only the anconeus muscle and joint capsule lying between the skin and the joint. After this area has been scrubbed with a surgical prep, an 18-gauge needle is inserted into the joint. Usually about 5 to 10 ml. of blood is aspirated; the patient has immediate relief of much of his pain.

Quigley in 1949[220] and later Wagner[298] suggested that one of the prime reasons for aspirating the joint was to also inject a small amount of local anesthetic into the joint, thereby permitting a more accurate examination of the elbow. They both noted that any limitation of motion, a mechanical block to motion, or palpable grating within the joint after anesthetic injection were indications for immediate excision of the radial head. Wagner further noted that the presence of a loose fragment in the joint was also an indication for surgery.

Type II

It is in the management of this type of radial head fracture that the most heated controversy arises. As noted above, Quigley[220] and Wagner[298] suggested using the physical examination after local infiltration of anesthetic agent into the joint to determine the indications for surgery. Most other authors rely upon the roentgenographic appearance, although Pike[215] has observed, as we have, that the degree of articular damage is usually much more extensive than suspected from the original roentgenograms. Because of his anatomical observations noted above, Mason[179] advocated excision of the radial head if more than one-fourth of the head was involved. McLaughlin's[184] indications were angulation greater than 30 degrees or depression greater than 3 mm. Radin and Riseborough[221] believed that involvement of two-thirds of the head was a definite indication for excision of the head.

The timing of radial head excision has been widely discussed and debated. Since Gaston, Smith, and Baab's article in 1949[104] many have believed that excision should be done within 24 hours of injury, in order to minimize the danger of myositis ossificans. There are others who do not accept this concept.

Charnley[54] wrote in 1968 that immediate excision of any radial head is contraindicated, believing that the physician cannot properly assess the need for excision until 2 weeks after the injury. His plan of management was to begin motion 2 to 3 days after the injury; limitation of motion after a 2-week trial of motion was his indication for surgery, and he reported that he had never seen ectopic bone following this delayed excision.

Adler and Shaftan[3] advocated a similar principle, but extended the period of observation to 8 weeks, excising the head only if a mechanical block to motion was present at that time.

To further confuse the issue, Mason's[179] conclusions as a result of his study of 100 fractures led him to state, "if in doubt, resect." Charnley[54] and Adler and Shaftan[3] arrived at precisely the opposite conclusion: if in doubt, leave it in.

Authors' Preferred Method of Treatment. It is difficult to put all of these rather divergent viewpoints into perspective and to come up with any consensus, because a consensus does not exist. In general, we tend to follow the indications for immediate excision as laid down by McLaughlin: angulation greater than 30 degrees, depression greater than 3 mm., and involvement of more than one-third of the head. Aspiration of the hemarthrosis and injection of local anesthetic into the joint, followed by passive range of motion, provides additional data upon which to base a surgical decision. If there is a definite mechanical block or crepitus within the joint, primary excision is probably indicated.

Our tendency is to agree with Adler and Shaftan, that if you are in doubt regarding the indications for excision, give the patient a trial of motion for a few months, and if pain and limitation of forearm rotation persist, remove the radial head.

We generally agree that if primary excision is elected, it should be done in the first 24 hours if possible. Occasionally, this is not possible, especially if the patient presents several days after injury. While the threat of myositis ossificans should always be considered, it is probably much more significant in the patient with a Type IV lesion, and some delay in excision of the *isolated* radial head fracture is probably not likely to lead to myositis.

Type III

With the exception of Charnley[54] and Adler and Shaftan,[3] there is fairly general agreement that primary excision of the radial head is indicated for comminuted fractures. Early excision is again advised.

It is universally agreed that if the radial head is excised, total excision is necessary. Keon-Cohen[144] noted that the tendency is to take too little rather than too much (probably because of the surgeon's respect for the posterior interosseous nerve, which winds around the neck of the radius, but sufficiently far distal to allow easy excision of the entire head without danger). Strachan and Ellis[276] studied the anatomical relationship between the proximal radius and the posterior interosseous nerve; they concluded that the safest approach for excision of the radial head is posterolateral, with the forearm in full pronation. We have found it advisable, especially in comminuted fractures, to reassemble the radial head on the Mayo stand at operation, to be sure that all fragments have in fact been removed. An additional safeguard is to take a roentgenograph in the operating room prior to wound closure. Even when the surgeon thinks that he has totally removed the head, he is occasionally surprised to discover a loose fragment remaining.

Type IV

In a patient with a posterior dislocation of the elbow with an associated radial head fracture, prompt reduction of the dislocation is the most important immediate treatment. The status of the radial head must then be assessed, and if it meets the criteria for excision, this should be done within the first 24 hours. This injury, with its extensive soft-tissue damage and loose fragments of bone lying among the shredded fibers of the brachialis muscle, provides the perfect nidus for the development of myositis ossificans, with or without operation. Additional trauma to the area in the form of operative intervention after a delay of days or weeks is probably not advisable, as suggested by Gaston *et al.*[104] and Thompson and Garcia.[287] If excision of the radial head cannot be done immediately, it probably should be delayed for several weeks to months, to watch for the development of myositis. Thompson and Garcia noted that it will usually be apparent on roentgenograms within 3 to 4 weeks after injury. Myositis is discussed in greater detail on page 533.

PROGNOSIS

Results from reported series of patients with radial head fractures has varied from 95 per cent good results[135] to Mason's[179] series, in which no patient had full range of motion following head excision (average loss—30 degrees). Mason postulated that this loss of extension may not be due entirely to the radial head fracture, but perhaps in part to concomitant injury to the articular surfaces of the trochlea, olecranon, and capitellum, which also bear the brunt of the initial impact of injury. Radin and Riseborough[221] noted that patients with fractures involving more than one-third of the head will likely have some limitation of motion; the actual limitation is related to the anatomical result.

Subluxation of the distal radioulnar joint following radial head excision has been reported by several authors.[91,182,221,282] In Radin and Riseborough's[221] series, 14 of 36 patients who had radial head excision developed subluxation of the distal radioulnar joint, but only three were symptomatic, and these mildly so. These authors also noted that three patients with radial head fractures who were treated nonoperatively also developed this same complication.

Despite these potential problems, which can develop at the wrist following radial head excision, they are not serious enough to contraindicate operative treatment if the criteria for excision are met. It is also our opinion that the degree of disability that might develop from distal radioulnar joint subluxation is not sufficient to justify the use of prosthetic replacement in the treatment of fractures of the radial head.

SIDESWIPE INJURIES

Various terms—sideswipe,[11,118,126,254] traffic elbow,[314] car window elbow[245]—have been used to describe this spectrum of injuries that have a common mechanism. Its seriousness is represented by the fact that in one series the amputation rate was 50 per cent.[314]

MECHANISM OF INJURY

The common denominator is the application of a force of great magnitude to an elbow protruding from a car window. It usually involves the left elbow of the driver. This force can be applied by a passing car or truck, when the car hits a fixed object, or overturns. With the advent of auto air conditioning, it has been our observation, at least in the Southwestern United States, that the incidence of this injury has decreased. Shorbe[245] grouped these injuries according to the severity of injury and the type of fractures seen. He felt that this grouping provided some insight into the mechanism of injury. In the first group only soft-tissue trauma occurs. This is usually the result of only a slight injury to the elbow. The second group usually occurs only when the tip of the elbow is injured. Fractures of the olecranon are common to this group. Application of the force to more of the protruding elbow can result in fractures of both the radius and ulna. In this third group the radius and fractured ulna may be dislocated anteriorly. Variations of fractures of the humerus comprise the fourth group. The force can be directed through the olecranon to the distal humerus, producing a comminuted intercondylar fracture. If the arm is forced posteriorly against the post on the car door, the humeral fracture may occur more proximally. The most severely injured comprise the fifth group. These patients have fractures of all the bones about the elbow with considerable soft-tissue injury.

Extensive open wounds are not unusual. Often bits of clothing and road dirt are forced into the depths of the wounds. It is this combination of massive tissue injury and contamination that makes them very vulnerable to serious infections.

METHODS OF TREATMENT

Since sideswipes create a spectrum of injuries, the treatments vary. The first decision may involve a consideration for primary amputation.[314] The primary indication for amputation appears to be circulatory impairment. Every effort should be made to preserve the hand and forearm. Debridement should be complete but not overzealous. Excessive debridement can lead to avascularity of many of the fracture fragments.[254] With the exception of stabilization of the ulna with an intramedullary rod, there appears little opportunity to use internal fixation. This is usually on the basis of comminution of the fractures. Once the soft tissues are stable, the elbow should be placed in as much flexion as possible, as this is the more desired position, should ankylosis develop. Fortunately, since the elbow joint bears no weight, instability is not too disabling. No attempt is made to recommend specific treatments for each of the varieties of this injury. Our general plan is to first obtain soft-tissue healing. Once this appears to be occurring satisfactorily attention can be directed to the bone injuries. One should be cautious in performing extensive resection of the bone fragments initially, because the final outcome of these injuries is often better than originally suspected. Almost any degree of functional recovery with intact sensation is better than a prosthesis.

COMPLICATIONS OF ELBOW INJURIES

Although many complications are discussed throughout this chapter as they relate specifically to a particular injury, a few general comments are noted here with regard to some of the complications that may potentially affect any injury of the elbow.

JOINT STIFFNESS

In some situations, joint stiffness may be the inevitable result of a severe fracture and associated soft-tissue injury rather than a true complication of treatment. Unfortunately, when the after care of a fracture becomes too intense, increasing amounts of joint stiffness can occur. It must be strongly reemphasized that passive stretching should never be done after elbow fractures. Even though it is tempting for the doctor, physical therapist, and patient to push and pull on an elbow that is slow in regaining extension, it should never be done passively. Stretching adhesions produces additional edema, and this causes more fibrous tissue response. Slow, methodical, active exercises and dynamic splinting will be effective in correcting, at least partially, many joint contractures resulting from elbow injury. These modalities should be prescribed and continued until one is certain that additional extension cannot be achieved. In the event that a fixed flexion contracture results which is unacceptable, a soft-tissue release and capsulectomy[312] may be considered. This is often an extensive procedure with inherent dangers and complications of its own, and it should not be done unless the contracture causes disability and is definitely refractory to properly applied nonoperative therapy.

MALUNION

Malunion in fractures about the elbow can occasionally result in a consequential loss of motion. On rare occasions, it may be advisable to remove a prominent or projecting portion of bone if it is causing consider-

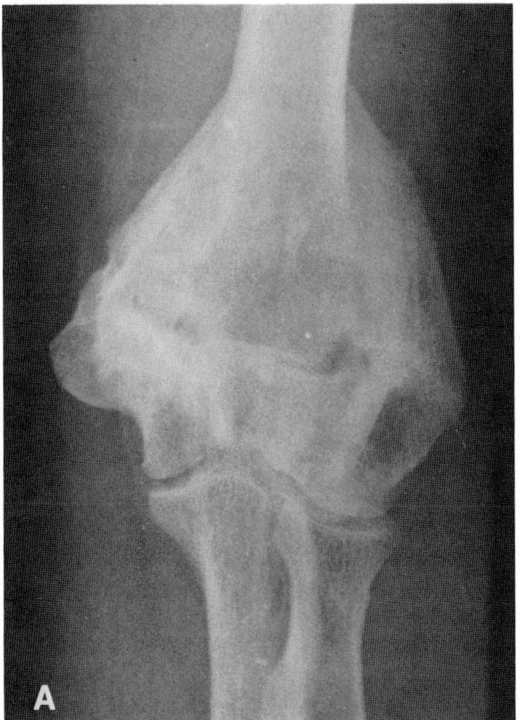

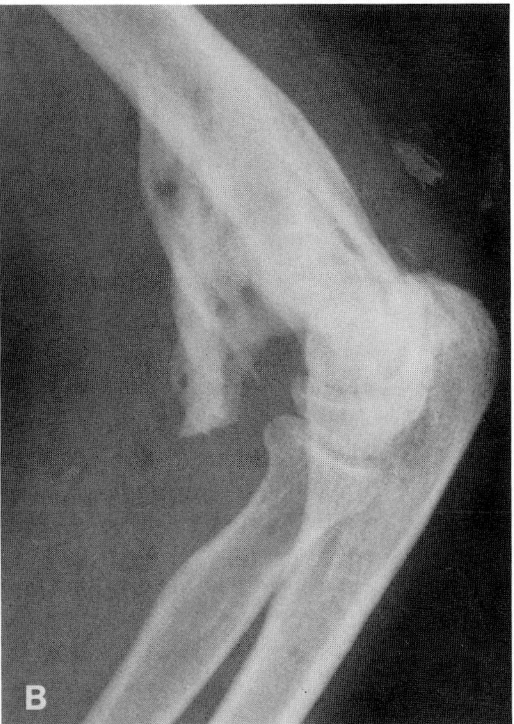

Fig. 9-41. (*A*) An anteroposterior view of a healed **T**-condylar fracture of the distal humerus, with a large amount of callus formation. (*B*) The lateral view reveals a large projection of bone anteriorly, which is limiting elbow flexion (probably myositis ossificans).

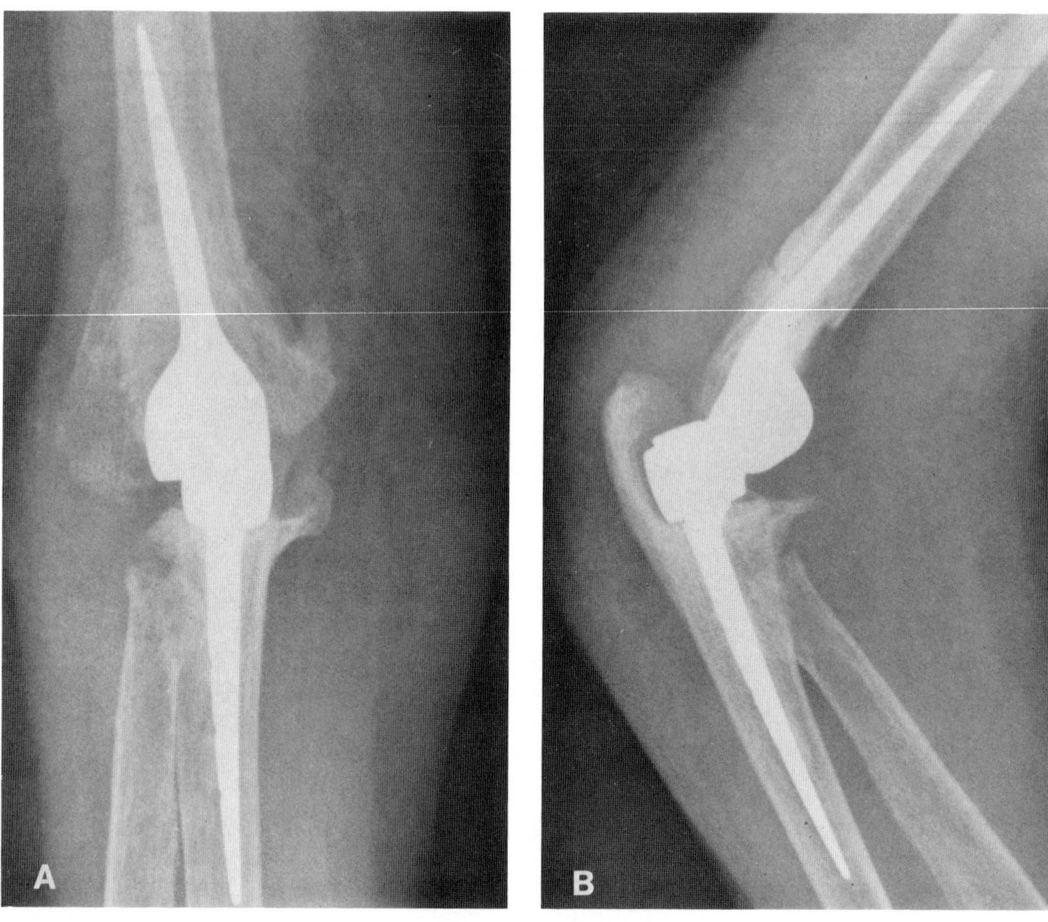

Fig. 9-42. Anteroposterior (*A*) and lateral (*B*) views of an elbow prosthesis used in a patient as a replacement for a painful arthroplasty.

able loss of flexion (Fig. 9-41). The foremost concern with this complication is being sure that the loss of motion is entirely due to the projecting fragment. It must be evaluated preoperatively to see how much of the loss of motion is due to joint irregularity and how much is due to actual soft-tissue contracture.

Cubitus varus or anterior angulation deformities of the distal humerus are uncommon in the adult patient after an elbow fracture. If the deformity results in loss of motion, it can occasionally be improved by an osteotomy of the humerus.

Fractures in close proximity to the elbow joint, such as a dicondylar fracture, are rarely amenable to operative correction to improve joint function. A properly selected arthroplasty should give a better probability of enhancing joint motion. At present, the replacement elbow prostheses (Fig. 9-42) have not had sufficient trial to justify their use other than as a salvage procedure.

LIGAMENT INJURIES

Extensive soft-tissue injuries of the elbow occurring with dislocations can result in recurrent dislocations. Obviously, lesser injuries occur and a major portion of the damaged ligament mends. Occasionally, the residua of a dislocation result in an attenuated ligament that causes the elbow to be unstable (Fig. 9-43). Since the elbow is

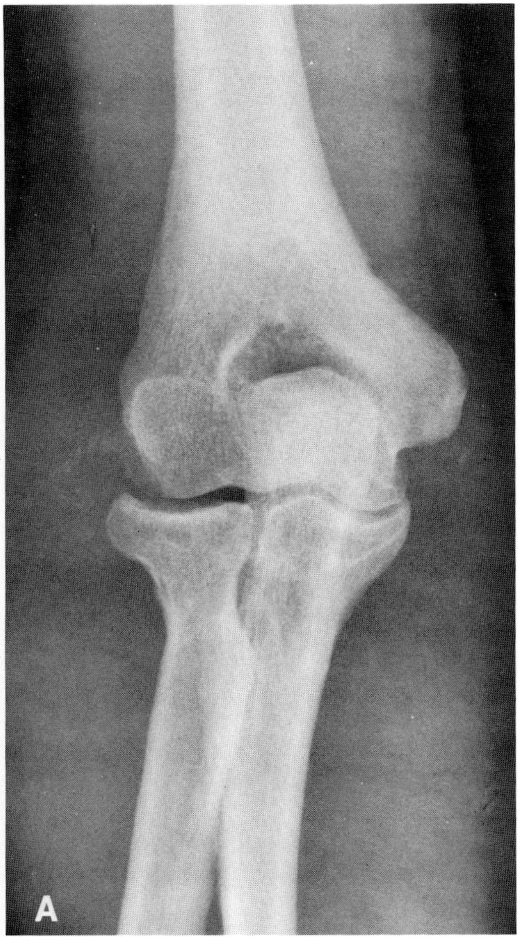

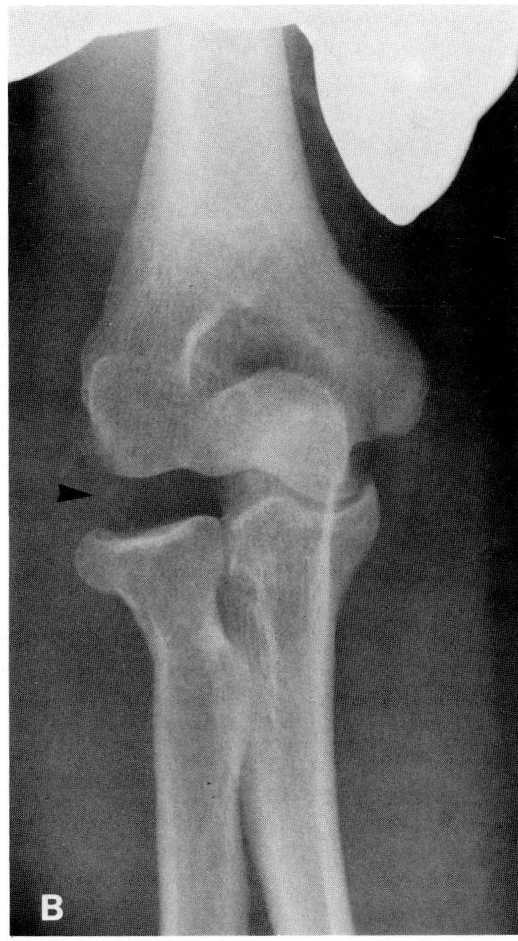

Fig. 9-43. (*A*) An anteroposterior view of the elbow in a 49-year-old male, 4 months after dislocation. He was complaining of pain over the radioulnar joint. (*B*) A varus stress film demonstrated attenuation of the radial collateral ligament (*arrow*).

not a weight-bearing joint, active resistive exercises can be of invaluable assistance in the treatment of the disability associated with relaxed ligaments. Rarely do these ligaments need repair.

NERVE INJURIES

It is possible for the median (or anterior interosseous), radial (or posterior interosseous), and ulnar nerves to be injured as they cross the elbow joint. The force of trauma may cause local contusion, stretching, or laceration of any of the three nerves. Fortunately, complete severance of the nerves is rarely seen, except in open wounds such as lacerations, gun-shot wounds, or sideswipe injuries. In closed injuries we have not encountered any injury of the median nerve except after supracondylar fractures, and all of these have recovered spontaneously. Injuries of the radial and posterior interosseous nerve have been associated with fractures and with anterior dislocation of the radial head. Recovery can be expected unless the nerve is caught in the fracture site.

The ulnar nerve is the one most frequently injured in association with elbow fractures. It can occur after fracture-dislocations, supracondylar fractures, and avulsion fractures of the medial epicondyle. If open reduction for displacement of a medial epicondyle fracture is necessary, the ulnar nerve should probably be transposed anteriorly at the same time. In incomplete ulnar nerve lesions complicating fractures about the elbow, it is usually best to delay treatment to allow sufficient time to detect signs of recovery. This means a waiting time of at least 3 to 4 weeks "lag time" plus 1 mm./day from the site of nerve injury to the first branches of the ulnar nerve below the elbow (i.e., to the flexor carpi ulnaris). If spontaneous return does not occur, then ulnar nerve neurolysis and transposition can be performed.

Delayed, or tardy, ulnar nerve palsy is not often seen as a complication of adult elbow fractures. However, small alterations in the region of the medial epicondyle, plus repeated minor trauma to this area, can cause sufficient adhesions around the nerve to produce symptoms. Anterior transposition of the nerve, with or without medial epicondylectomy, may alleviate the patient's symptoms.

VASCULAR INJURIES

Damage of a serious nature can occur to the brachial artery as it traverses the bony fragments of a severely displaced fracture. Spasm of the artery, due to vascular contusion or intimal damage, is probably the most common cause of absence of the radial pulse after elbow injuries. The spasm may be aggravated by a circular plaster cast or bandage that is too tight. This also can occur by positioning a swollen elbow in excessive flexion. The consequences of the loss of the vascularity of the arm can be avoided by careful assessment of the extremity, before and after initial treatment of the elbow injury.

Early recognition and treatment is imperative in vascular injuries around the elbow. Management of this complication is discussed on page 534.

MYOSITIS OSSIFICANS

Myositis ossificans is discussed on page 533.

REFERENCES

1. Ackerman, L. O.: Extra-osseous localized non-neoplastic bone and cartilage formation (so-called myositis ossificans). J. Bone Joint Surg., *40A*:279-298, 1958.
2. Adams, J. D.: A report on six cases of supracondylar fractures of the elbow. New Eng. J. Med., *216*:837-842, 1937.
3. Adler, J. B., and Shaftan, G. W.: Radial head fractures, is excision necessary? J. Trauma, *4*:115-136, 1964.
4. Adler, S., Fay, G. F., and MacAusland, W. R., Jr.: Treatment of olecranon fractures. Indication for excision of the olecranon fragment and repair of the triceps tendon. J. Trauma, *2*:597-602, 1962.
5. Aitken, A. P., and Childress, H. M.: Intra-articular displacement of the internal epicondyle following dislocation. J. Bone Joint Surg., *20*:161, 1938.
6. Albee, F. H.: Arthroplasty of the elbow. J. Bone Joint Surg., *15*:979-985, 1933.
7. Aldredge, G. N., Jr., and Gregory, C. F.: Triceps advancement in olecranon fractures. J. Bone Joint Surg., *51A*:816, 1969.
8. Allen, P. D., and Gramse, A. E.: Transcondylar fractures of the humerus treated by Dunlop traction. Amer. J. Surg., *57*:217-227, 1945.
9. Allende, G., and Freytes, M.: Old dislocations of the elbow. J. Bone Joint Surg., *26*:691-706, 1944.
10. Alonso-Llames, M.: Bilaterotricipital approach to the elbow. Acta Orthop. Scand., *43*:479-490, 1972.
11. Anderson, L.: Fractures. *In* Crenshaw, A. H. (ed.): Campbell's Operative Orthopaedics. ed. 5. St. Louis, C. V. Mosby, 1971.
12. Anderson, R.: Fractures of the humerus. Surg. Gynecol. Obstet., *64*:919-926, 1937.
13. Anson, B. J., and Maddock, W. G.: Callander's Surgical Anatomy. Philadelphia, W. B. Saunders, 1958.
14. Ashbell, T. S., Kleinert, H. E., and Kutz, J. E.: Vascular injuries about the elbow. Clin. Orthop., *50*:107-127, 1967.
15. Ashurst, A. P. C.: An anatomical and surgical study of fractures of the lower end of the humerus. Philadelphia, Lea & Febiger, 1910.
16. Aufranc, O. E., Jones, W. N., and Turner,

R. H.: Dislocation of the elbow with brachial artery injury. J.A.M.A., *197*:719-721, 1966.
17. ———: Dislocation of the elbow with brachial artery injury. J.A.M.A., *197*: 1092-1094, 1966.
18. Aufranc, O. E., Jones, W. N., Turner, R. H., and Thomas, W. H.: Dislocation of the elbow with fracture of the radial head and distal radius. J.A.M.A., *202*:131-134, 1967.
19. Aufranc, O. E., Jones, W. N., and Bierbaum, B. E.: Open supracondylar fracture of the humerus. J.A.M.A., *208*:682-685, 1969.
20. Babcock, W. W.: Textbook of Surgery. Philadelphia, W. B. Saunders, 1935.
21. Bakalim, G.: Fractures of radial head and their treatment. Acta Orthop. Scand., *41*: 320-331, 1970.
22. Bakalim, G., and Wilppula, E.: Fractures of the olecranon II. Excision of the fragment and reinsertion of triceps tendon in comminuted fractures. Ann. Chir. Gynecol. Fenn., *60*:102-104, 1971.
23. Balchandani, R. H.: Unreduced dislocations of the elbow. J. Bone Joint Surg., *51B*:781, 1969.
24. Barr, J. S., and Eaton, R. G.: Elbow reconstruction with a new prosthesis to replace the distal end of the humerus. J. Bone Joint Surg., *47A*:1408-1413, 1965.
25. Barrington, T. W.: Radial head replacement. J. Bone Joint Surg., *51B*:778, 1969.
26. Bennett, G. E.: Shoulder and elbow lesions of the professional baseball pitcher. J.A.M.A., *117*:510-514, 1941.
27. ———: Shoulder and elbow lesions distinctive of baseball players. Ann. Surg., *126*:107-110, 1947.
28. Berger, P.: Le traitement de fractures de l'olecrane et particiluerement la sutur de l'olecrane pa un procede (cedarg de l'olecranon). Ga 2 Hebd de Med. 193-199, 1902.
29. Bergmann, E.: Tardy ulnar palsy. Amer. J. Surg., *80*:371-372, 1950.
30. Bickel, W. H., and Perry, R. E.: Comminuted fractures of the distal humerus. J.A.M.A., *184*:553-557, 1963.
31. Böhler, L.: The Treatment of Fractures. Vienna, Wilhelm Maudrich, 1929.
32. ———: The Treatment of Fractures. vol. 1. 5th English Edition. New York, Grune and Stratton, 1956.
33. Bohrer, J. V.: Fractures of the head and neck of the radius. Ann. Surg., *97*:204-208, 1933.
34. Bonnin, J. G.: A Complete Outline of Fractures. London, William Heinemann, 1941.
35. Bontrous, T. A., Blain, A., and Chipman, W. A.: Non-splinting treatment of elbow joint injuries (report of its use in twenty cases). Amer. J. Surg., *68*:212-218, 1945.
36. Bowers, R. F.: Myositis ossificans traumatica. J. Bone Joint Surg., *19*:215-221, 1937.
37. Brown, R. F., and Morgan, R. G.: Intercondylar **T**-shaped fractures of the humerus. J. Bone Joint Surg., *53B*:425-428, 1971.
38. Bryan, R. S., and Bickel, W. H.: "T" condylar fractures of distal humerus. J. Trauma, *11*:830-835, 1971.
39. Buffington, C. B.: The treatment of simple and comminuted fractures of the head of the radius. West Va. Med. J., *43*:198-200, 1947.
40. Burton, A. E.: Fractures of the head of the radius. Proc. Roy. Soc. Med., *35*: 764-765, 1942.
41. Bush, L. F., and McClain, E. J., Jr.: Operative treatment of fractures of the elbow in adults. American Academy of Orthopaedic Surgeons, Instructional Course Lectures, *16*:265-277, 1959.
42. Buxton, St. J. D.: Fractures of the head of the radius and capitellum including fractures of childhood. Brit. Med. J., *2*:665-666, 1936.
43. ———: Ossification in the ligaments of the elbow joint. J. Bone Joint Surg., *20*: 709-714, 1938.
44. Callahan, J. J.: Dislocations. J.A.M.A., *132*:440-442, 1946.
45. Callander, C. L.: Surgical Anatomy. ed. 2. Philadelphia, W. B. Saunders, 1939.
46. Campbell, W. C.: Malunited fractures and unreduced dislocations about the elbow. J.A.M.A., *92*:122-128, 1929.
47. ———: Operative Orthopaedics. ed. 1. St. Louis, C. V. Mosby, 1939.
48. Caravias, D. E.: Forward dislocation of the elbow without fracture of the olecranon. J. Bone Joint Surg., *39B*:334, 1957.
49. Carstam, N.: Operative treatment of fractures of the upper end of the radius. Acta Orthop. Scand., *19*:502-526, 1950.
50. Cassebaum, W. H.: Operative treatment of **T**- and **Y**-fractures of the lower end of the humerus. Amer. J. Surg., *83*:265-270, 1952.
51. ———: Open reduction of **T**- and **Y**-fractures of the lower end of the humerus. J. Trauma, *9*:915-925, 1969.
52. Castberg, T., and Thing, E.: Treatment

of fractures of the upper end of the radius. Acta Chir. Scand., *105*:62-69, 1953.
53. Cave, E. F.: Fractures and Other Injuries. Chicago, The Year Book Publishers, 1958.
54. Charnley, J.: The Closed Treatment of Common Fractures. Edinburgh, E. & S. Livingstone, 1950.
55. Cherry, J. C.: Dislocations of the elbow. Practitioner, *160*:191-195, 1948.
56. Childress, H. M.: Transarticular pin fixation in supracondylar fractures of the elbow in children. J. Bone Joint Surg., *59A*: 1548-1552, 1972.
57. Christopher, F., and Bushnell, L. F.: Conservative treatment of fracture of the capitellum. J. Bone Joint Surg., *17*:489-492, 1935.
58. Cohn, I.: Forward dislocation of both bones of the forearm at the elbow. Surg. Gynecol. Obstet., *35*:776-788, 1922.
59. ———: Fractures of the elbow. Amer. J. Surg., *55*:210-227, 1942.
60. Colp, R., and Mage, S.: The treatment of joint fractures. Ann. Surg., *97*:177-188, 1933.
61. Colton, C. L.: Fractures of the olecranon in adults: classification and management. Injury, *5*:121-129, 1973.
62. Conn, J., and Wade, P. A.: Injuries of the elbow (a ten-year review). J. Trauma, *1*:248-268, 1961.
63. Conner, A. N., and Smith, M. G. H.: Displaced fractures of the lateral humeral condyle in children. J. Bone Joint Surg., *52B*:460-464, 1970.
64. Conwell, H. E., and Reynolds, F. C.: Key and Conwell's Management of Fractures, Dislocations and Sprains. ed. 7. St. Louis, C. V. Mosby, 1961.
65. Coonrad, R. W.: A review of severe elbow injuries. J. Bone Joint Surg., *38A*:1396, 1956.
66. Cotton, F. J.: Dislocations and Joint Fractures. ed. 2. Philadelphia, W. B. Saunders, 1924.
67. ———: Elbow dislocation and ulnar nerve injury. J. Bone Joint Surg., *11*:348-352, 1929.
68. Crenshaw, A. H. (ed.): Campbell's Operative Orthopaedics. ed. 5. St. Louis, C. V. Mosby, 1971.
69. Cutler, C. W.: Fractures of the head and neck of the radius. Ann. Surg., *83*:267-278, 1926.
70. Daland, E. M.: Fractures of the olecranon. J. Bone Joint Surg., *15*:601-607, 1933.
71. D'Ambrosia, R. D.: Supracondylar fractures of the humerus—prevention of cubitus varus. J. Bone Joint Surg., *54A*:60-66, 1972.
72. Darrach, W.: Open reduction of fractured external condyle of humerus. Ann. Surg., *63*:486-487, 1916.
73. ———: Open reduction of fractures of the capitellum. Ann. Surg., *63*:487-488, 1916.
74. ———: Surgical approaches for surgery of the extremities. Amer. J. Surg., *67*:237-262, 1945.
75. De Bakey, M. E., Beall, A. C., Jr., and Wukasch, D. C.: Recent developments in vascular surgery with particular reference to orthopedics. Amer. J. Surg., *109*:134-142, 1965.
76. DePalma, A. F.: The Management of Fractures and Dislocations. Philadelphia, W. B. Saunders, 1959.
77. Desault, P. J.: A treatise on fractures, luxations and other affections of the bones. Philadelphia, Kimber and Conrad, 1811.
78. Devine, J.: Shattering gunshot wounds of the elbow. Austral. New Zealand J. Surg., *13*:208-209, 1944.
79. Doane, C. P.: Fractures of the supracondylar process of the humerus. J. Bone Joint Surg., *18*:757-759, 1936.
80. Donchess, J. C.: Treatment of supracondylar fracture of the humerus. J. Indiana State Med. Ass., *42*:217-222, 1949.
81. Dunlop, J.: Traumatic separation of the medial epicondyle of the humerus in adolescence. J. Bone Joint Surg., *17*:577-587, 1935.
82. ———: Transcondylar fractures of the humerus in childhood. J. Bone Joint Surg., *21*:59-73, 1939.
83. Dunn, A. W.: A distal humeral prosthesis. Clin. Orthop., *77*:199-202, 1971.
84. Dunn, N.: Operation for fracture of the olecranon. Brit. Med. J., *1*:214-215, 1939.
85. Dupuytren, B. G.: On the Injuries and Diseases of Bones (Collected Edition of the Clinical Lectures). London, Sydenham Society, 1847.
86. Eastwood, W. J.: The T-shaped fracture of the lower end of the humerus. J. Bone Joint Surg., *19*:364-369, 1937.
87. Edman, P., and Lohr, G.: Supracondylar fractures of the humerus treated with olecranon traction. Acta Chir. Scand., *126*:505-516, 1963.
88. Eliason, E. L., and North, J. P.: Fractures about the elbow. Amer. J. Surg., *44*:88, 1939.
89. Eliot, E., Jr.: Fracture of the olecranon. Surg. Clin. N. Amer., *14*:487-492, 1934.
90. Eriksson, E., Sahlen, O., and Sandohl, U.: Late results of conservative and surgical treatment of fracture of the olecranon. Acta Chir. Scand., *113*:153-166, 1957.

91. Essex-Lopresti, P.: Fractures of the radial head with distal radio-ulnar dislocation. (Report of two cases). J. Bone Joint Surg., *33B*:244-247, 1951.
92. Evans, E. M.: Pronation injuries of the forearm, with special reference to the anterior Monteggia lesion. J. Bone Joint Surg., *31B*:578-588, 1949.
93. ———: Supracondylar **Y**-fractures of the humerus. J. Bone Joint Surg., *35B*:381-385, 1953.
94. Exarhou, E. I., and Antoniou, N. K.: Congenital dislocation of the head of the radius. Acta Orthop. Scand., *41*:551-556, 1970.
95. Fairbank, H. A. T.: Discussion of two cases of disability at the wrist joint following excision of the head of the radius. Proc. Roy. Soc. Med., *24*:904-905, 1930.
96. ———: Prognosis in injuries of the elbow joint. Lancet, *227*:263-264, 1934.
97. Farr, R. S.: Fractures of the elbow. New York State J. Med., *40*:1288-1291, 1940.
98. Fiolle, D. J.: Note sur les fractures de l'olécrane par projectiles de guerre. Marseille Medical, *55*:241-245, 1918.
99. Fitts, W. T., Jr.: Fractures of the upper extremity (a review of experience in World War II). Amer. J. Surg., *72*:393-403, 1946.
100. Flemming, C. W.: Fractures of the head of the radius. Proc. Roy. Soc. Med., *25*: 1011-1015, 1932.
101. Flint, C. P.: Fracture of the eminentia capitata. Surg. Gynecol. & Obstet., *7*:342-356, 1908.
102. Fowles, J. V., Kassab, M. T., and Said, K.: Supracondylar fractures in children, stabilization by two lateral percutaneous pins. Presented at the Canadian Orthopaedic Association Annual Meeting, Winnipeg, Manitoba, June 1973.
103. Garceau, G. J.: Fractures of the lower end of the humerus. J.A.M.A., *112*:623-626, 1939.
104. Gaston, S. R., Smith, F. M., and Baab, O. D.: Adult injuries of the radial head and neck (importance of time element in treatment). Amer. J. Surg., *78*:631-635, 1949.
105. Gay, J. R., and Love, J. G.: Diagnosis and treatment of tardy paralysis of the ulnar nerve. J. Bone Joint Surg., *29*:1087-1097, 1947.
106. Gejrot, W.: On intra-articular fractures of the capitellum and trochlea of humerus with special reference of treatment. Acta Chir. Scand., *71*:253, 1932.
107. Gellman, M.: Arthrodesis of the elbow. J. Bone Joint Surg., *29*:850-852, 1947.
108. Gosman, J. A.: Recurrent dislocation of the ulna at the elbow. J. Bone Joint Surg., *25*:448-449, 1943.
109. Goss, C. M. (ed.): Gray's Anatomy of the Human Body. ed. 26. Philadelphia, Lea & Febiger, 1954.
110. Gould, A. L.: A neglected danger in the treatment of elbow fractures. Maine Med. J., *27*:116-118, 1936.
111. Grant, J. C. B.: A Method of Anatomy. ed. 5. Baltimore, Williams & Wilkins, 1952.
112. Grossman, J.: Fracture of the head and neck of the radius. New York J. Med., *117*:472-475, 1923.
113. Groves, E. W. H.: Direct skeletal traction in the treatment of fractures. Brit. J. Surg., *16*:149-157, 1928.
114. Gunner, B. A.: Fracture of supracondyloid process. J. Bone Joint Surg., *41A*: 1333-1335, 1959.
115. Hamilton, F. H.: A Practical Treatise on Fractures and Dislocations. ed. 8. Philadelphia, Lea Brothers & Co., 1891.
116. Harmer, T. W.: Fractures and dislocations at the elbow. *In* Wilson, P. D. (ed.): Fractures and Dislocation. Philadelphia, J. B. Lippincott, 1938.
117. Harmon, P. H.: Treatment of fractures of the olecranon by fixation with stainless-steel screws. J. Bone Joint Surg., *27*:328-329, 1945.
118. Harris, W. H., Jones, W. N., and Aufranc, O. E.: Fracture Problems. St. Louis, C. V. Mosby, 1965.
119. Hart, G. M.: Subluxation of the head of the radius in young children. J.A.M.A., *169*:1734-1736, 1959.
120. Hasner, E., and Husby, J.: Fracture of the epicondyle and condyle of the humerus. Acta Chir. Scand., *101*:195, 1951.
121. Hein, B. J.: Fractures of the head of the radius. (An analysis of fifty-two cases with specific reference to disabilities). Indust. Med., *6*:529-532, 1937.
122. Henderson, M. S.: Fractures of hip, ankle, and elbow. Ann. Surg., *93*:968-983, 1931.
123. Henderson, R. S., and Robertson, I. M.: Open dislocation of the elbow with rupture of the brachial artery. J. Bone Joint Surg., *34B*:636-637, 1952.
124. Henry, A. K.: Extensile Exposure. Baltimore, Williams & Wilkins, 1945.
125. Higgs, S. L.: Fractures of the internal epicondyle of the humerus. Brit. Med. J., *2*:666-667, 1936.
126. Highsmith, L. S., and Phalen, G. S.: Sideswipe fractures. Arch. Surg., *52*:513-522, 1946.
127. Hitzrot, J. M.: Fractures at the lower end

of the humerus in adults. Surg. Clin. N. Amer., *12*:291-304, 1932.

128. ———: The treatment of simple fractures: a study of some end results. Ann. Surg., *55*:338-367, 1941.
129. Ho, K. C., and Marmor, L.: Entrapment of the ulnar nerve at the elbow. Amer. J. Surg., *121*:355-356, 1971.
130. Howard, J. L., and Urist, M. R.: Fracture-dislocation of the radius and the ulna at the elbow joint. Clin. Orthop., *12*:276-284, 1958.
131. Howorth, M. B.: Textbook of Orthopedics. Philadelphia, W. B. Saunders, 1952.
132. Hoyer, A.: Treatment of supracondylar fractures of the humerus by skeletal traction in an abduction splint. J. Bone Joint Surg., *34A*:623-637, 1952.
133. Jackman, R. J., and Pugh, D. G.: The positive elbow fat pad sign in rheumatoid arthritis. Amer. J. Roentgenol., *108*:812-818, 1970.
134. Jackson, J. A.: Simple anterior dislocation of the elbow joint with rupture of the brachial artery (case report). Amer. J. Surg., *47*:479-486, 1940.
135. Jacobs, J. C., and Kernodle, H. B.: Fractures of the head of the radius. J. Bone Joint Surg., *28*:616-622, 1946.
136. Jeanneney, J. P., and Vielle, J. J.: Luxation du coude chez un homme de 22 ans. rupture de l'artere et de la veina humerales. Syndrome de Volkmann. J. Med. de Bordeaux, *54*:522-524, 1927.
137. Jeffey, C. C.: Fractures of the neck of the radius in children. Mechanism of causation. J. Bone Joint Surg., *54B*:717-719, 1972.
138. Johansson, H., and Olerud, S.: Operative treatment of intercondylar fractures of the humerus. J. Trauma, *11*:836-843, 1971.
139. Johnston, G. W.: A follow-up of one hundred cases of fracture of the head of the radius with a review of the literature. Ulster Med. J., *31*:51-56, 1962.
140. Jones, K. G.: Percutaneous pin fixation of fractures of the lower end of the humerus. Clin. Orthop., *50*:53-69, 1967.
141. Jones, R.: A note on the treatment of injuries about the elbow. Prov. Med. J., *14*:28, 1895.
142. Kapel, O.: Operation for habitual dislocation of the elbow. J. Bone Joint Surg., *33A*:707-714, 1951.
143. Kelly, R. P., and Griffin, T. W.: Open reduction of T-condylar fractures of the humerus through an anterior approach. J. Trauma, *9*:901-914, 1969.
144. Keon-Cohen, B. T.: Fractures at the elbow. J. Bone Joint Surg., *48A*:1623-1639, 1966.
145. Kerin, R.: Elbow dislocations and its association with vascular disruption. J. Bone Joint Surg., *51A*:756-758, 1969.
146. Kettlekamp, D. B., and Alexander, H.: Clinical review of radial nerve injury. J. Trauma, *7*:424-432, 1967.
147. Key, J. A.: Treatment of fractures of the head and neck of the radius. J.A.M.A., *96*:101-104, 1931.
148. Kilburn, P., Sweeney, J. G., and Silk, F. E.: Three cases of compound posterior dislocation of the elbow with rupture of the brachial artery. J. Bone Joint Surg., *44B*:119-121, 1962.
149. King, B. B.: Resection of the radial head and neck (an end-result study of thirteen cases). J. Bone Joint Surg., *21*:839-857, 1939.
150. King, D., and Secor, C.: Bow elbow (cubitus varus). J. Bone Joint Surg., *33A*:572-576, 1951.
151. King, O. C.: Fractures and dislocations about the elbow. Surg. Clin. N. Amer., *20*:1645-1667, 1940.
152. King, T.: Recurrent dislocation of the elbow. J. Bone Joint Surg., *35B*:30-54, 1953.
153. Kini, M. G.: Dislocation of the elbow and its complications. J. Bone Joint Surg., *22*:107-117, 1940.
154. Knapp, M. E.: Physical therapy in fractures about the elbow joint. Arch. Phys. Therap., *21*:709-715, 1940.
155. Knight, R. A.: Fractures of the humeral condyles in adults. South. Med. J., *48*:1165-1173, 1955.
156. ———: Management of fractures about the elbow in adults. American Academy of Orthopaedic Surgeons Instructional Course Lectures, *14*:123-141, 1957.
157. Koch, M., and Lipscomb, P. R.: Arthrodesis of the elbow. Clin. Orthop., *50*:151-157, 1967.
158. Köhler, A., and Zimmer, E. A.: Borderlands of the normal and early pathologic in skeletal roentgenology. Amer. ed. 3. New York, Grune and Stratton, 1968.
159. Kohn, A. M.: Soft-tissue alterations in elbow trauma. Amer. J. Roentgenol., *82*:867-874, 1959.
160. Kolb, L. W., and Moore, R. D.: Fractures of the supracondylar process of the humerus: report of two cases. J. Bone Joint Surg., *49A*:532-534, 1967.
161. Ladd, W. E.: Fractures of the lower end of the humerus. Boston Med. Surg. J., *175*:220-225, 1916.
162. Lee, W. E., and Summey, T. J.: Fracture

of the capitellum of the humerus. Ann. Surg., 99:497-509, 1934.

163. Lewis, D., and Miller, E. M.: Peripheral nerve injuries associated with fractures. Ann. Surg., *76*:528-538, 1922.

164. Lewis, R. W., and Thibodeau, A. A.: Deformity of the wrist following resection of the radial head. Surg. Gynecol. Obstet., *64*:1079-1085, 1937.

165. Lindem, M. C.: Fractures of the capitellum and trochlea. Ann. Surg., *74*:78, 1922.

166. Linscheid, R. L., and Wheeler, D. K.: Elbow dislocations. J.A.M.A., *194*:1171-1176, 1965.

167. Loomis, L. K.: Reduction and after-treatment of posterior dislocation of the elbow. Amer. J. Surg., *63*:56-60, 1944.

168. Lou, I.: Olecranon fractures treated in the Orthopaedic Hospital, Copenhagen 1936-47. A follow-up examination. Acta Orthop. Scand., *19*:166-179, 1949-1950.

169. Lund, H. J.: Fracture of the supracondyloid process of the humerus: Report of a case. J. Bone Joint Surg., *12*:925-928, 1930.

170. MacAusland, W. R.: The treatment of fractures of the olecranon by longitudinal screw or nail fixation. Ann. Surg., *116*: 293-296, 1942.

171. ———: Replacement of the lower end of the humerus with a prosthesis. Western J. of Surg., *62*:557-566, 1954.

172. ———: Arthroplasty of the elbow. New Eng. J. Med., *236*:97-99, 1947.

173. MacAusland, W. R., Jr.: Personal communication.

174. Magnuson, P. B., and Stack, J. K.: Fractures. ed. 5. Philadelphia, J. B. Lippincott, 1949.

175. Mann, T. S.: Prognosis in supracondylar fractures. J. Bone Joint Surg., *45B*:516-522, 1963.

176. Mannefelt, L.: Median nerve entrapment after dislocation of the elbow (report of a case). J. Bone Joint Surg., *50B*:152-155, 1968.

177. Marnham, R.: Dislocation of the elbow with rupture of the brachial artery. Brit. J. Surg., *22*:181, 1934-1935.

178. Mason, J. A., and Shutkin, N. M.: Immediate active motion treatment of fractures of the head and neck of the radius. Surg. Gynecol. Obstet., *76*:731-737, 1943.

179. Mason, M. L.: Some observations on fractures of the head of the radius with a review of one hundred cases. Brit. J. Surg., *42*:123-132, 1954.

180. Maylaln, D. J.: Fractures of the elbow in children. Review of three hundred consecutive cases. J.A.M.A., *166*:220-228, 1958.

181. Mazel, M. S.: Fracture of the capitellum. J. Bone Joint Surg., *17*:483-488, 1935.

182. McDougall, A. M., and White, J.: Subluxation of the inferior radio-ulnar joint complicating fracture of the radial head. J. Bone Joint Surg., *39B*:278-287, 1957.

183. McKeever, F. M., and Buck, R. M.: Fracture of the olecranon process of the ulna. J.A.M.A., *135*:1-5, 1947.

184. McLaughlin, H. L.: Trauma. Philadelphia, W. B. Saunders, 1959.

185. Meekison, D. M.: Some remarks on three common fractures. (Carpal scaphoid, head of radius, and medial malleolus). J. Bone Joint Surg., *27*:80-85, 1945.

186. Mellen, R. H., and Phalen, G. S.: Arthroplasty of the elbow by replacement of the distal portion of the humerus with an acrylic prosthesis. J. Bone Joint Surg., *29*:348-352, 1947.

187. Milch, H.: Dislocation of the inferior end of the ulna, suggestions for a new operative procedure. Amer. J. Surg., *1*:141-146, 1926.

188. ———: Unusual fractures of the capitulum humeri and the capitulum radii. J. Bone Joint Surg., *13*:882, 1931.

189. ———: Fractures of the external humeral condyle. J.A.M.A., *160*:641, 1956.

190. ———: Fractures and fracture dislocations of the humeral condyles. J. Trauma, *4*:592-607, 1964.

191. Miller, O. L.: Blind nailing of the T-fracture of the lower end of the humerus which involves the joint. J. Bone Joint Surg., *21*:933-938, 1939.

192. Miller, W. A.: Comminuted fractures of the distal end of the humerus in the adult. J. Bone Joint Surg., *46A*:644-657, 1964.

193. Mohan, K.: Myositis ossificans traumatica of the elbow. Int. Surg., *57*:475-478, 1972.

194. Müller, M. E., Allgöwer, M., and Willenegger, H.: Manual of internal fixation. New York, Springer-Verlag, 1970.

195. Murray, J. M.: Traumatic flail elbow. J.A.M.A., *106*:282-283, 1936.

196. Murray, R. C.: Fractures of the head and neck of the radius. Brit. J. Surg., *28*:106-118, 1940.

197. Myers, M.: Dislocations: diagnosis, management, and complications. Surg. Clin. N. Amer., *48*:1391-1402, 1968.

198. Neuwirth, A. A.: Nonsplinting treatment of fractures of the elbow joint. J.A.M.A., *118*:971-972, 1942.

199. Neviaser, R. J., and LeFevre, G. W.: Irreducible isolated dislocation of the

radial head. A case report. Clin. Orthop., *80*:72-74, 1971.

200. Nicholson, J. T.: Compound comminuted fractures involving the elbow joint; treatment by resection of fragments. J. Bone Joint Surg., *38*:565, 1946.
201. Nicola, T.: Atlas of Surgical Approaches to Bone and Joints. New York, Macmillan Co., 1945.
202. Norell, H. G.: Roentgenologic visualization of extra-capsular fat; its importance in the diagnosis of traumatic injuries to the elbow. Acta Radiol., *42*:205-210, 1954.
203. O'Connor, B. T., and Taylor, T. K. F.: The conservative approach to radial head fractures. J. Bone Joint Surg., *44B*:743, 1962.
204. O'Donoghue, D. H., and Sell, L. S.: Persistent olecranon epiphysis in adults. J. Bone Joint Surg., *24*:677-680, 1942.
205. Ogilvie, W. H.: Discussion on minor injuries of the elbow. Proc. Roy. Soc. Med., *23*:306-322, 1930.
206. Osborne, G., and Cotterill, P.: Recurrent dislocation of the elbow. J. Bone Joint Surg., *48B*:340-346, 1966.
207. Osgood, G., and Penhallow, D. P.: A new apparatus for the treatment of fractures of the humerus. J.A.M.A., *53*:375-378, 1909.
208. Oury, J. H., Roe, R. D., and Laning, R. C.: A case of bilateral anterior dislocations of the elbow. J. Trauma, *12*:170-173, 1972.
209. Paradies, L. H., and Gregory, C. F.: The early treatment of close-range shotgun wounds to the extremities. J. Bone Joint Surg., *48A*:425-435, 1966.
210. Patrick, J.: Fracture of the medial epicondyle with displacement into the elbow joint. J. Bone Joint Surg., *28*:143-147, 1946.
211. Patterson, R. F.: A method of applying traction in **T**- and **Y**-fractures of the humerus. J. Bone Joint Surg., *17*:476-477, 1935.
212. Pawlowski, R. F., Palumbo, F. C., and Callahan, J. J.: Irreducible posterolateral elbow dislocation: report of a rare case. J. Trauma, *10*:260-266, 1970.
213. Perkins, G.: Fractures of the olecranon. Brit. Med. J., *2*:668-669, 1936.
214. Persson, M.: Treatment of supracondylar fractures of the humerus. Nord. Med. Tidshr., *15*:457-461, 1938.
215. Pike, W.: Fracture of the head of the radius. J. Bone Joint Surg., *51B*:198, 1969.
216. Pinder, I. M.: Fracture of the head of the radius in adults. J. Bone Joint Surg., *51B*:386, 1969.
217. Pollock, W. J., and Parkes, J. C., II: Early reconstruction of the elbow following severe trauma. J. Trauma, *10*:839-852, 1970.
218. Postlethwait, R. W.: Modified treatment for fractures of the head of the radius. Amer. J. Surg., *67*:77-80, 1945.
219. Purser, D. W.: Dislocation of the elbow and inclusion of the medial epicondyle in the adult. J. Bone Joint Surg., *36B*:247-249, 1954.
220. Quigley, T. B.: Aspiration of the elbow joint in treatment of fractures of the head of the radius. New Eng. J. Med., *240*:915-916, 1949.
221. Radin, E. L., and Riseborough, E. J.: Fractures of the radial head. (A review of eighty-eight cases and analysis of the indications for excision of the radial head and non-operative treatment). J. Bone Joint Surg., *48A*:1055-1064, 1966.
222. Railton, S. V.: Compound dislocation of elbow joint without fracture (case report). Canad. Med. Ass. J., *59*:367, 1948.
223. Reich, R. S.: Treatment of intercondylar fractures of the elbow by means of traction. J. Bone Joint Surg., *18*:997-1004, 1936.
224. Reichenheim, P. P.: Transplantation of the biceps tendon as a treatment for recurrent dislocation of the elbow. Brit. J. Surg., *35*:201, 1947.
225. Rhodin, R.: On the treatment of fracture of the capitellum. Acta Chir. Scand., *86*:475-486, 1942.
226. Rieth, P. L.: Fractures of the radial head (associated with chip fracture of the capitellum in adults: surgical considerations). South. Surg., *14*:154-159, 1948.
227. Riseborough, E. J., and Radin, E. L.: Intercondylar **T**-fractures of the humerus in the adult (a comparison of operative and non-operative treatment in twenty-nine cases). J. Bone Joint Surg., *51A*:130-141, 1969.
228. Roaf, R.: Foramen in the humerus caused by the median nerve. J. Bone Joint Surg., *39B*:748-749, 1957.
229. Roberts, J. B., and Kelly, J. A.: Treatise on Fractures. ed. 2. Philadelphia, J. B. Lippincott, 1921.
230. Roberts, N. W.: Displacement of the in-

ternal condyle into the elbow joint. Lancet, *2*:78-79, 1934.
231. Roberts, P. H.: Dislocation of the elbow. Brit. J. Surg., *56*:806-815, 1969.
232. Robertson, R. C., and Bogart, F. B.: Fracture of the capitellum and trochlea, combined with fracture of the external humeral condyle. J. Bone Joint Surg., *15*: 206-213, 1933.
233. Rocyn-Jones, A.: Fractures and dislocations at the elbow. Practitioner, *144*:589-597, 1940.
234. Rombold, C.: A new operative treatment for fractures of the olecranon. J. Bone Joint Surg., *16*:947-949, 1934.
235. Rowe, C.: The management of fractures in elderly patients is different. J. Bone Joint Surg., *47A*:1043-1059, 1965.
236. Rush, L. V., and Rush, H. L.: A reconstruction operation for comminuted fractures of upper third of the ulna. Amer. J. Surg., *38*:332-333, 1937.
237. Salter, R. B.: Problem fractures in children. American Academy of Orthopaedic Surgeons Instructional Course Lectures. Annual Meeting, Dallas, Texas, 1974.
238. Schultz, R. S.: The Language of Fractures. Baltimore, Williams & Wilkins, 1972.
239. Schwartz, R. P., and Young, F.: Treatment of fractures of the head and neck of the radius and slipped radial epiphysis in children. Surg. Gynecol. Obstet., *57*: 528-537, 1933.
240. Scudder, C. L.: Treatment of Fractures. ed. 10. Philadelphia, W. B. Saunders, 1922.
241. ———: Treatment of Fractures. ed. 11. Philadelphia, W. B. Saunders, 1939.
242. Seddon, H. J.: Volkmann's contracture: treatment by excision of the infarct. J. Bone Joint Surg., *38B*:152-174, 1956.
243. Sever, J. W.: Fractures of the head and neck of the radius (a study of end results). J.A.M.A., *84*:1551-1555, 1925.
244. Sherrill, J. G.: Direct suture of the brachial artery following rupture, result of traumatism. Ann. Surg., *58*:534-536, 1913.
245. Shorbe, H. B.: Car window elbows. South. Med. J., *34*:372-376, 1941.
246. Simon, M. M.: Complete anterior dislocation of both bones of the forearm at the elbow (review of recorded cases and literature with report of a case). Med. J. Rec., *133*:333-336, 1931.
247. Siris, I. E.: Supracondylar fracture of the humerus (an analysis of 330 cases). Surg. Gynecol. Obstet., *68*:201-222, 1939.
248. Smith, F. M.: Fractures and dislocations involving elbow joint. *In* Bancroft, F. W., and Marble, H. C. (eds.): Surgical Treatment of Motor-Skeletal System. ed. 1. Philadelphia, J. B. Lippincott, 1945.
249. ———: Displacement of the medial epicondyle of the humerus into the elbow joint Ann. Surg., *124*:410-425, 1946.
250. ———: Kirschner wire traction in elbow and upper arm injuries. Amer. J. Surg., *74*:770-787, 1947.
251. ———: Medial epicondyle injuries. J.A.M.A., *142*:396-402, 1950.
252. ———: Traction and suspension in the treatment of fractures. Surg. Clin. N. Amer., *31*:545-560, 1951.
253. ———: Fractures and dislocations involving elbow joint. *In* Bancroft, F. W., and Marble, H. C. (eds.): Surgery of the Motor-Skeletal System. ed. 2. Philadelphia, J. B. Lippincott, 1951.
254. ———: Surgery of the elbow. Springfield, Charles C Thomas, 1954.
255. Smith, J. E. M.: Internal fixation in the treatment of fractures of the shafts of the radius and ulna in adults. The value of delayed operation in the prevention of non-union. J. Bone Joint Surg., *41B*:122-131, 1959.
256. Smith, L.: Deformity following supracondylar fracture of the humerus. J. Bone Joint Surg., *42A*:235-252, 1960.
257. Smith, L.: Supracondylar fractures of the humerus treated by direct observation. Clin. Orthop., *50*:37-42, 1967.
258. Snedecor, S. T., and Graham, W. C.: Severe war injuries of the elbow. J. Bone Joint Surg., *27*:623-631, 1945.
259. Soeur, R.: Fractures of the true condyle of the humerus. Acta Orthop. Belg., *12*: 235, 1946.
260. Spear, H. C., and Jones, J. M.: Rupture of the brachial artery accompanying dislocation of the elbow or supracondylar fracture. J. Bone Joint Surg., *33A*:889-894, 1951.
261. Speed, J. S.: An operation for unreduced posterior dislocation of the elbow. South. Med. J., *18*:193-198, 1925.
262. ———: Surgical treatment of condylar fractures of the humerus. American Academy of Orthopaedic Surgeons Instructional Course Lectures, *7*:187-194, 1950.
263. Speed, J. S., and Boyd, H. B.: Fractures

about the elbow. Amer. J. Surg., *38*:727-738, 1937.

264. ———: Treatment of fractures of ulna with dislocation of head of radius (Monteggia fracture). J.A.M.A., *115*:1699-1705, 1940.
265. Speed, K.: Fracture of the head of the radius. Amer. J. Surg., *38*:157-159, 1924.
266. ———: A Textbook of Fractures and Dislocation. Philadelphia, Lea & Febiger, 1935.
267. ———: Ferrule caps for the head of the radius. Surg. Gynecol. Obstet., *73*:845-850, 1941.
268. Spinner, M., and Kaplan, E. B.: The quadrate ligament of the elbow—its relationship to the stability of the proximal radio-ulnar joint. Acta Orthop. Scand., *41*:632-647, 1970.
269. Starkloff, G. B.: Posterior dislocations at the elbow. J. Missouri State Med. Assoc., *45*:895, 1948.
270. Staunton, F. W.: Dislocation forwards of the forearm without fracture of the olecranon. Brit. Med. J., *2*:1520, 1905.
271. Stehman, M., and Delmotte, S.: La mobilisation immediate des fractures de la tete radiale. Acta Orthop. Belg., *26*:214-230, 1960.
272. Steiger, R. N., Larrick, R. D., and Meyer, T. F.: Median-nerve entrapment following elbow dislocation in children (a report of two cases). J. Bone Joint Surg., *51A*:381-385, 1969.
273. Steindler, A.: The traumatic deformities and disabilities of the upper extremity. Springfield, Charles C Thomas, 1946.
274. Stimson, B. B.: A Manual of Fractures and Dislocations. ed. 2. Philadelphia, Lea & Febiger, 1947.
275. Stimson, L. A.: A Treatise on Fractures. Philadelphia, Henry C. Lea's Son and Co., 1890.
276. Strachan, J. C. H., and Ellis, B. W.: Vulnerability of the posterior interosseous nerve during radial head excision. J. Bone Joint Surg., *53B*:320-323, 1971.
277. Strug, L. H.: Anterior dislocation of the elbow with fracture of the olecranon. Amer. J. Surg., *75*:700-703, 1948.
278. Sudder, C. L.: The Treatment of Fractures. Philadelphia, W. B. Saunders, 1926.
279. Sullivan, M. F.: Rupture of the brachial artery from posterior dislocation of the elbow treated by veingraft (a case report). Brit. J. Surg., *58*:470-471, 1971.
280. Swenson, A. L.: The treatment of supracondylar fractures of the humerus by Kirschner-wire transfixion. J. Bone Joint Surg., *30A*:933-997, 1948.
281. Taylor, T. K. F., and O'Connor, B. T.: The effect upon the inferior radio-ulnar joint of excision of the head of the radius in adults. J. Bone Joint Surg., *46B*:83-88, 1964.
282. Taylor, T. K. F., and Scham, S. M.: A posteromedial approach to the proximal end of the ulna for the internal fixation of olecranon fractures. J. Trauma, *9*:594-602, 1969.
283. Tees, F. J., and McKim, L. H.: Case reports. Anterior dislocation of the elbow. Can. Med. Ass. J., *20*:36-38, 1929.
284. Thomas, T. T.: A contribution to the mechanism of fractures and dislocations in the elbow region. Ann. Surg., *89*:108-121, 1929.
285. ———: Fractures of the head of the radius. An experimental study and report of cases. Univ. Penn. Med. Bull., *18*: 184-197, 221-234, 1905.
286. Thompson, C. F., and Kalayjian, B.: Madelung's deformity and associated deformity at elbow. Surg. Gynecol. Obstet., *69*:221-230, 1939.
287. Thompson, H. C., III, and Garcia, A.: Myositis ossificans (aftermath of elbow injuries). Clin. Orthop., *50*:129-134, 1967.
288. Thorndike, A., Jr.: Myositis ossificans traumatica. J. Bone Joint Surg., *22*:315-323, 1940.
289. Thornton, L.: Fractures of the humerus treated by means of the Hoke plaster traction apparatus. J. Bone Joint Surg., *12*:911-917, 1930.
290. Trynin, A. H.: Intercondylar **T**-fracture of elbow. J. Bone Joint Surg., *23*:709-711, 1941.
291. Van Gorder, G. W.: Surgical approach in supracondylar **T**-fractures of the humerus requiring open reduction. J. Bone Joint Surg., *22*:278-292, 1940.
292. Venable, C. S.: An elbow and an elbow prosthesis. Amer. J. Surg., *83*:271-275, 1952.
293. Vesley, D. G.: Isolated traumatic dislocations of the radial head in children. Clin. Orthop., *50*:31-36, 1967.
294. Villagrana, J. C.: Advantages of operative treatment of fractures of the elbow. J. Bone Joint Surg., *14*:65-72, 1932.
295. Voshell, A. F., and Taylor, K. P. A.: Regeneration of the lateral condyle of the humerus after excision. J. Bone Joint Surg., *21*:421-424, 1939.

296. Waddell, G., and Hyatt, T. W.: A technique of plating severe olecranon fractures. Injury, *5*:135-140, 1973.
297. Wade, F. V., and Batdorf, J.: Supracondylar fractures of the humerus (a twelve year review with follow-up). J. Trauma, *1*:269-278, 1961.
298. Wagner, C. J.: Fractures of the head of the radius. Amer. J. Surg., *89*:911-913, 1955.
299. Wainwright, D.: Fractures of the olecranon process. Brit. J. Surg., *29*:403-406, 1942.
300. Watson-Jones, R.: Primary nerve lesions in injuries of the elbow and wrist. J. Bone Joint Surg., *12*:121, 1930.
301. ———: Fractures and Joint Injuries. ed. 3. vol. 2. Baltimore, Williams & Wilkins, 1946.
302. ———: Fractures and Joint Injuries. ed. 4. Edinburgh, E. & S. Livingstone. vol. 1, 1952; vol. 2, 1955.
303. Wheeler, D. K., and Linscheid, R. L.: Fracture-dislocations of the elbow. Clin. Orthop., *50*:95-106, 1967.
304. Wickstrom, J., and Meyer, P. R., Jr.: Fractures of the distal humerus in adults. Clin. Orthop., *50*:43-51, 1967.
305. Wiley, J. J.: Traumatic dislocation of the radial head. J. Bone Joint Surg., *53B*: 773, 1971.
306. Wiley, J. J., Horwich, J., and Pegington, J.: Traumatic dislocation of the radius at the elbow. J. Bone Joint Surg., *54B*:768, 1972.
307. Wilppula, E., Bakalim, G.: Fractures of the olecranon III. Fractures complicated by forward dislocation of the forearm. Ann. Chir. Gynaecol. Fenn., *60*:105-108, 1971.
308. Wilson, J. N.: The treatment of fractures of the medial epicondyle of the humerus. J. Bone Joint Surg., *42B*:778-781, 1960.
309. Wilson, P. D., and Cochrane, W. A.: Fractures and Dislocations. Philadelphia, J. B. Lippincott, 1925.
310. ———: Fracture and dislocation in the region of the elbow. Surg. Gynecol. Obstet., *56*:335-359, 1933.
311. ———: Management of Fractures and Dislocations. Philadelphia, J. B. Lippincott, 1938.
312. ———: Capsulectomy for the relief of flexion contractures of the elbow following fracture. J. Bone Joint Surg., *26*: 71-86, 1944.
313. Winslow, R.: A case of complete anterior dislocation of both bones of the forearm at the elbow. Surg. Gynecol. Obstet., *16*:570-571, 1913.
314. Wood, C. F.: Traffic elbow. Kentucky Med. J., *39*:78-81, 1941.
315. Yancey, D. L.: Fractures about the elbow joint. J. Missouri State Med. Ass., *44*: 262-267, 1947.
316. Yelton, C. L.: Injuries about the elbow. J. Bone Joint Surg., *37A*:650, 1955.
317. Young, C., Jr.: Primary elbow arthroplasty. Arch. Surg., *101*:78-81, 1970.
318. Zeitlin, A.: The traumatic origin of accessory bones at the elbow. J. Bone Joint Surg., *17*:933-938, 1935.
319. Zeno, L. O.: Supracondylar fractures of the humerus. Rev. Ortop. Traumatol., *3*:452-462, 1934.

10 Fractures of the Shaft of the Humerus

Charles H. Epps, Jr., M.D.

The shaft of the humerus is capable of a wide range of responses when it is fractured. Closed methods of treatment are usually successful, although in some fractures union is difficult to obtain. Open methods are sometimes necessary.

ANATOMY

An understanding of the anatomy of the upper arm is essential for proper treatment of fractures of the shaft of the humerus. Anatomically, the shaft may be considered to extend from the upper border of the insertion of the pectoralis major muscle above to the supracondylar ridges below. The upper half of the shaft is cylindrical on cross section; it tends to become flat in the distal portion in an anteroposterior direction. Three borders and three surfaces are described. The anterior border extends from the front of the greater tuberosity above to the coronoid fossa below. The medial border begins with the crest of the lesser tuberosity and ends at the medial supracondylar ridge. The lateral border extends from the back of the greater tuberosity above to the lateral supracondylar ridge. The anterolateral surface presents the deltoid tuberosity, for the insertion of the deltoid, and below this the radial sulcus, which transmits the radial nerve and profunda artery. The anteromedial surface forms the floor of the intertubercular groove, but it has no outstanding surface markings. The posterior surface is the origin for the triceps and contains the spiral groove.[28]

There are medial and lateral intermuscular septa which divide the arm into anterior and posterior compartments. The biceps brachii, coracobrachialis, and brachialis anticus muscles are contained in the anterior compartment. The neurovascular bundle courses along the mesial border of the biceps and includes the brachial artery and vein and the median, musculocutaneous, and ulnar nerves. The posterior compartment contains the triceps brachii muscle and the radial nerve.[33] An interesting variation is the supracondylar process, a projection arising from the anteromedial surface, about 2 inches above the medial epicondyle.[64] When the process is present, the median nerve and the brachial artery take an abnormal course to pass behind it and then forward between a fibrous band connecting the process to the epicondyle.

An analysis of humeral shaft fractures is made possible by an appreciation of the muscle forces that act on the shaft at varying levels (Fig. 10-1). A fracture above the level of the pectoralis major allows the proximal fragment to abduct and rotate internally, owing to action of the rotator cuff (Fig. 10-1A). If the shaft is broken above the deltoid insertion, this muscle pulls the lower fragment outward, while the pectoralis major, latissimus dorsi, and

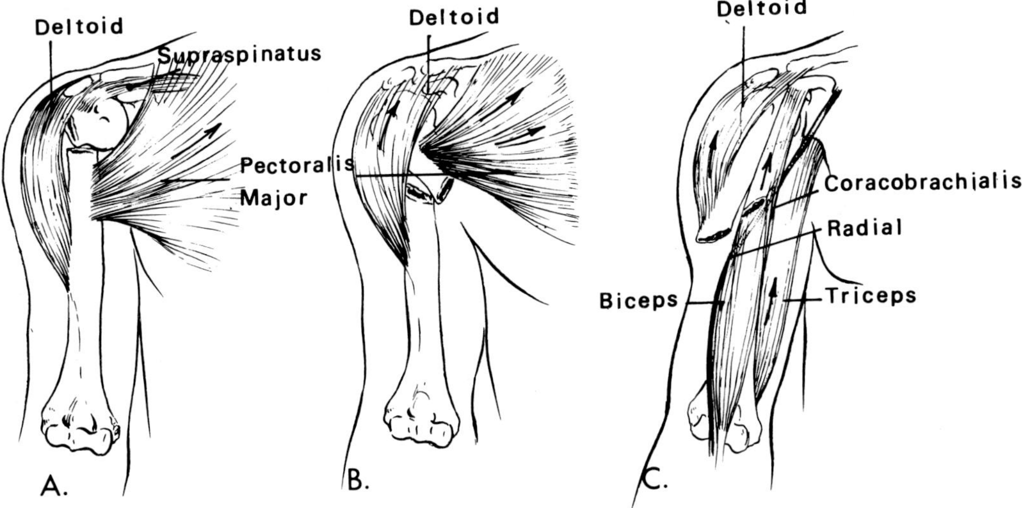

Fig. 10-1. Anatomical factors that influence deformities in typical fractures of the humeral shaft. (*A*) Fracture between rotator cuff and pectoralis major causing abduction and rotation of proximal fragment. (*B*) Fracture between pectoralis major insertion and deltoid producing adduction of proximal fragment. (*C*) Fracture below deltoid insertion causing abduction of proximal fragment.

teres major pull the proximal fragment inward (Fig. 10-1B). When the fracture line lies below the deltoid, this muscle and the coracobrachialis draw the upper fragment outward and forward while the lower fragment is drawn upward (Fig. 10-1C). Occasionally, the fracture ends remain in contact with varying degrees of angulation. It is more common for the ends to displace and override. This superior displacement is influenced to a considerable degree by muscle contraction, an observation that was probably responsible for the development of the hanging cast principle.

MECHANISMS OF INJURY

Fractures of the shaft of the humerus occur most frequently as the result of direct violence: falls, direct blows to the arm, automobile injuries, or crushing injuries from machinery. Missiles from firearms or shell fragments may pierce soft tissues and cause fractures. Therefore, many of these fractures are open. Indirect trauma, such as a fall on the elbow or the outstretched hand, or even violent muscle contraction, may cause fracture of the humeral shaft. There are reports of fractures incurred while throwing javelins, baseballs, or grenades violently and usually over-arm.[29] Typically, the injury occurs at the junction of the distal and middle thirds.

The common fractures of the adult humerus have been reproduced experimentally by simple mechanical means. Fractures at the proximal and distal ends are dependent on the anatomy of the bone itself, but shaft fractures vary according to the nature and degree of the trauma.[39] Compression forces acting on the humerus may affect either end but not the shaft. On the other hand, a bending force will produce a transverse fracture of the shaft, and a torsion force will result in a spiral fracture. A combination of bending and torsion will usually produce an oblique fracture and, possibly, a butterfly fragment.

The resulting angulation and displacement of the fracture fragments depend upon the fracturing forces, the level of fracture, and the influence of muscle pull. These factors have been analyzed above (Fig. 10-1).

CLASSIFICATION

Fractures of the shaft of the humerus may be conveniently classified on the basis of various factors. Several categories are utilized for full descriptive classification of individual fractures.

- I. Communication with external environment
  - A. Open
  - B. Closed
- II. Location of fracture
  - A. Above pectoralis major insertion
  - B. Below pectoralis major insertion but above deltoid insertion
  - C. Below deltoid insertion
- III. Degree of fracture
  - A. Incomplete
  - B. Complete
- IV. Direction and character of fracture line
  - A. Longitudinal
  - B. Transverse
  - C. Oblique
  - D. Spiral
  - E. Segmental
  - F. Comminuted
- V. Associated injury
  - A. Nerve
    - 1. Radial
    - 2. Median
    - 3. Ulnar
  - B. Blood vessel
    - 1. Brachial artery
    - 2. Brachial vein
- VI. Intrinsic condition of bone
  - A. Normal
  - B. Pathological
    - 1. Due to local bone changes
      - a. Bone atrophy
      - b. Inflammatory process
      - c. Neoplasm
        - (1) Benign
        - (2) Malignant
    - 2. Due to disorders affecting entire skeleton
      - a. Congenital abnormalities
      - b. Metabolic bone disease
      - c. Disseminated bone disorders of unknown etiology

CLINICAL SIGNS AND SYMPTOMS

When the fracture of the shaft of the humerus is complete with displacement, the diagnosis is usually obvious. The extremity is shortened, and there is abnormal mobility or crepitus on gentle manipulation associated with swelling and pain. The diagnosis is more difficult in incomplete fractures or fractures without displacement and is based on disability and point tenderness. The roentgenographic examination is confirmatory and must include both ends of the bone, the shoulder, and the elbow joint. The examiner must check for possible secondary or associated soft tissue injury carefully examining the entire extremity and the patient in general. The neurovascular status must be evaluated, and the initial examination must establish a baseline for comparison in the event of progressive vascular or neural complications.

ROENTGENOGRAPHIC FINDINGS

Roentgenographic examination must include not only two views of the entire bone, but the shoulder and the elbow joints. Anatomical variations in the shaft are uncommon. The supracondylar process, which arises from the anteromedial surface above the medial epicondyle, may be discovered initially on a roentgenogram made for trauma (Fig. 10-2). Median nerve symptoms resulting from fracture of the process have been reported by Newman.[52]

METHODS OF TREATMENT

Closed Methods

It was not many years ago that fractures of the shaft of the humerus were high on the list of injuries associated with delayed union and nonunion. Improved methods of closed treatment have reversed this tendency. The numerous methods available today allow considerable individuality in the election of a technique. The type and level of the fracture, the patient's age and

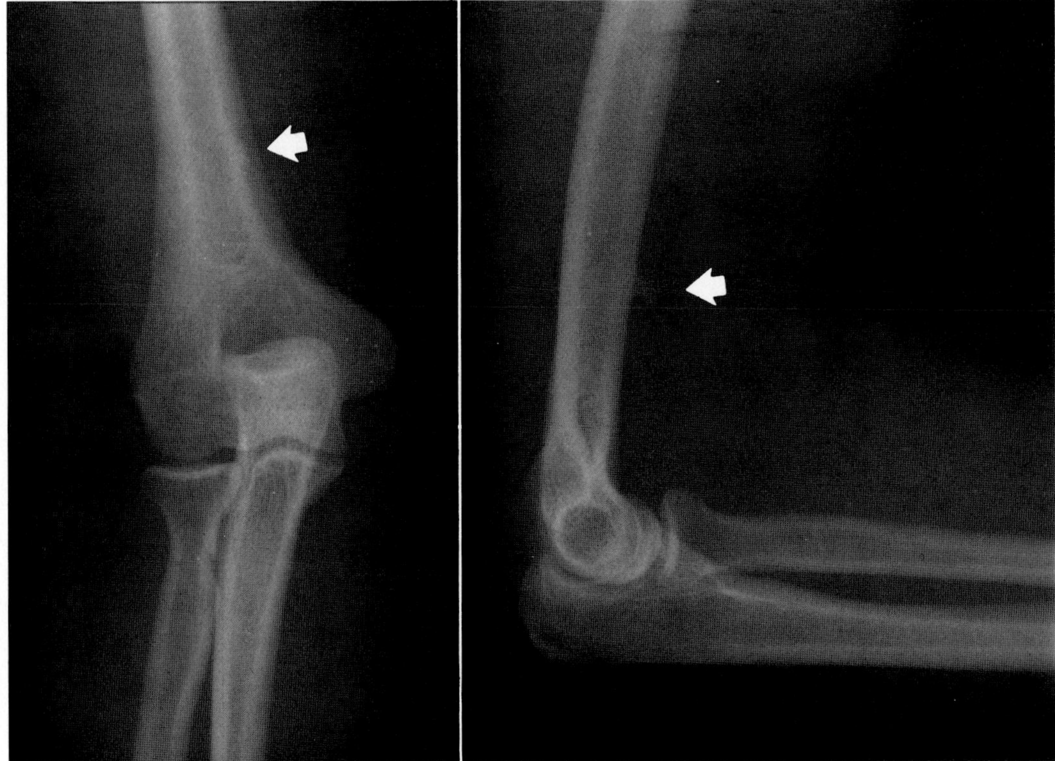

Fig. 10-2. Anteroposterior (*A*) and lateral (*B*) roentgenograms of distal humerus demonstrating a supracondylar process. This patient developed transient median nerve symptoms.

ability to cooperate, the degree of fracture displacement, and the presence of associated injuries are factors that influence the choice. The nonoperative means most frequently used have been (1) traction by means of a hanging cast, (2) coaptation or U-shaped brachial splint, (3) shoulder spica cast, (4) Velpeau or thoracobrachial casting, (5) abduction humeral splint, and (6) skeletal traction by means of a pin through the olecranon.

The Hanging Cast. Caldwell[8,9] introduced the hanging cast technique in 1933, and it has become one of the most widely accepted and successful methods for treatment of humeral shaft fractures. The cast is best applied to displaced fractures of the humeral shaft with shortening, and also to oblique and spiral fractures. However, it can be used in most instances, including comminuted fractures and those involving the distal shaft, when certain principles are carefully observed:[63]

1. The cast must be lightweight and must extend from at least 1 inch proximal to the fracture site to the wrist, with the elbow at a right angle and the forearm in neutral rotation (Fig. 10-3).

2. The arm must always be dependent so as to provide a traction force. The patient should sleep erect or semierect and must avoid supporting the elbow when seated.

3. The sling must be securely fixed at the wrist by a loop made of plaster or other material. To correct lateral angulation, place the loop on the dorsum of the wrist; to correct medial angulation, place it on the volar side.

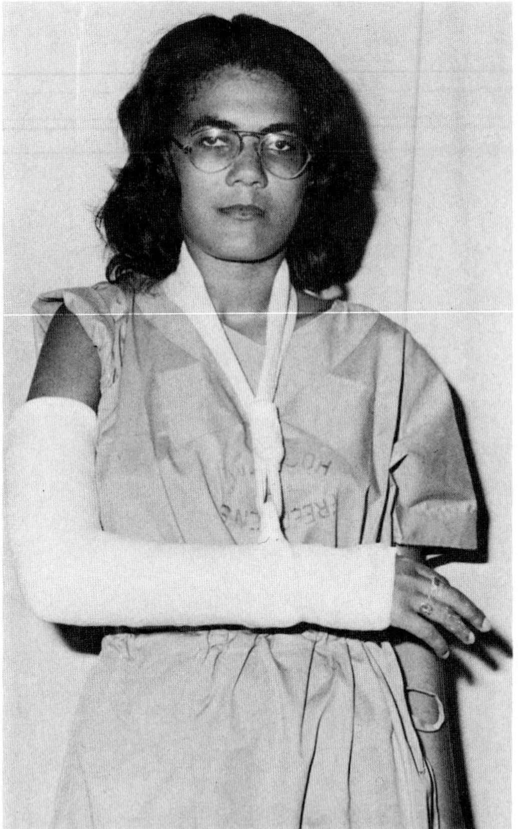

Fig. 10-3. Typical hanging cast.

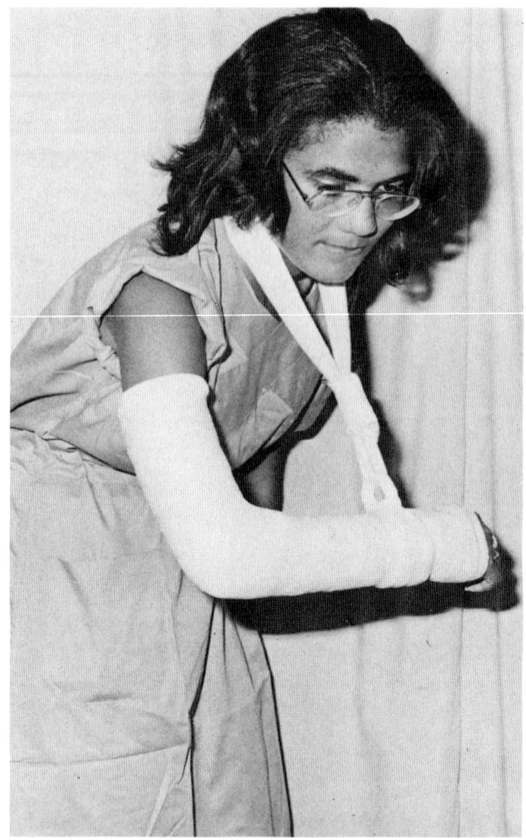

Fig. 10-4. Patient in forward flexed position with hanging cast swinging free for circumduction and pendulum exercises.

4. Posterior angulation should be corrected by lengthening the sling or suspension apparatus; shortening the sling corrects anterior angulation.

5. Roentgenograms of the fracture should be made at weekly intervals, or as frequently as indicated.

6. Exercises should be started immediately. Finger exercises will prevent a stiff hand. If the cast stops at the wrist, this joint is also exercised. As soon as comfort permits, or in a few days, circumduction exercises must be instituted to prevent distraction, shoulder subluxation, and particularly, adhesive capsulitis (Fig. 10-4). This is accomplished by having the patient bend forward at the waist, allowing the cast to hang free in order to perform circumduction and pendulum movements.

7. Isometric exercises are also helpful under these circumstances and can be done easily by the patient in the hanging cast or splint. It is felt that isometrics assist in the prevention of distraction and help to pull fragments together.

The requirement that the vertical position be maintained is regarded by some as a disadvantage. However, it can be accomplished easily if the patient is cooperative. Occasionally for an obese person a wedge or pad may be required at the medial aspect of the elbow where angulation occurs due to a pendulous breast or redundant tissue. The pad is added if dorsal placement of the wrist loop does not suffice. It is not essential to obtain perfect alignment and apposition. The musculature of the upper arm will accommodate 20 degrees of

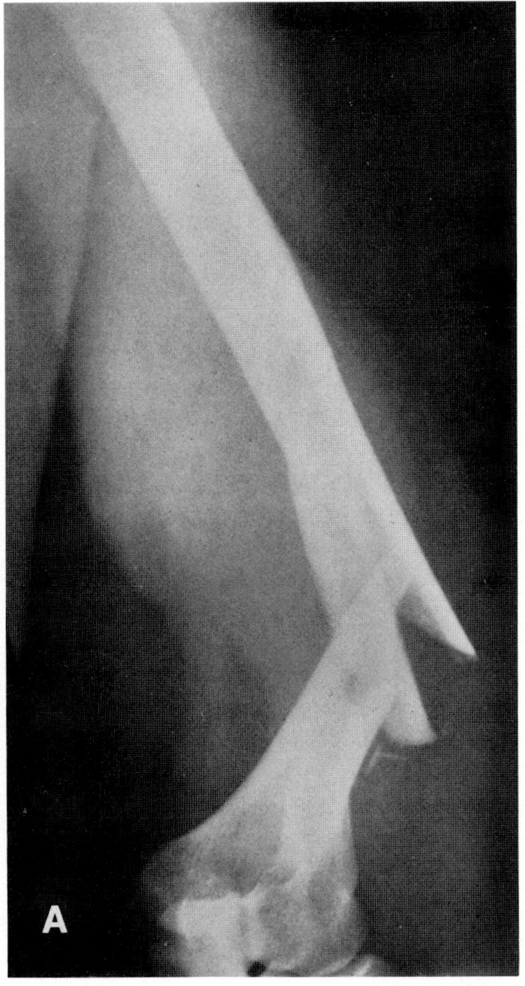

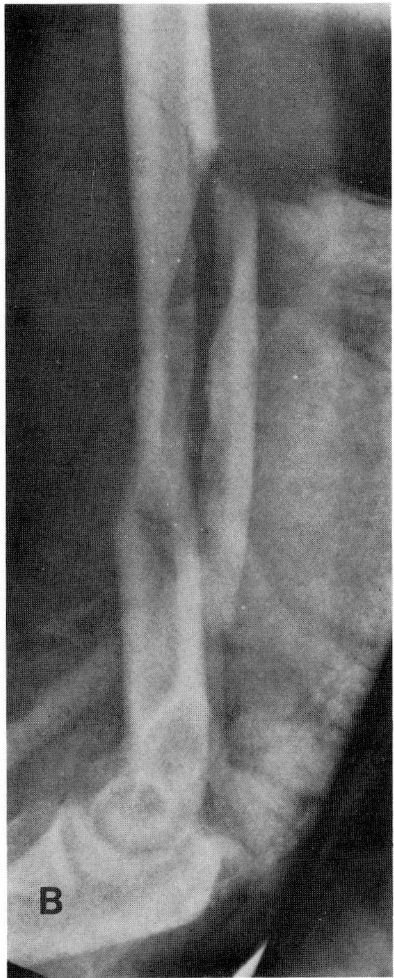

Fig. 10-5. (*A*) Comminuted fracture of the distal humerus. (*B, C on page 570*) Fracture in plaster. (*D, E*) The fracture was clinically solid after 2 months and function of the arm was excellent.

anterior angulation and 30 degrees of varus angulation without compromising function or appearance.[38] Similarly, bayonet position resulting in shortening up to 1 inch is not noticeable in the upper extremity and requires a minor adjustment in the sleeve lengths of clothing.

Spiral, comminuted, and oblique fractures have the advantage of generous fracture surface areas and tend to heal rapidly (Fig. 10-5). Simple transverse fractures without comminution in some instances fail to unite as promptly and require closer observation to avoid distraction and angulation. Fractures just distal to the insertion of the deltoid muscle are prone to abduction of the proximal fragment and also require special attention.

In the 40 years since its introduction, the hanging cast has enjoyed wide application by a great number of surgeons with outstanding success. Winfield and others[67] in 1942 reported 136 cases in which the hanging cast was used exclusively. Of this number 103 were available for analysis. There was one case of delayed union and one of nonunion. Stewart and Hundley,[62] in 1955, reported 107 fractures treated in hanging

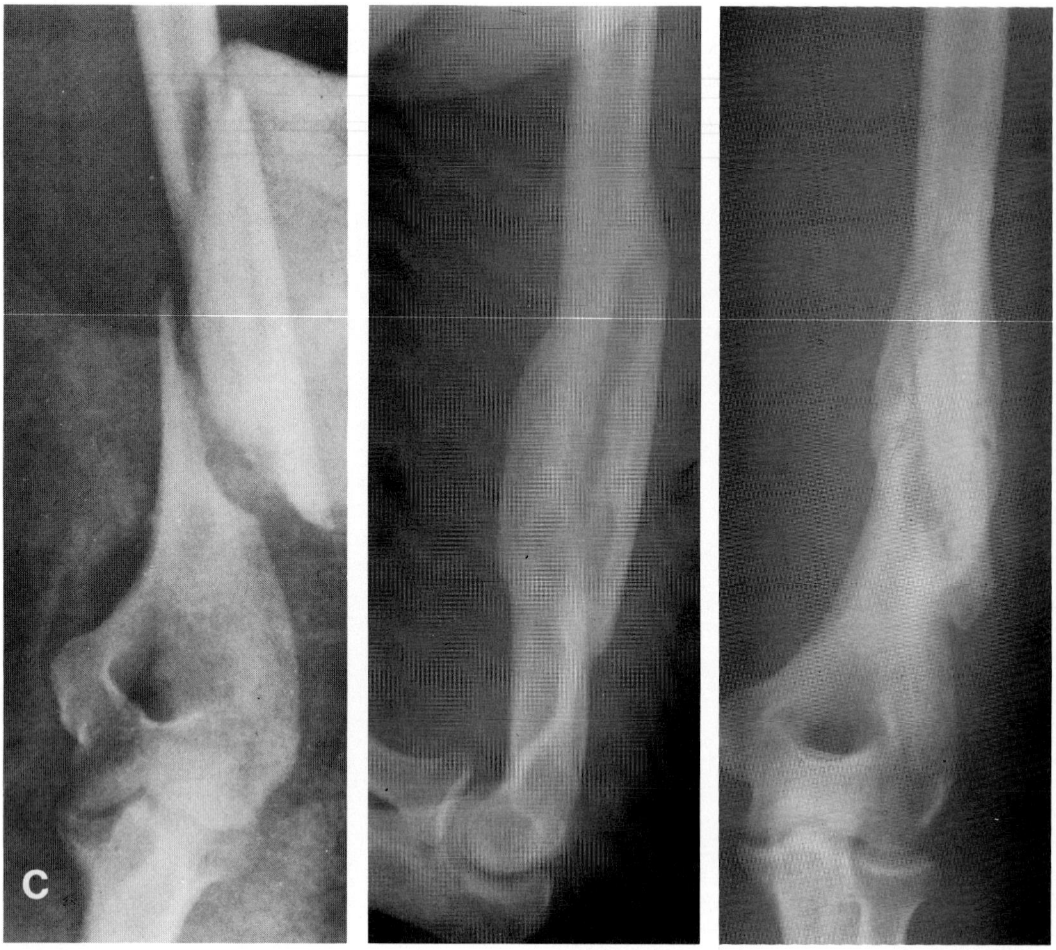

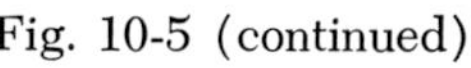

Fig. 10-5 (continued)

casts; 93.5 per cent of the patients experienced excellent or good results, and 6.5 per cent, fair or poor. In 1959, the Pennsylvania Orthopaedic Society[60] reported a study of 159 fractures of the humeral shaft. The hanging cast was used in 54 per cent of the patients, and of these 96 per cent attained union, in an average of 10 weeks' healing time. Stewart[63] cites a study by Louis Breck and members of the Trauma Committee of the American Academy of Orthopaedic Surgeons in 1961, in which 95.4 per cent of 174 patients with hanging cast treatment obtained good results. The last two reports concern cooperative studies by a number of surgeons and affirm the general applicability of this technique. The current literature[14,35,43,56] and many standard texts[1,12,17,37,45] contain reports of success with the hanging cast.

Coaptation Splint. The application of a U-shaped coaptation plaster splint with a collar and cuff is another acceptable method (Fig. 10-6). The prime candidate is the patient whose fracture might be distracted by even a light hanging cast. The slab of plaster is placed over thin but adequate layers of padding adhered to wet coatings of benzoin and secured by a Kling bandage to prevent slippage. The slab extends from the axilla around the elbow and over the deltoid. The collar and cuff may be shortened or lengthened to maintain alignment. This technique, sometimes called a "sugar-tong splint," may also be useful as secondary immobilization after a period of time in the hanging cast or other means. It has the distinct advantage of allowing exercises at the elbow, wrist, and hand, as well as the shoulder, during the entire period of immobilization. Bohler,[5] Charnley,[13] and DePalma[21] expressed a preference for this splint over the hanging cast.

Abduction Humeral Splint. Stewart[63] has advocated use of the humeral abduction splint in certain fractures of the shaft. Close and continued observation is required, but increased comfort is cited as an advantage. The splint supports the arm and cast in abduction and maintains the humerus in straight alignment. This method is best used as an adjunct only in the early stages of treatment, as it eliminates the possibility of shoulder exercises.

Shoulder Spica Cast. The shoulder spica has been recommended in the early healing stage of the unstable fracture and where delayed union or nonunion appears imminent. It is usually replaced by a simpler form of treatment as soon as the fracture fragments show signs of maintaining reduction. Its drawbacks are the difficulty encountered in applying it, its weight and awkwardness and patient discomfort in hot, humid climates. Additional problems are encountered if the patient is elderly or obese. From the practical standpoint, it is not clear that the shoulder spica provides better immobilization.

Open Velpeau-Type Cast. Holm[32] has advocated the open Velpeau-type cast for active and unmanageable children under 8 or 10 years of age and for some older patients unable to cooperate in the use of hanging casts. Axillary and forearm Webril or polyurethane forearm pads are inserted to maintain the desired degree of abduction and flexion of the arm. The elbow is flexed to 90 degrees. Coaptation splints are secured by circumferential turns of plaster, passing around the arm, shoulder, and trunk. The cast is windowed anteromedially to expose the axilla and antecubital fossa and molded carefully about the elbow, axilla, and the iliac crest. The cast is cut off around the wrist to allow active wrist and finger exercises. Once healing has progressed enough so that the cast can be removed, a less rigid support is substituted.

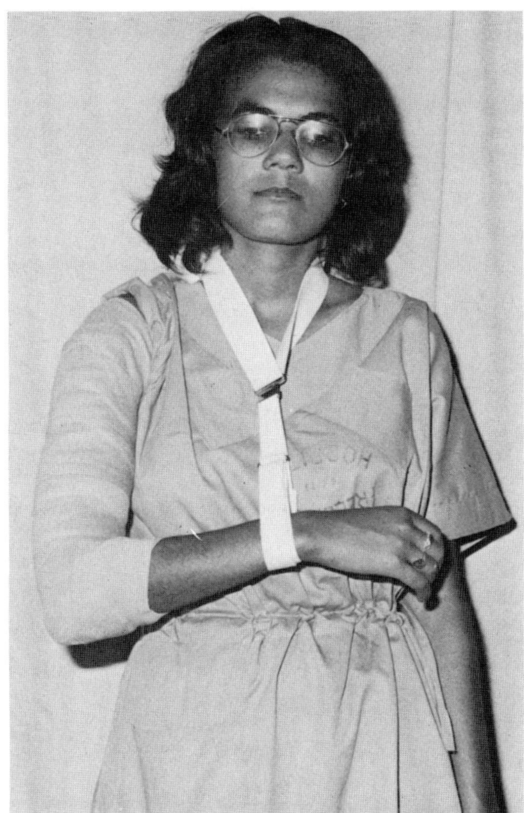

Fig. 10-6. U-shaped coaptation splint and wrist suspension appliance.

Skeletal Traction. Occasionally, in special circumstances when the patient cannot walk, skeletal traction must be used. Associated skeletal injuries that require the patient to remain recumbent and extensive compound fracture wounds are frequent indications. The method requires the patient's cooperation and close supervision by the surgeon. Traction is provided by a Kirschner wire (0.0625-inch) or a Steinmann pin (5/32- or 7/64-inch), inserted through the olecranon (Fig. 10-7).

The technique of traction is simple, but it should be applied under sterile skin prep-

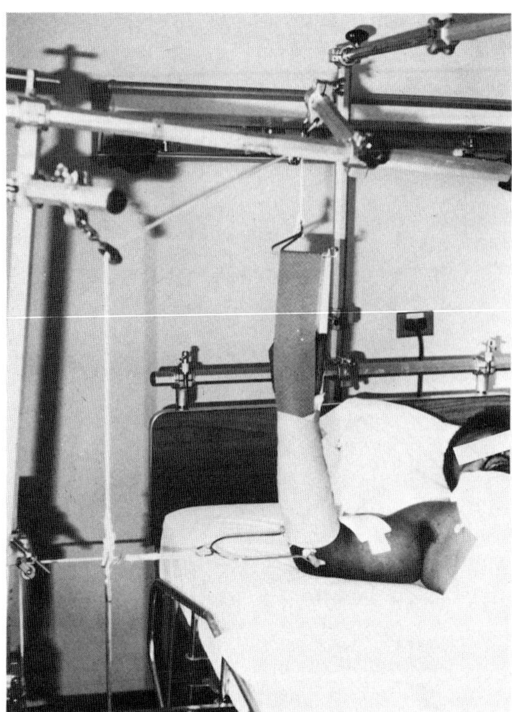

Fig. 10-7. Lateral traction with a Steinmann pin through the olecranon. Note dressing over the compound fracture wound on the anterior aspect of upper arm. Patient also sustained posterior dislocation of right hip in a vehicular accident.

aration and draping in order to minimize infection. The procedure may be performed in the emergency room, but the operating room is ideal. The site for insertion is selected where the olecranon joins the body of the ulna, and a tract down to the periosteum is infiltrated with a local anesthetic. A small nick is made in the skin, and, with a cannulated hand drill, the Kirschner wire or Steinmann pin is inserted in a plane perpendicular to the longitudinal axis of the ulna. The ulnar nerve is best avoided by drilling the wire from the medial to the lateral side. If circumstances demand another site, the wire may be inserted in the distal humerus. Soft tissues on the other side of the bone at the point of exit are also infiltrated, thus making the entire procedure relatively painless. The wire is usually drilled until equal lengths protrude from both sides of the elbow, and then sterile dressings are applied. The handle of the Kirschner wire bow should be tightened to minimize the tendency of the wire to bend. The Steinmann pin bow should not be used for a Kirschner wire, nor a Kirschner wire bow for a Steinmann pin. A disposable nylon bow is available that accepts both pins and wires.* The elbow is flexed to 90 degrees, and the forearm is supported by adhesive material or additional skeletal traction.

Active exercises of the hand and wrist are possible and should be encouraged while the arm is in traction.

Sling and Swathe. Certain elderly patients may be best managed in a sling and stockinette body swathe.[12] In these cases the reduction is not a critical consideration, but comfort of the patient and disadvantages of other forms of immobilization are major factors. A wedge-shaped axillary pad may be used to obtain a few degrees of abduction in the distal fragment. The apparatus requires frequent adjustment, but this is easy to do. The shoulder is freed for exercises in a week or two, or when comfort permits.

Operative Methods

Open Fractures. The open fracture is an orthopaedic emergency and requires operative treatment. In many cases patients have multiple injuries, and proper consideration must be given to treatment priority. Attention is given first to patency of the airway, hemorrhage, and shock. Tetanus toxoid or antitoxin is given as indicated. A sterile dressing covers the wound, and the limb is splinted until the patient reaches the operating theater.

The wound is cleansed and debrided in the standard orthopaedic manner. Care is exercised to avoid injuring blood vessels and nerves. Sterile saline is used in copious amounts, and cultures are taken to identify

* Salvatore Traction Bow. Wright Manufacturing Co., Memphis, Tenn.

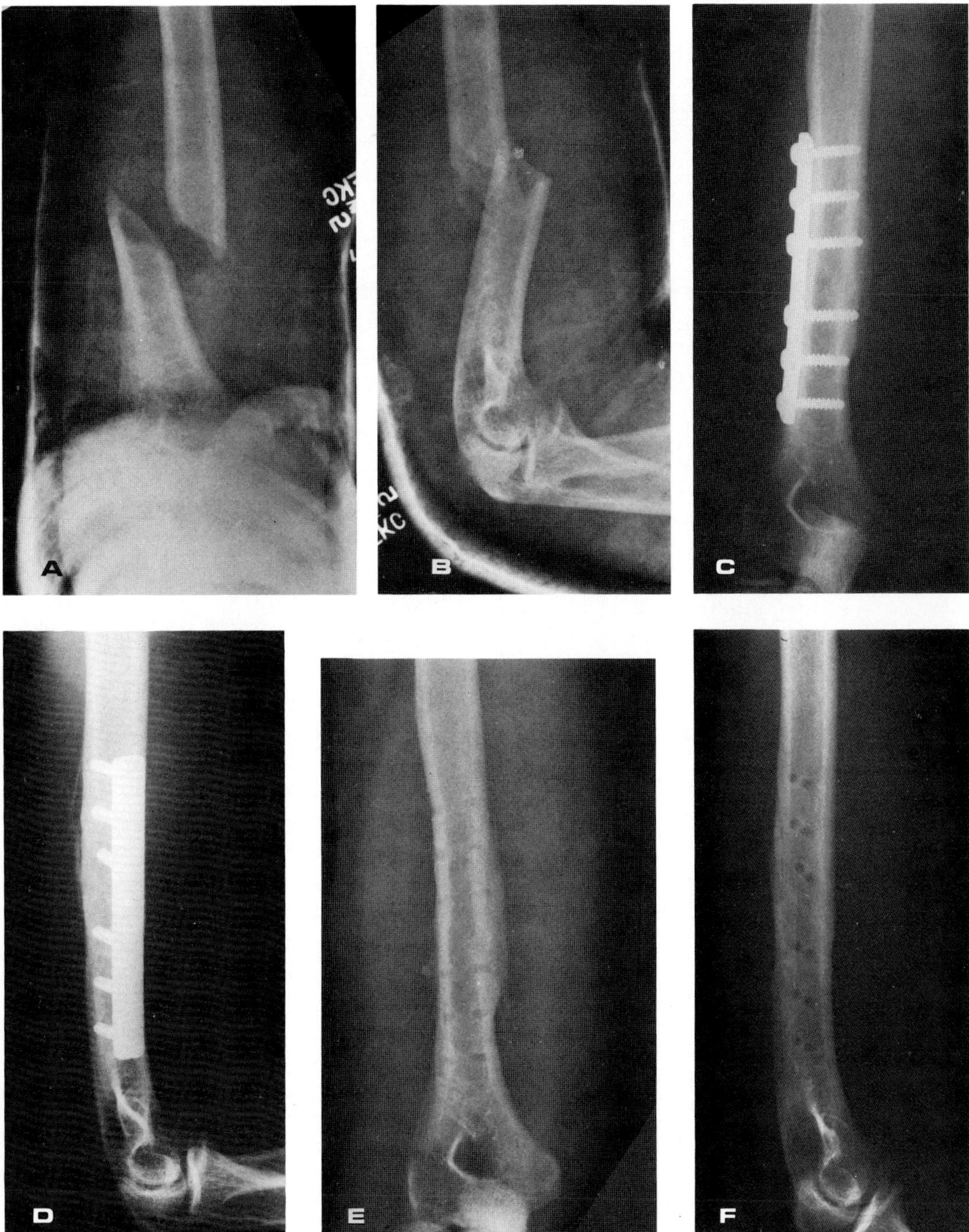

Fig. 10-8. (*A, B*) Roentgenograms of fracture at junction of middle and distal thirds showing poor position due to soft-tissue interposition. (*C, D*) Same fracture after application of an AO compression plate and cancellous bone graft. Union obtained at 6 weeks. (*E, F*) Roentgenograms of fracture after removal of plate and screws.

any pathogens that may be present. There are surgeons who elect primary closure for wounds that are seen in the first 6 to 8 hours after injury and that are considered "clean." On the other hand, some surgeons routinely leave open all wounds, particularly those seen after 8 to 12 hours, grossly contaminated wounds, and gunshot and combat wounds. Delayed primary closure, after 5 to 7 days, has been proved an excellent and safe means of wound care in daily practice as well as under war conditions.[15,25]

The election of internal fixation, if any, is a matter determined by the experience and judgment of the surgeon.

Closed Fractures. Because closed methods of treatment for humeral shaft fractures have a high rate of success, open reduction of closed fractures is rarely indicated. There are several situations in which open reduction and internal fixation may be indicated. First, there are certain segmental fractures in which satisfactory position and alignment cannot be achieved. Secondly, pathological fractures secondary to malignancy should be fixed. Certain of these also may be treated successfully by coaptation splints. Shaft fractures with associated injuries of the elbow that require early mobilization need internal fixation. Any fracture associated with a vascular injury should be fixed. Last, a spiral fracture of the distal humerus, of the type described by Holstein and Lewis,[34] in which a radial nerve palsy develops after hanging cast treatment or manipulation requires internal fixation. Similar indications for open reduction and internal fixation have been listed in Campbell's *Operative Orthopaedics.*[19] Another possible indication is Parkinson's disease or another neurological or systemic disease that would make the hanging cast or its equivalent inappropriate.

The shaft of the humerus is easily approached by medial displacement of the biceps and incision of the brachialis. This exposure avoids the radial nerve, but retraction must be done gently to avoid injury. The proximal shaft may be approached through the deltopectoral groove, and in the distal one-third a posterior incision is useful. Excellent descriptions of surgical approaches to this area are available in Campbell's *Operative Orthopaedics,*[19] Banks and Laufman's *Atlas of Surgical Exposures of the Extremities,* and Henry's *Extensile Exposure.*

Once the surgeon has decided that an open reduction is indicated, the techniques and the type of internal fixation device must be chosen. Plates provide rigid internal fixation for fresh fractures and nonunion. However, the AO type of plate, developed by Müller and associates,[49] is designed to provide not only rigid fixation but also compression (Fig. 10-8). The experiences of many surgeons have established this as one of the preferred methods in open reduction.[6,19,51] Cancellous bone graft can be added at the time of operation to promote osteosynthesis and minimize the predisposition to nonunion. Postoperatively, there is the advantage that external fixation is not needed, and active mobilization of the whole extremity can be pursued during the entire course of fracture healing. Even if the surgeon wishes to apply external immobilization in the form of a posterior splint for a few weeks or just during wound healing, the early mobility should reduce the tendency for stiffness in all joints.

Intramedullary rods and nails are used in humeral fractures to maintain alignment and length.[59] In general they do not provide as rigid internal fixation as plates. For this reason most rods require supplemental external immobilization, at least during part of the time required for healing. Küntscher[40,42] has described a technique of intramedullary nailing in which the length and circumference of the nails are carefully determined. This method, applied to properly selected cases, provides the rigid fixation needed for osteosynthesis. Küntscher specifically recommends that external support not be applied. Under these circumstances the patient is allowed active exercise. Multiple intramedullary rods inserted from below by the method of Hackethal[50] have been described as useful. Preliminary reports of a few cases show good results with an elastic plastic pin (of Supramid) inserted in the medullary canal.[53,54] The choice of a technique for intramedullary nailing will depend upon the training and experience of the surgeon. Infection is particularly unfortunate when it develops after intramedullary nailing or any open procedure that utilizes internal fixation.

Screw fixation inserted across a long spiral fracture has been utilized, but the internal fixation is less secure than with other methods. Circumferential wire loops and Parham bands have been used in the past, but, used alone, they seem to have no place in today's armamentarium.

Occasionally, one may wish to use autogenous or homogenous cortical bone grafts for internal fixation. In these circumstances, the plating material provides not only internal fixation but osteosynthesis as well. Such grafts are also useful in bridging defects in the shaft of the humerus.

The level of the fracture may also influence the choice of an internal fixation device. A fracture in the shaft may be suited to either an intramedullary rod or a plate, but fractures at the ends of the humerus demand careful selection of a device. A rod may be better applied proximally, while a plate would meet the requirements of a distal fracture.

Interesting and extremely revealing data is available through a comparison of the results obtained by closed treatment as opposed to open reduction in two reported series. Breck's[63] study reported 95.4 per cent good results in 174 treated closed in hanging casts, while 50 fractures, handled by open reduction, had 88 per cent good results. In the Pennsylvania Orthopaedic Society study,[60] the good results were 96 per cent for the closed cases treated in a hanging cast and 88 per cent for the open cases.

AUTHOR'S PREFERRED METHOD OF TREATMENT

Dependency Traction

It has been my experience that most closed fractures of the humeral shaft can be treated by nonoperative methods. Dependency traction is the treatment I prefer. Through the years the hanging cast has been used successfully by utilizing certain recognized mechanical principles (Fig. 10-9). Lengthening the sling helps to correct posterior bowing; shortening the sling helps correct anterior bowing. A valgus deformity of the distal fragment can be

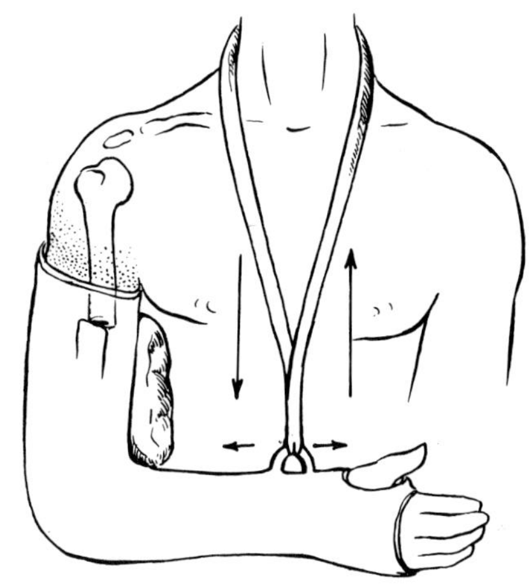

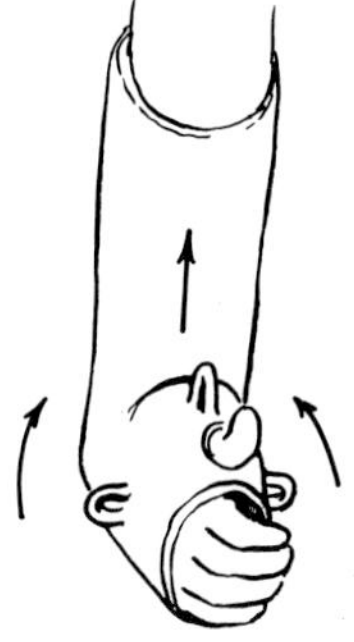

Fig. 10-9. Biomechanical factors of hanging cast technique. Shortening the suspension device corrects anterior bowing, while lengthening corrects posterior bowing. When moved toward the elbow the wrist loop reduces the traction force; when moved toward the wrist, it increases the force. A dorsal position of the loop reduces a varus deformity, and a more volar position reduces a valgus deformity. Note axillary pad to correct varus tendency.

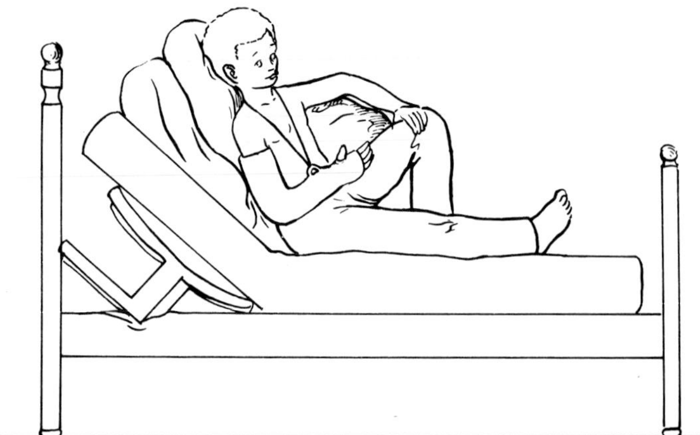

Fig. 10-10. A chair inverted and placed between the mattress and bedspring makes the semi-Fowler's position possible at home.

reduced by placing the plaster wrist loop in a more volar position. Conversely, a varus deformity of the distal fragment can be improved by placing a pad or roll of Webril at the elbow of the cast (medial wall), and by moving the plaster loop to a more dorsal position. The weight of the cast can be kept to a minimum by using two 4-inch plaster rolls. The hanging cast should remain in place 4 to 6 weeks; the degree of healing is easily determined by roentgenographic examination. One may apply a **U**-shaped coaptation splint if the surgeon wants to remove the hanging cast early. Usually, patients are comfortable in a collar and cuff or a sling for a week or two after cast removal, while the elbow joint is mobilized.

In recent times, I have used the **U**-shaped coaptation splint more frequently. The splint requires less plaster than the hanging cast and is lighter and has less tendency to distract the fragments. More importantly, this method allows not only circumduction of the shoulder, as can be done with the hanging cast, but active exercises of the elbow, wrist, and hand. If there is a disadvantage, it is the fact that the physician cannot control against possible varus or valgus deformity by changing the position of the wrist loop. As soon as the fracture has healed sufficiently to permit removal of immobilization, a vigorous exercise program designed to restore strength and range of motion is begun.

The dependency position can be maintained in bed by placing an inverted chair under the mattress (Fig. 10-10). Pillows are added to prop the patient in a comfortable position.

For complicated cases that require lateral traction, I prefer using a threaded Steinmann pin (5/32- or 7/64-inch) or a Kirschner wire (0.0625-inch) at the olecranon. This may be used in combination with coaptation humeral splints and a sling, if necessary, to control bowing. When conditions permit and the patient may walk about, the **U**-shaped splint or some other means is utilized.

Very few closed fractures require open reduction. When it is indicated, I prefer the compression plating technique in transverse or short oblique fractures. This method provides rigid internal fixation and compression. If for any reason open reduction has been postponed for several weeks, I add cancellous bone grafts at the primary procedure. When alignment is the critical requirement, a Rush nail or a Küntscher nail will suffice. I usually use the Rush rod. The indications for open reduction listed above have served me well.

Wound management is a most important consideration in open fractures. My preference is thorough debridement and irrigation with the wound left open. Cultures are taken before treatment and after the final irrigation. The patient is usually given a broad-spectrum antibiotic until a specific

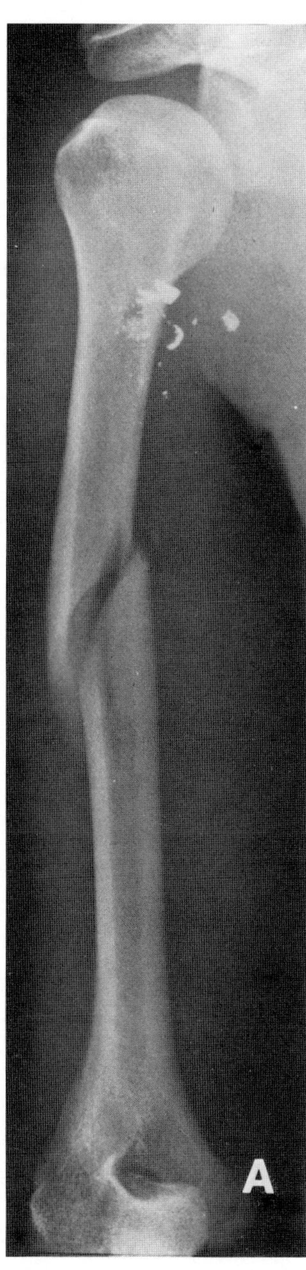

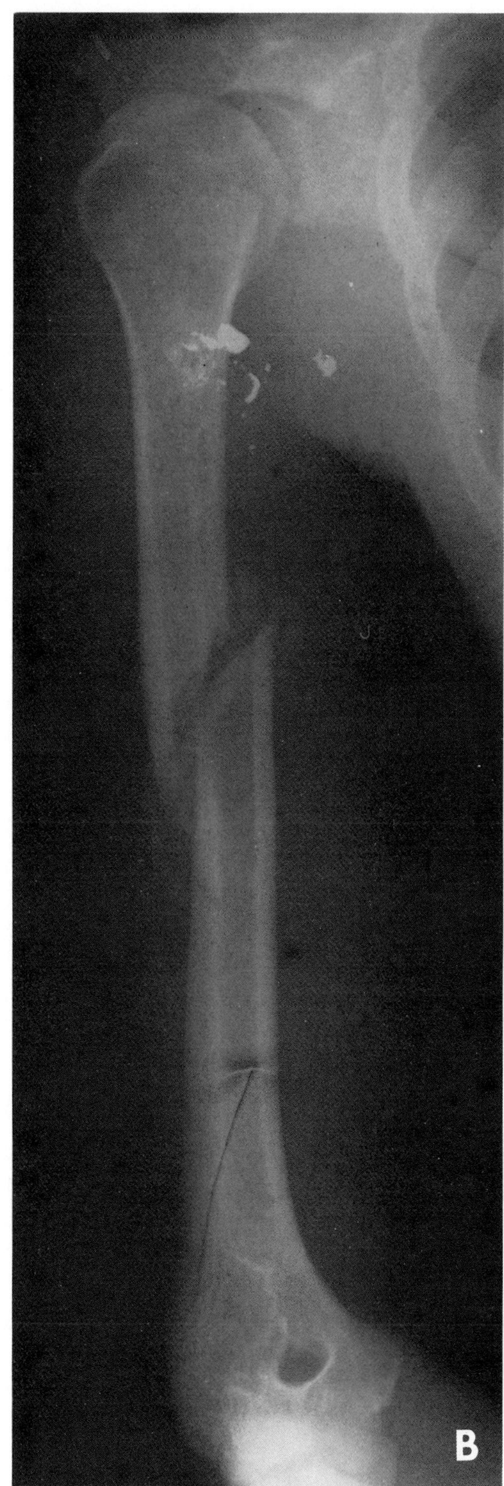

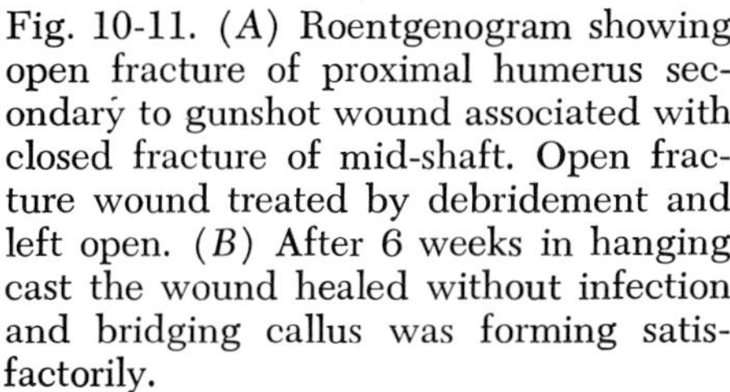
Fig. 10-11. (*A*) Roentgenogram showing open fracture of proximal humerus secondary to gunshot wound associated with closed fracture of mid-shaft. Open fracture wound treated by debridement and left open. (*B*) After 6 weeks in hanging cast the wound healed without infection and bridging callus was forming satisfactorily.

organism is cultured and the best antibiotic is determined by sensitivity studies. Under these circumstances, it is my usual practice to start intravenous administration of a broad-spectrum antibiotic in the Emergency Room and continue it for 5 to 7 days postoperatively. If the wound is clinically clean, delayed primary closure is done between the fifth and seventh days. A hanging cast or traction can be used as dictated by other circumstances (Fig. 10-11).

POSTFRACTURE CARE AND REHABILITATION

It is essential to remember that the rehabilitation of the patient begins immediately after the injury. Immobilization devices should be applied in a manner that will allow maximum active exercise. Early and vigorous movement of the hand is essential if stiffness is to be avoided. When the hanging cast is used and the wrist is immobilized, the plaster should be trimmed proximal to the metacarpophalangeal joints to allow full flexion of the fingers. The patient is started early on circumduction exercise for the shoulder (Fig. 10-4). This may not be possible the same day, but it usually can be accomplished by the second or third day after injury. In this manner, adhesive capsulitis of the shoulder can be prevented. The patient in skeletal traction is also instructed to move his fingers and wrist to maintain full mobility of these joints.

Once the cast, splint, or traction has been removed, the patient is started on a well planned and closely supervised program of exercise to regain strength and joint motion in the entire extremity. Stewart[63] made the observation that, barring mechanical interference in any joint, whether from trauma, infection, or other abnormality, the function will return in direct proportion to the strength of the musculature that controls that joint. The elbow merits special attention and should not be passively stretched. Myositis ossificans has been observed in elbows and is avoided by limiting the exercise to an active routine performed by the patient. The shoulder can be benefited by an assistive and passive program combined with the active routine.

It is vitally important that the surgeon make his patient aware of the importance of the rehabilitation program from the day of injury until maximum recovery has been realized.

PROGNOSIS

Careful consideration of at least eight factors will give the surgeon a fairly accurate prognosis for humeral shaft fractures. The first factor to be weighed is the type of fracture. Spiral and oblique fractures and those that are comminuted tend to heal better than transverse or segmental fractures.

Second, fractures that are in close proximity to either the shoulder joint or the elbow joint may have a compromised outcome, depending upon the degree of involvement of the soft tissues supporting the joint. Third, an open wound is a significant factor; the open fracture tends to heal more slowly, and there is always the additional risk of infection and osteomyelitis. Fourth, the interposition of soft tissue may make the attaining of a satisfactory reduction impossible by closed means, and open surgery involves entirely different considerations with regard to risk and management. Next, the outcome is affected substantially by the presence of either neural or vascular involvement. Naturally, if both components are injured, the prognosis is more serious. A sixth consideration is the complex situation in which associated fractures in the shoulder, elbow, or forearm may affect the end result. The mode of treatment is a factor. Patients who require thoracobrachial immobilization instead of the U-type splint or hanging cast, have a greater chance of joint stiffness. Finally, the degree of cooperation by the patient, especially as reflected by his willingness to exercise actively, affects the functional result. The surgeon who approaches his patient with an awareness of these prognostic considerations can make enlightened decisions.

COMPLICATIONS

Neural Complications

Among complications associated with fractures of the shaft of the humerus, injury to the radial nerve is probably the most common. Fortunately, the wrist drop usually makes this condition easy to recognize. However, in the patient with multiple severe injuries, the examiner may be preoccupied with other matters that are potentially life-threatening, or the patient's unresponsive state may make careful motor examination difficult or impossible. Under these circumstances, radial nerve injury may be overlooked. The examiner must be alert to this possible complication and return, when time and circumstances permit, to make a careful examination of the entire extremity, including its neurovascular status. This practice helps avoid the embarrassment of belated diagnosis of a radial palsy.

It has been estimated that 5 or 10 per cent of patients with humeral shaft fractures demonstrate radial nerve involvement. This is particularly true in spiral fractures in the distal third. The displaced fragments may trap the nerve in the fracture site. The anatomical features of this fracture have been analyzed and described by Holstein and Lewis[34] (Fig. 10-12), and Whitson.[66] This situation demands open reduction through the lateral approach and internal fixation.

Most radial nerve injuries are the result of stretching or bruising and are incomplete. Function will return within days or months. Where the radial nerve lesion is complete, delayed repair has achieved results as good or better than those of primary repair. Therefore, there is little or no need to explore the nerve unless there is another reason for open intervention. Stewart[63] feels that exploration of the nerve to determine the severity of injury is indicated only in an open fracture. Electromyography and nerve conduction study are important aids in determining the precise degree of nerve damage and are valuable in monitoring the rate of nerve regeneration. Seddon[61] made the astute clinical observation that the surgeon is justified in waiting until the calendar tells him that the axons regenerating at the rate of 1 mm.

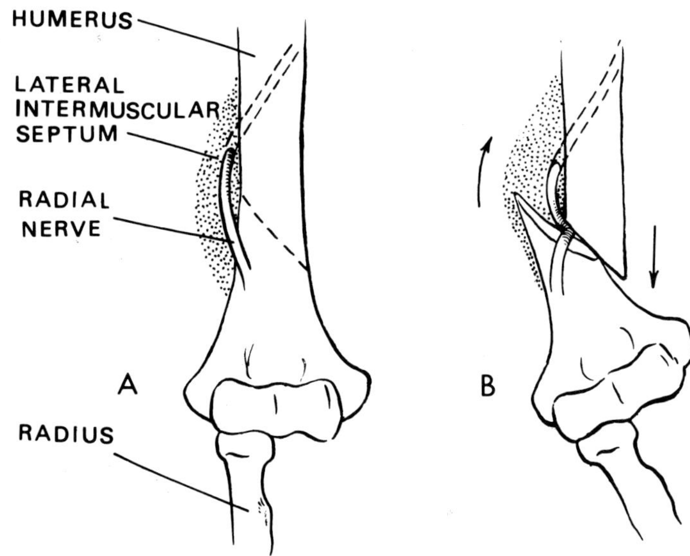

Fig. 10-12. Fractures of the distal third of the humerus may be particularly vulnerable to radial nerve injury. (*A*) The relationship of the radial nerve to the fracture. (*B*) with lateral displacement and overriding of the distal fragment. The nerve, fixed to the proximal fragment by the intermuscular septum, is trapped between the fracture surfaces when closed reduction is attempted. (Holstein, A. and Lewis, G. B.: J. Bone Joint Surg., *45A*:1382, 1963)

a day ought to have reached the most proximal muscle.

A sound program is to treat the fracture and support the fingers and wrist with a dynamic splint. After the fracture has healed, the nerve can be repaired if necessary. Usually nerve function will be returning by this time.

Palsy of the radial nerve can be seen after open reduction, as a result of too vigorous traction at operation. Transient palsy of the median and ulnar nerves is rare but may be seen with humeral shaft fracture.

Vascular Complications

Fractures complicated by vascular injury constitute severe orthopaedic emergencies and demand prompt restoration of blood supply if the limb is to be saved. Primary control of hemorrhage can be accomplished, usually by direct pressure, while the patient is readied for surgery. If the vascular injury is associated with an open fracture, the vessel should be explored and repaired after the fracture has been stabilized by internal fixation. On the other hand, angiography is an extremely valuable aid in determining the level of vascular impairment in injuries to the brachial artery. The choice of technique for definitive arterial repair in a particular case is governed by the type of injury and its location. Clean lacerations, involving short segments of arterial wall often can be managed by lateral repair. Jagged injuries and gunshot wounds may require excision of segments of artery, after which end-to-end anastomosis is performed, if it can be accomplished without too much tension. If not, a graft is required.

There are occasions when the artery is sufficiently traumatized to cause vascular spasm. This condition obliterates the vessel without thrombosis or laceration. The effects of spasm may be reversed by periarterial infiltration with Novocain or Xylocaine. The stellate ganglion block may be helpful in some cases. If the spasm persists, the vessel should be explored and the serosal coat, along with its innervation, totally stripped for a distance of at least 3 cm.[63] Most orthopaedic surgeons have not had extensive training or experience in repairing peripheral blood vessels, and in most instances, a consultant should be called.

Nonunion

Delayed union and nonunion of humeral shaft fractures occur most frequently in the transverse fracture, where there is only minimal bone contact between the fragments. Distraction of fractures and the interposition of soft parts are also significant factors. It is paradoxical that open reduction, even though it is performed with good justification, often contributes to nonunion. Treatment should be continued at least 4 months before the surgeon decides that a delayed union is frank nonunion.[63]

Vigorous and determined treatment is mandatory once the surgeon accepts the diagnosis of nonunion. The skin (especially the extent of any scar tissue) and the circulation of the extremity should be evaluated thoroughly. Essential to success is rigid internal fixation. Today this is perhaps best obtained by compression plating (Fig. 10-13). Intramedullary pinning is also an acceptable means of fixation. The fracture ends are cut back to good bone, and the medullary canal is drilled. If necessary the bone may be shortened an inch or more, and cancellous bone graft is a must, regardless of the means of fixation. There will be times when wisdom may dictate not disturbing the nonunion site. For example, a transverse fracture with a strong fibrous union being treated with a compression plate would be ideally suited for onlay cancellous bone grafting. Under these circumstances, I would prefer not to take down the fibrous union and cut back the ends of the bones. Often, stimulated by the grafts, such a fracture will go on to solid union.

It appears that good results can be pre-

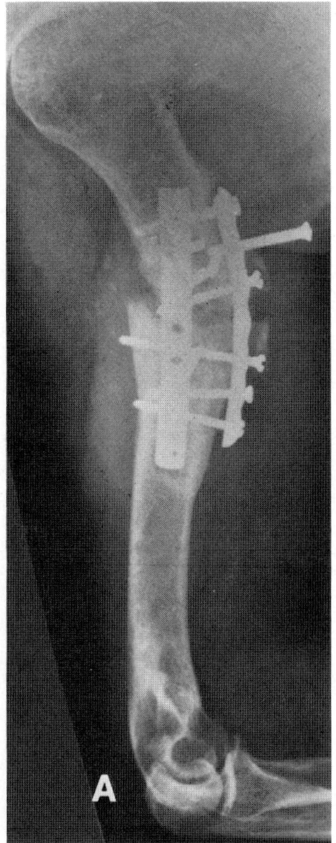

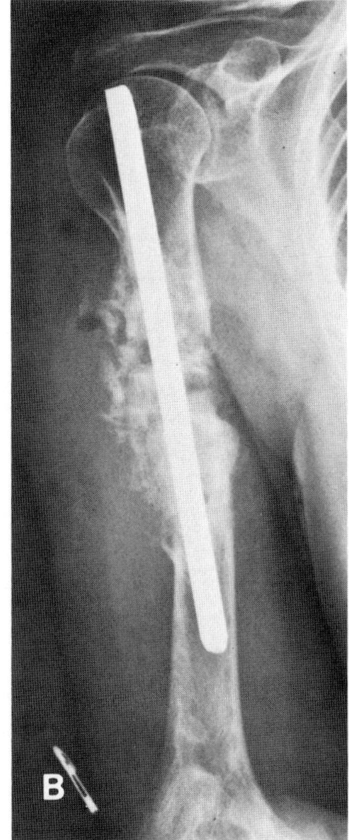

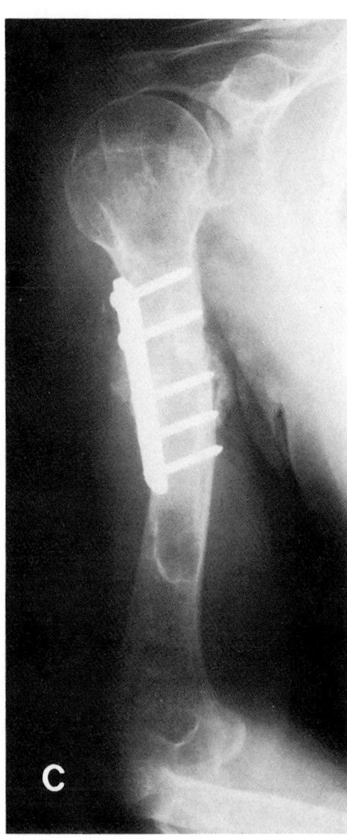

Fig. 10-13. (*A*) Roentgenogram of a fracture of the humerus with frank nonunion after multiple previous surgical procedures during a 3-year period. (*B*) Roentgenogram of same fracture following removal of plates and intramedullary nailing with bone graft. The fracture did not heal. (*C*) The nonunion finally healed after compression plating and cancellous bone grafts.

dicted from any one of several methods. In 1961 Boyd and others[7] reported 94 per cent union using medullary fixation and autogenous cancellous bone. Campbell[11] reported 93.8 per cent good results in 52 cases of humeral shaft fracture using massive onlay bone grafts. Müller[48] reported the use of rigid fixation by plate or intramedullary nail. Küntscher[41] used the intramedullary nail alone for 786 cases of nonunion, in which nailing was accomplished under roentgenographic control, without direct exposure of the fracture site. The nail was inserted so as to provide rigid fixation, and external support was not used in these cases.

Pathological Fractures

The humeral shaft is not uncommonly involved by metastatic disease, and pathological fractures may result. Parrish[55] has observed that displacement and comminution are rare in these neoplastic fractures. The gradual loss of continuity in the cortex of the bone causes some local reaction, including varying degrees of periostitis, osteoblastic activity, hemorrhage, edema, and increased blood supply. These condi-

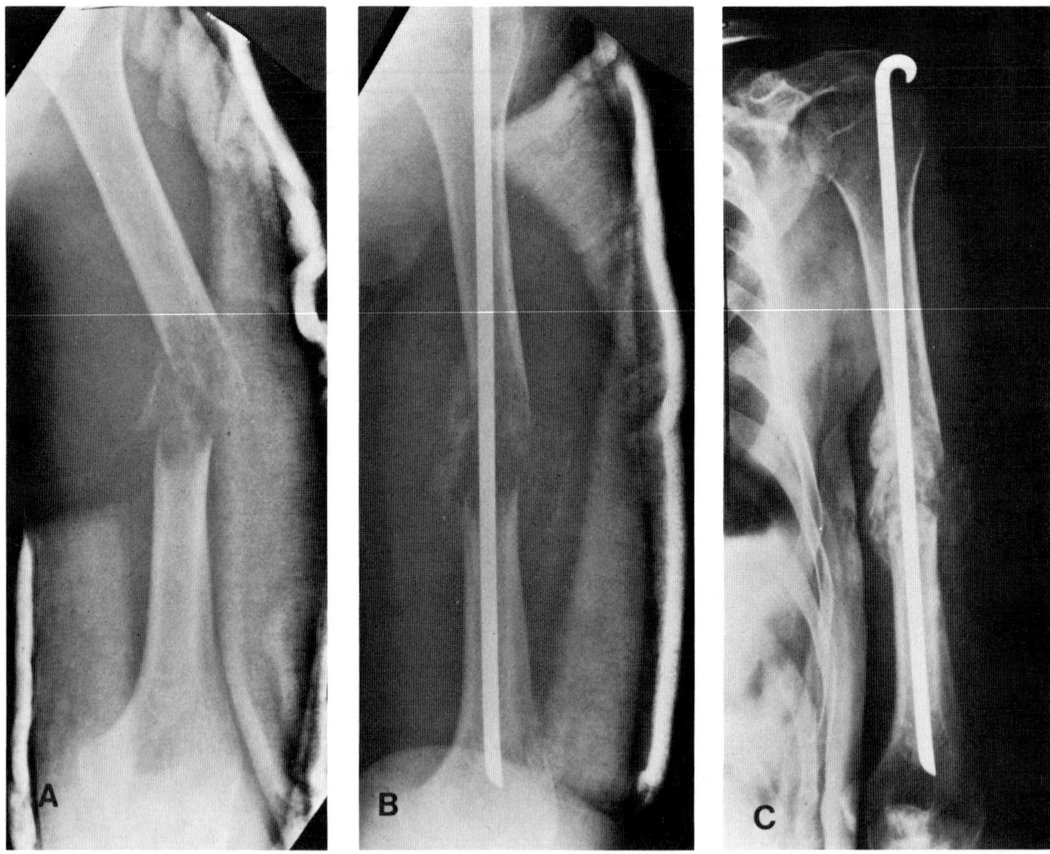

Fig. 10-14. (*A*) Roentgenogram showing pathological fracture through a metastatic lesion resulting from carcinoma of kidney. (*B*) Same fracture after intramedullary nailing. (*C*) Roentgenogram after 8 weeks showing healing of fracture.

tions may lead to sufficient tissue reaction and new bone formation to provide some stability in the region of the neoplastic process before the fracture occurs. In such cases, simple methods of immobilization have been used by Parrish.[55]

Operative procedures have been reserved for fractures that would otherwise confine the patients to bed or seriously restrict their function. The intramedullary nail is preferred by most surgeons for its stability and resulting relief of pain. The patient thus treated is able to remain mobile, if, his general condition is good. The presence of the nail does not preclude radiation or chemotherapy if either is indicated to treat or control the neoplastic process. Pathological fractures fixed in this manner go on to solid union in many instances (Fig. 10-14).

Late Complications

There are other complications that present less formidable problems. Once the fracture has proceeded to solid union, refracture has not been observed in the author's experience or reported to be a significant problem. In cases where there has been healing in bayonet position or shortening with comminution, the length discrepancy is not a serious problem. Myositis ossificans seems to be more frequently associated with injuries of the elbow than with those of the humeral shaft. Injuries to neighboring muscles and joints may result in stiffness and loss of function after the fracture has healed. However, proper use of the hanging cast or splint and a vigorous exercise program should minimize this complication.

REFERENCES

1. Adams, J. C.: Outline of Fractures. Edinburgh, E. & S. Livingstone, 1968.
2. American College of Surgeons Committee on Trauma: An Outline of the Treatment of Fractures. ed. 8. Philadelphia, W. B. Saunders, 1965.
3. Baker, D. M.: Fractures of the humeral shaft associated with ipsilateral fracture dislocation of the shoulder: report of a case. J. Trauma, *11*:532, 1971.
4. Bennett, G. E.: Fractures of the humerus with particular reference to nonunion and its treatment. Ann. Surg., *103*:994, 1936.
5. Bohler, L.: The Treatment of Fractures. Supplementary Volume. New York, Grune & Stratton, 1966.
6. Boyd, H. B., Anderson, L. D., and Johnston, D. S.: Changing concepts in the treatment of nonunion. Clin. Orthop., *43*:37, 1965.
7. Boyd, H. B., Lipinski, S. W., and Wiley, J. H.: Observation on nonunion of the shaft of the long bones with a statistical analysis of 842 patients. J. Bone Joint Surg., *43A*: 159, 1961.
8. Caldwell, J. A.: Treatment of fractures in the Cincinnati General Hospital. Ann. Surg., *97*:161, 1933.
9. ———: Treatment of fractures of the shaft of the humerus by hanging cast. Surg. Gynecol. Obstet., *70*:421, 1940.
10. Cameron, B. M.: Shaft Fractures and Pseudarthroses. Springfield, Charles C Thomas, 1966.
11. Campbell, W. C.: Ununited fractures of the shaft of the humerus. Ann. Surg., *105*: 135, 1937.
12. Cave, E. A.: Fractures and Other Injuries. Chicago, The Year Book Publishers, 1958.
13. Charnley, J.: The Closed Treatment of Common Fractures. Baltimore, Williams & Wilkins, 1961.
14. Christensen, S.: Humeral shaft fractures, operative and conservative treatment: Acta Chir. Scand., *133*:455, 1967.
15. Coates, J. B. (ed.): Orthopaedic Surgery in the European Theater of Operations. Washington, D. C., Office of the Surgeon General, Department of the Army, 1956.
16. Connolly, J.: Management of fractures associated with arterial injuries. Amer. J. Surg., *120*:331, 1970.
17. Conwell, H. E., and Reynolds, F. C.: Management of Fractures, Dislocations and Sprains. ed. 7. St. Louis, C. V. Mosby, 1961.
18. Coventry, M. B., and Laurnen, E. L.: Ununited fractures of the middle and upper humerus. Special problems in treatment. Clin. Orthop., *69*:192, 1970.
19. Crenshaw, A. H. (ed.): Campbell's Operative Orthopaedics. St. Louis, C. V. Mosby, 1971.
20. DeGeeter, L.: Treatment of diaphyseal humeral fractures by percutaneous pinning. Acta Chir. Belg., *69*:198, 1970.
21. DePalma, A. F.: The Management of Fractures and Dislocations. Philadelphia, W. B. Saunders, 1970.
22. Doran, F. S. A.: The problems and principles of the restoration of limb function following injury as demonstrated by humeral shaft fractures. Brit. J. Surg., *31*:351, 1944.
23. Doty, D. B., *et al.*: Prevention of gangrene due to fractures. Surg. Gynecol. Obstet., *125*:284, 1967.
24. Duthie, H. L.: Radial nerve in osseous tunnel at humeral fracture site diagnosed radiographically. J. Bone Joint Surg., *39B*: 746, 1957.
25. Epps, C. H., Jr., and Adams, J. P.: Wound management in open fractures. Amer. Surgeon, *27*:766, 1961.
26. Fenyo, G.: On fractures of the shaft of the humerus. Acta Chir. Scand., *137*:221, 1971.
27. Garcia, A., Jr., and Maeck, B. H.: Radial nerve injuries in fractures of the shaft of the humerus. Amer. J. Surg., *99*:625, 1960.
28. Goss, C. M. (ed.): Gray's Anatomy. ed. 25. Philadelphia, Lea & Febiger, 1950.
29. Gregersen, H. N.: Fractures of the humerus from muscular violence. Acta Orthop. Scand., *42*:506, 1971.
30. Hampton, O. P., Jr., and Fitts, W. T., Jr.: Open Reduction of Common Fractures. New York, Grune & Stratton, 1959.
31. Harris, W. H., Jones, W. N., and Aufranc, O. E.: Fracture Problems. St. Louis, C. V. Mosby, 1965.
32. Holm, C. L.: Management of humeral shaft fractures. Fundamentals of nonoperative techniques. Clin. Orthop., *71*:132, 1970.
33. Hollinshead, W. H.: Anatomy for Surgeons. vol. 3. New York, Hoeber-Harper, 1958.

34. Holstein, A., and Lewis, G. B.: Fractures of the humerus with radial nerve paralysis. J. Bone Joint Surg., *45A*:1382, 1963.
35. Hudson, R. T.: The use of the hanging cast in treatment of fractures of the humerus. South. Surgeon, *10*:132, 1941.
36. Kettlekemp, D. B., and Alexander, H.: Clinical review of radial nerve injury. J. Trauma, 7:424, 1967.
37. Key, J. A., and Conwell, H. E.: Fractures, Dislocations and Sprains. St. Louis, C. V. Mosby, 1956.
38. Klenerman, L.: Fractures of the shaft of the humerus. J. Bone Joint Surg., *48B*:105, 1966.
39. ———: Experimental fractures of the adult humerus. Med. Biol. Eng., *7*:357, 1969.
40. Küntscher, G.: The Küntscher method of intramedullary fixation. J. Bone Joint Surg., *40A*:17, 1958.
41. ———: Intramedullary surgical technique and its place in orthopaedic surgery: my present concept. J. Bone Joint Surg., *47A*: 809, 1965.
42. ———: Practice of Intramedullary Nailing. Springfield, Charles C Thomas, 1967.
43. LaFerte, A. D., and Nutter, P. D.: The treatment of fractures of the humerus by means of hanging plaster cast—"hanging cast." Ann. Surg., *114*:919, 1941.
44. Mann, R., and Neal, E. G.: Fractures of the shaft of the humerus in adults. Southern Med. J., *58*:264, 1965.
45. Mazet, R., Jr.: A Manual of Closed Reduction of Fractures and Dislocations. Springfield, Charles C Thomas, 1967.
46. McAusland, W. R., Jr., *et al.*: Management of Metastatic Pathological Fractures. Clin. Orthop., *73*:39, 1970.
47. McNamara, J. J., Brief, D. K., Stremple, J. F., and Wright, J. K.: Management of fractures with associated arterial injury in combat casualties. J. Trauma, *13*:17, 1973.
48. Müller, M. E.: Treatment of nonunions by compression. Clin. Orthop., *43*:83, 1965.
49. Müller, M. E., Allgower, M., and Willenegger, H.: Technique of Internal Fixation of Fractures. New York, Springer-Verlag, 1965.
50. ———: Manual of Internal Fixation, New York, Springer-Verlag, 1970.
51. Naiman, P. T., *et al.*: Use of ASIF compression plates in selected shaft fractures of the upper extremity. A preliminary report. Clin. Orthop., *71*:208, 1970.
52. Newman, A.: The supracondylar process and its fracture. Amer. J. Roentgenol. Radium Ther. Nucl. Med., *105*:844, 1969.
53. Nummi, P.: Supramid pin in medullary fixation. Acta Chir. Scand., *137*:67, 1971.
54. ———: Intramedullary fixation with compression for the treatment of fracture in the shaft of the humerus. Acta Chir. Scand., *137*:71, 1971.
55. Parrish, F. F., and Murray, J. A., *et al.*: Surgical treatment for secondary neoplastic fractures—a retrospective study of 96 patients. J. Bone Joint Surg., *52A*:665, 1970.
56. Raney, R. B.: The treatment of fractures of the humerus with the hanging cast. North Carolina Med. J., *6*:88, 1945.
57. Rich, N. M., Baugh, J. H., and Hughes, C. W.: Acute arterial injuries in Vietnam, 1000 cases. J. Trauma, *10*:359, 1970.
58. Rich, N. M., *et al.*: Internal versus external fixation of fractures with concomitant vascular injuries in Vietnam. J. Trauma, *11*: 463, 1971.
59. Rush, L. V., and Rush, H. L.: Intramedullary fixation of fractures of the humerus by the longitudinal pin. Surgery, *27*:268, 1950.
60. Scientific Research Committee, Pennsylvania Orthopaedic Society. Fresh midshaft fractures of the humerus in adults. Penn. Med. J., *62*:848, 1959.
61. Seddon, H. J.: Nerve lesions complicating certain closed bone injuries. J.A.M.A., *135*: 691, 1947.
62. Stewart, M. J., and Hundley, J. M.: Fractures of the humerus. A comparative study in methods and treatment. J. Bone Joint Surg., *37A*:681, 1955.
63. Stewart, M. J.: Fractures of the humeral shaft. *In* Adams, J. P. (ed.): Current Practice in Orthopaedic Surgery. St. Louis, C. V. Mosby, 1964.
64. Terry, R. J.: A study of the supracondyloid process in the living. Amer. J. Phys. Anthropol., *4*:129, 1921.
65. Watson-Jones, R.: Fractures and Joint Injuries. ed. 4. Baltimore, Williams & Wilkins, 1960.
66. Whitson, R. O.: Relation of the radial nerve to the shaft of the humerus. J. Bone Joint Surg., *36A*:85, 1954.
67. Winfield, J. M., Miller, H., and LaFerte, A. D.: Evaluation of the "hanging cast" as a method of treating fractures of humerus. Amer. J. Surg., *55*:228, 1942.

11 Fractures and Dislocations of the Shoulder

Charles S. Neer II, M.D.
Charles A. Rockwood, Jr., M.D.

Part 1: Fractures About the Shoulder, Charles S. Neer II, M.D.

FRACTURES OF THE PROXIMAL HUMERUS

Fractures of the upper end of the humerus are common and account for 4 to 5 per cent of all fractures.[63] They occur more frequently in older patients, after the cancellous bone of the humeral neck has become weakened by senility, but they are seen in patients of all ages, and merge with epiphyseal separations. In older patients the fracture often results from a minor fall and is usually minimally displaced. The most serious fractures and fracture-dislocations are more often seen in active, middle-aged patients (averaging 54 years of age) and these lesions can be extremely disabling. Their management often demands experienced surgical skill and judgment.

Previous classifications according to the level of the fracture[4,36] or mechanism of injury[9,68] were found inadequate to accurately identify the more difficult displaced lesions and have caused much confusion in the literature. In this discussion, the concept of the Four-Segment Classification[51] will be used. This system simply insists upon the accurate identification of the location and relationship of each of the four major groups of fragments by good initial roentgenographic studies. Nothing has to be memorized, but a knowledge of the anatomy and insertions of the tendons of the rotator cuff is essential.

Fortunately, in 80 per cent of upper humeral fractures none of the four major segments is significantly displaced, and the fragments are held together by the attachments of the tendons of the rotator cuff, joint capsule, and intact periosteum. These lesions are amenable to simple treatment by early functional exercises and can all, regardless of the number of fracture lines, be considered together because of similarity in treatment and prognosis. In 15 per cent of upper humeral fractures one or more of the major segments is displaced. These displaced fractures are associated with characteristic soft-tissue injuries. They are often unstable, may not be reducible by closed methods, and can be associated with distortion of the rotator mechanism or even loss of circulation to the head (articular segment). The pathology and treatment of each displaced lesion will be considered individually.

SURGICAL ANATOMY AND FUNCTION

The glenohumeral joint has a greater range of movement than any other joint in the body. This is made possible by its loose capsule, the stabilization of the humeral head by the rotator cuff and ligaments rather than a fixed bony socket, and an extensive lubricating system of bursae (see Figs. 11-47 to 11-50). Repair processes following injury and immobilization result in adhesions that interfere with the gliding mechanism. Therefore it is important to institute motion prior to the maturation of adhesions whenever possible.

In the case of most fractures with minimal displacement this can be accomplished by early gentle active assisted exercises, which are progressed to active exercises as the fracture heals. Unimpacted fractures require a period of immobilization or surgical repair, as the case may be, before exercises are begun. The objective is to first obtain a good passive range, working later for recovery of muscle tone and strength. The muscles of the shoulder comprise the

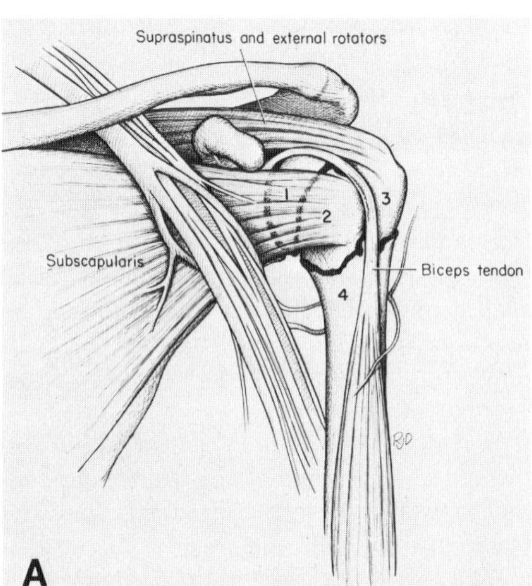

Fig. 11-1. (*A*) Humeral neck fractures occur between two or all of four major segments: (*1*) the head, (*2*) the lesser tuberosity, (*3*) the greater tuberosity, and (*4*) the shaft. All types of fractures with minimal displacement are classified together, regardless of the level or number of fracture lines. They present similar problems in management, in that the segments are impacted or held together by the periosteum and rotator cuff, permitting early functional exercises as soon as the head and shaft rotate as one. (*B*) The forces exerted by the rotator cuff on detached tuberosities. Retraction of both tuberosities displaces both the "anatomical neck" and "surgical neck" levels, a fact that renders previous classifications inadequate to describe displaced lesions. Note the long head of the biceps, an important surgical landmark and guide to the rotator interval, which is the key to accurate surgical repair. (Neer, C. S., II: J. Bone Joint Surg., *52A*:1077-1089, 1970)

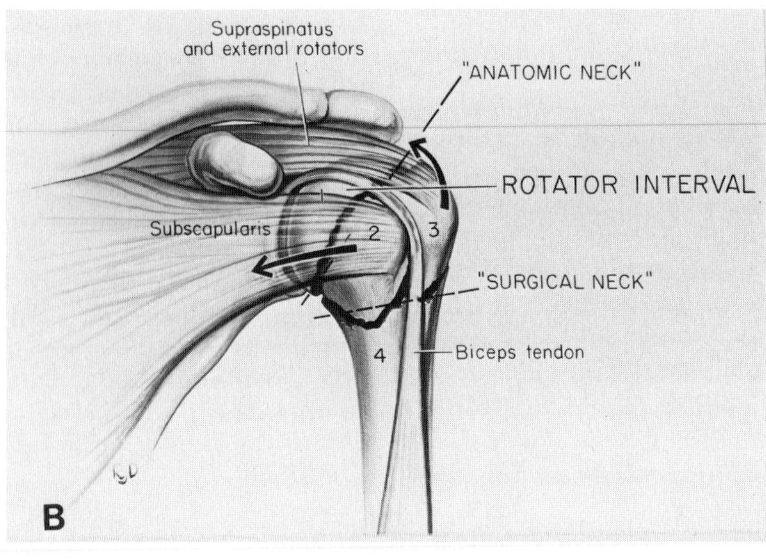

most complex functional unit of muscle couplings. These become atonic following injury. As fracture healing progresses their tone can be restored by isometric exercises followed later by active strengthening and resistive exercises. Coordination is eventually established by purposeful use.

Displaced fractures are usually treated best by closed or open reduction. They require a knowledge of the muscle forces acting upon the four major segments (Fig. 11-1). The greater tuberosity, for example, may be retracted by the supraspinatus and external rotators, and the lesser tuberosity by the subscapularis. The shaft tends to be displaced medially and anteriorly by the pectoralis major. These active forces and the status of the rotator cuff must be considered when reduction is being contemplated. Displaced fractures at the anatomical neck level separate the head from its blood supply and result in a high incidence of aseptic necrosis.

The neurovascular bundle is anteromedial, and the axillary nerve is just inferior to the glenohumeral joint (see Figs. 11-81—11-83). They are in greatest peril in anterior fracture-dislocations and displacements at the surgical neck level (see Fig. 11-82).

MECHANISM OF INJURY

A fall on the outstretched arm is the classical mechanism of injury. Lateral rotation is essential for full glenohumeral abduction. Continuing abduction when rotation has been blocked exceeds the check point of the ligaments. In younger patients, where the breaking strength of the bone exceeds the tensile strengths of the ligaments, a dislocation usually occurs. When the bone is weaker than the ligaments, as in older patients, a fracture of the humeral neck occurs. As might be expected, the most severe combination of injuries, fracture-dislocation, usually results from hard falls in middle-aged patients.

Upper humeral fractures can also result from a blow on the lateral side of the arm. Most patients are unable to recall the details of the injury, but the fact is that some of them fall while carrying an object in their arms and are still holding the object after the fracture has occurred. In this case the injury must have been a blow on the lateral side of the arm rather than on the outstretched hand.

FOUR-SEGMENT CLASSIFICATION

The key to understanding this system is to recognize it as a concept rather than a numerical classification. There is nothing to memorize, but accurate initial roentgen evaluation is essential.

It has been observed that upper humeral fractures occur between one or all of four major segments: (1) the articular segment or "anatomical neck" level, (2) the greater tuberosity, which often has been broken into a number of fragments, (3) the lesser tuberosity, and (4) the shaft or "surgical neck" level (Fig. 11-1). The relationships of each of these four major segments must be carefully identified in the initial roentgenograms. When any of the four major segments is displaced over 1.0 cm. or angulated more than 45 degrees, the fracture is considered to be displaced. Less displacement is categorized as minimal displacement, regardless of the number and level of the fracture lines. For clarity, a fracture with minimal displacement could be called a one-part fracture. A two-part fracture is one in which only one segment is displaced in relationship to the three that remain undisplaced. A three-part fracture is one in which two segments are displaced in relation to two other segments that are in apposition. In a four-part fracture, all four major segments are displaced. Thus there are four major categories of fractures based on the number of displaced segments rather than the number of fracture lines: minimal displacement, two-part displacement, three-part displacement, and four-part displacement.

The term fracture-dislocation implies that the articular segment is outside the joint space rather than subluxated or rotated. Both anterior and posterior fracture-dislocations are associated with characteristic

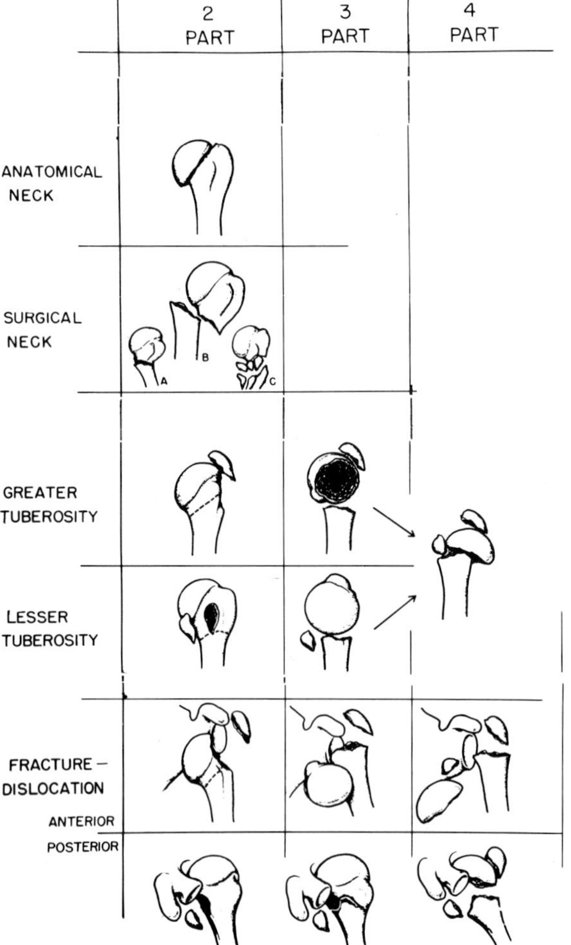

Fig. 11-2. The four-segment classification of displaced fractures. One or more of the four major segments has been displaced 1.0 cm. or angulated 45 degrees. Additional hairline components may or may not be present, but they are not considered because *this classification describes only displaced segments.* Two-part displacements include isolated displacements of the head (anatomic neck level), the shaft (surgical neck level), the greater tuberosity, and the lesser tuberosity. The three-part displacements are associated with an unimpacted surgical neck component which allows the head to be rotated by the muscles attaching to the tuberosity that remains in continuity with the head (e.g., the articular surface is rotated posteriorly in the greater tuberosity three-part displacement and anteriorly in the lesser tuberosity three-part displacement). Both tuberosities are displaced in the four-part lesions, in which there is serious loss of circulation to the articular segment. Fracture-dislocation implies damage outside the joint space, and segment distribution is important in estimating the circulation of the head. The articular surface fractures, in which portions of the head may be dislocated, include the "impression fracture" and the "headsplitting fracture." (Modified from Neer, C. S., II: J. Bone Joint Surg., *52A*:1077-1089, 1970)

two-, three-, and four-part lesions. Finally, fractures of the articular surface, the "impression fracture" or "headsplitting fracture," are given separate consideration (Fig. 11-2).

One of the advantages of this system is that it demands good initial roentgenograms prior to considering treatment and prognosis. It is important to have at least two views of the *upper humerus* made at right angles to each other. The technique of accomplishing this in an acutely injured and painful shoulder requires special consideration. A trauma series of roentgen views made in the scapular planes should be standardized for the first examinations of all fractures and will be described in detail (Fig. 11-3).

SIGNS AND SYMPTOMS

Since the upper humerus is well covered by soft tissue and the displacement is often minimal, early signs are usually limited to direct and indirect tenderness. The diagnosis depends upon roentgen studies, which should be made in any patient with continuing shoulder pain subsequent to an injury. Within a few days, ecchymosis, which may extend from the chest wall to the elbow, appears, and it strongly suggests the diagnosis.

Fracture-dislocations are more difficult to recognize clinically than simple dislocations,

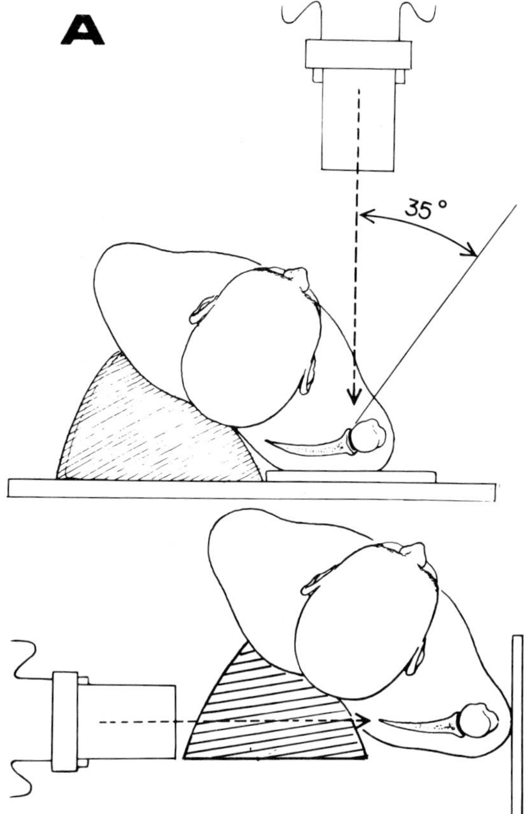

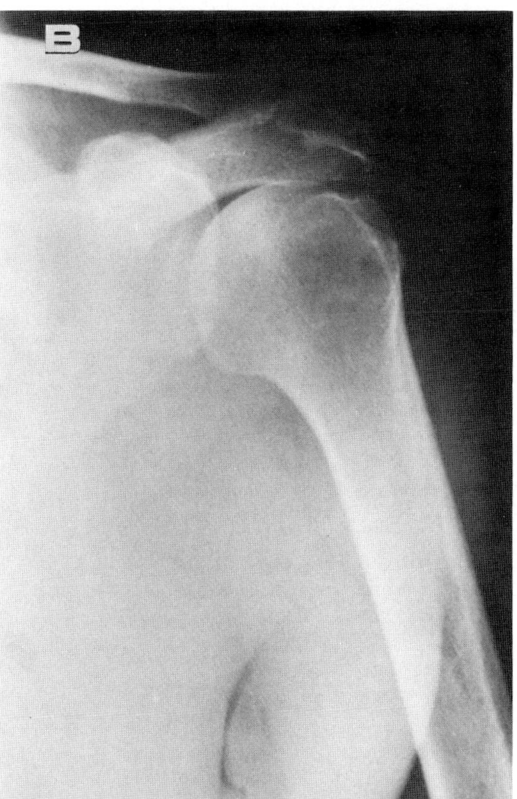

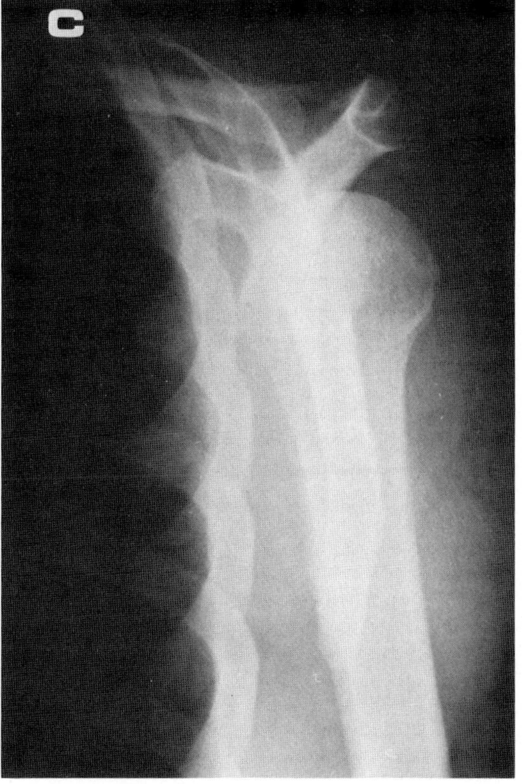

Fig. 11-3. The "Trauma Series" of roentgenographic projections consists of two views of the upper humerus made perpendicular and parallel to the scapular plane. (*A*) They can be made without removing the arm from the sling and without discomfort to the patient. The patient may be standing, sitting, or lying. The normal appearance of an intact left humerus is shown in each of these projections (*B, C*). These two initial survey views should be standardized in every hospital emergency service. (Modified from Neer, C. S., II: J. Bone Joint Surg., *52A*: 1077-1089, 1970)

because, while the contour of the shoulder may be flattened, the break in the continuity of the bone allows the shaft to fall into normal alignment and to be moved without the characteristic limitations of range. This is especially true of posterior fracture-dislocations, and, statistically, over 50 per cent of these are missed on initial examination. The true axillary view (Fig. 11-4) is the most reliable method for establishing the diagnosis of a posterior dislocation. This should always be obtained if the lesion is suspected

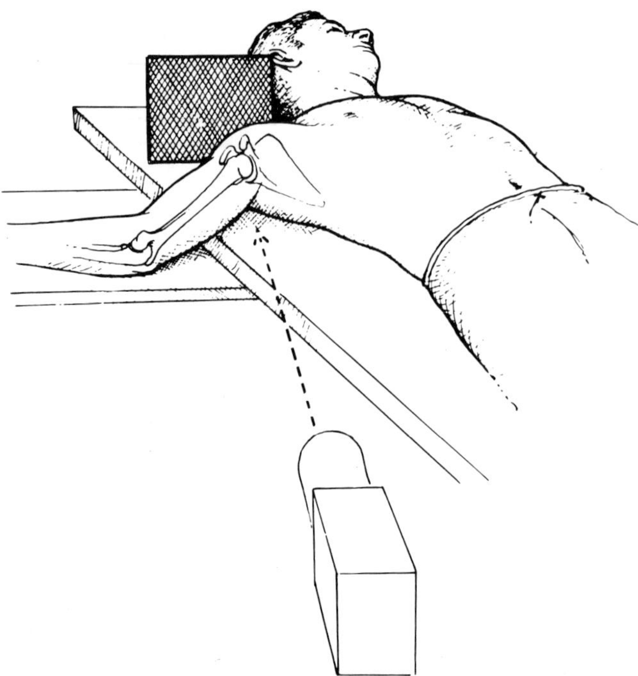

Fig. 11-4. The method of obtaining a true axillary view of the glenohumeral joint. The tube is placed near the patient's hip, and the film is held superior to the shoulder and firmly against the patient's neck. This exposure can be made with the patient prone, supine, or standing; minimal abduction of the injured arm is required.

from other views or from the physical findings. The physical signs of posterior dislocation include prominent coracoid, loss of external rotation, prominence of the head posteriorly, and altered axis of the arm so that it is directed posteriorly, but in fracture-dislocations these signs are less apparent than in posterior dislocations without fracture.

Upper humeral fractures are more frequently missed or underdiagnosed in patients with multiple injuries, because the physician is distracted by other more obvious injuries and because it is more awkward to obtain good roentgen evaluation of the shoulder. Even in this situation, however, it is possible to obtain views of the upper humerus in two planes and to supplement as needed with axillary views. Roentgen techniques are most important (Figs. 11-3, 11-4).

Associated injuries to the axillary nerve and brachial plexus are not rare, and the axillary vessels are occasionally torn. The status of these structures should be documented before and after instituting treatment. Displacements at the surgical neck level and anterior fracture-dislocations are especially apt to cause neurovascular damage. Violent trauma to the shoulder, capable of avulsing the roots of the plexus, can occur in the absence of a fracture.

ROENTGENOGRAPHIC FINDINGS

Oblique and poorly centered films of any fracture cause confusion and make logical treatment impossible. The glenohumeral joint lies neither in the coronal nor in the sagittal plane. Two-plane views of this joint and the upper humerus are best made by placing the beam vertical and then parallel to the scapular plane (Fig. 11-3), rather than in the coronal and sagittal planes. This can be done without removing the arm from the sling, and without discomfort to the patient. The patient may be standing, sitting or supine. These two initial survey views which we call the trauma series, should be standardized in every hospital emergency service.

Supplemental studies are made at the discretion of the surgeon, the most important of which is the axillary view. This can be made with minimal abduction of the injured arm by placing the x-ray tube near the patient's hip and holding the film superior to the glenohumeral joint (Fig. 11-4). The axillary view can be obtained with the patient standing or lying prone or supine. This is the most valuable method of diagnosing posterior dislocations and is also the best way to identify glenoid fractures.

Other supplemental studies may include transthoracic views, anteroposterior views with the humerus in various positions of rotation, and laminagrams. All are at times helpful in estimating the amount of displacement of specific segments. Laminagrams can be especially useful in judging the size of articular surface defects.

TREATMENT

Methods of Treatment

Early motion has long been one of the mainstays in treatment of shoulder injuries. Since the bone lesions will heal unless greatly displaced, the major goal in treatment of these injuries has been restoration of shoulder function and prevention of adhesions. The usual disability results from biceps tendon or rotator cuff scarring and adhesions.[5,8,11,18]

Abduction casts and splints were classically used in an attempt to bring the distal fragment to meet the proximal one. The rationale for this method was that the rotator cuff was believed to have abducted the proximal fragment, but in fact this is not the case. In actual practice, abduction of the arm increases the deforming force of the pectoralis major and, generally, any reduction obtained under anesthesia is usually lost. The use of traction in a similar manner also has these pitfalls. In addition, abduction splints and casts are heavy, cumbersome, uncomfortable, difficult to fit, and do not permit early motion of the shoulder, which is desirable in many of these patients.[11,14,29,56]

The hanging cast has been used by many authors to treat proximal humeral fractures.[6,7,28,29,68,69] The primary indication is an angulated, impacted surgical neck fracture in which the weight of the cast aids in reduction traction by gravity. Some authors have objected to the use of the hanging cast, believing that the weight of the arm alone (10 to 15 pounds), suspended by a loose sling or collar and cuff, is all that is necessary to reduce the deformity or at least maintain its position.[11] The excessive weight of the hanging cast may distract the fragments or increase inferior subluxation of the shoulder secondary to the muscle atony.

Traction is still employed by many to reduce and maintain reduction of surgical neck fractures.[7,34] It is best suited for a patient with multiple injuries who is confined to bed for treatment of other injuries, or it may be used when there is a fracture of the surgical neck with severe comminution distally. The pull of the traction should be with the arm adducted and flexed.[56]

Many different methods of open reduction and internal fixation have been used and are still employed. These include wire loops, simple screws, staples, blade plates, simple plates, and intramedullary nails. These are usually reserved for displaced and excessively rotated fractures of the surgical neck.[11,56] Open reduction and internal fixation has also been employed for fracture-dislocation of the shoulder.

Multiple techniques have been described in the treatment of four-segment fractures and four-segment fracture-dislocations of the humerus.[12,21,30,31,35,44,45,54] Treatment of these injuries has run the full gamut, including closed reduction, open reduction, *laissez faire,* removal of the head with or without plastic reconstruction, and primary arthrodesis of the shoulder. Attempts at open reduction met with difficulty, and there was a high incidence of aseptic necrosis of the humeral head. Because of the latter complications, the Jones procedure (resection of the head and reattachment of the greater and lesser tuberosities to the humeral shaft) was popularized.[30,31] This procedure resulted in a shoulder with limited range of motion, weakness, and lack of endurance. Pain was usually not a problem. Accompanying acromionectomy, biceps tendon suspension, and excision of the outer end of the clavicle did not improve the results in the series of Neer, Brown, and McLaughlin,[54] but they were helpful in Knight and Mayne's series.[35] A primary arthrodesis has been used, but it met with failure.[54]

Because of the disappointing results in the treatment of four-segment fractures and fracture-dislocations, plus the high incidence of avascular necrosis, prosthetic replacement of the humeral head was developed and has been recommended by many authors for these injuries.[13,37,47,48,49,50,54,58,66,67]

Author's Preferred Method of Treatment

There is some truth in the time-worn statement that perfect anatomical reduction is not necessary for a satisfactory functional result. The glenohumeral joint has so much movement that some motion can be lost without overwhelming handicap to older and less active patients. However, it is now well recognized that displaced fragments can block movement and cause sufficient

Table 11-1. Therapeutic Implications of the Four-Segment Classification*

	Approximate Incidence†	Problem	Author's Treatment
Minimal Displacement	80%	Adhesions	Passive exercises progressing to active exercises as continuity permits
2-Part	10%	Usually amenable to closed reduction	Closed treatment, except for greater tuberosity and some shaft displacements
3-Part	3%	Rotary forces of muscles prevent accurate closed reduction	Open reduction, buried wire-loop fixation, and cuff repair
4-Part	4%	Extremely high incidence of avascular necrosis	Prosthesis to replace the head but with accurate wire-loop fixation of the tuberosities and cuff repair
Articular Surface Fractures	3%		
"Impression" under 20%		Stable	Closed reduction, immobilization in external rotation
20% to 40%		Often unstable after closed reduction	Transplant lesser tuberosity
over 50%		Redisplace into head defect	Prosthesis
"Headsplitting"		Articular surface crushed	Prosthesis

* These generalizations apply only to active patients who are good operative risks and have reasonable life expectancy.

† Expressed as percentage of all upper humeral fractures and fracture-dislocations.

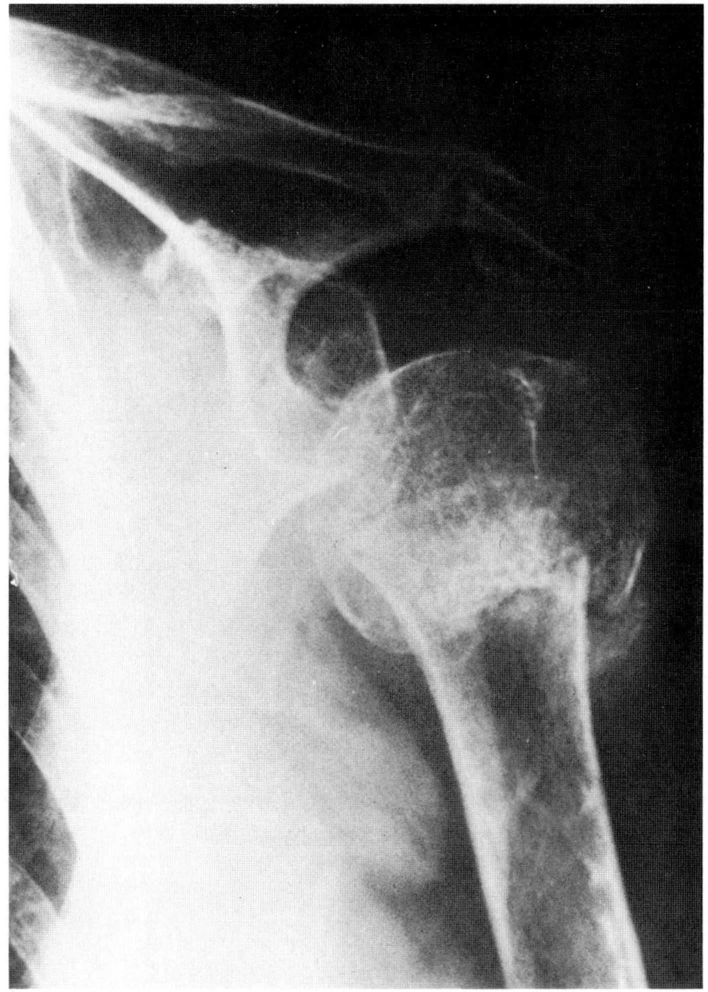

Fig. 11-5. A typical upper humeral fracture with "minimal displacement." There are hairline fracture components in the greater and lesser tuberosities and an impacted surgical neck component, none of which are significantly displaced. They are splinted by the intact rotator cuff and periosteum, permitting early functional exercises. The transitory subluxation disappeared when the muscles regained tone.

permanent pain to be quite disabling, especially in younger and more active patients. The type of displacement that causes significant functional loss can now be rather accurately identified. The method of treatment and the decision to accept or reduce the displacement, on the other hand, is a matter of judgment that is based not only on the anatomical problem but also on the age and activities of the patient.

In order to understand the terminology of the four-segment classification for displaced fractures, it should be clear that in each pattern only displaced segments are considered, and undisplaced fractures, which may also be present elsewhere in the upper humerus, are ignored. With this concept in mind, one can generalize on therapeutic indications as shown in Table 11-1. As previously stated, the treatment selected for displaced lesions depends on the patient involved, and the more complicated techniques apply only to patients who are good operative risks, are active, and have a reasonable life expectancy. It should be appreciated, however, that the average age of patients with displaced fractures is only 54 years, and the majority of these patients qualify for operative treatment when needed.

Minimal Displacement

This important group constitutes approximately 80 per cent of upper humeral fractures. No segment is displaced significantly (less than 1.0 cm. or less than 45 degrees; Fig. 11-5). They might well be called one-part fractures. Usually the fragments are held together by the intact rotator cuff and periosteum and move together as one piece when the humeral shaft is rotated. This allows early functional exercises which are increased as the patient can tolerate more. At times the shaft fragment is disimpacted so that false motion is present at the surgical neck level. This requires initial immobilization with a sling and swathe or similar appliance (Fig. 11-6) until sufficient clinical union has occurred for the head and shaft to rotate in unison before exercises can be started.

It is important to test for false motion as a guide to when functional exercises can be begun. The examiner stands behind the patient and with one hand palpates the outlines of the acromion and then slides his fingers down around the head of the humerus. With the other hand at the bent elbow he gently rotates the humeral shaft. When clinical continuity is present, the sling and swathe is removed for pendulum exercises, which progress as pain permits (Fig. 11-7). I believe the patient feels more secure and makes better progress when the early exercises are done lying supine. The good arm supplies the power for elevating and externally rotating the injured arm. Internal rotation exercises and the pulley are added after 2 weeks. As union progresses, stretching exercises, as from the top of a door, are very helpful. "Wall climbing" (creeping up the wall with the fingers) is not an effective exercise for regaining range.

The first objective is to establish a good range of motion with heat and passive exercises. Isometric exercises to preserve muscle tone should be introduced early. Active and resistive exercises to restore strength (Fig. 11-8) are not attempted until union is quite advanced and a good passive range has been accomplished (see p. 595). Fractures through cancellous bone heal with almost predictable regularity, and union can be expected at 6 weeks. However, optimal

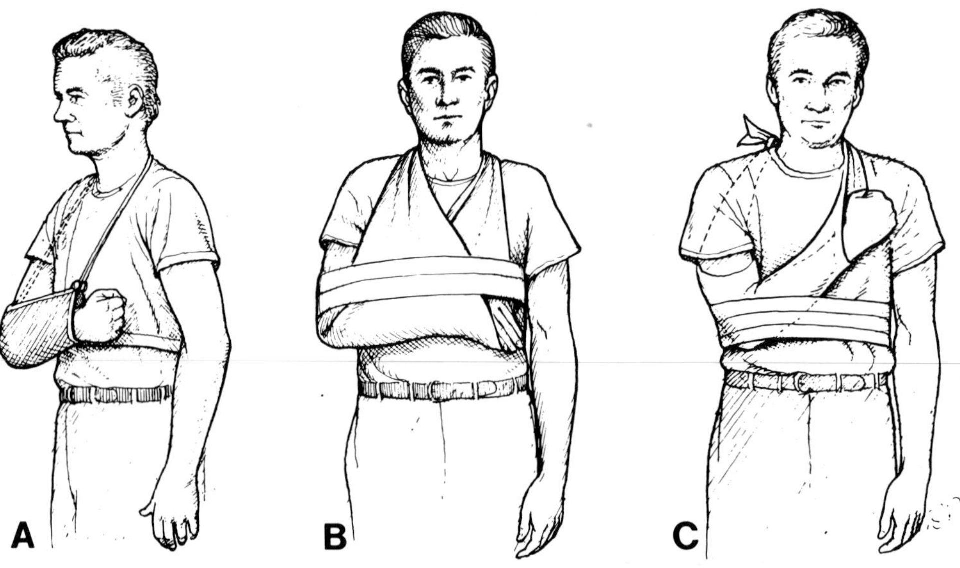

Fig. 11-6. The types of immobilizing dressings used for upper humeral fractures. (*A*) A commercial sling and swathe, which permits easy removal of the arm for exercises and is comfortable on the neck. (*B*) A conventional sling and swathe. (*C*) A stockinette Velpeau and swathe used when there is an unstable surgical neck component, because this position relaxes the pectoralis major.

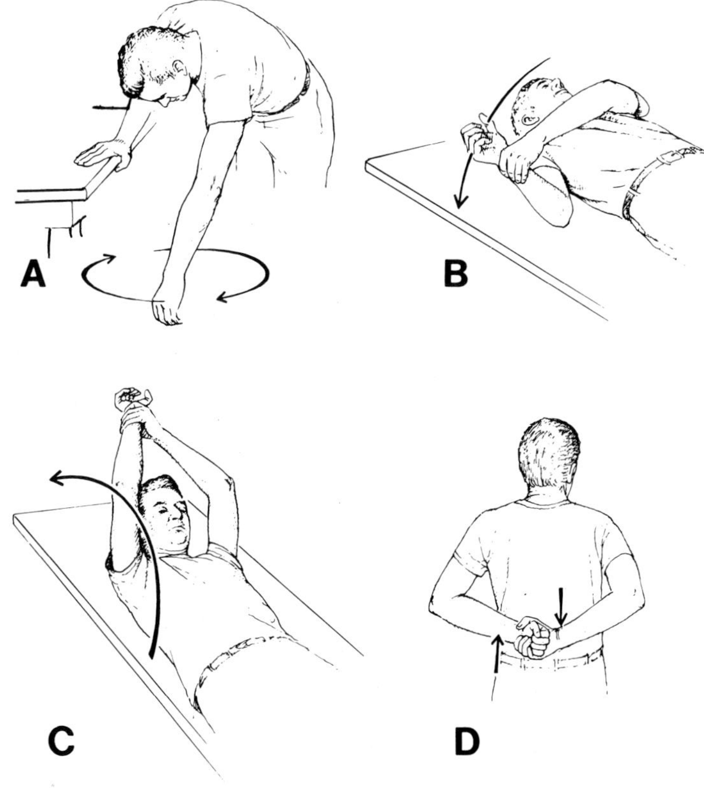

Fig. 11-7. Active assisted exercises. (*A*) Pendulum, using gravity with the muscles relaxed. (*B*) External rotation, using the good arm for power. (*C*) Elevation, using the good arm for power. (*D*) Internal rotation, using the good arm for power.

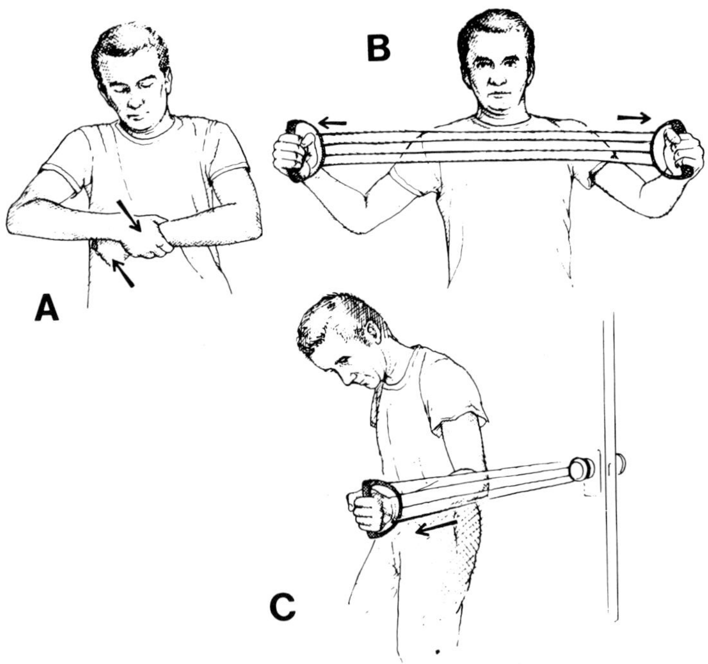

Fig. 11-8. Active exercises. (*A*) The good arm is resisting internal rotation or external rotation. (*B*) Rubber tubing or a spring exerciser is used for progressive strengthening of the external rotators and lateral deltoid as well as for the anterior deltoid (*C*).

functional recovery is usually best obtained when the exercises are continued for a number of months.

A "transitory subluxation" of the humeral head (Fig. 11-5) often follows upper humeral fractures of all types and can cause considerable concern to the inexperienced surgeon. It is best explained by two facts: (1) the deltoid and rotator cuff muscles are known to become atonic after these injuries and (2) the ligaments and capsule of the glenohumeral joint are normally loose enough to allow a wide range of motion. Thus, the weight of the arm can lead to a transitory subluxation which disappears as the muscles regain tone. Treatment consists of a sling to support the arm and isometrics between regular exercise periods.

Two-Part Displacement

In two-part displacements, since only one segment is displaced, it is usually possible to accomplish and maintain reduction by closed methods. There are exceptions to this generalization, however, and each lesion merits individual discussion.

Articular-Segment Displacement (Displaced Anatomical Neck Fracture). Isolated displacement of the articular segment at the anatomical neck, perhaps in association with hairline tuberosity components but without accompanying displacement of the tuberosities, is quite rare. Its presence is easily overlooked unless a good anteroposterior roentgenogram of the upper humerus is obtained (Fig. 11-3). In our experience the incidence of late avascular necrosis of the head has been very high regardless of the method of treatment (Fig. 11-9).

Since no surgeon has had a great deal of experience with these fractures it is not possible to be dogmatic about treatment. Because the tuberosities are in good position, it seems logical to treat an acute lesion in the way recommended for other large displaced fragments of articular surface in other major joints; namely, by open reduction and screw fixation. The alternative is to accept the displacement and hope for a comfortable malunion that does not go on to collapse of the head. If avascular necrosis occurs, it is usually sufficiently disabling to require prosthetic replacement.

Shaft Displacement. Displaced surgical neck fractures are common and occur in patients of all ages. Epiphyseal fractures

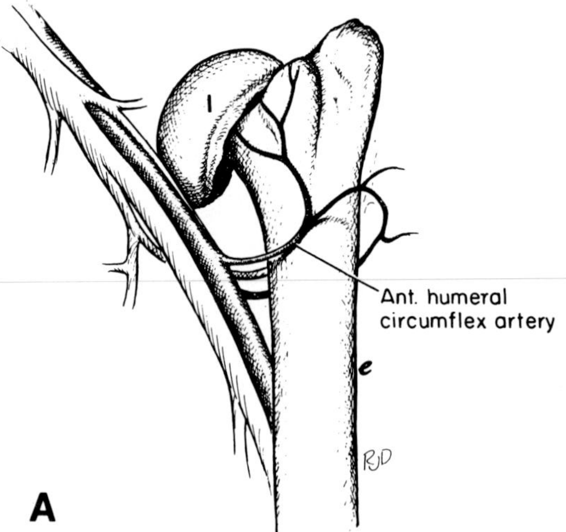

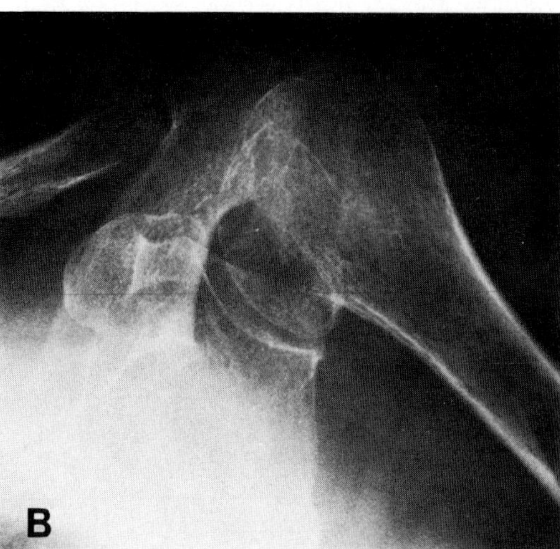

Fig. 11-9. The two-part articular segment displacement, or displaced anatomical neck fracture. (*A*) Diagram of the lesion and loss of circulation to the head. (*B*) Appearance of a malunion seen 3 months after injury. Subsequently there was collapse and resorption of the head.

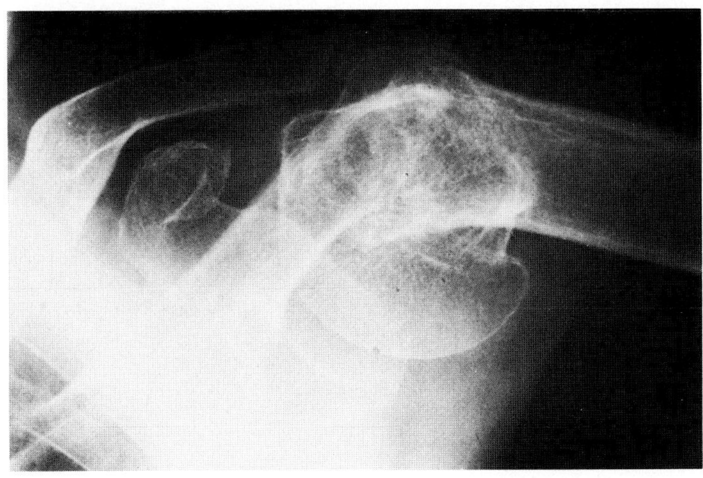

Fig. 11-10. An impacted two-part surgical neck displacement showing a malunion in maximum abduction. The shaft had been allowed to unite with 70 degrees anterior angulation. (Neer, C. S., II: J. Bone Joint Surg., 52*A*:1077-1089, 1970)

are of this type.[55] A displacement of more than 1.0 cm. or more than 45 degrees angulation is present at the surgical neck level just distal to the tuberosities. Although fissure fractures may exist proximally, the rotator cuff is intact and holds the head in neutral rotation. The head is only slightly abducted, unless tilted by an overriding shaft. Three variations are seen in adult patients:

Impacted and Angulated. The apex of the angle is usually anterior, and the posterior periosteum is intact (Fig. 11-10). If allowed to unite in this position, shoulder elevation will be permanently limited in direct proportion to the amount of residual angulation. Therefore I prefer to treat active patients by closed reduction. The periosteal sleeve posteriorly affords sufficient stability so that the fracture may be disimpacted with traction and the angulation corrected by full forward elevation beyond the pivotal position. After correcting the alignment the arm is immobilized in the Velpeau position across the chest. This position relaxes the pectoralis and is more effective and comfortable than an abduction cast or a hanging cast. I use a stockinette and swathe (Fig. 11-6C), until clinical union is strong enough to allow gentle exercises, usually about 3 weeks. Rehabilitation is then continued as for minimally displaced fractures.

Unimpacted. The shaft is displaced forward and medially by the pull of the pectoralis major while the head remains in neutral rotation (Fig. 11-11). This fracture is often unstable after closed reduction. An abduction cast increases the deformity by intensifying the pull of the pectoralis. A hanging cast levers the shaft forward when the patient lies supine and may lead to nonunion, especially if it distracts the fracture. A tight sling increases the anterior angulation. Closed reduction has usually been accomplished best by traction, pulling the shaft forward and adducting it to relax the pectoralis, and then displacing the upper end of the proximal humerus laterally to lock it under the tuberosities as the traction is released. The arm is then secured across the chest in the Velpeau position, because in this position the pectoralis major is relaxed. I prefer a stockinette Velpeau and swathe with an axillary pad (Fig. 11-6C). If the fracture can be reduced but is unstable, it is percutaneously transfixed with a stiff threaded Steinmann pin before applying the Velpeau dressing. The pin is removed within 3 weeks, prior to starting exercises. If the patient has multiple injuries requiring access to the chest, overhead olecranon traction is used. If the fracture cannot be reduced, interposition of the periosteal sleeve or the long head of the biceps must be suspected and an open reduction

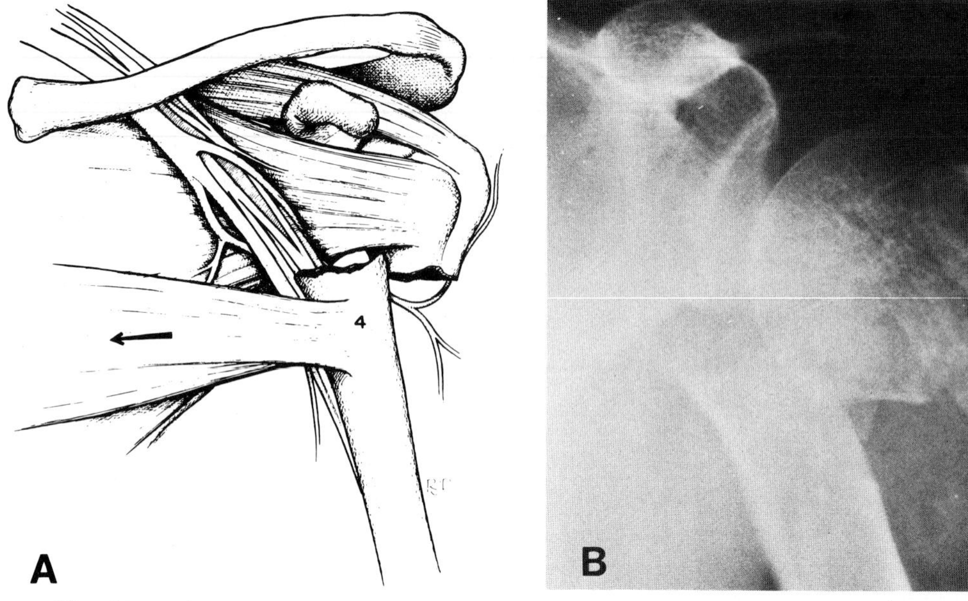

Fig. 11-11. An unimpacted two-part surgical neck displacement. (*A*) The rotator cuff is intact, and the pectoralis major is the deforming muscle. (*B*) Roentgenographic appearance of a typical lesion.

with internal fixation with a wire suture is performed.

As previously stated, this lesion is often associated with injuries of the infraclavicular part of the brachial plexus. Fortunately, the prognosis for spontaneous recovery of nerve function following infraclavicular injuries is generally good.

Comminuted. When the fragmentation extends distally for several centimeters, the fragments of bone undergo twist displacement if the arm is placed in internal rotation across the chest (Fig. 11-12). This occurs because the tuberosities and head are held in neutral rotation by the intact rotator cuff. Intermediate fragments may be retracted by the pectoralis. This fracture cannot be adequately aligned across the chest but is well aligned by overhead olecranon traction. Traction is applied in neutral rotation to accommodate the position of the proximal segments, and in forward flexion to relax the pectoralis. Care must be

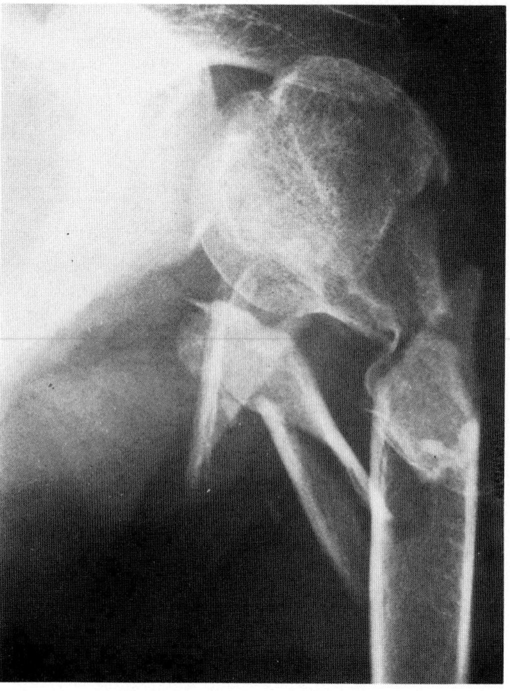

Fig. 11-12. A comminuted two-part surgical neck displacement which is slightly overriding and twisted by the arm having been placed across the chest in a sling. The pectoralis major has pulled some fragments medially. (Neer, C. S., II: J. Bone Joint Surg., *52A*:1077-1089, 1970)

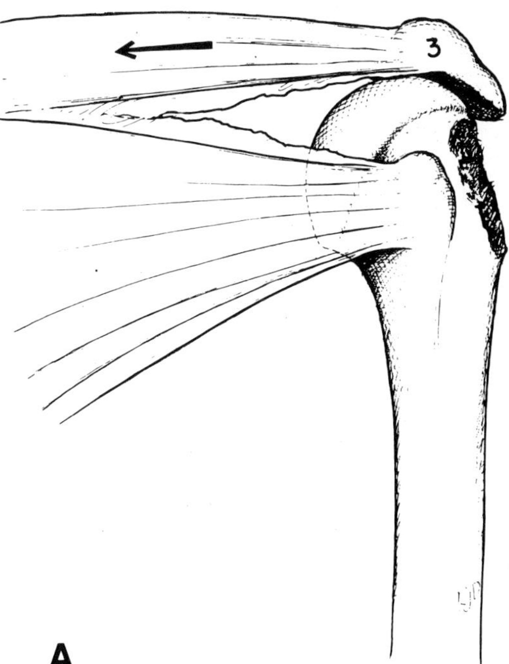

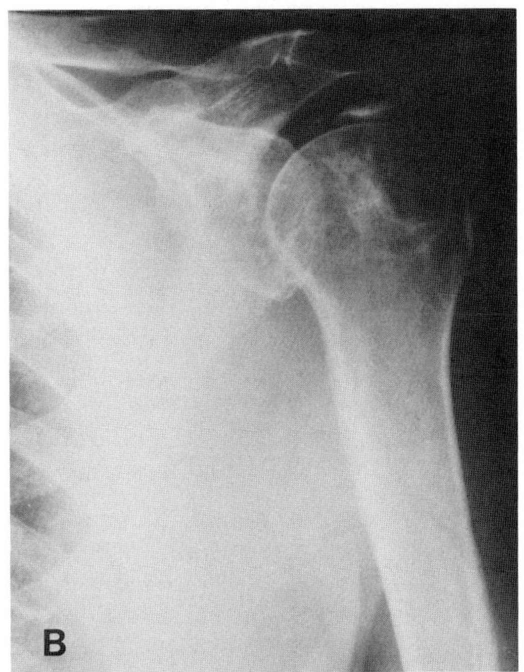

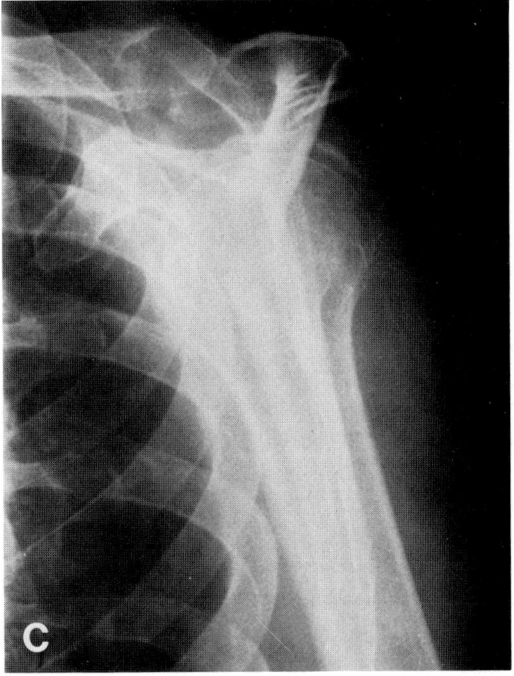

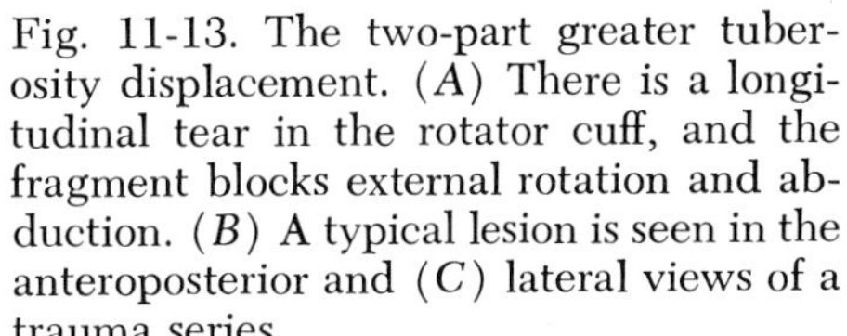
Fig. 11-13. The two-part greater tuberosity displacement. (*A*) There is a longitudinal tear in the rotator cuff, and the fragment blocks external rotation and abduction. (*B*) A typical lesion is seen in the anteroposterior and (*C*) lateral views of a trauma series.

taken to avoid distraction, which can interfere with union. Internal fixation is not necessary, and attempts to accomplish this have been unrewarding because of the comminution.

Greater Tuberosity Displacement. The greater tuberosity has three facets for the insertion of the supraspinatus, infraspinatus, and teres minor. Retraction of 1.0 cm. of the entire greater tuberosity or one of its facets is pathognomonic of a longitudinal tear in the rotator cuff (Fig. 11-13). In general, the tuberosity fragment is large in younger patients and smaller in older patients. In addition to the cuff deficiency, the retracted tuberosity further impairs motion by impinging under the acromion and against the posterior glenoid, where it blocks external rotation and abduction. It is now generally accepted that a 1.0-cm. displacement of this type in an active patient is best treated by open reduction and cuff repair.[3,11,41,46] This can be accomplished through a 2-inch deltoid splitting incision. I usually excise part of the fragment and

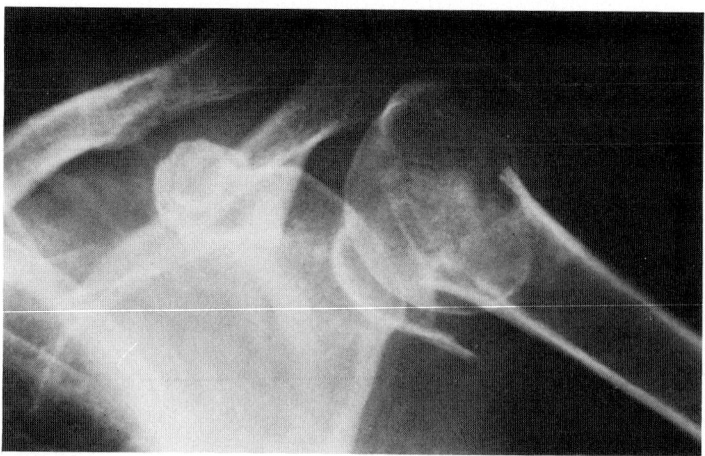

Fig. 11-14. A two-part lesser tuberosity displacement. The lesser tuberosity is retracted medially by the subscapularis, but the head remains in normal position, with or without a minimally displaced fracture at the surgical neck level.

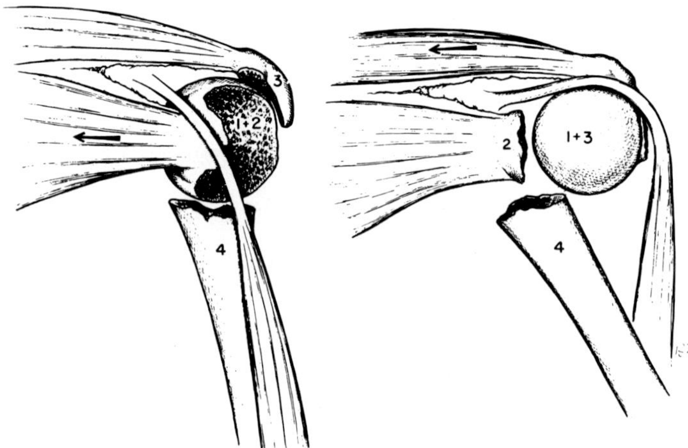

Fig. 11-15. The two types of three-part displacement. When the greater tuberosity is detached, the subscapularis rotates the head so that the articular surface faces posteriorly. When the lesser tuberosity is detached, the supraspinatus and external rotators cause the articular surface to face anteriorly. (Modified from Neer, C. S., II: J. Bone Joint Surg., *52A*:1077-1089, 1970)

prefer to suture it in place with nylon, using a similar suture material for repairing the cuff. If a minimally displaced fracture at the surgical neck level is also present, it is not disturbed.

Lesser Tuberosity Displacement. This is seen either as an isolated lesion (for example, following a seizure) or in association with an undisplaced fracture of the surgical neck (Fig. 11-14). While this displacement produces spreading of the anterior fibers of the rotator cuff and results in a bony prominence, neither of these defects has had clinical significance greater than slight loss of internal rotation. No special treatment is required.

Three-Part Displacement

The two types of three-part displacement are illustrated in Figure 11-15, which shows the muscle forces involved. An unimpacted surgical neck fracture is associated with detachment and retraction of one of the tuberosities. The other tuberosity remains attached to the articular segment and rotates it so as to open the defect in the rotator cuff. These lesions have been called rotary fracture-subluxations or rotary fracture-dislocations. The anatomical distortion is much greater than that of two-part fractures, and because of the opposing forces on the muscle attachments, they cannot be reduced by closed methods. However, since the articular segment retains soft-tissue attachments either in front or in back, it usually has sufficient blood supply to survive after carefully performed open reduction and internal fixation.

I prefer to treat both of these lesions by open reduction through a deltopectoral incision with detachment of the anterior deltoid from the clavicle.[52] After division of the clavipectoral fascia, the long head of the biceps serves as a guide to the interval between the lesser and greater tuberosities.

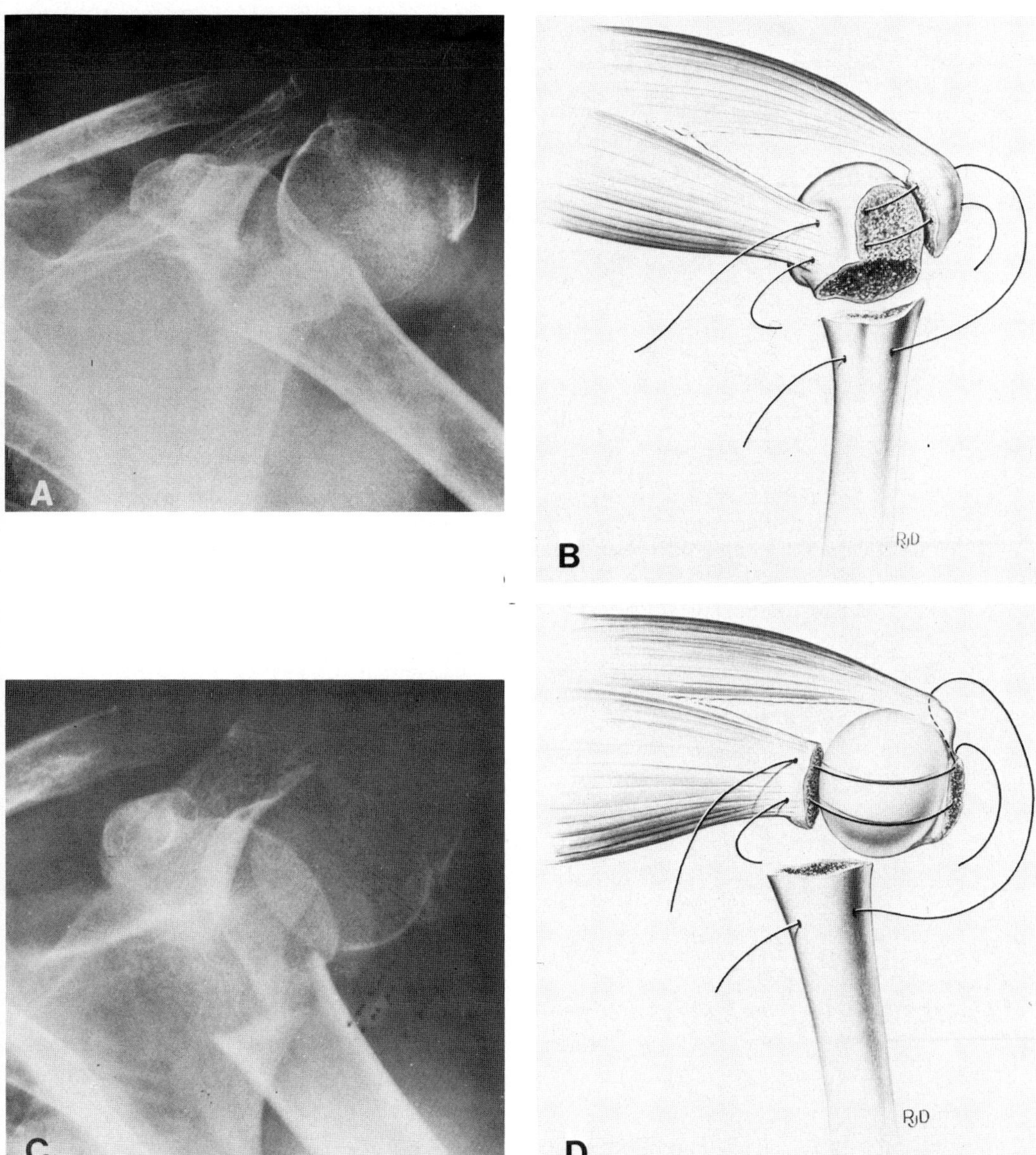

Fig. 11-16. The technique of buried wire repair used for the two types of three-part displacement: displacement of the greater tuberosity (*A*, *B*) and of the less tuberosity (*C*, *D*). In each case the head is derotated and the tuberosities are approximated. A second wire anchors the head and tuberosities to the shaft. The rotator cuff is then sutured (see Fig. 11-18).

Surgical trauma to the soft-tissue attachments on the articular segment is carefully avoided. The tuberosities are first brought into accurate approximation and secured with a buried 18- or 20-gauge wire loop. They are again fixed with a second wire loop, which is then carried down to anchor them to the shaft (Fig. 11-16). The tear in the rotator cuff is repaired and the deltoid is carefully reattached (Fig. 11-18). While I

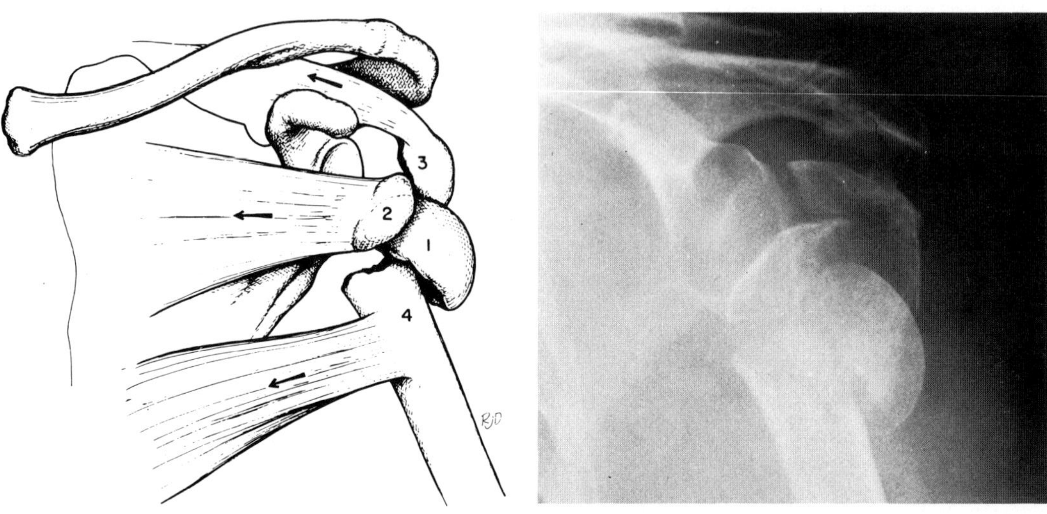

Fig. 11-17. The pathology and roentgenographic appearance of a typical four-part displacement. The articular segment is detached from its circulation and displaced out from under the tuberosities, which are usually retracted by muscle forces.

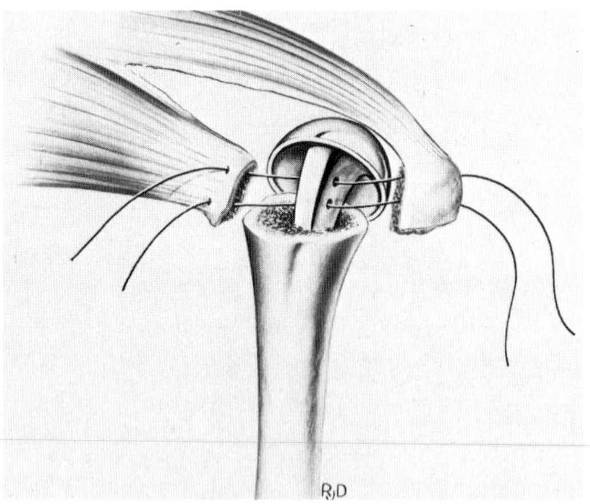

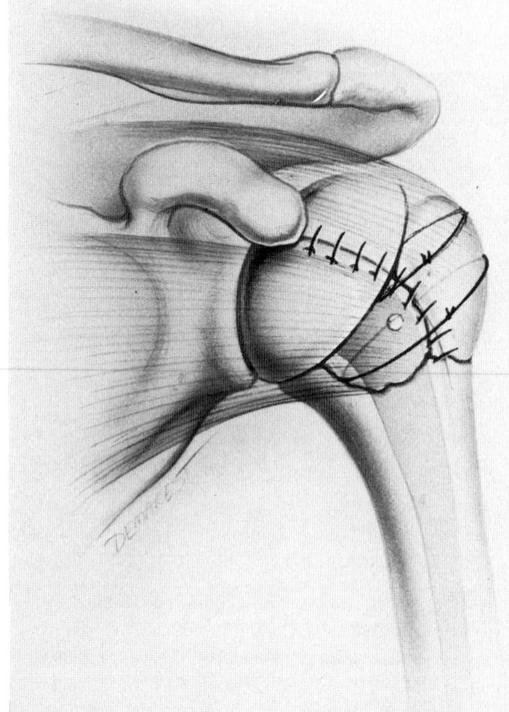

Fig. 11-18. The method of prosthetic replacement with buried wire repair of the tuberosities and suture of the cuff used for four-part fractures. The tuberosity segments are approximated in their normal anatomical positions and are not excised.

have found this method of internal fixation to be superior to screws, Kirschner wires, staples, or Rush rods, it is not rigid. An alternate method of fixation sometimes used is the AO buttress plate designed for the shoulder, but it is bulky, and because of the soft bone, it rarely achieves sufficient fixation for immediate exercises. Sling and swathe immobilization is usually needed for 2 or 3 weeks, until some early repair has occurred before beginning exercises. The rehabilitation program then follows the outline above for fractures with minimal displacement. The exercise program for these serious injuries is of key importance and should be expected to continue for many months, working first for passive range and later for strength.

Four-Part Displacement

When both tuberosities are detached and retracted (Fig. 11-17) the articular segment remains as a "shell fragment" devoid of soft-tissue attachments and without a blood supply. It is displaced laterally so the term "lateral fracture-dislocation" has been aptly applied. In our experience the incidence of avascular necrosis and resorption of the head following open reduction and internal fixation has been so high that we prefer to treat this lesion initially with a prosthesis[52] (Fig. 11-18). The prosthesis replaces the articular segment and provides a firm anchorage for an accurate wire-loop fixation of the tuberosities and repair of the cuff. This allows early gentle passive exercises and minimizes adhesions. Following this procedure it should be possible to begin passive exercises on the fourth day, first in the supine position and later erect. Active exercises are not attempted until the tuberosities have united. The importance of a good rehabilitation program cannot be overemphasized, and exercises should be continued for many months, working first for passive range and later for strength.

Fracture-Dislocation

In a fracture-dislocation the articular surface of the humerus is outside the joint space, either anterior or posterior. The associated humeral fracture is almost always displaced and can be a two-, three-, or four-part displacement (Figs. 11-19—11-27). It is of clinical value, in analyzing these lesions, to note that anterior dislocations are associated with displacement of the greater tuberosity while posterior dislocations are associated with displacements of the lesser tuberosity. Both tuberosities are displaced in either type of four-part fracture-dislocation.

Since fracture fragments and damaged soft-tissue are present outside of the joint space, these lesions are prone to cause unwanted pericapsular bone formation, which restricts motion and is usually referred to as myositis ossificans. Factors which appear to be related to the production of this complication are: (1) repeated unsuccessful attempts at manipulative reduction, (2) open reduction delayed beyond 5 or 6 days, and (3) possible variations in the tissue responses to repair in individual patients. This complication appears to be related to the effect of reinjury upon early repair responses. In any event, it is important to reduce fracture-dislocations within the first week, avoiding repeated manipulations and unnecessary trauma.

Anterior Fracture-Dislocations. *Two-Part Anterior Fracture-Dislocations.* The greater tuberosity is displaced in approximately 15 per cent of anterior dislocations (Fig. 11-19). This is the most common type of fracture-dislocation. The ligaments and capsule usually cause the fragment to fall in good position after closed reduction of the dislocation. The most atraumatic reduction possible should be used. I prefer traction with gradual abduction until the head can be gently lifted into the joint. Occasionally the greater tuberosity remains displaced and retracted after reduction of the dislocation; then the problem is that of a two-part greater tuberosity displacement as described above. This is best treated by open reduction of the tuberosity and cuff repair.

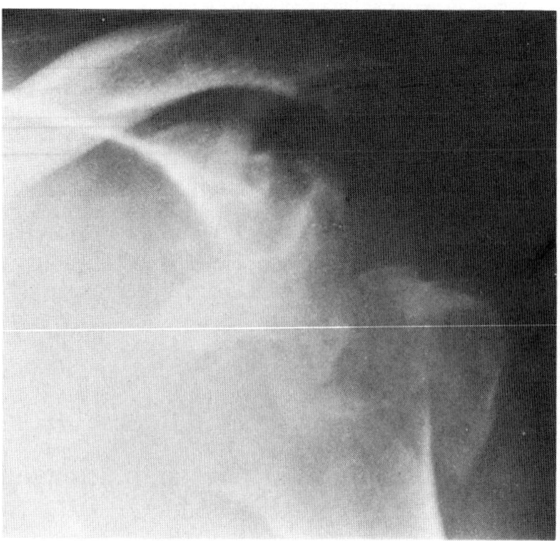

Fig. 11-19. Anteroposterior view of the two-part anterior fracture-dislocation with the entire greater tuberosity displaced.

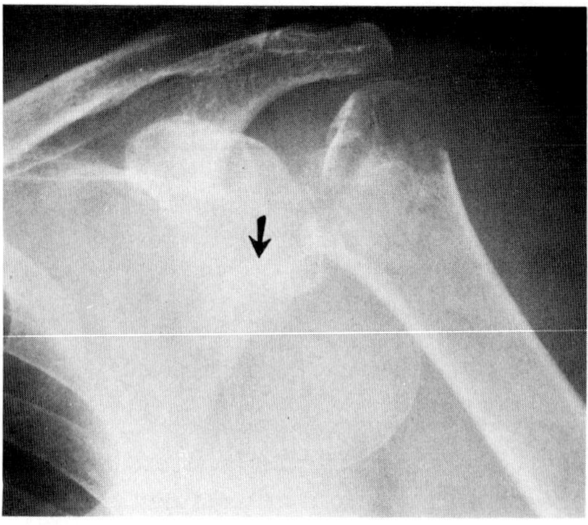

Fig. 11-20. Anteroposterior view of a three-part anterior fracture-dislocation. The arrow points to the lesser tuberosity, which remains in continuity with the articular segment. The greater tuberosity has been retracted backward by the external rotators.

Two common errors in assessing these lesions are failure to test for axillary nerve palsy, and mistaking a facet avulsion for "calcium deposits." Prognostically, it is of interest that dislocations associated with this fracture do not become recurrent dislocations.[42] This is explained by the fact that the anterior ligaments have not been torn, and once fracture healing occurs the joint is stable.

Three-Part Anterior Fracture-Dislocation. The articular segment and lesser tuberosity are in continuity so that the subscapularis and anterior capsule remain attached to provide circulation to the head (Fig. 11-20). I believe that a more gentle and accurate reduction can be accomplished surgically than by closed reduction. The subscapularis interferes with closed reduction and tends to rotate the head, even when it can be relocated into the joint. Residual internal rotation of the head after closed reduction may make it appear to be upside down on roentgenograms. Accurate wire loop fixation and cuff repair is preferred, as for three-part fractures without dislocation.

Four-part anterior fracture-dislocation is not uncommon. Both tuberosities are usually retracted, but at times the soft tissue holds the tuberosity fragments in contact, so that the head is dislocated out from under them (Fig. 11-21). In all four-part lesions, the head is detached from all soft tissue, and the incidence of late avascular necrosis is so high that I prefer prosthetic replacement and tuberosity repair, as discussed above for four-part fracture without dislocation.

Posterior Fracture-Dislocations. *Two-Part Posterior Fracture-Dislocations.* Avulsion of the lesser tuberosity often accompanies posterior dislocation because of the tension placed on the subscapularis tendon and anterior capsule (Fig. 11-22). This fracture *per se* is of no importance, and closed reduction is indicated. The method I prefer for reducing a posterior dislocation is to apply traction while the arm is held in 90 degrees forward flexion, gradually adducting it across the chest, causing the glenoid to lever the neck of the humerus laterally. This unlocks the head from behind the glenoid, so that the head can be relocated with minimal risk of further fracture. Following reduction the arm is immobilized at

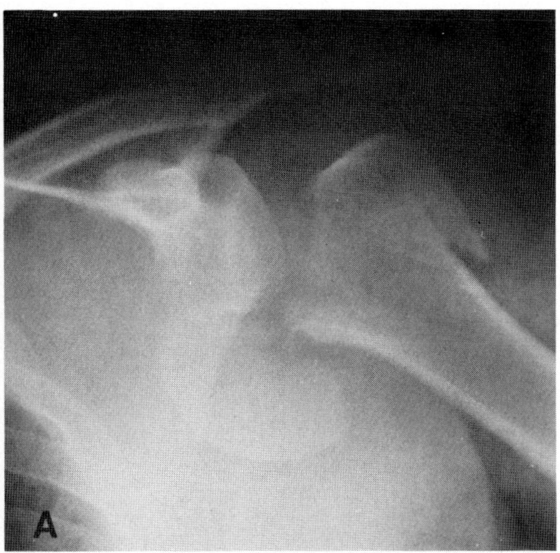

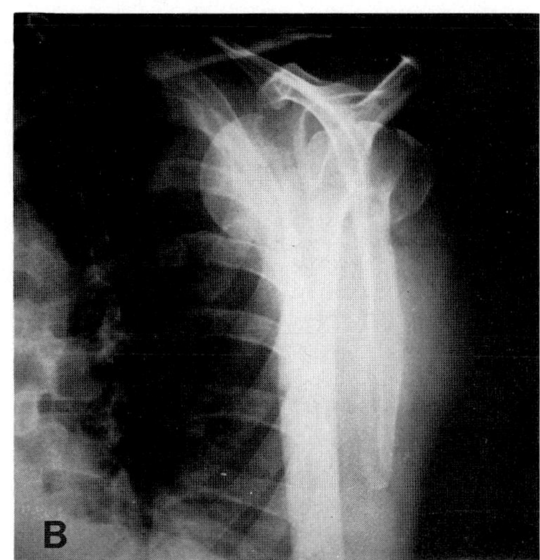

Fig. 11-21. The trauma series of a typical four-part anterior fracture-dislocation. (*A*) Anteroposterior view in the scapular plane showing the articular segment to be a "shell," devoid of soft-part attachments, dislocated beneath the coracoid and both tuberosities fractured. (*B*) Lateral scapular view showing the greater tuberosity retracted behind the glenoid and the lesser tuberosity in front of the glenoid but behind the head. In some atypical four-part lesions the tuberosities are held together by the soft tissue, and the head is displaced out from under them.

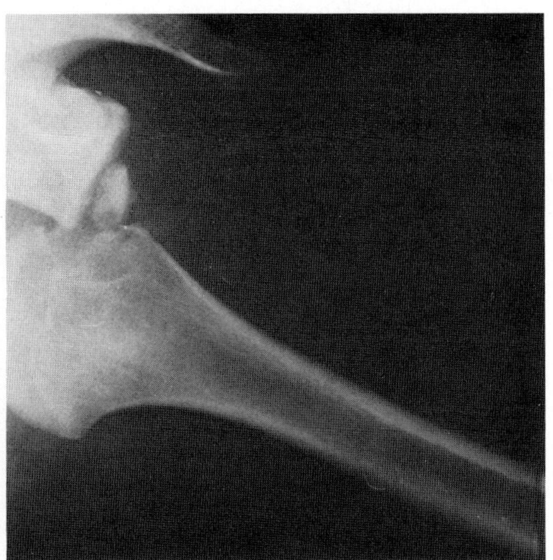

Fig. 11-22. Axillary view of a two-part posterior fracture-dislocation. The lesser tuberosity has been avulsed by the subscapularis, and the head is behind the glenoid.

the side but in slight external rotation for 4 weeks (Fig. 11-23).

Three-Part Posterior Fracture-Dislocations. This lesion (Fig. 11-24) is often missed because of inadequate roentgen studies. An

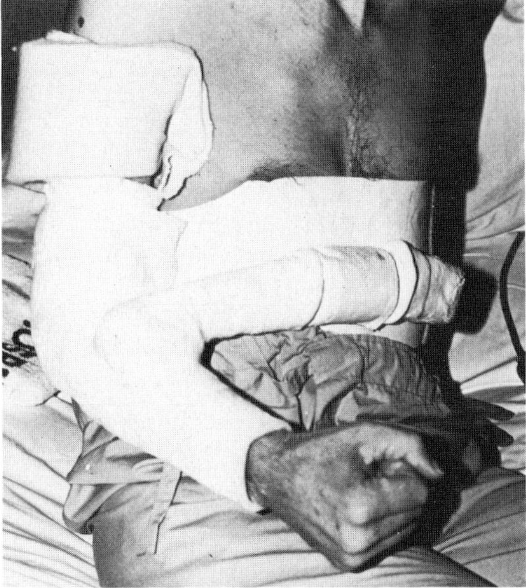

Fig. 11-23. An efficient method of immobilizing the shoulder in external rotation after reduction of a posterior dislocation suggested by Dr. William Kennedy. The elastic commercial arm immobilizer is used with a light circular cast on the forearm and elbow, which is held in external rotation by a strut of plaster over rolled paper. The axillary pad can be changed daily.

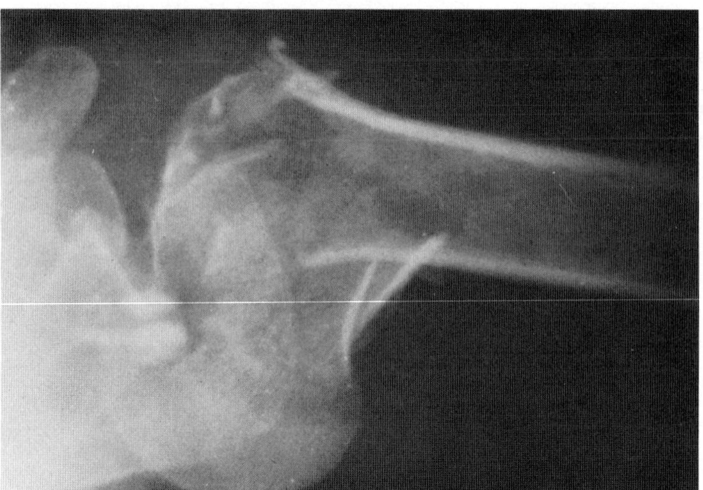

Fig. 11-24. Axillary view of a three-part posterior fracture-dislocation. The head, which is in continuity with most of the greater tuberosity, is dislocated behind the glenoid. The lesser tuberosity is detached and there is 90 degrees rotation of the shaft at the surgical neck level. This lesion is easily overlooked unless an axillary view is obtained.

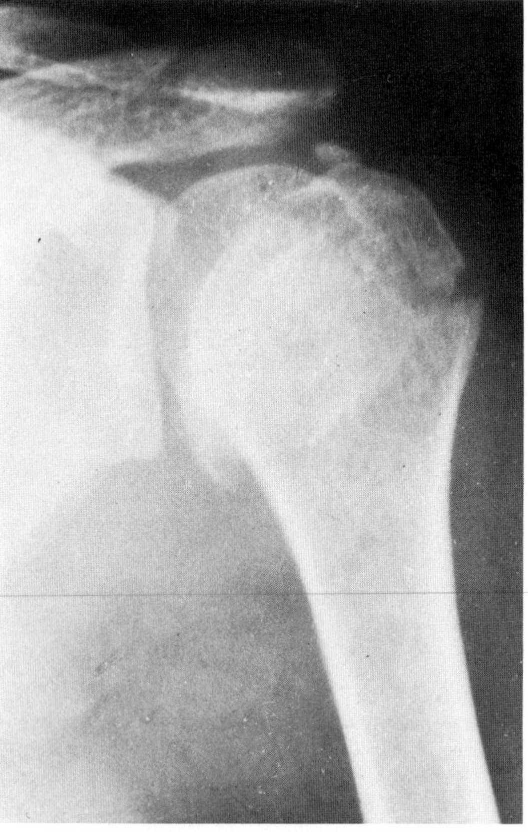

Fig. 11-25. Anteroposterior view of a four-part posterior fracture-dislocation. The posterior dislocation of the articular segment was proven by an axillary view.

axillary view roentgenogram is the best way to establish the diagnosis, and this should always be obtained if the lesion is suggested in other views. If recognized early, closed reduction by traction in forward flexion and gradual adduction may be successful, but I prefer open reduction and accurate wire loop fixation.

Four-Part Posterior Fracture-Dislocations. This rather rare lesion (Fig. 11-25) cannot be reduced by closed means, and because the incidence of avascular necrosis is very high, I prefer early prosthetic replacement and tuberosity repair, as illustrated above for four-part fracture without dislocation.

Fractures of the Articular Surface

Impression Fractures. Small lesions are often seen at the posterior edge of the articular surface in patients with recurrent anterior dislocation (Hill-Sachs defect). They may be the source of a loose osteochondral body that becomes detached to float free in the joint (see p. 642). Larger impression fractures result from acute dislocations when there is severe impact of the head against the rim of the glenoid, usually with posterior dislocations (Fig. 11-26). The bone beneath the indented cartilage is compressed and crushed. The indentation locks the head behind the glenoid, where it remains unless the posterior dislocation is recognized and reduced. Treatment varies with the age of the lesion and the size of the head defect. When recognized early, if less than 20 per cent of the articular surface is involved, the joint is stable after closed reduction. Reduction is accomplished by traction forward with adduction, and the arm is immobilized in slight external rotation (Fig. 11-23). If from 20 to 40 per cent of the articular surface is indented, the joint is often unstable after closed reduction. In this situation I prefer to transplant the lesser tuberosity with the attached subscapularis tendon into the head defect. This is a modification of the McLaughlin procedure.[41] When 50 per cent or more of the head is impressed, I prefer to use a prosthesis to replace the articular surface.

Headsplitting fracture, an uncommon injury, is produced by a violent central impact of the head against the glenoid. The articular surface is fragmented into a number of separate pieces (Fig. 11-27). The tuberosities may also be broken and retracted. This lesion is treated with a prosthesis, and the tuberosities and cuff are repaired.

POSTFRACTURE CARE AND REHABILITATION

A good exercise program is of key importance for optimum results following all upper humeral fractures, especially the displaced lesions. Gentle active assisted exercises using gravity (pendulum exercises) or the good arm are started as soon as healing or surgical repair of the fracture permits the fracture segments to be moved as one (Fig. 11-7). The first objective is to establish a good passive range of motion prior to the maturation of bursal and capsular adhesions. We stress the importance of the

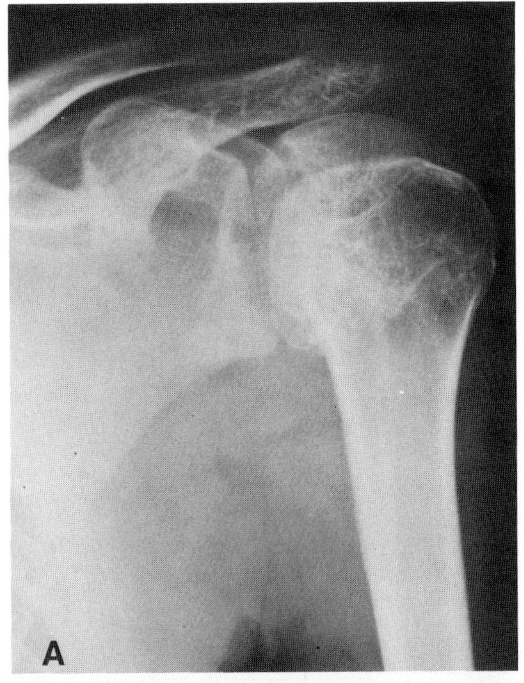

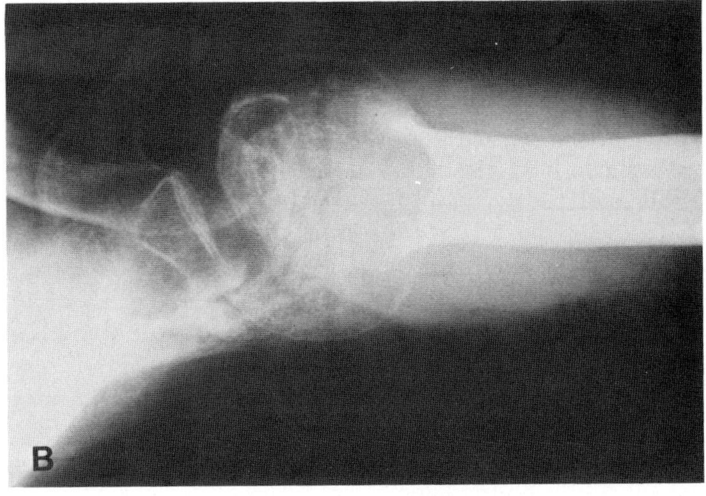

Fig. 11-26. The "impression fracture" usually occurs with a locked posterior dislocation and an axillary view should be obtained whenever it is suspected. (*A*) Anteroposterior view. (*B*) The same lesion is much better appreciated in the axillary view, which shows the head to be posterior to the glenoid.

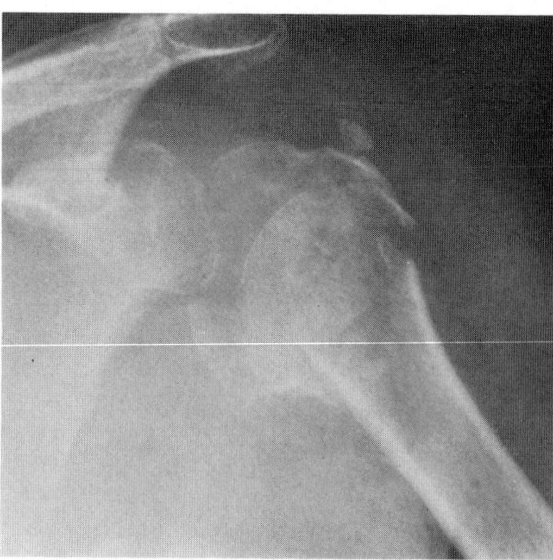

Fig. 11-27. The "headsplitting fracture" results from a central impact, which fragments the articular segment into a number of pieces.

early recovery of external rotation and believe this has been especially helpful.

As union progresses, or when repair permits, isometrics for the deltoid and external rotators are added. Active motion is not attempted until the fragments have united and a good passive range has been achieved, usually at about 6 or 7 weeks, and at this point a considerable lag between active and passive range of motion can be expected. With progressive resistive exercises, performed against the good arm or with a spring exerciser (Fig. 11-8) muscle strength usually returns to normal eventually. For optimum results one should continue stretching exercises for a number of months against any deficiency in range of motion. These are performed after the daily shower. Coordination is reestablished by purposeful use.

The shoulder has the greatest range of motion and the most complex muscle coupling of any joint in the body and is the most difficult to rehabilitate properly. We have found the plan outlined to be of the utmost importance. Displaced fractures require a realistic time schedule and an understanding physician if the best possible results are to be obtained.

PROGNOSIS

There has been a tendency in the literature to underestimate the disability time that follows fractures with minimal displacement. Some patients do recover motion and function within 2 months, but they are exceptional. Lingering stiffness, pain at the extremes of motion, and "weatherache" usually persist for at least 6 months. Strength and coordination return even more slowly.

Displaced lesions requiring tuberosity and cuff repair, with or without prosthetic replacement, can be expected to require much longer periods of recovery. Patients with the most serious injuries have, however, been seen to improve in range, strength, and comfort over several years, provided they continue with occasional stretching and strengthening exercises, which are best done after a shower or bath.

COMPLICATIONS

Joint Stiffness

Bursal and capsular adhesions that restrict range and cause pain at the extremes of motion can usually be overcome by warm applications and stretching exercises. Forceful manipulation may fracture the weakened and osteoporotic bone and are to be avoided. In rare instances, usually in patients treated surgically with inadequate aftercare, when conservative measures have failed to relieve marked restriction and motion has been on a plateau for a number of months, open release of adhesions can be helpful. It is of course mandatory that this latter procedure be followed by an adequate exercise regime.

Unless edema and immobilization of the hand have been avoided throughout the course of treatment, shoulder injuries may be complicated by stiffness of the finger joints. This can be overcome by range-of-motion exercises, but in fact it is best prevented by active and passive exercises of all finger joints during the period of shoulder immobilization.

Malunion

Reconstruction, which should be undertaken only by the most experienced shoulder surgeon, may be required for fixed retraction and malunion of the greater tuberosity which restricts external rotation and elevation and causes pain. The procedure may be technically difficult because of joint and bursal adhesions, adherence of the greater tuberosity to the posterior part of the articular surface, and fixed retraction of the external rotators. The reconstruction involves releasing the adhesions, detaching the greater tuberosity from the head of the humerus, reducing it, and often removing most of it, and repairing the defect in the cuff. The arm is temporarily immobilized on an airplane splint in abduction and external rotation until early healing has occurred. Passive exercises to assist external rotation are especially important during the recovery period.

Although malunion with marked anterior angulation at the surgical neck level permanently restricts elevation (Fig. 11-10), it has rarely been treated by an osteotomy.

Malunited three-part and four-part fractures can be very disabling and are formidable lesions because of fixed retraction of the rotator cuff and scar tissue. The choice of treatment lies between prosthetic replacement arthroplasty and arthrodesis. We usually attempt the replacement arthroplasty first but with the understanding that fusion may be indicated if it fails. Although several new types of total joint replacement are being tried on an experimental basis, failure is usually due to the inadequacy of the rotator cuff.

Old posterior fracture-dislocations have generally been more amenable to prosthetic reconstruction than old anterior fracture-dislocations because of less distortion of the soft tissues.

Avascular Necrosis

Untreated four-part fractures usually develop aseptic necrosis with resorption of the articular segment. As in other malunions, prosthetic reconstruction is unfortunately more difficult than in an acute lesion because of fixed retraction of the rotator cuff and adhesions.

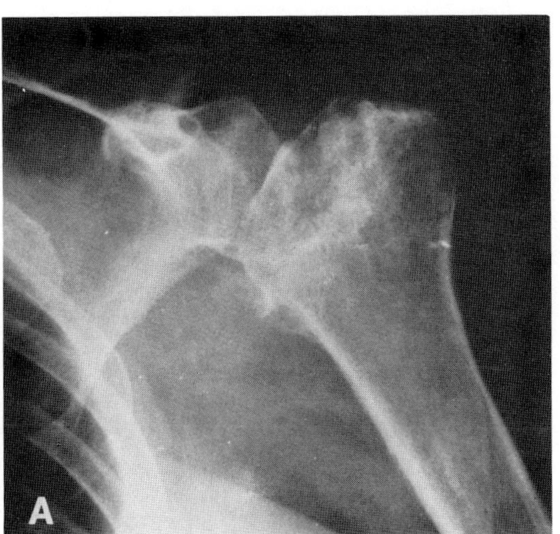

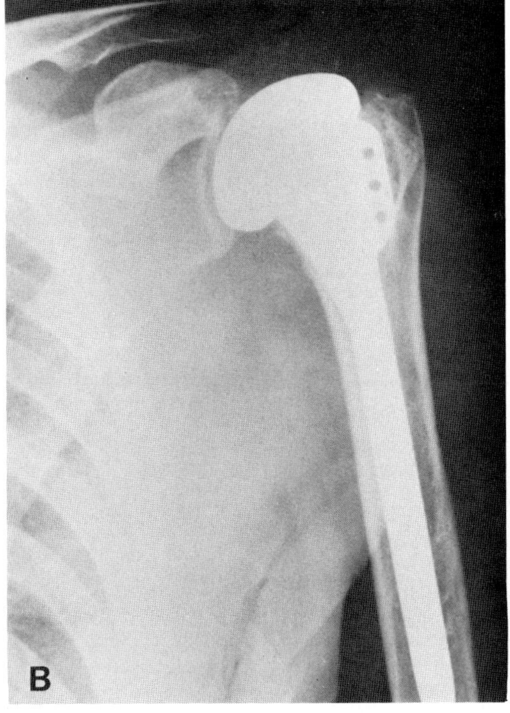

Fig. 11-28. Avascular necrosis of the articular segment following fracture. (*A*) Collapse and resorption of the head seen 2 years after injury. (*B*) The revised prosthesis currently used for repairing such lesions.

Fractures with minimal displacement are occasionally followed by collapse of the head, but these are rare and are easier to treat by prosthetic replacement because the tuberosities and cuff are intact[53] (Fig. 11-28).

Nonunion

Nonunion at the surgical neck is unusual, but it does occur. It usually follows treatment with traction or a hanging cast that distracts the fracture. It is occasionally due to a disregard for immobilization of an unimpacted fracture, such as in patients with multiple injuries or alcoholic patients. The lesion is usually painful, and characteristically the arm cannot be actively elevated to the horizontal. Repair by an overconfident surgeon often fails. The bone is too soft for plate or screw fixation. I prefer to fix this nonunion with an intramedually Rush nail used with a tension wire for compression, iliac bone grafts, and plaster spica for external fixation. I wait for roentgen evidences of consolidation, at least 3 months, before starting exercises.

Myositis Ossificans

As previously stated, this complication has been seen only after fracture-dislocations. The pericapsular bone usually diminishes with time and very rarely requires excision. In no case should an attempt to remove the unwanted bone be made before it has reached maturity. It is observed for at least one year after injury, and observation is continued as long as there are even gradual gains in motion.

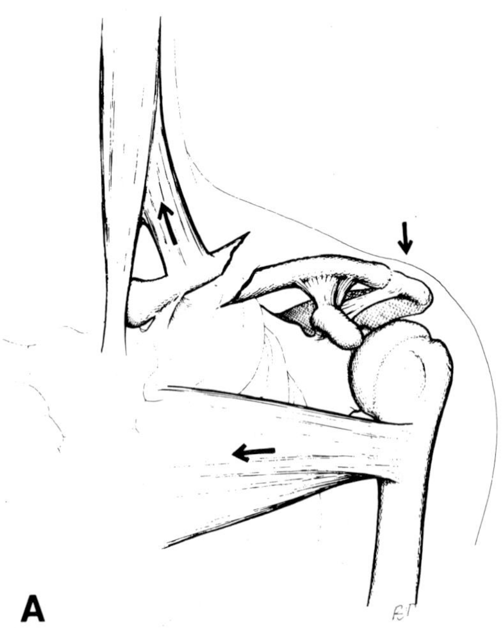

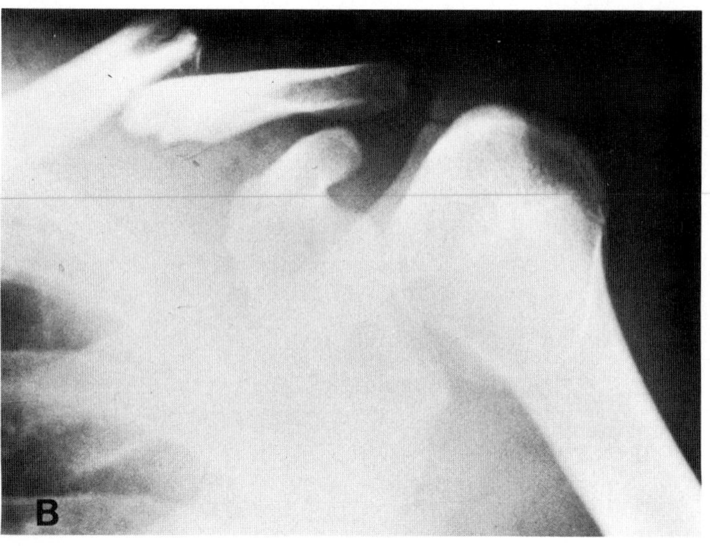

Fig. 11-29. Forces acting to displace fractures of the clavicle. (*A*) The distal segment is pulled downward by the weight of the arm and inward by the pectoralis major and latissimus dorsi. The proximal fragment is pulled upward by the sternomastoid. (*B*) Typical roentgenographic appearance.

FRACTURES OF THE CLAVICLE

The clavicle is the first bone to begin to ossify in the embryo. It is the bone most frequently fractured while passing through the birth canal, and it is among the bones most often fractured during childhood. Statistics indicate that one of every 20 fractures involves the clavicle, but the majority of these injuries occur in children. Surgeons who are accustomed to seeing the amazing healing qualities of this bone in children often fail to appreciate that similar lesions in adult patients usually result from much greater violence, are much slower to unite, and demand more care.

SURGICAL ANATOMY AND FUNCTION

Anchored securely to the scapula by the acromioclavicular and coracoclavicular ligaments and to the trunk by the sternoclavicular and costoclavicular ligaments, the clavicle serves as the only osseous strut to maintain the width of the shoulders. Fractures of the clavicle allow the shoulder to slump downward and forward owing to spasm of the muscles crossing from the thorax to the arm and to the effect of gravity (Fig. 11-29). The proximal fragment tends to be displaced upward by the sternomastoid muscle. With violent trauma the subclavian vessels may be torn and the brachial plexus contused or its roots avulsed.

While the mid-clavicle is tubular, the outer clavicle is flattened, and the coracoclavicular ligaments are attached to the entire length of the undersurface of this flattened portion. Fractures of the outer clavicle have been subdivided into three categories (Fig. 11-30)[109,110] based on anatomical considerations. Undisplaced fractures in the distal clavicle (Type I) are splinted by these ligaments and can be treated symptomatically. With Type II displaced fractures, however, the coracoclavicular ligaments are detached from the proximal fragment. This allows the proximal fragment to be withdrawn backward within the substance of the tapezius muscle (see Fig. 11-32C) while the distal fragment drops forward and downward. Because the distal fragment is anchored to the coracoid and acromion by ligaments, it is rotated by any movement of the scapula (Fig. 11-30). Thus displaced interligamentous fractures of the distal clavicle are prone to delayed union (Fig. 11-31).[108-110]

MECHANISM OF INJURY

Since the clavicle is an S-shaped bone, mechanical forces from the side cause a

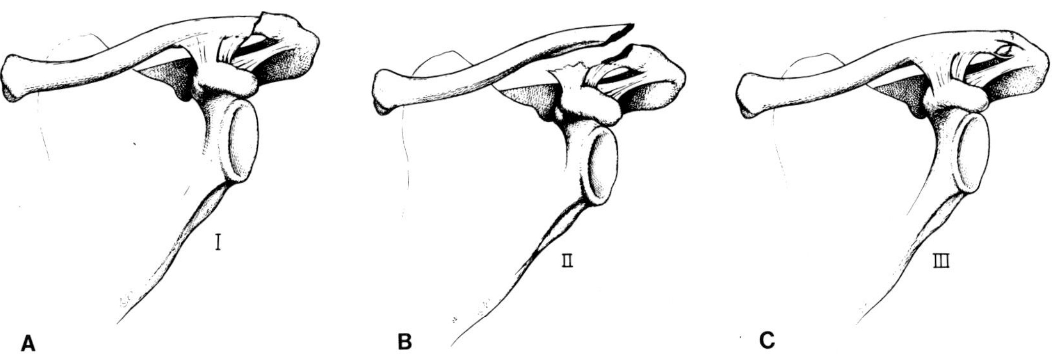

Fig. 11-30. Classification of fractures of the distal clavicle. (*A*) Type I, nondisplaced with intact ligaments. (*B*) Type II, displaced interligamentous fracture in which the coracoclavicular ligaments are detached from the proximal segment, rendering the lesion unstable. (*C*) Type III, articular surface fracture which is easily overlooked and may lead to posttraumatic arthritis.

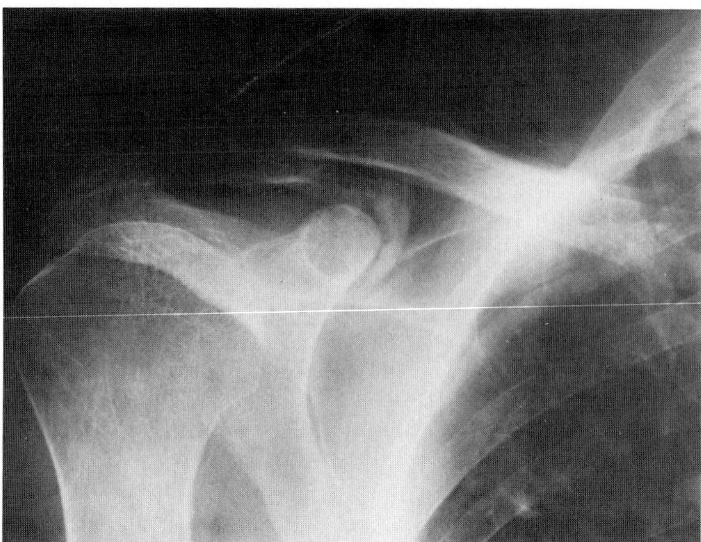

Fig. 11-31. Nonunion of a Type II fracture of the distal clavicle seen 2 years after closed treatment. Bone formed in the coracoclavicular ligament, making it possible to demonstrate that the portion of the ligament going to the distal fragment is intact while that going to the proximal fragment has been detached.

shearing effect on its middle third, where the majority of clavicle fractures occur.

Fractures of the distal portion of the clavicle result from a blow on the point of the shoulder from above downward, while acromioclavicular separations usually result from a force that strikes somewhat more posteriorly. The impact that produces displaced fractures of the outer clavicle may drive the scapula against the chest wall with such force as to produce rib fractures, and when this injury is sustained from a high fall, accompanying head and cervical spine injuries are not uncommon.

Fractures of the inner clavicle usually result from direct trauma. Articular surface fractures at either end are caused by compression of the joint surfaces.

CLASSIFICATION

It is customary to classify these lesions in three groups: (1) mid-third, 80 per cent; (2) distal or interligamentous, 15 per cent; and (3) inner-third, 5 per cent of clavicle fractures.

Because of differences in clinical behavior it has proven helpful to me to subdivide fractures of the distal clavicle as shown in Figure 11-30: Type I, minimal displacement with intact ligaments; Type II, displaced with detachment of the ligaments from the proximal fragment; and Type III, fractures of the articular surface. Type I is a minor injury, but Types II and III can be troublesome.[109,110]

Articular surface fractures are less common at the inner end than at the distal clavicle, but they do occur and can cause permanent symptoms because of subsequent arthritic changes.

SIGNS AND SYMPTOMS

When the fracture is displaced, the shoulder slumps downward and inward, and the patient holds his arm against the chest to protect against shoulder movements. Since the superior surface of the clavicle is subcutaneous, there is direct and indirect tenderness and often palpable deformity and crepitus at the fracture.

Undisplaced fractures and isolated fractures of the articular surfaces do not cause deformity and can easily be overlooked unless special roentgen views are obtained.

ROENTGENOGRAPHIC FINDINGS

Fractures of the middle and inner thirds are studied by an anteroposterior view and a 45-degree view which is made with the tube directed from below cephalad.

Fractures of the distal third require spe-

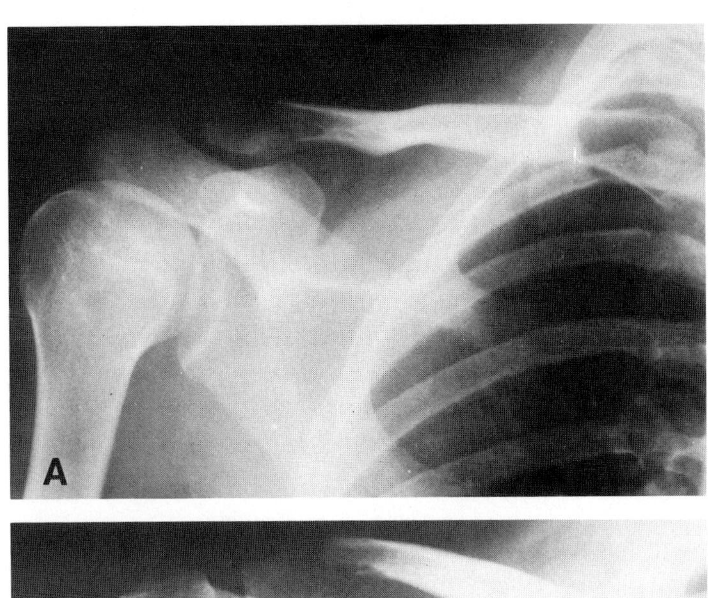

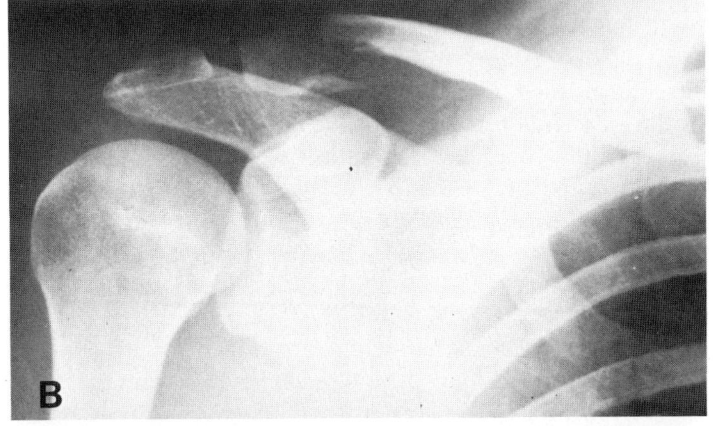

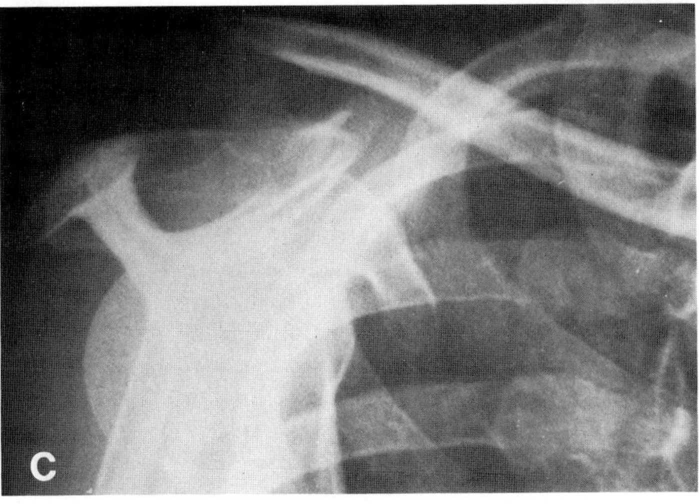

Fig. 11-32. Method of evaluating the coracoclavicular ligament in distal clavicular fractures. Anteroposterior view made (*A*) without weights and (*B*) with the patient erect and with 10 pounds weight in the hand which has caused widening of the coracoclavicular distance from the proximal fragment to the coracoid. The lateral scapular view (*C*) shows the typical displacement of the proximal fragment, which is pulled backward by the trapezius muscle.

cial studies to determine the integrity of the coracoclavicular ligaments (Fig. 11-32). The presence of displacement can be shown by anteroposterior and lateral views in the scapular plane (the "trauma series"). Disruption of the ligaments attaching on the proximal fragment can be further demonstrated by an anteroposterior view of both shoulders on a single large film made with the patient erect and holding 10 pounds of weight in each hand, which shows widening of the space between the coracoid and the clavicle on the injured side.[109,110]

Fractures of the articular surfaces in the acromioclavicular and sternoclavicular joints may require laminagrams for accurate diagnosis.

TREATMENT

Methods of Treatment

An extensive review of the literature on fractures of the clavicle would lead one to conclude that an ideal method of management has not yet been developed. Authors from Hippocrates[72] to the present have been dissatisfied with the results, regardless of the method of treatment. In 1929, Lester[97] reported that over 200 methods had been described for the management of clavicle fractures. Virtually all of these methods can be divided into two major groups: those that merely support the shoulder, such as a sling, sling and swathe, and the Velpeau bandage[97] and those that attempt to maintain a reduction achieved by closed manipulation, including the adhesive dressing of Sayre,[121] figure-of-eight bandages,[117] the Billington Yoke (basically a plaster figure-of-eight),[77] and various types of modified shoulder spicas.[92,113,118] Materials for these appliances also vary, including metal, leather, and plastic, in addition to muslin and plaster.[100,124]

Although many authors have written in support of specific types of methods, there is a familiar recurring theme throughout the extensive literature on unstable fractures of the clavicle i.e., that reduction is practically impossible to maintain, and a certain amount of deformity is to be expected, generally compatible with satisfactory return of function in the shoulder.

Open reduction has rarely been considered to be the preferred treatment for uncomplicated fractures of the shaft of the clavicle. Even the AO group[106] acknowledges that these fractures generally do well with nonoperative management, noting moreover that open reduction frequently results in an unsightly and occasionally painful scar, and that nonunion is not an uncommon complication after operative exposure of the fracture. Open reduction does have a place in the management of complicated fractures of the shaft and fractures of the outer end of the clavicle, as well as in nonunion. The specific indications for these situations are discussed in the following sections.

Author's Preferred Method of Treatment

Fractures of the Middle Third

Reduction can usually be accomplished by drawing the shoulders upward and backward as the ends of the fragments are manipulated into alignment. This may be done with the patient sitting on a stool between two tables to support the arms or supine on a canvas sling. Local anesthesia—10 ml. of 1 per cent Lidocaine may be used. Reduction is usually easy, but, as noted above, maintenance of reduction is not a simple matter. I prefer a modified shoulder spica ("clavicular cast"; Fig. 11-33), which presses backward against the anterior deltoid regions. Union of these fractures in adults requires at least 6 weeks in plaster, followed by a sling. In my experience, figure-of-eight dressings have been inadequate for adult patients.

Fractures of the Distal Clavicle

Group I fractures (Fig. 11-30A) with minimal displacement and intact ligaments require only a sling, and activities are extended as pain subsides.

Group II displaced fractures are unstable, because the coracoclavicular ligaments are detached from the proximal fragment (see Figs. 11-30B and 11-32). The proximal fragment is retracted upward and backward within the substance of the trapezius muscle, while the distal fragment drops

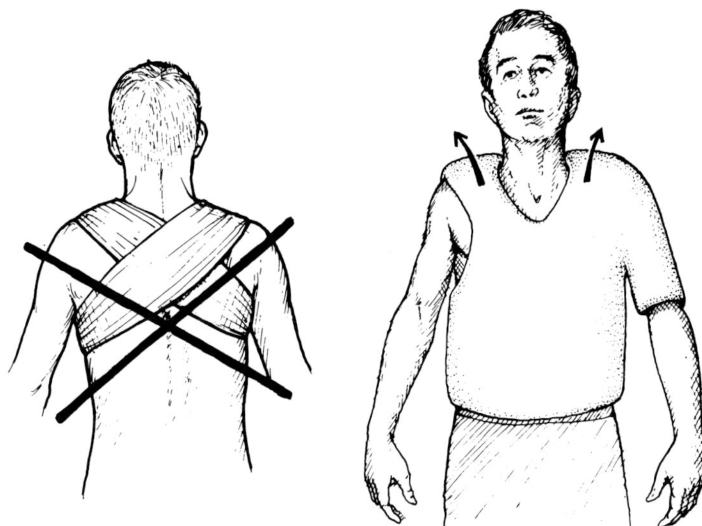

Fig. 11-33. The clavicular cast, a modified shoulder spica that exerts backward and upward pressure on the anterior deltoid regions, is preferred for clavicular fractures in adult patients. The figure-of-eight dressing, commonly used in children, provides less immobilization and comfort.

downward and forward and is rotated by any movements of the scapula. The usual figure-of-eight dressing should not be used, because it presses the proximal fragment backward and exaggerates this deformity. Closed treatment requires a type of strapping that draws the point of the shoulder upward and backward, and while closed treatment may succeed, it is difficult to maintain reduction, and union is usually slow and imperfect. For this reason I prefer internal fixation with a transacromial wire that transfixes the distal fragment between the acromion and the proximal fragment.[109,110] In doing operative fixation it is important to appreciate that the distal fragment retains intact ligamentous attachments which contribute to the strength of the repair, and this fragment should not be excised except in rare instances when its articular surface has been distorted by the injury. It is important to carefully position the patient semi-sitting with a sandbag under the scapula and the head turned away from the operating field. A stiff, smooth $\frac{3}{32}$-inch Steinmann pin is passed laterally out through the distal fragment, after the fracture site is exposed through a 3-cm. oblique incision. The blunt end of the wire is passed back into the proximal fragment, and the distal end of the pin is bent to prevent medial migration. It is cut off beneath the skin. A sling and swathe is worn for 6 weeks, at which time the pin is removed. A good alternative method of internal fixation is two No. 18 wire sutures passed under the coracoid behind the conjoint tendon attachment and around the shaft of the clavicle to hold it in close apposition to the distal fragment. These wires are also removed through a small incision after about 6 weeks.

Group III fractures of the articular surface of the clavicle (see Fig. 11-30C) frequently lead to symptomatic arthritic changes, and, apparently because of the abundant blood supply, they may be followed by extensive resorption of the end of this bone. When this injury is followed by persistent symptoms, it can be treated satisfactorily by excision of the acromioclavicular joint leaving most of the coracoclavicular ligament intact. It is important in acromioclavicular arthroplasty to suture the trapezius muscle to the deltoid muscle so that it covers the stump of the clavicle and fills the dead space.

Fractures of the Inner Clavicle

These fractures can be treated with a supporting sling, but occasionally, when the articular surface is involved, they lead to arthritic changes with persistent pain and disability. The latter complication is treated by excision of the inner clavicle. In doing sternoclavicular arthroplasty it is important to leave most of the costoclavicular ligament intact and to transfer the clavicular head of the sternomastoid into the dead space, to minimize hematoma formation and to reduce the tendency of the stump to ride upward.

Indications for Operative Treatment

The indications for operative treatment of acute fractures of the clavicle may be summarized as follows: (1) neurovascular involvement; (2) interposition of soft tissues; (3) open fractures; (4) electively for uncontrolled deformity, especially in young women; (5) electively for the management of selected patients with multiple injuries; and (6) electively for Group II distal clavicle fractures.

Unless the surgeon approaches internal fixation of clavicle fractures with the same precautions and scrupulous technique accorded any other long bone fracture, the incidence of complications is high. Short oblique incisions in Langer's lines (which parallel the curve of a necklace) are preferred and an intramedullary pin is passed retrograde as described by Rowe.[118] Through a 3.0-cm. incision a smooth, 3/32-inch Steinmann pin is inserted out through the distal fragment and skin. Then, after reducing the fracture, the blunt end is passed back into the proximal fragment. The wire is bent and cut off beneath the skin.

The indications and technique for late resection of the acromioclavicular or sternoclavicular joints have been discussed above.

PROGNOSIS

Nonunion of the clavicle is rare.[108] It is more likely to occur in poorly immobilized and neglected fractures, such as in patients with multiple injuries or in unstable Group II displaced fractures of the distal end. Malunion is common, and for this reason it seems justifiable to consider elective internal fixation in selected displaced fractures of the middle third in young women who require a good cosmetic result.

The time required for enough consolidation to permit adult patients to resume heavier activities is considerably greater than that for children—at least 3 months. The incidence of refracture is high in mature clavicles that are subjected to violent activities prior to that time.

COMPLICATIONS

Neurovascular

Exuberant callus, residual deformity, and scarring in the middle third may be associated with persistent neurological defects and circulatory changes due to compression of the subclavian vessels and brachial plexus against the first rib (see Fig. 11-81). The presence of anomalous cervical ribs predisposes the patient to this problem, and cervical spine roentgenograms should be obtained. When neurovascular symptoms are severe, decompression by excision of the middle third of the clavicle may be indicated. It is also important to consider the possibility that a cervical root avulsion or brachial plexus injury could have occurred at the time the fracture was sustained.

Malunion

An ugly prominence in the middle clavicle can be extremely disturbing to a young woman. Shaving away the bone is usually inadequate, and an osteotomy for realignment and internal fixation is usually required.

Nonunion

This less common complication, in my experience, is usually symptomatic and is treated by internal fixation and iliac grafts, which are placed posteriorly (away from the neurovascular bundle and subcutaneous surfaces).[108] Occasionally the patient has insufficient disability to require treatment, but most have pain and fatigue symptoms until the lesion is repaired.

Posttraumatic Arthritis

The acromioclavicular joint is much more frequently involved than the sternoclavicular joint. The articular surface defect has usually been overlooked at the time of the injury. Comparison roentgenograms of the normal side and laminagrams are helpful in establishing the diagnosis. A therapeutic test injection of 1 per cent Xylocaine into the joint should temporarily eliminate pain; this is done before recommending surgical excision of the joint.[127] In acromioclavicular arthroplasty, after excising the outer clavicle, the trapezius muscle is sutured to the deltoid muscle. In sternoclavicular arthroplasty the clavicular head of the sternomastoid is used to fill the dead space, as described above.

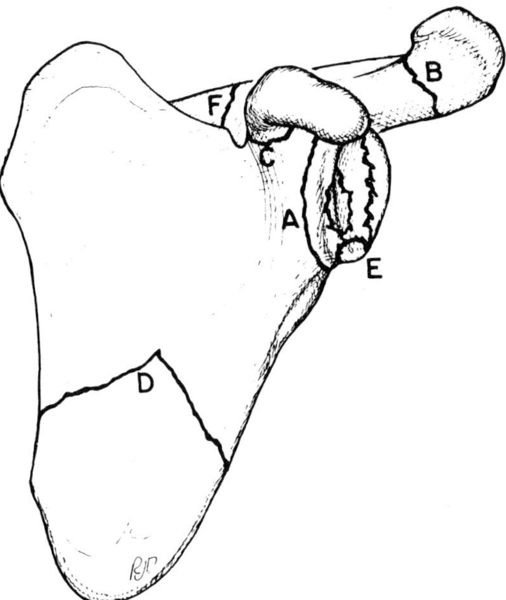

Fig. 11-34. The scapula is subject to a variety of fractures, (*A*) neck, (*B*) acromial process, (C) coracoid process, (*D*) body, (*E*) glenoid rim or articular surface, (*F*) spinous process.

FRACTURES OF THE SCAPULA

Fractures of the scapula are relatively uncommon and occur most frequently in persons between the ages of 40 and 60 years.[163] The scapula acts as a flat surface against the ribs for stabilization of the upper extremity against the thorax. Since it is firmly attached to the clavicle and articulates with the humerus, it is subjected to a large variety of injuries (Fig. 11-34). The surgical anatomy, mechanism of injury, and therapeutic implications of each of these injuries will be considered separately.

FRACTURE OF THE BODY AND SPINE OF THE SCAPULA

The body and spine of the scapula are surrounded by muscles and heal rapidly with little residual disability. The scapula's muscle coverage and ability to slide and recoil along the chest wall protect it from both direct and indirect trauma. Injury to the scapula, therefore, usually requires direct trauma of appreciable magnitude and should alert the surgeon to search for associated injuries (e.g., multiple rib fractures, pneumothorax, subcutaneous emphysema, vertebral compression fractures, and extremity fractures). Because of the gravity of associated injuries, fractures of the scapula are often missed initially.[166] Scapula fractures may also occur from indirect trauma, and there are even reports of avulsion fractures from psychiatric electroshock therapy.[164]

Clinical and Roentgenographic Findings

The patient with a fractured scapula usually holds his arm adducted and protects it from all movement, especially abduction. Tenderness, ecchymosis and hematoma are found overlying and adjacent to the fracture site. "Pseudorupture of the rotator cuff" may occur, as described by Neviaser.[157] This syndrome is caused by intramuscular hemorrhage into the supraspinatus, infraspinatus, and subscapularis, resulting in secondary spasm which produces loss of arm abduction and may mimic a rotator cuff injury. Abduction power returns as the hematoma and spasm resolve.

Roentgenograms should include anteroposterior and tangential oblique views of the scapula (trauma series).

Methods of Treatment

A method of skeletal traction through the scapula has been described to improve the alignment,[144] and surgery has been suggested to remove malaligned fragments,[143] but the primary objective of treatment is to make the patient comfortable. Infiltration of the fracture with local anesthesia and hyaluronidase has been recommended as providing prolonged relief.[154] Most authors recommend local ice and immobilization of the scapula for comfort. Skin condition permitting, the scapula of a nonambulatory patient can be immobilized by a criss-cross moleskin adhesive strapping across the shoulder and down over the patient's back to the level of his waist. Ambulatory patients may be treated with a sling and swathe or a simple sling. Pendulum exercises as tolerated should be started early. At 10 to 14 days, the sling is removed, and use of the shoulder within pain tolerance is encouraged. Full range of motion is usually regained, although discomfort may persist for several weeks.[138]

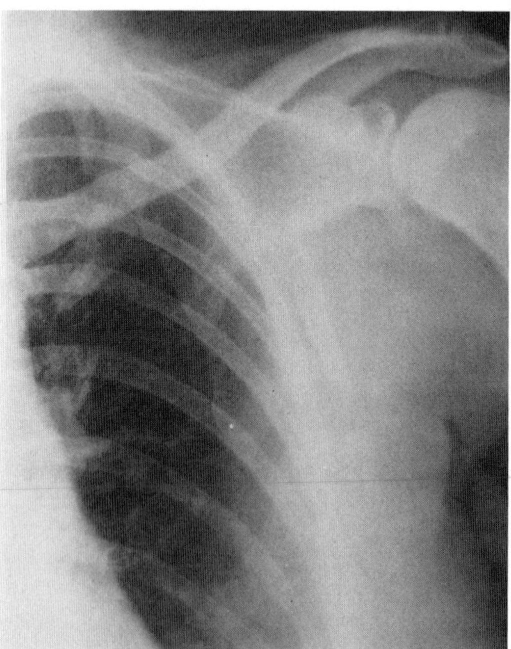

Fig. 11-35. A displaced fracture of the body of the scapula that was associated with fractures of ten ribs. It was allowed to unite in this position, and there was no residual functional or cosmetic impairment.

Tachdijan[167] believes that if displacement and deformity are marked, reduction attempts may be indicated, though rarely. This is accomplished with traction on the arm and abduction or adduction of the shoulder. If displacement recurs when the arm is lowered, immobilization in abduction may be necessary for a brief period. This can be done with an abduction splint, shoulder spica, or lateral traction with an olecranon pin.[167]

Author's Preferred Method of Treatment

I believe that fractures of the body and spine of the scapula can be treated in the same way that the surrounding soft-tissue injury is treated, by cold applications to minimize bleeding for the first 48 hours followed by low heat, to increase local resorption, and by continuing immobilization so long as needed to relieve pain. Considerable displacement is compatible with a good result (Fig. 11-35) and can be accepted.

Complications

Complications of these fractures are rare, but axillary artery injury[161] and partial brachial plexus palsy[159] have been reported. Fractures involving the vertebral border may heal with bony irregularities which cause soft-tissue to impinge on the vertebral bodies. Chronic irritation may cause pain, crepitus, and limitation of motion, which may necessitate excision of irregular areas on the scapula.[131] A large displaced fragment or a wad of callus may cause pressure symptoms by encroachment on the intrascapulothoracic space. Excision of the mass or irregularity may be required for relief.[154]

INTRATHORACIC DISLOCATION OF THE SCAPULA

Intrathoracic dislocation, also known as "locked scapula,"[156] is rare. The mechanism of injury is postulated by Key and Conwell[147] to be forceful outward traction on the arm or direct force applied to the posterior surface of the scapula. The entire body of the scapula is displaced forward and outward, and its lower angle is locked between the ribs. Usually the surrounding soft tissues tear, or the scapula or ribs fracture before this dislocation occurs.

Clinical and Roentgenographic Findings

The patient complains of shoulder or chest pain, and superior and lateral displacement of the scapula may be noted. However, the diagnosis may be masked by other injuries. A single case reported by Nettrour *et al.*[156] was associated with a sternoclavicular separation and a rib fracture on the same side. The diagnosis was not made until 6 weeks after injury, necessitating surgery to reef up the soft tissues before reduction could be maintained; full function returned. The dislocation in this case was not apparent on the anteroposterior chest film (although some lateral and superior scapular displacement was noted), but it could be seen readily; on an anterior oblique film of the chest (tangential view of the scapula).

Treatment

DePalma[11] states that the injury responds to closed reduction and that surgery is never indicated. His technique of reduction is as follows: while an assistant applies steady traction on the hyperabducted arm, the surgeon grasps the axillary border of the scapula and in one movement rotates it forward and pushes it directly backward. After reduction is obtained, the scapula is fixed to the chest wall with eight to ten lengths of 3-inch adhesive tape (padding the axilla) and the arm is suspended in a collar and cuff sling with a swathe around the chest and arm. This dressing is changed after 7 to 10 days, and free use of the arm is begun after 2 weeks.

FRACTURE OF THE NECK OF THE SCAPULA

Although fracture of the neck of the scapula is an uncommon lesion, one of the earliest fractures on record is of this type. A healed fracture of the neck of the scapula was noted on a skeleton exhumed from a neolithic burial chamber.[145]

Clinical and Roentgenographic Findings

Sir Astley Cooper[135] described what he thought was the classic clinical picture of this lesion over a century ago. He noted flattening of the shoulder, prominence of the acromion, easy reduction of downward displacement of the shoulder by supporting the elbow, and immediate return with crepitus when unsupported. Unfortunately, two of the three cases in which he made the diagnosis proved to be fractures of the neck of the humerus at autopsy. Even so, older fracture textbooks quoted his clinical description for years.

This injury usually occurs as the result of a blow that may be directed anteriorly, posteriorly, or directly on the point of the shoulder.[131,138] The fracture is usually impacted, and is the counterpart of the more common surgical neck fractures of the humerus on the other side of the glenohumeral joint.

The patient holds the arm in abduction. All movement is painful, as is lateral pressure over the humeral head. Flattening of the shoulder, with pain and fullness in the infraclavicular fossa may be noted. Ecchymosis may be absent.

Anteroposterior and tangential roentgenograms (trauma series) usually reveal that the typical fracture extends from the supraclavicular notch through the surgical neck to a point below the coracoid process. The glenoid and the coracoid constitute the distal fragment and may be a single fragment or comminuted. The articular surface of the glenoid is usually intact, and the capsule and ligaments of the shoulder remain unaffected.[131]

Tachdijan[167] states that if the coracoclavicular or acromioclavicular ligaments are intact, there is no displacement of the articular fragment. However, if the ligaments are torn or if the fracture line is lateral to the coracoid, then the weight of the limb and pull of the muscles displaces the fracture downward and inward. Restoration of the neck of the scapula to its anatomical position is not necessary for good functional results, but marked angulation of the articular surface may predispose to glenohumeral subluxation or dislocation.[138]

Methods of Treatment

DePalma[11] recommends that severely angulated fractures be treated with lateral traction. The patient is placed in the supine position, and skeletal traction of 6 to 12 pounds is applied through a threaded olecranon pin. Three to 6 pounds of skin traction is applied to the forearm to position the extremity with the shoulder in 90 degrees abduction and the elbow in 90 degrees flexion. The side of the bed supporting the injured extremity is elevated 4 inches. Traction is maintained for 3 weeks, followed by 2 weeks in an arm sling with a progressive physical therapy and exercise program. Bateman recommends closed manipulation of the fracture and 6 to 8 weeks in a shoulder spica.

Author's Preferred Method of Treatment

There is rarely an indication for open reduction of a fracture of the neck of the scapula unless the glenoid is involved (see next section). The functional results of these fractures are much better than the disturbing roentgenograms would indicate.[166]

When these fractures are minimally displaced and stable, I treat them by early functional exercises, as described above for upper humeral fractures.

FRACTURE OF THE GLENOID

The rim of the bony glenoid is avulsed in about 20 per cent of traumatic shoulder

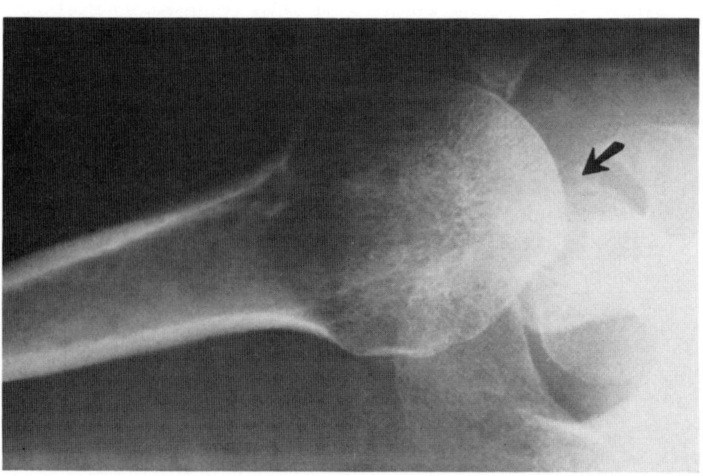

Fig. 11-36. Fracture of the anterior rim of the glenoid seen in the axillary view several months after an anterior, subcoracoid dislocation of the glenohumeral joint.

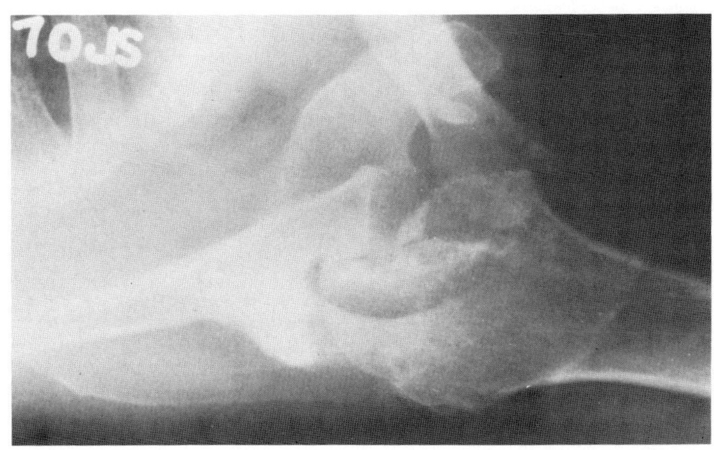

Fig. 11-37. Axillary view shows a displaced fracture of the articular surface of the glenoid. The posterior half of the glenoid is depressed in association with an impression fracture of the humeral head. This malunion required replacement arthroplasty.

dislocations (Fig. 11-36). These small fragments are best seen in axillary view roentgenograms made with the film held above the shoulder and the tube near the patient's hip (see Fig. 11-4). It is helpful to determine the presence of these fragments, because they confirm the diagnosis and may be useful in repairing recurrent subluxations or dislocations.[130] In posterior dislocations the posterior rim may be avulsed.

Large portions of the articular surface of the glenoid are occasionally depressed with either anterior or posterior fracture-dislocations, as illustrated in Fig. 11-37. These lesions are caused by a violent central impact of the head of the humerus, and they render the joint incongruous and unstable. They require open operative treatment.

The inferior lip of the glenoid may be avulsed by a violent contraction of the triceps muscle, as in throwing a baseball. Repeated episodes of this type can lead to an osteochondral prominence that has at times been quite disabling to professional athletes and is difficult to treat.

FRACTURE OF THE ACROMION

These lesions usually result from a direct downward blow on the shoulder. A careful neurological examination is important, because an impact of this magnitude may also produce avulsion of the roots of the brachial plexus.

Clinical and Roentgenographic Findings

The fracture line is usually lateral to the acromioclavicular joint, but it may occur at the base of the acromion, adjacent to the scapular spine. Attempted abduction of the arm is very painful, and motion is restricted. The shoulder may be flattened, and there is localized pain, swelling, and tenderness.

Diagnosis is confirmed on anteroposterior and axillary lateral views of the shoulder. An unfused acromial epiphysis, or os acromiale, may be confused with a fracture of the acromion. When in doubt, both shoulders should be x-rayed, the os acromiale being bilateral in about 60 per cent of the cases.[151,166] In compensation cases, distinguishing between an old fracture and an os acromiale may be important. According to Liberson,[151] such a distinction may be facilitated by a top-to-bottom axillary view of the acromion, placing the cassette in the axilla and shooting from above.

Methods of Treatment

Immobilization of the shoulder in an arm sling and a circular strapping that pushes the flexed elbow upward and the lateral part of the clavicle downward has been advocated.[140,167] Range-of-motion exercises are begun after 3 to 4 weeks. McLaughlin[154] stated that bony union is the rule, despite the presence or absence of immobilization, provided the fragments are in apposition.

Fibrous union occasionally occurs with failure to recognize interposition of soft tissue. He noted that symptomatic nonunion or malunion can be relieved by periosteal resection of enough acromion to include the offending lesion.

Author's Preferred Method of Treatment

The fracture is usually without significant displacement and can be treated symptomatically. Displaced fractures occasionally require elevation and Kirschner wire fixation to eliminate impingement on the subacromial space or derangement of the acromioclavicular joint.

The acromion may be fractured by an upward impact of the humeral head when the rare "superior dislocation" of the glenohumeral joint occurs. The powerful force that produces this lesion also causes extensive tearing of the rotator cuff, which requires surgical repair. The lesion is usually underdiagnosed, but it should be suspected if the acromial fragment is displaced upward and the subacromial space (acromiohumeral distance) is less than 5 mm. An arthrogram of the glenohumeral joint demonstrates the extent of the tear in the rotator cuff. Every effort should be made to repair the rotator tendons and the acromion. Acromionectomy should be especially avoided, because it weakens the deltoid muscle, which, in the face of cuff impairment, can be disastrous.

FRACTURE OF THE CORACOID

The coracoid process stands out from the anterosuperior aspect of the scapula, and its attached muscles and ligaments play an important role in stabilizing the scapula as well as contributing to flexion of the shoulder and elbow. The muscles that attach to it are the short head of the biceps, the coracobrachialis and the pectoralis minor. Its attached ligaments are the coracohumeral, coracoacromial, and coracoclavicular. A hard blow on the point of the shoulder, such as that which produces a displaced fracture of the distal clavicle of an acromioclavicular dislocation, may avulse the coracoid by exerting traction on the coracoclavicular ligament (see Fig. 11-143). It may also be avulsed by strong muscle pull,[131] and McLaughlin[154] stated that it is most often fractured by the impact of a dislocating humeral head. Others state that the coracoid process usually fractures at the base, most often secondary to direct trauma.[131,162] Serious displacement occurs only when the ligaments are torn.[154,162]

Clinical and Roentgenographic Findings

Acute injuries are associated with local pain and tenderness, as well as pain on forced adduction of the shoulder and flexion of the elbow. The patient may also complain of pain with deep inspiration, thought to be due to the pull of the pectoralis minor.[162] If the coracoid process is severely displaced, the fragment may be palpated close to the axillary fold.[162] Old injuries may cause vague symptoms aggravated by specific motions of the shoulder.[132] The initial force may cause the coracoid to contuse the cords of the brachial plexus which lie just beneath it. This can produce subtle and occult neurological defects which are easily overlooked initially.

Anteroposterior roentgenograms may demonstrate a fractured coracoid, but a good axillary lateral is essential to avoid missing the lesion. The distal fragment is usually displaced downward and medially.[131] Fractures may be confused with accessory ossification centers, which may occur at the proximal and distal aspects of the coracoid process. These are generally shell-like and are characteristically located medial to the base, or they may be small and located at the tip of the coracoid process.[148] An infracoracoid bone has been reported. This appears to lie free between the coracoid process and the glenoid fossa.[148]

Treatment

Bateman[131] stated that considerable disability may occur from weakness of the muscles and suspensory ligament. If the ligaments are involved in the injury, he recommended either fixation in a shoulder spica cast for 6 weeks, or transfixation of the acromioclavicular joint. Most authors state that no specific treatment is indicated other than what is required for the patient's immediate comfort.[132,134,147,154,166] McLaughlin[155] believed that fibrous union is not uncommon and is associated with no residual defect. Rowe[162] noted that if the fractured fragment is markedly displaced, open repair should give excellent results. Benton[132] stated that in fresh fractures internal fixation is not necessary, but in symptomatic old injuries, excision of the distal fragment and reattachment of the conjoined tendon is preferable.

In most instances I feel that no special treatment of the coracoid fracture is needed other than to insure decompression of the neurovascular bundle. Dislocation of the acromioclavicular joint, which may occur in association with fracture of the coracoid, is treated by open repair of the fracture and dislocation.

Part 2: Dislocations About the Shoulder

Charles A. Rockwood, Jr., M.D.

Dislocations about the shoulder include those of the glenohumeral joint and of the clavicle with its articulations. A working classification of dislocations of the shoulder complex is shown below:

Classification of Dislocations About the Shoulder

I. GLENOHUMERAL JOINT
- A. Anterior dislocation
  - 1. *Traumatic injuries*
    - Sprain
    - Subluxation
    - Acute dislocation—subcoracoid, subglenoid, subclavicular, or intrathoracic
    - Recurring dislocation
    - Unreduced dislocation
  - 2. *Atraumatic dislocation*
    - Voluntary or habitual dislocation
    - Congenital dislocation
- B. Posterior dislocation
  - 1. *Traumatic injuries*
    - Sprains
    - Subluxation
    - Acute dislocations—subacromial, subglenoid, or subspinous
    - Recurring dislocations
    - Unreduced dislocations
  - 2. *Atraumatic dislocation*
    - Voluntary or habitual dislocations
    - Congenital dislocations
- C. Superior dislocation
- D. Inferior Dislocation (luxatio erecta)

II. DISLOCATION OF THE CLAVICLE AND ITS ARTICULATIONS
- A. Acromioclavicular joint
  - Sprain
  - Subluxation—anterior, posterior, or superior
  - Acute dislocation—superior or inferior
  - Unreduced dislocation
- B. Sternoclavicular joint
  - 1. *Traumatic*
    - Sprain
    - Subluxation
    - Acute dislocation—anterior or posterior
    - Unreduced dislocation
  - 2. *Atraumatic dislocation*
    - Voluntary or habitual dislocation
    - Congenital dislocation
- C. Total dislocation of the clavicle

III. DISLOCATION OF THE SCAPULA

In this classification, I have tried to be as complete as possible, including each of the common and the uncommon types of dislocations in an appropriate category.

The most common dislocation about the shoulder is an anterior dislocation of the glenohumeral joint (80 to 85%). In fact, it is the most commonly dislocated major joint of the body. Second in frequency is dislocation of the acromioclavicular joint (10 to 15%). Dislocations of the sternoclavicular joint and posterior dislocations of the shoulder are quite rare (3 to 5%).

ANTERIOR DISLOCATION OF THE SHOULDER

HISTORICAL BACKGROUND

While the statement "nothing is new" has been made many times, it certainly is most appropriate for dislocations about the shoulder. The most detailed early description of anterior dislocations came from the father of medicine, Hippocrates, who was born in 460 B.C., on the Island of Cos. In his three texts on the skeleton, he beautifully described the anatomy and types of dislocations, discussed problems with recurrent dislocations, and described the first surgical procedure. In the translation by Adams,[169] it is interesting to note that Hippocrates saw and treated only the downward (into the armpit) type of dislocation. However, he did say that anterior, posterior, and upward dislocations can occur. Hence, all of his maneuvers to reduce the shoulder were a direct approach to the head of the humerus through the axilla to replace the humerus into the glenoid cavity. In one of his classical pro-

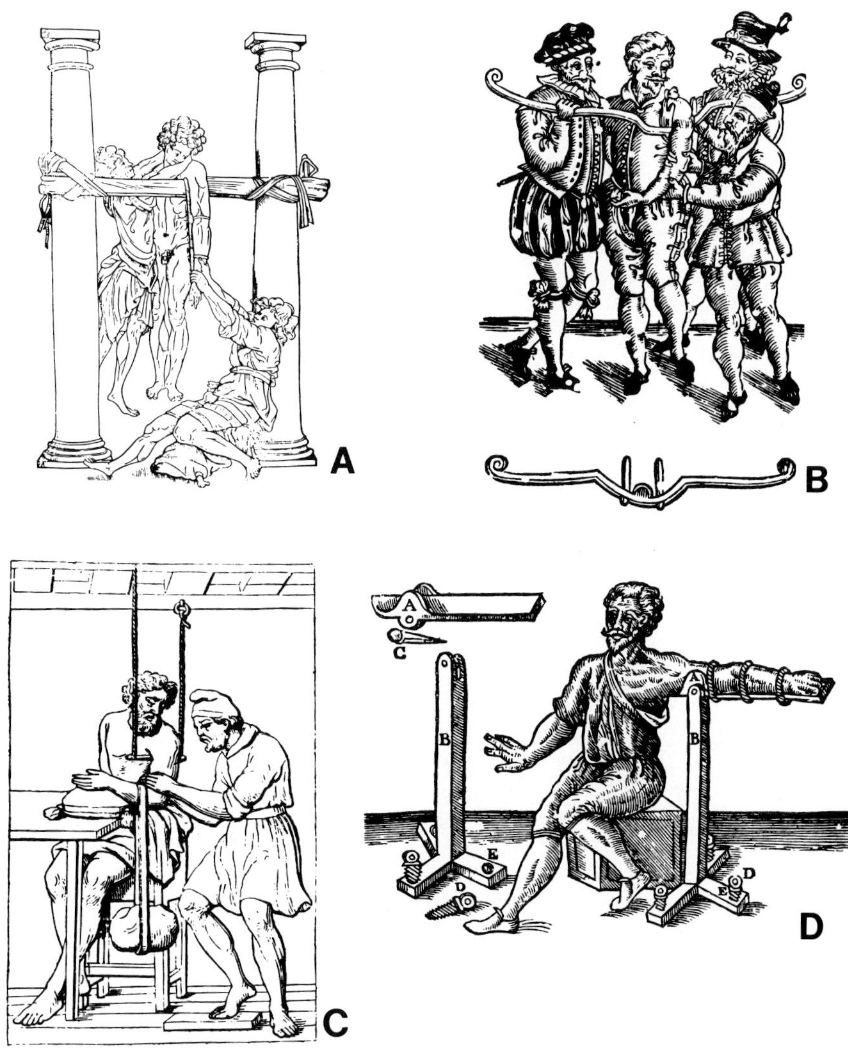

Fig. 11-38. Methods used to reduce dislocations of the shoulder during the 16th and 17th centuries. (*A*) Reduction over a beam with a wooden splint along the medial side of the arm. (*B*) Reduction over a padded wooden yoke. (*C*) Reduction over a wooden axillary frame along with manipulation of the arm. (*D*) Reduction through the use of a hinge fulcrum technique. (Brockbank, W., and Griffiths, D. L.: J. Bone Joint Surg., *30B*:365-375, 1948)

cedures for reduction, he stressed the need for suitable sized leather-covered balls to be placed into the axilla, for without them the heel could not reach the head of the humerus. Other techniques described by Hippocrates are reported by Brockbank and Griffiths,[205] who also studied woodcuts from the early texts of Cruce, Galen, Pare, Scultetus, Vidus, and Worthington (Fig. 11-38).

Hippocrates wrote, "It deserves to be known how a shoulder which is subject to frequent dislocations should be treated."[169] He stated, "I have never known any physician to treat a case properly." He went on to say that "some persons, owing to frequent dislocations, were obliged to give up gymnastic exercises. And some, because of their ineptness in war, had perished." Burning of the shoulder was popular at that time, and Hippocrates criticized his contemporaries for improper burning. In this, the first description of a surgical procedure for recurrent dislocation of the shoulder, he described how physicians had burned the top, anterior, and posterior aspects of the shoulder which only caused scarring in those areas and promoted the downward dislocation. He described the use of cautery in which an oblong, red-hot iron was inserted through the axilla to make eschars, but only in the lower part of the joint. He displayed considerable knowledge of the anatomy of the shoulder. (Adams infers that Hippocrates must have done anatomical dissections.) In his description, Hippocrates warned the surgeon not to let the iron come in contact with the major vessels and nerves, as that would cause great harm. Following the burnings, he bound the arm to the side, day and night for a long time, "for thus more especially will cicatrization take place, and the wide space into which the humerus used to escape will become contracted."

I don't think anyone can say just why all of the dislocated shoulders seen by Hippocrates were into the armpit. Quite probably many were the subcoracoid type which were interpreted, without the benefit of roentgenography, as a type of downward dislocation. However, Adams, who translated the original Greek text by Hippocrates in 1886, stated that after reviewing his 30 years of practice, he had reached the same conclusion (i.e., he had never seen the anterior or posterior dislocation).[169] He also noted that Galen, in the course of

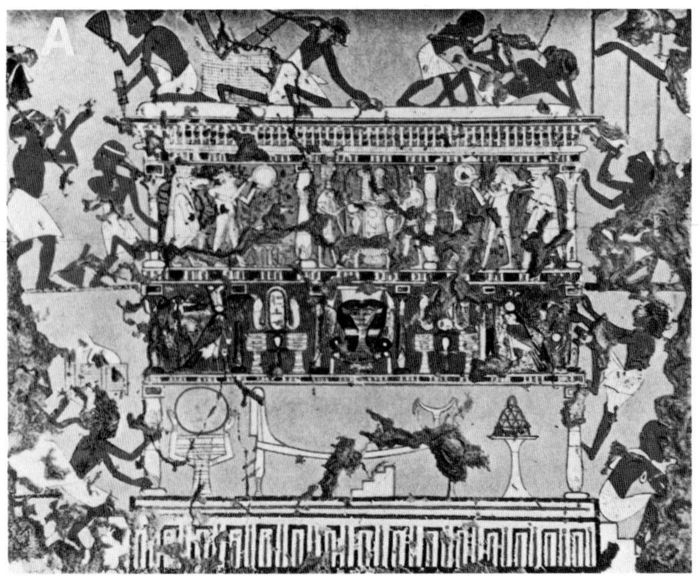

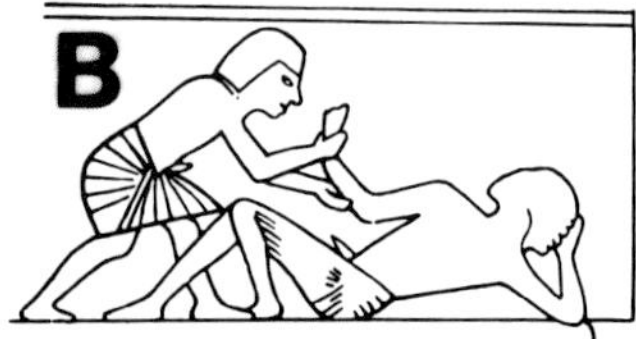

Fig. 11-39. The Kocher technique is 3,000 years old. (*A*) Drawing from the tomb of Upuy in the year 1200 B.C. (*B*) Schematic drawing of the picture in the upper right hand corner of the tomb painting depicting a patient on the ground while a man—possibly a physician is manipulating a dislocated shoulder in the technique of Kocher. (*A;* The Metropolitan Museum of Art. *B;* Hussein, M. K.: J. Bone Joint Surg., *50B*:669-671, 1968)

his life, had seen only five instances of the two uncommon anterior and posterior types of dislocations; that Paul of Aegena, in the seventh century A.D., had admitted to the reality of the rarer forms; that Scultetus described the forward dislocation; and that after 38 years of practice, Sir Astley Cooper had met with only two backward dislocations but had seen several forward dislocations. You should remember that x-rays were discovered by Wilhelm Roentgen in 1895.

There is a striking similarity between the discussion by Hippocrates and today's attitudes toward the operative repair of recurrent dislocations of the shoulder; that is, that you should be familiar with the anatomy, that you should scar down the area of the joint weakness, and that you should bind the arm to the side "for a long time." The main difference between now and then is that we use "cold steel" to scar down the joint and he used a "hot iron."

It is interesting to note that the first orthopaedic case, reported in mankind's oldest book, was a dislocation of the shoulder in an epileptic. The Edwin Smith Papyrus,[334,455] written some 2000 years before Hippocrates, was named after a pioneer American Egyptologist who purchased the scroll in 1862 from a native dealer in Luxor, Egypt. The original text, which dates back to 3000 to 2500 B.C., was not translated until 1930 and commented briefly on injuries, including those of the collarbone, humerus, and shoulder. The translation concerning the dislocation states, "The eagle of his shoulder has fled. Leave him alone for he will be well." Milgram[334] has interpreted the eagle to represent the three prominences of the scapula, which encircle the humeral head like an eagle's talons (i.e., the glenoid, coracoid, and acromion) assuming that, at the time of dislocation, the bony projection would be evident (the eagle) and that following reduction a normal contour would occur—therefore, "the eagle has fled."

Hussein[292] reported that in 1200 B.C., in the tomb of the Upuy, who was an artist and sculptor to Ramses II, there was a drawing of a scene that was strikingly similar to Kocher's method of reduction (Fig. 11-39).

In the centuries that followed, we begin to see refinements of the problems. If you are interested in history, I urge you to refer to the text by H. F. Moseley,[350] a classic that has a particularly good section on the historical aspects of the problems.

Cuff Injuries, Posterolateral Defects in the Humeral Head, and Anterior Capsule Defects

Cuff Ruptures

In 1880, Joessel[299] reported on four cases of known recurrent dislocations of the shoulder on which he did careful postmortem studies. In all cases, he described a rupture of the posterolateral portion of the rotator cuff from the greater tuberosity and a greatly increased shoulder joint capsule volume. He also noted fractures of the humeral head and the anterior glenoid rim. He concluded that the cuff disruption which did not heal predisposed recurrence of the problem; that recurrences were facilitated by the enlarged capsule; and that a fracture of the glenoid or head of the humerus resulted in a smaller articular surface, which may tend to produce recurrent dislocation. However, his four patients were elderly, and they probably presented degenerative cuff changes, which are so common in older people.

Following Joessel's report, Kuster,[309] Cramer,[222] Popke,[385] and Volkmann managed recurrent dislocations by resecting the head of the humerus.[309] I suppose their thinking was: if the cuff does not heal and the shoulder will continue to dislocate, you might as well go ahead and remove the head of the humerus. This operation was short-lived, but some beautiful specimens of the humeral head with large posterior notch defects were obtained.

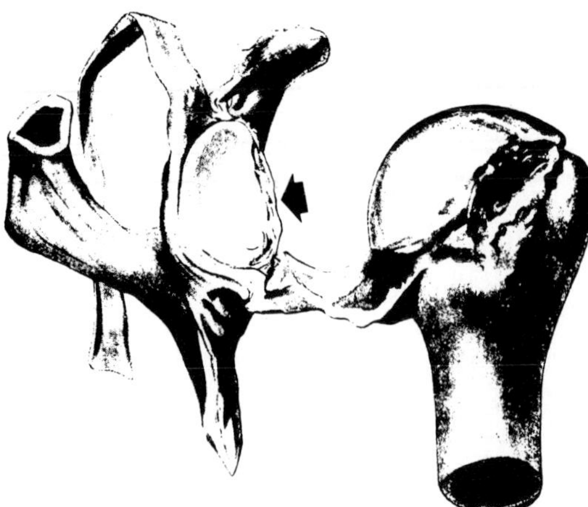

Fig. 11-40. Drawing of a specimen presented by Caird[208] in 1887 depicting avulsion of the anterior portion of the glenoid labrum (*arrow*) and a posterolateral fracture defect produced by the acute dislocation.

Posterolateral Defects in the Humeral Head

In 1880, Joessel[299] commented on the defect and Ev[254] first proved that the posterolateral defect in the humeral head was associated with anterior dislocation and that it can occur with an acute anterior dislocation. He performed an autopsy on a patient 12 hours after an acute anterior dislocation and found the deep groove in the posterolateral aspect of the head.

In 1887, Caird[208] of Edinburgh concluded that in the true subcoracoid dislocation there must be an indentation fracture of the humeral head which is produced by the dense, hard anterior lip of the glenoid fossa. In cadaver experiments, he was able to produce the head defect (Fig. 11-40). He said that the hard, dense glenoid lip would cut into the soft cancellous bone like a knife.

Anterior Capsule Defects

Following the description of the humeral head defect, the next anatomic consideration was to the soft tissue in the front of the shoulder. Broca and Hartmann[203] published two articles in 1890 describing the previously described posterolateral head defect and a new finding of detachment of the anterior labrum, periosteum, and capsule from the scapula (Fig. 11-41). They stressed that the anterior dislocation, or

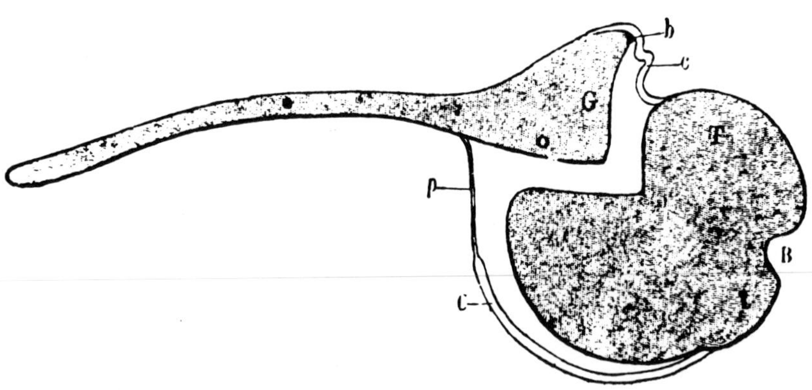

Fig. 11-41. A cross-section through the glenohumeral joint, showing that the anterior capsule has been detached from the anterior glenoid. Note the large posterolateral defect in the humeral head created by the worn and deformed anterior rim of the glenoid. G—anterior glenoid rim, O—neck of glenoid, p—periosteum, c—capsule, t—lesser tuberosity, B—bicipital groove, T—greater tuberosity, b—posterior attachment of labrum. (Broca and Hartmann[203])

subluxation, was really an intracapsular problem and was the product of forward displacement of the head, which sheared off the anterior soft-tissue structures from the glenoid. This fact was later stressed by Perthes[380] and Bankart[185] (Fig. 11-42).

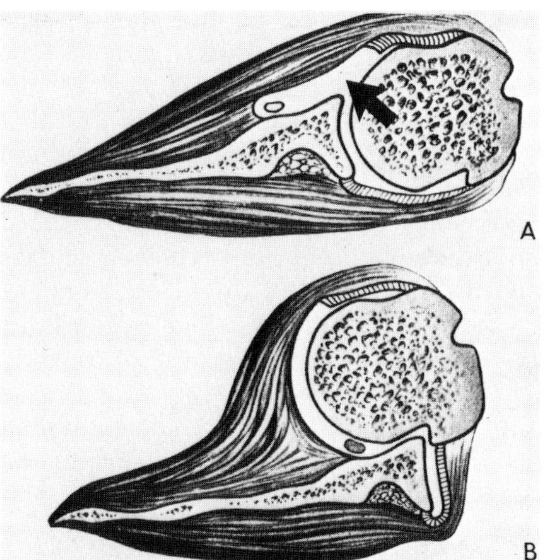

Fig. 11-42. (*A*) Perthes' concept of the detached anterior capsule and labrum with formation of a subscapular pouch (*arrow*).[380] Note the loose body anterior to the neck of the glenoid. (*B*) Diagram of the anatomical relations during anterior dislocation. Note the posterolateral notch in the humeral head.

Early Operative Repairs

On the basis of the posterolateral defect and the soft-tissue disruptions on the front of the shoulder, other authors described various operative techniques. Bardenheuer,[188] in 1886, and Thomas,[429,430] from 1909 to 1926, discussed capsular plication or shrinking; in 1888 Albert[172] performed arthrodesis; and in 1901 Hildebrand[287] deepened the glenoid socket. These operations were also short-lived.

In 1906, Perthes[380] reported a classic paper on the operative treatment of recurrent dislocations (Fig. 11-43). He stated that the operation should be directed to a repair of the underlying lesion (that is the capsule or cuff from the greater tuberosity) or a repair of the detached glenoid labrum from the anterior bony rim. He even used staples in several cases to repair the anterior capsular structures operatively. This was the first descriptive series of anterior labral and soft-tissue repairs to the anterior glenoid rim. There were no recurrences. Two patients were followed for 17 years, one for 12 years, two for 3 years, and one for 1 year and nine months. All had excellent function.

The muscle-sling myoplasty operation was used in 1913 by Clairmont and Ehrlich.[213] The posterior one-third of the deltoid, with its innervation left intact,

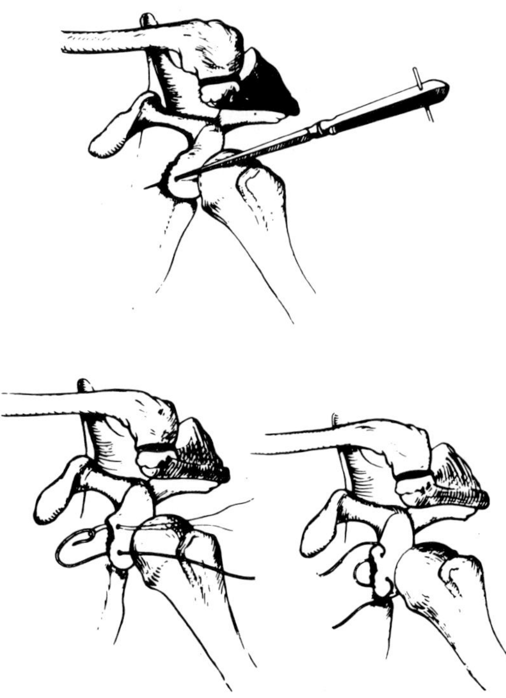

Fig. 11-43. Method of repair used by Perthes in 1906.[380] The labrum and anterior capsule were reattached using either suture, as shown, or using small staples in the anterior rim of the glenoid.

was removed from its insertion on the humerus and was passed through the quadrilateral space and sutured to the coracoid process. The principle was that when the arm was abducted the deltoid contracted, which held up the humeral head. Finsterer,[259] in a similar but reversed procedure, utilized the coracobrachialis and the short head of the biceps from the coracoid and transferred them posteriorly. Both operations failed because of high recurrence rates.

In 1923 when Bankart[185] first published his now famous operative technique, he stated that there were only two classes of operations being used at that time for recurrent dislocations of the shoulder (i.e., operations designed to diminish the size of the capsule by plication or pleating, as described by Thomas,[429,430] and the operation designed to give inferior support to the capsule, such as the Clairmont-Ehrlich[213] myoplasty). Bankart condemned them both.

Beginning in 1929, Nicola[360] published a series of articles on management of recurrent dislocations of the shoulder (Fig. 11-44). He used the long head of the biceps tendon and the coracohumeral ligament as a checkrein to the front of the shoulder. Because of technical difficulties and the high rate of recurrences, most practitioners have abandoned the procedure.

Another checkrein operation was described by Henderson.[283,284] The so-called tenosuspension operation used half of the peroneus longus tendon to loop through drill holes in the acromion and the greater tuberosity (Fig. 11-45). The Henderson operation has been practically abandoned.

The Gallie-LeMesurier[262] operation for recurrent dislocations of the shoulder was introduced in 1927 by Gallie of Canada. He used autogenous fascia lata as living suture to form new ligaments and, in the 1948 series, reported a recurrence rate of only 2.4 per cent (Fig. 11-46). This procedure has been modified and is still being

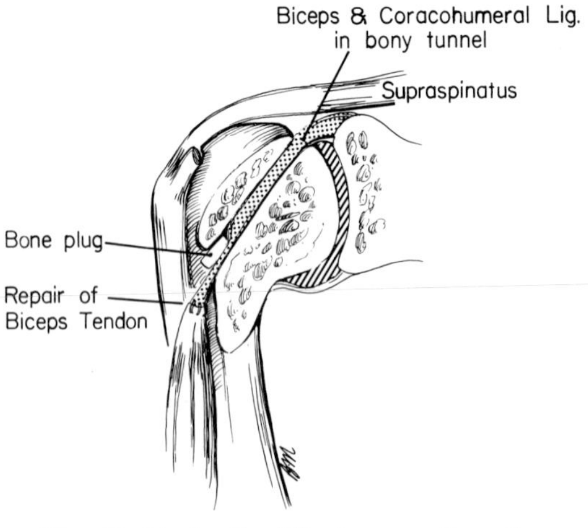

Fig. 11-44. In the Nicola operation, the long head of the biceps and the coracohumeral ligament are passed through a bony tunnel in the head of the humerus to act as a "checkrein" ligament.[360]

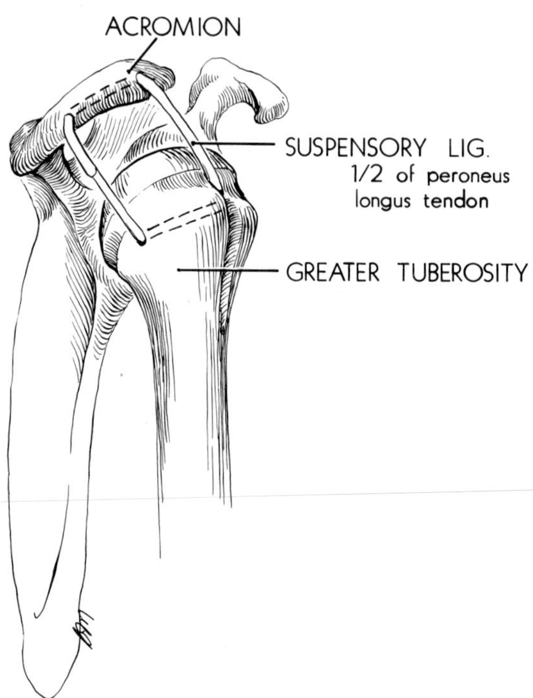

Fig. 11-45. In the Henderson tenosuspension operation, the peroneus longus tendon was passed through drill holes in the acromion and the greater tuberosity, which acted as a type of checkrein ligament.[283]

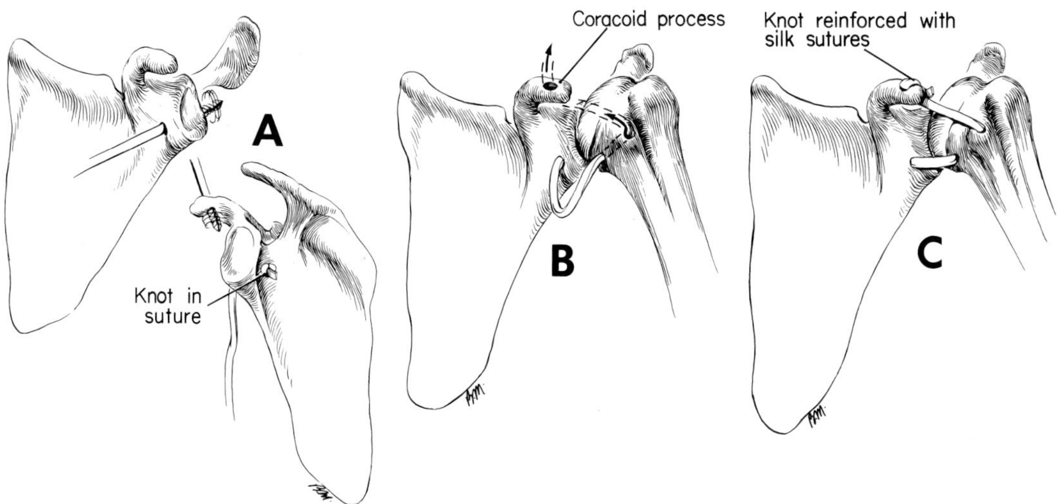

Fig. 11-46. Gallie and LeMesurier used autogenous fascia latae to form new anterior ligaments of the shoulder. (*A*) The living suture is anchored posteriorly in the neck of the glenoid by a knotted end. (*B*) Suture is anchored in the neck of the humerus through two drill holes medial to the bicipital groove. (*C*) The end of the fascia latae is anchored into the tip of the coracoid process.[262]

used today by Bateman,[190] with a low recurrence rate of 2.1 per cent.

The "Essential Lesion" of Recurring Dislocations: Bone Defects Versus Soft-Tissue Defects and Others

With the discovery of x-ray by Roentgen[455] in 1895 came new evaluations and studies on the anatomy and on humeral head defects. This gave impetus to the theory that the essential lesion that produced recurrent anterior dislocations was the osseous posterolateral defect of the head. Bankart,[185] following the concepts of Perthes,[380] continued to claim that the essential lesion was the detached labrum and soft tissues from the anterior glenoid. (This has been referred to by subsequent authors as the Bankartarian lesion.) In some respects, the argument still rages on. Some authors report that the labral defect is present in 80 to 90 per cent of the recurrent dislocated shoulders, and others report that 90 per cent of the time there is a posterolateral humeral defect.

A more realistic point of view might be that *there is no single essential lesion* as the cause for recurrent dislocations of the shoulder. The term, essential lesion, is a poor one, because many factors have been shown to cause recurring dislocations of the shoulder (e.g., aplasia of the glenoid socket, variations of the contour of the socket, excessive anteversion of the glenoid tilt, increased anteversion of the head, insufficiency of the posterior short rotators, fracture of the anterior glenoid rim, stretching of the anterior capsule, detachment of the anterior capsule from the glenoid, insufficiency, overstretching or avulsion of the subscapularis muscle, posterolateral osseous defect in the humeral head, and muscle imbalances).

All in all, the theories of recurrent dislocation of the shoulder have stimulated other theories and a general interest in the shoulder. Entire texts have been written on recurrent dislocations; general shoulder texts have been written by Codman,[215] Moseley,[346,350] Bateman,[189,191] Saha,[406] and DePalma.[239,241] It was only natural that newer operative reconstructions were developed (e.g., Eden-Hybbinette, Magnuson-Stack, modified Gallie, Putti-Platt, Saha, and Bristow). I am sure that as long as there are orthopaedists new reconstructions will be created.

ANATOMY

Developmental Anatomy

Gardner[265] has shown that a differentiation of bones and joints of the upper extremity from a general cellular blastema to structures having a form and arrangement similar to those of the adult occurs between 4.5 weeks and 7 weeks from fertilization. The limb bud occurs at 4 weeks, and at 5 weeks individual muscles are forming, and the humerus is preformed in mesenchyme. Chondrification begins first in the humerus and then forms in the scapula. Initial bone formation occurs in the primary ossification center of the humerus at 6.5 weeks. Joint cavitation begins at 6 or 7 weeks, and by the end of the seventh week, the shoulder has assumed the characteristics of the adult joint, including most of the bursae.

At 3 to 4 months, blood vessels begin an extensive invasion of ligaments, tendons, and bones. Gardner[265] took particular time to study the glenoid labrum and found that it was formed of fibrous tissue, not fibrocartilaginous tissue. However, at the transition area between the glenoid lip and the hyaline articular cartilage of the glenoid fossa there were occasional small areas of fibrocartilage. (Details of this are presented on p. 637.) Even at term, the glenoid labrum consisted of only a dense fibrous tissue with some elastic fibers.

After the seventh week, the anterior capsule with the glenohumeral ligament becomes increasingly fibrous, and there is a variation in size and distinctiveness of the glenohumeral ligaments.

Development of the Clavicle

Most bones of the body develop from condensation of mesenchymal cells, which then proceed to preform the bone in cartilage and then undergo ossification. This process is known as enchondral bone formation. The major part of the clavicle, is not preformed in cartilage, and the mesenchymal cells are simply mineralized directly into bone in a process known as intramembranous ossification. There are two separate ossification centers in the clavicle which develop at 5½ weeks. The lateral center is usually more advanced than the medial one, and soon the two masses join to form a long mass of bone. Failure of the two masses to join is thought by some to result in a congenital pseudoarthrosis of the clavicle.

Gardner[265] has shown that the clavicle and the mandible are the first bones in the body to ossify. The cells at the acromial and sternal end of the clavicle mass take on a chondrogenous pattern and form the acromioclavicular and sternoclavicular joints. A marrow cavity is produced, and from this point on, the clavicle grows like a long bone of the cartilaginous type; that is, it increases in diameter by periosteal ossification (intramembranous), and it grows in length through activity at the cartilaginous ends. While early fetal growth of the clavicle may occur at both ends, usually only one secondary epiphyseal center develops. The medial clavicle epiphysis first undergoes ossification at age 18 and fuses with the clavicle at approximately age 25.[274,443] Occasionally, a lateral clavicle epiphysis occurs, and it fuses with the clavicle during adolescence.

Development of the Scapula

The scapula,[239] at birth, has advanced ossification of its body. During the first year, the coracoid develops an ossification center, and at 10 years, a second ossification center occurs at its base. These two centers unite at age 15, with the center at the base contributing to the formation of the upper glenoid cavity. The acromion process has two (sometimes three) ossification centers. They appear at puberty and fuse about the 22nd year. Two ossification centers form the glenoid. The one at the base of the coracoid at 10 years, which fuses with the scapula at 15, and a horseshoe-shaped lower epiphysis which forms the lower three-fourths of the glenoid. The vertebral border and the inferior angle of the scapula each have an ossification center, which appears at puberty and fuses before the 22nd year.

Tilt of the Glenoid Fossa. In 1966 Das, Saha, and Roy[227] reported on their observations of the tilt of the glenoid fossa of the scapula. They reported that in a majority of men, the tilt is directed posteriorly from 2 to 12 degrees. The amount of tilt is measured on a modified axillary roentgenogram and is the angle formed by the line through the axis of the scapula, which meets a line drawn through the maximum glenoid diameter.

Development of the Proximal End of the Humerus

At birth, an ossification center may be present in the humeral head. Usually there are three ossification centers to the proximal end of the humerus: the first one for the head of the humerus, which appears between the first week and 6 months; a second for the greater tuberosity, which appears usually in the second year; and a third one for the lesser tuberosity, which appears during the fifth year. The two epiphyses of the tuberosities fuse into a single mass about the fifth year. This, in turn, unites with the epiphysis of the head, usually before the seventh year, but it may be delayed as long as the fourteenth year. The head and shaft unite during the nineteeth year. According to Kuhns *et al.*,[306] patients with meconium aspiration and uncorrected transposition of the great vessels commonly have an ossification center in the humeral head at birth.

Comparative Anatomy

The evolution of the shoulder girdle is a complex subject, and the reader should refer to the classic articles by Watson,[444] Lewis,[319] and Jones[300] and the texts by Montagu,[345] Howell,[291] and Kingsley.[304]

It suffices to say that there is little, if any, resemblance between human shoulders and those of fish, amphibians, birds, or reptiles. The scapula, more than any other bone in the evolution of the shoulder girdle, has made momentous morphological changes to accommodate the change in posture of man to an upright position and the need for a functional, freely movable prehensile upper extremity.[239] The scapula has gradually migrated from the high cervical spine region to its present position and is longer, more narrow, and less massive. The long and narrow scapula is due almost exclusively to the relative extension and increase in size of the infraspinatus' fossa. According to Inman, Saunders, and Abbott,[295] the extension of the infraspinatus fossa is due to a change in the functional requirements of the attached muscles and the extraordinary significance of the infraspinatus muscle in helping the shoulder joint attain its great range of motion. The supraspinatus fossa has remained unchanged in size. Whereas man's scapula has become less massive in some respects, it has gained mass in the form of the spine and the acromion process. In the lower mammals, the coracoid process was a rather large and massive structure which articulated with the sternum leaving a rather large foramen similar to the obturator foramen seen in the pelvis. Man's coracoid is only represented as a small rudimentary process.

The humerus has undergone several changes that affect the shoulder joint. In keeping with the increase in size, shape, and mass of the acromion process of the scapula, there is an increase in the size, bulk, and power of the deltoid muscle. In addition, the insertion deltoid muscle has migrated distally on the shaft of the humerus. The relationship of the head, neck, and shaft angle of the humerus has changed from 90 degrees retroversion in quadrupeds to 30 degrees retroversion in man. This change in torsion of the shaft has affected the size and shape of the tuberosity of the humerus and the position of the long head of the biceps tendon. In primitive form, the tuberosities were of equal size, and the bicipital groove was directly over the top of the humeral head. In modern man, the bicipital groove is displaced medially, and the lesser tuberosity is much smaller.

The clavicle, while it used to be a part of the scapula, is now, in man, the only bony connection between the shoulder girdle and the axial skeleton. Animals that have the best prehension of the upper extremity have the best-developed clavicles. Animals that run and get their driving force from their powerful hind extremities absorb the shock of the landing on their front extremities, which have, by necessity, no bony connection to the scapula, only a free-floating shoulder girdle suspended by muscles.

Anatomy of the Glenohumeral Joint

Stability of the Glenohumeral Joint

The glenohumeral joint is an unstable mechanism at best. The large spherical head of the humerus articulates against, and not within, a small, shallow glenoid fossa of the scapula (Fig. 11-47). Actually, the glenoid has one-third of the articular surface of the humeral head. While this makes for a very unstable joint, it allows for the remarkable range of motion so important for prehensile activities. Saha[406,409] has demonstrated that there is considerable variation in the radii of the curvature of the glenoid fossa. The contour may be almost flat, slightly curved, or it may have a definite socket-like appearance. He has demonstrated that the deeper the socket, the less to-and-fro gliding of the head there is, and the greater the tendency for subluxation. According to Saha,[409] the dynamic stability of the glenohumeral joint is achieved by the size, shape, and tilt of the glenoid, the power of the surrounding muscles, and the amount of retroversion of the humeral head on the shaft of the humerus.

Joint stability is obtained through a joint capsule with varying ligamentous thickenings, an overhead roof formed by the acromion process, the lateral end of the clavicle, the acromioclavicular joint, the coracoacromial ligament, and by a cuff of musculotendinous units that reinforce

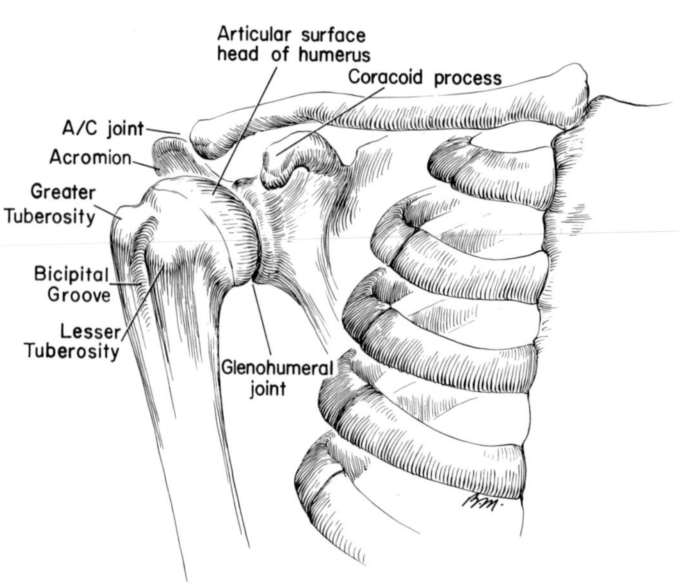

Fig. 11-47. Normal bone architecture of the shoulder joint.

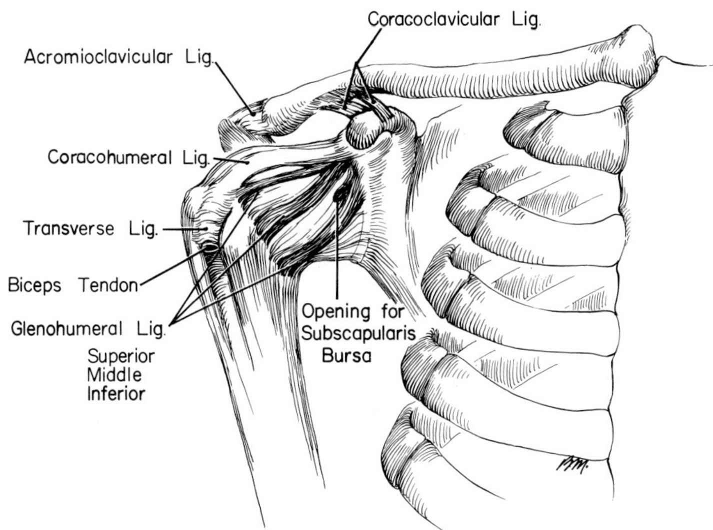

Fig. 11-48. Normal ligaments about the shoulder joint.

the capsule anteriorly, superiorly, and posteriorly (that is, the subscapularis in the front, the supraspinatus on top, and the infraspinatus and teres minor in the back; Figs. 11-48 to 11-50).

Capsule, Ligaments, Bursae, and Synovial Recesses

Capsule. The joint capsule is large, loose, and redundant and has twice the surface area of the humeral head. The capacity of the glenohumeral joint capsule obviously has to be larger than the humeral head, to allow for the full and free range of motion of the shoulder. The capsule, lined with synovium, offers some protection against dislocation at its anterior and anteroinferior reinforcement by the glenohumeral ligaments (Fig. 11-49).

Glenohumeral Ligaments. There are three ligaments in the anterior capsule which were first described by Schlemm[413] in 1853 (Fig. 11-48). Many authors, including Codman,[215] believe that the ligaments are represented only by a thickening of the capsule, and many have shown great variation in the size and shape of the ligaments. The three ligaments of the capsule are called the superior, middle, and inferior glenohumeral ligaments.

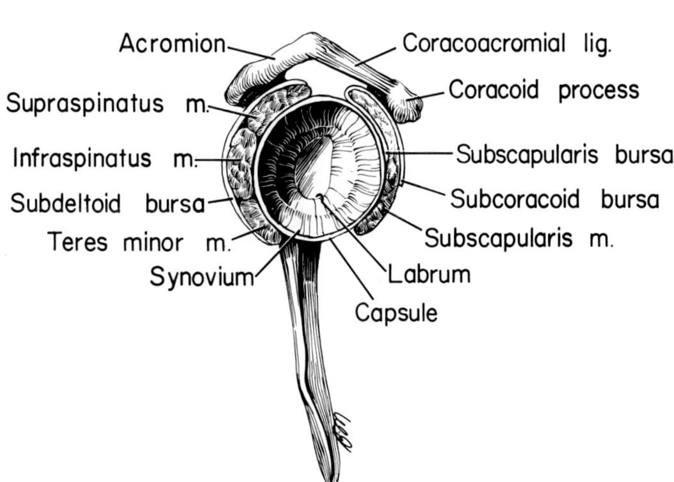

Fig. 11-49. Cross-section through the shoulder joint, showing the anatomical relationships of the labrum, capsule, muscles, bursae, and bone structures. (Redrawn from Moseley, H. F., and Overgaard, B.: J. Bone Joint Surg., *44B*:913-927, 1962)

The superior glenohumeral ligament extends from the anterosuperior edge of the glenoid, near the tendon of the long head of the biceps, to the top of the lesser tuberosity of the humerus.

The middle glenohumeral ligament extends from almost the same place on the glenoid, but just below the superior glenohumeral ligament, and attaches on the lesser tuberosity of the humerus with the posterior aspect of the subscapularis muscle. The tendon of subscapularis blends with the anterior capsule at the humeral attachment.

The inferior glenohumeral ligament extends from the anteromedial labrum and glenoid lip to the lesser tuberosity of the humerus just inferior to the middle glenohumeral ligament. Delorme[234] has found these ligaments to vary considerably in size and thickness. They may be 1 to 2 cm. wide and up to 4 mm. thick.

Accessory Glenohumeral Ligaments. *The coracohumeral ligament* serves to strengthen the superior glenohumeral capsular ligament and works as a suspensory ligament of the humeral head (Fig. 11-48). Medially, the ligament attaches to the lateral border of the horizontal arm of the coracoid process, below the coracoacromial ligament, and extends laterally to the greater and lesser tuberosities and capsule in the interval between the supraspinatus and subscapularis tendon insertions. The ligament acts as a checkrein to external rotation.

The coracoacromial ligament is a heavy, broad, quadrangular structure that helps to form the roof of the glenohumeral joint (see Figs. 11-49, 11-125). Medially, it attaches by two fasciculi from the posterolateral surface of the base of the coracoid above the coracohumeral ligament to the anterior medial surface of the acromion.[443] The function of the coracoacromial ligament is undetermined. The ligament, along with the acromion and coracoid processes, constitutes the coracoacromial arch. This is located between the subacromial bursa and the acromioclavicular joint. The posterior fasciculus attaches at the base of the coracoid, just lateral to the coracoclavicular ligament and the anterior fasciculus attaches more distally onto the mid-lateral coracoid process. Occasionally (15%), the ligament is continuous with the tendon of the pectoralis minor muscle and is thought to represent the old insertion of the tendon into the proximal humerus.[322,443]

Bursae. The subacromial bursa is the largest and most important bursa of the shoulder and is sometimes known as the subdeltoid bursa (Fig. 11-49). It has been thoroughly described by Codman[215] and Fahey.[258] The floor of the bursa sac is the greater tuberosity of the humerus and the tendons of the rotator cuff and the bicipital groove. The roof is formed by the undersurface of the acromion, the coracoacromial arch, and the deltoid muscle. Anteriorly it extends to the subcoracoid position. The subscapularis bursa is an out-pouching of the synovial membrane of the glenohumeral joint, usually between the superior and middle glenohumeral ligaments.

Synovial Recesses and Subscapularis Muscles. DePalma[239] has found the glenohumeral ligaments to vary quite a bit in size and thickness. They are sometimes poorly—if at all—defined. He has demonstrated a great variation in size and number of synovial recesses that form in the anterior capsule above, below, and between the glenohumeral ligaments. He has shown from dissections that, if the capsule arises at the labrum and glenoid border of the scapula, there are few, if any, synovial recesses (i.e., there may be a generalized blending of all three ligament structures, which leave no room for synovial recesses or weaknesses, and hence there will be a stronger anterior glenohumeral capsule). However, he points out that the farther medially the capsule arises from the glenoid (i.e., from the anterior scapular neck) the larger and more numerous will be the synovial recesses. The end result of this can be a thin, weak anterior

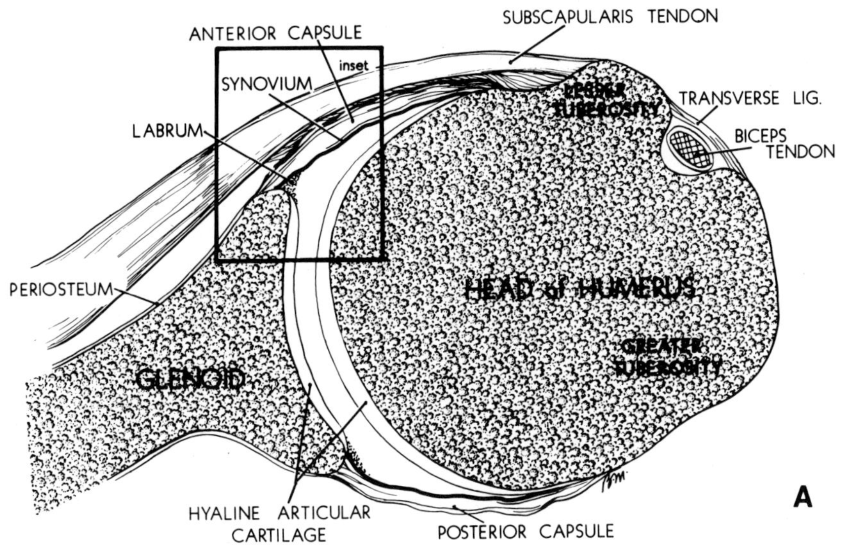

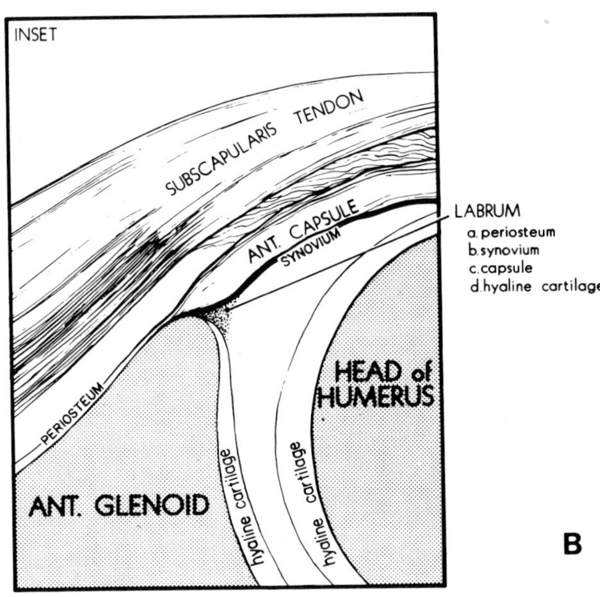

Fig. 11-50. Normal shoulder anatomy. (*A*) Drawing of a horizontal section through the middle of the glenohumeral joint demonstrating normal anatomical relationships. Note the close relation of the subscapularis tendon to the anterior capsule. (*B*) A close-up view in the area of the labrum. The labrum is essentially devoid of fibrocartilage, and is composed of tissues from the nearby hyaline cartilage, capsule, synovium, and periosteum. (Redrawn from Moseley, H. F., and Overgaard, B.: J. Bone Joint Surg., *44B*:913-927, 1962)

capsule. In some cases because of the large size of the synovial recesses, there may be no more than a remnant of the anterior capsule, and the stability of the anterior joint has to rely on the subscapularis muscle. Moseley and Overgaard[352] are in agreement with these findings. The inference to be drawn from these anatomical findings is that, in some patients, there will be only a very thin capsule without ligament thickenings, which may predispose the patient to the initial anterior dislocation and contribute to the high incidence of recurrent dislocations.

Glenoid Labrum

The glenoid labrum has been the subject of great controversy over the years and many contributions in the literature describe its significance, its structural composition, and its function. It has been mistakenly likened to a meniscus in the knee, a strong fibrocartilaginous rim of the glenoid fossa. Bankart deemed its detachment the essential lesion responsible for the high incidence of recurrent anterior dislocations. Although at surgery the labrum is noted to be detached in the majority of cases, it is not detached in all cases. DePalma[239] and Olsson[369] have shown that in patients in the later decades of life, when the labral detachment is more common, the incidence of severe recurrent dislocations is uncommon. Further, Townley,[432] through a posterior approach, removed the glenoid and found that the anterior capsular mechanism remained as a strong structural unit.

Extensive studies have been performed by Moseley and Overgaard,[352] Townley,[432] and Gardner,[265] who concluded that the labrum does *not* consist entirely of fibrocartilage. Microscopic studies have shown that in a very small area, at the junction of the hyaline cartilage of the glenoid and fibrous capsule, there might be a nidus of fibrocartilage, but the vast majority of the labrum consists of dense fibrous tissue with a few elastic fibers. Anatomically, then, the labrum appears to be no more than a rim of fibrous tissue which is formed at the glenoid rim by the interconnection and joining of the periosteum of the anterior surface of the glenoid, the hyaline articular cartilage of the glenoid fossa, and the anterior capsule and synovium (Fig. 11-50).

MOVEMENTS OF THE SHOULDER

Joint Movements

Older literature states that the motion of the shoulder was quite simple, inferring that the first 90 degrees of abduction was in the glenohumeral joint and that the remaining 90 degrees came from scapular elevation and rotation. However, in 1944, in a classic article on shoulder function, Inman, Saunders, and Abbott[295] demonstrated that motion was a complex action.

Motion of the upper extremity involves motion of four separate joints about the shoulder complex: the glenohumeral joint, the acromioclavicular joint, the sternoclavicular joint, and the so-called scapulothoracic joint, which effects movement between the scapula and the thoracic cage. Complete elevation of the arm, in either flexion or abduction, is dependent on the *free* motion in *all* of the joints of the shoulder complex.

Glenohumeral Motion

Between the humerus and the glenoid fossa 120 degrees of passive motion is possible without moving the scapula. Beyond this point motion is blocked by the neck of the humerus against the acromion process. The glenohumeral joint is capable of only 90 degrees of active abduction. If the arm is in full internal rotation, only 60 degrees of glenohumeral motion is possible, because the greater tuberosity impinges on the acromion process. In external rotation, the greater tuberosity is rotated behind the acromion.

Scapulothoracic Motion

In full abduction or flexion, the scapula rotates outward 60 degrees (Fig. 11-51). The rotation begins after the first 30 degrees of abduction or 60 degrees of glenohumeral flexion and then moves smoothly and synchronously with the movement of the glenohumeral joint.

Scapulohumeral Motion

During the first 30 to 60 degrees of elevation, the motion of the scapula varies. Beyond that, however, and up to full abduction or flexion, there is a 2:1 ratio of glenohumeral motion to scapulothoracic motion (i.e., for every 15 degrees of elevation, 10 degrees occurs at the glenohumeral joint and 5 degrees at the scapulothoracic joint). This is known as scapulohumeral rhythm.

Sternoclavicular Motion

During full elevation, motion of the sternoclavicular joint occurs early and is almost complete during the first 90 degrees of motion. For every 10 degrees of abduction of the arm, 4 degrees of elevation of the clavicle

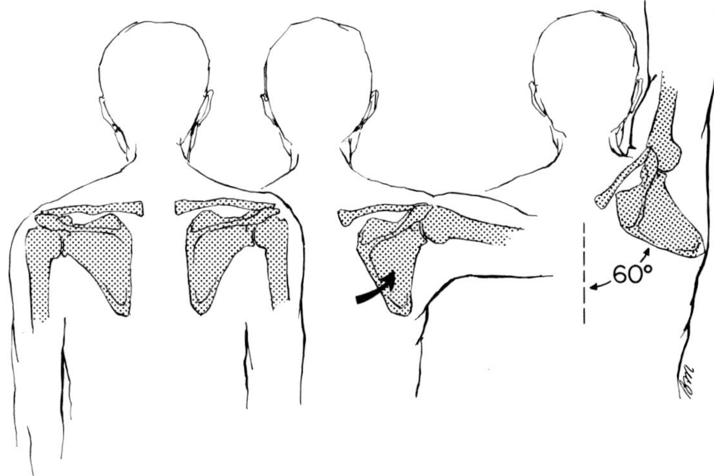

Fig. 11-51. During full elevation of the upper extremity, the scapula rotates outward 60 degrees. In general, the scapula rotates on the thorax 1 degree for every 2 degrees of glenohumeral elevation.

occurs at the sternoclavicular joint (i.e., *approximately* 40 degrees).

Acromioclavicular Motion

The total range of 20 degrees occurs both early (in the first 30 degrees of abduction) and late (during the last 60 degrees of elevation of the arm). The sum of motion of the sternoclavicular and the acromioclavicular joints is equal to the range of motion permitted by the scapula (see p. 638).

Clavicular Motion

The continuous rotation of the scapula on the thoracic wall during elevation of the upper extremity is possible only through rotation of the clavicle and motion occurring at its proximal and distal articulation. With full elevation of the arm, the clavicle rotates upward 40 to 50 degrees.

Interaction of the Deltoid and Short Rotators During Elevation of the Arm

The deltoid is the primary abductor of the arm. However, without the short rotators, which act as depressors of the arm, the deltoid is helpless. Saha[406,408-410] has confirmed the work of Inman, Saunders, and Abbott[295] and has shown that the short rotators function as horizontal stabilizers and steering muscles: they hold the head in the glenoid during abduction, and during abduction the power of the subscapularis is primarily between 120 and 150 degrees of abduction and acts to glide and roll the head posterior in the glenoid, to counteract the tendency toward anterior subluxation. The large infraspinatus and the smaller teres minor act to prevent anterior displacement of the head and to pull the head down and backward, while the deltoid abducts the arm. Saha has shown by electromyography that the latissimus dorsi is most active from 60 to 180 degrees.[407,409]

Other Abduction Mechanisms

Biceps Tendon

In the anatomical position, the long head of the biceps tendon is ineffective to abduct the arm, because it is anterior to the center of the head of the humerus. However, when the arm is externally rotated 90 degrees, the line of the long head, from its insertion through muscle belly and through the tendon to its origin, is across the top of the humeral head. In this position, with biceps contraction, the head rotates beneath the tendon and is prevented from riding upward by the hood-like action of the biceps tendon. This mechanism is a weak one and may be used to abduct the arm of a patient who has paralysis of the deltoid muscle.

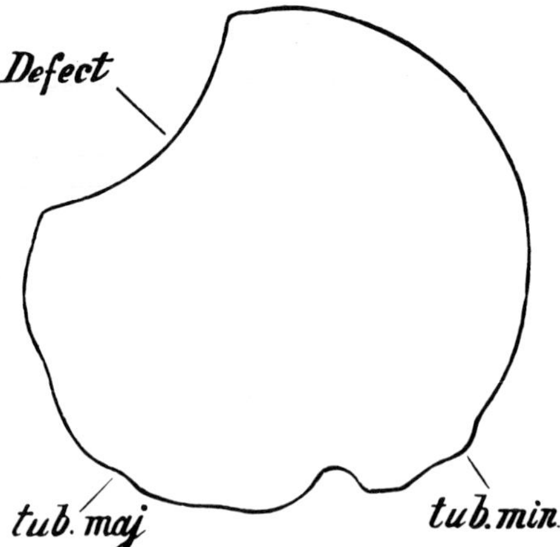

Fig. 11-52. Drawing of a dissected humeral head showing posterolateral notch defect as published by Cramer in 1882.

Supraspinatus Mechanism

Lucas[322] has pointed out that the supraspinatus mechanism is similar to the biceps mechanism, except that the muscle motor is on the scapula and the insertion is on the greater tuberosity of the humerus. In addition, the tendon in the anatomical position is more nearly over the center of the head. Electromyographic studies reveal that the supraspinatus acts with the deltoid muscle throughout the entire range of motion of arm elevation.

Summary of Shoulder Motion

In summary, then, motion of the shoulder is complex. All four joints of the shoulder (i.e., glenohumeral, scapulothoracic, acromioclavicular, and sternoclavicular) must be freely movable. There is keen interaction between the deltoid and the upper short rotator depressors (i.e., subscapularis, infraspinatus, and teres minor). The short rotators guide, steer, and maintain the humeral head in the glenoid fossa. They depress or hold down the humeral head, so that, while the deltoid elevates the arm primarily, the subscapularis, along with the infraspinatus and teres minor, prevent anterior subluxation of the head. The infraspinatus and the teres minor externally rotate the humerus to prevent impingement of the greater tuberosity into the acromion during abduction.

Full elevation of the arm is accomplished by a 2:1 ratio of glenohumeral to scapulothoracic motion; scapular rotation of 60 degrees; and clavicular upward rotation of 40 to 50 degrees and elevation of 30 to 40 degrees. Rotation and upward displacement occur in the sternoclavicular joint, and some motion occurs at the acromioclavicular joint.

Should the reader desire more detailed information on the function, movements, and biomechanics of the shoulder joint, I recommend the articles by Inman, Saunders, and Abbott,[295] Lucas,[322] and Saha.[406,409]

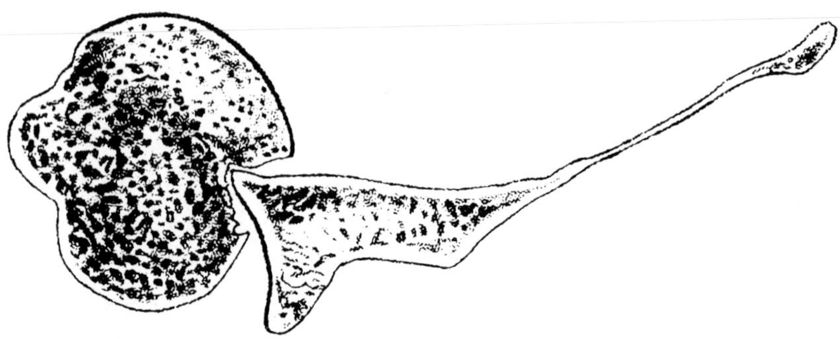

Fig. 11-53. Coronal section showing Caird's understanding of the production of the posterolateral defect by impaction on the anterior bony rim in a dislocation that was artificially produced.[40]

MECHANISM OF INJURY

Direct Force

Direct force can be a cause of anterior dislocation of the shoulder. A sharp blow on the lateral or posterolateral aspect of the shoulder sprains or tears the supporting structure of the joint and may force the shoulder out anteriorly (e.g., being kicked in the back of the shoulder by a mule or falling onto the lateral or posterolateral shoulder).

Indirect Force

Forces applied indirectly to the arm can sprain or tear the supporting structure of the joint, allowing anterior displacement of the head. This is the most common cause of anterior sprain or dislocation. The common denominator in this mechanism is abduction and external rotation forces on the arm. Mild forces do not produce any joint displacement, whereas moderate forces produce subluxation of the joint, and severe forces produce the complete dislocation. The combination of the abduction and external rotation forces drives the head into the anterior capsule, which is either strained, stretched, disrupted in its substance, or disrupted from the glenoid.

Classifications of Injuries to the Anterior Shoulder

I. Classification based on the anatomy of the dislocation
  - A. Subcoracoid
  - B. Subglenoid
  - C. Subclavicular
  - D. Intrathoracic

II. Classification based on the etiology of the dislocation (traumatic or atraumatic)
  - A. Traumatic injuries
    1. Sprains to anterior shoulder joint
    2. Acute subluxation of joint
    3. Acute anterior dislocation
    4. Recurring anterior dislocation
    5. Unreduced anterior dislocation
  - B. Atraumatic injuries
    1. Voluntary or habitual subluxation or dislocation
    2. Congenital or developmental subluxation or dislocation

CLASSIFICATION OF INJURIES OF THE ANTERIOR SHOULDER

In general there are two ways to classify anterior dislocations of the shoulder, (1) by the anatomical position that the dislocation assumes and (2) by the etiology of the dislocation (traumatic or atraumatic).

Rowe[394] carefully analyzed 500 dislocations of the glenohumeral joint and determined that 96 per cent were caused by trauma, and the remaining 4 per cent were atraumatic. He further noted the incidence of dislocations was the same for persons over the age of 45 years as for younger people.

ROENTGENOGRAPHIC FINDINGS

Historical Review

The defect created by the anterior margin of the glenoid in the posterolateral aspect of the humeral head has long been recognized. In 1880, Joessel[299] had observed the defect and Ev[254] had proved that the defect was the result of a traumatic anterior dislocation (see p. 627). Joessel reported on the postmortem studies of four patients with known recurring anterior dislocations of the shoulder, in each of whom he found a rupture of a portion of the rotator cuff and an increase in the shoulder joint volume. This report may well have been responsible for the discovery of the humeral head defect, because it stirred the interest of Joessel's colleagues. They began resecting the humeral heads, because he had theorized that the disrupted soft tissue would not heal.

At any rate, according to Hill and Sachs,[288] beginning in 1882 publications appeared by Kuster (1882), Cramer (1882), Popke (1882), Loebker (1887), Schuller (1890), Staffell (1895), Francke (1898), and Wendell (1903) which described the pathoanatomic findings of the posterolateral defect in the humeral heads that were resected for relief of chronic or habitual dislocation (see Figs. 11-50–11-52).

It was not so many years later that a review of Joessel's[299] cases revealed that the patients had been in the older age group, among whom cuff degeneration is prevalent. Hence, his observations were accurate, but had he studied shoulders in young individuals, he would have had totally different conclusions which would have had a different influence on his colleagues and on subsequent authors.

In 1887, Caird[40] of Edinburgh published an important paper in which he described in detail and with illustrations the posterolateral humeral head defect (see p. 628; Figs. 11-40, 11-53).

Hidden away in the transactions for the Pathological Society of London in 1861 is an article by Flower[260] in which he described the anatomical and pathological changes found in 41 traumatically dislocated shoulders on specimens in London museums. He described, "where the head of the humerus rests upon the edge of the glenoid fossa absorption occurs, and a groove is evacuated, usually between the articular head and the greater tuberosity." Earlier theories proposed to explain the cause of the humeral head defect; (i.e., an avulsion fracture of the humeral head, a grinding erosion, osteochondritis dissecans, a congenital abnormality, and chronic inflammation) were all disproved.

Hermodsson's[285] text on radiographic studies of anterior dislocations of the shoulder offers the best review of the changes associated with anterior dislocation of the shoulder that are detectable by roentgenography. The text was first published in German (Acta Radiologica; Suppl. 20, 1934). Largely through the efforts of Dr. Fred Moseley of Montreal the text was translated into English in 1963. Hermodsson's work has shown the posterolateral humeral head defect is the result of a compression fracture by the anterior glenoid rim during the exit of the humeral head from the glenoid fossa. He also made several observations about fresh, acute traumatic anterior dislocations. (1) The defect is seen in the majority of cases. (2) The

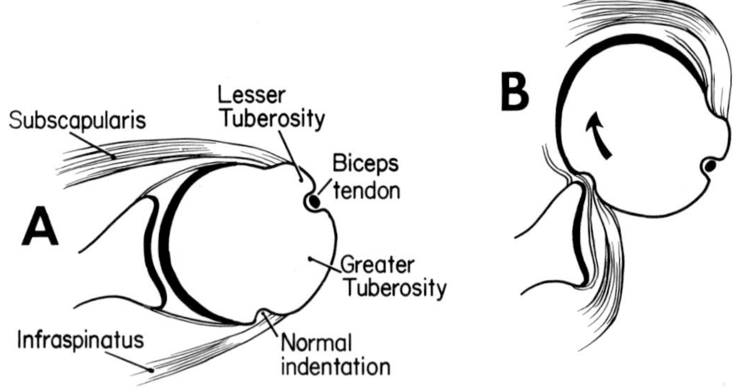

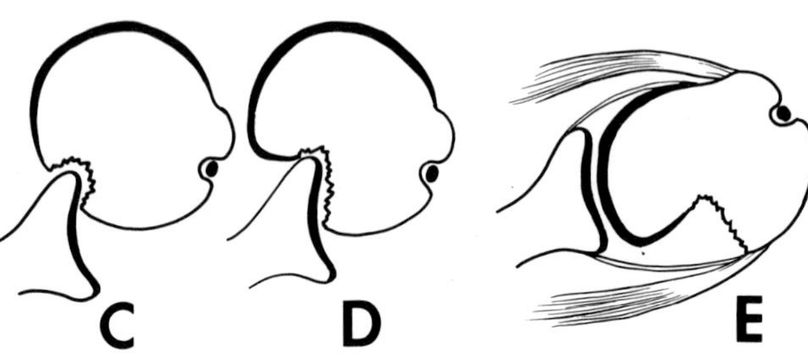

Fig. 11-54. A horizontal section through the glenohumeral joint shows the formation of a posterolateral humeral head defect. (*A*) Normal anatomical relationships. (*B*) Anterior dislocation without a compression fracture defect. (*C*) A small posterolateral defect. (*D*) A large compression fracture defect. (*E*) Following reduction, the defect is quite evident and has deformed the normal articular surface of the humeral head.

longer the head is dislocated, the larger the defect will be. (3) The defects are generally larger with antero-inferior dislocations than with anterior dislocations. (4) The defect is generally larger in recurrent anterior dislocations of the shoulder (Fig. 11-54).

Hermodsson reports that the first mention of the reoentgenographic changes in the humeral head associated with recurrent dislocation of the shoulder was made by Francke in 1898. In 1925, Piltz[382] gave the first detailed description of the technique for roentgenographic examination of recurrent dislocation of the shoulder and stated that routine roentgenograms were of little help. He stressed the need for an angled beam projection to observe the defect. Currently, practically all of the special views that roentgenographically demonstrate the posterolateral humeral head defect involve an angled projection of the x-ray beam.

I might add at this point that Hermodsson's text is not only a classic for radiographic techniques and changes associated with recurrent anterior dislocations of the shoulder; it offers a classical view for the entire literature of the subject. Most of the earlier publications were in German, and his review of these articles in his own language is superb.

An article by Hill and Sachs,[288] published in 1940, attributed the head defect to a compression fracture produced by the dense cortical bone of the anterior glenoid rim. Very clear and concise, this was the first review of the subject in the English language. The defect now carries their names.

Routine Roentgenograms of the Shoulder

Patients who have acute anterior dislocation of the shoulder should have roentgenograms made in two views: an anteroposterior of the shoulder, and a true lateral of the scapula (see Figs. 11-77, 11-82). Patients who have recurrent dislocation or a history of recurrent subluxations should have views made of the shoulder with the humerus in internal and external rotation and axillary lateral and true lateral views of the scapula. When subluxation is suspected, a modified axillary lateral (West Point) view should be made. The technique for this view is described on page 678). Special views, which will be described, are required to demonstrate the posterolateral defect in the humeral head.

Characteristic Roentgenographic Changes in Anterior Dislocation of the Shoulder

Acute Anterior Dislocation

The humeral head may be displaced to the subcoracoid, subglenoid, subclavicular, or intrathoracic position (Fig. 11-55). Routine anteroposterior films are diagnostic, but lateral views are recommended.

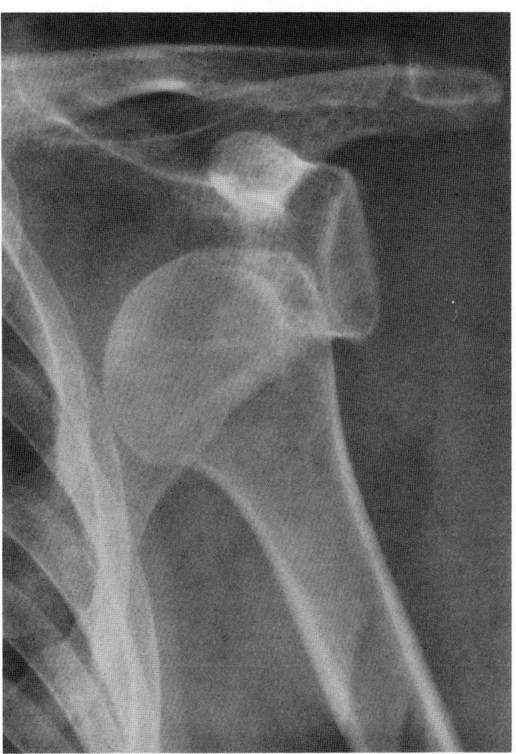

Fig. 11-55. A typical subcoracoid anterior dislocation of the left shoulder. The superior aspect of head of the humerus is below the coracoid process, and the entire articular surface of the head of the humerus is displaced medial to the glenoid fossa.

Recurring Anterior Dislocation

Bone changes on routine anteroposterior roentgenograms may include a slight flattening of the contour, sclerosis, and cyst formation of the posterolateral aspect of the humeral head. I personally am of the opinion that the presence of a posterolateral head defect indicates that a complete dislocation has occurred.

Technique for Roentgenography to Observe a Posterolateral Defect in the Humeral Head

The defect in the head will be demonstrated only in approximately 50 per cent of standard anteroposterior views, and then only on the internal rotation view and when the defect is huge. Special views must be taken to reveal the defect. According to Hermodsson,[285] Hill and Sachs,[288] and Hall Isaac, and Booth,[278] the hallmark position is internal rotation. The location of the defect is so characteristic that it has been referred to as the typical defect (Fig. 11-56). Whether or not the roentgenogram demonstrates the lesion depends, to a great extent, upon the care and deliberation used by the radiologic technician.

Hermodsson's Internal Rotation Technique —Anteroposterior Roentgenogram in Internal Rotation

Hermodsson recommends that the patient be supine and that a sandbag be placed under the elbow to put the humerus horizontal to the table top. The arm is adducted to the side of the patient, the humerus is internally rotated 45 degrees, and the forearm lies across the anterior trunk. The x-ray beam is tilted 15 degrees toward the feet and is centered over the humeral head.[285]

Hermodsson's Tangential View Technique

To obtain marked internal rotation of the humerus, the elbow is flexed 90 degrees, and the dorsum of the hand is placed behind the trunk, over the upper lumbar spine. The thumb points upward. The film cassette is

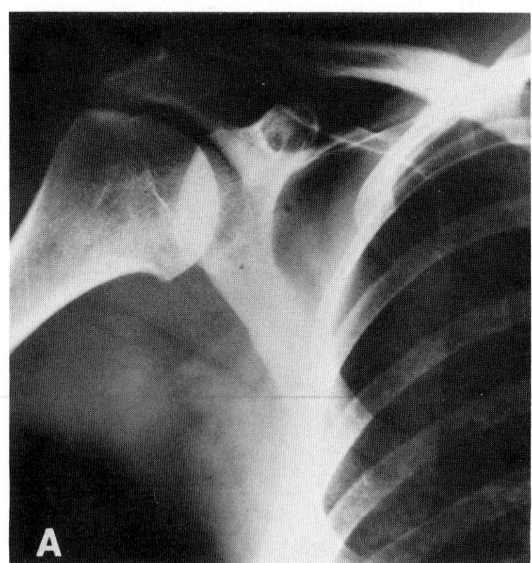

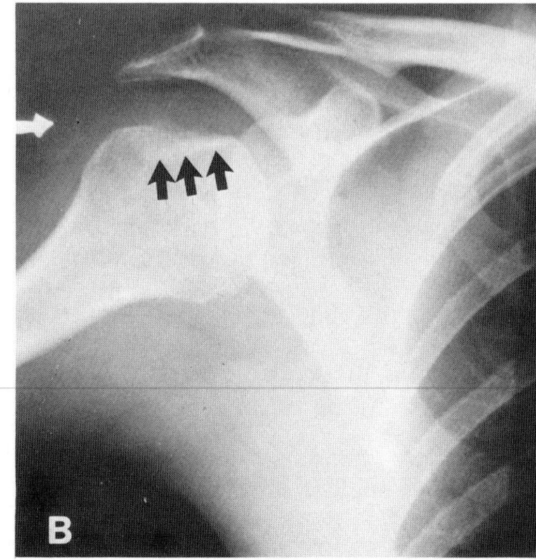

Fig. 11-56. The Hill-Sachs sign. (*A*) An anteroposterior roentgenogram of the right shoulder in 45 degrees of abduction and external rotation. There is some sclerosis in the superior aspect of the head of the humerus. (*B*) In full internal rotation, the posterolateral head defect, the Hill-Sachs sign is evident. Note the dense line of condensation marked by the three arrows.

held superior to the adducted arm, and the x-ray tube is placed posterior, lateral, and inferior to the elbow joint. The beam is aimed at the shoulder joint and makes a 30-degree angle with the humeral axis.[350]

Hill and Sachs' View

An anteroposterior roentgenogram is made of the shoulder with the arm in marked internal rotation. According to Hill and Sachs, the roentgenographic findings with the internal rotation view are: (1) flattening of the contour of the articular surface of the humeral head; (2) varying degrees of defect on the level of the greater tuberosity (i.e., the wedge-shaped defect may be an indentation, and evacuation, or a groove), and (3) a sharp dense line running downward from the top of the humeral head parallel to the axis of the shaft somewhat lateral to the mid-line—"a line of condensation," the result of the impaction fracture. The longer this line of condensation, the larger the defect. The size of the defect varies in length (cephalocaudal), 5 mm. to 3 cm.; in width, 3 mm. to 2 cm.; and in depth, 10 to 22 mm.[288]

Adams' Modification of the Internal Rotation View

Adams' modification[2] is essentially the same view recommended by Hermodsson,[119] but internal rotation is increased to 70 to 100 degrees.

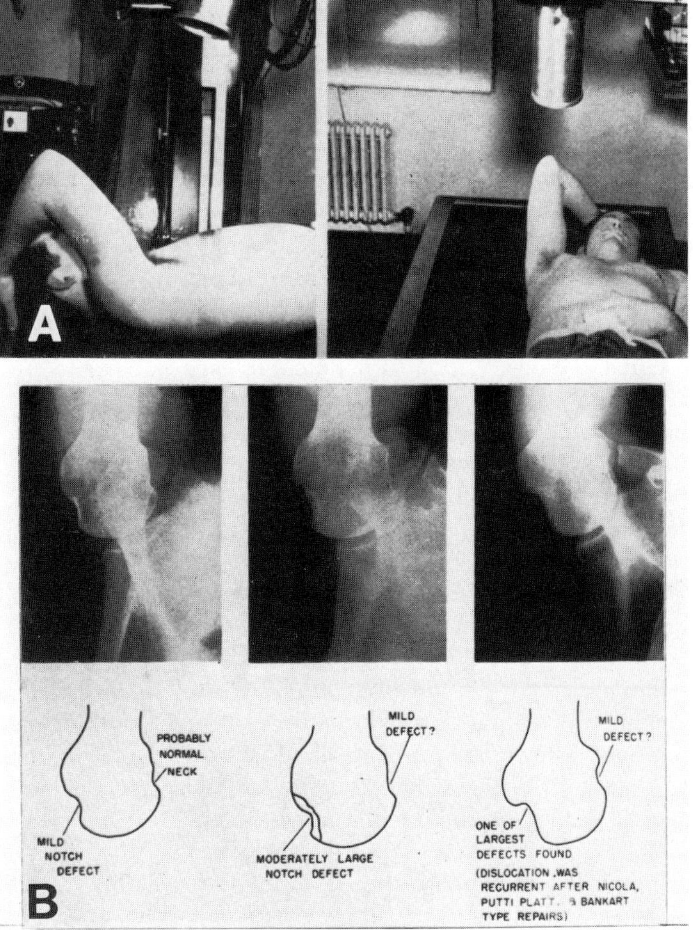

Fig. 11-57. Technique of making the Stryker notch view. (*A*) Position of the patient and the x-ray tube for making the notch view of the humerus. (*B*) Bone contour defects seen in the notch view roentgenograms of three different patients with recurrent anterior dislocations. (Hall, R. H. *et al.*: J. Bone Joint Surg., *41A*:489-494, 1959)

Stryker Notch View

The patient is supine on the table with the cassette under the shoulder.[278] The palm of the hand of the affected shoulder is placed on top of the head, and the fingers are directed toward the back of the head. The elbow of the affected shoulder should point straight upward. The x-ray beam is tilted 10 degrees toward the head and is centered over the coracoid process (Fig. 11-57). This technique was developed by William S. Stryker, and reported by Hall, Isaac, and Booth.[278] They stated that they could demonstrate the humeral head defect in 90 per cent of 20 patients with a history of recurring anterior dislocation of the shoulder.

Didiee View

The patient is prone on the table with the cassette under the shoulder.[245,350] The forearm is behind the trunk, as for the tangential view of Hermodsson. The arm is parallel to the table top with a 3-inch pad under the elbow. The dorsum of the hand is on the iliac crest with the thumb directed upward. The x-ray tube is directly lateral to the shoulder joint, and the beam is angled 45 degrees.

Incidence of the Posterolateral Defect

Hill and Sachs[288] report the defect in only 27 per cent of 119 acute anterior dislocations and in 74 per cent of 15 recurrent anterior dislocations. However, they state that the incidence of the groove defect was low, undoubtedly because it was only in the last 6 months of their 10-year study (1930 to 1940) that they used the special roentgenographic views.

In 1972, Symeonides,[427] using the Adams technique, reported the humeral head defect in 23 of 45 patients who had recurrent anterior dislocations of the shoulder, an incidence of 50 per cent. However, at the time of surgery he could confirm only 18 out of 45, bringing the incidence of the defect down to 40 per cent. In the remaining five cases, he was only able to palpate the groove, which is normally located between the greater tuberosity and the humeral head.

Eyre-Brook[257] reported an incidence of the defect in 64 per cent of 17 recurrent anterior dislocations; Brav,[201] 67 per cent of 69 recurrent dislocations. Rowe[394] noted the defect in 38 per cent of 125 acute dislocations and in 57 per cent of 63 recurrent dislocations. Adams[170] noted that the defect was found at the time of surgery in 82 per cent of 68 patients. Palmer and Widen[375] noted the defect at surgery in all of 60 cases. Strauss[423] has demonstrated in a prospective roentgenographic evaluation study of 68 patients with anterior shoulder instability that, when a combination of Hermodsson's tangential view and the Stryker notch view were used, the posterolateral humeral head defect was visualized in 87 per cent of the patients. The anteroposterior internal rotation was positive in 48 per cent; Hermodsson's tangential view in 77 per cent, and the Stryker notch view in 69 per cent.

SPRAINS OF THE ANTERIOR SHOULDER JOINT

Three distinct types of sprains can occur in the anterior shoulder. The mechanism of the sprains is essentially the same; the forces that produce each injury are of different magnitudes.

Mild Sprain

The fibers of the ligament and surrounding structures are stressed but remain intact; the ligaments are not lengthened and the joint, therefore, remains stable.

Signs and Symptoms

The joint is painful. There is mild anterior shoulder pain to palpation—which is worse with external rotation or abduction. Swelling is not noted.

Treatment

Ice may be used for 12 hours or so, followed by heat, if pain persists. A sling for 3 to 7 days usually is sufficient to allow the soft-tissue pain to subside. Gradual range-of-motion exercises can be started after 5 days. The shoulder should be protected for 10 to 14 days from contact activities and until a full range of motion is accomplished without pain. Elderly patients should begin range-of-motion exercises after 1 to 2 days' rest in a sling. The patients should not have any disability.

Moderate Sprain—Subluxation of the Glenohumeral Joint

The fibers have been partially separated or stretched, and the joint will be lax. At the time of injury, there is sufficient force to push the joint into subluxation. The recognition of this entity is very important and is covered in detail on pages 677-680.

Severe Sprain—Dislocation of the Glenohumeral Joint

The ligaments and capsule have been either disrupted in their substance, detached from the anterior glenoid or have been stripped sufficiently from the anterior glenoid and labrum to allow the head to completely displace anterior to the glenoid fossa. The signs, symptoms, treatment, and prognosis of acute anterior dislocation are discussed completely in the following section.

ACUTE ANTERIOR DISLOCATIONS OF THE SHOULDER

Traumatic Acute Dislocations

The methods of treating this problem are as ancient as medicine itself. Hippocrates,[169] discussed in detail at least six different techniques to reduce the dislocated shoulder (remember that he saw and treated only downward-into-the-axilla-type dislocations). Woodcuts, drawings, redrawings, and modifications of Hippocrates' teachings have been reported from century to century in the literature of Pare, de Cruce, Vidius, and Scultetus, and some of his techniques are still in use today (Fig. 11-58).

Theodore Kocher,[305] a Nobel Prize winner for medicine in 1909, reported in 1870 his technique for levering in the anterior dislocation instead of the direct head pressure described by Hippocrates. His article is quite confusing, and his illustrations are difficult to interpret because they were turned sideways or upside down. Had Kocher not been so famous as a thyroid surgeon, his article might have received only scant attention.

Classification Based on Anatomy

Subcoracoid dislocation is the most common type, not only in the shoulder but in the body. It accounts for the majority of anterior dislocations of the shoulder. It is far more common than the subglenoid type of dislocation. The head of the humerus is displaced anteriorly with respect to the glenoid fossa and is inferior to the coracoid process.

Subglenoid dislocation is the second most common type of acute anterior shoulder dislocation. The head of the humerus is located anterior *and* below the inferior glenoid fossa.

Subclavicular dislocation is a rare type of acute anterior shoulder dislocation. The head of the humerus is medial to the coracoid process and just inferior to the lower border of the midclavicle.

Intrathoracic dislocation is a very rare type of acute anterior shoulder dislocation, in which a lateral force has driven the head of the humerus medially between the ribs and into the thoracic cavity.

Mechanism of Injury

Subcoracoid. The mechanism that produces subcoracoid dislocation is usually a combination of indirect abduction and external rotation forces (see p. 641). With forced abduction, the greater tuberosity abuts the acromion process, and with con-

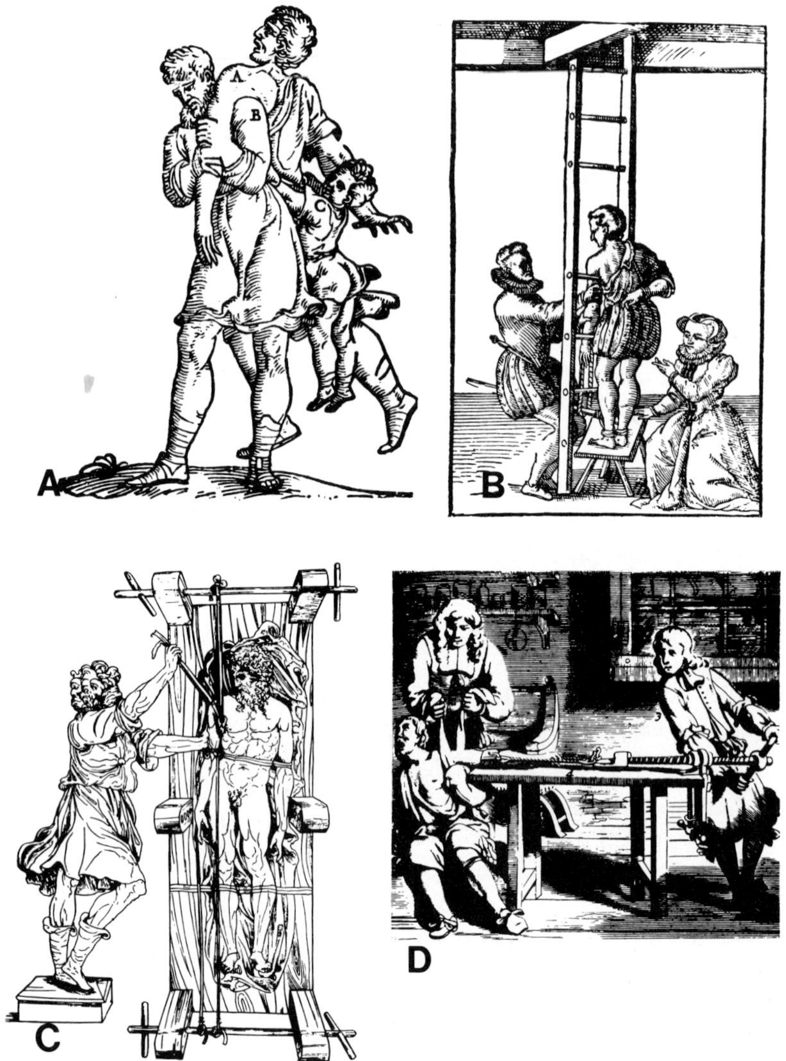

Fig. 11-58. Modified techniques of Hippocrates to reduce dislocations of the shoulder. (*A*) Reduction over the operator's shoulder (from the Venice edition of Galen in 1625[37]). (*B*) Reduction over the rung of the ladder. When the step stool on which the patient is standing is withdrawn, the weight of the patient's body produced by the fall, produces a reduction of the dislocation (from deCruce in 1607). (*C*) The use of the rack to reduce the shoulder dislocation (Vidius). (*D*) Reduction of the dislocation by a medieval type of screw traction from Scultetus in 1693. (Brockbank, W., and Griffiths, D. L.: J. Bone Joint Surg., *30B*:365-375, 1948)

tinued external rotation force, there is combined anterior stress on the capsule. When the pressure exerted by these forces overcomes the strength of the capsule, the head is dislocated anteriorly. Pure external rotation forces on the arm at the side alone may produce anterior dislocation of the shoulder (e.g., "hyper-external" rotation stress in football during arm tackling). Other mechanisms of subcoracoid anterior dislocation include a direct blow on the posterior aspect of the shoulder, which pushes the head out anteriorly, and violent muscle contractures, as are seen in convulsions.

Subglenoid. If the usual anterior dislocation mechanism has a stronger abduction component than the external rotation force, the head is levered out anteriorly and inferiorly by the impingement of the neck of the humerus on the acromion process (Fig. 11-59). Moseley[351] reports that with the subglenoid dislocation there is a higher incidence of fracture of the greater tuberosity of the humerus. There also is a higher incidence of rotator cuff avulsion.

Subclavicular and intrathoracic dislocations are produced by the same abduction —external rotation forces that produce the subglenoid dislocation. However, there is a strong accompanying direct lateral force, which displaces the head medially. So, the final resting place of the head may be medial to the coracoid and under the clavicle, or the force may drive the head farther medially to lie within the chest cavity.

Signs and Symptoms

The patient with an acute traumatic anterior dislocation is in severe pain. The dislocated arm is slightly abducted and externally rotated and is firmly held by the normal extremity. Viewed from the front, the acromion process is quite prominent. The usual subacromial roundness on the lateral aspect of the shoulder is absent, and the shoulder assumes a squared-off appearance (Fig. 11-60). There may be an anterior shoulder fullness, and the coracoid process is no longer a distinct projecting mass. The patient seems to lean away from the affected side, bending at the waist. While the dislocated arm is held in slight abduction of 10 to 15 degrees in the subcoracoid type of dislocation, the affected arm is held in moderate to marked amounts of abduction in the subglenoid type of dislocation. On palpation, the lateral border of the acromion is prominent, and a vacancy is felt below the acromion process. The cor-

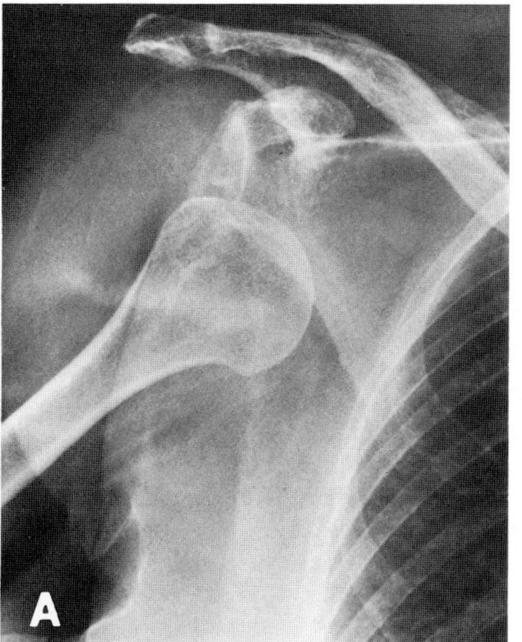

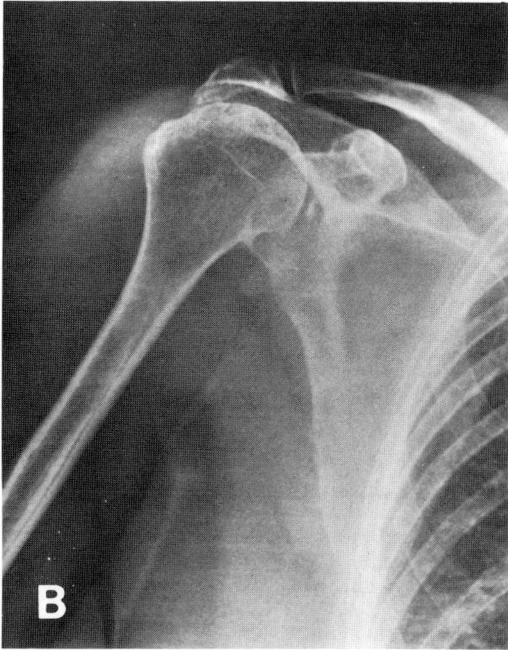

Fig. 11-59. (*A*) Subglenoid anterior dislocation of the right shoulder. Note that the superior aspect of the head is impinging on the inferior aspect of the glenoid. In addition, the arm is abducted farther than is usually seen with the common anterior subcoracoid type of dislocation. (*B*) Postreduction check film.

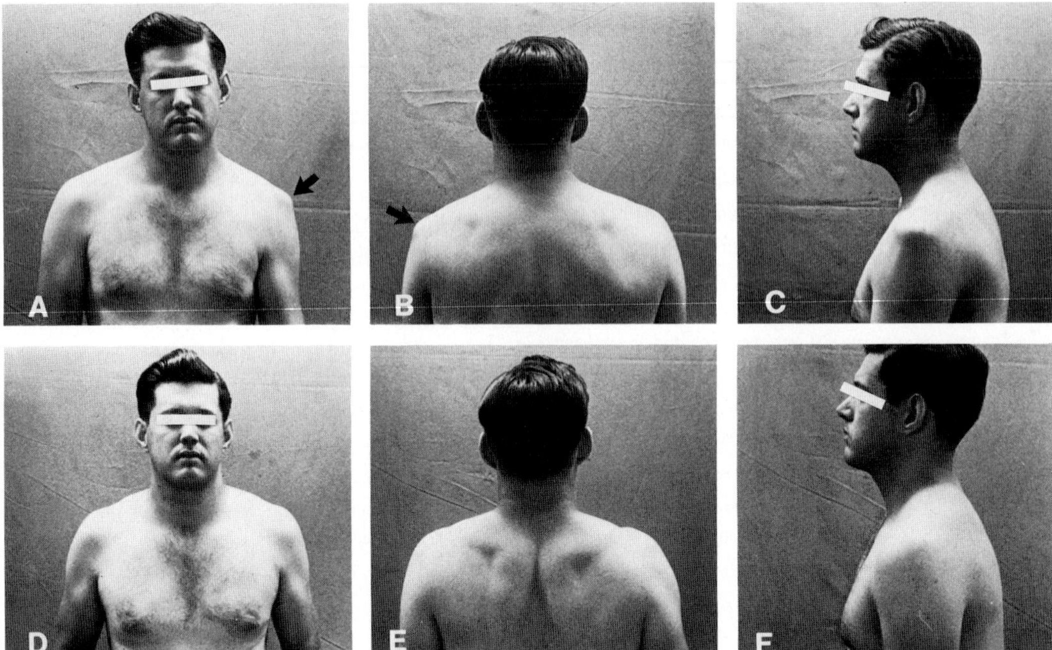

Fig. 11-60. Comparison of the clinical signs of an anterior dislocation of the shoulder before (*A-D*) and after (*D-F*) reduction. (*A*) The acromion process (*arrow*) is quite prominent on the left shoulder, giving the shoulder a squared-off appearance. There appears to be a shortening of the left shoulder, and the patient seems to be leaning away from the left side. The arm is in slight abduction. (*B*) A posterior view reveals the shortening of the left shoulder and again the prominence of the left acromion process (*arrow*). (*C*) A lateral view of the left shoulder reveals the marked prominence of the acromion process. (*D*) There is normal contour to both shoulders. (*E*) The left shoulder is not shortened. (*F*) There is normal fullness of the lateral aspect of the left shoulder.

acoid process may not be identified because of soft-tissue swelling and because of the anterior position of the humeral head. Any movement of the arm is painful and limited, especially attempted adduction or internal rotation. Obviously, many of the visual signs described are most marked on thin, asthenic individuals, and they may be absent in obese patients. With the patient undressed, however, you can always observe a difference between the shoulder with the suspected anterior dislocation and the normal shoulder.

Method of Treatment

Regardless of the technique used, the dislocated shoulder should be reduced as soon as possible. The dislocation produces considerable pain, and muscle spasm, and as the spasm increases, so does the difficulty of reduction. If the reduction is performed immediately (e.g., on the athletic field), the shoulder may be replaced without medications. Usually, the patient is seen an hour or so after dislocation and is having a considerable amount of pain and spasm. Reduction should then be accomplished only after a careful history and physical examination. The history should include such data as the mechanism of injury, the exact time of injury, whether it is the first dislocation, and whether any tingling or numbing is associated with the dislocation. The physican should take careful note, particularly in patients over age 50, of the status of the circulation to the extremity, and he should look for damage to the brachial plexus (see pp. 680-686).

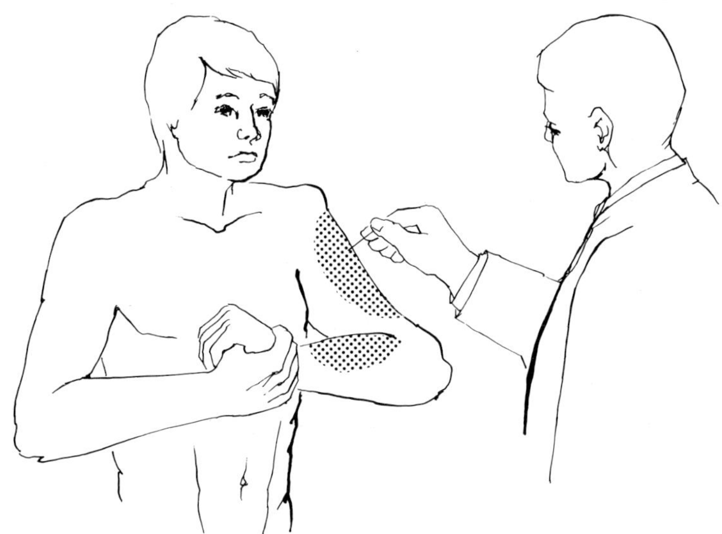

Fig. 11-61. The examiner is testing skin sensation for damage to the axillary nerve before reduction of the anterior dislocation of the left shoulder. The other area to be tested is the dorsal aspect of the forearm, which is supplied by the musculocutaneous nerve. Blom[194] has shown that testing the skin for abnormalities may be unreliable.

We have all been taught the importance of examining for damage to the axillary nerve by checking the skin sensation overlying the lateral shoulder just above the insertion of the deltoid muscle (Fig. 11-61). However, it has been demonstrated recently by Blom[194] that skin sensation abnormalities are unreliable. In his series, three patients who showed total axillary denervation on electromyography had normal sensation, and three patients who had loss of skin sensation had normal axillary nerve function. Partial denervation is probably more common than is appreciated. Blom's experience suggests that delayed recovery of function of the shoulder, particularly full range of motion, should suggest partial deltoid muscle paralysis (see p. 684).

Simple observation may tell you the type of dislocation, and gentle palpation of the shoulder may confirm your observations. The neurovascular status must always be evaluated before reduction is accomplished.

Roentgenography not only confirms your observations as to the type of dislocation, but determines whether there are any associated fractures. Roentgenograms should always be taken from three views: anteroposterior and true lateral of the glenohumeral joint (the co-called tangential scapula or posterior oblique view of the shoulder) and the axillary lateral view of shoulder (see Figs. 11-99, 11-106-108). Following reduction, the patient should again have a neurovascular check and roentgenograms to confirm the reduction of the entire humeral head.

Anesthesia. If the patient is seen immediately, the reduction may be accomplished without anesthesia or analgesia. After several hours after injury, the dislocation can usually be reduced using only narcotics. DePalma[239] and other authors prefer to use general anesthesia when the dislocation is over 2 hours old. Edeland and Stefansson[250] have reported successful reductions after blocking the suprascapular nerve with local anesthetic.

General anesthesia has some advantages over the "local and vocal" technique, in that there is total relaxation of the muscles and no real force is required to reduce the joint. One should remember that general anesthetics do not immediately relieve the muscle spasm, and it may be necessary to use a curare-like medication.

Methods of Reduction. The oldest techniques of Hippocrates or modifications thereof are still being used throughout the world to reduce shoulders. Essentially there are two different principles, traction and leverage (Fig. 11-62). Practically all of

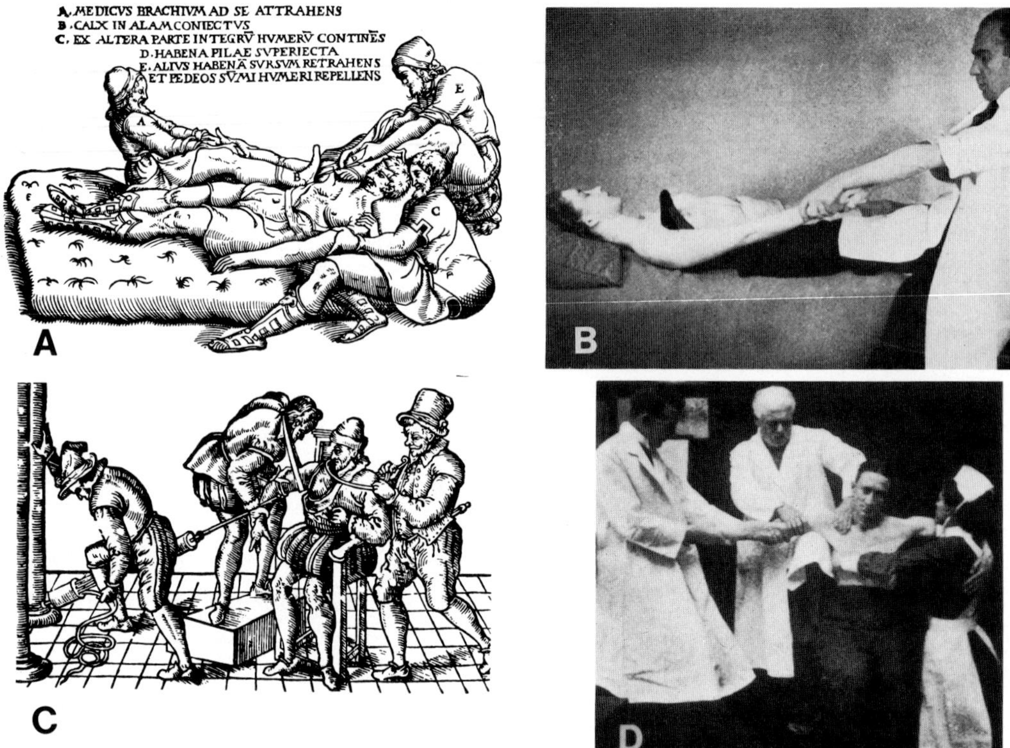

Fig. 11-62. Similarities among several techniques of closed reduction of anterior dislocations of the shoulder. (*A*) This is taken from Galen in the year 1562 and is one of the original techniques described by Hippocrates. (*B*) Sir Reginald Watson-Jones demonstrating Hippocratic technique to reduce the dislocation of the right shoulder. (*C*) Three assistants are being used to reduce an anterior dislocation of the right shoulder as depicted by Pare in 1678. (*D*) Three assistants are assisting Sir Robert Jones in reduction of an anterior dislocation of the left shoulder. (*A, C*: Brockbank, W., and Griffiths, D. L.: J. Bone and Joint Surg., *30B*:365-375, 1948; *B*, Watson-Jones, R.: Fractures and Joint Injuries. vol. II. ed. 4. Edinburgh, Churchill Livingstone, 1952-55; *D*, Jones, R.: Joints. Oxford University Press, London, 1917)

the older texts and some of the more current ones prefer the Kocher leverage techniques, but more recently authors have not recommended its use because of the possibility of increasing damage to the capsule and injuring the axillary vessels and the brachial plexus by the required leverage.

Simple Traction. With a dislocation that is only a few minutes old, straight traction on the arm in line with the shaft of the humerus, with some gentle rotation, is usually successful.

Traction with Countertraction. Traction and countertraction are applied in line with the position of the arm. The countertraction may be the hands of an assistant to stabilize the chest and shoulder, or a folded sheet can be used to loop across the front of the chest through the axilla of the dislocated shoulder and then across the back in the form of an axillary swathe. The traction should begin very gently and should be increased very gradually. Gentle internal and external rotation maneuvers can be applied to the arm to disengage the head from the glenoid (see Fig. 11-67).

Traction with Lateral Traction. Traction is applied in line with the position of the arm while lateral traction is applied to the

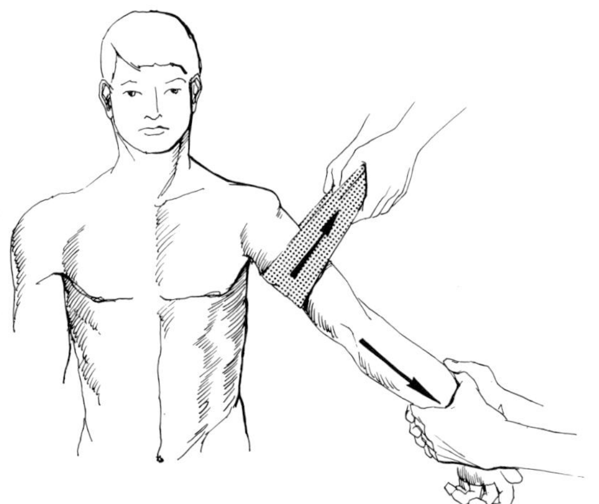

Fig. 11-63. A technique of closed reduction of an anterior dislocation of the left shoulder with traction combined with lateral traction.

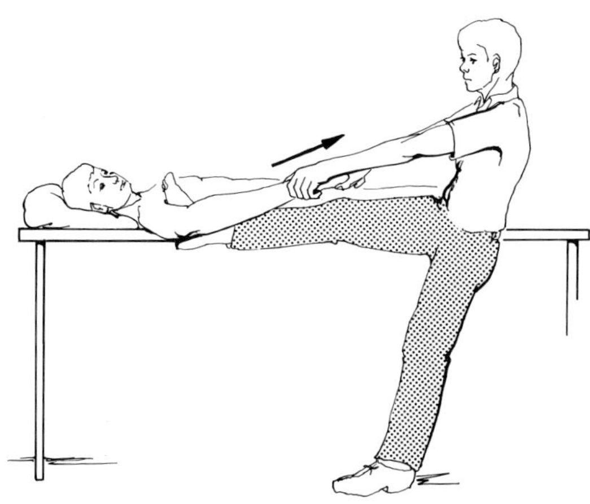

Fig. 11-64. Hippocratic technique of closed reduction. Note that the heel of the physician is not in the axilla and that the foot extends anteriorly and posteriorly across the axillary folds of the axilla.

upper arm with a folded sheet or towel (Fig. 11-63).

Hippocratic Technique. This is one of Hippocrates' original techniques[1] and is still effective when there is only one person available to reduce the shoulder. The stocking foot of the physician is used as countertraction. The heel should *not* actually go into the axilla (that is, up between the anterior and posterior axillary folds), but it should extend across the folds and against the chest wall (Fig. 11-64). Traction should be slow and gentle, and, as with all traction techniques, the arm may be gently rotated internally and externally to disengage the head.

Stimson's Technique. The patient is placed prone on the edge of the examining table.[422] Appropriate weights are taped to the wrist of the dislocated shoulder, which hangs free off the edge of the table. Five pounds is usually sufficient, but more or less weight may be used, depending upon the size of the patient (Fig. 11-65). McLaughlin felt that the weight of the arm may be sufficient to reduce the shoulder. When using this technique, you should not be in a hurry (i.e., you should leave the patient alone for a minimum of 15 to 20 minutes. Mild narcotics can be used in heavily muscled individuals).

Milch's Technique. In 1938, Milch described a technique that employed abduction, external rotation, and pulsion.[345] With

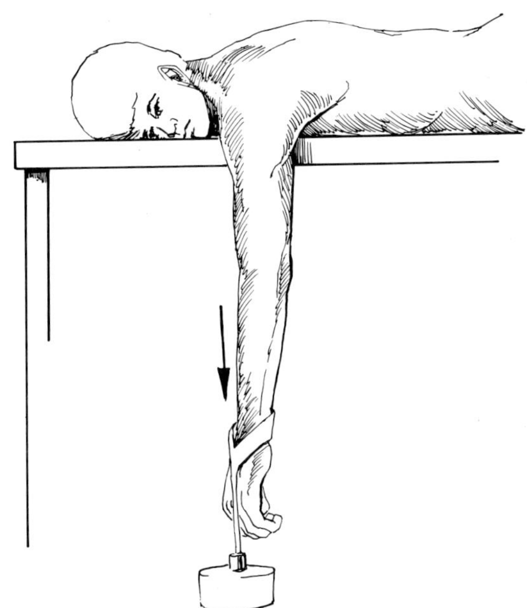

Fig. 11-65. The modified Stimson technique of closed reduction. The amount of weight that is hung from the hand depends on the size of the patient.

the patient supine, the arm is abducted in external rotation. Then, using his thumb, the physician gently pushes the head over the glenoid rim into the fossa. Milch reported no neurovascular complications and stated that this technique might be particularly advantageous in a fracture-dislocation of the shoulder. The technique never became popular.

Leverage Technique of Kocher. There are essentially four steps to this maneuver.[305] (1) With the elbow flexed 90 degrees, traction is applied in line with the humeral shaft. This should be gentle and steady for a minute or so. (2) The arm is slowly and smoothly brought into full external rotation. (3) The humerus is adducted across the front of the chest, approximately to the mid-line. (4) The arm is rotated internally until the hand is placed on the opposite shoulder. During this maneuver, the humeral head is levered on the anterior glenoid, and the shaft is levered against the anterior thoracic wall until the reduction is completed. If the technique fails, Key and Conwell[219] recommend a folded towel in the axilla to act as a fulcrum to increase the leverage during the fourth maneuver. DePalma[239] uses the standard Kocher technique only if less traumatic techniques of reduction fail. He warns that undue forces utilized in rotation leverage can damage the soft tissues of the shoulder joint, the vessels, and the brachial plexus. Others report spiral fractures of the upper shaft of the humerus, and further damage to the anterior capsular mechanism resulting when the Kocher leverage technique of reduction was used.

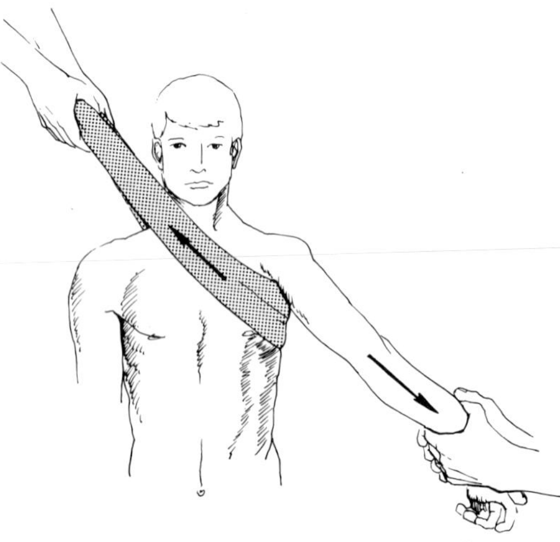

Fig. 11-66. Closed reduction of the left shoulder with traction against countertraction.

Author's Preferred Method of Reduction

I prefer the use of traction and countertraction with the axillary swathe combined with analgesics, tranquilizers, or muscle relaxants. I prefer to use a combination of narcotics, with muscle relaxants or tranquilizers in the emergency department. An IV is routinely established. Half of the narcotics are given intramuscularly, and half are given intravenously into the IV tubing, followed by a tranquilizer or a muscle relaxant. If this fails to produce sufficient relief of pain and muscle spasm, use general anesthesia. A sheet folded to form a 5-inch swathe is used as countertraction to stabilize the chest (Fig. 11-66). Half of the narcotic is given subcutaneously and half is given in an intravenous infusion. Once the patient begins to become drowsy and the pain is diminished, the muscle relaxant is injected into the running intravenous infusion. After 5 to 6 minutes have passed, very gentle traction is applied to the arm and increased gradually against the countertraction. With very gentle traction, the reduction will be accomplished without pain and without any palpable sensation of reduction. Occasionally gentle internal and external rotation is used to disengage the head from the glenoid rim. In some larger patients, the reduction may be so atraumatic that neither the physician nor the patient feels or sees the reduction. It is only after you have discontinued your traction that the patient moves his arm about, stating that everything is all right. If this technique is unsuccessful and there are no other contraindications, I prefer to use general anesthesia, again with traction-countertraction maneuvers, instead of the leverage type of reduction.

Treatment of Intrathoracic Dislocations. The injury is usually associated with severe trauma. Following abduction and external rotation forces which dislocate the humeral head anteriorly, a strong lateral force displaces the humeral head medially through the ribs and into the thoracic cavity. There may be an associated fracture of the anatomical neck of the humerus, so that, with reduction, the head may actually remain in the chest. Either the greater tuberosity or the rotator cuff is avulsed (Fig. 11-67). The patient presents with a shortened arm, which is abducted. Neurologic and vascular complications can occur, as can subcutaneous emphysema. Reduction should be accomplished under general anesthesia with gentle lateral traction. West[450] reported a case in which with reduction, the humerus was felt to slip out of the chest cavity with a sensation similar to slipping a large cork out of a bottle. His patient, who had an avulsion fracture of the greater tuberosity and no neurological deficit, regained a functional range of motion and returned to his previous job as a carpenter.

Patel, Pardee, and Singerman[378] reported a case of intrathoracic dislocation in which there was a fracture of the humeral head at the anatomical neck. After reduction, because of the general condition of the patient, the head was left in the chest cavity. The case reported by Glessner[272] was similar, except that the head was removed from the chest cavity.

Irreducible Acute Anterior Dislocations

In the absence of fractures of the humeral head or tuberosities, or the glenoid or coracoid processes, the problem probably lies with interposed soft tissues (i.e., a curtain of the rotator cuff, capsule, or biceps tendon). The posterolateral groove of the head of the humerus, located in the interval between the articular surface and the posterior aspects of the greater tuberosity, may be held firmly against the anterior glenoid rim by the tightly stretched subscapularis muscle. In this condition, the subscapularis may be so tight that it may have to be divided, at surgery, before reduction can be accomplished.

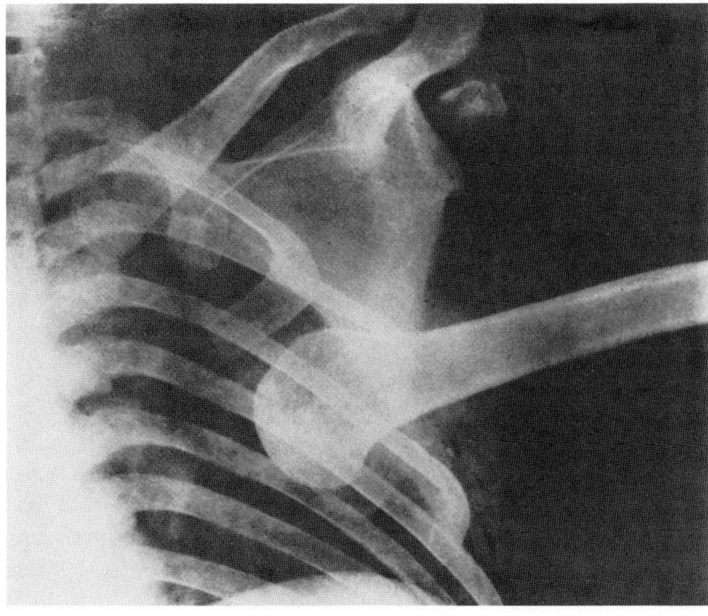

Fig. 11-67. An intrathoracic anterior dislocation of the left shoulder. Note the wide interspace laterally between the third and the fourth ribs and the avulsion fracture of the greater tuberosity, which remained in the vicinity of the glenoid fossa. (West, E. F.: J. Bone Joint Surg., *31B*:61, 1949)

Indications for Surgery with Acute Anterior Dislocations.

Soft-Tissue Interpositions. The rotator cuff, capsule, or biceps tendon may prevent closed reduction, and operative reduction will be required. The severe types of displacement (subglenoid and subclavicular in a young, active patient) indicate a complete cuff disruption, and consideration should be given to operative repairs. The more active the patient, the more likely the need for operative repair.

Fracture of the Greater Tuberosity. Occasionally with anterior dislocation of the shoulder, the greater tuberosity fragment displaces up under the acromion process and does not reduce into its bed. This requires surgical replacement.

Glenoid Rim Fracture. The mechanism may be a fall on the lateral shoulder which drives the shoulder anteriorly and knocks off a fragment, or it could occur during dislocation and as a result of a combination of forces produced by direct pressure from the head and an avulsion force from the capsule (Fig. 11-68). Aston and Gregory[178] reported three cases in which a large anterior fragment of the glenoid occurred as a result of a fall on the lateral aspect of the adducted shoulder. Most authors agree that an anterior dislocation combined with a fracture of the anterior glenoid lip is always associated with a recurring subluxation or recurrent anterior dislocation. Chip-sized fragments (5 mm.) should be treated with the usual conservative techniques but larger fragments require operative repair. DePalma[239] not only recommends replacement of the fragment but in addition, an operative procedure that would ordinarily cure the problem of recurrent dislocation.

"Selective" Repairs. The incidence of recurrent dislocation following an acute anterior dislocation, regardless of the treatment, is quite high (see p. 660). In special selected circumstances, such as an acute anterior dislocation that occurs late in the season in a valuable and talented athlete, surgical repair may be justified so that he can be ready for the next season and not have to worry himself, his coach, or the team about another dislocation.

Management After Reduction

For patients less than 40 years old, one of the oldest techniques is the use of a Velpeau dressing to bind the arm to the chest wall. In my experience and in the experience of others, this can be uncomfortable for the patient. There are a variety of immobilizers available, and all have one thing in common: they prevent abduction and external rotation. One of the simplest is a combination of the old standard tri-

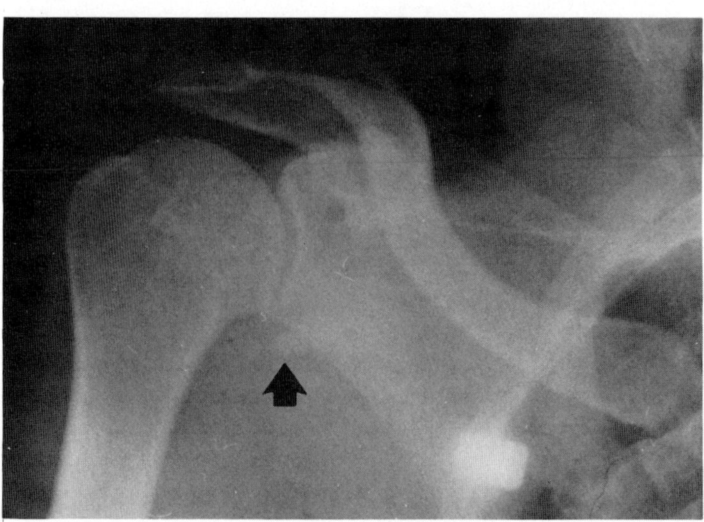

Fig. 11-68. A large fracture of the anterior glenoid rim (*arrow*) associated with an acute primary anterior dislocation of the shoulder produces recurrent dislocations. This fracture is an indication for a surgical repair and/or reconstruction.

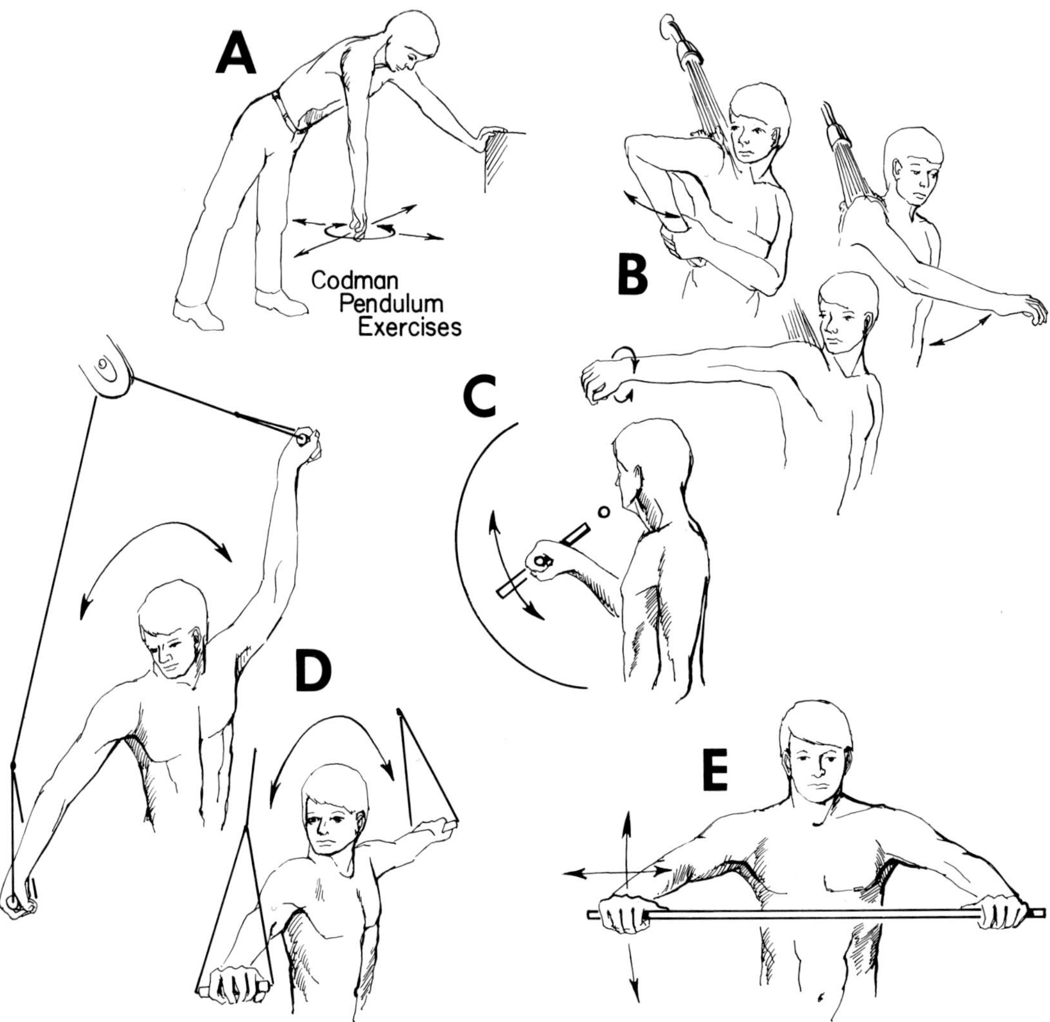

Fig. 11-69. Rehabilitation routines used after postreduction immobilization for anterior dislocation of the shoulder.

angular sling with a swathe about the arm and chest. Nicola[239] and others have devised various slings, and harness devices. Commercial immobilizers with Velcro fasteners are available, and are, in many instances, very comfortable.

The length of time the shoulder is immobilized after reduction varies considerably —from 2 to 3 days to 8 weeks.[191,239,328,448] Essentially, the purpose of the immobilization is to allow the anterior capsule and ligaments and the subscapularis muscle unit to heal. If they do heal and they are not lengthened, stretched, or detached, the healing process prevents the complication of recurrent dislocation. After reconstruction Rowe uses only a sling for 2 to 3 days and then allows the patient to use the arm to regain an early range of motion.*

Following immobilization, the patient should be instructed in gentle range-of-motion exercises. They should begin with the Codman pendulum maneuvers, followed by active regaining of motion through the use of active range of motion, passive assistance with the normal arm, and others. The use of pulleys with rope and broomstick are all helpful (Fig. 11-69). The increase in

* Personal communication.

motion should be slow and easy, and the patient should be instructed that pain associated with any forced motion only delays recovery. Moist heat may be used with exercise, or a method I like is to have the patient do his active range of motion while standing in a hot shower with the stream directed onto the involved shoulder. Only after the patient has regained 80 to 90 degrees of motion should a resistive exercise routine be instituted. Strenuous exercises or a return to sports should be delayed until there is a full range of motion in the shoulder and no discernible muscle atrophy or weakness to the shoulder or arm.

For patients over age 40, acute traumatic dislocation should be protected with a sling or a collar and cuff for 1 to 2 weeks. McLaughlin[328] recommends the use of a sling and swathe while sleeping, for 1 to 2 weeks, to protect against reinjury. A gentle active range of motion program should begin within a few days of reduction. A general rule is—the older the patient, the sooner the shoulder should be moved. Codman pendulum shoulder maneuvers should be done several times during the day, followed by a gentle and graduated range-of-motion routine, but abduction and external maneuvers should be avoided for the first 2 weeks. The use of overhead pulley and broomstick handle are helpful to regain motion. Very active people should be cautioned against vigorous activities for at least 6 weeks (see Fig. 11-69).

Patients, regardless of their age, should be given instructions on how to keep their axilla clean and dry. While both age groups should exercise their elbow, wrist, and fingers, it is particularly important for older patients.

Author's Method of Care After Reduction

I prefer to immobilize the patient in a sling and swathe or a commercially available immobilizer. Young and active patients are immobilized for 3 weeks. After reduction, gentle and gradual range-of-motion exercises are instituted. Pulleys and rope and other devices are used to gain the full range of motion before a resistive weight program is instituted. Active physical use of the arm and contact sports should ordinarily be avoided until there is a painless full range of motion and until normal muscle strength has been achieved. However, under *certain circumstances,* before the 3-week immobilization and the rehabilitation are completed, an athlete may be allowed to return to competition. It may be necessary to restrain the shoulder in a harness of some sort that limits abduction and external rotation.

Prognosis Following Acute Anterior Dislocations

There are two types of recurrent anterior dislocations, traumatic and atraumatic. The atraumatic type includes dislocations that recur because of congenital bone and muscle abnormalities about the shoulder and habitual or voluntary dislocations. The prognosis following a traumatic dislocation depends upon the amount of force that produced the initial dislocation, the age of the patient, and whether there are associated fractures and soft-tissue injuries. (The factors relating to the incidence of recurrence are discussed on p. 674.)

Atraumatic Dislocations

Voluntary or Habitual Anterior Dislocations of the Shoulder

In atraumatic dislocation of the shoulder —in which the patient can voluntarily displace the joint anteriorly, posteriorly, or inferiorly and, in some instances, into all three positions—there is usually no history of trauma, but should there be, it is only very minor. Most voluntary dislocations begin in childhood or adolescence, and the condition may be unilateral or bilateral. Most cases of bilateral dislocation of the shoulder are the atraumatic type. The dislocations and spontaneous reductions are painless, and the patient may continue the maneuver as a habit. He may demonstrate his trick to the marvel of his family or perform for his friends at parties.

While a significant number of patients with habitual dislocations have emotional disorders, there may be anatomical and pathological reasons for the problem (e.g., hypoplastic bone structures about the shoulder, excessive anterior tilt of the glenoid fossa, congenital joint laxity as associated with Ehlers-Danlos syndrome, and muscle weakness, imbalances, or paralysis). There may be a familial predisposition.[239]

The association of voluntary dislocations of the shoulder with emotional instability and definite psychiatric problems has been noted by several authors. Rowe, Pierce, and Clark[402] have studied extensively 26 patients with voluntary dislocations of the shoulder and have separated the patients into two distinct groups. Group I (8 patients) were those with significant psychiatric, emotional, or character problems, and Group II (18 patients) were those in which no psychological or social disorders could be demonstrated. The authors reported that the 8 patients with emotional problems paid little attention to any conservative therapeutic regime and did poorly following various operative procedures. Only two of the 13 dislocated shoulders in the eight patients in Group I had a good result, regardless of the type of treatment. The remainder of the patients had poor results. Five of the patients in Group I had 37 operative procedures, practically all of which were unsuccessful. When, after three or four anterior reconstructions, one finally is successful, the emotionally disturbed patient works and practices and finally learns to dislocate the shoulder posteriorly (Fig. 11-70). Then after repeated posterior reconstructions, he may learn to dislocate inferiorly, and the end result is a shoulder so degenerated that the only operative procedure left to perform is arthrodesis.

The emotionally disturbed patient seems to enjoy spoiling the work of the surgeon. I have seen one patient, who, after eight unsuccessful anterior and posterior reconstructions, had a successful arthrodesis (Fig. 11-71). He then "fell" from a ladder onto the arthrodesed shoulder and fractured his humerus.

Rowe *et al.* have shown that the patients who do not have psychological problems respond remarkably well to a rehabilitation program that strengthens the shoulder abductors and the external and internal ro-

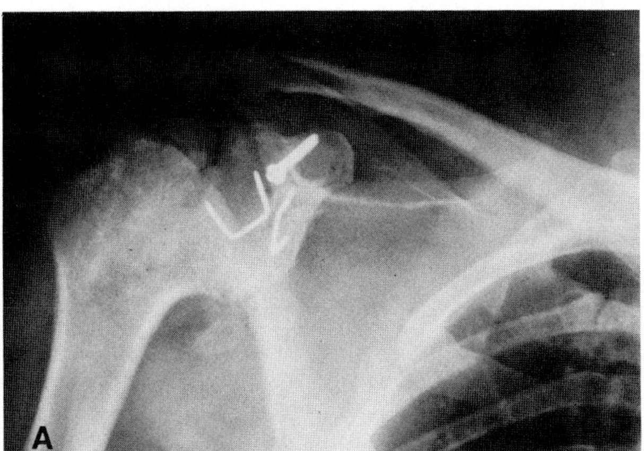

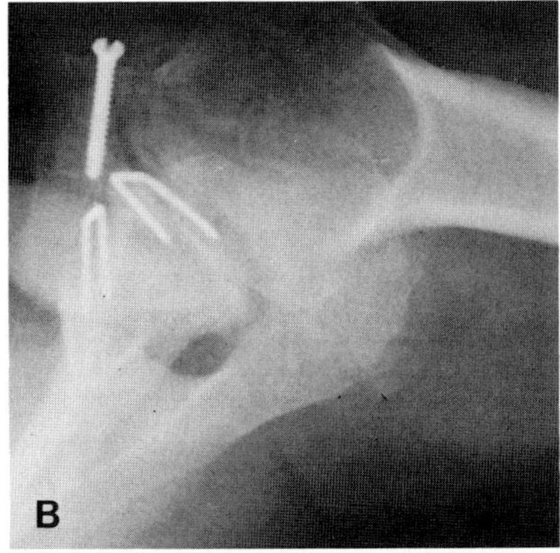

Fig. 11-70. Pitfalls associated with voluntary dislocations. (*A*) Severe traumatic arthritis following six reconstructions of the right shoulder in a patient who had voluntary dislocations of the shoulder. Note the irregularity of the joint, the loose bodies, and the floating metal. (*B*) In the axillary lateral roentgenogram, note the degenerative changes and the irregular contour of the humeral head.

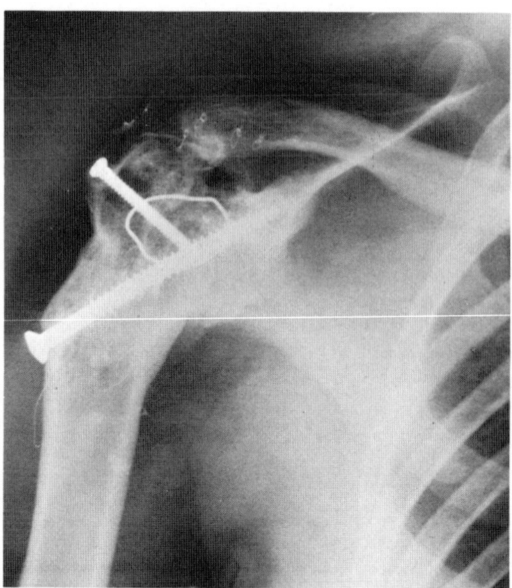

Fig. 11-71. Arthrodesis of the right shoulder was the final operation for a patient who had voluntary anterior dislocations and eight unsuccessful attempts at reconstruction.

tators. Further, they report that operative procedures can be performed successfully in this group, *when they are indicated.*

In summary then, patients with voluntary dislocations of the shoulder are in a completely distinct and different category from those with the involuntary or traumatic type of recurrent dislocations. Those patients with significant emotional problems should not have surgical reconstructions and should receive psychiatric help.

Congenital Dislocations of the Shoulder

According to Greig[275] and Cozen,[221] who have reviewed the literature on congenital dislocation quite extensively, the condition was first described in 1901 by Wunsch. The abnormality is uncommon. There are *many* possible defects, and the treatment varies. I urge you to read the articles by Cozen and Greig.

Complications of Anterior Dislocations of the Shoulder

Complications that can occur with anterior dislocation include detachment of the rotator cuff, injuries to the axillary artery or vein, injuries to the brachial plexus (particularly the axillary nerve), damage to the biceps tendon, and various fractures to the joint including the glenoid rim, the humeral head, the tuberosity, and assorted fractures to the humeral head. Recurring anterior subluxations should also be considered complications of acute traumatic anterior dislocations.

TRAUMATIC RECURRENT ANTERIOR DISLOCATIONS OF THE SHOULDER

Recurrent dislocation is the most common complication following a traumatic anterior dislocation of the shoulder. Most authors agree that the incidence of recurrence of the traumatic dislocation in younger age groups is very high. Under the age of 20, the incidence is reported by Rowe,[394] McLaughlin and Cavallaro[330] and others[239,350] to be between 80 and 92 per cent. Under the age of 30, the incidence is approximately 60 per cent, and over the age of 40, the incidence drops sharply down to 10 to 15 per cent. Moseley,[350] Rowe,[394] DePalma,[239] and McLaughlin[330] state that the majority of all recurrences occur within the first 2 years after the first traumatic dislocation, and only 25 per cent occur between the second and fifth years. Whereas anterior dislocations associated with fracture of the anterior glenoid rim carry a high recurrence rate (>95%), anterior dislocations associated with fracture of the greater tuberosity cause a low recurrence rate (5 to 30%).

In other words, the damage seems to be done at the time of the traumatic dislocation, and healing will not occur in a high percentage of cases. In general, the younger the patient, the higher the incidence of recurrent dislocations. There are many orthopaedists who are not in agreement with the reported recurrence rates. However, all of the published data points to the fact that recurrence in younger patients is very common—in the 80 to 90 per cent range.

The strongest opponent to the high recurrence rate concept is Watson-Jones. In the fourth edition of his classic text, published in 1956, he states, "None of the several hundred primary dislocations that I have treated with strict immobilization of the shoulder for at least 3 weeks have recurred." He states further that dislocations of the shoulder are just like dislocations of every other joint. Then (in a personal communication reported in Moseley's text,[350] published in 1961) he stated that his views had not changed.

While there may be indications for doing a primary repair of the acute traumatic anterior dislocation of the shoulder, most authors recommend a 3- to 4-week immobilization period. The usual indication for doing a reconstruction is after the second or third dislocation, when the operation can be scheduled most conveniently with respect to the patient's job or profession or school vacation.

Recurrences are definitely more common in men than in women. Moseley[350] quotes several series, and the ratios vary from 4:1 to 6:1. Rowe[394] reports that recurrent dislocations are neither more nor less common in the dominant shoulder, nor does the weaker shoulder tend to suffer primary or recurrent dislocations more frequently than the stronger, dominant, one.

Rowe has stated that the most consistent and significant factor influencing the prognosis in shoulder dislocation is the age of the patient at the time of the initial or primary dislocation. Rowe also has pointed out that the recurrence rate varies inversely with the severity of the original trauma; another way of saying this is: the easier it occurred primarily, the easier it recurs. He has stated further that the incidence of recurrence seems to be affected very little by the type and length of immobilization of the shoulder following initial dislocation. In his series, patients were immobilized anywhere from 1 to 6 weeks. In the series of 573 dislocations of the shoulder reported by McLaughlin and Cavallaro,[330] they concluded the length of time that the shoulder was immobilized after initial anterior dislocation was of little importance. The age of the patient and the site and nature of the damage done to the joint at the time of the dislocation were of primary importance.

Anatomical Factors

Before proceeding to a discussion of recurring anterior dislocation of the shoulder, I think it is important to mention the theories that have been credited for the cause of the condition. The two theories that have been *cussed and discussed* are the role of the "essential lesion" and the relative deficiencies of the subscapularis muscle and tendon. The works of Moseley and Overgaard,[352] Townley,[432] and Gardner[265] have shown that the labrum itself is not the entire problem. Certainly, with the anterior displacement of the humeral head, there will be changes in the anatomy of the anterior glenoid. However, this is not the only cause of the dislocation.

Many authors, including Moseley and Overgaard,[352] Jens,[298] DePalma *et al.*,[241] and Symeonides[427] have found laxity and deficiencies in the subscapularis muscle tendon unit at the time of surgery. Moseley and Overgaard found laxity in 25 consecutive cases, and DePalma reported laxity and decreased muscle tone of the subscapularis in 38 consecutive cases. Several of their cases revealed a definite defect along the inferior aspect of the subscapularis tendon, as if it had been partially torn from its bone attachment, along with separation of those muscle fibers that insert into the humerus directly below the lesser tuberosity. McLaughlin,[329] DePalma,[241] and Jens[298] have noted, at the time of surgery but before arthrotomy, that with abduction and external rotation, the humeral head would dislocate under the lower edge of the subscapularis tendon.

DePalma *et al.*[241] say that the subscapularis muscle is the most important buttress against dislocations of the shoulder joint. It is their opinion that at the time of initial dislocation the muscle is severely stretched, and some of its fibers even rupture. This is followed by an increased laxity, loss of tone, volume, and power. Symeonides biopsied the subscapularis muscle tendon unit at the time of surgery and found microscopic evidence of "healed posttraumatic lesions." He states that the lengthening of the subscapularis muscle, which leads to a decrease in power, is the prime factor producing instability of the shoulder.

These investigations on the subscapularis muscle tendon unit seem quite logical and reasonable. However, so do the more recent investigations (i.e., deficiencies of the posterior short depressor or steering muscles) by Saha and his associates.[406-411] What role does the posterolateral humeral head compression fracture play? Debevoise, Hyatt, and Townsend[232] have shown that the average value for humeral torsion in the repeatedly dislocating shoulder is greater than that in the normal shoulder. What about other fractures about the glenohumeral joint and the congenital bone and muscle problems that produce recurring anterior dislocations?

Reasonably, there have to be many possible etiologies that can produce recurring anterior dislocation of the shoulder. Hence various etiologies require selective and special operative reconstructions, which are designed to correct the problem. I believe it is an error to consider that only one basic lesion can be responsible for all recurring anterior dislocations of the shoulder.

Mechanism of Recurrent Anterior Dislocations

The mechanisms of recurrent dislocations of the shoulder are similar to the mechanisms that produce the acute dislocation, except that less force is required. In some patients, the dislocation may occur during their sleep, or it may occur when the arm is raised overhead. In other patients considerable force may be required to produce the dislocation.

Signs and Symptoms

The signs and symptoms of recurrent anterior dislocation vary with each patient. Some require manipulative assistance and analgesia by the physician, and some patients reduce the dislocation, with and without help. There is far less pain with a recurring dislocation than with the acute dislocation. The anterior shoulder may be tender to palpation, and instability usually is present.

Roentgenographic Findings

Degenerative changes may be noted in the glenohumeral joint, particularly with a long history of multiple dislocations. The posterolateral humeral head defect can usually be seen on various special roentgenographic views described above. Usually, loose bodies or angular ossification or fragments of bone can be noted at the anteroinferior glenoid rim on the modified axillary view.

Treatment of Recurrent Anterior Dislocation of the Shoulder

Most of the published literature on shoulder dislocations is concerned with the problem of recurrent anterior dislocations. Beginning with Hippocrates,[169] who described, over 2300 years ago, the use of a white-hot poker to scar the capsule of the shoulder, there have been more than 100 different operative procedures described to manage the recurrent anterior dislocation of the shoulder. The reader who has a yearning for the detailed history should read the classic texts by Moseley[350] and Hermodsson.[285]

Of the many procedures that have been described for reconstructing the anterior shoulder, only a handful are still popular today. They are directed to repair of the anterior capsular mechanism (Bankart[186,187]), subscapular muscle shortening (Putti-Platt),[370] subscapular transfer (Magnuson-Stack),[210,333-335] bone block procedures (Eden-Hybbinette),[252,293] and transfer of the tip of the coracoid process with muscle attachments (Bristow[282]).

Other procedures used less often include autogenous fascia lata used as a free graft (Gallie-Bateman[190,263]), osteotomy of the proximal humerus (Weber[449]), latissimus dorsi muscle used to reinforce the action of the subscapularis and the posterior short depressor muscle (Saha),[406-408] transfer of the infraspinatus muscle into the posterolateral defect in the humeral head Connolly),[218] and bicipital tendon used as a checkrein ligament (Nicola).[360-364] Anterior glenoid bone pegs (Speed,[420] Noordenbos,[365] and Leguit)[316] have been used in the past.

Many authors, particularly Watson-Jones,[446] are of the opinion that the common denominator of all of the reconstructions is the anterior approach, with the resultant anterior scarring to the capsule and subscapularis, which limits external rotation and thus prevents future recurrences. Other authors specifically utilize operative procedures that do not limit external rotation. In those cases where there is a large posterolateral defect in the head of the humerus, some authors recommend the use of an anterior bone block, and Connolly[218] recommends the use of a transfer of the infraspinatus muscle into the defect, a reverse of the procedure described by McLaughlin for posterior dislocation of the shoulder when there is a large anteromedial defect in the humeral head.

It is not the intent of this chapter to vividly portray all of the operative procedures, but the principles involved in each will be described briefly. Familiarity with the different common types of reconstruction is important, as the anatomy and surgical pathology is not the same for all patients. In other words, use the proper reconstruction for each individual problem.

Repair of Anterior Capsular Mechanism

This repair was first done by Perthes[380] in 1906, who, even then, recommended the use of staples for fixation. However, the popularity of the technique is due to Bankart,[185] who first performed the operation in 1923 on one of his former house surgeons. The procedure is now universally referred to as the Bankart operation. Essentially, the operation was designed to reattach the anterior capsule to the anterior glenoid. This defect of the capsule from the anterior glenoid is commonly referred to as the Bankartarian lesion. The subscapularis muscle, which is carefully divided to expose the capsule, is reapproximated without any overlap or shortening. Modifications have come from Moseley,[348] who utilized a Vitallium rim to the anterior glenoid in selected cases; DuToit,[247] who uses special staples; Boyd and Hunt,[199] who approach the capsule by splitting the subscapularis muscle instead of detaching it; Viek, Bell, and Mawr[442] and Luckey,[323] who utilize a pull-out wire technique to repair the capsule; Delitala,[233] who uses a special nail to repair the capsule; Metcalfe,[341] a screw and one plate; and M. E. Müller,[449] who uses screws. While many authors assert that it is technically a difficult procedure to perform, others declare it the best procedure available.

Subscapularis Muscle Procedures

Muscle Shortening. Osmond-Clarke[370] described this procedure, which was being used by Sir Harry Platt of England and by Vittorio Putti of Italy. Platt evolved his technique after he found no single and constant Bankartarian lesion and first used it in an operation in November, 1925. Some years later H. Osmond-Clarke saw Putti perform essentially the same operation, which had been his standard practice since 1923. Scaglietta,[370] one of Putti's pupils, revealed that the operation may well have been performed first by Codivilla, Putti's teacher and predecessor. Neither Putti nor Platt ever described the technique in the literature. We are indeed indebted to Osmond-Clarke for this important contribution.

In the Putti-Platt procedure, the subscapularis tendon is divided 2.5 cm. from its insertion. The anterior shoulder joint capsule, which adheres to the posterior surface of the subscapularis tendon, may be opened at this point. If not, the capsule is opened in the same plane as the tendon is divided, so that the joint can be inspected. The lateral stump of the tendon is attached to the "most convenient soft-tissue structure along the anterior rim of the glenoid cavity." If the capsule and labrum have been stripped from the anterior glenoid and the neck of the scapula, the tendon is sutured to the deep surface of the capsule, and "it is advisable to raw the anterior surface of the neck of the scapula, so that the sutured tendo-capsule will adhere to it." After the lateral tendon stump is secured, the medial muscle stump is lapped over the lateral stump, producing a substantial shortening of the subscapularis muscle.

In those instances when the medial capsule can be separated from the medial muscle tendon unit, the capsule is sutured on top of the secured lateral tendon, then the medial muscle tendon unit is secured over the capsule laterally in the area of the greater tuberosity of the humerus. The exact placement of the lateral stump into the anterior soft tissues and of the medial stump into the greater tuberosity is predetermined, so that, after conclusion of the procedure, the arm should rotate externally to the neutral position.

Watson-Jones[446] and other authors have recommended that the Bankart and the Putti-Platt procedures be combined (i.e., following the meticulous repair of the capsule to the glenoid, they "double-breast" the subscapularis rather than merely reapproximating it). M. E. Müller[449] reattaches the capsule with screws and then shortens the subscapularis. Certainly one should consider the Putti-Platt procedure when, during the performance of a Bankart operation, the capsule is found to be very thin or atrophic.

Author's Comment on the Putti-Platt Operation. Since the publication of the Putti-Platt technique by Osmond-Clarke in 1948, authors have described the technique as securing the lateral tendon into the *"rawed" anterior glenoid rim of the scapula.* In effect, this would create a tenodesis of the subscapularis tendon. I do not believe that this was the intent of the authors. In essence, they shortened the subscapularis muscle unit by doubling it anteriorly over the joint. They "rawed" only the "anterior surface of the neck of the scapula" and not the glenoid, and only when the capsule was stripped away from that area. The purpose was to cause the anterior capsule to readhere to the anterior scapular neck, which decreases the large anterior joint space.

Another point to remember is that with a 2.5-cm. lateral stump of the tendon to work with, there is no way that you can attach it to the anterior glenoid or the neck of the scapula and be able to externally rotate the arm to the neutral position or flex, extend, abduct, or elevate the upper extremity. If the lateral stump of the subscapularis tendon is attached to the raw bone of the anterior glenoid and if the patient develops a functional range of motion, this suggests to me that the tendon was disrupted from the glenoid and the double-breasting of the muscle tendon unit is in effect. In essence then, the primary objective in the Putti-Platt operation is to shorten the subscapularis muscle tendon unit, which produces a double layer of subscapularis muscle and tendon anterior to the shoulder joint.

Muscle Transfer. Transfer of the subscapularis tendon from the lesser tuberosity across the bicipital groove to the greater tuberosity was originally described by Paul Magnuson and James Stack in 1940.[334] In 1955, Magnuson[200] recommended that in some cases the tendon should be transferred not only across the bicipital groove but distally into an area between the greater tuberosity and the upper shaft. In this manner, when the arm is abducted the subscapularis muscle tendon unit would act more effectively as a sling to support the head of the humerus. DePalma[239] recommends that the tendon be transferred to the upper shaft below the greater tuberosity. He interprets this procedure as being designed to strengthen the anterior muscle barrier to the front of the shoulder and to produce a dynamic force, which, on elevation of the arm, forces and holds the head of the humerus in the glenoid fascia. When the tendon is transferred laterally, the laxity of the muscle is taken out. When the tendon is transferred distally, the tendon remains anterior, even when the arm is in 90 degrees of abduction. The tendon cannot displace upward under the coracoid and allow the head of the humerus to dislocate under the tendon. The tendon may be attached to the shaft into a bone trough with sutures, a staple, or a boat nail.

Badgley and O'Connor[182] and Bailey[184] have reported on a combination of the Putti-Platt and the Magnuson-Stack operations; they use the upper half of the subscapularis muscle to perform the Putti-Platt procedure and the lower half of the muscle to perform the Magnuson-Stack procedure. In their earlier series, Badgley and O'Connor also used the principles recommended by Nicola.[360-364]

Anterior Glenoid Bone Block

The Eden-Hybbinette procedure was performed independently by R. Eden,[251] in 1918, and S. Hybbinette,[293] in 1932. Eden first used tibial grafts, but both finally recommended the use of iliac grafts (Fig. 11-72). This procedure has the effect of extending the anterior buttress of the anterior glenoid and has been shown by Palmer and Widen[375] to be particularly valuable when there is a large posterolateral defect in the humeral head. Alvik[412] has modified the Eden-Hybbinette by inserting the graft into the substance of the anterior glenoid rim.

In 1924, Oudard[373] reported the use of the coracoid process as an anterior buttress which acted as a bone block to prevent recurrent dislocations. He also shortened the subscapularis tendon.

Authors Comment on the Eden-Hybbinette Operation. I have used this procedure when there has been destruction or erosion of the anterior glenoid rim. The autogenous bone graft is taken from the ilium and is trimmed to fit anteriorly between the bone and the capsule. I prefer to fix the graft with small screws.

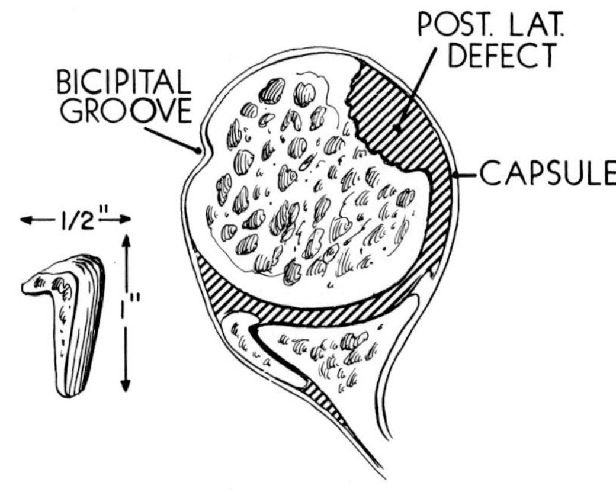

Fig. 11-72. Technique of the Eden-Hybbinette reconstruction utilizing anterior bone block from the iliac crest.[251,293]

Transfer of the Coracoid Process to the Glenoid

This procedure, first reported by Arthur Helfet[282] in 1958, was named the Bristow operation, after W. Rowley Bristow of South Africa. There is some question as to whether or not Bristow ever performed the procedure. In any event, Helfet originally described detaching the coracoid process from the scapula just distal to the insertion of the pectoralis minor muscle, leaving the conjoined tendons (i.e., the short head of the biceps, and the coracobrachialis) attached. Through a vertical slit in the subscapularis tendon, the joint is exposed, and the anterior surface of the neck of the scapula is "rawed up." The coracoid process with its attached tendons is then passed through the slit in the subscapularis and kept in contact with the raw area on the scapula by suturing the conjoined tendon to the cut edges of the subscapularis tendon.

In 1958, Mr. T. B. McMurray (son of the T. P. McMurray of hip osteotomy fame) visited Dr. Newton Mead[340] of Chicago and described modifications of the Bristow operation that were being used in Capetown, Johannesburg, and Pretoria. Since that time, Mead and Sweeney[340] have employed the modifications in over 100 cases. They consist of splitting the subscapularis muscle and tendon unit in line with its fibers to open the joint and firmly securing the coracoid process to the anterior glenoid rim with a screw. Virgil May[339] has modified the Bristow procedure further by taking down the subscapularis tendon, attaching the coracoid to the anterior glenoid with a screw, and reattaching the split subscapularis tendon, half above and half below, around the transferred conjoined tendon.

Helfet[282] claimed that the procedure not only "reinforced the defective part of the joint" but has a "bone block" effect. Mead,[340] however, does not regard the bone block as being a very important part of the procedure. He believes that the transfer adds a muscle reinforcement at the lower anterior aspect of the shoulder joint that prevents the lower portion of the subscapularis muscle from displacing upward as the humerus is abducted. Bonnin[196,197] has modified the procedure; he does not shorten or split the subscapularis muscle tendon unit. For exposure, he divides the subscapularis muscle at its muscle-tendon junction, and following the attachment of the coracoid process to the glenoid with a screw, he reattaches the subscapularis on top of the conjoined tendon.

Artz and Huffer[176] have reported a complication of using a screw to secure the coracoid process. The screw became loose and caused a false aneurysm of the axillary artery with a subsequent compression of the brachial plexus and paralysis of the upper extremity.

Author's Comment on Bristow Operation. Ordinarily the musculocutaneous nerve, which supplies the coracobrachialis and the short head of the biceps brachii, enters the posterior medial aspect of the coracobrachialis muscles 6.25 cm. distal to the tip of the coracoid process. However, when performing this procedure, the surgeon should always be mindful of the fact that musculocutaneous nerve may have an abnormally high penetration into the conjoined muscles (Fig. 11-73). Therefore, in freeing up the medial and posterior aspect of the conjoined muscles, care should be taken. In addition, you should be careful not to put unlimited distal traction on the detached coracoid process, for it may put tension on the nerve. Helfet[282] described one case in which the nerve had a high penetration into the coracobrachialis and became impinged where the conjoined tendon entered the slit in the subscapularis tendon. In order to prevent the screw from working loose and migrating, it is suggested that the screw be long enough to gain cortical fixation on the posterior glenoid rim.

Fascial Repairs

Gallie and Le Mesurier[262,263] originally described the use of autogenous fascia lata to create new ligaments between the anterior inferior aspect of the capsule and the anterior neck of the humerus in 1927 (see Fig. 11-46). James E. Bateman[190] of Toronto has continued to do this procedure and has made modifications in it. Bateman states, "It is an operation for the skilled surgeon requiring good assistance and all the proper equipment." The published end results of this procedure are quite successful (i.e., comparable to those with the Bankart, Putti-Platt, and Magnuson procedures).

Use of the Biceps Tendon

Toufick Nicola's name is usually associated with this operation, but the procedure was first described by Rupp[404] in 1926 and Heymanowitsch[286] in 1927. In 1929, Nicola[360] published his first article and described the use of the long head of the biceps tendon as a checkrein ligament (see Fig. 11-44). While the procedure was modified several

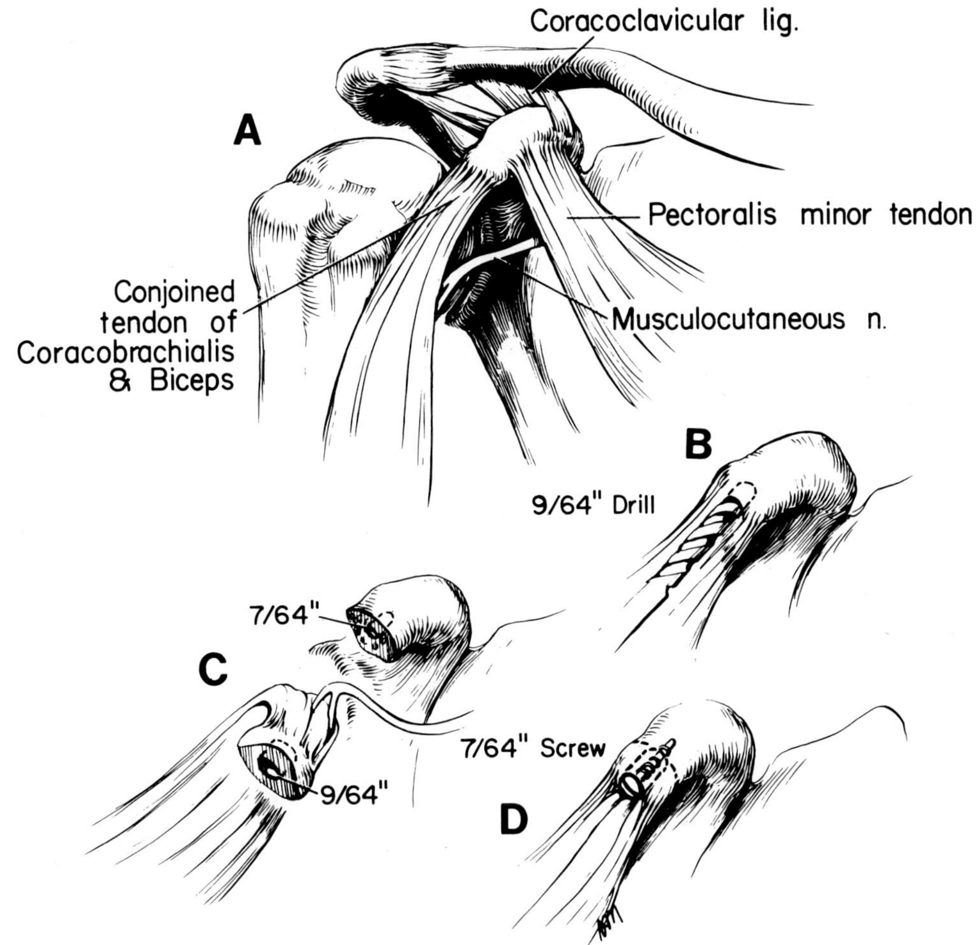

Fig. 11-73. Caution should be taken in detaching the conjoined tendon with the tip of the coracoid process. (*A*) Normal anatomy showing the musculocutaneous nerve entering the posterior aspect of the coracobrachialis and the short head of the biceps muscles. (*B*) The tip of the coracoid is located and a hole is drilled about 13 mm. into the center of the coracoid process with a 9/64-inch bit. (*C, D*) Before, during, and after the coracoid process is divided, care should be taken to avoid injury to the musculocutaneous nerve, which *may* have a high penetration into the posterior aspect of the coracobrachialis muscle. If the distal tip of the coracoid process is to be reattached to the coracoid, the base of the coracoid should be drilled with a 7/64-inch bit, which will create a lag effect of the screw through the distal fragment. Obviously this step is unnecessary if the coracoid is to be transplanted to the neck of the glenoid, as in the Bristow operation.

times by Nicola,[361-364] the recurrence rates have been so high that it has essentially been abandoned as an independent procedure. However, some authors continue to use it in conjunction with other reconstructions about the shoulder. The most significant complication of the Nicola procedure is its very high recurrence rate, reported to be between 30 and 50 per cent.[170,388,394]

Other Muscle Tendon Transfers

Latissimus Dorsi. A. K. Saha[406-411] has reported on the transfer of the latissimus dorsi posteriorly into the site of the infraspinatus insertion on the greater tuberosity. He reports that, during abduction, the transferred latissimus reinforces the subscapularis muscle and the short posterior steering and depressor muscles by pulling the humeral head backward. He has used the procedure for traumatic and atraumatic dislocations, and in 1969, he reported 45 cases with no recurrence.

Infraspinatus Muscle Tendon Transfer. When the recurrent anterior dislocation is associated with a large posterolateral humeral head defect, John Connolly of Nebraska has transferred the tendon insertion of the infraspinatus into the defect. This serves to keep the defect from sliding anteriorly over and onto the glenoid, which would result in anterior dislocation, and converts the defect into an extraarticular structure. In addition, he reports that this diminishes the postoperative symptoms of instability due to impingement of the defect on the articular surface of the glenoid. This operation is essentially a mirror image of the McLaughlin procedure used in posterior dislocations of the shoulder when there is a large anterior bone defect in the humeral head.

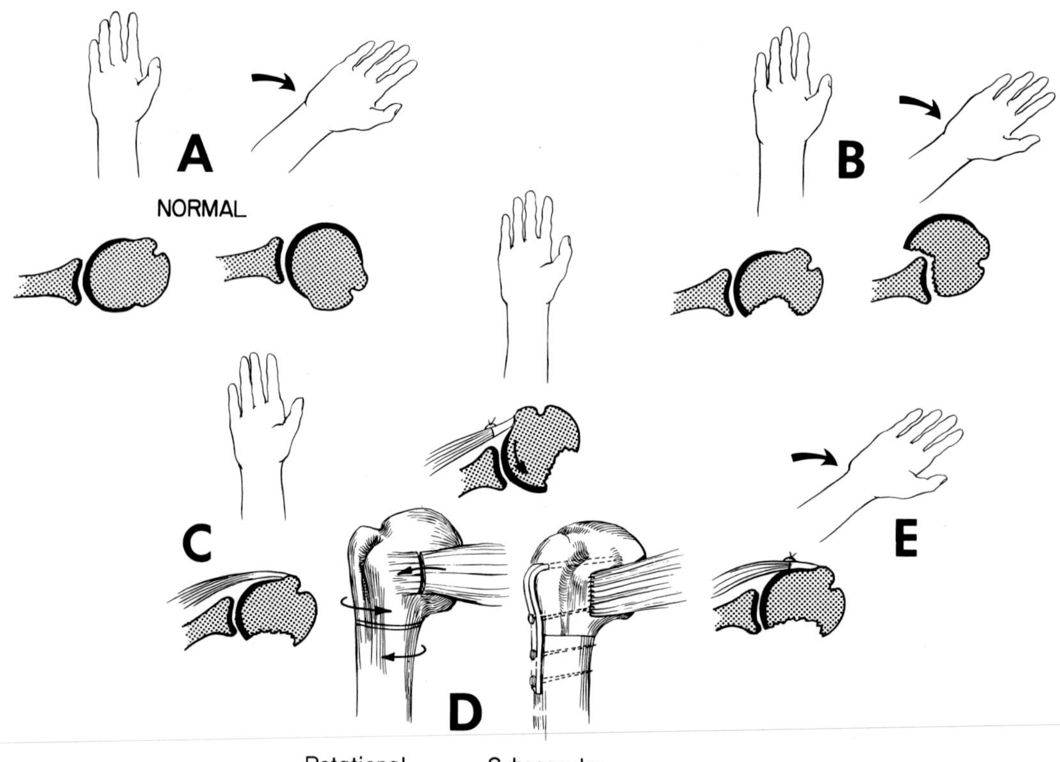

Fig. 11-74. Weber osteotomy of the proximal humerus to prevent recurrent anterior dislocation. (*A*) Normally when the arm is externally rotated, the posterior articular surface of the humerus stays in contact with the glenoid fossa. (*B*) However, during external rotation, when there is a large posterolateral humeral head defect, the articular surface of the head is decreased, which causes the recurrent anterior dislocation. The humerus is then held impinged by the anterior glenoid rim. (*C, D, E*) With external rotation, according to Weber, if the normal retroversion of the humeral head is increased by proximal humeral osteotomy and subscapularis shortening, the defect does not come in contact with the anterior glenoid rim, and recurrences are prevented. (Redrawn from Weber, B. G.: Injury, *1*:107-109, 1969)

Osteotomy of the Proximal Humerus

B. G. Weber,[449] of Switzerland, uses a rotational osteotomy, and he increases the retroversion of the head–neck shaft angle and shortens the subscapularis muscle (Fig. 11-74). This procedure was designed for cases when there is a large posterolateral defect in the humeral head, which, with external rotation, allows the defect to slip over and onto the anterior glenoid lip. By increasing the retroversion, the posterolateral defect is delivered more posteriorly, and the anterior and undisturbed portion of the articular surface of the humeral head then articulates against the glenoid. Following the procedure, even with external rotation of the arm, the posterolateral defect no longer engages the glenoid cavity.

Osteotomy of the Neck of the Glenoid

In 1933, Meyer-Burgdorff reported on decreasing the anterior tilt of the glenoid by a posterior wedge resection osteotomy (Fig. 11-75).[406] Sen is reported by Saha[406] to perform an anterior opening wedge osteotomy with bone graft, into the neck of the glenoid to decrease the tilt. Saha has described a modified Meyer-Burgdorff procedure that achieved excellent results in six cases. This is an appealing procedure when it is determined that there is a deficiency of the anterior glenoid or when there is excessive anterior tilt of the glenoid fossa.

Author's Preferred Method of Treatment

Practically all of the more commonly used standard operative procedures yield

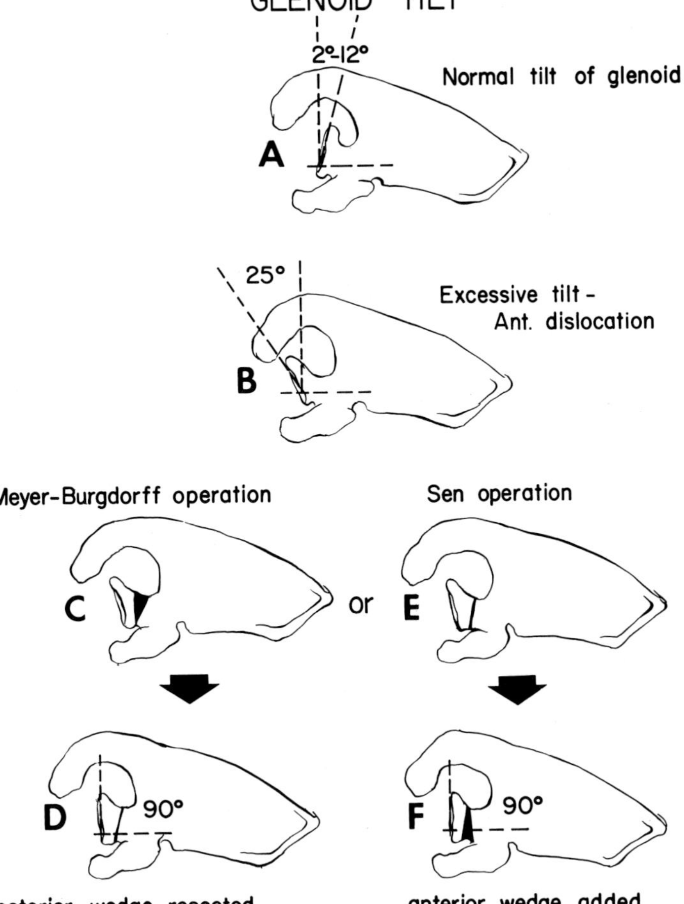

Fig. 11-75. Osteotomy of the neck of the glenoid. (*A*) Normal tilt of the glenoid fossa is 2 to 12 degrees and is directed posteriorly. (*B*) One of the etiologies of recurrent anterior dislocation of the shoulder may be excessive anterior tilt to the glenoid fossa. (*C*, *D*) When there is excessive anterior tilt of the glenoid fossa; Meyer-Burgdorff has described a posterior wedge resection of the glenoid neck. (*E*, *F*) Sen has also described correcting an excessive anterior tilt of the glenoid fossa by creating an anterior opening wedge osteotomy in the glenoid neck and inserting a bone graft. (Redrawn from Saha, A. K.: Theory of Shoulder Mechanism. Springfield, Ill., Charles C Thomas, 1961)

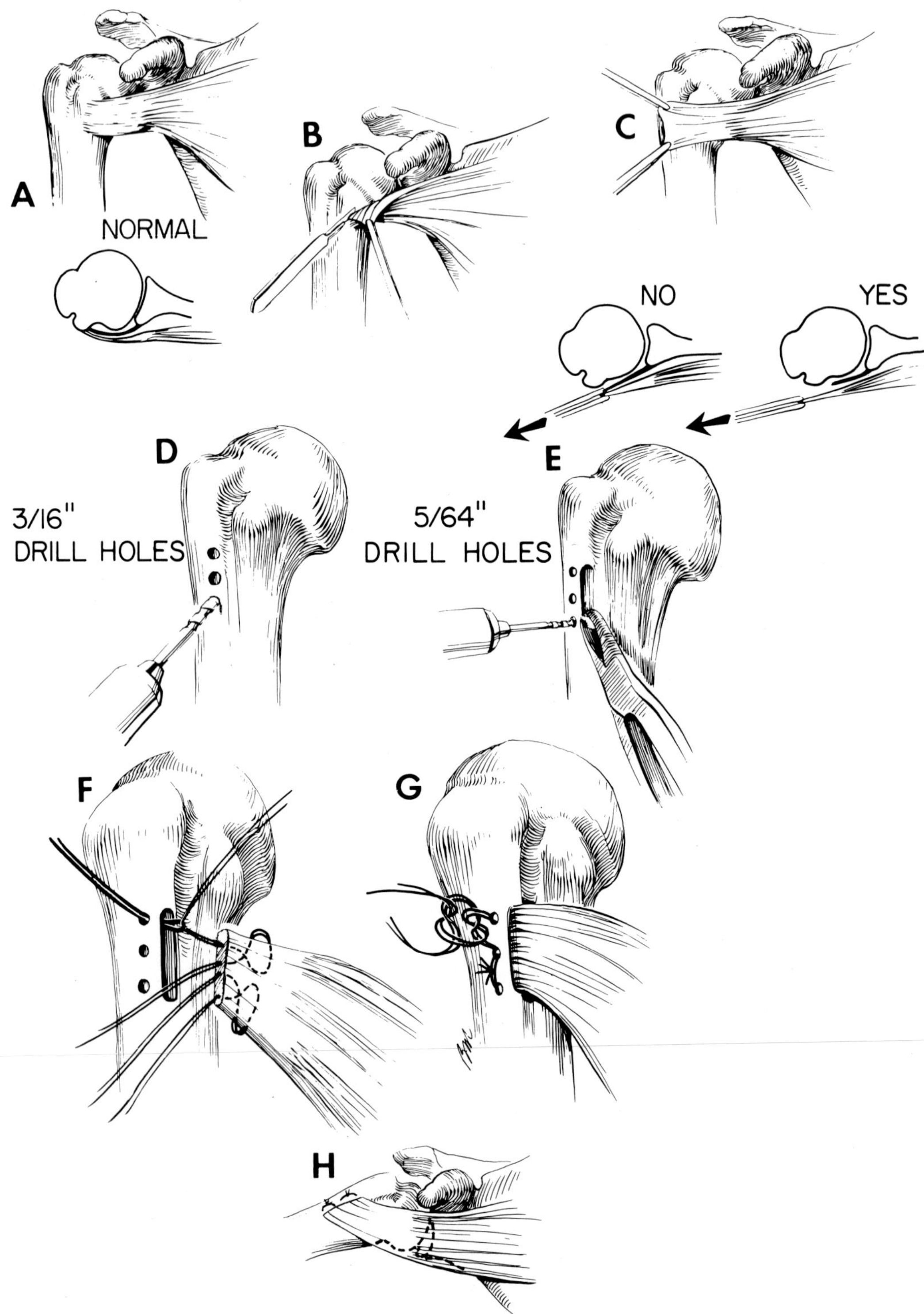

Fig. 11-76. Caption opposite page.

results in the 90-per-cent range (Table 11-2). I have used the modified Magnuson-Stack primarily (i.e., transfer of the subscapularis tendon across the bicipital groove and down into the upper shaft of the humerus). This procedure provides excellent visualization of the joint, allows for capsule repairs, removes laxity of the subscapularis muscle tendon unit, and prevents further recurrence in abduction by protecting the inferior aspect of the joint. A standard anterior incision is used, which begins above the coracoid process and extends down toward the axillary crease as reported by Levy.[318] Only in large, muscular men does the incision curve proximally, so that some of the origin of the deltoid can be detached. I prefer to not detach the deltoid from the clavicle and usually do not take down the coracoid process. In women, I use the axillary incision described by Leslie and Ryan.[317]

The deltoid is entered just lateral to the deltopectoral groove, and about 8 mm. of the medial deltoid is left to protect the cephalic vein. The tendon of the subscapularis muscle is sharply detached from the lesser tuberosity. Care should be taken to avoid damaging the transverse ligament or the long head of the biceps tendon. Special care should be taken to dissect the subscapularis tendon and muscle free from the capsule, so that when you pull on the clamps holding the tendon, you get a rubbery bounce from the stretching of the muscle. If a resistance or checkrein effect is noted, the posterior surface of the tendon and muscle is adhering to the anterior capsule, which is still attached to the anterior glenoid (Fig. 11-76). This must be separated. After the capsule is free, the joint is thoroughly explored and debrided. If the capsule is a sound structure, it is reattached. The subscapularis tendon is transferred across the bicipital groove to a trough created by using 3/16-inch drill holes connected by small rongeurs and currettes (Fig. 11-76D, E). The exact position of the trough is below the greater tuberosity and lateral to the bicipital groove in a location that allows the arm, when the tendon is secured, to reach a neutral position of rotation. Heavy nonabsorbable sutures are used to secure the tendon into the trough (Fig. 11-76F, G).

Fig. 11-76. Author's technique for modified Magnuson Stack operation. (*A*) The normal relationships of the subscapularis to the bony architecture. (*B*) The tendon of the subscapularis muscle is sharply detached from the lesser tuberosity. Care is taken not to damage the transverse ligament or the long head of the biceps tendon. (*C*) The capsule must be separated from the posterior edge of the subscapularis tendon until traction on the tendon produces a rubbery bounce. Failure to remove the capsule from the tendon does not allow for a dynamic functioning subscapularis transfer. (*D*) Drill holes are created lateral to the bicipital groove and distal from the original insertion of the subscapularis on the lesser tuberosity. The exact location of the trough is predetermined by being sure, with the insertion of the tendon into the trough, that the arm rotates externally to a neutral position. When it is noted that the subscapularis muscle tendon unit is not long enough to be transferred across the bicipital groove, it is usually because the posterior capsule still adheres to the posterior edge of the subscapularis, which produces a "checkrein" effect. (*E*) A small rongeur is used to enlarge the trough to receive the transferred tendon. Three 5/64-inch drill holes are placed lateral to the trough to be used to anchor the tendon in the bone trough. (*F*) A loop of 24- or 25-gauge stainless steel wire is passed through the 5/64-inch drill holes into the trough. The heavy No. 1 nylon suture is then passed through the loop in the wire suture, which then is passed out through the 5/64-inch drill holes when the wire loop is withdrawn. (*G*) With the arm in internal rotation, the transferred subscapularis tendon is held down in the trough with a bone awl while the sutures are tied as shown. (*H*) By transferring the insertion of the subscapularis muscle across the bicipital groove and distally, the lower edge of the glenohumeral joint is protected when the arm is abducted.

Table 11-2. Incidence of Recurrence Following Various Reconstructions for Anterior Dislocations of the Shoulder

Procedure	Authors	Year	Number of Cases	Recurrence Per Cent
Putti-Platt	Adams[170]	1948	37	5.4%
	Brav[201]	1955	41	7.3%
	Jeffery[296]	1959	34	3%
	H. Osmond-Clarke[371]	1965	140	1.4%
	Truckly[437]	1968	102	0%
			354 Total	3.4 Average
Nicola	Raney and Miller[388]	1942	26	34.6%
	Adams[170]	1948	59	35.6%
	Rowe[394]	1956	32	53.1%
			117 Total	41.7 Average
Magnuson-Stack and Modified Magnuson-Stack	Giannestras[269]	1948	31	6.4%
	Polumbo and Quiring[376]	1950	13	0%
	Vare[441]	1953	30	0%
	Alldred[173]	1958	10	0%
	DePalma and Silberstein[240]	1963	75	2.7%
	Jen[298]	1964	42	9%
	Bryan, DeMichele, Ford, and Cary[207]	1969	53	7.5%
			254 Total	3.8 Average
Bankart and Modified Bankart	Adams[170]	1948	18	5.5%
	Townley[432]	1950	26	0%
	Rowe[394]	1956	75	1.3%
	DuToit and Roux[247]	1956	150	5%
	Dickson and Devas[244]	1957	50	4%
	Boyd and Hunt[199]	1965	49	4.1%
			368 Total	3.3 Average
Saha	Saha[408]	1967	45	0%
			45 Total	0 Average
Bankart, Putti-Platt Combination	Watson-Jones[446]	1948	52	2%
	Viek and Bell[442]	1959	39	2.5%
	Weber[449]	1969	62	1.6%
	Lambdin, Young, Unsicker[313]	1971	50	5%
			203 Total	2.8 Average
Bristow	Helfet[282]	1958	30	3%
	McMurray[332]	1961	73	2.7%
	May[339]	1970	16	0%
			119 Total	1.9 Average

Table 11-2. Continued.

Badgley Combination (i.e., Putti-Platt, Nicola, and Magnuson-Stack)	Bailey[184]	1967	115	1.7%
			115 Total	1.7 Average
Eden-Hybbinette and Modifications	Palmer and Widen[375]	1948	128	6.3%
	Oster[372]	1969	78	18%
	Said and Medro[412]	1970	21	0%
	Bonnin[196]	1973	27	0%
			254 Total	6.0 Average
Gallie	Gallie and LeMesurier[262]	1948	175	4%
	Bateman[190]	1963	102	1.9%
			277 Total	2.9 Average
Weber	Weber[449]	1969	27	0%
			27 Total	0 Average

Total number of studies: 37
Total number of cases: 1751

Total number of cases without Nicola procedure: 1634
Average % of recurrence without Nicola procedure: ±3%

I also like the modified Bristow as described by Virgil May[339] and Newton Mead.[340] I prefer to detach the subscapularis tendon by leaving a 6-mm. stump at its insertion. After the coracoid has been transferred to the neck of the scapula, the subscapularis tendon is divided horizontally in line with the fibers. The bottom half passes under the conjoined tendon, and the top half passes over it. The arm is then held in the neutral rotation position, and the tendon is reattached at its insertion to the stump under tension. Occasionally, there may be so much slack in the subscapularis muscle that a segment of the tendon is resected before it is reattached. I prefer the modified Bristow procedure in the athlete who needs to use his arms for overhead movements, because it is not only a strong repair, but it offers an earlier return of motion and function than does the Magnuson-Stack operation.

I suggest that in the first modified Bristow operation that any surgeon performs he take down the subscapularis muscle, attach the coracoid process to the scapula, then split the subscapularis tendon and muscle horizontally into upper and lower halves and pass the upper half superior and anterior and the lower half inferior and posterior to the conjoined tendons as described by May.[339] The two halves are then reattached to the stump of the subscapularis. This allows better visualization of the glenoid and the joint space and better appreciation of the operative procedure.

Certainly, not all patients with recurrent anterior dislocations of the shoulder can be managed with one or two operative procedures. Selected problems, such as a deficient anterior glenoid, an extremely large posterolateral defect, or muscle imbalance, require the specific reconstructions that have been described. In other words, as with any other reconstruction, you plan the individual operative procedure on the individual problem.

Postoperative Management

Obviously, the length of time of postoperative immobilization varies, not only with the type of reconstruction but with modifications of one basic operation. Some authors recommend 6 weeks in a sling and swathe to allow for soft-tissue healing (i.e., transplanted subscapularis tendon to bone or the shortened subscapularis muscle and tendon). Some authors wait for the skin to heal and then begin motion, and some begin range of motion exercises before the skin has healed.

Author's Preferred Postoperative Management. As a general rule: the older the patient, the shorter the postoperative immobilization, and the younger and more active, the longer the postoperative immobilization. I prefer the use of a sling and swathe, because it is quite comfortable and readily available. Some of the newer commercially available shoulder immobilizers are quite effective to prevent abduction and external rotation. Competitive athletes are held 4 to 6 weeks; people with athletic inclinations are held 3 to 6 weeks, and nonathletes are held 3 to 4 weeks. Older patients —from 55 to 70—are held 2 to 4 weeks.

Following the discontinuation of the sling and swathe, a gentle rehabilitation program is instituted, as was described under the rehabilitation following the acute anterior dislocation (Fig. 11-69). In general, however, patients can return to light types of work after 7 to 14 days from surgery. The subcuticular suture is removed at 14 days, and then the patient can shower or bathe. However, the patient should be taught how to clean and care for the axilla before the sutures are removed. During axilla care the patient should avoid external rotation, and abduct the arm no more than 15 to 20 degrees. During the entire immobilization period, they should perform gentle isometric exercises of the upper extremity and shoulder and actively move the hand, wrist, and elbow. Athletes are not permitted to return to competition until they have a completely functional range of motion and have regained muscle strength and muscle mass in the involved extremity.

Incidence of Recurrence Following Reconstruction

The surprising fact is that all of the reconstructions currently in vogue give approximately 97 per cent excellent results. The results may even be better as some of the recurrences following reconstruction are produced by a force equal to the force that produced the acute dislocation.

A review of 1634 reconstructions compiled from the literature reveals that the incidence of recurrence is approximately 3 per cent (Table 11-2). This includes 354 Putti-Platt operations; 254 Magnuson-Stack or modifications; 368 Bankart or modifications; 45 Saha operations; 203 Bankart–Putti-Platt combinations; 119 Bristow operations; 115 Badgley combination operations; 254 Eden-Hybbinette operations; 277 Gallie or modifications; and 27 Weber operations. If only the more commonly performed procedures were analyzed (i.e., Putti-Platt, Magnuson-Stack, Bankart, Bristow, and modifications of these), the incidence is still approximately 3 per cent. A series of 117 Nicola operations were not included, as the average incidence of recurrence was 41 per cent.

UNREDUCED ANTERIOR DISLOCATIONS

Old, persistent dislocation is usually a very difficult problem to handle, particularly in the elderly, and it points out the need for a very careful history and physical examination. It is not uncommon to be called to the emergency department to see an elderly patient with pain in the shoulder whose roentgenograms reveal an anterior dislocation. It is only after very careful questioning that you may determine the injury occurred anywhere from a week to several months earlier.

The condition is noted most commonly in elderly persons whose general mental status prevents them from seeking help at the time of the injury. Ten of the 14 patients presented by Bennett[192] were over the age of 50. In addition, the dislocation may be produced by a trivial injury, because with increasing age there is weakness and degeneration of the soft-tissue structure about the joint (i.e., rotator cuff and subscapularis

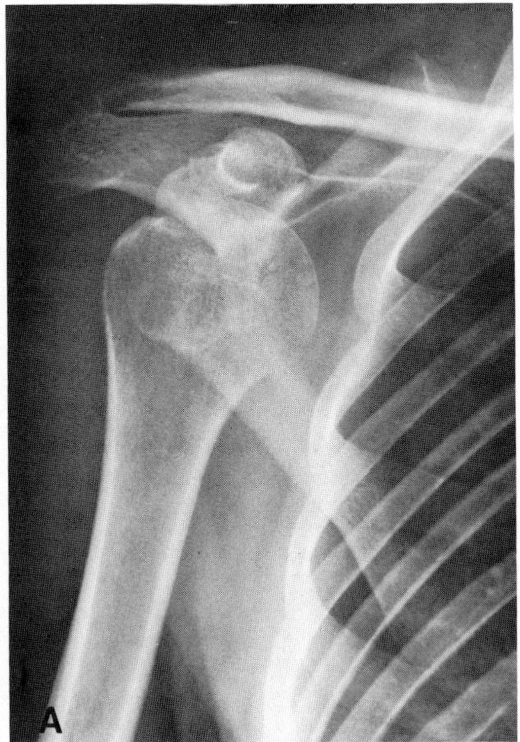

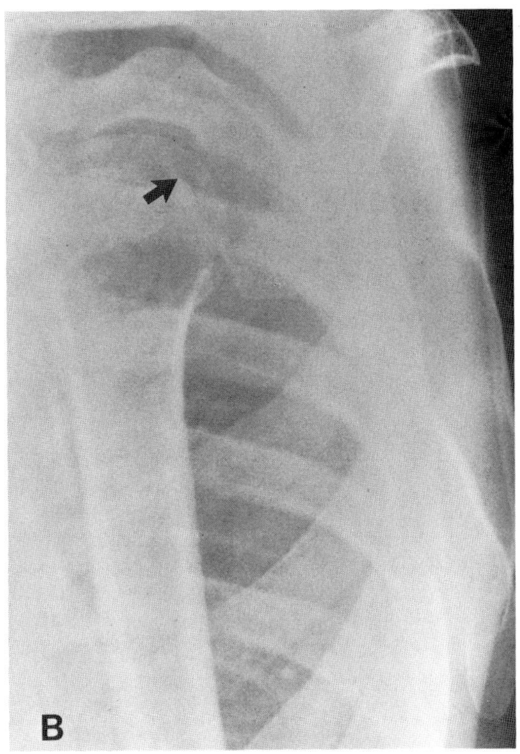

Fig. 11-77. Unreduced anterior dislocation of the shoulder of four months duration. (*A*) The head is in the subcoracoid position, and there appears to be erosion of the superior aspect of the head by the glenoid rim. (*B*) A true lateral view of the humeral joint reveals that there is a compression fracture (*arrow*) of the posterolateral head by the anterior rim of the glenoid.

tendon;[239] Fig. 11-77). In younger patients, the late diagnosis of an old unreduced anterior dislocation of the shoulder may occur when the patient is unconscious for a while with severe multiple injuries.

A very comprehensive article on unrecognized dislocations has been written by Schulz, Jacobs, and Patterson.[414] In their series of 61 shoulders in 58 patients, 17 (24%) were posterior dislocations and 44 (76%) were old anterior dislocations. This excellent article makes other important points: The condition occurs primarily among elderly persons. More than half of the dislocations were associated with fracture of the tuberosities, head or neck of the humerus, or the glenoid or coracoid process. More than one-third had neurological deficits. Treatment consisted of closed reduction in 20, open reduction in 20, and humeral head excision in six. Eight patients were not treated, and five were irreducible. Closed reduction was attempted in 40 shoulders and was successful in 20. Of the 20 shoulders successfully reduced (three posterior and 17 anterior), the duration of dislocation exceeded 4 weeks in only one instance. Good results can be achieved with either closed reduction or open reduction, or by leaving the shoulder unreduced.

Signs and Symptoms

Surprisingly, the elderly patient may have a completely functional and comfortable upper extremity. The limited glenohumeral motion combined with the scapulothoracic motion may allow 70 to 90 degrees of ab-

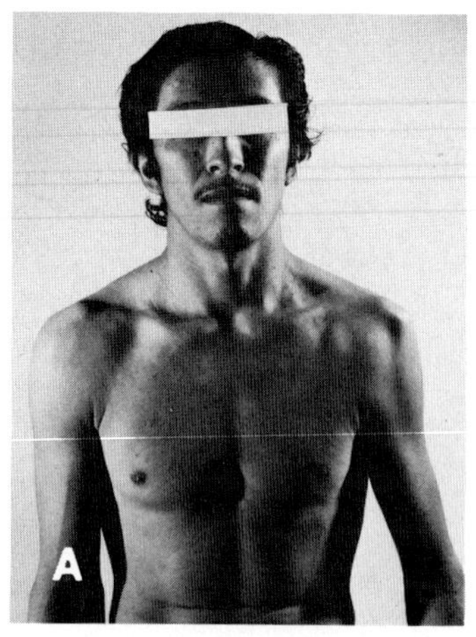

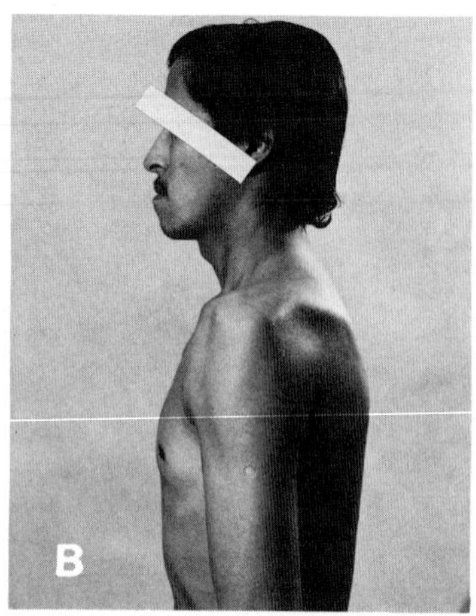

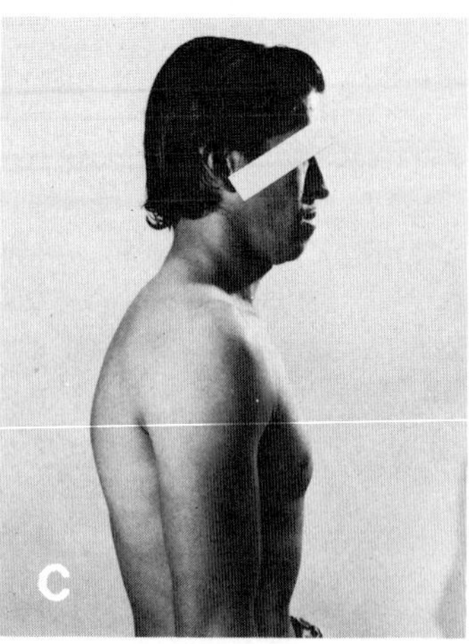

Fig. 11-78. Permanent anterior dislocation in a young patient. (*A*) Frontal view of a 23-year-old man with a 4-month history of permanent subcoracoid anterior dislocation of the left shoulder. The acromion process is quite prominent, and there is an extra bulge anteriorly produced by the humeral head. The glenohumeral joint was fixed, and the arm was constantly maintained in an abducted position. (*B*) A lateral view of the left shoulder reveals not so much an anterior fullness but a void in the posterior aspect of the shoulder. (*C*) A side view of the normal shoulder with normal contours for a comparison.

duction and/or forward flexion. In general, the longer the interval since dislocation, the less pain there is and the better the range of motion.

Younger patients, because their muscles, ligaments, and capsule tissues are in better condition, have a fixed position of the glenohumeral joint. Any type of motion to the shoulder produces severe pain (Fig. 11-78).

Treatment

McLaughlin[325] describes this type of dislocation of the shoulder as the most difficult of all. It is difficult to establish criteria for when you should try to perform a closed reduction, when you should operate and reduce the shoulder, and when you should simply rehabilitate it. As a general rule, the young and active patient should have the shoulder relocated, and the older patient should be rehabilitated. There are no hard and set rules, because conditions—the age of patient, the length of time from dislocation, the degree of symptoms, the range of motion, roentgenographic findings, and general stability of the patient—can vary so much. If a closed reduction is being considered, it should be done with minimal traction, without leverage, and always with total muscle relaxation under general anesthesia. If the closed reduction fails, then an open procedure should follow. Usually by 2 to 3 weeks after the dislocation, the humeral head is firmly impinged on the anterior glenoid, and there is so much soft-tissue contraction that it is impossible to perform a gentle closed reduction. Only after an anterior approach and release of the subscapularis is it possible to perform an open reduction. As mentioned, some of the older patients with 6- to 9-month-old dislocations do quite well with conservative measures directed to rehabilitation and increasing the patient's range of motion.

Operative reductions are based on cleaning out the glenoid fossa, returning the head into the fossa, and possibly stabilizing the reduction with temporary internal fixation. The subscapularis is the door of entry to the joint, and it should be snug at the completion of the procedure. Neviaser[356,357] has recommended a stripping operation performed through a superior approach. Occasionally, because of the extensive destruction of the humeral head, a prosthesis will have to be inserted.

Complications

The complications are related to scarring and the contracture of the soft tissues about the shoulder; that is, the brachial plexus, the capsule, and the arteriosclerotic condition of the axillary artery. The worst complication of attempting a forceful closed reduction of a permanent anterior dislocation is rupture of the axillary artery. Anatomically the artery is divided into three parts. The first part is medial to the pectoralis minor muscle, the second part is behind the pectoralis minor, and the third part is lateral to the muscle-tendon unit. The traction that is required on the arm in an old anterior dislocation must be greater than usual, and this force on an old arteriosclerotic artery securely held down by the pectoralis minor muscle may rupture the artery or avulse one of its branches (see pp. 680-686).

TRAUMATIC ANTERIOR SUBLUXATION OF THE SHOULDER

If the abduction-external rotation force is great enough to produce more than a mild strain to the joint but not great enough to frankly disrupt the joint, the capsule is stretched or partially detached, and the result is partial dislocation or subluxation. This should not be confused with habitual dislocation of the shoulder.

Signs and Symptoms

The signs and symptoms of the entity have been presented in detail only in recent years. We are indebted to the orthopaedists who devote a great deal of time to sports medicine for emphasizing the recognition, incidence, signs and symptoms, and management of this problem. In many ways, it is more of a problem than recurrent dislocation of the shoulder, because the dislocation presents with a clear-cut diagnosis, which can be managed by a clear-cut operative procedure. The disability from subluxation of the shoulder can be as incapacitating as that from dislocation.

Blazina and Satzman[193] reported their findings in 34 patients to the American Academy of Orthopaedic Surgeons in 1969. In their series, football was the major initiating activity responsible for the symptoms. In most instances, patients can describe the initial injury, and most commonly this was reported as a forced external rotation of the shoulder. Every patient in their series described a predominant complaint: recurrent sensations of the shoulder "slipping out." Among the other symptoms were the following: They could feel the shoulder voluntarily slip back in, after which there was a residual anterior aching shoulder pain. They could feel a click, or snapping, or "clunking" in the shoulder. After the injury the entire upper extremity felt numb, or tingled, or felt limp (which indicates that the axillary nerve has been stretched).

Physical examination reveals a distinct tendency either to actively resist external rotation of a shoulder or to exhibit a marked apprehension when external rotation of the shoulder is attempted. In some cases, the shoulder can be moved into anterior subluxation. Pain can be elicited with palpation over the anterior aspect of the shoulder, sometimes in the proximity of the long head of the biceps tendon in the intertubercular groove and sometimes over the anterior inferior glenoid area.

I have been impressed, when standing behind the seated patient with both of his arms abducted 90 degrees to the sides, that the patient with the recurrent subluxation of the shoulder will not allow you to extend or externally rotate the involved arm as far as the normal one. The normal shoulder will, at least, extend to the mid-line and beyond and the patient will allow external rotation of the arm until the forearm is directed straight up. The injured shoulder frequently will not allow full extension or external rotation. Another point worth mentioning is that many patients complain of pain in the posterior shoulder joint region—both on palpation and during examination for limitation of abduction and external rotation. With the shoulder held in abduction and external rotation, palpation of the anterior aspect of the shoulder joint may be quite painful.

Roentgenographic Findings

The routine roentgenograms of the shoulder (i.e., anteroposterior in internal and external rotation, and axillary lateral) may reveal anterior glenoid fractures or calcification. However, a modified axillary view (West Point) has been described by Rokus, Feagin, and Abbott[393] that demonstrates bony abnormality, if it is present, on the anteroinferior glenoid rim.

Technique of the West Point View

The patient is prone on the x-ray table with the involved shoulder on a pad raised 7.5 cm. from the table top (Fig. 11-79). The head and neck are turned away from the involved side. With the cassette held against the superior aspect of the shoulder, the x-ray beam is centered at the axilla with 25 degrees downward beam from the horizontal and 25 degrees medial beam from the midline. The resulting roentgenogram is a tangential view of the anteroinferior rim of the glenoid.

Rokus and his colleagues demonstrated bony abnormalities of the anterior glenoid rim in 53 of 63 patients whose histories indicated recurrent subluxation of the shoulder. In addition, at the time of surgery, they found bony abnormalities in the anterior glenoid rim in all but one of 51 patients. They point out that, while the bony changes may represent a small fracture, they most likely represent an abortive calcified repair process (Fig. 11-80).

Blazina and Satzman[193] reported avulsed anteroinferior glenoid rim fractures in nine of their cases. They also reported that in some cases radiopaque arthrography demonstrated redundant axillary folds and irregularity of the anterior glenoid rim.

Kummel[308] has reported on the use of arthrograms to diagnose anterior capsule derangements. In some cases, cineradiography may demonstrate a potential for anterior subluxation. Blazina and Satzman[193]

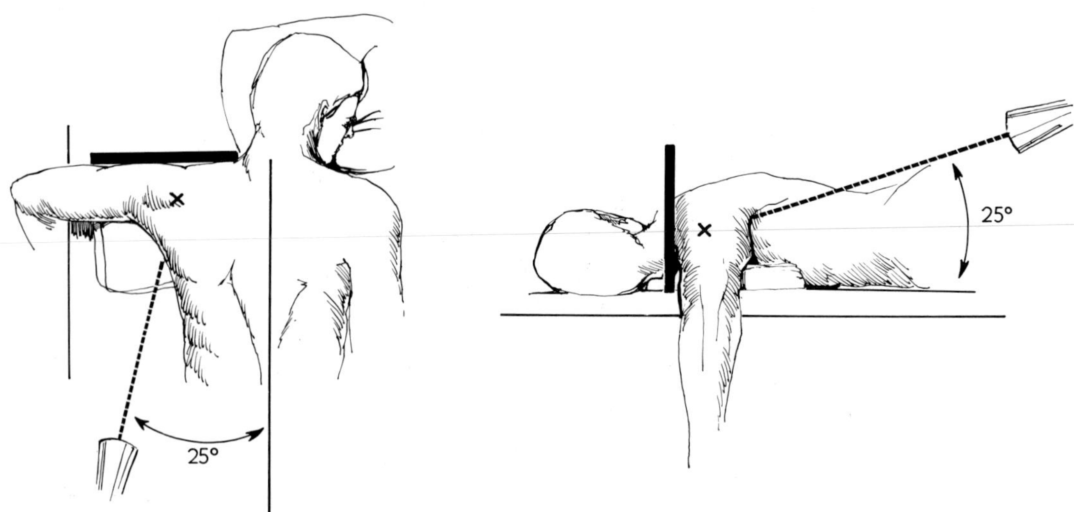

Fig. 11-79. Positioning of the patient for taking the West Point View (a modified axillary view) to visualize the anterior-inferior glenoid rim in subluxations of the shoulder.

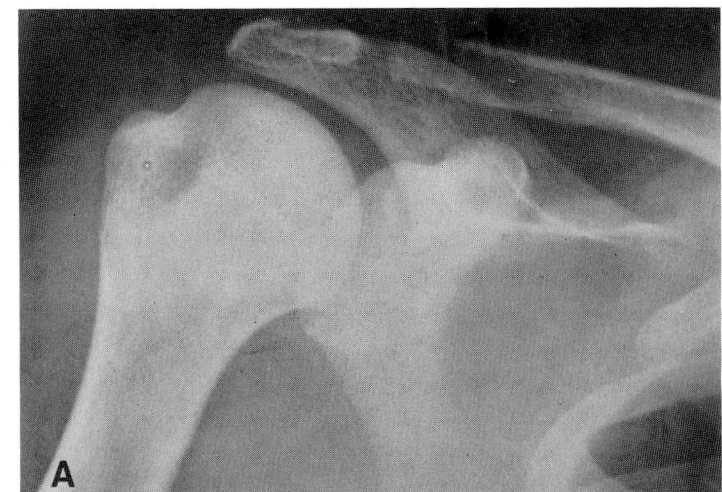

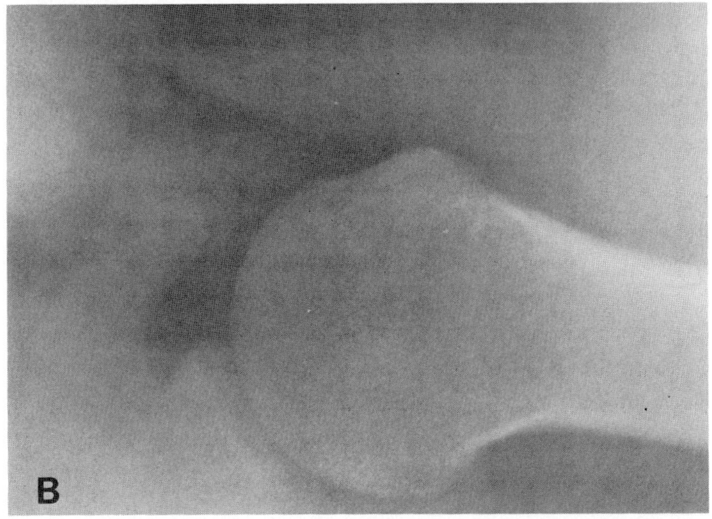

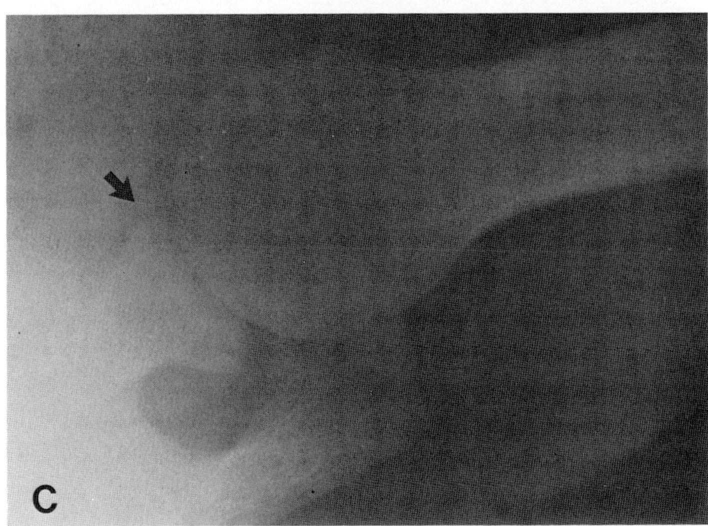

Fig. 11-80. Subluxation of the right glenohumeral joint. (*A*) Anteroposterior roentgenogram of the shoulder shows no bony abnormalities. (*B*) Axillary lateral shows no abnormalities of the anterior glenoid rim. (*C*) West Point View depicts a fragment or calcification (*arrow*) located in front of the anterior rim of the glenoid.

and Rokus, Feagin, and Abbott[393] mention seeing the posterolateral humeral head defect in some of their patients with subluxation of the shoulder. This implies that at one time the shoulder had been completely dislocated (the anterior glenoid rim created the compression fracture defect in the head). Certainly it is reasonable to assume that a recurrent shoulder subluxation could be the end result of an unrecognized and untreated acute anterior dislocation or of a recognized and treated but incompletely healed primary dislocation.

Treatment

One of the most significant conclusions to come from recent studies of this problem is that if the physician can document sufficient evidence for a diagnosis of chronic anterior subluxation of the shoulder, then the treatment is the same as that for a chronic dislocating shoulder—surgical reconstruction.

Rehabilitation to strengthen the anterior shoulder internal rotator muscles does not resolve the basic problem. I personally have found exercises useful while I am trying to document a difficult case. Blazina is of the opinion that it offers little lasting benefit.

In years past, it was in vogue to examine the questionable anterior dislocation, or the subluxing shoulder, under general anesthesia. Today, however, with our current knowledge of the art concerning shoulder subluxation, this should rarely be required. I personally feel, that if the physician is armed with a very precise and careful history and a careful physical examination with the indicated roentgenograms, examination under general anesthesia is seldom indicated.

The type of operative repair does not appear to be as important as making the decision to operate. Blazina and Satzman[193] have reported using the Putti-Platt, Bankart, Magnuson, and Bristow—all successfully. Rokus, Feagin, and Abbott[393] used primarily a modified Putti-Platt in their repairs, with good results.

Postoperative Care and Rehabilitation, Prognosis, and Complications

Since the operative repairs for recurrent subluxation of the shoulder are essentially the same as the ones done for recurrent anterior dislocations of the shoulders, the postoperative care, prognosis, and complications are discussed in detail in that section (see p. 673).

COMPLICATIONS OF ANTERIOR DISLOCATION OF THE SHOULDER

Bone Injuries

Bone injuries have been discussed briefly in this section and thoroughly in Part 1 of this chapter. Essentially they consist of compression fracture of the humeral head (the Hill-Sachs lesion), fracture of the anterior glenoid lip, fracture of the greater tuberosity, and fracture of the acromion or coracoid process associated with the superior dislocation of the shoulder.

Soft-Tissue Injuries

While it is not my intent to discuss the general subject of rupture of the rotator cuff, injuries of this type can occur with anterior dislocation of the shoulder. According to McLaughlin and MacLellan,[331] posterior cuff damage is common in nonrecurring anterior dislocation. Reeves[389] has reported an incidence of five in 27 cases of acute anterior dislocation, and Petterson[381] has reported an incidence of tendon cuff rupture in the nonrecurring dislocation of about 50 per cent. Reeves[390] has demonstrated that rupture of the capsule and subscapularis tendon occurs most commonly in elderly patients. With severe displacement of the humeral head—subclavicular, intrathoracic, or luxatio erecta—the cuff is always disrupted. Patients who have poor return of function following an anterior dislocation of the shoulder may have had an associated cuff tear, which can be diagnosed best by arthrogram. Other soft-tissue complications associated with anterior dislocation include rupture of the transverse ligament across the intertubercular groove of the humerus with lateral dislocation of the biceps tendon. Recurring anterior subluxations and dislocations should also be considered as complications of acute traumatic anterior dislocations.

Vascular Injuries

Vascular Damage at the Time of Dislocation

This almost always occurs in elderly patients or those who have marked arteriosclerosis of the vessels. The injury is to the axillary artery or vein or to the branches of the axillary artery, the thoracoacromial trunk, subscapular, circumflex, and rarely, the long thoracic branch. Approximately 200 cases have been reported in the literature.

Anatomy. The axillary artery is divided into three parts that lie medial to, behind, and lateral to the pectoralis minor muscle (Fig. 11-81). The damage to the axillary artery can be a complete transsection rupture, a linear tear of the artery caused by avulsion of one of its branches, or an intravascular thrombus. The sites most commonly injured are in the second part, where the thoracoacromial trunk is avulsed, and the third part, where subscapular and circumflex branches are avulsed and where the axillary artery is totally ruptured.

Signs and Symptoms. The findings of damage to the axillary artery are very typical: The dislocation usually occurs in elderly patients. There is a rapid expanding hematoma and marked pain in the axilla. The involved arm may be numb or paralyzed. There is no radial pulse. The ex-

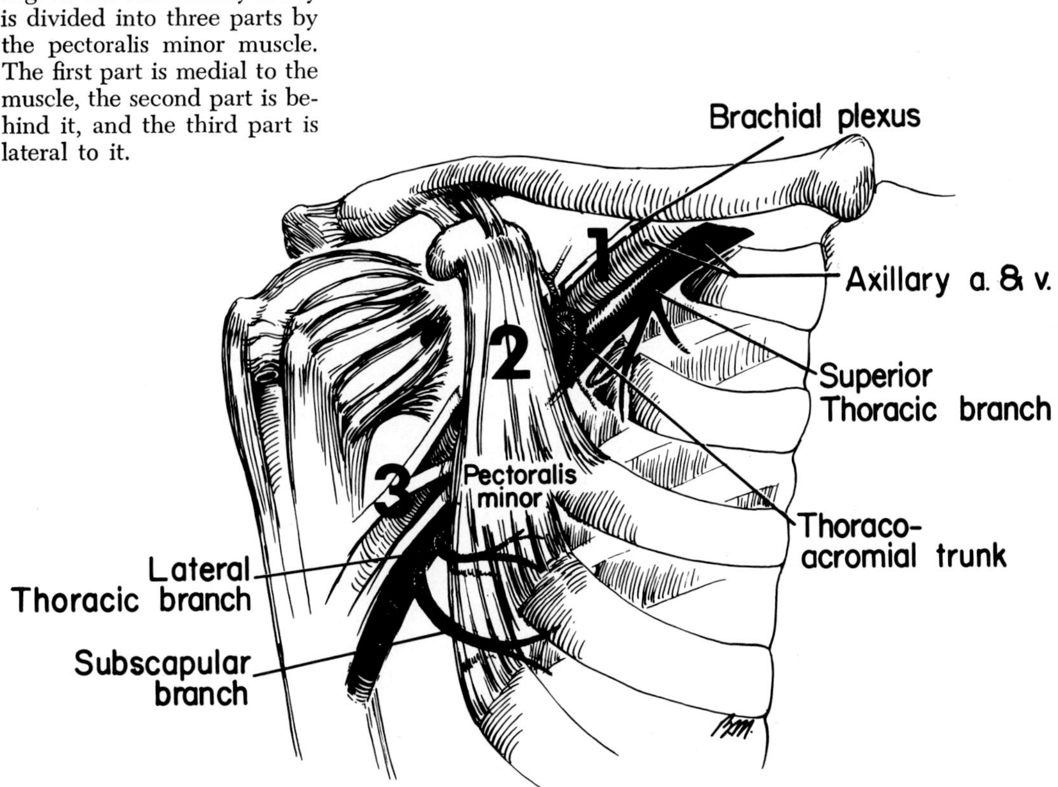

Fig. 11-81. The axillary artery is divided into three parts by the pectoralis minor muscle. The first part is medial to the muscle, the second part is behind it, and the third part is lateral to it.

tremity is cold, and the hands may be pale, the fingers cyanotic. Or the patient may present with all of the signs and symptoms of profound shock. An arteriogram should be used to confirm the diagnosis and to locate the exact site of injury.

Mechanism of Injury. Three mechanisms have been proposed:

Brown and Navigato[465] believe that the artery is relatively fixed at the lateral margin of the pectoralis minor muscle. With abduction and external rotation, the artery is taut, and when the head dislocates, it displaces the axillary artery forward, and the pectoralis minor border acts as a fulcrum over which the artery is deformed and ruptures.

Milton[489] proposed that the axillary artery was fixed in its third part by the circumflex and subscapular branches, and they hold the axillary artery in place and prevent it from escaping injury as the humeral head displaces forward (Fig. 11-81).

Jardon, Hood, and Lynch[482] reported two cases in which the axillary artery was fixed by scar to the pericapsular tissues and was transected during displacement of the capsule. In support of this theory, Watson-Jones[501] has reported the case of a man who had multiple anterior dislocations which he reduced himself. Finally, when the man was older, the axillary artery was ruptured during one of the dislocations, and he died.

I think it would be safe to say that one or all of the proposed theories could be responsible for damage to the axillary artery during dislocation.

Treatment and Prognosis. When the diagnosis is confirmed, by clinical findings or arteriogram, the artery must be repaired surgically. Jardon *et al.*[482] report that the bleeding can be controlled before operation by digital pressure compressing the axillary artery over the first rib. The treatment of choice is an end-to-end anastomosis. Excellent results have been reported by Henson,[481] Cranley, and Krause,[470] Stevens,[499] McKenzie and Sinclair,[487] Brown and Navigato,[465] Gibson,[478] Rob and Standeven,[493] and Jardon, Hood, and Lynch.[482] In order to prevent a late thrombus from occurring, the authors agree that it is most important to resect the damaged artery back to normal intima before the vessel is repaired. Jardon *et al.*[482] have recommended that the axillary artery be explored through the subclavicular operative approach, as described by Steenburg and Ravitch.[497] Ligation has been performed by van der Spek,[500] Johnston and Lowry,[483] and Kirker,[484] but the functional end results were disappointing. Ligation should never be performed in elderly patients, because they have such poor collateral circulation and severe arteriosclerotic heart disease. Even when ligation has been performed in younger patients with good collateral circulation, approximately two-thirds of these patients have lost some of the function of the upper extremity. Teflon grafts have been used by Antal.[456]

Vascular Damage at the Time of Reduction

This complication also occurs primarily in the elderly, and particularly when an old permanent anterior dislocation is mistaken for an acute injury and a closed reduction is performed. The axillary artery is bound down by the pectoralis minor muscle and frequently by anterior pericapsular scarring. It is bound down by its branches, and it is old and brittle and cannot stand the traction that is required to reduce an old dislocation. The injury can also occur during any forceful manipulation in younger patients who, because of a locked acute dislocation, have excessive forces applied during reduction. If the dislocated shoulder cannot be reduced atraumatically with analgesia, then general anesthesia should be used. If the dislocation does not reduce easily under anesthesia, open reduction should be used (Fig. 11-82).

The largest series of vascular complications associated with closed reduction of the shoulder has been reported by Calvet, Leroy, and Lacroix,[468] who, in 1941, collected 90 cases. This paper, revealing the tragic end results, accomplished its purpose: there have been very few reports in the literature since then dealing with the complications that occur during reduction. In their series, in which 64 of 91 reductions were performed many weeks after the initial dislocation, the mortality rate was 50 per cent. The other patients either lost

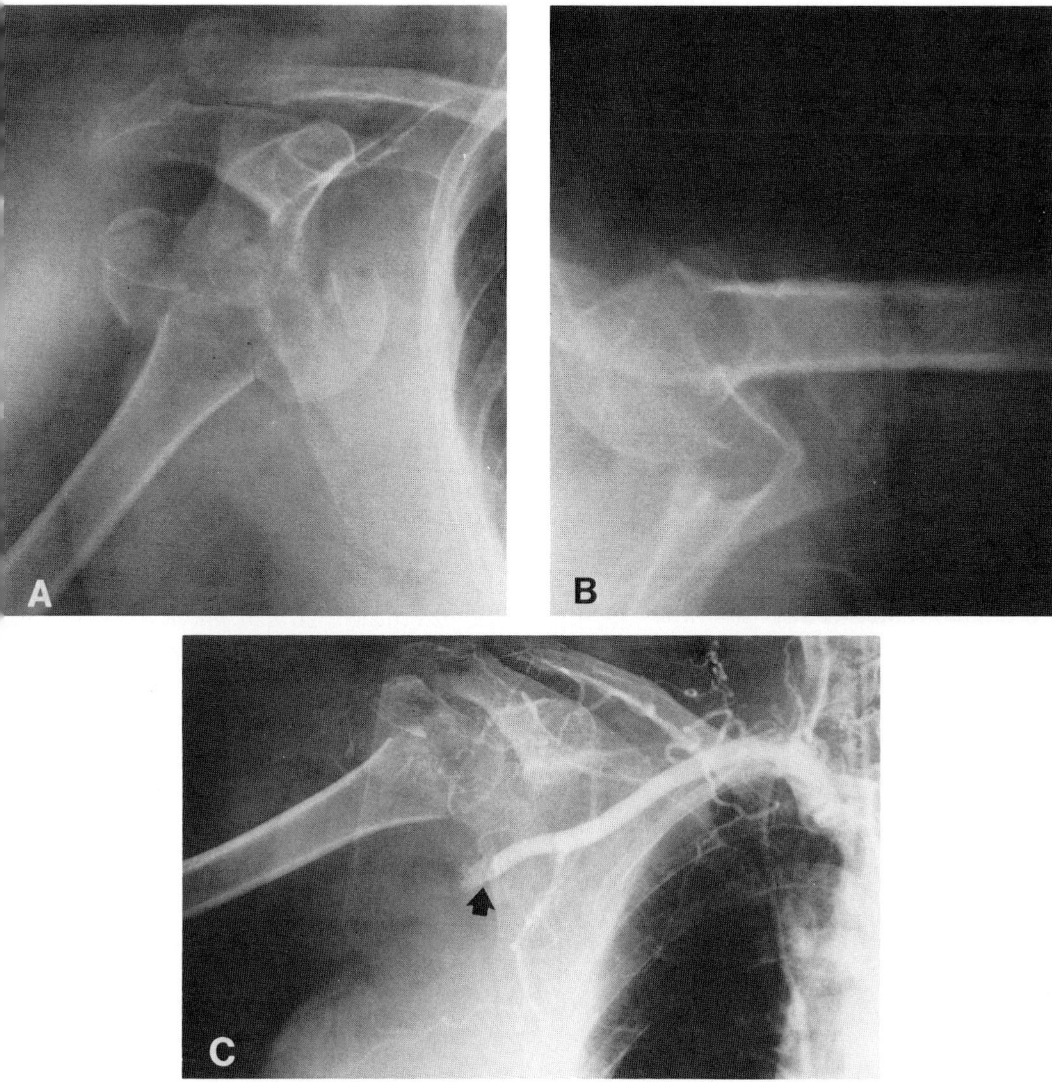

Fig. 11-82. Fracture-dislocation of the right shoulder associated with thrombosis of the axillary artery in a 71-year-old woman. (*A*) An anteroposterior view reveals a 7-day-old fracture-dislocation of the right shoulder. Note the communition of the proximal end of the humerus and the location of the articular surface of the humerus—anterior in the subcoracoid position. (*B*) An axillary lateral view demonstrates the displacement of the head anterior to the glenoid. Manipulation was unsuccessful in accomplishing reduction, and the surgeon elected to resect the head of the humerus, which was a free fragment. Following excision of the fragment, the right hand was pale, and there was no palpable brachial or radial pulse. (*C*) Arteriogram was interpreted as showing a thrombus (*arrow*) 3 cm. distal to the subscapular artery. The shoulder was reexplored immediately, and through an arteriotomy, an intimal tear approximately 3.8 cm. long was identified. Following the removal of the intimal tear there was prompt return of back bleeding. Following closure of the artery and release of the vascular clamps, the radial and normal pulses returned and the hand immediately became pink. The postoperative course was uneventful.

their arm or the function of the arm. Besides the long delay from dislocation to reduction, Guibe[480] (also reporting on the 19th century methods in 1911) stated that excessive forces were commonly used to reduce difficult dislocations of the shoulder. He quotes Delpeche, who observed a reduction in which the force of ten men was used to accomplish the shoulder reduction, which, incidentally, also damaged the axillary vessel. Kirker[484] described a case of rupture of the axillary artery, axillary vein, and brachial plexus palsy, but he was uncertain as to when the complication occurred (i.e., at the time of dislocation or at the time of reduction). Stener[498] has also reported a case of axillary artery damage in which he could not determine when the injury occurred.

In summary then, one should beware of dislocations of the shoulder that occur in the elderly for two reasons. First, the dislocation itself may damage the axillary artery; or attempts at reduction may damage it. One should always perform a gentle reduction, particularly in the elderly patient. Finally, when performing a closed reduction in an elderly person, be certain that it is not an unrecognized old dislocation.

Neural Injuries

The most common neural injuries associated with anterior dislocation of the shoulder are transient or complete denervations of the axillary nerves. Other nerves injured are the radial, musculocutaneous, median, ulnar, and the entire brachial plexus. Injuries can be of three types:

Neurapraxia is transient denervation produced by a mild contusion of the nerve in which recovery is complete in 1 to 2 months.

Axonotmesis is complete denervation produced by a moderate to severe contusion of the nerve, in which the nerve cells die but regeneration can be accomplished through the intact nerve sheaths. Recovery rate is approximately 2.5 cm. per month.

Neurotmesis is complete denervation that occurs when the axons and the sheaths are transsected. Recovery is poor and requires nerve repair. This rarely occurs as a result of anterior dislocation of the shoulder.

Incidence

The incidence of nerve injury associated with anterior dislocation of the shoulder, as reported in the literature, is quite variable. McLaughlin[331] reported nerve injuries in 2 per cent of recurrent dislocations and in 10 per cent of acute dislocations. Watson-Jones[445] reported 14 per cent and Rowe,[394] 5.4 per cent, DePalma[239] reports 5 per cent; Mumenthaler and Schliach,[490] 15 per cent; and Brown[466] reported an incidence of 25 per cent in 76 cases. Gariepy[477] states that the nerve injury is more common than is realized.

Blom and Dahlback,[463] in a very careful electromyographic study of 73 patients with anterior dislocation or fracture of the humeral neck, showed that the incidence of nerve injury was 35 per cent. Of the 73 patients studied, 26 had nerve damage (19 partial injuries and nine complete denervations). In seven of the nine denervation of the axillary nerve was produced by dislocation. Of the 26 nerve injuries, 22 were confined to the axillary nerve. In the remaining four, the breakdown was as follows: axillary and musculocutaneous nerves, one; axillary and radial nerves, one; radial nerve, one; and musculocutaneous and median nerves, one. In their series, over half of the patients over the age of 50 had damage to the axillary nerve. They observed that the transient, partial denervations of the axillary nerve were responsible for the poor recovery following an anterior dislocation and pointed out that, if a patient is still having delayed recovery beyond 1 to 3 months, it may well be secondary to an unrecognized partial axillary nerve injury. The average time from the date of injury to the electromyography was 36 days, and the authors pointed out that there must be at least a 3-week delay from injury until electromyographic findings can be noted.

Blom, *et al.*,[463] have also demonstrated that the usual sensory testing of the axillary nerve (i.e., checking the skin sensation just above the deltoid insertion on the lateral shoulder) is completely unreliable (see Fig. 11-61). According to the authors, most of the patients who had axillary nerve damage have no sensory loss, not even three patients who, by electromyography, showed complete denervation of the axillary nerve. In addition to this they stated that there were three other patients who had sensory loss but normal electromyographic patterns. They stressed that the patient who has somewhat delayed functional recovery probably has partial damage to the axillary nerve.

Mechanism of Injury to the Axillary Nerve

According to Milton,[488,489] McGregor has postulated that the nerve is crushed between the head of the humerus and the axillary border of the scapula. However, most authors do not agree with this theory and have accepted Stevens'[499] theory (described in the text by Codman). Stevens pointed out that in normal anatomy the path of the axillary nerve is directly across the anterior surface of the subscapularis tendon. Proximally the nerve arises from and is firmly attached to the brachial plexus and distally, the nerve angulates posterior and sharply around the lower border of the subscapularis tendon to exit from the axilla through the quadrangular space; then it wraps around the posterior aspect of the neck of the humerus (Fig. 11-83). He points out that, since the head of the dislocating humerus displaces the subscapularis tendon and muscle forward, thus creating traction and direct pressure on the nerve, it is a wonder that the nerve is not always injured at the time of anterior dislocation.

Treatment and Prognosis

There is general agreement that both transient and complete axillary nerve injuries secondary to anterior dislocation will recover completely. Blom and Dahlback[463] have shown full functional and electromyographic recovery at 3 to 5 months in 26 cases of partial and complete axillary nerve denervation, and Brown[466] has shown almost complete recovery in 76 cases. His

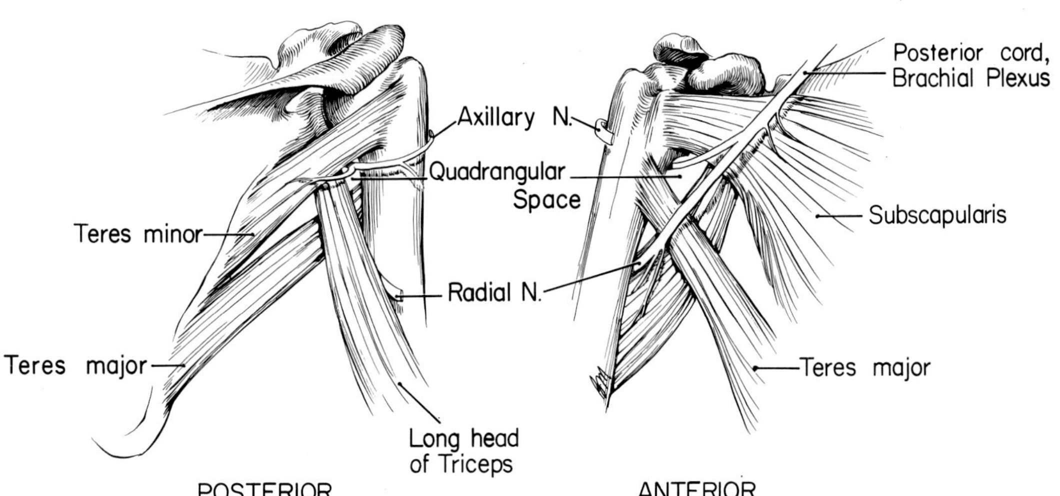

Fig. 11-83. Relations of the axillary nerve to the subscapularis muscle, the quadrangular space, and the neck of the humerus. With anterior dislocations the subscapularis is displaced forward, which creates a traction injury to the axillary nerve. The nerve cannot move out of the way because it is held above by the brachial plexus and below where it wraps around behind the neck of the humerus.

treatment consisted of "watchful expectancy," without galvanic stimulation or exploration of the nerve.

In summary then, damage to the axillary nerve is the most common complication of anterior dislocations of the shoulder, and regardless of whether the damage is transient or complete, the end result should yield a normal, functioning shoulder. The incidence of axillary nerve denervation is higher in elderly patients, and the overall incidence is probably in the range of 30 per cent. The classically described technique of checking the lateral shoulder for abnormal skin sensation indicating axillary nerve damage is unreliable.

POSTERIOR DISLOCATION OF THE SHOULDER

The history of posterior dislocation of the shoulder, as compared to that of anterior dislocation, is rather unexciting. Whereas many books and over a thousand articles have been written about anterior dislocation, less than 250 publications have appeared on the subject of posterior dislocations of the shoulder. I believe that little attention has been directed to posterior dislocation of the shoulder because it is a rare injury, and when it does occur, it is often unrecognized. In his 1832 text, Sir Astley Cooper[530] describes in detail many types of anterior dislocation, but he does not mention the posterior problem. However, in 1839, in a Guy's Hospital report,[531] he described in detail a dislocation of the os humeri upon the dorsum scapulae. This report is a classic, for Sir Astley presented most of the characteristic problems which today are associated with posterior dislocations (i.e., the dislocation occurred during an epileptic seizure; there was more pain than with the usual anterior dislocation; outward rotation of the arm was entirely impeded, and the patient could not elevate his arm from his side; there was an anterior void or flatness to the shoulder and a posterior fullness, and the patient was "unable to use or move his arm to any extent"). In the report of a case in which he had acted as a consultant, a reduction could not be accomplished, and the patient never recovered the use of his shoulder. A postmortem examination of the shoulder, performed 7 years later, revealed that the subscapularis tendon was detached, and the infraspinatus muscles were stretched posteriorly about the head of the humerus. It was suggested in the report that the detached subscapularis was "the cause of the symptoms." He further described a resorption of the anterior aspect of the humeral head where it was in contact with the posterior glenoid —probably the first description of the so-called reversed Hill-Sachs lesion.

Another classic article on the subject is by Malgaigne,[583] who reported on 37 cases in 1855; three were his own and 34 were from the literature. This was 40 years before the discovery of x-rays, and it points out that with adequate physical examination of the patient the correct diagnosis can be made. I say this, because most of the current literature reveals that the diagnosis of posterior dislocation, subacromial type, is missed in over half of the cases, and the most likely reason is that the physician has grown accustomed to relying on roentgenograms, and not on his physical examination, to make or confirm the diagnosis.

INCIDENCE OF POSTERIOR DISLOCATION OF THE SHOULDER

The incidence of posterior dislocation from the four largest published series is 45 dislocations in 1933 dislocations of the glenohumeral joint, or 2.17 per cent (Table 11-3). My own experience leads me to concur with Rowe,[526] who reports it as the rarest form of shoulder dislocation—even rarer than the dislocation of the sterno-clavicular joint. Rowe demonstrated that, in a series of 1600 shoulder injuries, 394 were dislocations; 84 per cent were anterior glenohumeral dislocations; 12 per cent, acromioclavicular; 2.5 per cent, sterno-

Table 11-3. Incidence of Posterior Dislocations of the Shoulder

Authors	Dislocations of the Glenohumeral Joint	Number of Posterior Dislocations	Per Cent of Posterior Dislocations
Ellerbroek[542]	404	4	.99
McLaughlin[579]	581	22	3.78
Wilson and McKeever[640]	260	4	1.53
Wood[641]	200	5	2.50
Rowe[612]	488	10	2.04
	1933	45	Average 2.17

clavicular; and only 6 of the 394, or 1.5 per cent, were posterior dislocations. Thomas[629] reported seeing only four cases of posterior dislocation in 6000 x-ray examinations of the shoulder.

SURGICAL ANATOMY

The anatomy of the glenohumeral joint was described on pages 634-638, but there are several points that deserve discussion. There is some built-in protection against posterior displacement of the humeral head by a direct blow to the anterior shoulder or indirect leverage forces through the upper extremity. First, the scapula is positioned on the thorax at an angle of 45 degrees. This places the posterior half of the glenoid behind the humeral head, which, to some degree, acts as a shelf to prevent posterior displacement of the head (see Fig. 11-99). Secondly, the acromion process and spine of the scapula act as a bone buttress to the posterior joint.

There are many anatomical similarities between the anterior and posterior shoulder. Actually, the posterior anatomy is simpler, because the surgeon does not have to contend with the brachial plexus, the major vessels, and the coracoid process and its attaching muscles. Anteriorly the subscapularis acts as the "front door" to the shoulder in the exposure of the anterior joint; the infraspinatus serves as the "back door" to the shoulder and is the key to the posterior approach (Fig. 11-84). When the infraspinatus is divided to expose the posterior capsule of the joint, care should be taken to avoid damage to the suprascapular nerve and artery, which are entering its substance on the deep surface. The suprascapular nerve, after leaving the supraspinatus fossa, passes around the greater scapular notch of the spine and into the infraspinatus fossa to supply the infraspinatus muscle (Fig. 11-85). As the surgeon must avoid too much distal traction on the conjoined tendon in the anterior shoulder approach (see Fig. 11-73), he must also avoid too much medial traction on the infraspinatus muscle in the posterior approach. If one is tempted to use the teres minor tendon with the infraspinatus tendon in posterior reconstruction, he should remember that its lower

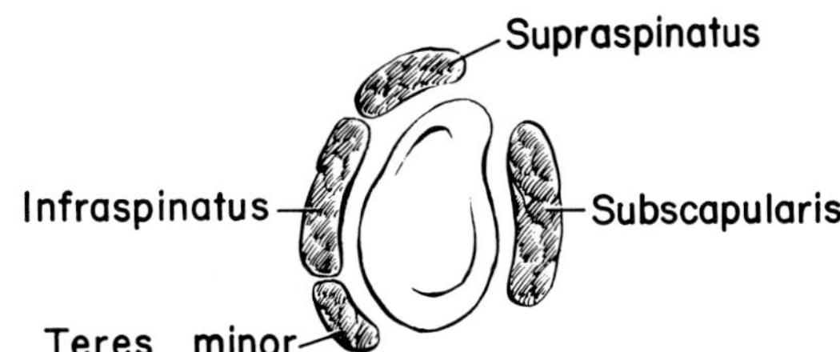

Fig. 11-84. A cross-section through the glenohumeral joint shows the muscles that make up the rotator cuff. The subscapularis is the muscle most commonly used in anterior reconstructions of the shoulder, whereas the infraspinatus is the muscle most commonly used to perform posterior soft-tissue reconstructions.

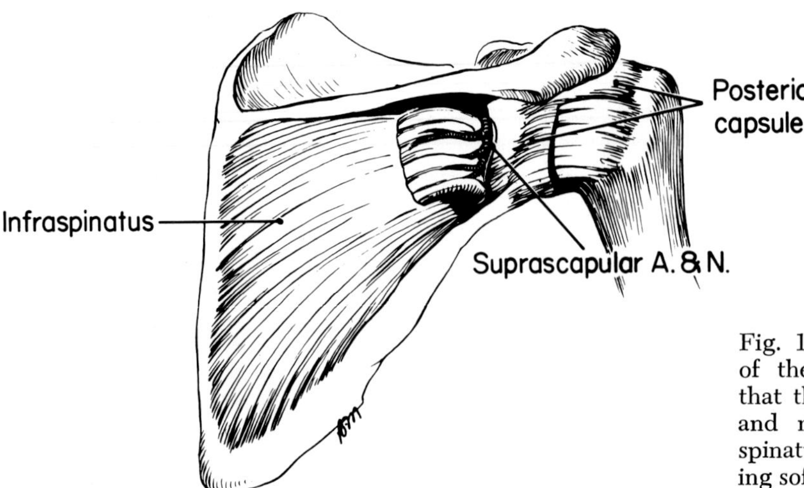

Fig. 11-85. A posterior view of the shoulder joint. Note that the suprascapular artery and nerve enter the infraspinatus muscle. In performing soft-tissue reconstructions, care should be taken to avoid excessive medial traction on the muscle, which could damage these structures.

border forms the upper boundary of the quadrangular space, through which the axillary nerve and the posterior humeral circumflex artery exit (Fig. 11-83).

CLASSIFICATION

In general, there are two ways to classify posterior dislocations. The first is a classification based on the etiology of the dislocation (traumatic or atraumatic), and the second is a classification based on the anatomical position that the dislocation assumes.

Classifications of Posterior Dislocations

I. *Classification of Posterior Dislocation of the Shoulder Based on Etiology*
   A. Traumatic injuries
      1. Sprains to posterior shoulder joint
      2. Acute subluxation of joint
      3. Acute posterior dislocations
      4. Recurring posterior dislocations
      5. Unreduced posterior (locked, persistent, or fixed) dislocations
   B. Atraumatic injuries
      1. Voluntary or habitual dislocations
      2. Congenital or developmental dislocations
II. *Classification Based on Anatomical Position of the Dislocation*
   A. Subacromial
   B. Subglenoid
   C. Subspinous

Classification Based on the Etiology of the Dislocation

Traumatic Injuries

Sprain to the Posterior Shoulder Joint

Type I is a mild strain to the posterior capsule and ligament with no resultant instability to the joint. *Type II (subluxation)* is a moderate strain to the posterior capsule and ligament with moderate laxity to the joint, which is in subluxation. With adequate conservative treatment, there should be no residual joint problems. *Type III (dislocation)* is a disruption of the posterior capsule and ligaments which produces complete joint instability—the result of severe injury. This type of injury requires the proper conservative care to insure proper ligament healing.

Acute Posterior Subluxation of the Shoulder is analogous to the Type II sprain.

Acute Posterior Dislocation of the Shoulder is analogous to the Type III sprain.

Recurrent Posterior Dislocation to the Shoulder. There is insufficient healing and strength in the posterior capsule and soft tissues, so that with internal rotation and adduction maneuvers, the shoulder dislocates again and again.

This condition follows successful recognition and reduction of an acute posterior dislocation of the shoulder or late reduction of an unreduced posterior dislocation of the shoulder. It is not a common problem, and without careful investigation, it can be confused with the atraumatic voluntary or habitual dislocation, which is not associated with an initial traumatic dislocation.

Unreduced Posterior Dislocation of the Shoulder. When the acute posterior dislocation is not immediately recognized, the humeral head remains engaged on the posterior glenoid rim. The length of time the head may be dislocated varies from days to months or years. Unfortunately, and often, many patients are in this category when the correct diagnosis is finally made. This gives posterior dislocations the distinction of being the most commonly missed major joint dislocation in the body.

Atraumatic Posterior Dislocation of the Shoulder

Voluntary or Habitual Dislocation. The most common type of atraumatic posterior dislocation is the voluntary or habitual type. The patient can voluntarily achieve posterior subluxation or dislocation in either or both shoulders. Some patients can even dislocate the shoulder anteriorly and posteriorly.

Congenital or Developmental Dislocation. The abnormality may be due to congenital deformities (i.e., absence of the proximal humerus or glenoid; excessive retroversion of the head or neck of the humerus; malformation of the posterior glenoid; or excessive posterior tilt to the glenoid). Congenital laxity of the capsule, as seen in Ehler-Danlos syndrome, may be the cause. Percy[604] reported a developmental cause of dislocation in a woman who, following encephalitis, developed a posterior dislocation. Kretzler and Blue[574] have discussed the management of posterior dislocations of the shoulder which occur in children with cerebral palsy.

Classification Based on Anatomical Position of the Dislocation

The anatomical positions that the proximal end of the humerus can assume in posterior dislocation of the shoulder are similar in many aspects to the positions seen in anterior dislocations of the shoulder. As the humeral head is traumatically displaced, its final place of rest is dependent upon the direction and the amount of the forces and the surrounding local anatomy.

Subacromial Posterior Dislocation of the Shoulder

While statistics are not available, probably 98 per cent of all posterior dislocations of the shoulder are subacromial. Only rarely do subglenoid and subspinous dislocations occur. The articular surface of the head of the humerus is directed posteriorly, so that it rests behind the glenoid and beneath the acromion process. The subscapularis tendon is stretched tightly across the anterior glenoid rim to its insertion on the lesser tuberosity, which occupies the glenoid fossa (see Fig. 11-117). The anatomical sulcus between the anterior articular surface and the lesser tuberosity becomes engaged on the posterior glenoid rim, and the engagement is held secure by the spasms of the strong internal rotator muscles. Either at the time of initial dislocation or, if the dislocation is missed, at a later date, the sharp posterior glenoid rim may produce a hatchet-like or V-shaped compression fracture defect into the anterior head and neck of the humerus—a reverse Hill-Sachs lesion.

Subglenoid Posterior Dislocation of the Shoulder

The proximal humerus is displaced posteriorly and inferiorly with respect to the glenoid fossa. This has been reported only rarely in the literature.[599]

Subspinous Posterior Dislocation

A force of greater magnitude further displaces the proximal humerus down under the posterior edge of the acromion and then medially to assume a position medial to the acromion process and inferior to the spine of the scapula. This also is a very rare type of posterior shoulder dislocation.

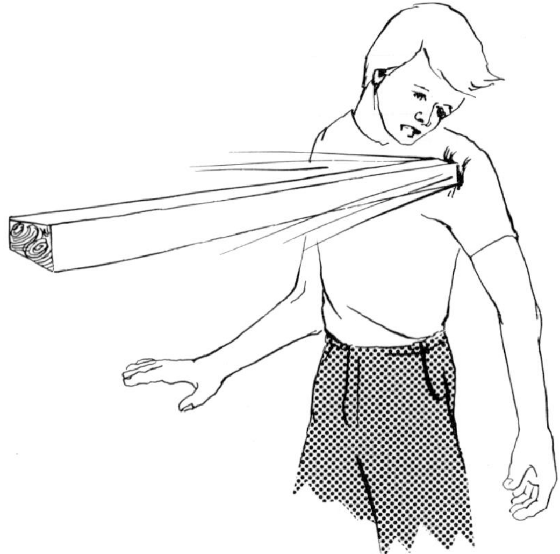

Fig. 11-86. Mechanism of injury for posterior dislocation of the shoulder. A direct force to the anterior shoulder pushes the humeral head out posteriorly.

Pathological Findings That Can Be Associated with Posterior Dislocations of the Shoulder

With posterior displacement of the humeral head from the glenoid cavity, many pathological possibilities can exist.

Pathology Associated With Posterior Dislocation of the Shoulder

1. Large and stretched posterior capsule
2. Detached posterior glenoid and capsule
3. Fracture of the posterior glenoid
4. Flattening or erosion of the posterior glenoid rim
5. A false posterior glenoid rim
6. A stretched subscapularis muscle and tendon across the anterior glenoid
7. A subscapularis tendon detached from the lesser tuberosity
8. An avulsion type fracture of the lesser tuberosity of the humerus by the subscapularis muscle

---

MECHANISM OF INJURY

Direct Force

A blow or a kick applied directly to the anterior shoulder forces or pushes the humeral head posteriorly out of the glenoid (Fig. 11-86). Dislocations produced by direct force are rare.

Indirect Force

The most common cause of posterior dislocation of the shoulder is a combination of internal rotation, adduction, and flexion forces which are applied indirectly to the shoulder (e.g., when the pullman conductor pushes closed the upper berth on a train or when falling onto the outstretched hand; Fig. 11-87). A common cause of posterior dislocation of the shoulder is the indirect forces produced with accidental electrical shock or convulsive seizures. During electrical shock or seizures, there is a sudden stimulation of the musculature about the shoulder with an overpowering of the weak external rotators by the stronger internal rotators. The combined strength of the latissimus dorsi, pectoralis major, and subscapularis muscles simply overpulls the infraspinatus and teres minor muscles. Obviously, other factors, such as the position of the arm, congenital abnormalities, and muscle weaknesses, must be considered, because some of the dislocations that occur with convulsions are noted to be anterior.

SIGNS AND SYMPTOMS

McLaughlin[579] stated that the posterior dislocations of the shoulder are sufficiently uncommon so that their occasional occurrence creates a "diagnostic trap." Other comments extracted from the literature con-

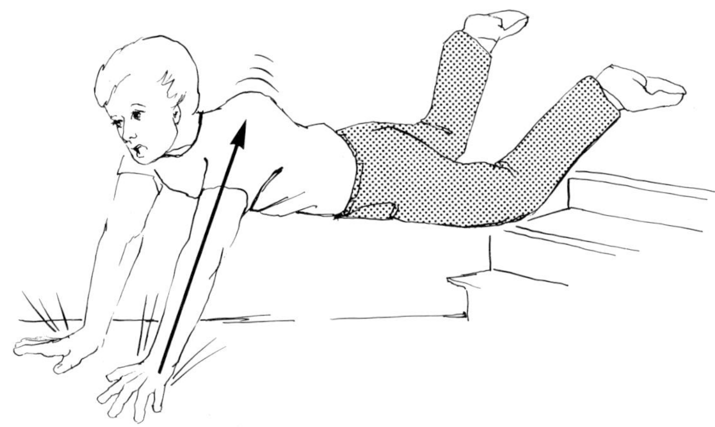

Fig. 11-87. Mechanism of injury of posterior dislocation of the shoulder. An indirect force is applied up through the upper extremity to the shoulder. This is particularly true when the upper extremity is in flexion, adduction, and internal rotation.

cerning signs and symptoms are: "whereas the average orthopaedist will see, diagnose, and treat many anterior dislocations, few will ever see a posterior dislocation"; "posterior dislocations are infrequently seen but frequently missed"; and "posterior dislocations of the shoulder are misdiagnosed, misinterpreted, mistreated, and misunderstood."

Despite all of these comments, there are classical signs and symptoms that all patients with posterior dislocations of the shoulder exhibit. Like any other diagnosis in medicine, this one requires some thought. Dimon[537] has said "seek, seek, seek, and ye shall find," and points out that if you are *aware* of the diagnosis and are *thinking* about it and are *looking* for it, then you will *correctly diagnose* the problem.

Most cases of posterior dislocations of the shoulder reported in the literature were missed at the first examination. The reported incidence of missed diagnosis is as high as 60 per cent, which gives posterior dislocation of the shoulder the distinction of being the most commonly missed major joint dislocation in the body. I should point out that it is the subacromial type of posterior dislocation of the shoulder that is missed—not the subglenoid or the subspinous types. The diagnosis is missed for several reasons. First, the entity is so rare

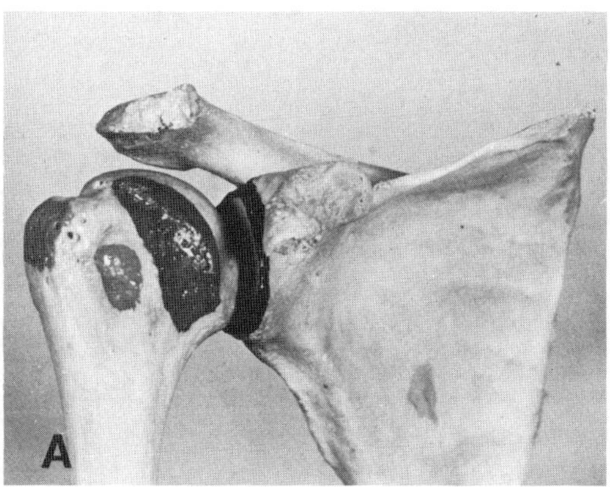

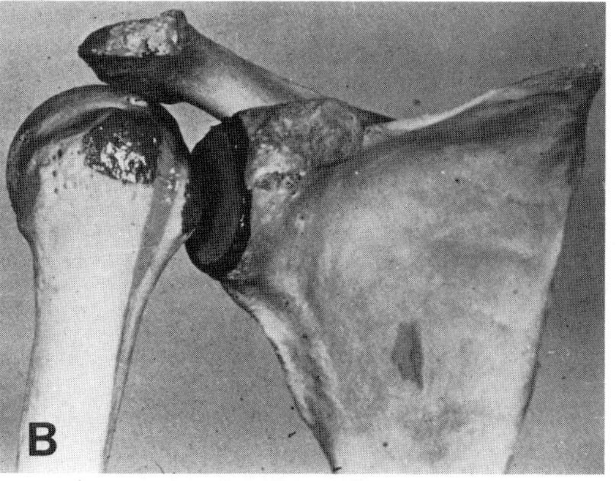

Fig. 11-88. The subacromial posterior dislocation can appear so deceptively normal on roentgenograms. (*A*) Normal position of the humeral head in the glenoid fossa. (*B*) In the subacromial type of posterior shoulder dislocation, the arm is in full internal rotation, and the articular surface of the head is completely posterior leaving only the lesser tuberosity in the glenoid fossa. This positioning explains why abduction—and particularly external rotation—are blocked in posterior dislocations of the shoulder.

that many physicians have never seen a case and, hence, do not think about it. Second, an adequate physical examination is not performed. Third, physicians tend to rely too much on routine anteroposterior roentgenograms of the shoulder, which may look deceptively normal.

Remember that the largest reported series of posterior dislocations of the shoulder was reported by Malgaigne[583] in 1855, 40 years before the discovery of x-rays. He and his colleagues made the diagnosis by performing a good physical examination and recognizing the characteristic physical findings, findings that led Sir Astley Cooper,[531] to call it "an accident which cannot be mistaken." It can be categorically stated that *if one is aware of the diagnosis and if he physically examines the patient, then he will not miss the diagnosis of posterior dislocation of the shoulder.*

Subacromial Posterior Dislocation of the Shoulder

When you can visualize the articular surface of the head of the humerus sitting posterior to the glenoid fossa and the lesser tuberosity of the humerus in the glenoid fossa, certain clinical signs become apparent (Figs. 11-88–11-90, 11-93, 11-94).

Cardinal Clinical Findings of Posterior Dislocation of the Shoulder

1. The arm is positioned in adduction and internal rotation.
2. External rotation of the shoulder is blocked.
3. Abduction is severely limited.
4. The posterior aspect of the shoulder is more pronounced as compared to the normal shoulder.
5. The anterior aspect of the shoulder is flat as compared to the normal shoulder.
6. The coracoid process is more obvious on the dislocated side than on the normal side.

The patient presents with the arm held tightly against the chest and the forearm held tightly to the front of the trunk. Any attempt at abduction or external rotation is blocked and produces an inordinate degree of pain (Fig. 11-90). *Blocking of external rotation and limitation of abduction is present in all cases of posterior dislocation of the shoulder.* In keeping with the locked internal rotation deformity of the humerus, Rowe has described that, in patients with posterior dislocation, when the arms are flexed forward, the hand of the dislocated

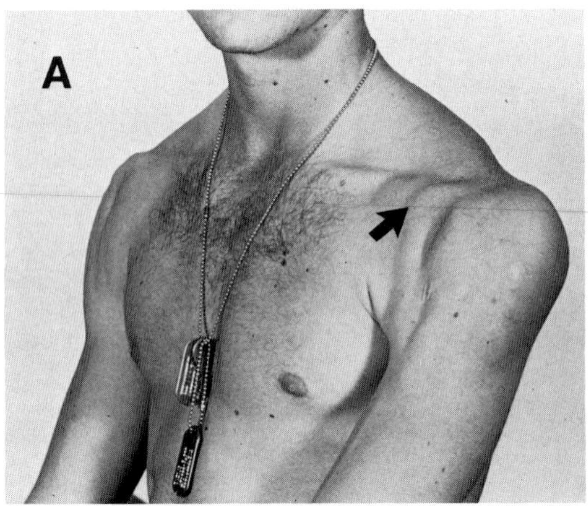

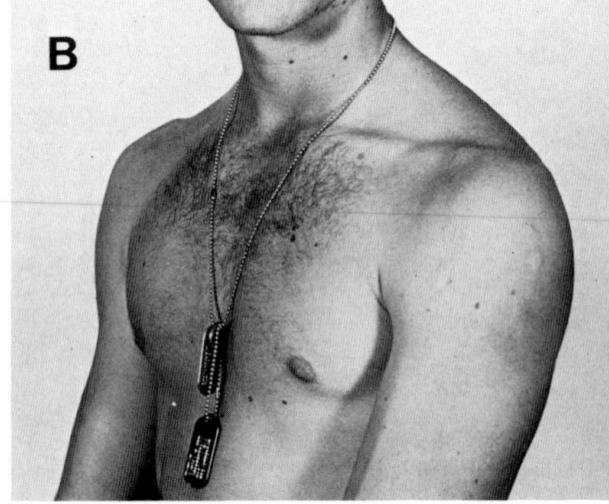

Fig. 11-89. Prominence of the coracoid process in posterior dislocations. (*A*) Note in this patient with a voluntary posterior dislocation of the left shoulder, the anterior prominence of the coracoid process and the conjoined tendon (*arrow*). (*B*) With the shoulder in the normal position, the coracoid process is not visible.

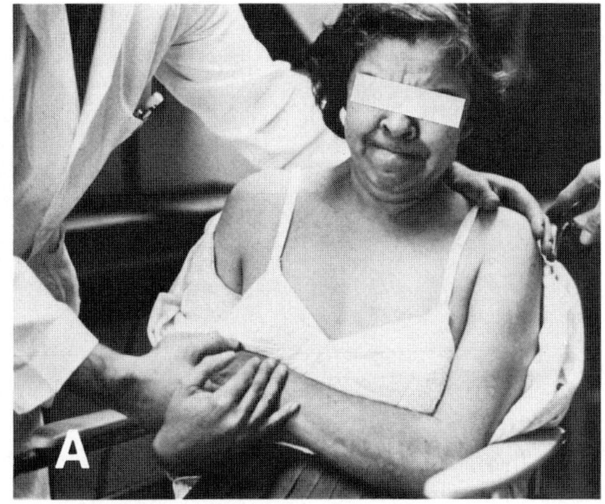

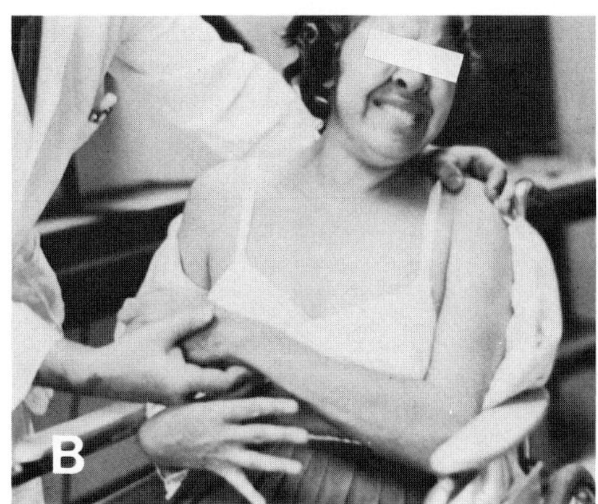

Fig. 11-90. Posterior dislocation of the left shoulder. (*A*) The patient is in severe pain and presented with the arm in full internal rotation and adduction with the forearm held tightly across the front of her trunk. (*B*) Any attempt to externally rotate or abduct the arm is blocked, as these movements severely increase the pain and muscle spasm.

shoulder cannot be fully supinated. (Try this yourself by holding your right arm in flexion and full internal rotation with your left arm and trying to supinate your right hand.) The posterior shoulder fullness and the anterior shoulder flatness can best be visualized standing behind the patient, who sits on a low stool. In this position, front and back of both shoulders are easy to see and compare (Figs. 11-91, 11-94).

Subglenoid and Subspinous Dislocations

The exceptions to the cardinal clinical findings are noted in these two rare types of posterior dislocations. The arm is not held in the usual adducted position but is locked in about 30 degrees of abduction and in internal rotation. Further abduction or external rotation from the fixed position is impossible. Clinically, however, it is quite obvious that something is wrong, and the diagnosis cannot be missed—even the roentgenograms indicate dislocation.

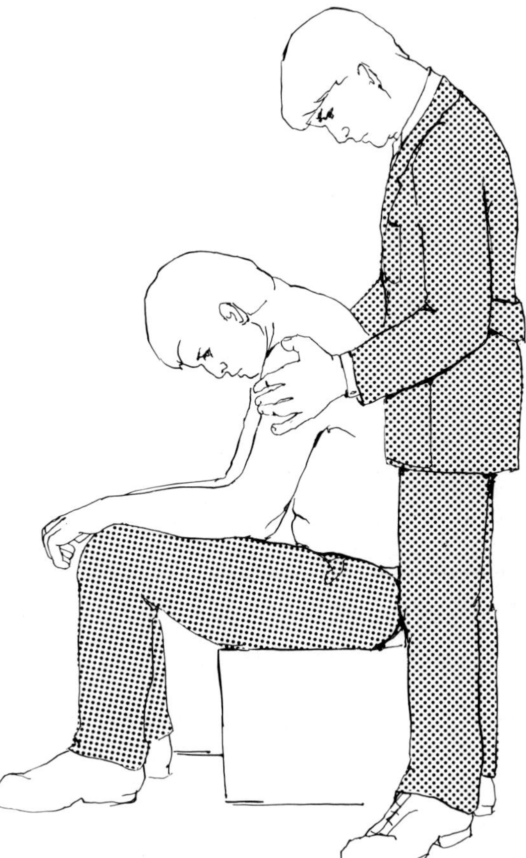

Fig. 11-91. Visualization of the anterior and posterior aspects of the shoulders can best be accomplished by having the patient sit on a low stool, with the examiner standing behind him. Then the injured shoulder can easily be compared to the uninjured one.

Noble[599] reported on one case of the rare posterior subglenoid type of dislocation where the acromion-olecranon distance was shortened by 1.5 inches (in the anterior subglenoid dislocation, the acromion-olecranon distance is usually lengthened). This may be the first case reported of this rare type of dislocation, or certainly one of the few that have ever been reported in the English language.

Unreduced Posterior Dislocation of the Shoulder

Locked, fixed, permanent, and persistent posterior dislocation are terms that have been used to describe the condition wherein the proximal humerus is unreduced and displaced posterior to the glenoid fossa. This type of posterior dislocation of the shoulder is almost always associated with the subacromial position of the humeral head, for it is the subacromial type of posterior dislocation that is missed at the time of the initial examination and on routine roentgenograms (Fig. 11-92). Initially, the head of the humerus is fixed in the posterior position by muscle forces, or there may be a fracture of the anterior portion of the head and neck of the humerus caused by the posterior glenoid rim. With the passage of time, the posterior rim of the glenoid may further impact the fracture of the humeral head and produce a deep hatchet-like defect or V-shaped compression fracture, which engages the head even more securely onto the posterior glenoid. Patients with old, unreduced posterior dislocation of the shoulder still present with the cardinal clinical findings. However, if they have had 2 to 3 months of physical therapy, they may have 30 to 40 degrees of abduction and yet be unable to rotate externally beyond the mid-line (Fig. 11-93). Because of disuse of the muscles about the shoulder, atrophy will be present, which accentuates the flattening of the anterior shoulder, the prominence of the coracoid, and the fullness of the posterior shoulder (Figs. 11-91, 11-94).

The missed diagnosis may have gone unrecognized for weeks or months or years. Hill and McLaughlin[560] reported that in their series the average time from injury to diagnosis was 8 months. In the interval before the diagnosis of posterior dislocation of the shoulder is made, the injury may be misdiagnosed as "frozen shoulder"[560,581] for which vigorous therapy may be instituted

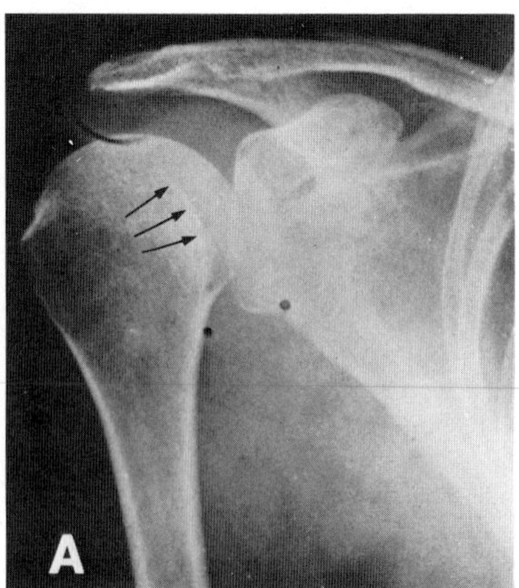

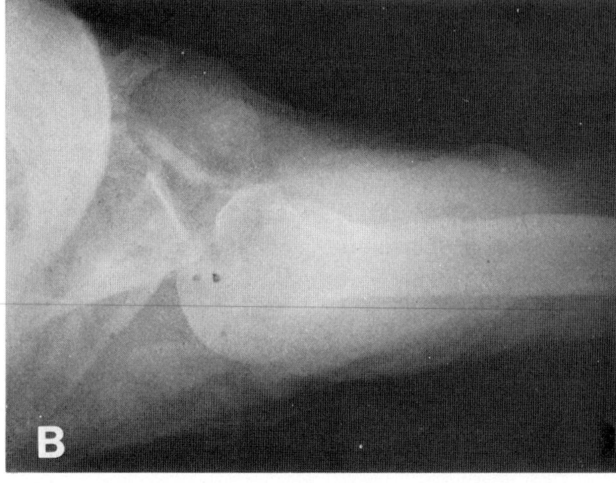

Fig. 11-92. (*A*) An anteroposterior roentgenogram of an unreduced subacromial posterior dislocation of the shoulder is deceptively normal in appearance. However, the anterior two-thirds of the glenoid fossa is vacant and the dense vertical line lateral to the head of the humerus is suggestive of an impaction fracture (*arrow*). (*B*) An axilliary lateral view confirms the anteromedial impaction fracture of the humeral head. Note that the entire articular surface of the head of the humerus is posterior to the glenoid fossa.

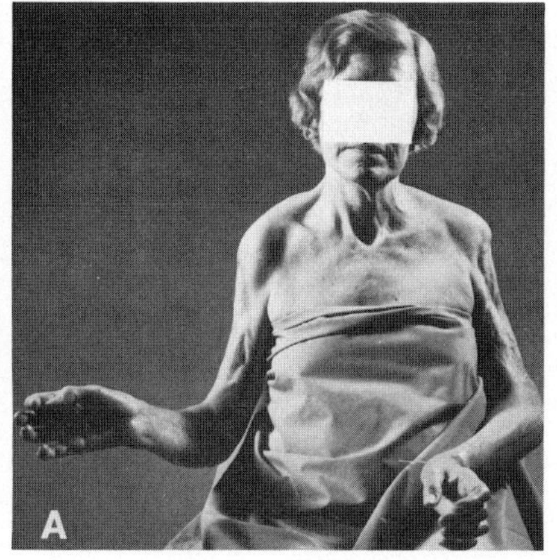

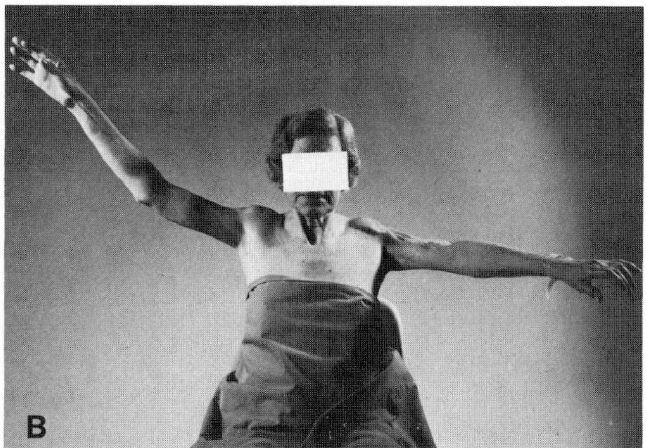

Fig. 11-93. Clinical characteristics of permanent posterior dislocation of the shoulder. (*A*) This patient has had an unreduced posterior dislocation of the left shoulder for the past 8 months. Notice that she still has marked limitation of external rotation, and note the flatness of the anterior shoulder compared to the normal right shoulder. (*B*) As a result of extensive physical therapy, she attained 80 degrees of abduction, but with so much destruction of the humeral head that a replacement prosthesis was inserted.

to restore the range of motion. If that is accomplished, the joint is destroyed. I repeat: *the key to correct clinical diagnosis in the unreduced posterior dislocation is severe limitation of external rotation and abduction.*

Bilateral Posterior Dislocation of the Shoulder

As you might expect, bilateral posterior dislocation of the shoulder is a very rare entity. However, it should be suspected in all patients who have bilateral shoulder pain following a convulsive episode or an electrical shock. Mynter[594] first described the condition in 1902, and, according to Honner,[562] there were only 20 cases reported up until 1969. The signs and symptoms are those of posterior dislocation, but the physician does not have the advantage of comparing the injured shoulder with the normal one. However, all of the cardinal features of posterior dislocation are present in both shoulders. The prognosis depends upon the interval of time from injury to the diagnosis and its treatment. As with acute posterior dislocation, the initially recognized and treated case will produce an excellent result, and a delay in treatment will produce a poor one.

ROENTGENOGRAPHIC FINDINGS

Whereas the routine anteroposterior shoulder film is enough to diagnose the various types of anterior dislocations and

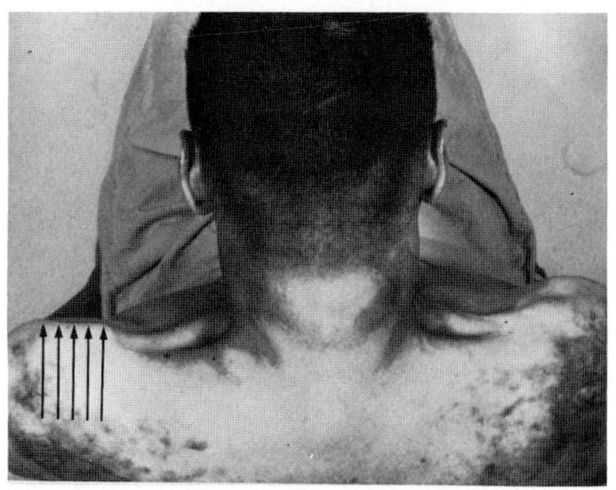

Fig. 11-94. Photograph viewing both shoulders from above in a patient with permanent posterior dislocation on the left. Note the flat anterior left shoulder (*arrow*) compared to the full anterior right shoulder. Patient has burns on both shoulders which occurred at the time of initial dislocation.

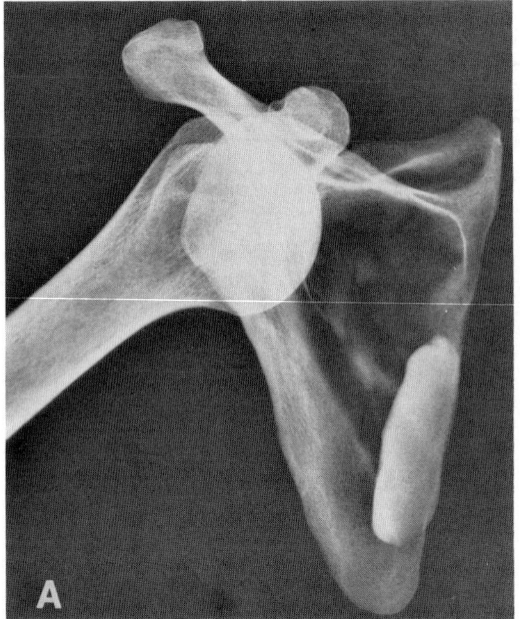

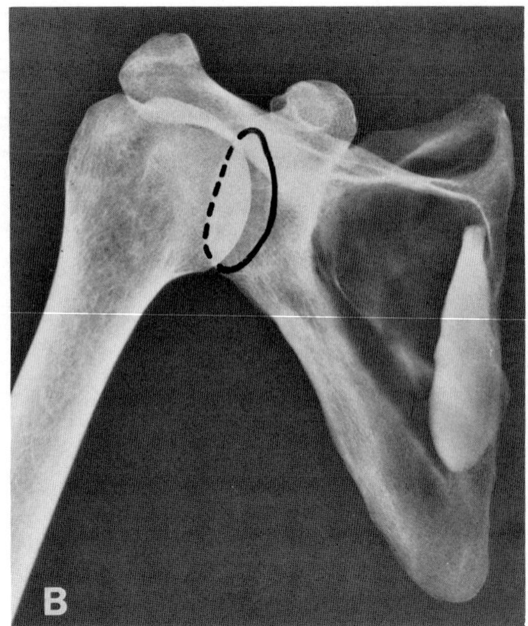

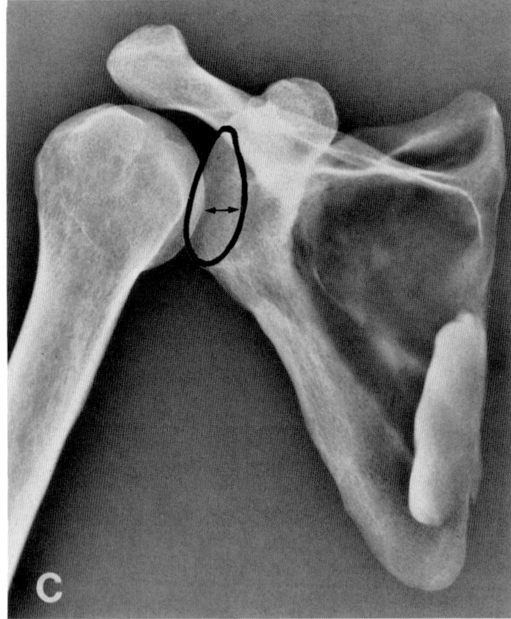

Fig. 11-95. Comparison roentgenograms of dislocations of the glenohumeral joint using cadaver bones. (*A*) Typical subcoracoid anterior dislocation. (*B*) Normal shoulder joint showing the seating of the humeral head into the glenoid fossa. (*C*) Posterior subacromial dislocation showing a very small overlap shadow of the humeral head with the posterior rim of the glenoid. Note the vacancy in the glenoid fossa between the anterior glenoid rim and the humeral head (*arrows*).

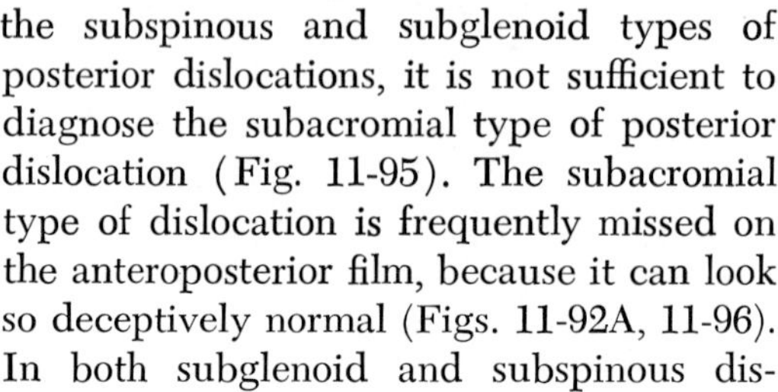

the subspinous and subglenoid types of posterior dislocations, it is not sufficient to diagnose the subacromial type of posterior dislocation (Fig. 11-95). The subacromial type of dislocation is frequently missed on the anteroposterior film, because it can look so deceptively normal (Figs. 11-92A, 11-96). In both subglenoid and subspinous dislocations, the routine anteroposterior film reveals an obvious joint dislocation (Figs. 11-97, 11-98). To anatomically differentiate the posterior subglenoid from the anterior subglenoid dislocation and the posterior subspinous dislocation from the anterior subclavicular type, axillary lateral or true lateral scapular films are required.

Keep in mind that the routine frontal anteroposterior shoulder film is not a true anteroposterior view of the glenohumeral joint, because the scapula lies on the posterolateral chest wall at an angle of 45 degrees from the frontal plane. Hence the glenoid is open or faces anteriorly 45 de-

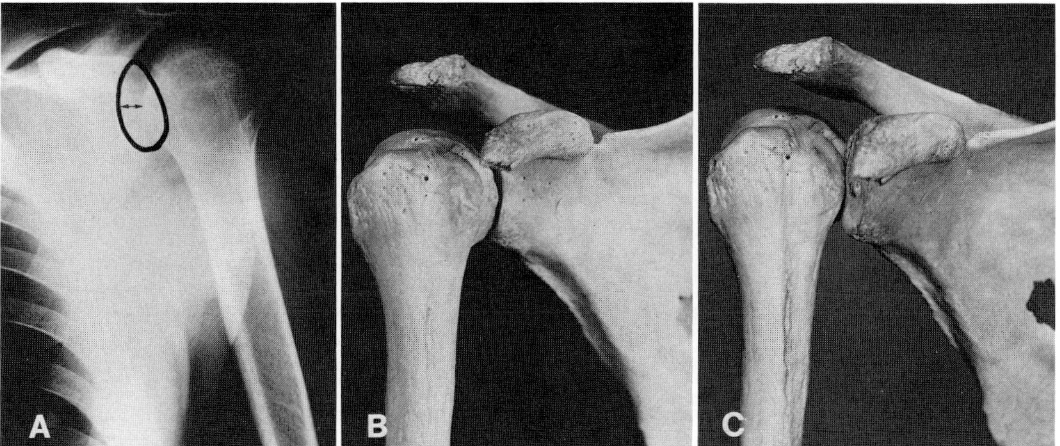

Fig. 11-96. Appearance of subacromial posterior dislocation. (*A*) Posterior dislocation of the left shoulder. Note that because the arm is in full internal rotation, only the lesser tuberosity is in full profile medially. The overlap shadow created by the lesser tuberosity and the posterior glenoid fossa is irregular in shape. There is also a vacancy in the anterior portion of the glenoid cavity. (*B*) The skeleton shows the normal position of the humeral head in the glenoid fossa. (*C*) Posterior skeleton depicts subacromial posterior dislocation. The head of the humerus is directed posteriorly from the glenoid, and only the lesser tuberosity is in the glenoid cavity. These three figures again demonstrate why so many subacromial posterior dislocations of the shoulder are interpreted as normal.

grees. In order to take a true anteroposterior roentgenogram of the shoulder joint, the direction of the x-ray beam must be perpendicular to the plane of the scapula. This is accomplished by directing the x-ray beam approximately 45 degrees lateral (Fig. 11-99). The routine anteroposterior film of the shoulder projects a significant overlap shadow of the humeral head superimposed on the posterior three-fourths to seven-eighths of the glenoid. As the beam is moved medially, the size of the overlap shadow decreases, until, at 45 degrees lateral deviation from the mid-line, there is no overlap and the articular surface of the humeral head is clearly separated from

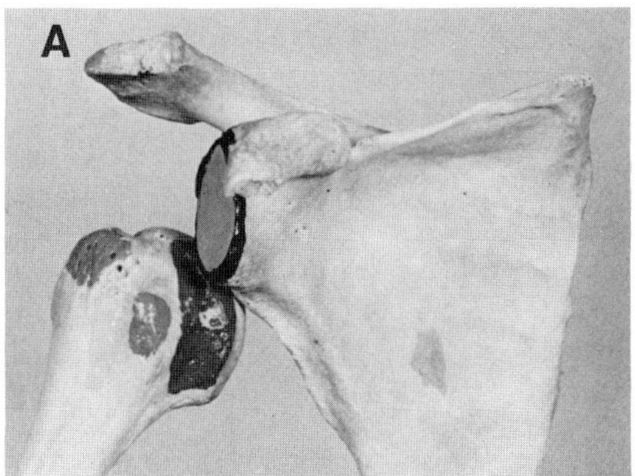

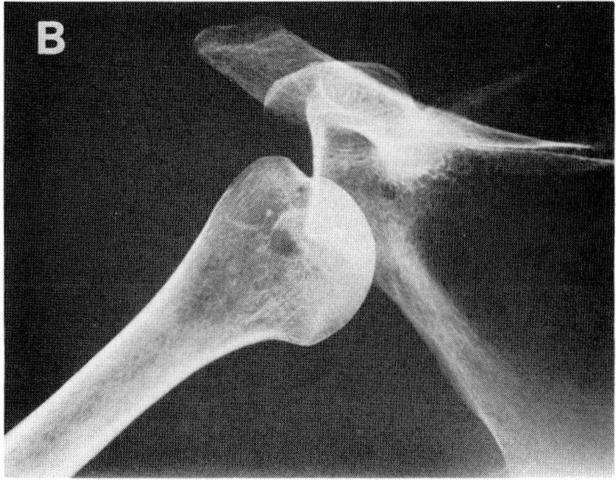

Fig. 11-97. Subglenoid posterior dislocation of the shoulder. (*A*) The head of the humerus is impinged posteriorly and inferiorly to the glenoid fossa. (*B*) A roentgenogram of cadaver bones shows the typical appearance of a dislocation. However, it cannot be determined whether or not the position of the head is anterior or posterior to the glenoid fossa.

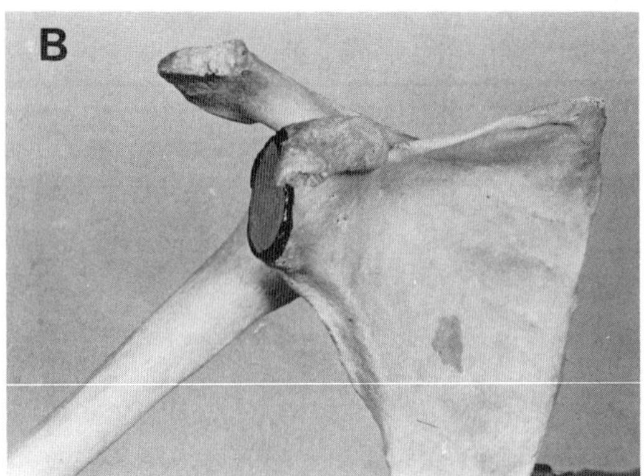

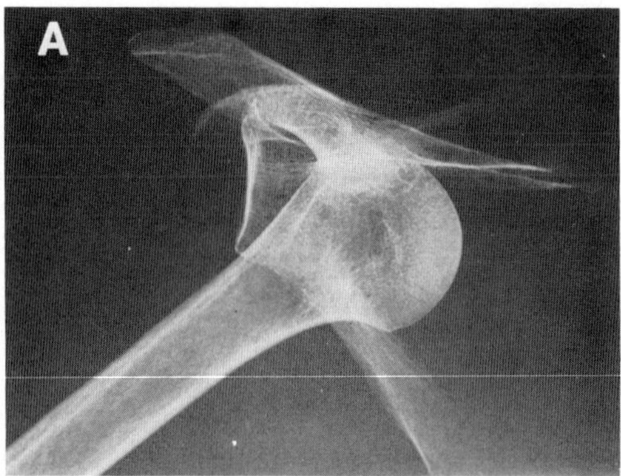

Fig. 11-98. In a subspinous posterior dislocation of the shoulder the head and the neck of the proximal humerus are completely behind the glenoid and displaced to a position inferior to the spine of the scapula (*A*). On the anterior posterior view (*B*) the dislocation is evident, but it is difficult to determine whether or not the head is posteriorly beneath the spine of the scapula or anteriorly underneath the clavicle.

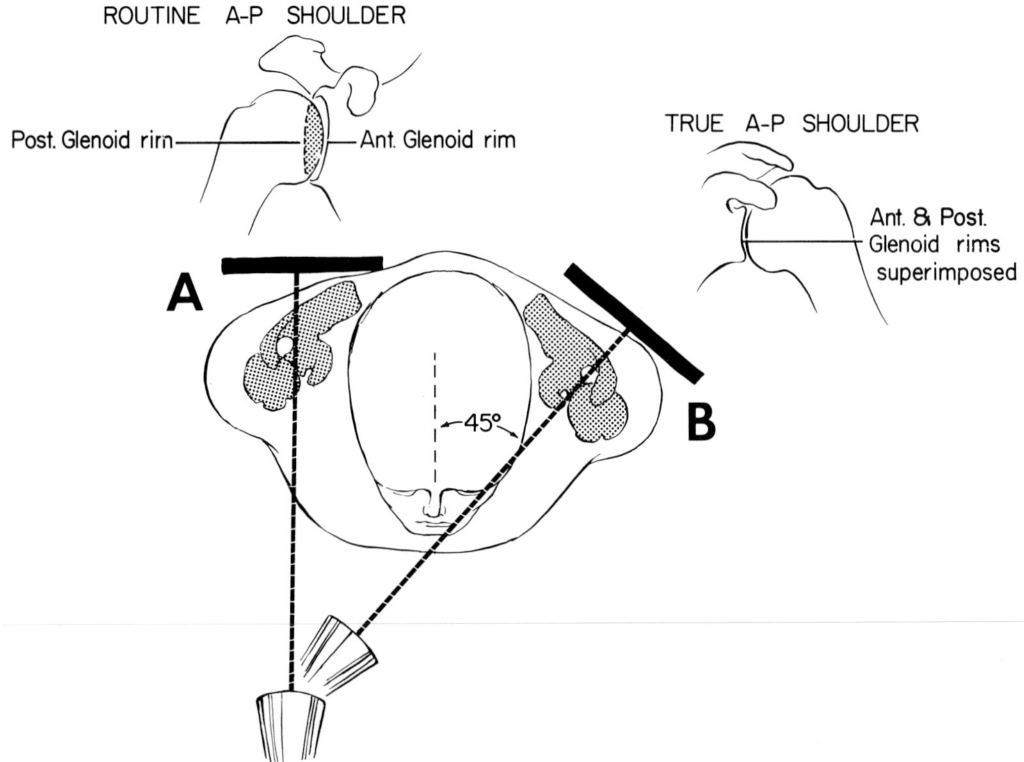

Fig. 11-99. Positioning of the patient for a routine anteroposterior roentgenogram and for the true anteroposterior view of the shoulder. (*A*) In the routine view of the shoulder, the glenoid fossa faces anteriorly, because the scapula is sitting on the posterolateral aspect of the thoracic cavity. Both the anterior and posterior rims of the glenoid fossa are visualized on the roentgenogram, as well as the head of the humerus. (*B*) In a true anteroposterior roentgenogram of the shoulder, the anterior and posterior glenoid rims are superimposed on each other into a single articular surface.

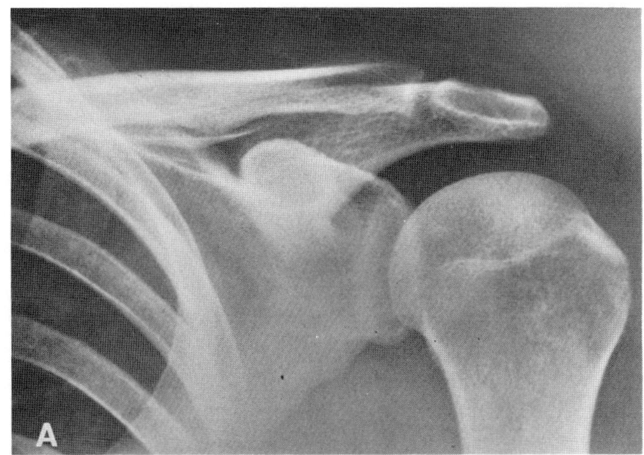

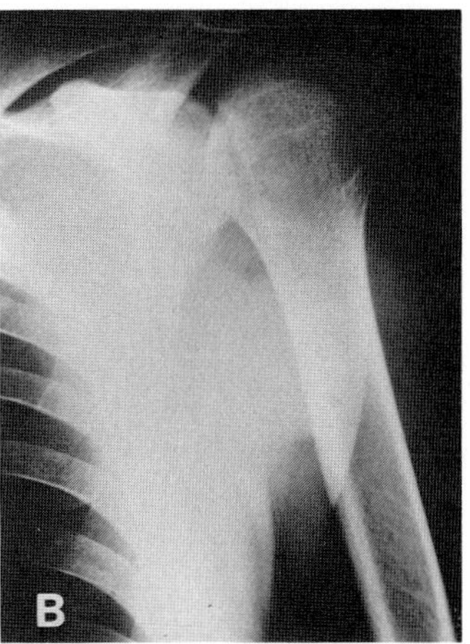

Fig. 11-100. Absence of the normal elliptical shadow in posterior dislocation of the shoulder. (*A*) In the anteroposterior view of a normal left shoulder, note that the humeral head in the glenoid fossa creates an elliptical overlap shadow with the posterior glenoid fossa. The head of the humerus is parallel to the anterior glenoid rim. (*B*) With posterior dislocation of the right shoulder, note that, because the arm is in full internal rotation, only the lesser tuberosity is in full profile medially. The overlap shadow created by the lesser tuberosity and the posterior glenoid fossa is irregular in shape. There is also a vacancy in the anterior portion of the glenoid cavity.

the glenoid fossa by a joint space (i.e., the anterior and posterior glenoid rims are superimposed and appear as a single articular surface. (See p. 702 for use of the roentgenogram.)

Signs Noted on Routine Anteroposterior Roentgenograms of the Shoulders That Suggest Subacromial Posterior Dislocation

Absence of the Normal Elliptical Overlap Shadow

Normally on the routine anteroposterior view, there is an overlap shadow created by the head of the humerus superimposed on the posterior glenoid fossa of the scapula (Figs. 11-100, 11-101A). The shadow is a smooth-bordered ellipse. In posterior dislocations, the articular surface of the humeral head is posterior to the glenoid and the elliptical overlap shadow is distorted (Figs. 11-100B, 11-101B).

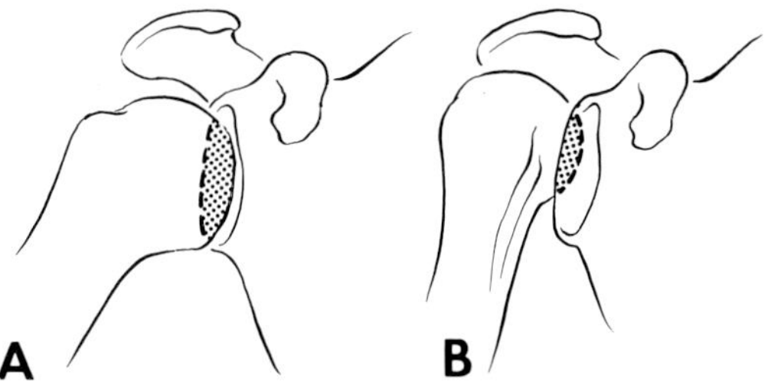

Fig. 11-101. Schematics of a normal shoulder and of a posterior dislocation. (*A*) and posterior dislocation of the shoulder (*B*). In the normal joint the head of the humerus almost fills the glenoid fossa, and the anterior rim of the glenoid fossa is parallel to the head of the humerus. The superimposition of the head of the humerus with the posterior glenoid fossa produces a smooth elliptical shadow. (*B*) In the subacromial posterior dislocation of the shoulder, the overlap shadow created by the posteroglenoid rim and the lesser tuberosity of the humerus produces a rather irregular shape. There is a loss of parallelism between the head of the humerus and the anterior glenoid fossa; there is a void in the anterior half of the glenoid fossa, and there may be a void in the inferior portion.

Vacant Glenoid Sign

Normally on the routine anteroposterior

view, the head fills the majority of the glenoid cavity (Fig. 11-101A). However, in posterior dislocations with the head resting behind the glenoid, the glenoid fossa appears to be partially vacant (Fig. 11-101B). Arndt and Sears[507] refer to this as a positive rim sign and state that if the space between the anterior rim and the humeral head is greater than 6 mm., then it is highly suggestive of a posterior dislocation (Fig. 11-102). Dimon[538] has pointed out that this sign is obliterated on a true anteroposterior view of the shoulder (that is, the more nearly the roentgenogram is a true anteroposterior projection, the less glenoid fossa will be visualized—hence the less discrepancy between the humeral head and the anterior rim of the glenoid fossa).

Some authors have noted that in the subacromial dislocation the normal parallelism between the humeral head and the anterior rim of the glenoid fossa is lost.

Cystic or Hollow Appearance of the Humeral Head

In posterior dislocation, with the arm in full internal rotation, the head may appear hollow, because the beam passed through both the greater and lesser tuberosities (Fig. 11-102B). However, this cystic or hollow appearance is often seen in normal shoulders held in full internal rotation.

No Profile to the Neck of the Humerus

Because the arm, with posterior dislocations of the shoulder, is in internal rotation, a profile of the neck of the humerus is not seen. However, the same is true for the normal shoulder when the roentgenogram is made in internal rotation (see Fig. 11-116A). If you order anteroposterior films of an injured shoulder in internal and external rotation and you do not see the profile of the neck of the humerus on either view, then you should suspect posterior dislocation of the shoulder. Occasionally the x-ray technician will give you a clue to posterior dislocation of the shoulder when he tells you that he cannot rotate the arm externally for the routine views.

Void in the Inferior Glenoid Fossa

With posterior dislocation, the head is occasionally displaced upward, leaving a

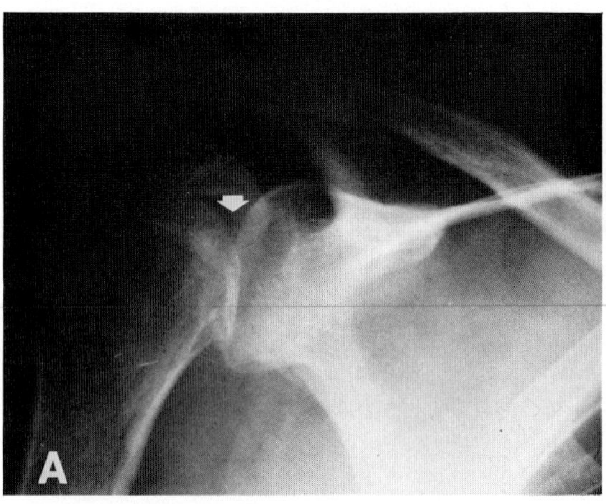

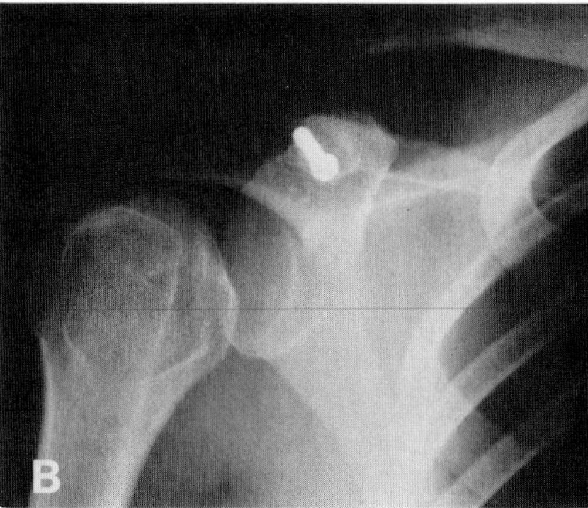

Fig. 11-102. Vacant glenoid sign. (*A*) The anterior three-fourths of the glenoid is vacant, as only the lesser tuberosity is in the glenoid fossa. The impaction fracture in the humeral head is impinged on the posterior edge of the glenoid rim (*arrow*). (*B*) Practically the entire glenoid fossa is vacant. Only a small edge of the lesser tuberosity is visible in the lower posterior fossa.

void in the inferior one-third of the glenoid fossa (see Figs. 11-101B; 11-103). In the normal shoulder, with internal rotation, the sign is not present.

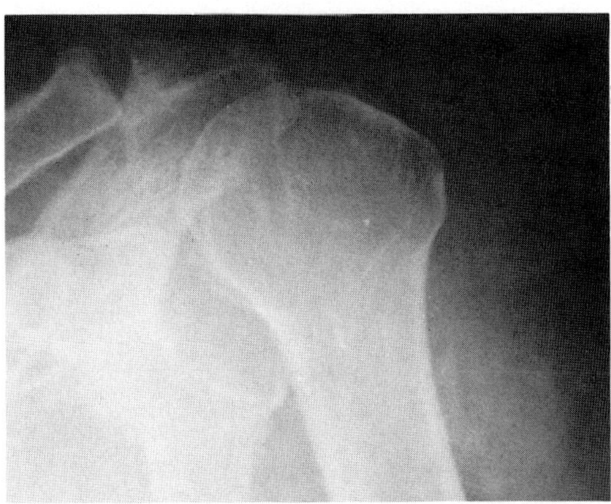

Fig. 11-103. Occasionally, in posterior dislocation of the shoulder, not only is there a space in the anterior aspect of the glenoid fossa, but the head seems to be displaced upward, creating a space in the inferior one-third of the glenoid.

Special Roentgenographic Techniques for Diagnosing Subacromial Posterior Shoulder Dislocation

Of all of the major joints of the body, the shoulder receives the least consideration and attention when it comes to x-ray evaluation. If we observed the age-old rule in orthopaedics of always obtaining roentgenograms of the injured part in two views at right angles to each other, few, if any, shoulder injuries would be missed. When was the last time you saw a true lateral of the glenohumeral joint—not axillary lateral, but a true lateral? In most cases, the shoulder is x-rayed from the frontal anteroposterior plane in internal and external rotation. That only gives you two oblique views of the shoulder. None of us would try to interpret or treat a patient with an injury of the ankle, hip, elbow, or wrist with only two oblique roentgenograms. In other words, if anteroposterior films *and* either a true lateral or an axillary lateral view (or both) were made of all shoulder joint injuries, the diagnosis of subacromial posterior dislocation of the shoulder and assorted other injuries would not be missed.

True Anteroposterior Roentgenograms of the Glenohumeral Joint

The true anteroposterior view of the shoulder should be taken with the tube angled 45 degrees laterally from the midline (Fig. 11-99). This presents a picture showing the humeral head clearly separated from the superimposed anterior and posterior glenoid rim (Fig. 11-104). But the *true* anteroposterior view is difficult to take consistently, because an error of being just a few degrees off the 45-degree angle does not project the glenoid fossa as a *single line* (Fig. 11-104B). However, this is an important view to request for any injured shoulder, as it produces a clearer anteromedial projection of the shoulder joint.

True Lateral View of the Shoulder Joint

For some reason, as has been discussed, lateral roentgenograms of the shoulder are not taken routinely. McLaughlin[579,581] and Neer[595] have repeatedly advocated this view, but their exhortations have, for the most part, fallen on deaf ears and closed minds. The axillary technique is most common, but it may be difficult or impossible to obtain when the patient has an acute posterior dislocation, because severe pain will not permit much abduction (Fig. 11-99). The true lateral of the glenohumeral joint can be taken without having to move the upper extremity, and it is diagnostic of posterior dislocations (Fig. 11-105).

Technique for Making the True Lateral Roentgenogram of the Shoulder. The anterior lateral portion of the injured shoulder is placed against the cassette, and the adducted, internally rotated arm is left undisturbed (Fig. 11-106). The x-ray beam passes tangentially across the posterolateral chest parallel to and down the spine of the

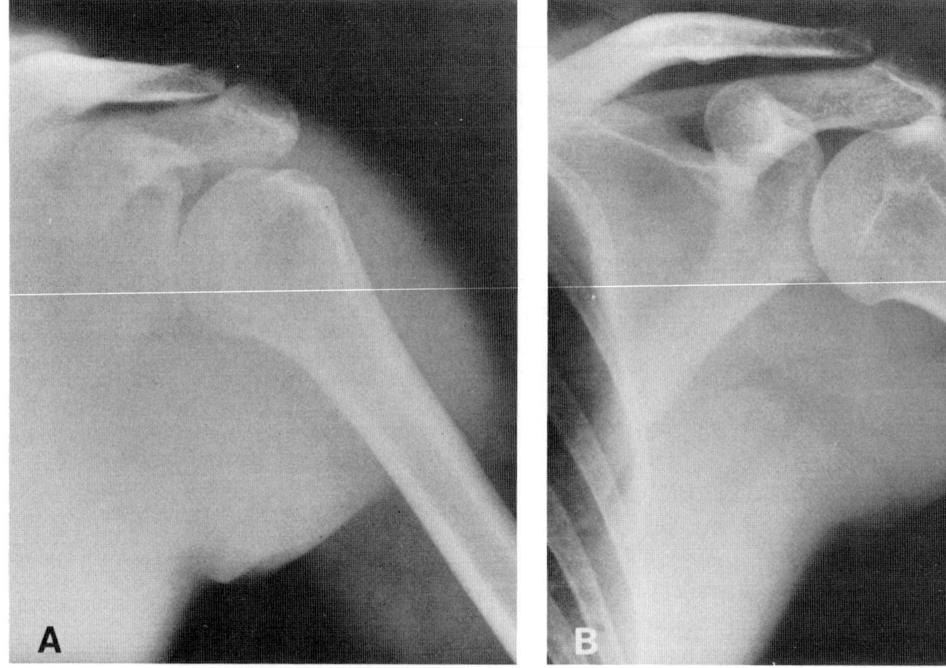

Fig. 11-104. (*A*) This anteroposterior view of the glenohumeral joint was taken from an angle of 45 degrees laterally from the mid-line. Note that there is a clear space between the humeral head and the glenoid fossa, because the anterior and posterior glenoid rims are superimposed and appear to be a single line. (*B*) An attempted true anteroposterior view of the glenoid humeral joint failed because there is superimposition of the head and the glenoid fossa. These two roentgenograms point out that it is virtually impossible to make a true anteroposterior view of the glenohumeral joint with only one roentgenogram (see Fig. 11-99).

scapula onto the cassette, which is perpendicular to the beam. The projected image is then a true lateral of the scapula, and hence, of the glenohumeral joint.

Interpretation of the True Lateral Roentgenogram of the Shoulder. In the true lateral roentgenogram of the glenohumeral joint, the contour of the scapula projects as the letter **Y**[615] (Fig. 11-107). The vertical stem of the **Y** is projected by the body of the scapula, and the upper fork of the **Y** is projected by the coracoid process and the spine-acromion process of the scapula. The glenoid is located at the junction of the stem with the two arms of the **Y** and appears as a dense circle of bone (Fig. 11-107B, C). In heavy people the circular density may not be appreciated, but it is always located at the intersection of the three branches of the **Y**. In the normal shoulder, as seen on the true lateral roentgenogram, the humeral head is centered about the center of the arms of the **Y**; that is, about the glenoid fossa (Fig. 11-107D). Accordingly, then, in posterior dislocations the head is seen posterior to the glenoid, and in anterior dislocations it is located anterior to the glenoid (Fig. 11-107E, F).

Technique for Making an Axillary Lateral Roentgenogram

Ideally, to take this view the patient lies supine on the x-ray table and the arm is abducted 90 degrees from the trunk (Fig. 11-108A). The cassette is placed above the shoulder, and the tube is positioned near the hip region. If the arm cannot be fully abducted, a curved cassette or a rolled

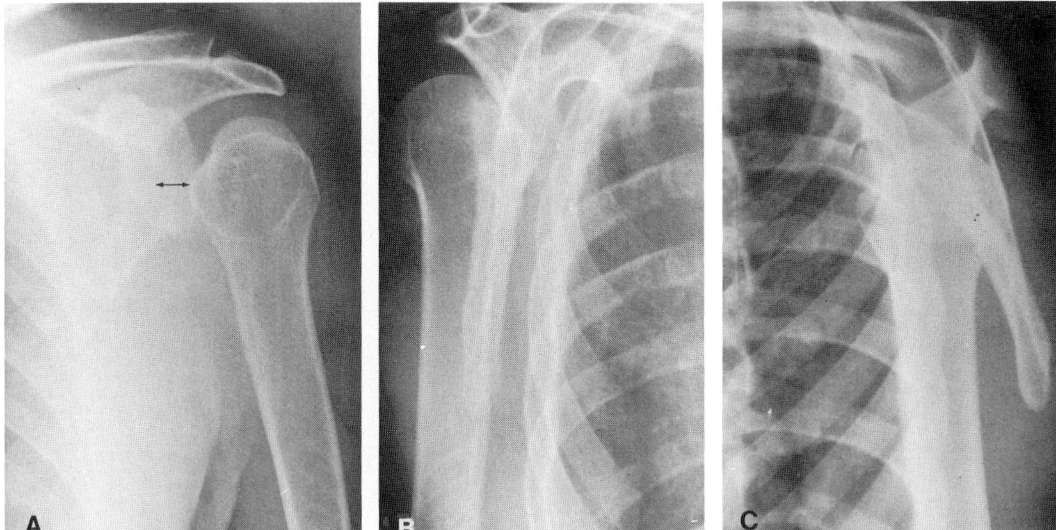

Fig. 11-105. The importance of true lateral roentgenograms of the shoulder. (*A*) Subacromial posterior dislocation of the left shoulder is visualized on the anteroposterior view. Note the vacant glenoid sign and anteromedial humeral head defect. (*B*) A true lateral view of the glenohumeral joint with posterior dislocation reveals that the articular surface of the humerus is directed posteriorly away from the glenoid fossa. (*C*) The true lateral of the normal and opposite shoulder reveals that the humeral head is centered about the glenoid fossa, which is located at the junction of the base of the coracoid process, the base of the spine, and the acromion process with the vertical body of the scapula (see Fig. 11-107).

cardboard cassette can be placed in the axilla with the tube located above the shoulder (Fig. 11-108B). In posterior dislocations, this technique has a disadvantage, in that the upper extremity must be moved away from the trunk. Bloom and Obata[515] have modified the axillary technique, so that the arm does not have to be abducted. (They call this the Velpeau axillary lateral view.) In their technique, the patient, in a Velpeau dressing, leans backward 30 degrees over the cassette on the table (Fig. 11-109). The tube is then placed above the shoulder, and the beam is projected vertically down through the shoulder onto the cassette. In his text on radiographic positioning, Jordan demonstrates the various techniques for obtaining axillary lateral views.[570]

An effort should always be made to take the axillary roentgenogram, for it is not only diagnostic of the dislocation but offers a special premium in that it will demonstrate the anterior head compression fracture (that is, the so-called reverse Hill-Sachs lesion) as well as fractures of the

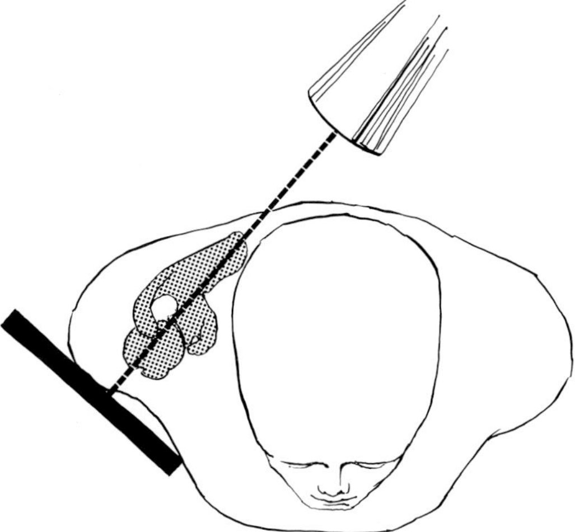

Fig. 11-106. Positioning of the patient for making the true lateral roentgenogram of the glenohumeral joint. This is sometimes referred to as the transscapular.

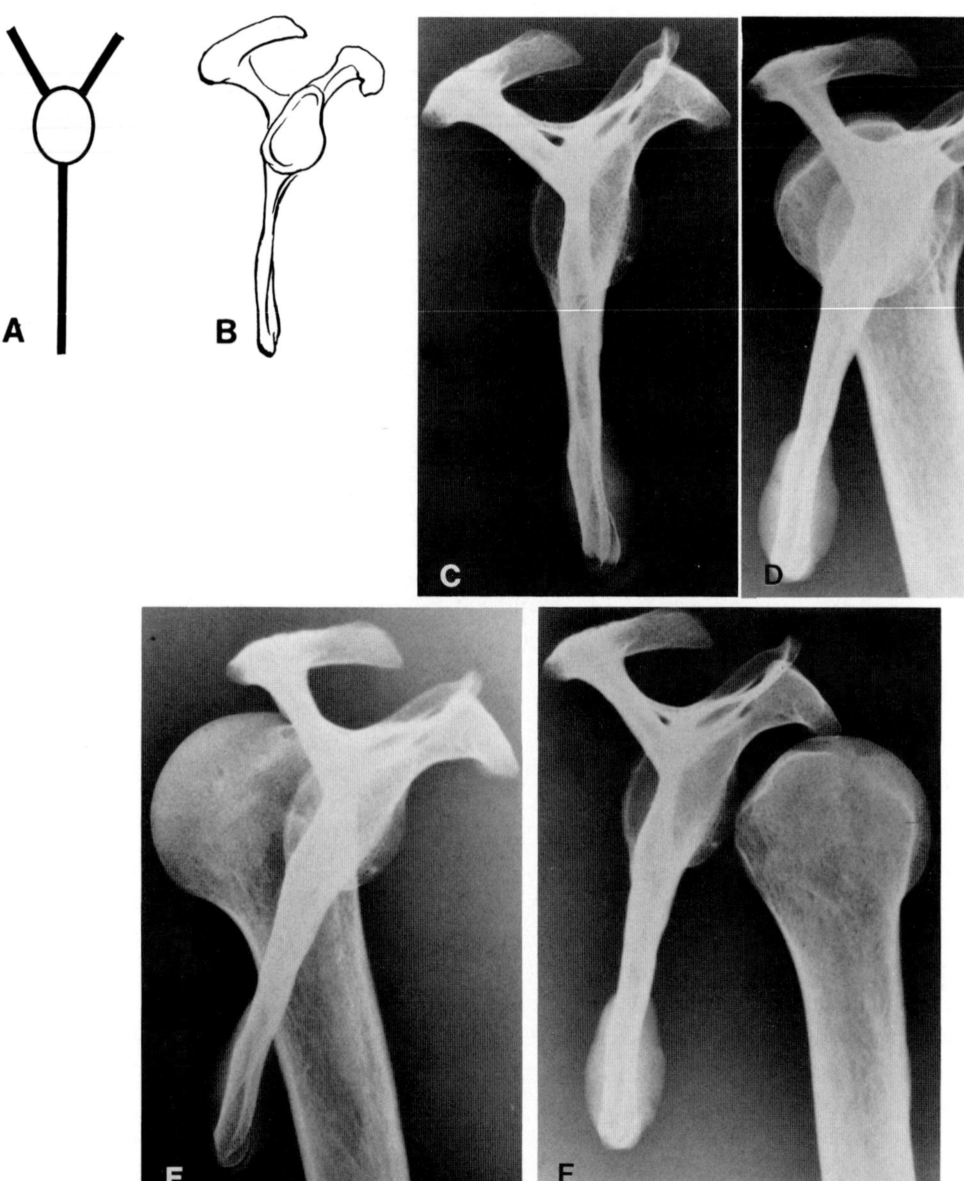

Fig. 11-107. Interpretation of a true lateral roentgenogram of the shoulder. (*A*) The schematic drawing illustrates how a lateral view of the scapula projects as the letter **Y**. (*B*) Drawing of the lateral view of the scapula. (*C*) True lateral roentgenogram of the scapula. Note that the glenoid fossa is located at the junction of the base of the spine and the base of the coracoid, with the body of the scapula projecting vertically. (*D*) The true lateral view of the glenohumeral joint shows the humeral head well centered about the glenoid fossa. (*E*) In the subacromial posterior dislocation of the shoulder, as seen on true lateral view, the articular surface of the head of the humerus is directed posterior to the glenoid fossa. (*F*) In anterior subcoracoid dislocations of the shoulder, as seen on the true lateral roentgenogram, the humeral head is anterior to the glenoid fossa and below the coracoid process.

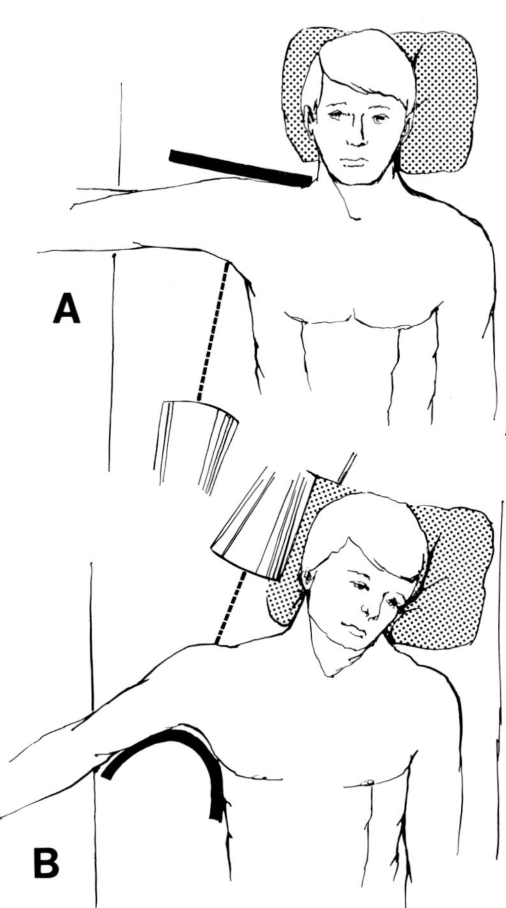

Fig. 11-108. Positioning of the patient for taking an axillary roentgenogram of the glenohumeral joint. (*A*) If the patient can abduct the arm 90 degrees, the cassette is placed above the shoulder. (*B*) If the injured shoulder cannot be abducted 90 degrees a curved cassette can be placed below and the tube above the shoulder.

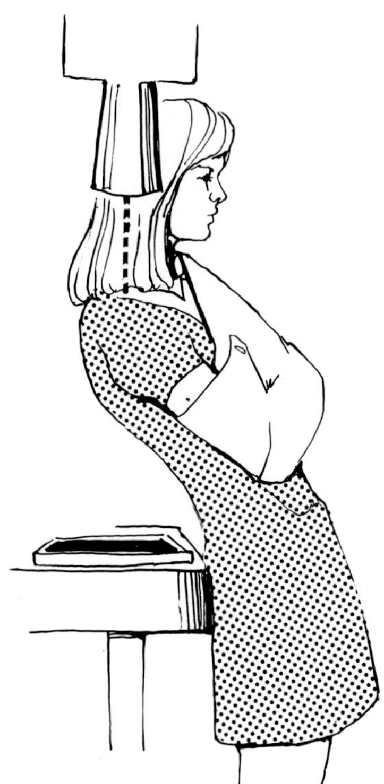

Fig. 11-109. Positioning of the patient for the Velpeau axillary lateral view as described by Bloom and Obata. (Redrawn from Bloom, M. H., and Obata, W. G.: J. Bone Joint Surg., 49A:943-949, 1967)

glenoid or fractures of the lesser tuberosity of the humerus (Fig. 11-110).

Transthoracic Lateral Roentgenogram

Like the true lateral of the glenohumeral joint, the transthoracic lateral view can be taken without having to move the upper extremity. However, since the scapula sits on the posterolateral chest wall, the transthoracic lateral is an oblique view of the glenohumeral joint.

Technique. The lateral aspect of the involved arm and shoulder is placed against the cassette, and the beam passes laterally through the chest from the opposite side while the uninvolved arm is raised overhead (Fig. 11-111). The roentgenogram is very difficult to interpret if the patient is large or obese, because of the sheer mass of the thorax which is superimposed on the glenohumeral joint. It is difficult to see how —before the work by Moloney, reported by Dorgan[540]—much, if any, detail of the glenohumeral joint could be interpreted from this technique.

Interpretation of Moloney's Line in the Transthoracic Lateral Technique. Dorgan[540] reported that, in addition to obesity, technical factors may prevent accurate identification of the glenohumeral joint in the transthoracic lateral view. He credits Dr. Albert Moloney of Boston with interpreting a "break in the normal scapulohumeral arch" (Moloney's line). Normally there is

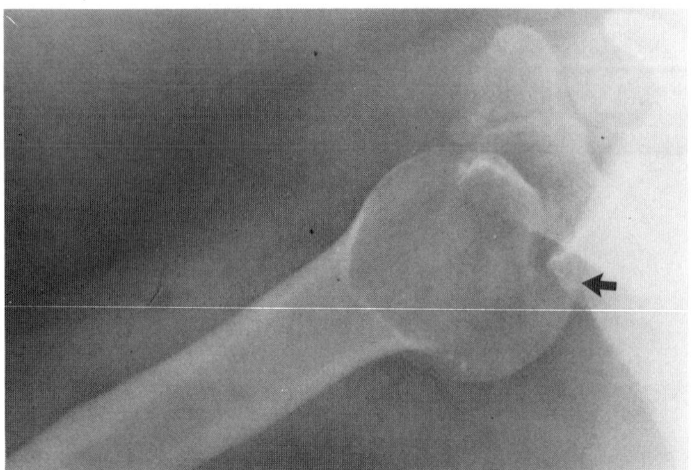

Fig. 11-110. An axillary lateral roentgenogram shows a subacromial posterior dislocation of the shoulder. Note that the articular surface of the humeral head is posterior to the glenoid rim (*arrow*). Note also the impaction fracture of the humeral head caused by the posterior glenoid rim.

a smooth or rounded dome type of arch created by the shoulder girdle in the transthoracic lateral film (Fig. 11-112A). For example, in a transthoracic lateral roentgenogram of the left shoulder, the arch is created by the following structures: the anterior upright of the arch is formed by the shaft of the humerus; the dome, rounded and smooth, is formed by the inferior neck and head of the humerus, which articulates with the inferior neck of the scapula; and the posterior upright of the arch is created by the lateral or axillary border of the scapula (Fig. 11-112A). Moloney's line is comparable to the arch in the hip region formed by the proximal shaft and neck of the femur and the upper border of the obturator foramen known as Shenton's line.

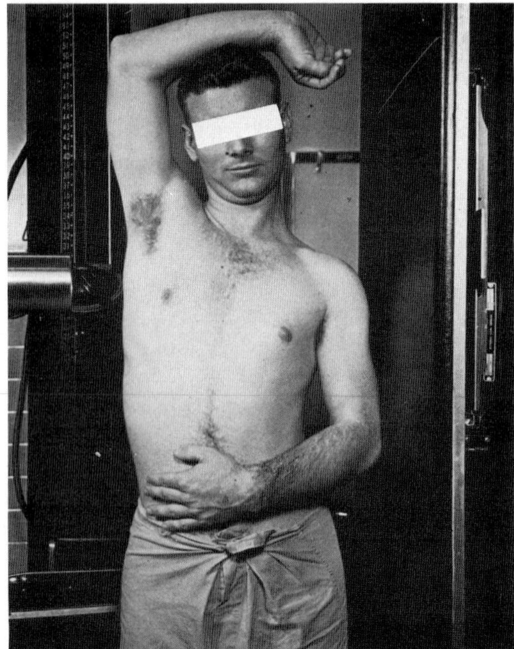

Fig. 11-111. Positioning of the patient to take the transthoracic lateral roentgenogram of the left glenohumeral joint.

In posterior dislocations of the shoulder, the head and neck of the humerus are behind and superimposed on the glenoid fossa, hence the smooth dome shape is obliterated (Fig. 11-112B); the result is that the top of the arch comes to a narrow apex created by the shaft of the humerus, which meets the axillary border of the scapula.

In anterior dislocations, the opposite is true; that is, the dome of the arch becomes quite wide (Fig. 11-112C). This occurs, first, because the head is displaced anteriorly and, second, because the arm is in external rotation and places more of the neck on profile, which widens the arch. Dorgan has found the interpretation of Moloney's line to be quite diagnostic.

Stereoscopic Views

Many authors have reported on the use of the stereoscopic examination to diagnose posterior dislocations, but Arden,[506]

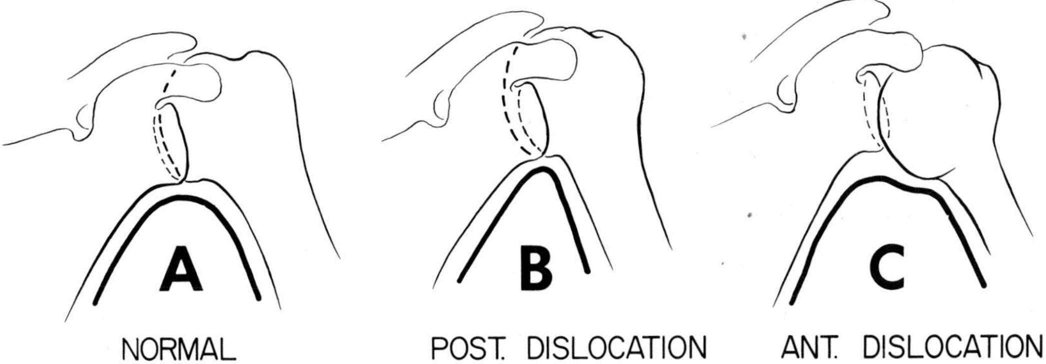

Fig. 11-112. Interpretation of Moloney's line on transthoracic lateral roentgenogram of the left shoulder. (*A*) In the normal shoulder, Moloney's line as depicted produces a smooth arch. (*B*) In posterior dislocation, the head is displaced behind the glenoid, thereby obliterating the smooth dome of the arch. (*C*) In anterior dislocation, because the head of the humerus is anterior to the glenoid rim, the dome of the arch is widened.

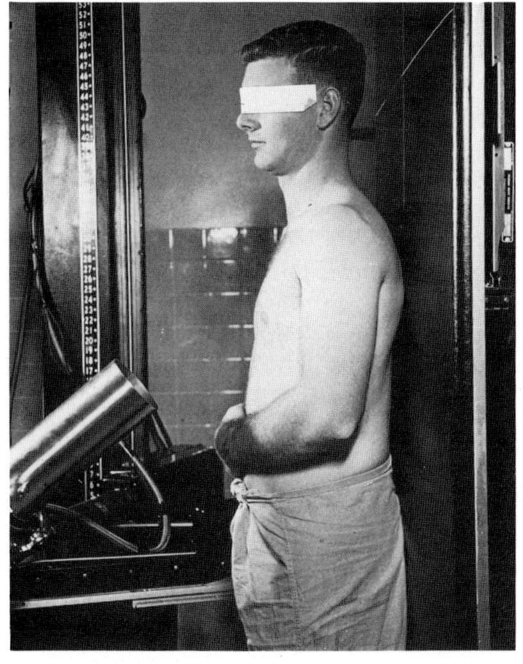

Fig. 11-113. Positioning of the patient to make the cephalic tilt roentgenogram of a posterior dislocation of the shoulder.

Thomas,[629] and others have reported that it may fail to document the diagnosis. This is particularly true if the stereos are made with both arms in full internal rotation. Thomas[629] does recommend that if stereos are made the arms be placed in maximum external rotation, which makes the diagnosis quite evident. Dorgan[540] has pointed out that, while this may be of benefit to the radiologist, it is of little benefit and difficult to interpret on an acute injury in the emergency department.

Cephalic Tilt Views

Langford,[575] in 1965, presented a technique in an exhibit where the posteriorly dislocated shoulder and the normal shoulder were both compared in 30-degree cephalic tilt anteroposterior roentgenograms (Fig. 11-113). In the shoulder with the posterior dislocation, the top of the upper humerus is lower in relation to the glenoid fossa than on the normal side. Bloom and Obata[515] referred to this view as the angle-up view. They pointed out that in posterior dislocations, the articular surface of the humeral head is low in relation to the glenoid fossa.

Compression Fracture of the Anteromedial Portion of the Humeral Head

The defect in the humeral head, which can best be visualized on the axillary lateral film, is actually a compression fracture of the anteromedial part of the head produced by the posterior cortical rim of the glenoid

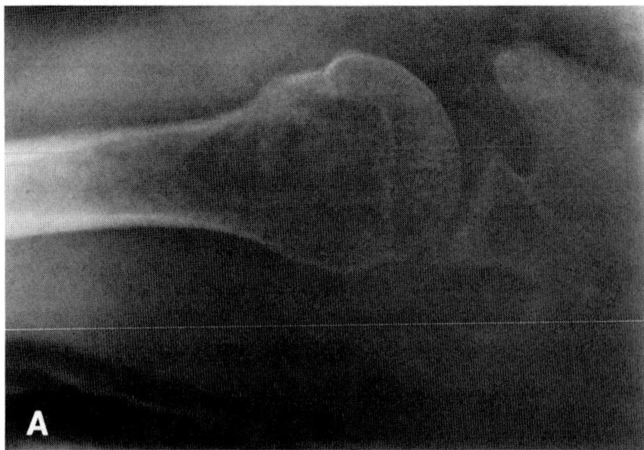

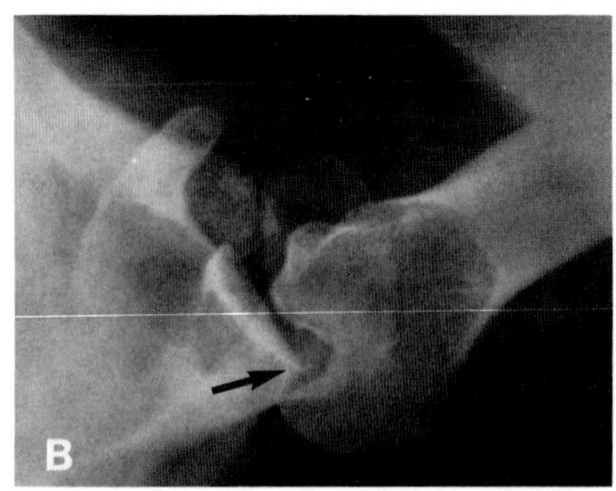

Fig. 11-114. (*A*) An axillary lateral view of the normal left shoulder shows the normal articulation of the humeral head with the glenoid fossa and normal relations of the humeral head to the coracoid process and the acromion process. (*B*) The axillary lateral roentgenogram of the right shoulder shows a subacromial posterior dislocation of the right shoulder with a large anteromedial compression fracture defect of the humeral head, the so-called reverse Hill-Sachs sign (*arrow*).

fossa (Fig. 11-114). It is analogous in practically all respects to the posterolateral defect in the humeral head, the Hill-Sachs sign, which is seen with anterior dislocation of the glenohumeral joint. It is readily noted on the axillary roentgenogram in a patient with an unreduced posterior dislocation of the shoulder (i.e., the wedge-shaped impaction fracture in the humeral head is impaled by the sharp posterior glenoid rim with the articular surface of the humeral head completely posterior to the glenoid fossa).

It is very important to know whether or not the impaction fracture defect is present before surgical reconstructions are planned. The compression fracture can occur at the time of the original posterior dislocation, may become larger with multiple posterior dislocations, and certainly is larger in unreduced posterior dislocation of the shoulder. Probably the most common cause of a very large defect is the unrecognized posterior dislocation that has received several months of grinding and grating in physical therapy. Figiel[548] *et al.* report that the anterior humeral head impaction fracture defect, seen on axillary views, was present in all of their 14 cases.

Other Roentgenographic Characteristics Associated with Posterior Dislocations

It would appear that the incidence of fractures of the posterior glenoid rim and fractures of the proximal humerus (i.e., upper shaft, tuberosities, as well as the compression fracture of the humeral head) are quite common in posterior dislocations of the shoulder. Thomas,[629] Wilson and McKeever,[640] and O'Connor and Jacknow[600,601] report that the incidence of associated fractures of the tuberosity and/or fractures of the upper shaft of the humerus is over 50 per cent.

Fracture of the Posterior Glenoid Rim

With posterior dislocation, the posterior rim of the glenoid may be knocked off. This occurs not only with direct anterior forces, which push the humeral head out posteriorly, but with indirect types of dislocations, which occur during seizures or accidental electrical shock. Occasionally when a large fragment has been displaced posteriorly, a pseudo-posterior glenoid fossa may develop.

Fracture of the Lesser Tuberosity of the Humerus

With posterior dislocations, the subscapularis muscle, which inserts into the lesser tuberosity, is under considerable tension, and it may avulse the lesser tuberosity from the humerus. Therefore, I believe that an isolated fracture of the lesser tuberosity of the humerus represents a posterior dislocation of the shoulder until proven otherwise. While the fracture can be seen on the routine anteroposterior and true lateral roentgenograms of the glenohumeral joint, the exact source of the fragment can best be seen in the axillary lateral view (Fig. 11-115).

Comminuted Fracture of the Proximal Humerus

When the roentgenogram reveals a comminuted fracture of the proximal humerus, you should be aware that the head fragment may be displaced posteriorly. Because of the distortion of the fragments, it is impossible to determine the exact position of the head without axillary lateral roentgenograms. In the series of 16 cases reported by O'Connor and Jacknow,[601] 12 had comminuted fractures of the proximal humerus, of which 8 had been incorrectly diagnosed initially as only fractures.

TREATMENT OF POSTERIOR DISLOCATION OF THE SHOULDER

Traumatic Injuries

Acute Posterior Dislocation

Patients with acute traumatic posterior dislocation of the shoulder have more pain than those with acute traumatic anterior dislocation. Therefore, the use of intravenous narcotics combined with muscle relaxants or tranquilizers to reduce the posterior dislocation may be unsuccessful.

Method of Reduction. Closed reduction under general anesthesia can be accomplished by applying traction in the line of the adducted deformity and concomitant direct posterior pressure on the humeral head. If the maneuver is done gently and

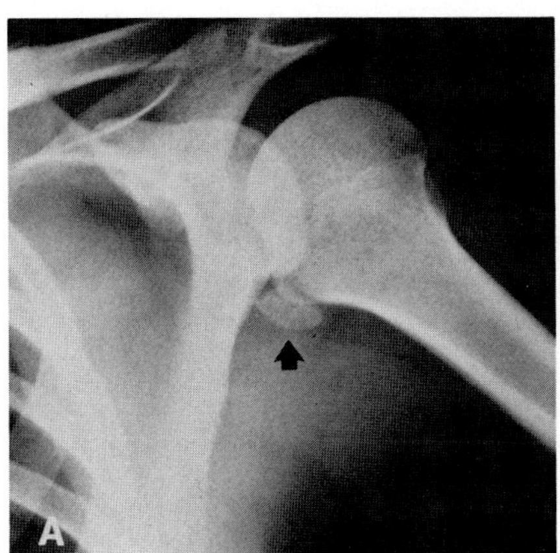

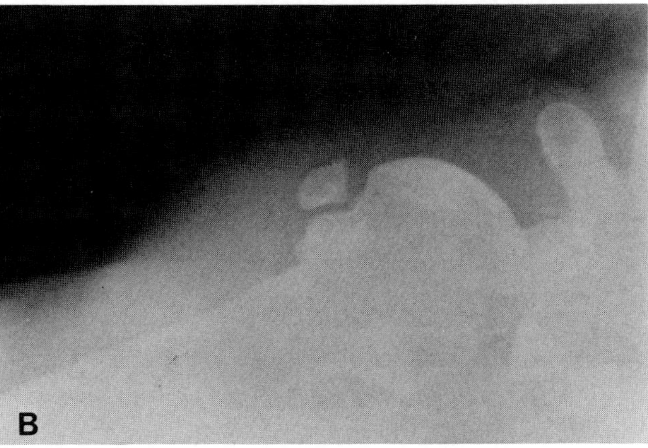

Fig. 11-115. Avulsion fracture of lesser tuberosity associated with posterior dislocation. (*A*) An axillary lateral view of the left shoulder reveals the old smooth-bordered fragment of the lesser tuberosity. (*B*) An anteroposterior view of the left shoulder taken with the arm in 45 degrees of abduction and full internal rotation. Note the avulsion fracture of the lesser tuberosity (*arrow*). The patient had a history of acute traumatic posterior dislocation in the past which was reduced on the playing field.

after total muscle relaxation has been accomplished, the reduction is very atraumatic. A modification of this technique is to apply traction to the adducted arm with the elbow flexed and use a slight internal rotation maneuver to dislodge the head from the posterior glenoid rim, followed by traction in external rotation to replace the articular surface in the glenoid fossa.

Recurrent Posterior Dislocation

With repeated recurring posterior dislocations, the pain and muscle spasm are less severe than with the first acute traumatic dislocation. Therefore, general anesthesia is usually not required. Sedation and pain relief, followed by traction to the adducted arm with posterior head pressure, will accomplish the reduction.

Unreduced Posterior Dislocation

The maneuvers for reducing an old unreduced posterior dislocation are the same as those for acute and recurrent posterior dislocations. However, if the dislocation has been missed for several weeks, or if a large anteromedial humeral head defect is seen on the axillary film, an open reduction is usually required (Fig. 11-116). I concur with DePalma, who recommends open reduction if the condition has existed longer than 2 weeks. Open reduction is required, because the shoulder is fixed so rigidly in its posterior position or because of the large size of the anteromedial defect in the humeral head, which is engaged on the posterior glenoid rim.

Atraumatic Injuries

Voluntary or Habitual Posterior Dislocation

Because of the very definition of this type of dislocation, the patient does not seek help for the reduction. The patient simply manipulates his shoulder into posterior subluxation or dislocation and reduces it at his own discretion. If the shoulder should become locked during one of these parlor tricks, a reduction like that described for recurrent posterior dislocations of the shoulder should be used.

Congenital or Developmental Posterior Dislocation

If any treatment is indicated, usually it will be in the nature of surgical reconstruction to restore muscle balance to the shoulder girdle or a realignment of the glenoid fossa. In the posterior subluxations or dislocations that occur with upper brachial plexus injuries caused at birth, multiple procedures have been described by Sever,[621] Fairbank,[547] L'Episcopo,[576] and Zachary.[642] Wickstrom[638] has reported on seven cases of posterior dislocation of the shoulder caused by upper brachial plexus birth injuries.

Indications for Surgery

Acute Posterior Dislocation

The need for surgery in the acute posterior dislocation of the shoulder is very unlikely, because with closed reduction the joint is quite stable. Indications would include a major displacement of an associated lesser tuberosity fragment or a locked or irreducible posterior dislocation. Adequate roentgenograms—particularly the anteroposterior, true lateral of the glenohumeral joint, and axillary lateral films—must be obtained, to determine the extent of the injury before surgery can be planned.

Recurrent Posterior Dislocation

The incidence of recurrent posterior dislocation of the shoulder has not been established, but it is an infrequent problem. If recurring posterior dislocation becomes a frequent problem, then surgical reconstruction should be performed.

Posterior Reconstruction. Most of the procedures utilized for posterior reconstruction are the reverse of the anterior glenohumeral reconstruction. The indications for each procedure depend upon a careful

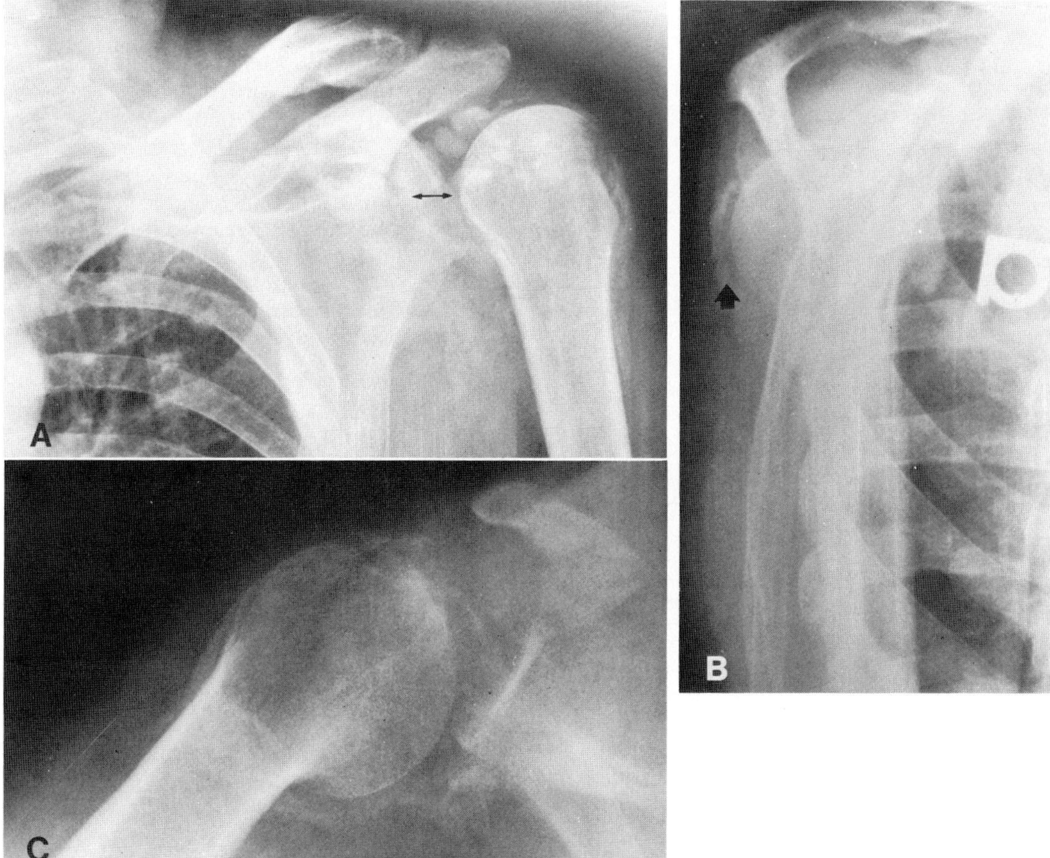

Fig. 11-116. Unreduced posterior dislocation of the left shoulder of 14 months duration. (*A*) An anteroposterior view shows that the left humerus is in marked internal rotation, and there is no profile of the neck of the humerus; the glenoid fossa is completely vacant of the humeral head. Note the marked amount of new bone formation about the shoulder joint as a result of physical therapy. (*B*) A true lateral view of the glenohumeral joint shows that the articular surface of the head of the humerus is posterior to the glenoid fossa. Note new bone formation posterior and superior to the humeral head (*arrow*). (*C*) An axillary lateral view taken with only 40 degrees of abduction also reveals heterotrophic bone formation about the glenohumeral joint and posterior displacement of the articular surface of the humerus.

evaluation of the etiology of the dislocation and complete roentgenographic studies.

Reverse Bankart. Only the posterior soft-tissue capsule structures are repaired.

Reverse Putti-Platt. The infraspinatus muscle and tendon is used in this muscle-shortening or muscle-plication procedure. In some cases, the infraspinatus and teres minor tendon may be used together in the plication.

The Boyd-Sisk[521] *Procedure.* A posterior capsulorrhaphy is performed with a posterior transfer of the long head of the triceps to the posterior glenoid rim.

Combined Soft-Tissue Repairs. These may be repairs of the posterior capsule, plication or double-breasting of the infraspinatus and/or teres minor muscles, and possibly using the long head of the biceps as an added suspensory ligament.

Reverse Eden-Hybbinette. This posterior bone-block procedure uses bone graft from the ilium, tibia, rib, spine, or the acromion process of the scapula.

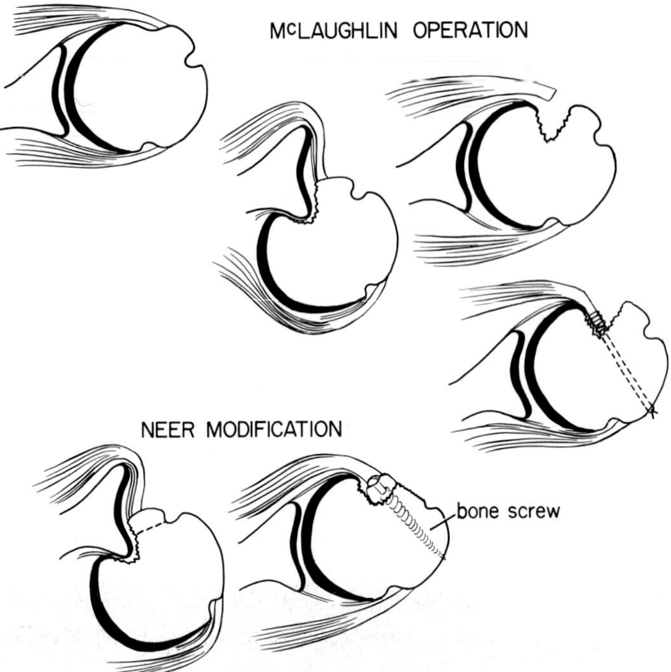

Fig. 11-117. When there is a large anteromedial humeral head defect, McLaughlin recommended that following reduction that through an anterior approach the tendon of the subscapularis be transferred into the humeral head defect. Neer has modified the procedure by transferring the lesser tuberosity with the attaching subscapularis tendon into the defect.

Glenoid Osteotomy. Kretzler and Blue,[574] Scott,[618] Kretzler,[573] and English and McNab[543] have all reported good results in using an opening, posterior wedge, glenoid osteotomy in recurrent posterior dislocations of the shoulder. In 1966, Kretzler and Blue[574] reported on the use of a posterior opening glenoid osteotomy in six patients with cerebral palsy. They used the acromion as the source of the graft, to hold the wedge open. Kretzler[573] reported on 31 cases of the posterior glenoid osteotomy in voluntary (15 cases) and involuntary (16 cases) posterior dislocations with recurrences in four patients, two from each category. English and McNab[543] have pointed out that, while there is a tendency for the humeral head to go into anterior subluxation during the osteotomy of the glenoid, it is unnecessary to supplement the procedure with an anterior soft-tissue reconstruction.

Combined Bone- and Soft-Tissue Reconstructions. Either the posterior bone block or the glenoid osteotomy can be combined with the various soft-tissue reconstructions.

McLaughlin Procedure. The specific indication for this operation is the presence of a large anteromedial humeral head defect. Through an anterior approach, the subscapularis is detached from the lesser tuberosity; the shoulder is reduced, and the subscapular tendon is transferred into the head defect (Fig. 11-117).[579,580] Neer* has modified this operation by transferring the lesser tuberosity with the tendon into the defect. The added fragment of the lesser tuberosity helps fill the space in the defect, and it is simpler to perform because the lesser tuberosity can be secured into the defect with a bone screw.

Unreduced Posterior Dislocation

If a patient, particularly an elderly patient, has had an unreduced posterior dislocation for years and it is not associated with pain and there is a functional range of motion, surgery is usually contraindicated. However, if disability exists and there is good bone stock to the glenohumeral joint, then a reconstruction is indicated. If the disability is severe with pain, poor range of motion, and a *large* humeral head defect (40% or more of the head destroyed)

* Personal communication.

but functioning muscles, a prosthesis can be used. If the patient has a poor range of motion, poor bone stock, and nonfunctioning muscles, an arthrodesis should be considered.

Before any of the operative reconstructions are performed, it is very important to determine whether or not the posterior glenoid rim is intact or has eroded into and produced a large anterior humeral head defect.

Reconstruction Without an Anteromedial Humeral Head Defect. In those cases where the humeral head defect compression fracture is small or nonexistent, the posterior approach should be utilized to perform the posterior reconstruction or posterior glenoid osteotomy as has been described.

Reconstruction With a Large Anteromedial Humeral Head Defect. If a large humeral head defect is present then several operative possibilities exist. Through a posterior approach, the head can be disengaged and a posterior reconstruction performed. Through an anterior approach, after the head is disengaged, the subscapularis is detached and implanted into the humeral head defect as described by McLaughlin[579,580] or as modified by Neer (Figs. 11-117, 11-118).

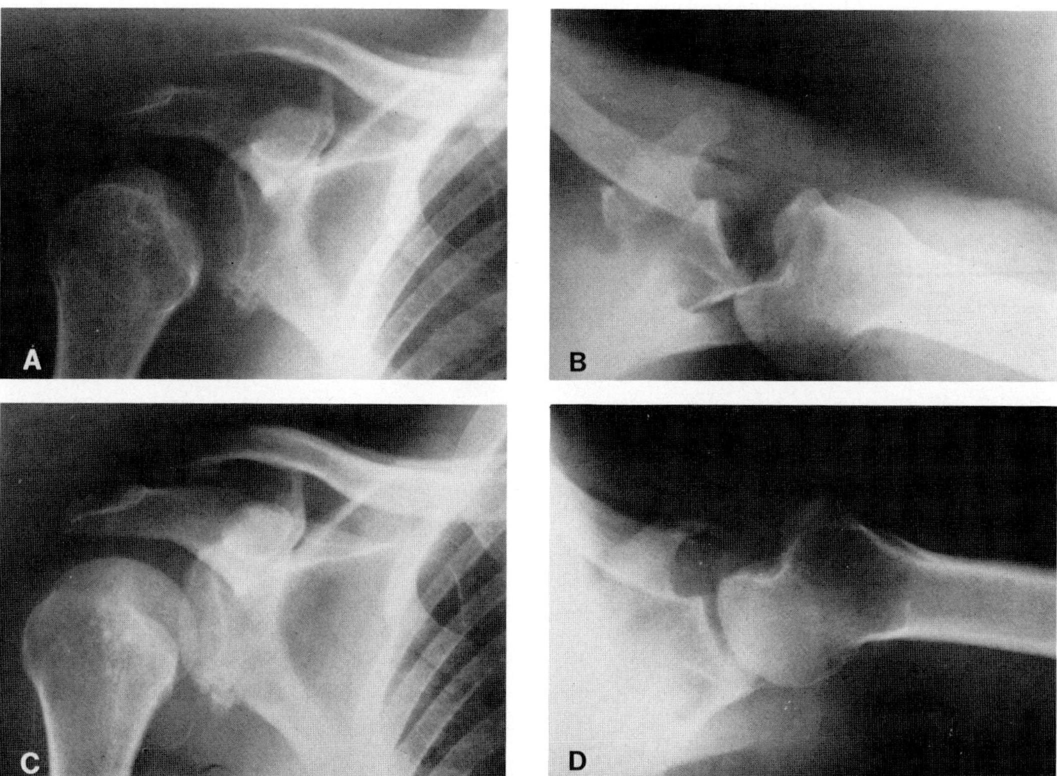

Fig. 11-118. Management of permanent posterior dislocation of the shoulder (*A, B* prereduction; *C, D* postreduction). (*A*) Subacromial permanent posterior dislocation of the right shoulder reveals a vacant glenoid sign and the appearance that the posterior glenoid rim has created a large defect in the humeral head. (*B*) The axillary lateral confirms the large anteromedial compression defect in the humeral head. Note the majority of the articular surface of the humeral head is posterior to the glenoid fossa. (*C*) The anteroposterior view shows that following the McLaughlin reconstruction, through an anterior approach, the humeral head is well within the glenoid fossa. (*D*) An axillary lateral roentgenogram confirms that the head of the humerus is relocated to the glenoid fossa. The subscapularis tendon has been transferred into the depth of the anteromedial defect, which blocks recurrent dislocations during internal rotation on the shoulder.

Neviaser[596-597] has described using a superior approach to perform the stripping operation of the upper humerus. This procedure can be used for either the unreduced anterior or posterior dislocation. In this procedure, the head and upper neck of the humerus are subperiosteally stripped of their capsule and muscle attachments. This allows for sufficient mobility to reduce the head into the cleared glenoid fossa, and it is held in place with a heavy pin.

Voluntary or Habitual Posterior Dislocation

The patient may be able to voluntarily dislocate the shoulder anteriorly as well as posteriorly. The dislocation usually is first noted at an early age. It is not preceded by trauma; it just happens. The patient, by voluntarily contracting some muscles about the shoulder and relaxing others, can induce subluxation or complete dislocation of the shoulder. It does present an unusual sight, and the patient may perform his feat as a party trick.

Rowe, Pierce, and Clark[614] have demonstrated in patients who do not have emotional or psychiatric disturbances that, with adequate conservative measures, the problem may subside. Conservative measures include a full explanation as to why the problem exists; a recommendation that the patient stop performing his trick or he will develop degenerative changes in the shoulder; and instruction in a rehabilitative program designed to strengthen the muscles about the shoulder. Occasionally, symptoms of the dislocation do persist and if the patient is judged to be emotionally stable, operative reconstructions can be performed successfully. In general, soft-tissue reconstructions in the voluntary or habitual dislocations have not given results as good as those from posterior bone block or posterior opening wedge osteotomy of the neck of the scapula.

Surgical reconstructions in the patient with voluntary posterior dislocation of the shoulder who has psychiatric or emotional disturbances are practically always a failure (Fig. 11-119). After three or four posterior procedures, you may succeed in

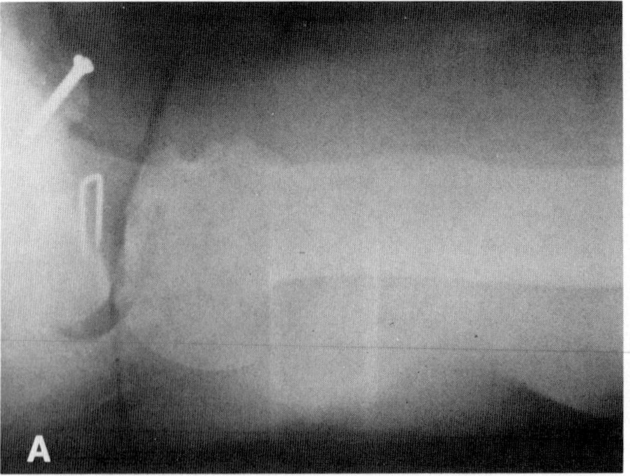

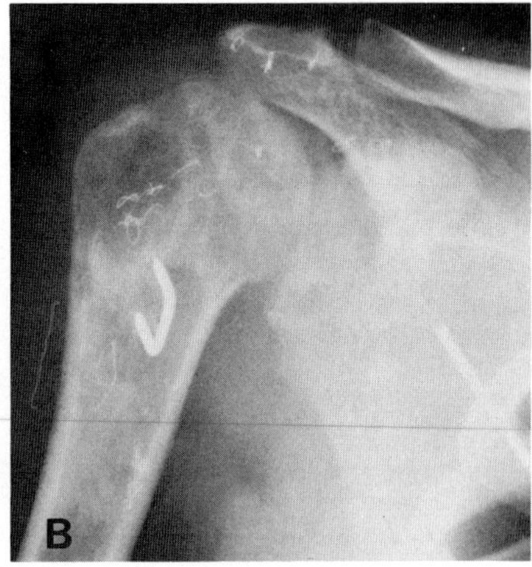

Fig. 11-119. Surgical failure in voluntary posterior dislocation of the shoulder. (*A*) Axillary lateral roentgenogram of a patient with voluntary dislocations of the shoulder who, after three anterior reconstructions, could no longer dislocate anteriorly and began to dislocate posteriorly. Note the loose staple anteriorly in the joint. (*B*) Anteroposterior roentgenogram of a patient with voluntary anterior and posterior dislocations of the shoulder who has had 8 attempts at reconstruction. The shoulder is still posteriorly dislocated; note the foreign bodies about the shoulder and the anterior chest wall. The end result of this problem was an arthrodesis.

preventing posterior dislocations, but then the patient will begin to dislocate the shoulder anteriorly. The usual end result, after six to eight anterior and posterior reconstructions, is a joint so degenerated that the final operation is an arthrodesis. So a word of warning: beware of surgery in the patient who has voluntary posterior dislocations who also has emotional or psychiatric disorders.

POSTOPERATIVE CARE

Acute Posterior Dislocation

The recommended techniques of post-reduction immobilization are quite varied. Three completely different types of immobilization have been recommended: (1) a sling and swathe position, which immobilizes the arm in internal rotation; (2) a shoulder spica or modifications thereof, which immobilize the arm in external rotation; and (3) pins placed down from the acromion into the humeral head.

If, after reduction, the shoulder is stable, then the sling and swathe immobilization is simplest and has been shown by McLaughlin[579] to be quite effective. However, if the shoulder tends to redislocate in the sling and swathe position, then a shoulder spica should be used. The amount of external rotation is determined by applying the cast with the arm in its most stable position. Wilson and McKeever[640] state that many of the acute traumatic posterior dislocations are unstable and recommend the use of external pins to maintain their closed reduction. In their technique, after the shoulder has been reduced, the arm is placed into the sling and swathe position. The head is then manually held reduced by a direct posterior pressure while two pins are drilled, in cruciate fashion, down from the acromion process into the reduced humeral head. The pins are removed after 3 weeks, and rehabilitation is instituted.

A large anterior humeral head defect, as is occasionally seen on axillary lateral roentgenograms, may predispose to recurrent dislocations, and the shoulder can best be immobilized with the arm in external rotation to allow posterior capsular healing. Scougall[620] has shown experimentally in monkeys that a surgically detached posterior glenoid and capsule heal soundly without repair. He concluded that the best position of immobilization, to allow healing for all of the posterior structures, was in abduction, external rotation, and extension, and that the position should be maintained for 4 weeks.

Stable reductions should be held 2 to 3 weeks, and unstable reductions should be held 3 to 4 weeks. As with anterior dislocations of the shoulder, the length of time of immobilization decreases with the increasing age of the patient.

Rehabilitation consists of essentially the same routine described for anterior dislocations (i.e., first the gravity-free Codman-type pendulum exercises to loosen up the joint, followed by gentle active assisted range-of-motion exercises, then exercises to strengthen muscles, particularly the external rotators of the shoulder). Overhead pulleys and heat, among others, should be used to restore function of all of the muscles about the shoulder girdle (see Fig. 11-69).

Recurrent and Voluntary Posterior Dislocation

After posterior soft-tissue or bone reconstructions, the shoulder should be immobilized for 4 to 6 weeks. The type of immobilization device varies from a sling and swathe to a shoulder spica. This is followed by Codman-type joint-loosening exercises for 1 to 2 weeks. Then the active assistive program is used to restore motion, and muscle-strengthening programs are instituted.

Unreduced Posterior Dislocation

McLaughlin[579] recommended the use of a sling and swathe position following the subscapularis transfer, and he begins gravity-free, Codman pendulum exercises when the wounds have healed. Others recommend plaster casts, which hold the arm in external rotation, for 2 to 4 weeks. The postoperative rehabilitation program is essentially the same as that for reconstructions following chronic posterior dislocations of the shoulder. Because of the fact that unreduced dislocations usually have been dislocated for weeks or months, the postoperative course is prolonged. Range of motion is limited, and prognosis is guarded. If a proximal humeral replacement prosthesis is used, then early passive assistive exercises, using the opposite upper extremity, are instituted, particularly flexion and external rotation (see p. 607).

AUTHOR'S PREFERRED METHOD OF TREATMENT

Acute Posterior Dislocation

I prefer to try the closed reduction first without general anesthesia. After an intravenous infusion is started, the patient is given a standard narcotic, half intramuscularly and half subcutaneously. In addition, a muscle relaxant or tranquilizer is given through the intravenous tubing. When the patient is tranquil and pain and muscle spasm have subsided, gentle traction is applied in line with the adducted and internally rotated humerus. Posterior pressure on the humeral head may be required. If traction and posterior pressure do not accomplish the reduction, I use gentle internal rotation to the arm to disengage the head from the posterior glenoid and, with continued traction and posterior head pressure, gently rotate the arm externally, which replaces the head in the glenoid fossa. It must be a gentle and gradual reduction. Force is not used. If the reduction cannot be accomplished easily without force and without significant pain to the patient, then a general anesthetic is used with the same maneuvers described above.

Recurrent Posterior Dislocation

If a large humeral head defect is not present, I prefer a combined posterior reconstruction primarily relying on a bone block with back-up support from soft-tissue reconstruction. The graft is taken from the posterior edge of the acromion, for it is in the operative field and has a gentle curve that seats very nicely on the posterior glenoid. If the acromion process is too small, bone graft is obtained from the posterior ilium. The graft should be applied on the lower half of the glenoid and should extend a few millimeters below the inferior lip of the glenoid fossa (Fig. 11-120A, B). The graft, 2.5 by 1.5 cm., is placed between the periosteum and the neck of the glenoid and held in place with two screws or two threaded pins which are long enough so that they can be removed under local anesthesia after 4 weeks (Fig. 11-120C, D). Following the insertion of the bone graft, the capsule is repaired or reefed, and the tendon of the infraspinatus muscle, which has been divided to expose the posterior capsule and joint, is effectively shortened by double-breasting the lateral edge of the tendon over the medial edge. I have had no experience in using the posterior glenoid opening wedge osteotomy as described by Kretzler and Blue,[574] Scott[618] and Kretzler,[573] or English and McNab.[543]

If a large anteromedial defect is present in the humeral head, I would perform the McLaughlin procedure as described below in the next section.

Unreduced Posterior Dislocation

Before reconstructing the unreduced dislocated shoulder, it is critical to ascertain whether or not there is a large anterior humeral head defect. If, on an axillary lateral roentgenogram, a large defect is apparent (and usually it is), then through a routine anterior operative approach I transfer the lesser tuberosity with the subscapularis tendon into the defect in the humeral head. If an anterior defect in the head is not

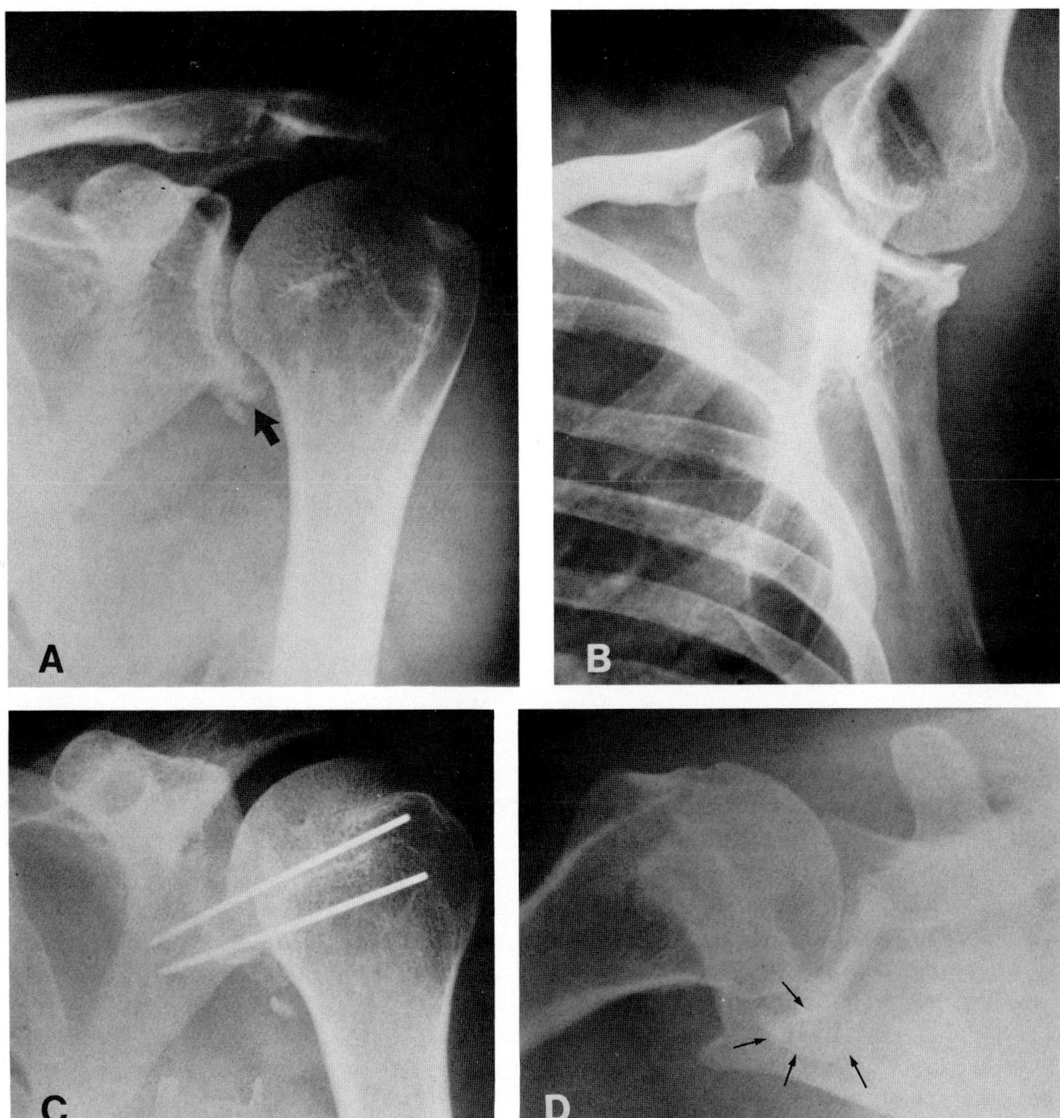

Fig. 11-120. Recurring posterior dislocation of the shoulder treated by posterior bone-block. (*A*) An anteroposterior roentgenogram 4 years after operation reveals that the posteroinferiorly placed bone graft is well incorporated (*arrow*). (*B*) At 160 degrees of abduction, the head is well seated in the glenoid fossa. (*C*) The bone graft, removed from the posterior acromion, is held in place with two threaded pins. (*D*) Axillary lateral reveals that posterior graft has incorporated to the scapula to form the posterior glenoid fossa (*arrow*). Note that the bone graft was taken from the posterior edge of the acromion process.

visualized on the axillary lateral roentgenograms, then a posterior approach is used to reconstruct the joint as described above under recurrent dislocations (i.e., combined bone block and soft-tissue reconstruction). In either the anterior or the posterior operative reconstruction, it may be necessary to maintain the glenohumeral relationship by inserting two large 5/32-inch smooth Steinmann pins through the humeral head into the glenoid for 10-14 days.

When it is noted at surgery that the humeral head is essentially destroyed (i.e., 40% or more of the articular surface has been eroded), I use the Neer humeral head replacement prothesis. Because the glenoid is usually undamaged, only a humeral head replacement is required. I have not seen a case with severe total joint destruction associated with nonfunctioning muscles about the shoulder, but if I saw one, I am sure I would consider either a total shoulder joint replacement or an arthrodesis.

Voluntary Posterior Dislocation

I concur completely with the outline for treatment as described by Rowe *et al.*[614] (p. 658).

Care After Operation

I am, essentially, in agreement with the routines that have been outlined. Ordinarily, the day following the McLaughlin reconstruction, I place the patient in a shoulder spica with the arm in 20 degrees external rotation. Following any of the reconstructions, when there is a tendency for the humeral head to displace posteriorly, I prefer the use of pins drilled laterally from the humerus into the glenoid rather than pins drilled down from the acromion process and into the humeral head.

PROGNOSIS

Unfortunately because posterior dislocation of the shoulder is such a rare entity, statistics are not available as they are with anterior dislocations of the shoulder. In general the following comments can be made:

Most acute traumatic posterior dislocations of the shoulder that are recognized and reduced primarily do not develop recurrent problems and have an excellent prognosis. Recurring posterior dislocations remain as recurring problems and require operative reconstructions. The soft-tissue procedures do not offer as good a result as the combined posterior bone block and soft-tissue reconstructions. Old unreduced posterior dislocation of the shoulder does not have as good a prognosis as either acute or recurring posterior dislocation. In general the longer the dislocation has been missed, the larger the humeral head defect will be—and the poorer the end result. Patients with a voluntary or habitual type of posterior dislocation, who have emotional or psychiatric problems, should not have surgical reconstructions, as they have a poor prognosis. Patients who are emotionally stable tend to have the same response to posterior reconstructions as the patients who have recurring-posterior dislocations.

COMPLICATIONS

Neurovascular problems are rare with all types of posterior dislocations of the shoulder. If subglenoid and subspinous dislocations were more common, I am certain that neurovascular complications would be reported.

INFERIOR DISLOCATION OF THE GLENOHUMERAL JOINT (LUXATIO ERECTA)

The incidence of this type of dislocation is so low that statistics are not available for review. However, in my experience, it is more common than superior dislocation of the glenohumeral joint and certainly more common than subclavicular, intrathoracic, and subspinous dislocations. Some authors have categorized luxatio erecta as a type of anterior dislocation, but I believe, because of the anatomical relationships, that this type of dislocation belongs in a separate category (i.e., the humerus is turned—upside down—with the entire humeral head below the glenoid fossa, Fig. 11-121A). It differs from the anterior and posterior subglenoid dislocations of the glenohumeral joint in that, with the luxatio erecta dislocation, the superior aspect of the articular

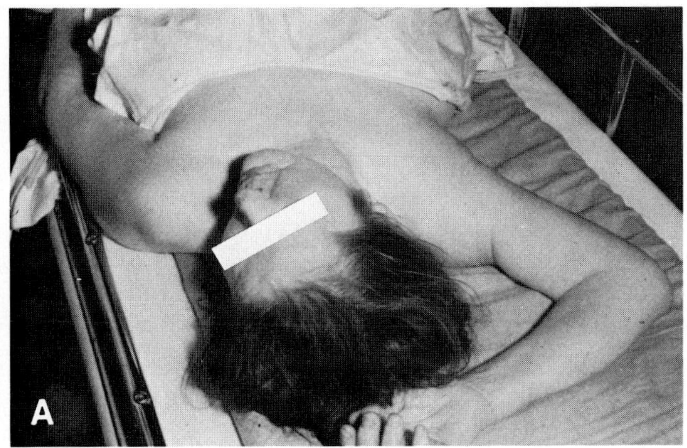

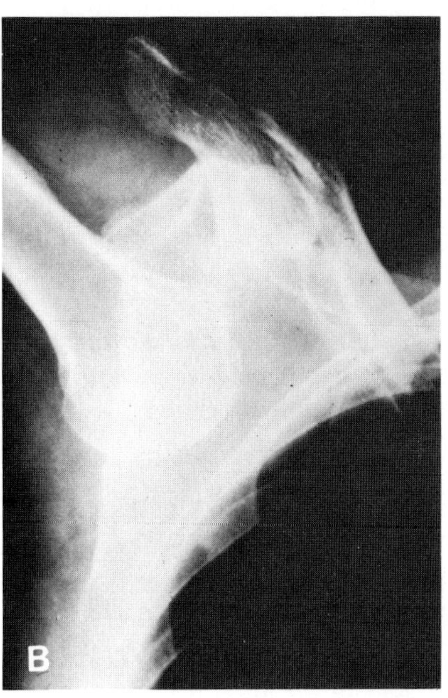

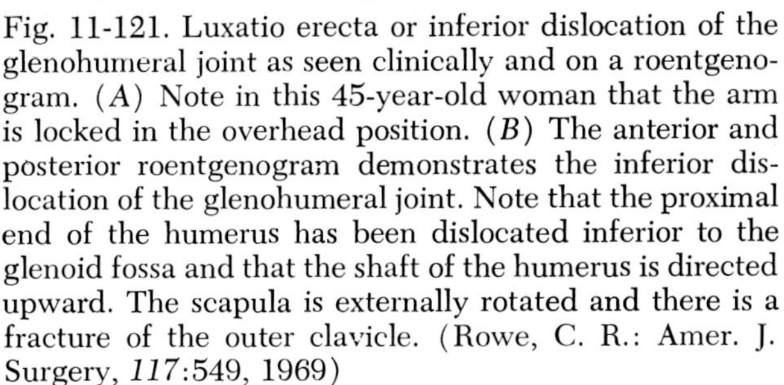

Fig. 11-121. Luxatio erecta or inferior dislocation of the glenohumeral joint as seen clinically and on a roentgenogram. (*A*) Note in this 45-year-old woman that the arm is locked in the overhead position. (*B*) The anterior and posterior roentgenogram demonstrates the inferior dislocation of the glenohumeral joint. Note that the proximal end of the humerus has been dislocated inferior to the glenoid fossa and that the shaft of the humerus is directed upward. The scapula is externally rotated and there is a fracture of the outer clavicle. (Rowe, C. R.: Amer. J. Surgery, *117*:549, 1969)

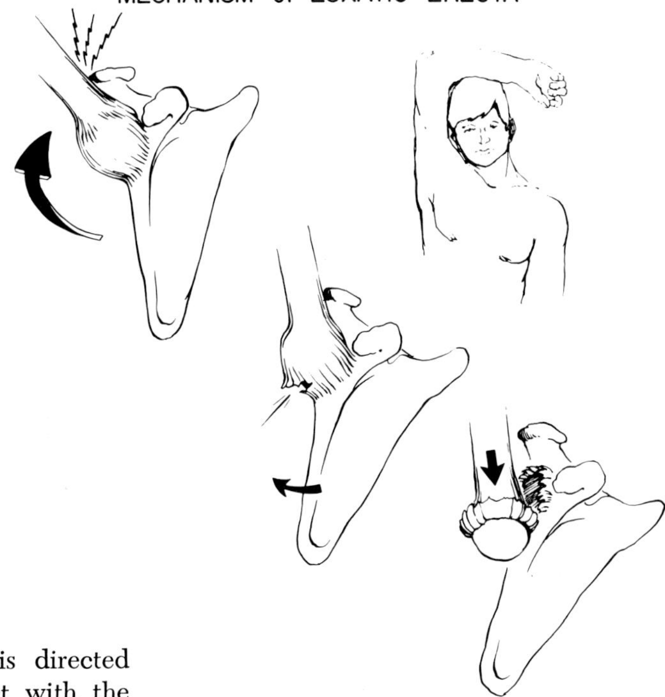

Fig. 11-122. With hyperabduction of the humerus, the shaft abuts the acromion process, which stresses and then tears the capsule inferiorly and levers the head out inferiorly. The head and neck may be buttonholed through a rent in the inferior capsule, or the entire capsule may be separated. The rotator cuff muscles are always detached and there may be an associated fracture of the greater tuberosity.

surface of the humeral head is directed inferiorly and is not in contact with the inferior glenoid rim.

The dislocation was first described by Middledorpf and Scharm[651] in 1859. Through cadaver work they also described the pathology involved. Lynn,[649] in 1921, reviewed 34 cases, and since that time only a few cases have been reported. Laskin[648] reported on luxatio erecta in infancy in 1971.

MECHANISM OF INJURY

Hyperabduction force produces an impingement of the neck of the humerus against the acromion process, which levers the head out inferiorly (Fig. 11-122). The humerus is then locked with the head below the glenoid fossa and the humeral shaft pointing overhead.

SIGNS AND SYMPTOMS

The clinical picture of a patient with luxatio erecta is so clear that it can hardly be mistaken for any other condition. The humerus points up overhead, and the arm is locked in this position. The elbow is usually flexed, and the forearm is lying on or behind the head (Fig. 11-121B). The head of the humerus may be palpated on the lateral chest wall. Pain is quite severe, and neurovascular complications may be present. The condition is more common among the elderly.

TREATMENT

Reduction is accomplished by traction and countertraction maneuvers. Traction should be applied in line with the arm (upward and outward) while countertraction is applied through a folded sheet up over and across the top of the shoulder by an assistant (Fig. 11-123). The line of countertraction is from across the top of the dislocated shoulder across the chest to the opposite side of the patient and, in general, is kept in line with the traction being applied to the arm of the dislocated shoulder. Occasionally, because the head and neck of the humerus have ruptured through the inferior capsule, closed reduction cannot be accomplished.[650] The buttonhole rent in the capsule must be enlarged at surgery before reduction can occur.

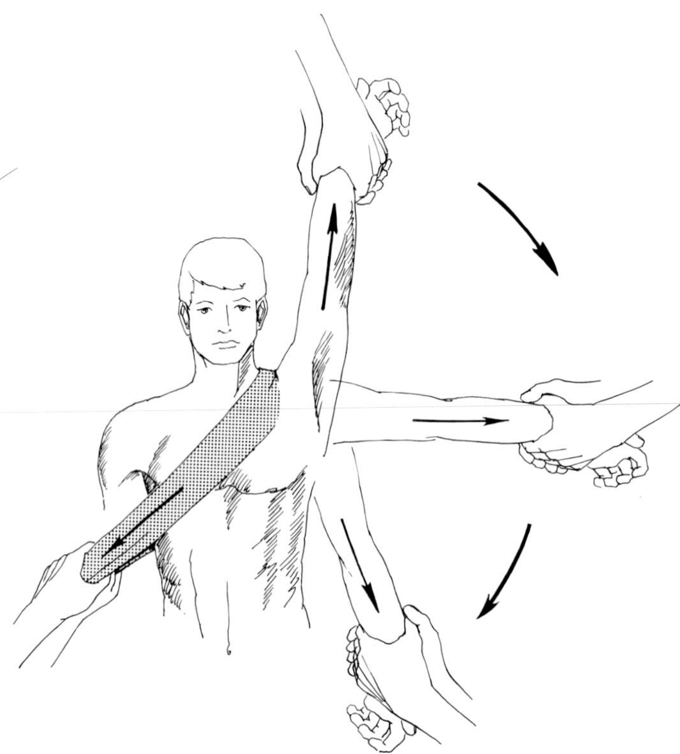

Fig. 11-123. Technique of reduction of an inferior dislocation (luxatio erecta) of the glenohumeral joint. Countertraction is applied by an assistant using a folded sheet across the superior aspect of the shoulder and neck. Traction on the arm is first applied upward and then gradually the arm is brought into less abduction and finally placed at the patient's side as demonstrated.

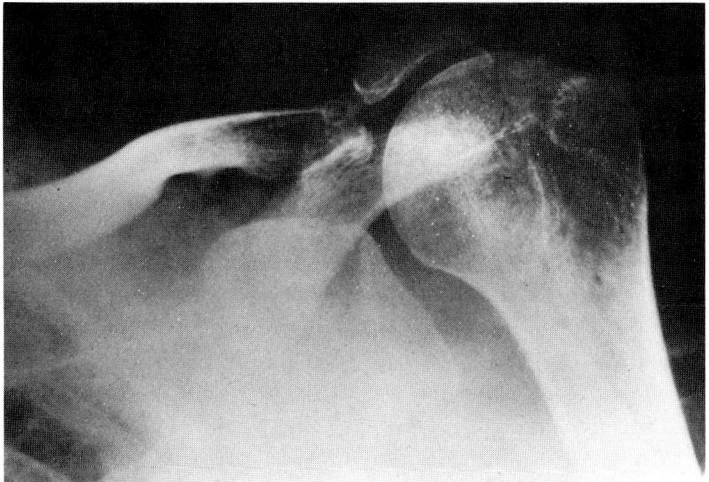

Fig. 11-124. Superior dislocation of the left shoulder. Note that the head of the humerus is displaced superiorly from the glenoid fossa and that the fracture of the acromion process has also been displaced upward.

COMPLICATIONS

Fractures may occur in the acromion process, the inferior glenoid fossa, or the greater tuberosity. The rotator cuff is detached, and possibly even the subscapularis tendon. Neurovascular damage may occur.

SUPERIOR DISLOCATION OF THE GLENOHUMERAL JOINT

Speed[652] reports that, in 1834, Langier was the first to record a case of superior dislocation of the glenohumeral joint, and Stimson[653] has reviewed 14 cases that had been reported in the literature prior to 1912. In current literature, little is mentioned of this type of dislocation, but undoubtedly occasional cases occur. The usual cause is an extreme forward and upward force on the adducted arm (Fig. 11-132). With displacement of the humerus upward, fractures may occur in the acromion, the acromioclavicular joint, the clavicle, the coracoid process, or the humeral tuberosities (Fig. 11-124). Extreme soft-tissue damage occurs to the capsule rotator cuff, the biceps tendon, and surrounding muscles. Clinically the head rides clearly above the level of the acromion, and the arm is shortened. The arm is adducted to the side, and shoulder movement is restricted and quite painful. Neurovascular complications are usually present. Treatment consists of closed reduction and restoration of the damaged tissues.

ACROMIOCLAVICULAR DISLOCATION

Dislocation of the acromioclavicular joint, and particularly the treatment of the injuries, has from the earliest medical writings been a subject of controversy. Hippocrates[655] (460 to 377 B.C.) said, "Physicians are particularly liable to be deceived in this accident (for as the separated bone protrudes, the top of the shoulder appears low and hollow), so that they may prepare as if for dislocation of the shoulder; for I have known many physicians otherwise not expert at the art who have done much mischief by attempting to reduce shoulders, thus supposing it as a case of dislocation." Galen[655] (129 to 199 A.D.) obviously had paid closs attention to Hippocrates, for he diagnosed his own acromioclavicular dislocation received from wrestling in the palestra. I think it is appropriate that one of the earliest reported cases in the literature was related to sports, as certainly today sports participation is one of the most common causes of acromioclavicular dislocations. This famous physician of the Graeco-Roman period treated himself in the manner of Hippocrates (that is, tight bandages to hold the projecting clavicle down while keeping the arm elevated).

From these earliest of publications on through the time of Paul of Aegina (7th century A.D.), the acromioclavicular joint became better recognized and the treatment remained essentially unchanged. Hippocrates[655] has said that no impediment, small or great, will result from such an injury. However, he went on to say that there would be a "tumefaction" or deformity, "for the bone cannot be properly restored to its natural situation." I suppose that this statement was, has been, and will be received by the orthopaedic world as a challenge, for there is probably not another small joint in the body that has been treated in so many different ways as the acromioclavicular joint in attempts to "properly restore" it to "its natural situation."

SURGICAL ANATOMY

The acromioclavicular joint is classified as a diarthrodial joint, and the articular surfaces are covered with fibrocartilage. Bosworth[685] states that the average size of the adult acromioclavicular joint is 9 mm. by 19 mm. The joint exists between the lateral end of the clavicle and the medial margin of the acromion process of the scapula (Fig. 11-125). Codman[697] relates that the acromioclavicular joint was only slightly movable, that it might swing a little, rock a little, twist a little, slide a little, and act like a hinge. DePalma[705] has shown that there is marked variability in the plane of the joint. Viewed from the front, the inclination of the joint may be almost vertical, or it may be inclined from downward medially, with the clavicle overriding the acromion by as much as an angle of 50 degrees (Fig. 11-126). Moseley[764] states that there may be an underriding type of inclination with the clavicle facet under the acromion process. In his experience, the vertical and underriding type of facets appear to be most prone to prolonged disability after injury. Urist[823] has shown that in 100 random roentgenograms of the shoulder, the articular surface of the clavicle overrides the articular surface of the acromion approximately 50 per cent of the time.

There may be two types of the fibrocartilaginous interarticular discs—complete and partial (meniscoid). The disc has great variation in its size and shape. DePalma[703] has demonstrated that with age the meniscus undergoes rapid degeneration until it is essentially no longer functional beyond the forth decade. The nerve supply to the acromioclavicular joint is from branches of the axillary, suprascapular and lateral pectoral nerves.

The Acromioclavicular Ligament

The joint is surrounded by a thin, weak capsule which is reinforced above and below by the superior and inferior acromioclavicular ligaments and even by the still weaker anterior and posterior acromioclavicular ligaments (Fig 11-127). The fibers of the superior acromioclavicular ligament blend with the fibers of the deltoid and trapezius muscles, which are attached onto the superior aspect of the clavicle and the acromion process. These muscle attachments are important, in that they strengthen the weak and thin ligament and add stability to the acromioclavicular joint.

Coracoclavicular Ligament

The coracoclavicular ligament is a very strong ligament whose fibers run from the outer inferior surface of the clavicle to the posteromedial aspect of the coracoid process of the scapula (Figs. 11-125, 11-127, 11-128). The coracoclavicular ligament has two parts, the conoid and the trapezoid ligaments.

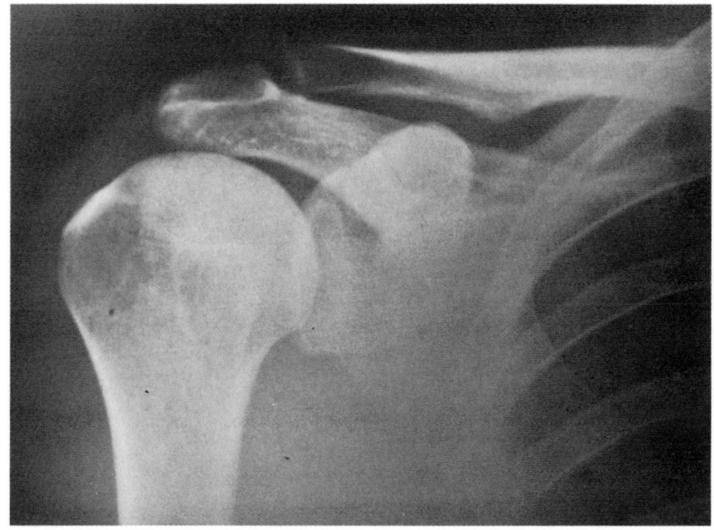

Fig. 11-125. Anteroposterior view of the normal shoulder. Note the acromioclavicular joint, the coracoid process, and the coracoclavicular interspace.

The conoid ligament[737] is cone-shaped with the apex of the cone attaching on the posteromedial side of the base of the coracoid process. The base of the cone attaches onto the conoid tubercle on the posterior undersurface of the clavicle. The conoid tubercle is located at the apex of the posteroclavicular curve, which is at the junction of the lateral third of the flattened clavicle with the medial two-thirds of the triangular-shaped shaft.

The trapezoid[737] arises anterior and lateral to the conoid ligament on the coracoid process and just behind the attaching pectoralis minor tendon. It extends superiorly to a rough line on the undersurface of the clavicle, which extends anteriorly and laterally from the conoid tubercle.

Function of the Coracoclavicular Ligament

Most authors agree that the primary function of the coracoclavicular ligament is to shore up and strengthen the nearby acromioclavicular articulation.[654,659,671,673,675,682,691,730,732,736,738,764,779,798,801,817] Owing to the medial and downward direction, the fibers of the ligament prevent the acromion process from being driven downward and medially.

According to Bosworth,[685] the average space between the clavicle and the coracoid process is 1.3 cm., and Bearden, Hughston, and Whatley[673] have found variations from 1.1 to 1.3 cm.

The only connection of the upper extremity with the axial skeleton is through the clavicular articulations at the acromio-

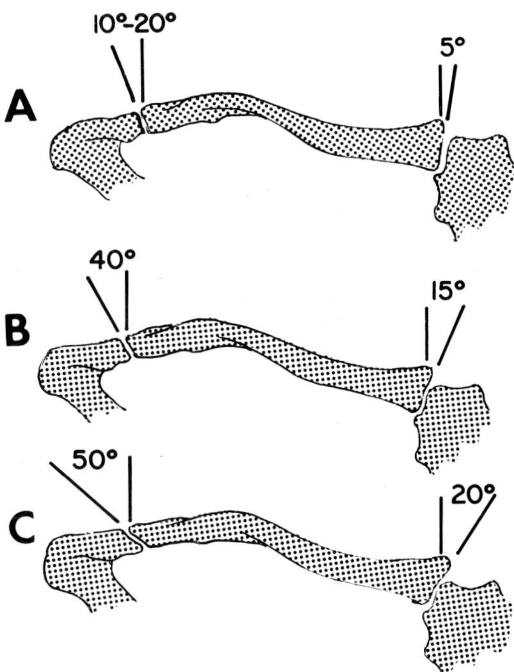

Fig. 11-126. Variations of the inclination of the acromioclavicular and the sternoclavicular joints. (Redrawn from DePalma, A. F.: Surgery of the Shoulder. Philadelphia, J. B. Lippincott, 1973)

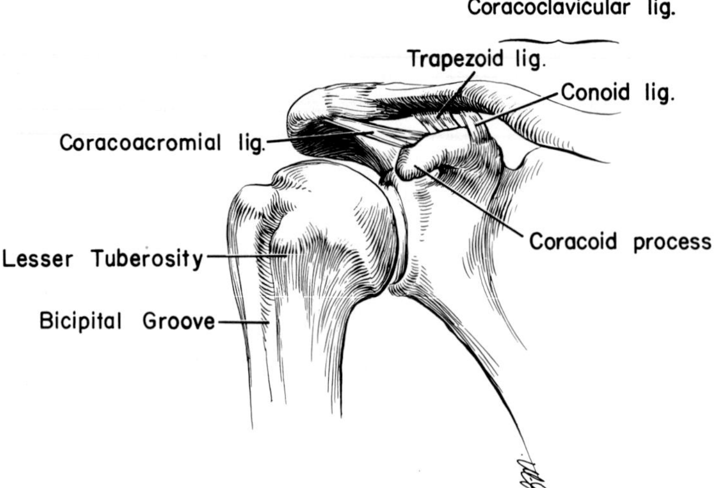

Fig. 11-127. Normal anatomy of the acromioclavicular joint.

clavicular and sternoclavicular joints. Therefore, the coracoclavicular ligament becomes the prime suspensory ligament of the upper extremity. The attachment of the coracoclavicular ligament on the apex of the posterior curve of the clavicle aids in clavicular rotation with abduction and elevation of the arm. Some authors feel that this is the prime importance of the coracoclavicular ligament.[704,705]

Cadenat,[691] in 1917, very carefully studied the importance of the coracoclavicular ligament in stabilizing the acromioclavicular joint. He concluded that a moderate blow to the acromion process would rupture the acromioclavicular ligament and produce an incomplete acromioclavicular dislocation and that a heavier blow would then rupture the coracoclavicular ligament and produce a complete dislocation. He then, with his own experiments, agrees with the studies of Poirier and Rieffel[788] and Delbet[691] and Mocquot,[691] which confirm that both the trapezoid and conoid portions of the coracoclavicular ligament must be divided to produce a complete dislocation of the acromioclavicular joint. He further pointed out that before the functional and clinical end results of a given injury can be evaluated, the physician must determine whether or not the dislocation was incomplete (a mild sprain to the joint) or complete (a complete dislocation of the joint).

Experimental Studies by Urist. Urist[823] concluded, after an extensive series of experiments, that *complete dislocation* of the acromioclavicular joint can occur without rupture of the coracoclavicular ligament. In a cadaver shoulder with the coracoclavicular ligament intact, he divided the superior acromioclavicular ligament and the entire joint capsule and detached the deltoid and trapezius muscles from the region of the acromioclavicular joint. He then demonstrated that under these conditions, the distal clavicle could be completely dislocated anteriorly and posteriorly away from the acromion process (i.e., in a horizontal plane). Since the coracoclavicular ligament was intact, upward displacement or subluxation of the acromioclavicular joint was minimal. Only after the coracoclavicular ligament was transected did a complete upward or vertical dislocation of the acromioclavicular joint occur.

I have repeated some of the cadaver studies of Urist[823] and agree with his anatomical findings, but I disagree with his terminology. The term *dislocation* of the acromioclavicular joint should be (and is) used to describe the *upward* or *vertical* displacement of the distal clavicle from the acromion, and not the anterior or posterior horizontal displacement.[656,658-660,662,673,682-685,691,694,704,705,730,734,738,739,743,749,756,764,765,767,768,793,801,812,813] Indeed, with the muscles and acro-

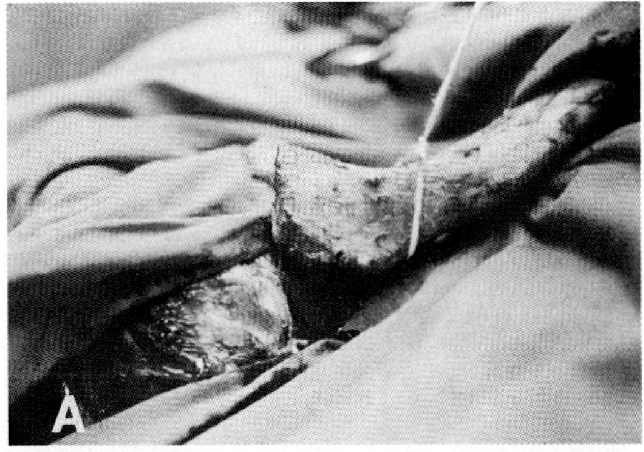

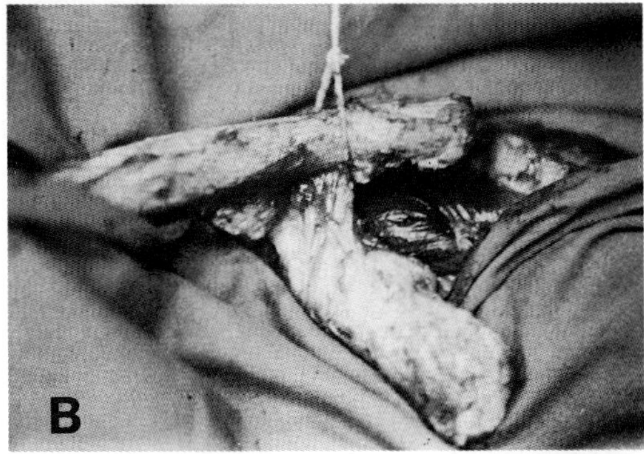

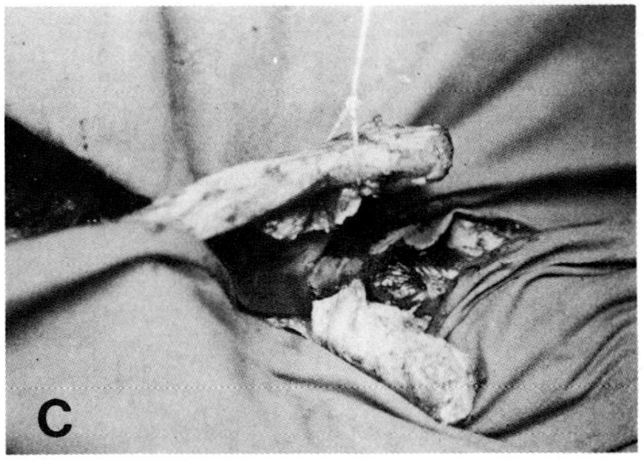

Fig. 11-128. The importance of the acromioclavicular and coracoclavicular ligaments for stability of the acromioclavicular joint, using a fresh cadaver. (*A*) With the muscles and acromioclavicular capsule and ligaments resected and with the coracoclavicular ligaments intact, the clavicle can be displaced anteriorly as shown or posteriorly from the articular surface of the acromion. (*B*) However, since the coracoclavicular ligaments are intact, the clavicle cannot be displaced significantly upward. (*C*) Following the transsection of the coracoclavicular ligaments the clavicle can be displaced completely above the acromion process. This suggests that the horizontal stability of the acromioclavicular joint is accomplished by the acromioclavicular ligaments, and vertical stability is obtained through the coracoclavicular ligaments.

mioclavicular ligaments detached, the clavicle can be dislocated in a horizontal position, either anterior or posterior to the acromion process (Fig. 11-128A). However, only a very slight upward displacement could be noted in the vertical plane (Fig. 11-128B). When the conoid and trapezoid ligaments have been cut, the lateral clavicle can be vertically and totally dislocated above the acromion process (Fig. 11-128C). These experiments have led to the conclusion that the horizontal stability of the acromioclavicular joint is controlled by the acromioclavicular ligaments, and the vertical stability is primarily dependent upon the coracoclavicular ligaments.

Coracoclavicular Articulation

The existence of a joint between the clavicle and the coracoid process is rare. Gradoyevitch[723] reported in 1939 that only 15 cases were known to medical science. Ten had been proven anatomically, and five were demonstrated by roentgenography. He reported one case with bilateral coracoclavicular joints. The patient's shoulders were asymptomatic and symmetrical, and he had normal range of motion. There were no abnormal findings of either the acromioclavicular or sternoclavicular joints.

Roentgenographic Appearance. Roentgenograms reveal a bony outgrowth from the undersurface of the clavicle. The outgrowth is triangular with the base of the triangle on the inferior surface of the clavicle and the lateral border of the triangle forming the articular surface with the tubercle with the dorsomedial surface of the coracoid process (Fig. 11-129). Not only does it look like a typical joint on the roentgenogram, but Schlyvitch[723] has dissected specimens and found a diarthrodial joint (that is, articular surfaces, a true capsule, and an intraarticular synovial membrane).

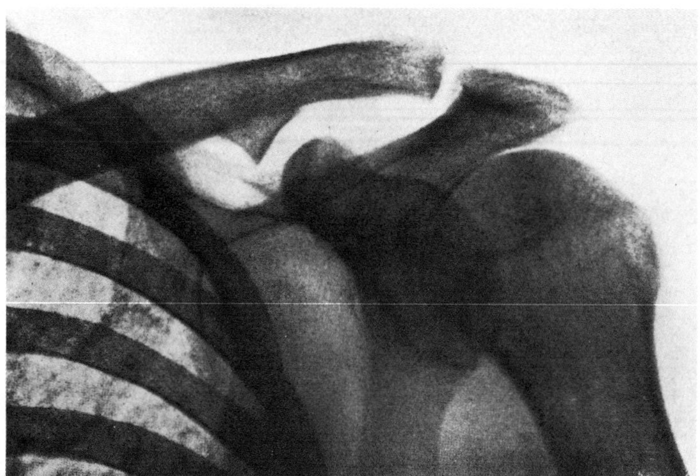

Fig. 11-129. Coracoclavicular articulation. This roentgenogram demonstrates the triangular bony outgrowth from the inferior clavicle and the general appearance of an articular surface with the dorsal medial aspect of the coracoid process. (Gradoyevitch, B.: J. Bone Joint Surg., *21*:918-920, 1939)

Incidence. In an attempt to determine the frequency of the coracoclavicular joint, Nutter[777] reviewed 1,000 roentgenograms of adult shoulders at random and found 12 cases, an incidence of 1.2 per cent. Six of the 12 cases were bilateral, and 11 of the 12 were in men. Liberson[743] reported an incidence of nine patients in 1800 shoulders studied; five had bilateral coracoclavicular joints. According to Wertheimer,[836] Poirier found one case in 2300 shoulders. Frassetto[836] is of the opinion that a coracoclavicular articulation predisposes to fracture of the neck of the humerus. His reasoning is that a fall on an outstretched hand is normally buffered somewhat by the rotation of the scapula about the thorax, and this is not possible when there is an extra articulation between the coracoid process of the scapula and the clavicle. Wertheimer[836] has excised the coracoclavicular joint of a manual laborer because of pain.

MOTIONS OF THE ACROMIOCLAVICULAR JOINT

The basic article by Inman, Saunders, and Abbott[733] showed that the total range of motion of the acromioclavicular joint is 20 degrees. It occurs in the first 30 degrees of abduction of the arm and after 135 degrees of elevation of the arm. They also demonstrated that with full elevation of the arm, the clavicle rotates upward 40 degrees. When they manually held the pin, which prevents clavicular rotation, abduction of the arm was restricted to 110 degrees, and they concluded the clavicular rotation was the fundamental feature of shoulder motion. Further, they concluded that an arthrodesis of the acromioclavicular joint would limit clavicular rotation and hence severely limit abduction of the arm. Authors since 1944 have condemned the use of the coracoclavicular screw, because, essentially, it produced an extraarticular acromioclavicular arthrodesis, which prevented normal clavicular rotation, the end result of which was limitation of elevation or abduction of the arm. However, in 1943 Caldwell[693] reported on two cases of acromioclavicular dislocation treated by arthrodesis of the acromioclavicular joint. One patient gained a full free range of motion of the shoulder, and the other had abduction to 165 degrees. Kennedy[738] and Kennedy and Cameron[739] have demonstrated that patients who have a coracoclavicular screw in place have an arthrodesis between the clavicle and the coracoid and are capable of full abduction. They also have demonstrated that patients, who have a coracoclavicular screw, can still have full abductions.

I have drilled Kirschner wires anteriorly into both clavicles of patients who have a

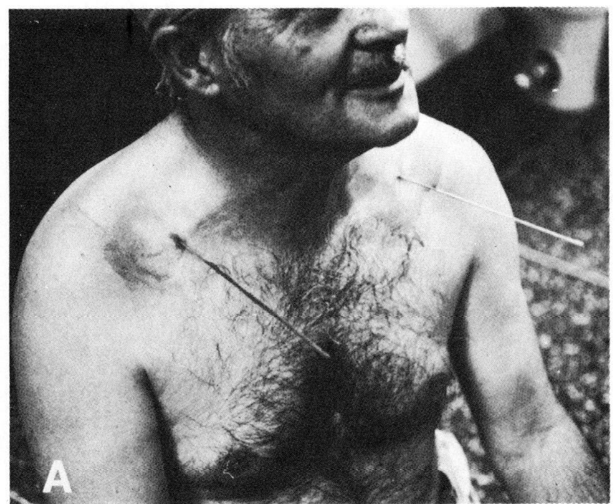

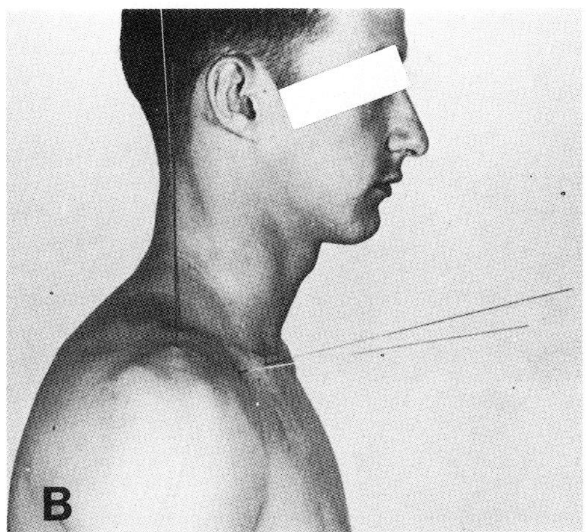

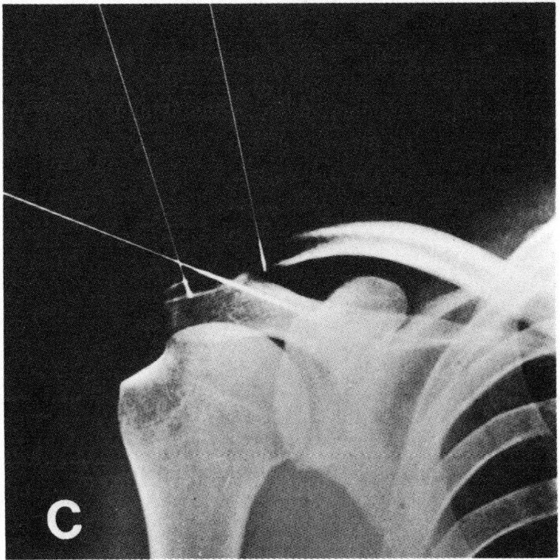

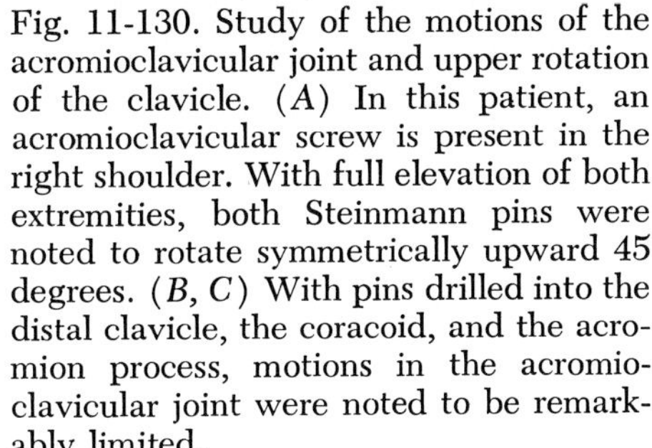

Fig. 11-130. Study of the motions of the acromioclavicular joint and upper rotation of the clavicle. (*A*) In this patient, an acromioclavicular screw is present in the right shoulder. With full elevation of both extremities, both Steinmann pins were noted to rotate symmetrically upward 45 degrees. (*B, C*) With pins drilled into the distal clavicle, the coracoid, and the acromion process, motions in the acromioclavicular joint were noted to be remarkably limited.

screw across the coracoclavicular space (Fig. 11-130A). The degree of upward rotation of each pin during shoulder abduction and forward flexion was essentially the same—40 degrees. This is in complete agreement with the work of Kennedy and Cameron,[739] who concluded that with screw fixation, a new movement has been introduced into the abduction mechanism of the shoulder. They call this "synchronous scapuloclavicular rotation."

In further studies of motion of the clavicle and the scapula, Kennedy and Cameron[739] showed that with the coracoclavicular screw in place, the degree of elevation of the clavicular wires corresponds to the degree of depression of pins drilled into the scapular spine. I have made similar determinations, but in the normal shoulder. Pins were placed anteriorly into the clavicle and superiorly into the acromion process, and the amount of displacement of the pins was measured during abduction and forward flexion (Fig. 11-130B, C). The results of these preliminary studies indicate that the amount of upward clavicular rotation is essentially the same as the amount of downward displacement of the acromion. This has led me to believe that the motion in the acromioclavicular joint is very limited.

MECHANISM OF INJURY

Direct Force

Injury by direct force is produced by the patient falling onto the point of the shoulder with the arm at the side in the adducted position (Fig. 11-131). This is the most common cause of acromioclavicular dislocations. The force drives the acromioclavicular joint downward and medially until the clavicle rests against the first rib. The rib prevents further downward displacement and the clavicle or the first rib

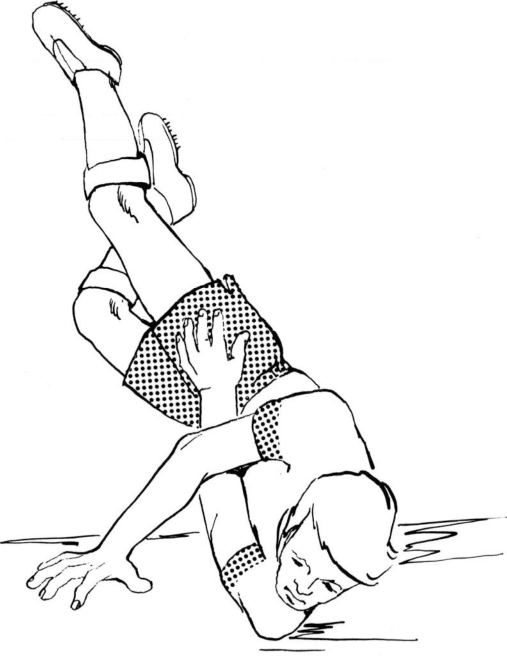

Fig. 11-131. The most common mechanism of injury is a direct force that occurs from a fall on the point of the shoulder.

fractures or the forces are transmitted directly to the acromioclavicular joint. If no fracture occurs, the force sprains first the acromioclavicular ligaments (a mild sprain), then tears the acromioclavicular ligaments (a moderate sprain), then stresses the coracoclavicular ligament, and finally—if the downward force continues—tears the deltoid and trapezius muscle attachments from the clavicle and ruptures the coracoclavicular ligament (a severe acromioclavicular sprain which completes the dislocation). At this point, the upper extremity has lost its ligament support and hence its articulations to the axial skeleton, and it droops from the high-riding clavicle.

Indirect Force

Upward Indirect Force on the Upper Extremity

Force from a fall on the outstretched hand is transmitted up the arm through the humeral head into the acromion process. The strain is referred only to the acromioclavicular ligaments and not to the coracoclavicular ligaments, as the coracoclavicular space is actually decreased (Fig. 11-132). This indirect force then can produce mild, moderate, or severe acromioclavicular joint injury. If the force were severe enough, it could fracture the acromion and cause a superior dislocation of the glenohumeral joint.

Downward Force Through the Upper Extremity

Forces can be applied indirectly to the acromioclavicular joint by a pull through

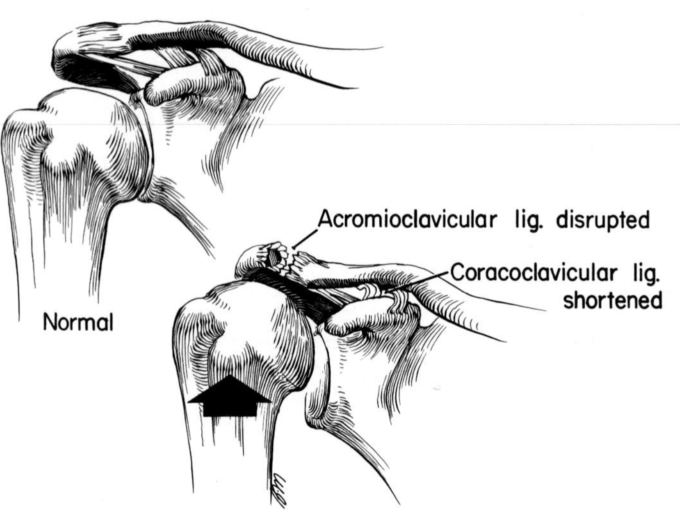

Fig. 11-132. An indirect force applied up through the upper extremity (e.g., a fall on the outstretched hand) may superiorly displace the acromion from the clavicle, producing injury to the acromioclavicular ligaments. However, stress is not placed on the coracoclavicular ligaments.

the upper extremity. Liberson[743] reported a case in which the scapula was forcibly drawn downward and anteriorly by a sudden change in the position of a heavy burden being carried.

CLASSIFICATIONS OF INJURY

Acromioclavicular joint injuries are best classified according to the amount of damage that is done by a given force. However, unlike other joints, the differential diagnosis of sprains of the acromioclavicular joint is based on the amount of injury to the ligament of the joint *and* on the amount of damage that has been done to the ligaments that are accessory in nature and that are anatomically separated from the acromioclavicular joint (that is, the coracoclavicular ligaments). Therefore, injuries to the acromioclavicular joint are graded upon the amount of injury to the acromioclavicular and the coracoclavicular ligaments.

Type I (Mild Sprain)

A mild force to the point of the shoulder produces a minor strain to the fibers of the acromioclavicular ligaments. The ligaments remain intact, and the acromioclavicular joint remains stable (Fig. 11-133A, B).

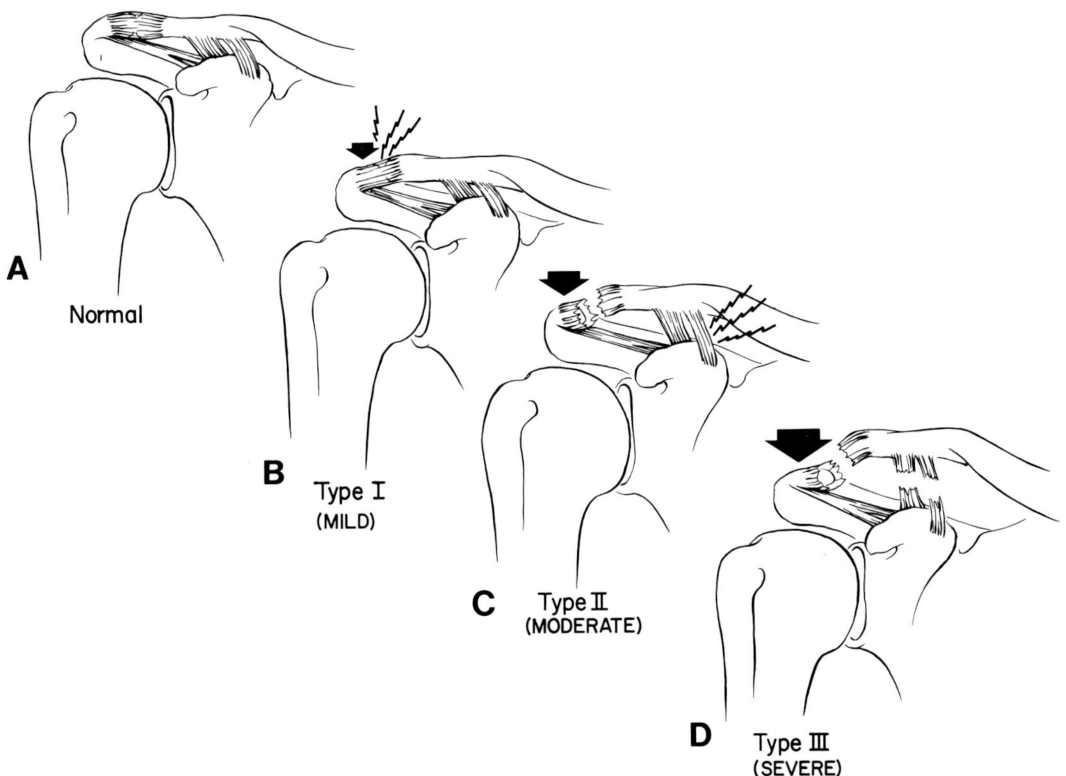

Fig. 11-133. These schematic drawings illustrate the ligamentous injuries that occur to the acromioclavicular joint. (*A*) Normal anatomical relationships. (*B*) In Type I injury, a mild force is applied to the point of the shoulder, which stretches only the acromioclavicular joints but does not disrupt the fibers of the joint. (*C*) In Type II injury, a moderate force applied to the point of the shoulder displaces the acromion process distally, disrupts the acromioclavicular ligaments, and may partially stretch the coracoclavicular ligaments. (*D*) In Type III injury, the severe force applied to the point of the shoulder drives the acromion and accompanying coracoid process downward, disrupting both the acromioclavicular and coracoclavicular ligaments. (Modified from Allman, F. L.: J. Bone Joint Surg., *49A*:774, 1967)

Type II (Moderate Sprain)

A moderate force to the point of the shoulder is severe enough to separate the ligaments of the acromioclavicular joint (Fig. 11-133C). The lateral clavicle is unstable, in that it may be displaced posteriorly or even may be thrown into slight subluxation upward from the acromion. The fibers of the coracoclavicular ligament may be strained slightly, but the ligaments remain intact. This is known as subluxation of the acromioclavicular joint.

Type III (Severe Sprain)

When a severe force is applied to the point of the shoulder, the acromioclavicular and the coracoclavicular ligaments are disrupted (Fig. 11-133D). Occasionally the coracoclavicular ligaments remain intact and produce an avulsion fracture of the coracoid process.

Possible Pathology in Acromioclavicular Injuries

Sprain of the acromioclavicular ligaments
Tear of the acromioclavicular ligaments
Sprain or tear of the coracoclavicular ligaments
Detachment of the deltoid and trapezius muscles from the clavicle
Fracture of the acromion or clavicle
Fracture of the coracoid process
Upward or inferior displacement of the clavicle

Superior Dislocation

In a superior dislocation of the acromioclavicular joint the lateral end of the clavicle is superiorly displaced in relationship to the acromion process. The deltoid and trapezius muscles are completely detached from the clavicle, or the periosteal sleeve with muscle attachments may be separated from the outer clavicle.

Injuries to the acromioclavicular joint can be further classified as to whether they are acute injuries or old chronic injuries. A classification based on the anatomical location of the dislocations seems unjustified, as practically all of the total dislocations consist of the clavicle riding above the acromion process.

Inferior Dislocation

Rarely, the physician may see an inferior dislocation, as reported by Patterson,[783] in which the clavicle was displaced under the coracoid process and behind the intact conjoined biceps and coracobrachialis tendons. The patient did not have any neurovascular problems. The author theorized that the mechanism was wide abduction of the arm and retraction of the scapula. Interestingly, before an open reduction was performed, the patient had a nearly normal range of motion of the upper extremity and no pain in his shoulder.

Incidence of Acromioclavicular Injuries

Rowe[526] (in a review of 1600 injuries to the shoulder in which there were 394 dislocations) has demonstrated that dislocations of the acromioclavicular account for 12 per cent of dislocations of the shoulder (85% glenohumeral and 2 to 3% sternoclavicular). Most authors report that the incidence of injury to the acromioclavicular joint is 5 males : 1 female. In some series, the proportion is 10 males : 1 female. Most authors also agree that incomplete injuries are twice as common as complete dislocations of the acromioclavicular joint.

SIGNS AND SYMPTOMS OF ACROMIOCLAVICULAR DISLOCATION

When an acromioclavicular joint injury is suspected, the patient should be examined, whenever possible, in the standing or sitting position. The weight of the arm stresses the acromioclavicular joint and may make a deformity more apparent.

Type I Injury

There is minimal to moderate joint tenderness and swelling over the acromioclavicular joint without palpable displacement of the joint. Usually there is only minimal pain with arm movements. Pain is not present in the coracoclavicular interval.

Type II Injury

With subluxation of the acromioclavicular joint, moderate to severe pain is noted at the joint. If the patient is seen soon after the injury, the outer end of the clavicle may be noted to ride higher than the acromion. Any motion of the arm produces pain referred to the acromioclavicular joint. With gentle palpation, the outer end of the clavicle may appear to be unstable and free-floating. If you grasp the mid-clavicle and stabilize the shoulder, you can detect a to-and-fro motion of the clavicle in the horizontal plane. Pain usually is felt when the physician palpates anteriorly in the coracoclavicular interspace.

Type III Injury

The patient with Type III injury, a dislocation of the acromioclavicular joint, characteristically presents with the upper extremity held abducted close to his body and upward to relieve the pain in the acromioclavicular joint. The shoulder appears depressed when compared to the normal shoulder, and the clavicle may be riding high enough to tent the skin. Severe pain is the rule, and any motion of the arm, particularly abduction, increases the pain. With palpation, pain is noted at the acromioclavicular joint, at the coracoclavicular interspace, and along the superior aspect of the lateral third of the clavicle. The lateral clavicle is quite unstable and seems to be floating free (Fig. 11-137D). Delbet[691] has stated that the clavicle in this situation may be so raised and prominent that it can be depressed like a piano key. Occasionally, instead of upper displacement, the clavicle is displaced so far posteriorly that it is trapped in the trapezius muscle.

Sir Astley Cooper,[699] in 1832, described a technique that could be used even by a blind man to detect the complete acromioclavicular dislocation: "The easiest mode of detecting this accident is to place the finger upon the spine of the scapula and to trace this portion of the bone forward to the acromion in which it ends; the finger is stopped by the projection of the clavicle, and so, as the shoulders are drawn back, the point of the clavicle sinks into place, but it reappears when the shoulders let go."

ROENTGENOGRAPHIC FINDINGS IN ACROMIOCLAVICULAR JOINT INJURIES

In most instances, roentgenograms of the acromioclavicular joint are made by using the same x-ray exposure settings used for penetrating the more dense glenohumeral joint. This produces a very dark, overpenetrated film of the acromioclavicular joint which is impossible to interpret (Fig. 11-134A). Therefore, you must request of the radiologist, not "shoulder" films, but specifically, films of the acromioclavicular joint. Quality films of the acromioclavicular joint require about one-third the beam intensity that is required for a quality roentgenogram of the glenohumeral joint (Fig. 11-134B). Even good quality anteroposterior films of the acromioclavicular joint are not always sufficient to diagnose the injuries. Unless there is a slight upward tilt to the x-ray beam, the acromioclavicular joint will be superimposed upon the acromion process, and small fractures will be missed (Fig. 11-134C, 11-135). Zanca,[840] therefore, has recommended that a 15-degree upward tilt view of the acromioclavicular joint be made routinely.

Patients who present clinically with the obvious high-riding clavicle of total dislocation have the obvious and characteristic roentgenographic findings of a complete dislocation. However, it is impossible to differentiate clinically all cases of Type II subluxations from a Type III complete dislocation. Therefore, stress films of both shoulders, which test the integrity of the coracoclavicular ligaments, should be made routinely when an injury of the acromioclavicular joint is suspected.

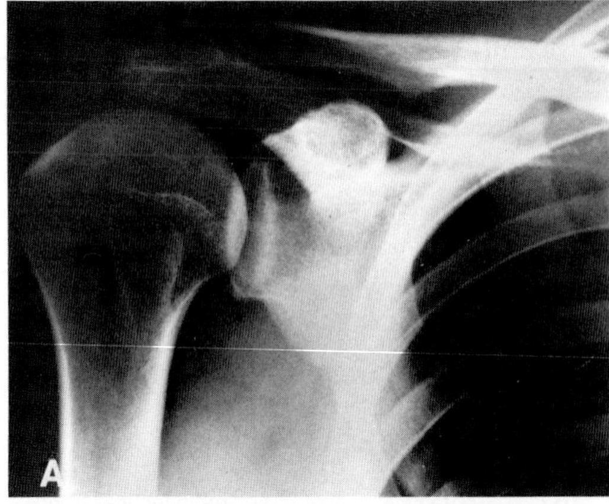

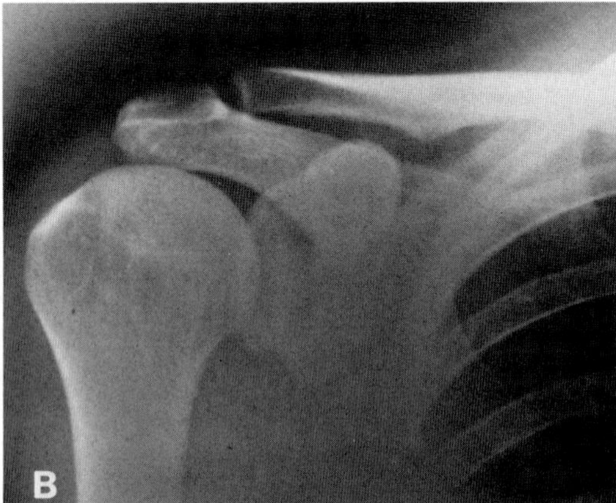

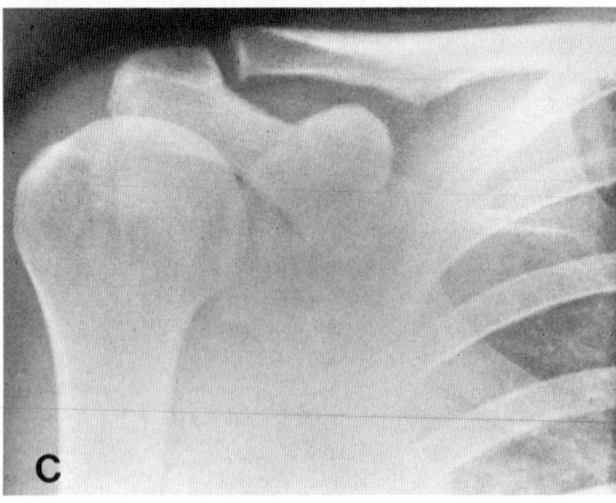

Fig. 11-134. Explanation of why the acromioclavicular joint is poorly visualized on routine shoulder roentgenograms. (*A*) This routine anteroposterior roentgenogram of the shoulder shows the glenohumeral joint well. However, the acromioclavicular joint is too dark to interpret, because that area of the anatomy has been overpenetrated by the x-ray technique. (*B*) When the exposure usually used to take the shoulder films is decreased by two-thirds, the acromioclavicular joint is well visualized. However, the inferior corner of the acromioclavicular joint is superimposed on the acromion process. (*C*) Tilting the tube 15 degrees upward clearly visualizes the acromioclavicular joint.

Technique of Stress Film

The patient should be standing or sitting with his arms hanging free and his back against a cassette large enough to visualize both shoulders (Fig. 11-136A). Five to 15 lbs. of weight—not held in the hand, but suspended by a loop of webbing around the wrists—allows for total relaxation of the muscles of the upper extremity and prevents any muscle forces from lifting the arm upward, which could alter the amount of coracoclavicular separation (Fig. 11-136A). The average distance between the superior aspect of the coracoid process and the inferior aspect of the clavicle varies from 1.1 to 1.3 cm.[673,685] However, the important detail is the comparison of the measured distances in the coracoclavicular space between the injured shoulder and the intact one (Fig. 11-136B). A difference of 3-4 mm. or less in the two measurements suggests only a moderate sprain with stretching of the ligaments. According to Bearden *et al.*,[673] an increase of the coracoclavicular distance of the injured shoulder over the normal shoulder by 40 to 50 per cent can be considered a complete coracoclavicular ligament disruption. I have documented that a difference of 5 mm. has been diagnostic of a complete disruption of the coracoclavicular ligaments (Fig. 11-147).

The routine use of stress films in doubtful cases prevents the patient from holding up his injured arm while the roentgenogram is being taken. I have seen normal roentgenograms of the acromioclavicular joint in patients who have total dislocations because the patient has reduced the joint

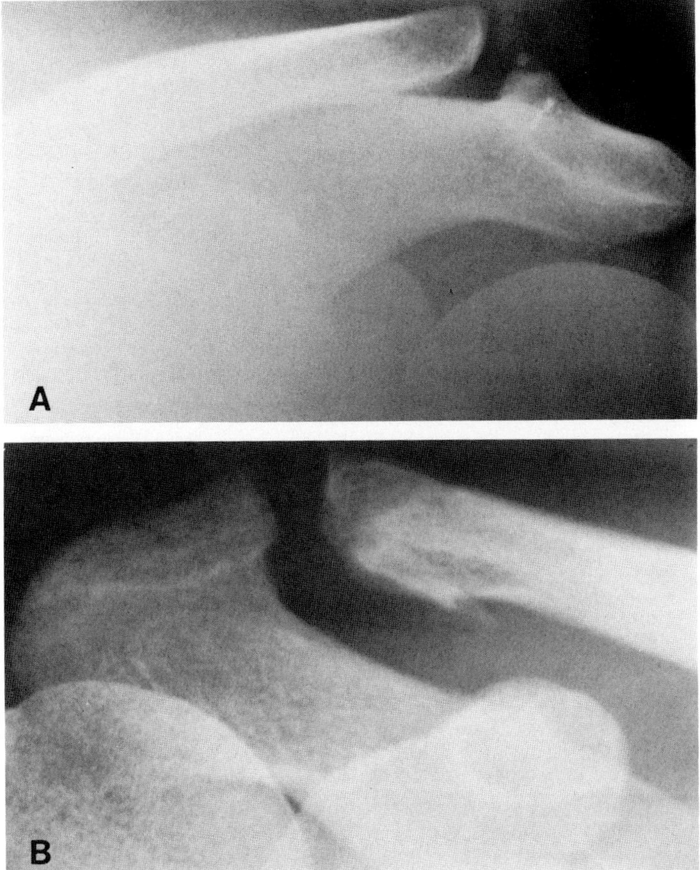

Fig. 11-135. Intraarticular fractures of the acromioclavicular joint. (*A*) An anteroposterior roentgenogram of the acromioclavicular joint with a small intraarticular fracture of the superior corner of the acromion. (*B*) An intraarticular fracture in the acromioclavicular joint involving the inferior portion of the distal clavicle.

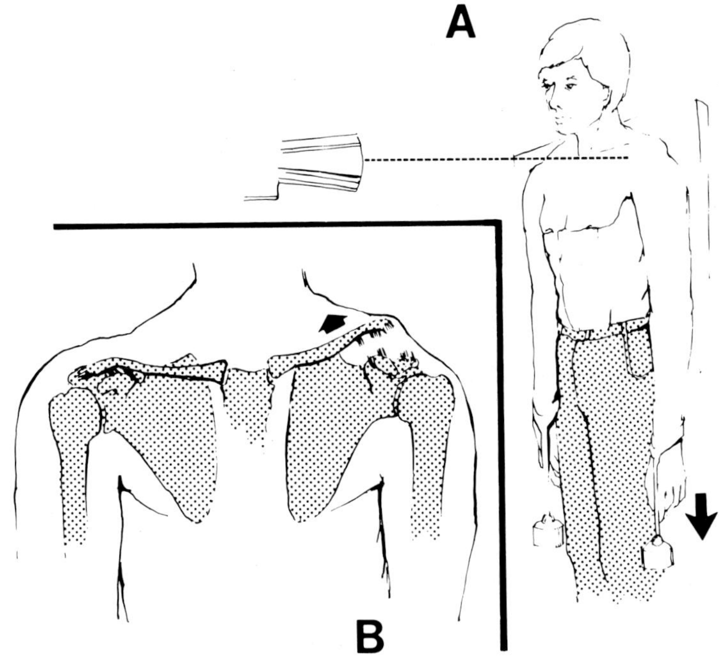

Fig. 11-136. Technique of obtaining stress films of the acromioclavicular joint. (*A*) Anteroposterior roentgenograms are made of both acromioclavicular joints with 10 to 15 lbs. of weight hanging from the wrists of both upper extremities. (*B*) The distance between the superior aspect of the coracoid process and the undersurface of the clavicle is measured to determine whether or not the coracoclavicular ligaments have been disrupted.

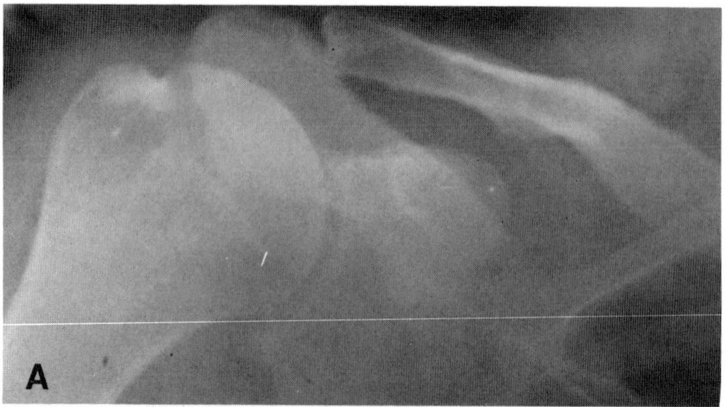

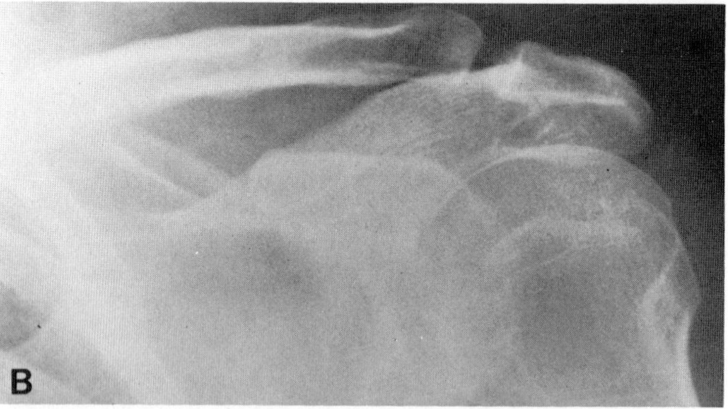

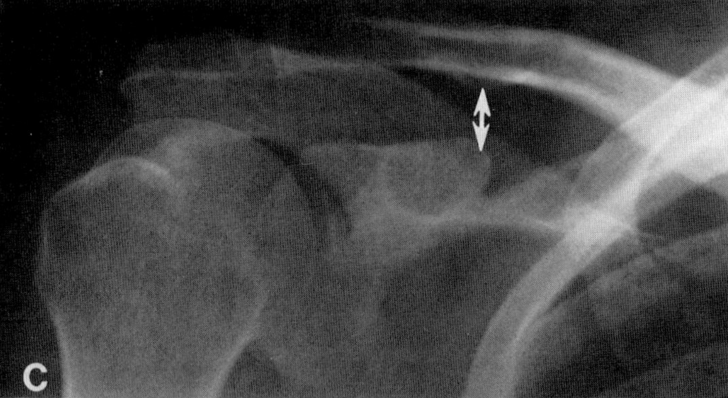

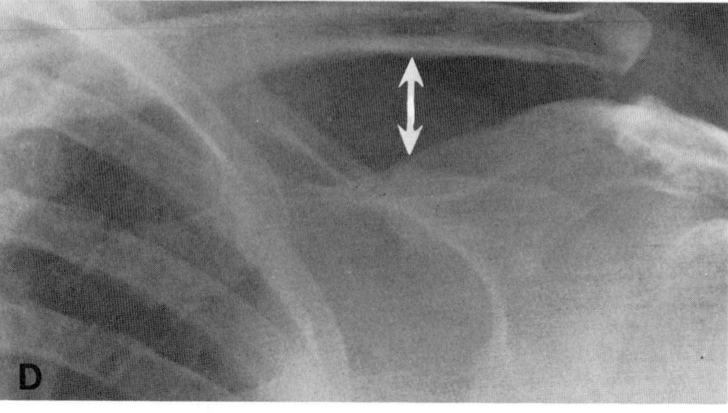

Fig. 11-137. Stress films of the normal right shoulder and the injured left shoulder. (*A*) An anteroposterior film of the normal right shoulder without stress shows no displacement of the acromioclavicular joint. (*B*) An anteroposterior view of the injured left shoulder is only suggestive of injury in that the acromioclavicular joint is widened as compared to the normal side. (*C*) Stress film (15 lbs.) of the normal right shoulder again shows no displacement of the acromioclavicular joint. (*D*) Stress film (15 lbs.) of the injured shoulder reveals that the end of the clavicle is elevated above the acromion process. More important, the distance between the superior border of the coracoid process and the inferior border of the clavicle is significantly greater than on the normal side. This indicates a Type III complete separation of the coracoclavicular ligaments and a Type III injury.

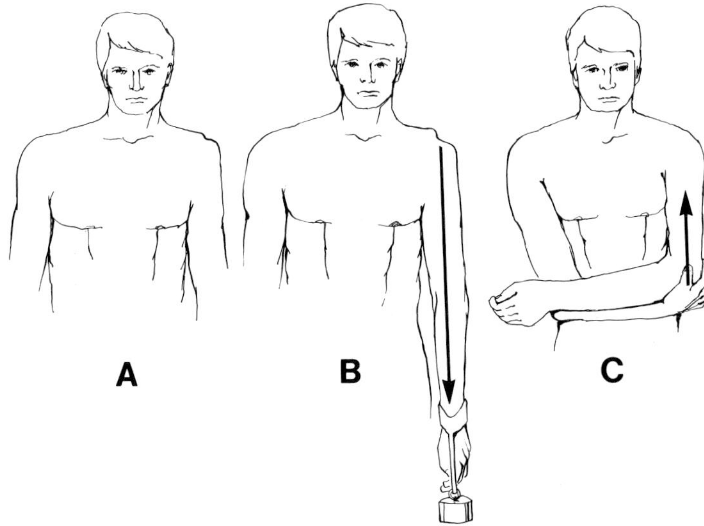

Fig. 11-138. Importance of obtaining stress roentgenograms of the acromioclavicular joint. (*A*) The patient presents only a mild deformity in the vicinity of the acromioclavicular joint. (*B*) With weight added to the wrist of the upper extremity, the deformity is exaggerated. (*C*) If the roentgenogram is taken of the acromioclavicular joint without weights attached to the upper extremity, the patient may, in an effort to relieve the pain, lift the shoulder upward, presenting a view that shows minimal separation of the acromioclavicular joint.

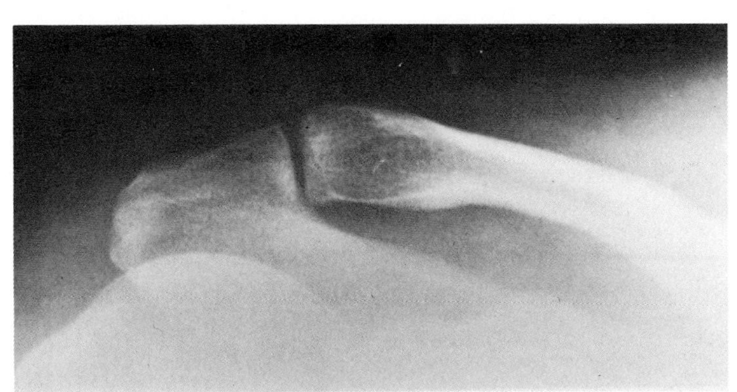

Fig. 11-139. Type I acromioclavicular joint injury. An anteroposterior view of the acromioclavicular joint reveals that there is no widening of the joint space, nor is there any separation of the joint surfaces.

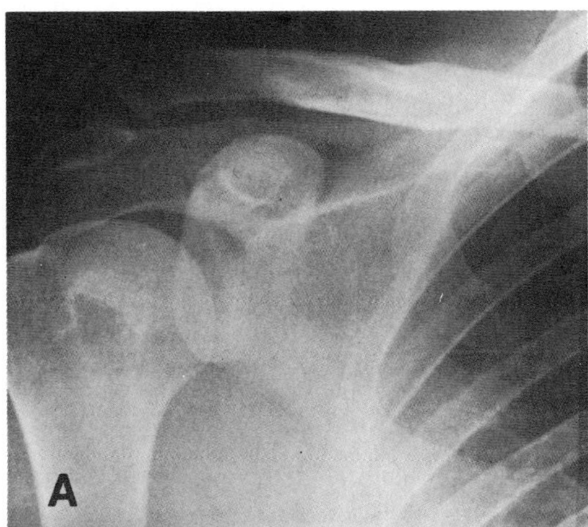

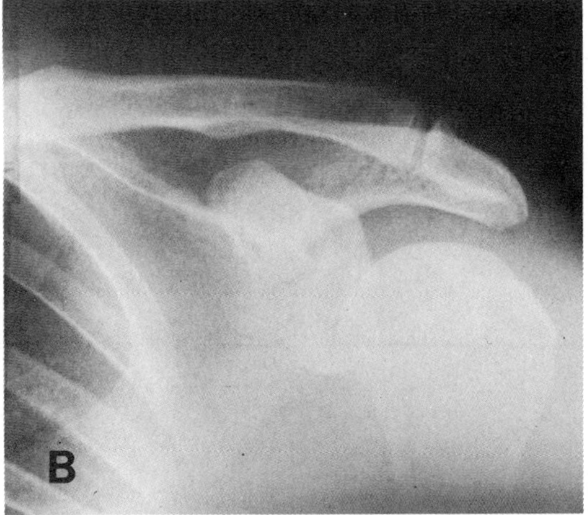

Fig. 11-140. Type II acromioclavicular joint injury. (*A*) In this stress film of the right acromioclavicular joint, appears to be slightly wider than the normal left side, and the distal end of the clavicle appears to be slightly elevated. The coracoclavicular distance as compared with the normal side is not appreciably changed. Note the difference in slope of inclination of the acromioclavicular joint of the injured right side with that of the normal left side. Compare the stress film of the normal left shoulder (*B*).

when he held up the arm as the films were being made (Fig. 11-138).

Alexander[657] has recommended the use of a "shoulder forward view" to demonstrate dislocations of the acromioclavicular joint. The patient is positioned as if you were going to take a true lateral roentgenogram of the scapula; then he is asked to thrust his shoulders forward, which, in dislocations of the acromioclavicular joint, projects the medial end of the acromion completely beneath the lateral end of the clavicle.

Roentgenographic Findings in Type I Injury

The roentgenograms of the acromioclavicular joint are essentially normal (i.e., no widening, no separation, and no deformity; Fig. 11-139).

Roentgenographic Findings in Type II Injury

The lateral end of the clavicle may be slightly elevated and the acromioclavicular joint, as compared to the normal side, may appear widened. Stress films of both shoulders to test the integrity of the coracoclavicular ligament are negative (i.e., the coracoclavicular space of the injured shoulder is the same as that of the normal shoulder; Fig. 11-140). A small fracture may be noted on the lateral clavicle or acromion process. Chronic or old injuries may reveal some calcification within the acromioclavicular joint or in the region of the coracoclavicular ligament.

Roentgenographic Findings in Type III Injury

In obvious cases, the joint is totally displaced. The lateral end of the clavicle rides completely above the superior border of the acromion, and the joint space is wide (Fig. 11-137D). In doubtful cases, stress films comparing the injured and normal shoulders reveal a major discrepancy in the coracoclavicular distances. Fractures may be noted on the outer clavicle of the acromion process. Rarely, instead of the coracoclavicular ligaments disrupting, there may be a fracture of the coracoid process, and it will be noted to be displaced upward (Fig. 11-143).

Occasionally, because of other major injuries that occur at the time of acromioclavicular joint dislocation, the acromioclavicular dislocation may be missed. Roentgenograms of the unreduced case will reveal varying degrees of degenerative arthritis of the joint and ectopic calcification about the joint and in the coracoclavicular interspace.

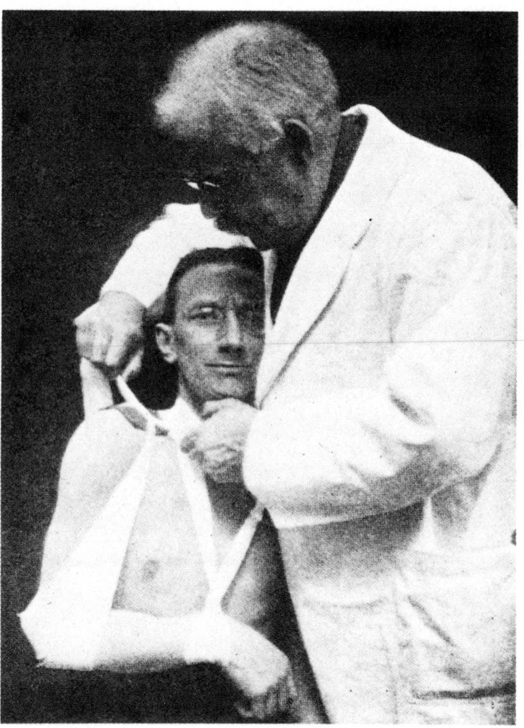

Fig. 11-141. Closed treatment of dislocations of the acromioclavicular joint. Sir Robert Jones is seen applying a sling and bandage which holds the arm elevated while depressing the lateral end of the clavicle. (Jones, R.: Injuries of Joints. London, Oxford University Press, 1917)

TREATMENT OF ACROMIOCLAVICULAR JOINT INJURIES

One of the interesting things revealed in a review of this subject is that about half of the authors of the 200 articles have contributed a new technique or a new twist to an old technique on how to manage dislocations of the acromioclavicular joint. There are two basic and fundamentally different schools of thought in the management of the acute complete acromioclavicular dislocation: the conservative, no-operation-is-necessary school, and those who recommend surgical repair. Each school thinks the other radical.

Some authors tend to lump mild injuries, subluxations, and dislocations together under one form of treatment and quote statistics for all of the cases. Only if the injuries to the acromioclavicular joint are graded according to severity and if the final results are also graded according to the severity, can you adequately evaluate the adequacy of a given form of treatment for a given type of injury.

Both the operative and the conservative schools basically agree on conservative management of Type I and Type II sprains. However, there are a few authors who advocate surgical repair of the Type II injury. It is in the complete dislocation where there are the greatest differences of opinion.

Treatment of Type I Injury

The ligaments are intact, but they have been strained. Usually, with ice for 12 hours followed by heat and then a sling for 3 to 7 days, the symptoms disappear. However, the shoulder should be protected from further injury until there is a painless full range of motion.

Treatment of Type II Injury

The damage with a Type II sprain is primarily localized to the acromioclavicular joint with coracoclavicular ligaments remaining intact. There may be some associated partial detachment of the deltoid and trapezius muscles from the clavicle, which increases the pain and discomfort.

Closed Treatment

Most authors agree that nonsurgical measures are indicated to treat this injury (Fig. 11-141). However, there are marked differences of opinion as to which type of conservative measures are indicated. Some authors routinely use the sling for 10 to 14 days to rest the injured shoulder, and this is followed by a gradual rehabilitation program. From this point on, things get pretty complicated, with various types of bandages and slings, adhesive tape strapping, braces, harnesses, traction techniques, and many, many types of plaster casts. Urist[823-825] has reviewed the literature extensively and has summarized beautifully the more than 35 forms of conservative treatment. Currently, it appears that the most commonly used type of conservative treatment, along with the sling, is an elastic compressive dressing over a clavicular pad or a sling-harness type of apparatus with a strap passing over and around the elbow, which, in effect, holds the arm up and the clavicle down. Allman[659] recommends the use of the sling harness immobilizing device for 3 weeks. Some authors continue to advocate a plaster cast device as described by Urist,[823] which holds the humerus up while an elastic strap depresses the clavicle.

Whether adhesive tape, elastic strapping, cast, or harness is used, it must have uninterrupted continuous pressure on the superior surface of the outer clavicle to allow ligament healing. Some authors recommend 3 weeks and some recommend 6 weeks. The shoulder must be protected for a minimum of 3 weeks to prevent another injury from converting the weakened Type II subluxation into a Type III total dislocation. Heavy lifting or contact sports should be avoided for 6 to 8 weeks until the ligament has healed completely.

In the elderly or debilitated patient, most authors manage a Type II sprain with only a sling for a few days and then encourage active use of the arm. A compression bandage on the top of the clavicle may be used for comfort.

Open Treatment

In some instances, following the Type II sprain, pain persists in the acromioclavicular joint, and the injury could rightly be called internal derangement of the acromioclavicular joint. Since fibers of the joint were initially disrupted, it is possible that shreds of the ligament or flakes of the articular cartilage are loose in the joint, causing symptoms. The meniscus may have been detached, and it will be noted, with motion, to pop and displace in and out of the joint like a torn meniscus in the knee. This internal derangement has been described by Bateman.[671] Brosgol[688] has described the technique of performing an arthrogram of the acromioclavicular joint, which may help to determine the integrity of the joint.

Ultimately it may be necessary to do an arthroplasty of the acromioclavicular joint, a do-what-is-needed-when-you-get-there type of operation—that is, debridement and meniscectomy and perhaps, if the degenerative arthritis is marked, excision of the outer 2 cm. of the clavicle. The clavicle does not displace upward, because the coracoclavicular ligaments are still intact. This procedure has been described by Mumford.[767]

Treatment of Type III Injury

Historical Review

The controversy over the conservative versus the operative treatment of complete dislocation of the acromioclavicular joint seems to have had cyclic turns in the literature. Obviously, in the earliest writings on the subject, closed reductions followed by strappings and bindings were practiced. The concept developed by the fathers of medicine (Hippocrates, Galen, and Paul of Aegina) are still valid. Hippocrates[655] recommended that the projecting part of the shoulder (the clavicle) be pushed down with compresses while the arm is kept elevated. He went on to say that the end result would be good, but that there would always be a deformity to the joint.

Following the discovery of anesthesia by Long, Wells, and Morton[842] in 1844, and following the development of antiseptic principles of surgery by Lister[842] in 1867 a great many operative procedures were described. Cadenat,[691] in his classic article of 1917, implies that the first operation on the acromioclavicular joint was performed by Samuel Cooper of San Francisco in 1861. Dr. Cooper used a loop of silver wire in the acromioclavicular joint. In 1886 Baum[691] used sutures of the acromioclavicular ligaments through the skin without an incision (a technique he learned from Volkmann); Paci,[691] in 1889, performed an arthrodesis of the acromioclavicular joint; Poirier and Rieffel,[788] in 1891, used sutures in the joint and the acromioclavicular ligament; Budinger,[691] a screw across the joint; Tuffier,[691] silk sutures in the acromioclavicular joint; Delbet[691] and Lambotte, acromioclavicular nailing; Morestin,[691] resection of the outer 2.5 cm. of the clavicle; and Bouchet,[691] ankylosis of the acromioclavicular joint. Cadenat[691] gives Baum credit for the first repair of the coracoclavicular ligaments in 1886 but states that he did it as an accessory step, because he felt repair of the acromioclavicular ligament was of primary importance. Delbet[691] is credited with the first coracoclavicular reconstruction when, in 3 cases, he passed a loop of suture from under the coracoid through an anteroposterior drill hole in the clavicle. In the first case, he used a single strand of silver wire, but he had to explore it in 45 days when the deformity reappeared. He found that the wire had broken. He replaced the wire with two silk sutures and concluded that wire should not be used because it breaks. In two subsequent cases, he used two strands of silk sutures tied over the top of the clavicle.

Cadenat[691] used a strip of the short head of the biceps tendon to reconstruct the coracoclavicular ligament in cadavers, but did not perform the operation on any patients, because the tip of the coracoid was too far anterior from the base of the coracoid, which is directly beneath the clavicle. However, in 1917, Cadenat did use the coracoacromial ligament to reconstruct the coracoclavicular ligament. He noted that the coracoacromial ligament had an anterior and a posterior attachment on the coracoid process and that the posterior attachment was in close proximity to the trapezoid ligament attachment. Therefore, after detaching the coracoacromial ligament from the acromium process and after dividing the anterior fasciculus from the coracoid process, he sutured the remaining posterior fasciculus from the base of the coracoid into the old conoid ligament and then onto the superior aspect of the clavicle.

In 1924, Henry[728] reported using autogenous fascia lata graft to replace the coracoclavicular ligaments and repair and stabilize the acromioclavicular joints with two Kirschner wires. Bunnell,[690] in 1928, used fascia lata to reconstruct the acromioclavicular joint. Murray,[768] in 1940, recommended the use of one or two Kirschner wires across the acromioclavicular joint, and Phemister,[785] in 1942, recommended the use of heavier threaded pins across the joint. Bloom,[679] in 1945, recommended two 1/32-inch Steinmann pins. Caldwell,[693] in 1943, reported good results from an arthrodesis of the acromioclavicular joint in two patients.

In the 1930's and 1940's, the trend began to swing away from the surgical repairs and back to conservative forms of treatment, old and new.

Plaster casts became particularly popular, and a sentence from Urist's[824] article of 1959 is worth quoting: "They range from the neatest and smallest to the largest and most grotesque seen in the whole field of traumatic and orthopaedic surgery."

Despite the five new splints and harnesses that were developed in the 1940's by Gibbens,[719] Morrison,[762] Batchelor,[670] Brandt,[687] and Varney, Coker, and Cawley,[828] there again seemed to be a decline in the conservative treatment in favor of operative procedures.

Conservative Forms of Treatment for Acromioclavicular Dislocation Reported in the Literature

1. Adhesive strapping—Rawlings,[795] Thorndike and Quigley,[816] Benson[676]
2. Sling or bandage—Sir Robert Jones and Watson-Jones[833]
3. Brace and harness—Giannestras,[718] Warner,[831] Currie,[702] Anderson and Burgess[661]
4. Figure-of-eight bandage—Usadel[826]
5. Sling and pressure dressing—Goldberg[722]
6. Abduction traction and suspension in bed—Caldwell[692]
7. Casts—Urist,[823] Howard,[731] Shaar,[804] Hart,[727] Trynin,[820] Stubbins,[813] Dillehunt,[708] Key and Conwell,[740] Gibbens,[719] Hunkin[838]

In 1941, Boardman M. Bosworth[682] described the technique of using a screw directed from the clavicle down into the coracoid process. Stewart[812] described a screw across the acromioclavicular joint, and there was a resurgence of the use of coracoclavicular sutures of various sorts. Pins across the acromioclavicular joint continued to be popular, and Mumford[767] and Gurd[724] both described the technique of excising the outer 2 cm. of the clavicle in 1941.

In the 1940's, 1950's, and 1960's there appeared to be more agreement by authors that the complete dislocation should be managed by operative means. Powers[789] states that the operative era (at least among orthopaedic residency program chairmen) continues today. In 1973, he sent a questionnaire to all of the chairmen of the approved residency programs in the

United States and drew the following conclusions from his analysis of the responses:

1. The majority of program chairmen treat Type III injury by open reduction.
2. Surgical treatment varied, but 60 per cent used temporary acromioclavicular fixation, and 35 per cent used coracoclavicular fixation.
3. Nonoperative treatment is rarely advocated and is often inadequate.

Nonoperative Management

Currently the three most commonly used forms of nonoperative treatment are a sling and harness immobilization device, plaster casts, and "skillful neglect." The sling and harness and the cast have two things in common: both elevate the arm and depress the clavicle.

Sling and Harness Immobilization Device

A sling and harness is advocated by Allman[659] and others. The sling supports and lifts the forearm and arm and thereby elevates the acromion, while a strap over a felt pad holds the clavicle down; the halter around the opposite side of the trunk keeps the sling pulled inward over the clavicle. The sling and harness must be worn for 6 weeks tightly enough to maintain the reduction. If at first the reduction cannot be accomplished, or if reduction cannot be maintained in the device, or if the patient will not wear and keep the device in position constantly, operative repairs are utilized. Allman* reports that one out of five patients, for reasons described above, cannot be treated with the sling and harness.

Plaster Casts

Many types of plaster casts have been used in the past, notably by Gibbens,[719] Shaar,[804] Key and Conwell,[740] Hart,[727] Trynin,[820] Dillehunt,[708] and Urist.[823] The Urist[823] cast remains the most popular and incorporates the most desirable features of the casts devised by other authors. Whereas the casts applied by Hart and Key and Conwell were basically modifications of the shoulder spica with the arm kept abducted, Urist applies his cast with the arm in adduction.

Technique of Applying Urist Cast. After a cylinder torso cast is applied, which will bear weight on the padded iliac crests, a cylinder cast is applied to the ipsilateral elbow. While the involved arm is pushed up, the elbow cast is attached to the torso cast with plaster, and the entire shoulder is held in an elevated position supported by the torso cast on the iliac crests. After a felt pad is placed over the top of the outer clavicle, a strip of rubber (inner tube from an automobile tire) is placed over the top of the felt pad. The rubber strip is incorporated anteriorly and posteriorly into the torso cast, producing a constant downward depression on the clavicle. Urist recommended uninterrupted immobilization for 6 weeks as a complete trial of conservative treatment, and only after the 6 weeks would he consider surgery. However, in 1963, Urist[825] recommended that surgery be considered when the closed treatment appeared to be failing, when the appearance of the shoulder was unacceptable to the patient, or when the joint was painful.

"Skillful Neglect"

Sometimes this method of treatment is brought about by the patient's insistence, sometimes by the circumstances of the time, and sometimes by the physician who is dissatisfied with the results achieved by either the operative or the nonoperative techniques. The treatment may consist of nothing more than a bulky compressive dressing over the top of the clavicle and a sling, or it may consist of only a sling. Nicol[774] states that conservative treatment cannot achieve the unattainable and that operative procedures are unwarranted. He recommends a sling for only 1 to 2 weeks, followed by exercises. However, in the annotation, he presented only his philosophy. I am sure that there are many physicians around the world who share Nicol's philos-

* Personal communication.

ophy. However, to my knowledge nothing has been published on the end results of this form of treatment.

Operative Methods of Treatment for Type III Injuries of the Acromioclavicular Joint

During the 1800's, practically every conceivable operation was done to the acromioclavicular joint, the coracoclavicular ligaments, and to both areas at the same time. Today most surgeons use various combinations of the older procedures described above. Four basic operations currently are being done (Fig. 11-142). Each of the four procedures is modified in many ways, and some authors have combined modifications (see outline below).

Acromioclavicular Repairs

This remains probably one of the most popular procedures. Strictly speaking Kirschner wires should not be used, because there are only three sizes of Kirschner wires—0.035, 0.045 and 0.062-inch—and they are all too small! Most authors use the smaller, 3/32-inch, Steinmann pins, smooth or threaded. They can be inserted from the acromion through the joint and on into the clavicle, or they can be drilled retrograde from the joint out through the acromion and then back across the joint and into the clavicle. The portion of the pin that protrudes through the lateral acromion process should always be bent to prevent migration of the pin. Blind pinning of the acromioclavicular joint has been mentioned occasionally in the literature, but I do not recommend it. It is hard enough to drill a pin across the acromioclavicular joint under direct vision.

Steinmann pins across the acromioclavicular joint have been used to stabilize the

---

Operative Repairs

I. Acromioclavicular Joint Repair, Fixation, or Reconstruction (Bateman,[671] Bundens and Cook,[689] Allman,[659] Ahstrom,[656] DePalma,[705] McLaughlin,[749] O'Donoghue,[780] Sage and Salvotore,[801] Rowe,[798] Inman,[734] Stephens,[811] Zaricznyj,[841] Neviaser,[773] Moshein and Elconin[766])
   - A. With or without coracoclavicular ligament and/or acromioclavicular ligament repair or reconstruction

II. Coracoclavicular Ligament Repair, Fixation or Reconstruction (Vere-Hodge,[833] Kennedy and Cameron,[739] Weitzman,[835] Orofinio and Stein,[782] Baker and Stryker,[667] Laing,[741] Bateman,[671] Jay and Monnet,[736] Alldredge,[658] Bearden, Hughston and Whatley,[673] Mumford,[767] Vargas[827])
   - A. Screw from clavicle to coracoid
     1. With or without coracoclavicular ligament repair or reconstruction
     2. With or without acromioclavicular ligament repair or reconstruction
   - B. Suture from clavicle to coracoid
     1. Fascia
     2. Wire, cotton, nylon sutures
     3. Reconstruction of new coracoclavicular ligament with coracoacromial ligament or short head of the biceps tendon or long head of the biceps tendon.

III. Excision of the Distal Clavicle (Gurd,[724] Mumford,[767] Bateman,[671] Urist,[825] Weaver,[834] Dewar and Barrington,[707] Moseley[764])
   - A. With or without imbrication of the deltoid and trapezius
   - B. With or without coracoacromial ligament transfer
   - C. With or without attachment of coracoid process to clavicle
   - D. With or without coracoclavicular ligament repair with fascia or suture

IV. Dynamic Muscle Transfers—with or without excision of the distal clavicle (Dewar and Barrington,[707] Bailey[665,666])

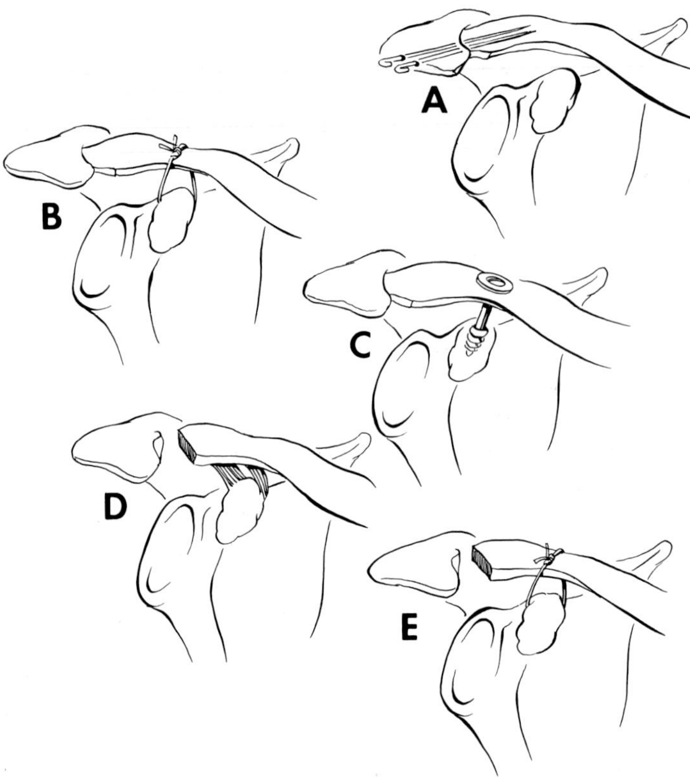

Fig. 11-142. Various operative procedures for injuries to the acromioclavicular joint. (*A*) Steinmann pins across the acromioclavicular joint. (*B*) Suture between the clavicle and the coracoid process. (*C*) A lag screw between the clavicle and the coracoid process. (*D*) Resection of the distal clavicle when the coracoclavicular ligaments are intact. (*E*) Resection of the distal clavicle with suture, fascia, or ligament between the clavicle and the coracoid process when the coracoclavicular ligaments are missing.

joint in a Type III injury when the coracoclavicular ligaments remain intact and when there is an avulsion fracture of the coracoid process (Fig. 11-143).

Sage and Salvatore repair the acromioclavicular ligament whenever possible.[801] They use temporary pins across the joint and use the fibrocartilaginous meniscus to reinforce the superior acromioclavicular ligament when feasible. Stevens[801] stabilizes the acromioclavicular joint with a Stuck nail. Bundens and Cook,[689] after stabilizing the acromioclavicular joint with two pins, stress the importance of reefing the attachment of the trapezius and deltoid muscles over each other on the top of the clavicle. Ahstrom[656] transfixes the acromioclavicular joint with one 9/64-inch threaded pin and then turns up a segment of the short head of the biceps to reinforce the coracoclavicular ligament. Zaricznyj[841] stabilizes the acromioclavicular joint with Kirschner wires and reconstructs the acromioclavicular ligament and the coracoclavicular ligament using the fifth toe extensor tendon. For the Type II sprain, Bateman[671] stabilizes the acromioclavicular joint with Kirschner wires, and for complete dislocation he creates a new suspensory ligament using fascia lata that passes from the coracoid around the clavicle and back to the spine of the acromion. If degenerative arthritis is present, he advises excision of the distal end of the clavicle. O'Donoghue,[780] Rowe,[798] and Inman *et al.*[734] recommend acromioclavicular stabilization with pins and repair of the coracoclavicular ligaments. Neviaser[770-773] stabilizes the acromioclavicular joint with one pin and then reconstructs a new superior acromioclavicular ligament by detaching the coracoacromial ligament from the coracoid process and swinging it up on top of the lateral clavicle. He does not repair the coracoclavicular ligaments. Moshein and Elconin[766] stabilize the acromioclavicular joint temporarily with Kirschner wires and repair the coracoclavicular ligament with

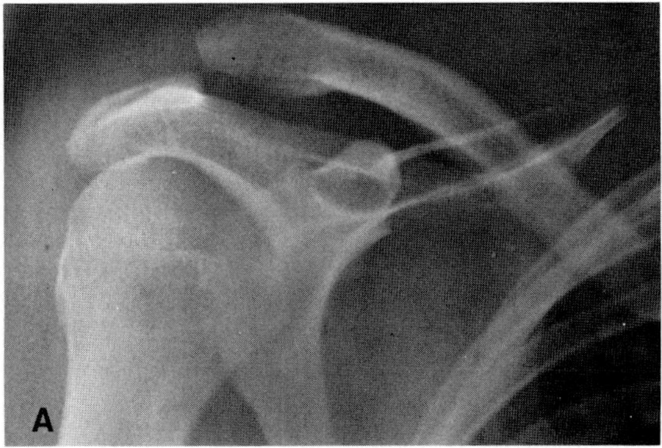

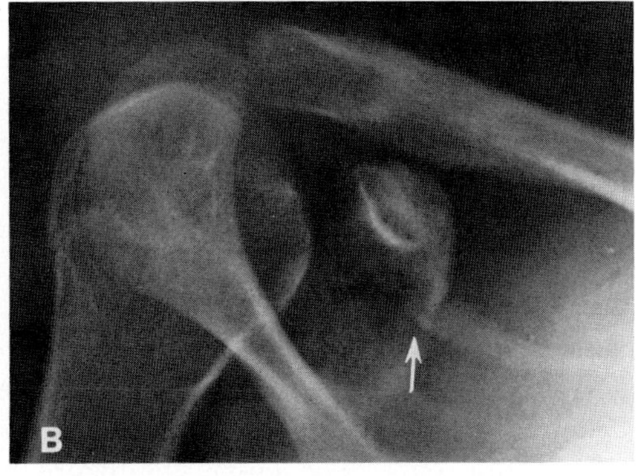

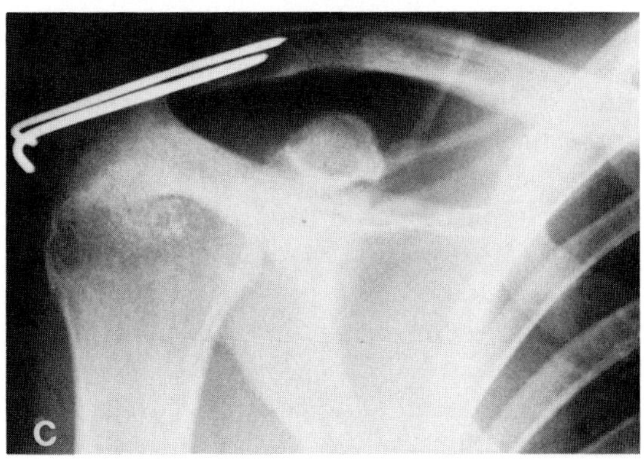

Fig. 11-143. Dislocation of the acromioclavicular joint associated with an avulsion type fracture of the coracoid process. (*A*) The distal end of the clavicle is completely dislocated away from the acromion process, but the coracoclavicular distance as compared to the normal shoulder was the same. (*B*) The 45-degree cephalic tilt roentgenogram of the shoulder reveals a fracture (*arrow*) at the base of the coracoid process, indicating that the coracoclavicular ligaments are intact and have displaced the coracoid process upward with the clavicle. Note that the fracture of the coracoid extends to include the superior border of the scapula. (*C*) Open reduction of the acromioclavicular joint and stabilization with two pins has effectively reduced the fracture of the coracoid process.

the coracoacromial ligament from the coracoid process.

Care After Acromioclavicular Joint Repairs. Patients are encouraged to move the hand and elbow but are discouraged from abducting the shoulder. Motion must be limited to prevent breakage or migration of the pins across the acromioclavicular joint. Rowe[798] recommends that abduction motion be limited to 40 degrees, and DePalma[705] recommends no abduction until the pins are removed. Most authors recommend that the pins be removed after 6 to 8 weeks. After pins are removed, patients are instructed in range of motion and strengthening exercises.

Coracoclavicular Repairs

The technique of placing a screw across the coracoclavicular space was described by Boardman M. Bosworth[682] in 1941. The operation was performed under local anesthesia. With the patient in a seated position, a stab wound was made on the superior shoulder 3.8 cm. proximal to the lateral end of the clavicle. Under fluoroscopy and after a drill hole was made in the clavicle, an assistant depressed and reduced the clavicle with a special clavicle depressor instrument and elevated the arm to reduce the acromioclavicular joint. Under fluoroscopy, an awl was used to develop a hole in the superior cortex of the base of the coracoid, and the screw was inserted. The screw was left indefinitely, unless specific indications developed. In the original article,[682] Bosworth reported on a newly developed lag screw with a broad head, which he preferred to the original regular bone screw. He referred to the procedure as a screw suspension operation, not a fixation (i.e., the screw suspends the scapula from the clavicle).

Bosworth, in all of his publications,[682-685] did not recommend repair of the coracoclavicular ligaments nor did he recommend exploration of the acromioclavicular joint. More recently, Kennedy and Cameron,[739] and Kennedy,[738] have popularized a modified Bosworth technique. Under general anesthesia, Kennedy debrides the acromioclavicular joint, preserves but does not repair the coracoclavicular ligament, internally overcorrects the dislocated acromioclavicular joint by compressing the clavicle down onto the top of the coracoid process with the lag screw, and repairs the trapezium and deltoid muscle detachments from the clavicle. In acute cases, he places the bone dust created by drilling the clavicle into the coracoclavicular joint space, and in chronic cases he uses refrigerated bone in an effort to gain a more permanent fixation of the clavicle to the coracoid process. Kennedy and Cameron[739] state that the screw fixation of the clavicle to the coracoid process with calcification and ossification creates an extraarticular fusion of the acromioclavicular joint, which does not interfere with the functional or normal clavicular rotation and produces an essentially normal range of motion in the shoulder. Weitzman[835] reports the use of a Bosworth screw, which he inserts under general anesthesia. He neither exposes nor repairs the coracoclavicular ligament, but he does expose and debride the acromioclavicular joint and imbricates the deltoid and trapezius muscle attachments.

Bearden, Hughston, and Whatley[673] recommend two coracoclavicular loops of wire, repair of the coracoclavicular ligament, debridement of the acromioclavicular joint, and repair of the trapezius and deltoid muscles (Fig. 11-144). Alldredge[658] recommends ligament repair and uses two loops of stainless steel wire between the coracoid and the clavicle. Jay and Monnet,[736] in an excellent series of 31 cases from the University of Oklahoma Medical Center, debrided the acromioclavicular joint, repaired the coracoclavicular ligaments, used a Bosworth screw, and repaired the trapezius and deltoid muscle attachments (Fig. 11-145). They recommended that a roentgenogram be taken on the operating table, to insure that the screw is in the vertical position and that it is engaging both cortices of the coracoid process.

Laing[741] reported on 30 cases in which he reconstructed a new coracoclavicular ligament by transferring the long head of the biceps up through a drill hole in the coracoid process into a drill hole in the clavicle. He states that this new ligament with its own nerve and blood supplies is

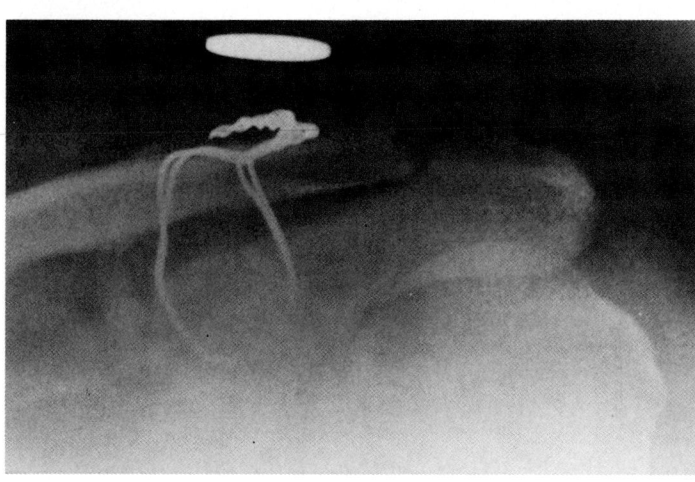

Fig. 11-144. A postoperative anteroposterior roentgenogram of the acromioclavicular joint shows two loops of wire used to reduce the acromioclavicular joint. The loops of wire passed beneath the coracoid process and over the clavicle. Note the coin that has been taped to the skin on the superior aspect of the shoulder to aid in the location of the loop of wire (or screw) when it is to be removed.

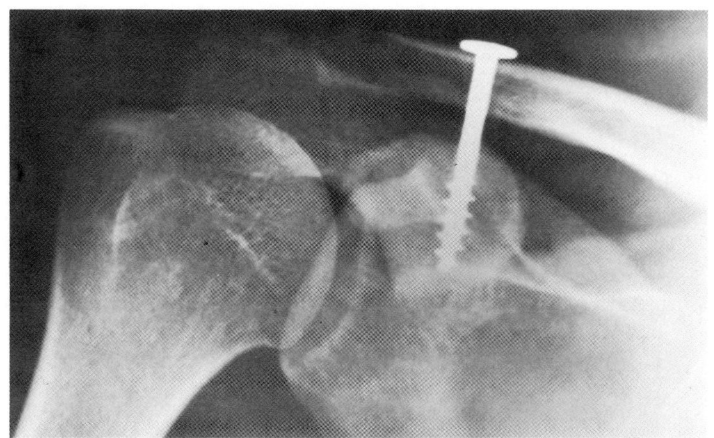

Fig. 11-145. Postoperative anteroposterior roentgenogram of the shoulder with Bosworth screw in place. Note that the acromioclavicular joint has been reduced and the coarse lag threads of the screw are well seated into the coracoid process.

sensitive to stress and is able to protect itself against stretching.

Postoperative Course After Coracoclavicular Fixations. Bosworth[682] recommended a sling until the soft tissues are healed. However, he encouraged the patient to remove the sling daily to perform pendulum- and crawling-up-the-wall exercises. He allowed the patient to bathe, dress, feed, and in general care for himself from the day of surgery. The patient was restricted from heavy work for 8 weeks. Kennedy[738] uses no form of external splintage and encourages a gradual range of motion. He looks for full abduction 7 to 10 days after the operation and returns the patient to vigorous athletic activities at 6 to 8 weeks. The screw is not removed.

Weitzman[835] recommends a sling and swathe immediately after surgery, but on the first day after the operation he applies a plaster shoulder Velpeau cast. This is worn for 4 weeks and then removed to allow active exercises. He recommends removal of the screw under local anesthesia after 3 months. Bearden, Hughston, and Whatley[673] support the arm in a sling for 10 to 14 days after surgery. The patient is instructed to avoid strenuous activity such as lifting weights. After the skin sutures are removed, the patient is encouraged to regain range of motion. The wire loops are removed at 6 to 8 weeks. They are removed in the hospital under local anesthesia, if possible, or general anesthesia, if necessary. They recommend removing all of the fragments if the wires are broken. Alldredge[658] recommends no postoperative immobilization beyond the second day and limits the patient's activities for 5 to 6 weeks. If the wires are broken and there is a full range of motion, the wires are not removed; otherwise, loops are removed after 6 to 8 weeks. Jay and Monnet[736] recommend a sling for 4 weeks after operation, at which time active exercises are started. They remove the screw under local anesthesia at 8 weeks.

Excision of the Distal Clavicle

Exactly who performed the first excision of the outer end of the clavicle is not known. McLaughlin[749] states that it was first recommended by Facassini in 1902 but gives no reference, and Cadenat[691] states that it was first performed by Morestin but gives no reference or date. Gurd[724] of Montreal, and Mumford[767] of Indiana, described their results of lateral clavicle excisions independently in 1941. Mumford[767] recommended his operation for the incompletely dislocated but symptomatic acromioclavicular joint, and Gurd[724] recommended his operation for the symptomatic, completely dislocated acromioclavicular joint (Figs. 11-142D, E; 11-146). For the complete

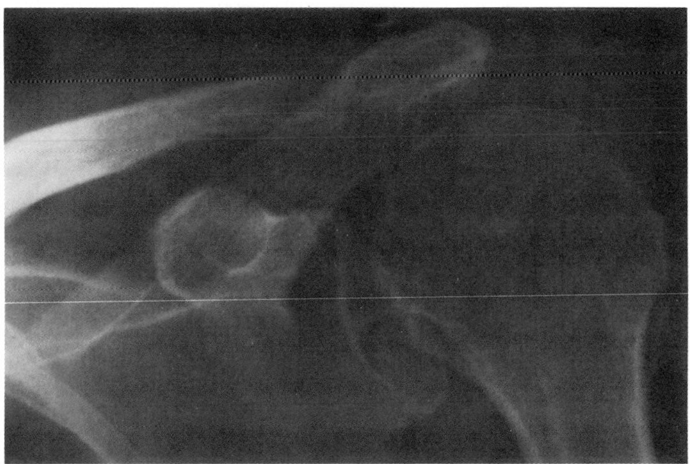

Fig. 11-146. Degenerative arthritis of the left shoulder particularly involving the acromioclavicular joint. Because the coracoclavicular ligaments are intact, a simple excision of the distal clavicle lateral to the coracoclavicular ligaments as described by Mumford should result in adequate relief of symptoms.

acromioclavicular separation, Mumford recommended a fascial suture between the clavicle and the coracoid.

Interestingly enough, in both of Gurd's cases with "complete dislocation of the acromioclavicular joint," the coracoclavicular ligaments were found at surgery to be intact. In one case that did not respond to conservative measures, the injury was 1 month old, and it is entirely possible either that the ligaments were stretched, or as has been shown by Urist,[823] that the coracoclavicular ligaments were healing. In the second case, the lateral clavicle excision was done 5 days after injury. Gurd again found that the coracoclavicular ligament was intact, which probably indicates that the injury was a subluxation of the acromioclavicular joint, a Type II sprain. Gurd[724] was of the opinion that the clavicle is "practically functionless, that it does not act as a strut, nor does it support the shoulder." He stated that its major function was to act as an attachment for muscles.

Currently, excision of the outer end of the clavicle is referred to as the Mumford[767] operation or the Gurd[724] operation or by both eponyms combined. What name is attached to the procedure is not nearly as important as realizing that there are two different types of resection procedures done on the outer end of the clavicle. If the indication is a degeneration of a Type II injury or joint subluxation, simple excision of the outer 2 cm. of the clavicle is sufficient to give a good result. However, the simple excision of 2 cm. of the outer clavicle for a completely dislocated joint where the clavicle is riding high enough to tent the skin only produces a "shortened high-riding clavicle." There is still deformity and tenting of the skin, and the lateral clavicle is still allowed to flop about in the trapezius muscles and surrounding structures. Various techniques have been suggested to hold the clavicle down in its normal position after excision of its distal end. Urist[824] recommends that the deltoid and trapezius muscles be imbricated over the top of the clavicle. Moseley[764,765] recommends a combination of loops of suture and fascia between the coracoid and the clavicle, and Weaver[834] recommends a reconstruction of the coracoclavicular ligament with the coracoacromial ligament.

Essentially, then, following the excision of the outer end of the clavicle in a Type III injury, a reconstruction of some sort has to be done to hold the clavicle down in normal approximation to the coracoid process.

Postoperative Course. Gurd[665] recommended that the hand of the patient be tied to the head of the bed for 5 days after which time range-of-motion exercises are begun. Mumford[767] recommended Velpeau dressings for 1 week, followed by active use of the arm. Weaver[834] recommends a Velpeau or a sling and begins circumduction exercises on the first day after operation. At the end of 4 weeks, the patient is allowed full active use of the shoulder.

Dynamic Muscle Transfers

In 1965, Dewar and Barrington[707] published results of a new procedure for old complete acromioclavicular dislocations in which the coracoid process, with its attachments to the short head of the biceps, coracobrachialis, and a segment of the pectoralis minor tendon, is transferred and fixed with a screw to the undersurface of the clavicle in the vicinity of the old coracoclavicular ligament attachments. This serves as a dynamic muscle transfer to hold the clavicle down. In two of five chronic acromioclavicular dislocations, he accompanied the coracoid transfer with lateral clavicular excision, and in three, he did not mention whether or not clavicular excision was performed. They recommend a Velpeau dressing after operation and mobilization of the shoulder starting at 4 weeks.

In 1964, Bailey[665] reported on the transfer of the coracoid process with the coracobrachialis and the short head of the biceps to the clavicle in nine cases with acute complete acromioclavicular dislocation. He reported that the operation acts as a dynamic depressor of the clavicle. He does not state whether he ever excises the lateral end of the clavicle. He stated that in lower vertebrate forms the coracobrachialis and short head of the biceps muscles arise from the clavicle and that in a sense the operation is a step backward in comparative vertebrate anatomy. In 1972, Bailey, O'Connor, Tilus, and Baril[666] reported on 38 cases.

AUTHOR'S PREFERRED METHOD OF TREATMENT

Type I Injury

Ice is used whenever it is convenient during the first 24 hours, and then moist heat, to decrease the pain and swelling. The arm is carried in a sling, to remind the patient that something is wrong with his shoulder, which seems to encourage him to rest the shoulder for 3 to 5 days. Usually by that time, the symptoms have subsided, so that the patient can regain range of motion in the shoulder. Heavy stresses, such as lifting and contact sports, should be delayed until there is a full range of motion and only minimal pain, if any.

Type II Injury

As with Type I injury, rest is the important factor. Ice is recommended during the first 12 to 24 hours, and is followed by 24 to 48 hours of moist heat. Initially, if a mild

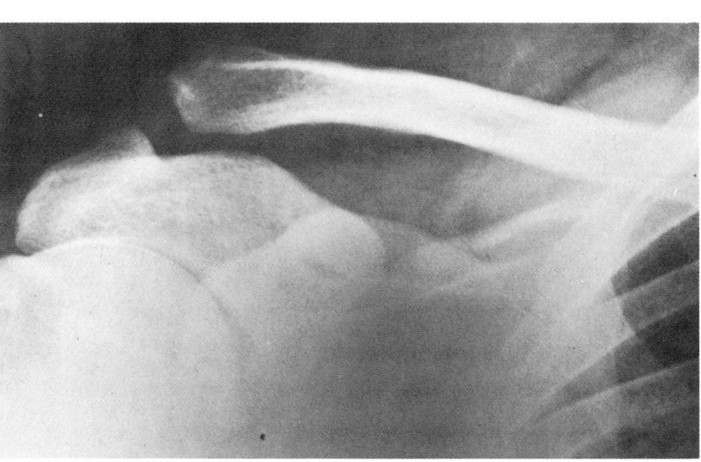

Fig. 11-147. In this complete acromioclavicular dislocation, the coracoclavicular distance in the injured shoulder measures 20 mm.; whereas the normal opposite shoulder measured 15 mm. Because of the significant posterior displacement of the right distal clavicle, surgery was performed and the coracoclavicular ligaments were disrupted completely.

compression to the outer clavicle gives the patient relief, I use folded compresses over the end of the clavicle held in place by elastic tape along with a sling to hold up the arm. The sling is worn for 7 to 21 days, depending on the age of the patient and the symptoms. Patients who are over 50, chronologically or physiologically, are urged to begin pendulum exercises as soon as possible and are instructed in range-of-motion exercises on the third to the fifth day. Beyond 3 weeks, the active patient can use his arm in everyday living activities, but patients who do heavy labor and athletes are held from vigorous activities or weight lifting or contact sports for 6 weeks—I do not want the patient to convert a subluxation into a total dislocation with another injury.

Should symptoms persist and interfere with function beyond 6 to 9 months, an arthroplasty is performed. Excision of the lateral clavicle should not be skimpy, for I have seen patients who, after excision of 1 cm. of the lateral clavicle, have continued pain in the joint. Films taken with the arm at the side revealed a clear acromioclavicular joint, but with 90 degrees of abduction there was impingement of the clavicle onto the acromion process. As a general rule, I recommend excision of a minimum 2 cm. of the lateral clavicle, or excision to where the strong coracoclavicular ligaments hold the remaining clavicle down to the coracoid process.

After the operation, the arm is carried in a sling until the sutures are removed, and then the patient is instructed in pendulum exercises, followed by range-of-motion exercises and finally strengthening exercises. Laborers and athletes in contact sports may return to their activities after 8 to 10 weeks.

Type III Injury

I have two indications for surgery for the acromioclavicular dislocation, and one indication for skillful neglect. Surgery is indicated in acute complete acromioclavicular dislocation in active patients (Fig. 11-147) and in those patients with pain, disability, and arthritis, for whom conservative measures or previous operative procedures have failed.

Elderly and very inactive patients may be treated with skillful neglect. I do not deny that good results can be obtained by conservative means. However, braces, casts, harnesses, and slings are bulky and uncomfortable and must be kept in place continuously. I do not use adhesive strapping for complete dislocation, as it is ineffective and only tends to irritate the skin. It seems unreasonable and impractical to immobilize the shoulder and the upper extremity of a young active person for the required 6 weeks. However, I admire the physicians who have the tenacity to achieve good results with nonoperative techniques.

I manage patients who are chronologically and physiologically over 60 with the skillful neglect routine (i.e., sling, ice bag, gentle active range-of-motion exercises). I also use the conservative routine for patients in their late 40's and 50's who lead essentially inactive lives; that is, they do not participate in any sports, do not do any work in the yard, and have desk jobs. Inactive women around the mid-40's who are not concerned with the cosmetic appearance of their shoulder are also managed without surgery.

Operative Procedure

I do not feel that the clavicle and the acromioclavicular joints are accessory parts of our anatomy which can be done away with indiscriminately. Therefore, I strongly believe that the totally dislocated acromioclavicular joint in the active young patient should be reduced primarily and repaired and allowed to heal. Primary excision of the outer end of the clavicle in the young active patient tends to be unphysiological.

The operation I have used for the past 13 years is not one that has been described in the literature. It is not necessarily a new operation; with a few minor variations it is the same operation that I learned as a resident from Dr. James Amspacher at the University of Oklahoma Medical Center. The operation encompasses the best ideas and qualities of several recommended procedures, and they are as follows: The acromioclavicular joint is exposed and debrided as is required. The coracoclavicular ligament is repaired. A vertical and horizontal reduction of the acromioclavicular joint is performed; temporary internal (screw) fixation is used to take the tension off of the coracoclavicular ligament repair. Finally, the deltoid trapezius muscles are repaired. I perform the operation through an incision on the top of the shoulder. It is cosmetically acceptable, because there is no anterior scar.

Exposure and Debridement of the Acromioclavicular Joint. Almost always there will be "gurry and junk" in the joint—flakes of cartilage, frayed ends of ligaments, remnants of ruptured meniscus. This must be resected to prevent further acromioclavicular joint symptoms, arthralgia, and arthritis.

Repair of the Coracoclavicular Ligament. The injury is a complete dislocation of the acromioclavicular joint, because this ligament has been ruptured. In some cases, it may be detached from the clavicle or from the coracoid, but in the majority of cases in my experience, the rupture is in the body of the ligament itself. The purpose of the suture is to bring the ruptured ends of the ligament fibers together, so that the ligament can heal primarily, without a gap of irresponsible scar tissue, which produces a weak repair and/or an elongated ligament. There are always ligament fibers that can be brought into approximation, and the type of suture that is used is unimportant, because the temporary internal fixation device takes the tension off the zone of repair.

Reduction of the Acromioclavicular Joint. The purpose of this step is to hold the acromioclavicular joint reduced and to take tension off the healing "coracoclavicular ligament." There are several ways to accomplish this:

Loop of Suture, Fascia, or Wire. This technique holds the clavicle down in a vertical plane but does not control horizontal stability of the acromioclavicular joint. In this type of fixation, unless you are careful to put the loop of suture back at the base of the coracoid process, the clavicle may tend to be displaced forward away from its articulation with the acromion.

Acromioclavicular Joint Screws or Steinmann Pins. This technique holds the acromioclavicular joint reduction and takes tension off the repaired coracoclavicular ligament. However, insertion of two 3/32-inch pins or a nail or a screw across a joint with a very small articular surface (9 mm. × 19 mm.) would seem to disrupt that joint and subject it to arthritis—the very thing we are trying to prevent by operative repair. Another drawback to fixation across the acromioclavicular joint is that the pins, nails, or screws must stick out of the lateral edge of the acromion process far enough so that they can be removed 6 to 8 weeks after surgery. Also, during the postoperative period, the patient must avoid moving his arm, particularly abducting it, or the pins may break. Even if he wanted to move his arm, he couldn't because of the irritation of the two pins protruding from the acromion into the deltoid muscle.

Coracoclavicular Screw. This screw depresses the clavicle vertically, holds the acromioclavicular joint reduced in the horizontal plane, does not interfere with motion postoperatively, does not disturb the acromioclavicular articulation, and can be removed in one piece under local anesthesia at 6 weeks (Fig. 11-148). Therefore, it seems to have all of the advantages of the acromioclavicular fixation and of the coracoclavicular loop fixation, but none of the disadvantages of either technique.

The biggest problem I have had with the Bosworth screw is difficulty working with it. The broad head cannot be held with a self-retaining screwdriver, and the point of the screw is too blunt to find the hole drilled into the base of the coracoid process easily and consistently. Modifications have been developed, and the one currently being used has the following

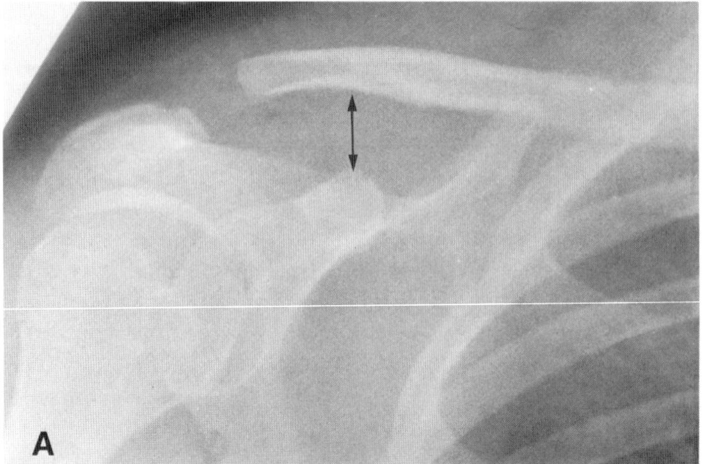

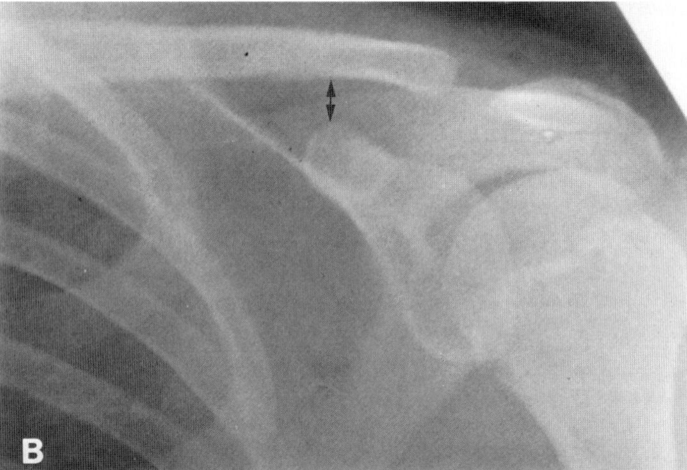

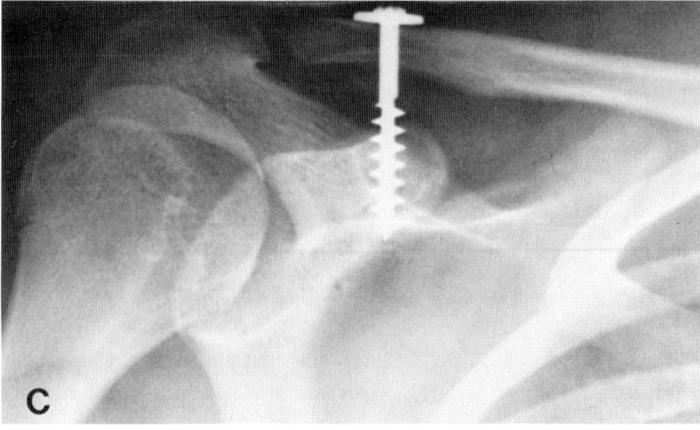

Fig. 11-148. Use of modified coracoclavicular lag screw. (*A*) Anteroposterior stress roentgenogram of the right shoulder in a patient who fell on the point of the right shoulder demonstrates a wide and displaced acromioclavicular joint and 18 mm. coracoclavicular space. (*B*) A stress film of the normal left shoulder reveals that the coracoclavicular space (the distance between the upper border of the coracoid process and the lower border of the clavicle) is 10 mm. (*C*) On this postoperative anteroposterior view of the right shoulder with the acromioclavicular joint reduced and held temporarily in place by a special coracoclavicular lag screw, note that the special screw has a regular screw head which is seated into a washer. Also note that the tip of the screw has a 5- to 6-mm. smooth nipple. This enables the surgeon to use the tip of the screw as a probe to locate the drill hole in the base of the coracoid process.

characteristics: (1) The screw head is a size that fits the standard self-retaining screwdriver. The screw head nestles into a washer, which has the same effect as the broad head of the Bosworth screw and which allows for some rolling and toggle motion of the head in the inside beveled washer. The shank of the screw is smooth and has no purchase on the clavicle. A smooth nipple extends 5 mm. beyond the tip of the coarse lag threads of the screw and seeks out the hole in the coracoid process and guides the screw (Fig. 11-149).

Repair of the Deltoid and Trapezius Muscles. During dislocation of the acromioclavicular joint, the trapezius and the deltoid muscles are stripped from the anterior and posterior superior border of the acromioclavicular joint and the distal portion of the clavicle. Following the reduction and internal fixation with the screw, the muscles are repaired firmly to each other on top of the clavicle and the acromioclavicular joint.

Details of the Author's Technique

Through the superior incision, the acromioclavicular joint, the lateral 6.4 cm. of the clavicle, and the coracoid process are exposed (Fig. 11-150A). The acromioclavicular joint is debrided. The coracoclavicular ligaments are identified, and the sutures are placed into the ligaments, but they are not tied (Fig. 11-150B).

A 3/16-inch hole is drilled in the superior clavicle, directly above the coracoid process (Fig. 11-150C).

A towel clip is used to grasp the clavicle anteriorly and posteriorly to hold the acromioclavicular joint reduced. A 9/64-inch drill bit is placed through the 3/16-inch hole in the clavicle and a hole is drilled into the coracoid process (Fig. 11-150D). When the acromioclavicular joint is held reduced, the hole will be properly made into the base of the coracoid process.

A screw of appropriate length, held firmly in a self-retaining screwdriver, is twisted through the clavicle, and the smooth nipple at the end of the screw is used as a probe to locate the hole in the coracoid process (Fig. 11-150E).

The screw is seated until the clavicle is held depressed down to the level of the acromion (Fig. 11-150F). The sutures in the coracoclavicular ligaments are tied. The screw is turned one-half turn more, which overcorrects the deformity slightly and takes the tension off the repaired coracoclavicular ligament. Finally, the deltoid and trapezius muscles are repaired (Fig. 11-150G).

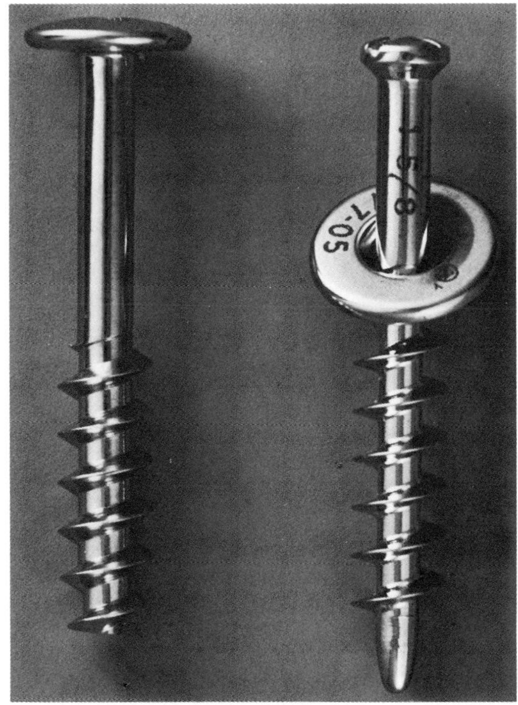

Fig. 11-149. A Bosworth screw is characterized by the large flat head, a smooth shank, and coarse lag threads that form a rather dull, broad surface at the tip of the screw. In the modified screw, the regular-sized head may be held by a standard self-retaining screwdriver. The same advantage of a broad head is accomplished through the use of a washer with a beveled inside diameter that allows toggle motion between the screw head and the washer. The other modification is the 6-mm. smooth nipple at the tip of the screw, which is used like a probe to locate the drill hole placed in the base of the coracoid process.

Care After Operation

The patient wears a sling until the skin sutures are removed after 10 to 14 days. He then is allowed and encouraged to use his arm to perform everyday activities and

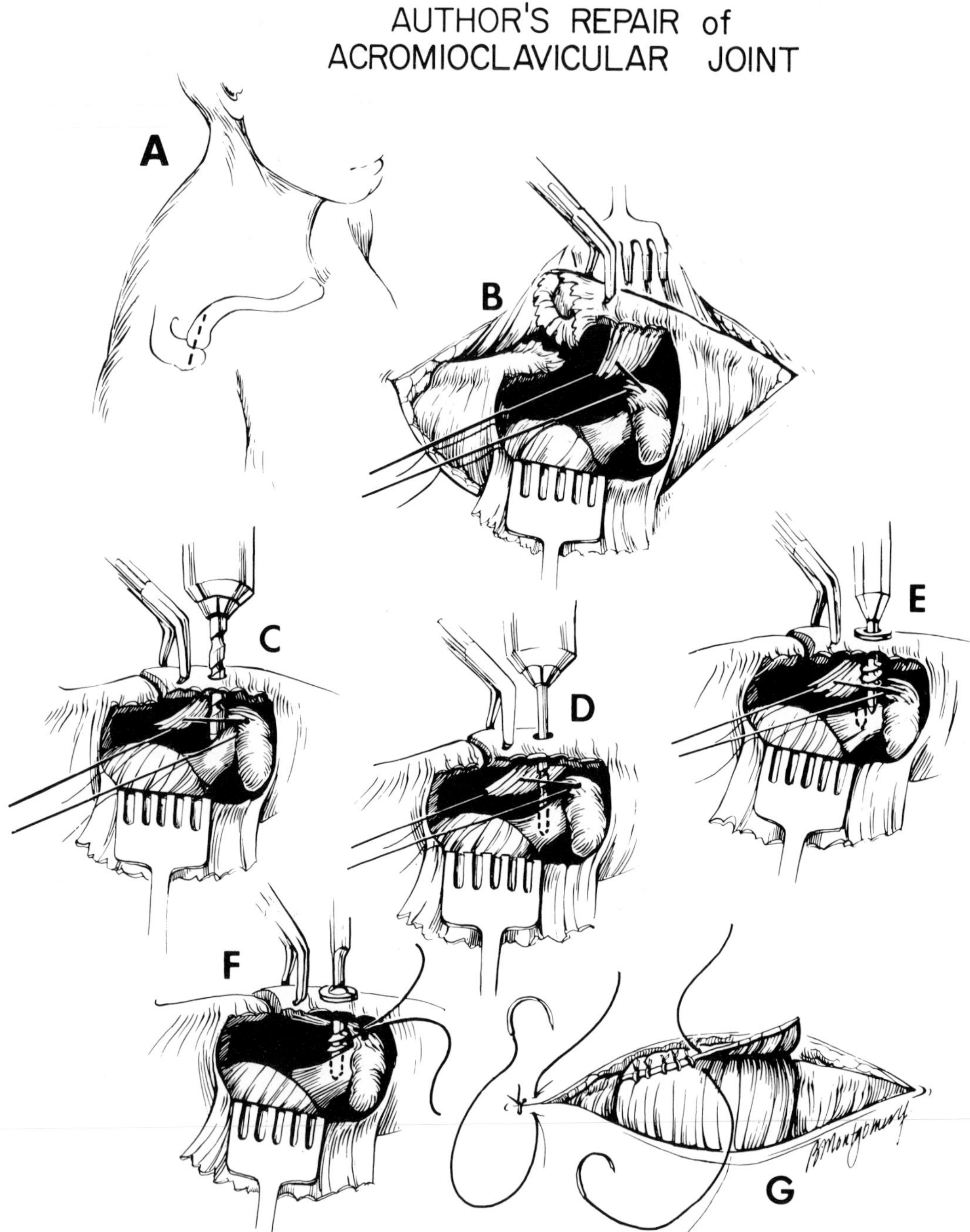

Fig. 11-150. (*A*) Author's repair of a complete acromioclavicular dislocation. The skin incision is in a straight line on top of the shoulder and helps to avoid cosmetic problems produced by anterior incisions. (*B*) The distal end of the clavicle is lifted upward with a towel clip to place sutures through the disrupted coracoclavicular ligament. The sutures are only tagged. The deltoid is usually detached from the distal clavicle or subperiosteally stripped away from the distal clavicle, which aids in the visualization of the repair of the coracoclavicular ligaments. (*C*) The acromioclavicular joint is thoroughly debrided of the meniscus, flecks of cartilage, and bone fragments. Usually the torn fibers of the acromio-

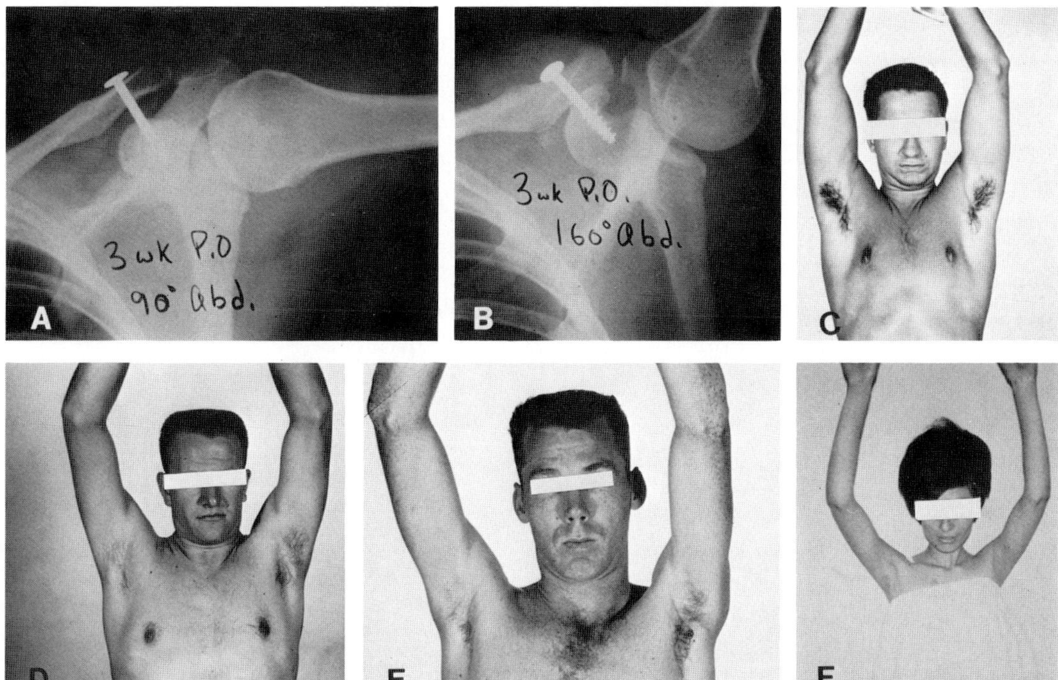

Fig. 11-151. A functional range of motion can be attained with the coracoclavicular screw in place. (*A*) Three weeks after operation, the patient is actively abducting 90 degrees. (*B*) Abduction to 160 degrees with screw in place. (*C*) Functional range of motion is demonstrated in patients with the screw in place.

to gain range of motion, but physical activities such as lifting and pushing are forbidden. After 6 weeks, the screw is removed through a stab wound under local anesthesia. The exact location of the head of the screw can be detected by taking an anteroposterior roentgenogram with a marker on the superior aspect of the shoulder (Fig. 11-144). By seeing the relation of the marker to the screw head, you can determine exactly where the stab wound should be made to excise the screw. Patients develop a very functional range of motion—in the range of 160 degrees of elevation—with the screw in place. Even girls attain this functional range of motion. In my experience, only a very few patients regain full and normal abduction, flexion, and elevation of the extremity with the screw in place. Most, however, develop at

---

clavicular ligament are debrided. With the acromioclavicular joint held reduced with the towel clip, a 3/16-inch drill bit is used to make a hole in the clavicle directly above the base of the coracoid process. (*D*) Through the 3/16-inch hole in the clavicle, a 9/64-inch drill bit is used to drill a hole into the base of the coracoid. (*E*) A specially designed screw of the appropriate length is twisted through the clavicle until the smooth shank of the screw is in the hole in the clavicle. With the screw held rigid in the screwdriver, the smooth nipple at the end of the screw is used as a probe, to locate the hole in the base of the coracoid process. (*F*) The screw is then drilled into the coracoid, and when the distal end of the clavicle is depressed by the screw until it is almost at the level of the acromion process, the tagged sutures in the coracoclavicular ligament are tied. Another half turn is then applied to the screw, taking tension off of the repaired ligaments. (*G*) The muscle attachments of the trapezius and the deltoid are imbricated over the repair of acromioclavicular joint.

least 160 degrees of forward flexion (Fig. 11-151). Usually, within a week of removing the screw, the patient has a full active range of motion. Occasionally I have noted that the patient gains the final few degrees of elevation immediately after the screw is removed. Patients are not allowed to return to vigorous activities, weight lifting, and competitive sports until 8 weeks from the time of initial surgery.

PROGNOSIS

Type I Injury. The prognosis is excellent. Essentially all patients recover full range of motion and have no pain by the end of the 2-week period.

Type II Injury. Better than 90 per cent of the patients recover fully, leaving only a very small percentage who require debridement and/or excision of the outer end of the clavicle because of arthritis in the joint.

Type III Injury. A review of the literature suggests that good results are attainable by either operative or conservative methods with a slight edge in favor of operative techniques. Approximately 80 per cent regain a normal range of motion with minimal symptoms. Twenty per cent have varying degrees of disability, which, in some instances, require reconstructive procedures.

COMPLICATIONS OF OPERATIVE AND NONOPERATIVE TREATMENT OF ACROMIOCLAVICULAR JOINT INJURIES

Obviously, each type of treatment has advantages and disadvantages. The following list includes the various complications associated with each form of treatment.

Complications of Nonoperative and Operative Treatment of Acromioclavicular Dislocations

Nonoperative Technique

1. Tissues interposed in the acromioclavicular joint
2. Joint stiffness as a result of immobilization
3. Requires close supervision and adjustments
4. Restrictive and uncomfortable
5. Skin irritation, maceration, or ulcers on the shoulder
6. Patient can remove the external device
7. Patient cannot bathe
8. Restricts everyday activities
9. Pressure sores on other parts of the body that are in contact with the immobilization device
10. Deformity may occur
11. Soft-tissue calcification
12. Acromioclavicular arthritis
13. Recurrence of deformity

Operative Technique

1. Wound infection
2. Acromioclavicular arthritis
3. Soft-tissue calcification
4. Erosion of bone by metal
5. Late fracture through the implant holes in the bone
6. Requires second operative procedure to remove the metals
7. Migration of pins or wires
8. Metal failure
9. Unsightly scar
10. Postoperative pain and loss of motion
11. Inadequate purchase of the fixation
12. Recurrent deformity

Complications of the Initial Injury

Associated Fractures

There may be fractures associated with the dislocation—fractures of the midclavicle, of the distal clavicle into the acromioclavicular joint, of the acromion process, and fracture of the coracoid process as the result of traction avulsion by the intact coracoclavicular ligaments.

Coracoclavicular Ossification

This has been referred to as ossification and calcification, and Urist[823] has demon-

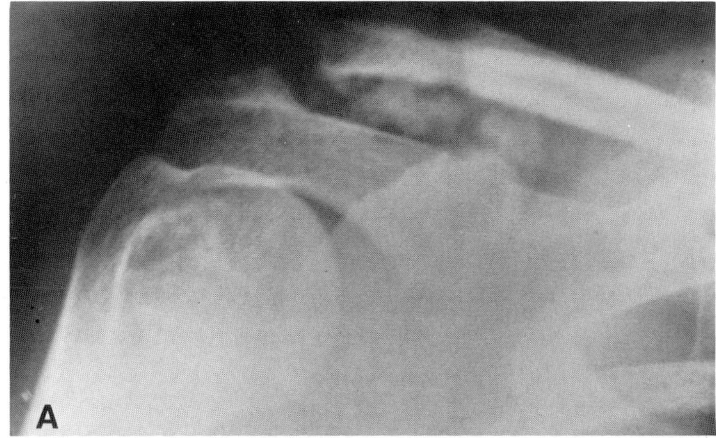

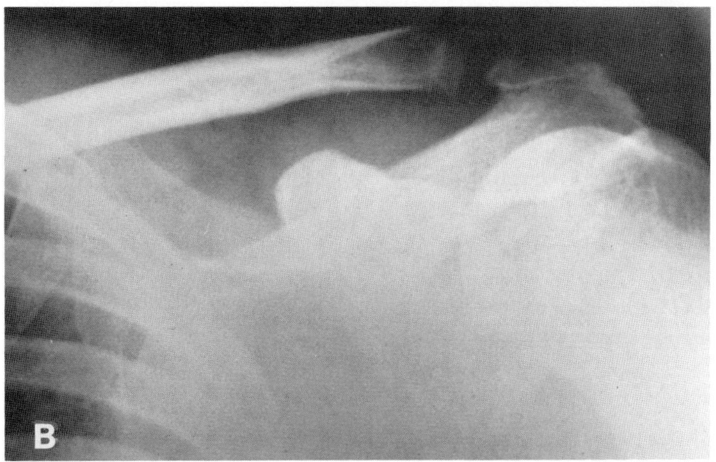

Fig. 11-152. (*A*) Ossification in the coracoclavicular inner space. An anteroposterior roentgenogram reveals marked ossification in the coracoclavicular inner space 12 months after operation. However, the patient, a laborer, has a normal range of motion and no complaints. Note the previous track of the coracoclavicular screw down through the distal clavicle. (*B*) In comparing the normal left shoulder, note that the coracoclavicular distance in the two shoulders is essentially the same.

strated that bone does indeed form in the coracoclavicular interval (Fig. 11-152). While some authors have felt that the ossification was the result of operative treatment, most have shown that the ossification occurs regardless of whether the lesion is treated by conservative or operative means. Arner, Sandahl, and Ohrling[662] report that calcification or ossification of the acromioclavicular or coracoclavicular ligament is the rule rather than the exception. They report the incidence of calcification in their series and others as 14 of 17 cases, 62 of 109 cases, and 15 of 22 cases respectively. Milburn[758] states that calcium appears in the mild or severe sprain, whether the treatment is conservative or operative, and that it can be observed as early as the third or fourth week. It may be a bone structure, and it may form a bridge from the coracoid to the clavicle, whether the treatment is operative or conservative. The ossification does not seem to affect the late functional results. In Weitzman's[835] series, 16 of 19 had calcification, and he could not correlate the end results with the presence of calcification. Alldredge[658] reported calcium in half of his operative cases, and there was no correlation with the end results.

Complications of Operative Technique

Obviously the most worrisome complications of any operative procedure are the risks associated with anesthesia and the possibility of a postoperative infection. However, with proper care, both can be avoided. Migration of the pins into various parts of the body has been reported (Fig. 11-153). Mazet[755] reported migration of a 6-cm. Kirschner wire into the lung 76 days after its insertion into the right acromioclavicular joint. Norrell and Llewellyn[776] reported migration of a Steinmann pin from the right acromioclavicular joint into the spinal cord. The pin was found in the subarachnoid space anterior to the spinal cord. It extended transversely across the spinal canal at the level of the first thoracic vertebra. It was easily removed in the direction from which it came. In most instances, migration of the pin can be prevented by bending a hook on the portion of the pin that protrudes from the acromion process. In addition, the patient must be prepared and forewarned of the possible necessity of pin removal and the complications if pins are not removed.

There are no reports of migration of loops of broken wire, and Bosworth states that he knows of no case of migration of a screw into another part of the body. Jay and Monnet[736] reported a Bosworth screw that broke during removal; the tip of the screw was left in the coracoid process.

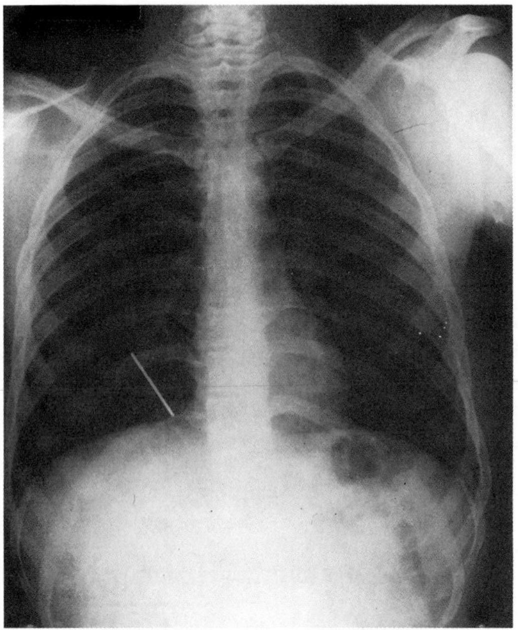

Fig. 11-153. A broken, threaded Steinmann pin has migrated into the right lung field from the right acromioclavicular joint.

There are no reports of neurovascular complications associated with injuries or with treatment of the injuries to the acromioclavicular joint. Madsen[754] has reported on a rare complication known as posttraumatic osteolysis of the lateral clavicle. In his seven cases, insufficiency and lack of treatment seem to be the predisposing causes. The most prominent roentgenographic finding is a tapering of the distal clavicle up to 2 to 3 cm., which has been noted as early as 4 weeks after injury. Symptoms usually are self-limiting within 1 to 2 years.

Complications of Nonoperative Treatment

The biggest complication with the nonoperative care of complete acromioclavicular dislocations is having to wear the immobilization apparatus continuously, day and night for 6 weeks. A harness and sling, cast, and similar devices become very uncomfortable and hot. It is difficult to bathe, and the patient may develop skin problems or stiff joints. Such treatment, to be successful, requires a very, very conscientious patient who will follow your instructions absolutely and to the letter and who is reliable enough to keep appointments for any adjustments that may be necessary. Some patients' personalities simply make them unsuitable candidates for confinement of this type in an external device.

DISLOCATION OF THE STERNOCLAVICULAR JOINT

A review of the early literature on this subject indicates that in the 19th century dislocations of the sternoclavicular joint were managed essentially the same way as fractures of the clavicle.[870,899] Sir Astley Cooper,[870] in his 1824 text, recommended that the injury be treated not only with a clavicle bandage, but also with a sling "which through the medium of the os humeri and scapula supports it and prevents the clavicle from being drawn down by the weight of the arm."

Cooper reported that he had never seen a posterior dislocation of the sternoclavicular joint that resulted from violence, but suggested that it might happen from excessive force.[870] However, he did describe a posterior dislocation of the sternoclavicular joint in a patient who had such a severe scoliosis that, as the scapula advanced laterally, it pushed the medial end of the clavicle behind the manubrium. The patient finally developed so much pressure on the esophagus and difficulty swallowing that Mr. Davie, a surgeon in Suffolk, resected the proximal clavicle. He must have been an excellent surgeon; he resected 1 inch of the proximal clavicle using a saw! He protected the vital structures in the area from the saw by introducing "a piece of well beaten sole leather under the bone whilst he divided it." The patient recovered and had no more problems with swallowing. This case probably represents the first resection of the medial end of the clavicle, either for dislocation or for arthritis.

Rodrigues[932] may have published the first case of traumatic posterior dislocation of the sternoclavicular joint in the literature, "a case of dislocation inward of the internal extremity of the clavicle," in 1843. The patient's left shoulder was against a wall when the right side of the chest and thorax were compressed and rolled forward almost to the mid-line by a cart. Immediately the patient experienced shortness of breath, which persisted for 3 weeks. When first seen by the physician, he appeared to be suffocating, and his face was blue. The left shoulder was swollen and painful, and there was "a depression on the left side of the superior extremity of the sternum." Pressure on the depression greatly increased the sensation of suffocation. Rodrigues observed that when the outer end of the shoulder was displaced backward, the inner end of the clavicle was displaced forward, which relieved the asphyxia. Therefore, treatment consisted of binding the left shoulder backward with a cushion between the two scapulae (but only after the patient had been bled twice within the first 24 hours). Rodrigues may have seen other cases of posterior dislocation, as he stated that the patient "retained a slight depression of the internal extremity of the clavicle; such, however, is the ordinary fate of the patients who present this form of dislocation."

In the late 19th century, a number of articles appeared from England, Germany, and France, and it wasn't until the 1930's that articles by Duggan,[875] Howard,[895] and Lowman[908] appeared in the American literature.

Incidence of Sternoclavicular Dislocations

Sternoclavicular injuries are rare, and many of the authors apologize for reporting only three or four cases. Attesting to this, there are some orthopaedists who have never treated the various dislocations of the sternoclavicular joint.[893,933]

The incidence of sternoclavicular dislocation, based on the series of 1603 injuries of the shoulder girdle reported by Rowe,[865] is 3 per cent (glenohumeral dislocations, 85%; acromioclavicular 12%; and sternoclavicular 3%). In the series by Rowe and in my own experience, dislocation of the sternoclavicular is not as rare as posterior dislocation of the glenohumeral joint.

Ratio of Anterior to Posterior Dislocations of the Sternoclavicular Joint

Undoubtedly, anterior dislocations of the sternoclavicular joint are much more common than the posterior retrosternal type. However, the ratio of anterior to posterior dislocations is reported only rarely. Theoretically, one could survey the literature and develop the ratio of anterior dislocations to posterior dislocations, but most of the published material on sternoclavicular dislocations is on the rare posterior dislocation. Of the references listed at the end of this chapter that deal with injuries of the sternoclavicular joint, over 60 per cent discuss only the rare posterior dislocation of the sternoclavicular joint and the various complications associated with it. The largest series from a single institution is reported by Nettles and Linscheid.[920] They reported on 60 patients with sternoclavicular dislocations—57 anterior and 3 posterior. This gives a ratio of anterior dislocations to posterior dislocations of the sternoclavicular joint of approximately 20:1. Waskowitz[942] reviewed 18 cases of sternoclavicular dislocation; none were posterior. However in my personal series of 30 cases there have been 20 cases of anterior dislocation and 10 cases of posterior dislocation.

Bilateral Dislocations of the Sternoclavicular Joint

In 1896, Hotchkiss[894] reported a bilateral traumatic dislocation of the sternoclavicular joint. A 28-year-old man was run over by a cart and received an anterior dislocation of the right shoulder and a posterior dislocation of the left one.

Most Common Cause of Sternoclavicular Dislocations

The most common cause of dislocation of the sternoclavicular joint is vehicular accidents; the second is sports.[920,922,942] Omer,[922] in his review of 14 military hospitals, accumulated 82 cases of dislocation to the sternoclavicular joint. He reported that almost 80 per cent occurred as the result of vehicular accidents (47%) and athletics (31%).

SURGICAL ANATOMY

General Considerations

The sternoclavicular joint is a diarthrodial type of joint and is the only true articulation between the upper extremity and the trunk (Fig. 11-154). The articular surfaces are covered with fibrocartilage. The enlarged bulbous medial end of the clavicle is concave, front to back, and convex vertically and, therefore, creates a saddle-type joint with the clavicular notch of the manubrium.[882,883] Cave[864] has demonstrated in 2.5 per cent of patients that, on the inferior aspect of the medial clavicle, there is a small facet which articulates with the superior aspect of the first rib at its synchondral junction with the manubrium.

Because only half of the proximal clavicle articulates with the upper angle of the manubrium, the sternoclavicular joint has the distinction of having the least amount of bony stability of the major joints of the body. Grant[882] remarks, "the two [make] an ill fit."

The sternoclavicular joint functions like a ball-and-socket joint, but with limits of excursion. The joint has motion in all planes, including rotation. It is most likely the most frequently moved joint of the long bones in the body. With your finger in the superior manubrial notch, you can feel that, with motion of the upper extremity, half of the inner clavicle is completely above the articulation with the manubrium.

Ligaments of the Sternoclavicular Joint

There is so much joint incongruity that the integrity of the joint has to come from its surrounding ligaments i.e., the intraarticular disc ligament, the extraarticular costoclavicular ligament [rhomboid ligament], the anterior and posterior sternoclavicular capsular ligaments, and the interclavicular ligament.

Intraarticular Disc Ligament

This is a very dense fibrous structure that arises from the synchondrosis junction of the first rib to the manubrium, passes through the sternoclavicular joint, and divides it into two separate joint spaces[882,883] (Fig. 11-155A). The upper attachment is

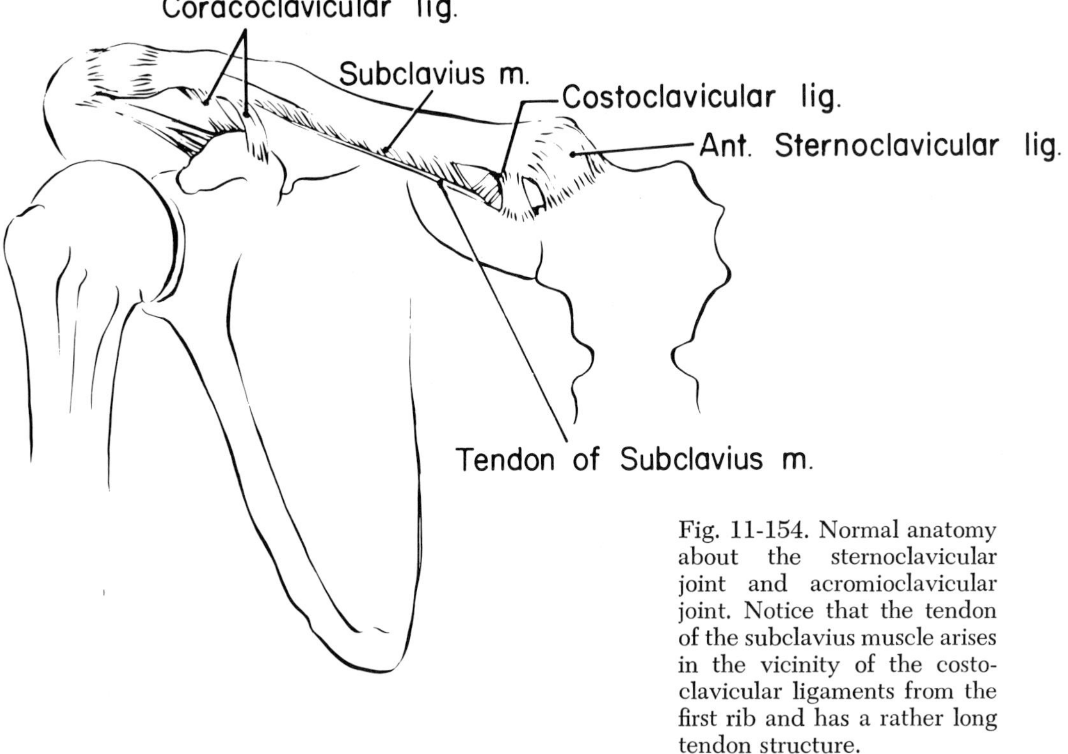

Fig. 11-154. Normal anatomy about the sternoclavicular joint and acromioclavicular joint. Notice that the tendon of the subclavius muscle arises in the vicinity of the costoclavicular ligaments from the first rib and has a rather long tendon structure.

on the superior and posterior aspects of the medial clavicle. DePalma[873] has shown that the disc is perforated only rarely; perforation allows a free communication between the two joint compartments. Anteriorly and posteriorly the disc blends into the fibers of the anterior and posterior capsular ligaments. The disc acts as a checkrein against medial displacement of the inner clavicle (Fig. 11-155B). While some authors say that the intraarticular disc ligament greatly assists the costoclavicular ligament in preventing upward displacement of the medial clavicle, Cave[864] believes that the costoclavicular ligament primarily prevents upward displacement of the clavicle. However, Bearn[852] has shown that the capsular ligament is the most important structure in preventing upward displacement. In experimental postmortem studies, he evaluated the strength and the role of each of the ligaments at the sternoclavicular joint, to see which one would prevent a downward displacement of the outer clavicle. Earlier he had shown by electromyographic studies that the trapezius does not hold up the lateral end of the clavicle, and he therefore attributed the "poise of the shoulder" to a locking mechanism of the ligaments at the sternoclavicular joint.

To accomplish his experiments, Bearn[852] resected the clavicle, the manubrium, and the first rib and left all of the ligaments attached. He secured the manubrium to a block in a vise (Fig. 11-156). He then loaded the outer end of the clavicle with 10 to 20 lbs. of weight and cut the ligaments of the sternoclavicular joint, one at a time and in various combinations, to determine each ligament's effect on maintaining the clavicle poise (i.e., which ligament was most important to hold up the lateral end of the shoulder—or, thinking of it in another way, which ligament would rupture first when the medial end of the clavicle was forced upward by the downward force on the outer end of the clavicle as it pivoted over the first rib).

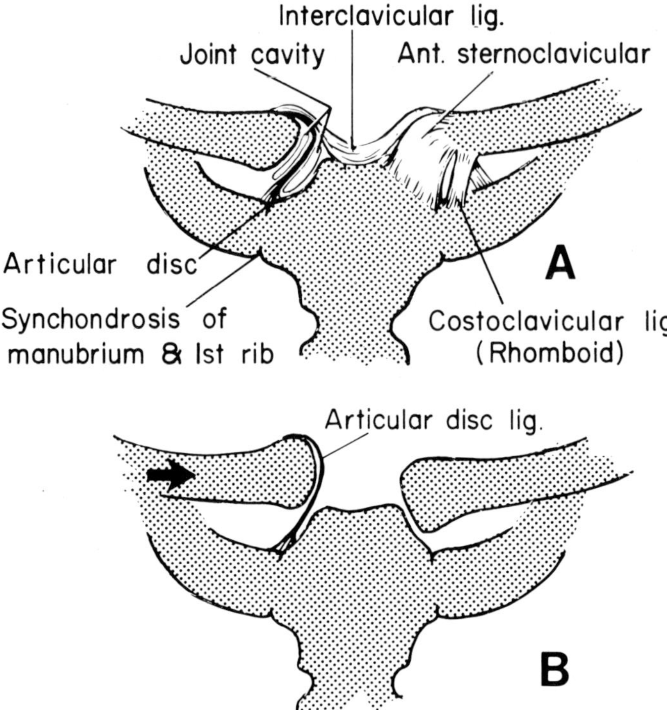

Fig. 11-155. (*A*) Normal anatomy about the sternoclavicular joint. Note that the articular disc ligament divides the sternoclavicular joint cavity into two separate spaces and inserts on the superior and posterior aspect of the medial clavicle. (*B*) The articular disc ligament acts as a checkrein for medial displacement of the proximal clavicle.

He determined, after cutting the costoclavicular ligament, the intraarticular disc ligament, and the interclavicular ligament, that they had no effect on clavicle poise. However, the division of the capsular ligament alone resulted in a downward depression on the lateral end of the clavicle about an axis of the costoclavicular ligament. He also noted that the intraarticular disc ligament tore under 5 lbs. of weight, once the capsular ligament had been cut. This article has many clinical implications for the mechanisms of injury of the sternoclavicular joint.

Cave[864] had previously stated that the costoclavicular ligament is the effective inferior ligament of the sternoclavicular joint, and that it is capable of maintaining clavicle stability even after division of the joint capsule and its meniscus: "it resists upward displacement of the clavicle head of the muscle sternomastoideus and the lateral pull of the clavicle portion of the muscle pectoralis major." I do not see any real disagreements with the comments of Bearn[852] and Cave,[864] as the costoclavicular ligament is an effective ligament of the sternoclavicular joint that resists forces that tend to displace it anteriorly, posteriorly, upward, or laterally. The work by Bearn[852] simply states that the capsular ligament is the first and strongest resistive force against depression of the outer clavicle and hence of the upward displacement of the inner end of the clavicle as it is levered over the first rib.

Costoclavicular Ligament

This ligament, also called the rhomboid ligament, is short and strong and consists of an anterior and a posterior fasciculus (Fig. 11-154).[852,864,883] Cave[864] reports that the average length is 1.3 cm., with 1.9 cm. maximum width; it is 1.3 cm. thick. Bearn[852] has shown that there is always a bursa between the two components of the ligament. Because of the two different parts of the ligament, it has a twisted appearance.[883] The costoclavicular ligament attaches below to the upper surface of the first rib and

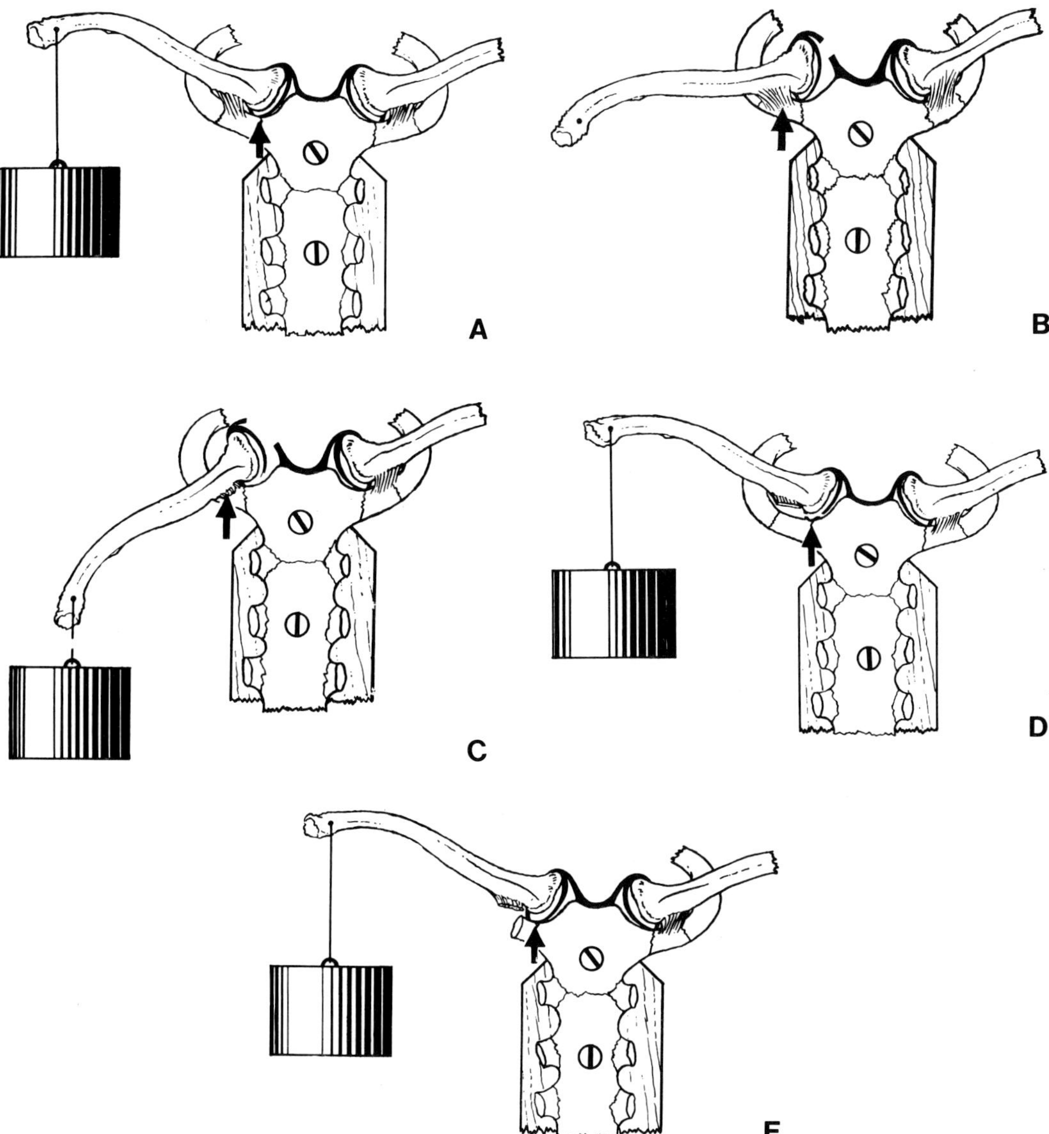

Fig. 11-156. The importance of the various ligaments about the sternoclavicular joint in maintaining normal clavicular poise. (*A*) The lateral end of the clavicle is maintained in an elevated position (clavicle poise) through the sternoclavicular ligaments. The arrow indicates the fulcrum. (*B*) When the capsule was divided completely, the lateral end of the clavicle descended without any loading under its own weight until it was lower than the medial end. The clavicle was then seen to be supported by the intraarticular disc ligaments. (*C*) After division of the capsular ligament, it was determined that a weight of less than 5 lbs. was enough to tear the intraarticular disc ligament from its attachment on the costal cartilage junction of the first rib. The fulcrum was transferred laterally so that the medial end of the clavicle hinged over the first rib in the vicinity of the costoclavicular ligament. (*D*) After division of the costoclavicular ligament, and the intraarticular disc ligament, the lateral end of the clavicle could not be depressed, as long as the capsular ligament was intact. (*E*) After resection of the medial first costal cartilage along with the costoclavicular ligaments, there was no effect on the poise of the lateral end of the clavicle, as long as the capsular ligament was intact. (Bearn, J. G.: J. Anat., *101*:159-170, 1967)

at the adjacent part of the synchondrosis junction with the manubrium, and above to the margins of the impression on the inferior surface of the medial end of the clavicle, sometimes known as the rhomboid fossa.[882,883] Cave[864] has shown, from a study of 153 clavicles, that the attachment to the costoclavicular ligament can be any of three shapes—a depression (the rhomboid fossa) in 30 per cent; flat in 60 per cent; and, in 10 per cent of the cases, an elevation.

Anterior Fasciculus. The fibers of the anterior fasciculus arise from the anterior medial surface of the first rib and are directed upward and laterally.

Posterior Fasciculus. The fibers of the posterior fasciculus are shorter and arise lateral to the anterior fibers on the rib and are directed upward and medially.

The fibers of the anterior and posterior components cross and allow for stability of the joint during rotation and elevation of the clavicle. The two-part costoclavicular ligament is in many ways similar to the two-part configuration of the coracoclavicular ligament on the outer end of the clavicle. Bearn[852] has shown experimentally that the anterior fibers resist upward rotation of the clavicle and the posterior fibers resist downward rotation. Specifically the anterior fibers also resist lateral displacement, and the posterior fibers resist medial displacement.

Anterior and Posterior Sternoclavicular Capsular Ligaments

These ligaments cover the anterior and posterior aspects of the joint and are thickenings of the joint capsule (Fig. 11-155). The anterior sternoclavicular ligament is heavier and stronger than the posterior ligament. According to the original work of Bearn,[852] these may not be the strongest ligaments of the sternoclavicular joint, but they are the first line of defense against the upward displacement of the inner clavicle caused by a force on the lateral aspect of the shoulder. Attachment of the anterior and posterior is primarily onto the epiphysis of the medial clavicle with some secondary blending of the fibers into the metaphysis. This has been demonstrated by Poland,[927] Denham and Dingley,[871] Brooks and Henning,[859] and myself.

Interclavicular Ligament

The interclavicular ligament connects the superior and inner aspects of each clavicle with the capsular ligaments and the upper manubrium (Fig. 11-155). According to Grant,[882] this band may be homologous with the wishbone of birds. This ligament acts to assist the capsular sternoclavicular ligaments to produce "shoulder poise," to hold up the outer end of the shoulder. You can test this by putting your finger in the superior manubrial notch; with elevation of the arm, the ligament is quite lax, but as soon as both arms hang at the side, the ligament becomes tight.

Motions of the Sternoclavicular Joint

The joint is freely movable. Inman, Saunders, and Abbott[898] and Lucas[909] have shown that for every 10 degrees of abduction of the arm up to 90 degrees, the clavicle is elevated 4 degrees. Beyond 90 degrees of abduction of the arm, clavicular elevation is negligible. At full abduction of the arm, the clavicle has been noted by the same authors to rotate 40 to 50 degrees, and to move slightly forward, backward, and downward.

In summary, then, the clavicle is capable of elevating 36 degrees and rotating upward 50 degrees, and it has slight forward, backward, and downward motions.

Epiphysis of the Medial Clavicle

While the clavicle is the first long bone of the body to ossify (fifth intrauterine week), the epiphysis at the inner end of the clavicle is the last of the long bones in the body to close[882,883,927] (Figs. 11-161C; 11-169). The medial clavicular epiphysis does not ossify until the 18th to the 20th year, and it fuses with the shaft of the clavicle around the 25th year. This knowledge of the epiphysis is important, for I believe that many of the so-called sternoclavicular dislocations are fractures through the epiphyseal plate. This text does not cover fractures and dislocations in children, but in this situation the epiphyseal injury occurs in an adult.

Applied Surgical Anatomy

The surgeon who is planning an operative repair of the sternoclavicular joint should be completely knowledgeable about the vast array of anatomical structures immediately behind the sternoclavicular joint. There is a "curtain" of muscles, the sternohyoid and sternothyroid, posterior to the sternoclavicular joint and the inner third of the clavicle, which blocks the view of the vital structures (among them the innominate artery, innominate vein, vagus nerve, phrenic nerve, internal jugular vein, trachea, and esophagus) (Fig. 11-157). If you are considering the possibility of stabilizing the sternoclavicular joint by running a pin down from the clavicle and into the manubrium, you might remember that the arch of the aorta, the superior vena cava, and the right pulmonary artery are very close at hand.

Another structure that may give you some bad moments is the anterior jugular vein, which is between the clavicle and the curtain of muscles. The anatomy books state that it can be quite variable in size; I have seen it as large as 1.5 cm. in diameter. This vein has no valves, and when it is nicked, it looks like someone has opened up flood gates.

MECHANISM OF INJURY

Because the sternoclavicular joint is subject to every motion of the upper extremity and because the joint is so incongruous, you would think it would be the most commonly dislocated joint in the body. However, its ligament structure is so designed that it is one of the least commonly dislocated joints in the body. The traumatic dislocation of the sternoclavicular joint usually occurs only after tremendous forces —direct or indirect—have been applied to the shoulder.

Direct Force

A direct force is one applied directly to

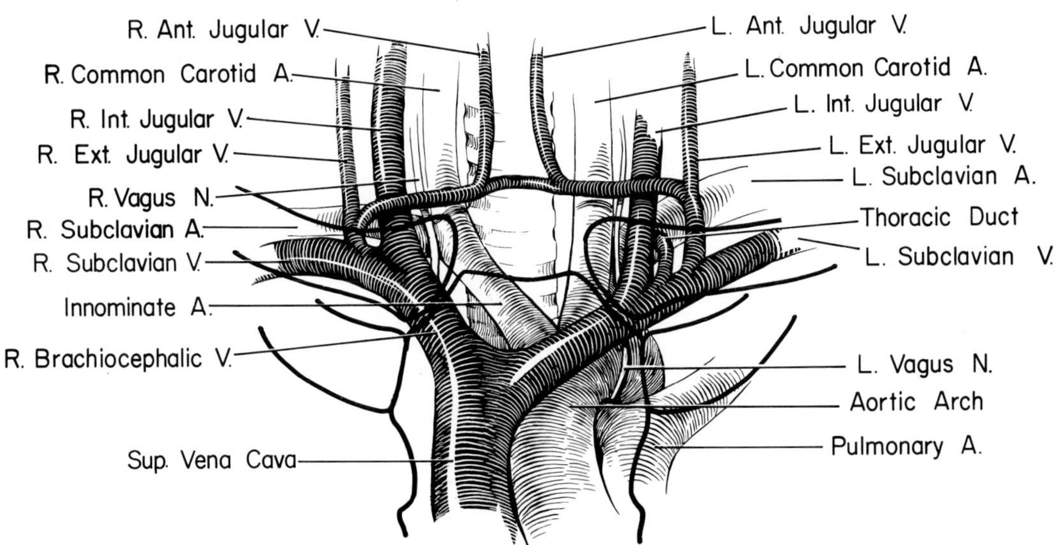

Fig. 11-157. Applied anatomy of the vital structures posterior to the sternoclavicular joint.

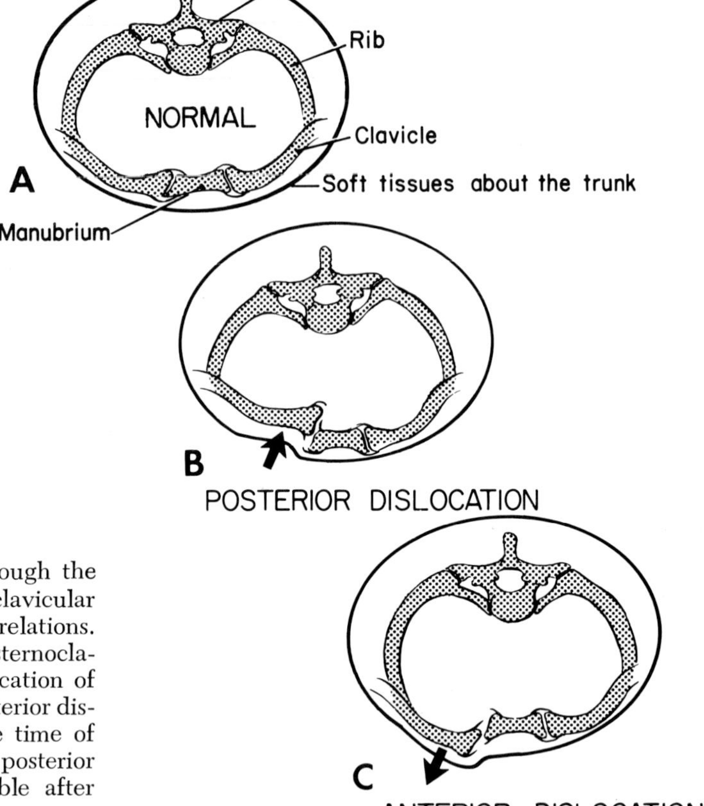

Fig. 11-158. A cross-section through the thorax at the level of the sternoclavicular joint. (*A*) Normal anatomical relations. (*B*) Posterior dislocation of the sternoclavicular joint. (*C*) Anterior dislocation of the sternoclavicular joint. The anterior dislocation may be unstable at the time of closed reduction, whereas the posterior dislocation is usually quite stable after reduction.

the anteromedial aspect of the clavicle which pushes the clavicle out posteriorly and behind the manubrium (Fig. 11-158B). This may occur in a variety of ways; an athlete lying on his back on the ground may be jumped on in a pile-on; a person may receive a kick to the front of the inner clavicle by a mule; or any type of crushing force, such as being run over by a vehicle or being pinned between a vehicle and a wall will do similar damage. Because of our anatomy, direct force can produce only posterior sternoclavicular dislocation.

Indirect Force

Force may be transmitted indirectly to the sternoclavicular joint from the anterolateral and posterolateral aspects of the shoulder. This is the most common cause of dislocations of the sternoclavicular joint. Mehta[915] reported that three of four posterior sternoclavicular dislocations were produced by indirect force, and Heinig[890] reported that indirect force was responsible for eight of nine cases of posterior sternoclavicular dislocations. If the shoulder is compressed and rolled forward, an ipsilateral posterior dislocation results; if the shoulder is compressed and rolled backward, an ipsilateral anterior dislocation results.

One of the most common causes that I have seen is a pile-on in a neighborhood football game, wherein the patient falls on the ground, landing on the lateral shoulder, and then before he can get out of the way, several boys pile on top of the opposite shoulder, which applies significant compressive force on the clavicle down toward the manubrium. If during the compression the shoulder is rolled forward, the dislocation of the sternoclavicular joint is posterior; if the shoulder rolls backward during the compressive force, the dislocation is anterior (Fig. 11-159). Other types of indirect forces that have been reported to produce dislocation are a cave-in on a ditch digger, with lateral compression of the shoulders by the falling dirt; lateral compressive forces within the shoulder when a patient was pinned between a vehicle and a wall; and (an even more indirect force) a patient falling on the outstretched abducted arm, which then drove the shoulder medially in the same manner as a lateral compression on the shoulder.

CLASSIFICATION OF DISLOCATIONS OF THE STERNOCLAVICULAR JOINT

There are two types of classifications. One is based on the etiology of the dislocation, and one, on the anatomical position that the dislocation assumes.

Classification Based on Anatomy

Many complicated categories and subcategories can be—and have been—used. However, detailed classifications are confusing and hard to remember. The following classification is suggested:

Anterior Sternoclavicular Dislocation

This is the most common sternoclavicular dislocation. The medial end of the clavicle is displaced anteriorly or anterosuperiorly to the anterior margin of the manubrium (Fig. 11-158C).

Posterior Dislocation

Posterior dislocation is uncommon. The medial end of the clavicle is displaced posteriorly or posterosuperiorly with respect to the posterior margin of the manubrium (Fig. 11-158B).

Some authors have, on occasion, reported superior dislocation of the sternoclavicular joint, so that could be considered a third type of dislocation. However, in most authors' experience, including my own, the dislocation is either anterosuperior or posterosuperior, and not purely superior.

Classification Based on Etiology

Traumatic Injuries of the Sternoclavicular Joint

Acute sprains to the sternoclavicular joint can be classified as mild, moderate or severe.

In a mild sprain all of the ligaments are intact. The joint is stable and not displaced.

In a moderate sprain there is subluxation of the sternoclavicular joint. The capsular ligaments and the interarticular disc ligament are usually ruptured. The subluxation may be anterior/superior or posterior/superior. The costoclavicular ligaments remain intact but may be stretched.

Severe sprain is analogous to acute dislocation.

Acute Dislocation. In a dislocated sternoclavicular joint the capsular and interarticular ligaments are ruptured, and usually the costoclavicular ligament as well. Occasionally the costoclavicular ligament is intact but stretched enough to allow the dislocation. Upward displacement of the dislocation—anterior or posterior—signifies rupture of the costoclavicular ligament.

Recurrent Dislocation. If the initial acute traumatic dislocation does not heal, mild to moderate forces may produce recurrent dislocations. This is a rare entity.

Unreduced Dislocation. The initial dislocation has not been reduced. The original dislocation may go unrecognized, or it may be irreducible, or the physician may decide not to reduce certain dislocations.

Atraumatic Sternoclavicular Dislocation

Voluntary or Habitual Dislocation. Patients may learn, by moving the arms overhead, to place one or both medial clavicles in subluxation or dislocation. This phenomenon may be associated with laxity in other joints.

Congenital or Developmental Dislocation. Congenital defects with loss of bone substance on either side of the joint can predispose to subluxation or dislocation. Cooper[870] described a patient with scoliosis so severe that the shoulder was displaced forward enough to posteriorly dislocate the clavicle behind the manubrium.

Spontaneous Dislocation. *Normal Degenerative Changes in the Elderly.* Bremner[858] and Bonnin[856] both have reported on this condition. The characteristics of the spontaneous subluxation are very clear-cut. The condition is the result of normal degeneration of a frequently moved joint. It usually occurs in elderly women and in the sternoclavicular joint of the dominant hand. It is almost without symptoms; a lump develops at the sternoclavicular joint, and, occasionally, a vague ache. There is no previous history of injury or disease. Roentgenograms reveal erosion of the articular surface of the clavicle and subluxation of the joint. The pathological changes are those of degenerative arthritis.

Joint Disease Processes. Spontaneous dislocation may be associated with subacute or acute bacterial arthritis and even with rheumatoid arthritis. Higoumenakis[880] has reported that unilateral enlargement of the sternoclavicular joint is a diagnostic sign of congenital syphilis. The enlargement of the sternoclavicular joint can be mistaken for an anterior dislocation. He reported the sign to be positive in 170 of 197 cases of congenital syphilis. Glickman and Minskey[880] have reported on the same condition. The enlargement is a hyperostosis of the medial clavicle occurring in the sternoclavicular joint of the dominant extremity, which reaches its permanent stage and size at puberty. The theory of why it affects the sternoclavicular joint relates it to spirochete invasion of the sternal end of the clavicle at the time of its early ossification.

SIGNS AND SYMPTOMS OF STERNOCLAVICULAR INJURIES

Acute Sprain of the Sternoclavicular Joint

Mild Sprain

The ligaments of the joint are intact. The patient complains of a mild to moderate amount of pain, particularly with movement of the upper extremity. The joint may

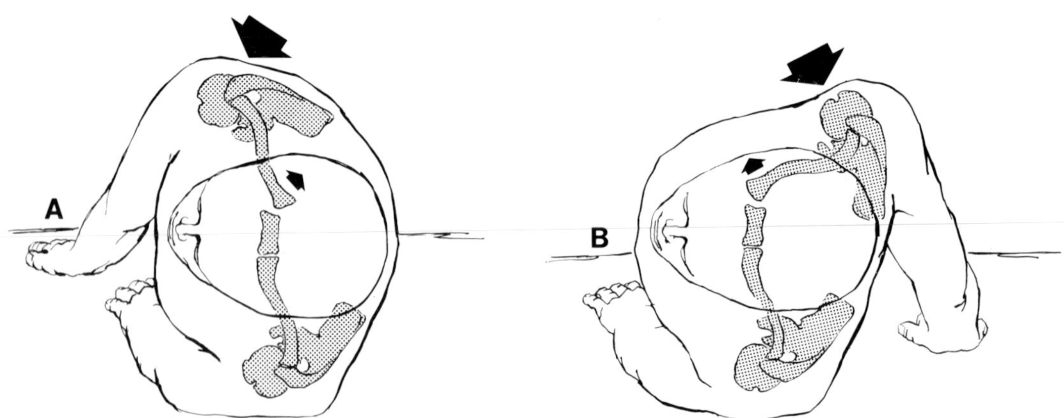

Fig. 11-159. Mechanisms that produce anterior and posterior dislocations of the sternoclavicular joint. (*A*) When the patient is lying on the ground, and a compression force is applied to the posterior lateral aspect of the shoulder, the medial end of the clavicle is displaced posteriorly. (*B*) When the lateral compression force is directed from the anterior position, the medial end of the clavicle is dislocated anteriorly. The same mechanism could apply with any type of lateral compression injury of the shoulder.

be swollen slightly and is tender to palpation, but instability is not noted.

Moderate Sprain

A moderate sprain is a sternoclavicular joint subluxation. Fibers of the capsule and the intraarticular disc are usually ruptured, but they may be only severely stretched. Swelling is noted and pain is marked, particularly with any movement of the arm. Anterior or posterior subluxation may be obvious to the eye when the injured joint is compared to the normal sternoclavicular joint. The medial clavicle may be lax when it is gently manipulated.

Severe Sprain

Dislocations of the sternoclavicular joint can be anterior or posterior. The capsular ligament and the intraarticular disc ligament are ruptured. The costoclavicular ligaments are usually ruptured, but one or both of the components may be intact but stretched. Regardless of whether the dislocation is anterior or posterior, there are characteristic findings of sternoclavicular joint dislocation (see below).

Signs Common to Both Anterior and Posterior Dislocations of the Sternoclavicular Joint

The patient has severe pain. This pain is increased with any movement of the arm, particularly when the shoulders are pressed together by a lateral force. The patient usually supports the injured arm across his trunk with his normal arm. The shoulder appears to be shortened and thrust forward, when compared to the normal shoulder. The head may be tilted toward the side of the dislocated joint. The patient's discomfort increases when he is put into the supine position. When the patient assumes the supine position, the involved shoulder will not lie back flat on the table top.

Signs of Anterior Sternoclavicular Dislocation

The medial end of the clavicle is visibly prominent anterior to the joint (in obese patients, this may not be seen). The medial end of the clavicle can be palpated anterior to the manubrium, even in the obese patient. The anteriorly displaced medial end of the clavicle may be fixed or it may be quite mobile. The medial anteriorly displaced clavicle may be riding quite high, which indicates complete disruption of the costoclavicular ligaments. (See Fig. 11-160.)

Signs of Posterior Sternoclavicular Dislocation

The patient has more pain than that associated with anterior sternoclavicular dislocations. The anterosuperior fullness of the chest produced by the clavicle is less

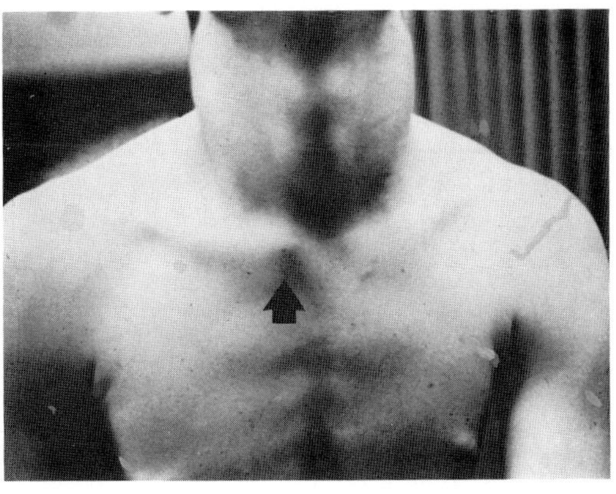

Fig. 11-160. Clinically evident anterior dislocation of the right sternoclavicular joint (*arrow*).

prominent when compared to the normal side. The usually prominent medial end of the clavicle is not visible and cannot be palpated. Venous congestion may be present in the neck. The patient may have breathing difficulties, shortness of breath, or a choking sensation. Circulation in the ipsilateral arm may be decreased. The patient may complain of difficulty in swallowing or a tight feeling in the throat. The patient may be in a state of complete shock or he may have a pneumothorax (see Fig. 11-167).

ROENTGENOGRAPHIC FINDINGS

The literature almost uniformly reflects that roentgenograms of the sternoclavicular joint, regardless of the special views, are difficult to interpret. Special oblique views of the chest have been recommended, but because of the distortion of one of the clavicles over the other, interpretation is almost impossible (Fig. 11-161). Most of the literature on dislocation of the sternoclavicular joint indicates that the diagnosis is made clinically and not by roentgenograms. Baker[848] reported that the fingers of his orthopaedic colleagues were far more accurate in diagnosing sternoclavicular dislocations than were his roentgenograms; however, he went on to say that tomography offered more detailed information, often showing small fractures in the vicinity of the sternoclavicular joint. Occasionally the routine anteroposterior or posteroanterior roentgenogram of the chest or sternoclavicular joint suggests that something is wrong with one of the clavicles, because it appears to be displaced as compared with the normal side. It would be ideal to take a view at right angles to the posteroanterior plane, but because our anatomy is the way it is, it is impossible to take a true 90-degree cephalic-to-caudal lateral. Lateral roentgenograms of the chest are at right angles to the anteroposterior plane, but they cannot be interpreted because of the density of the chest and the overlap of the medial clavicles with the first rib and the manubrium.

Special Views

Kattan[901] has recommended a special projection, as have Ritvo and Ritvo.[931] Kurzbauer[905] has recommended special lateral projections. Hobbs,[891] in 1968, recommended

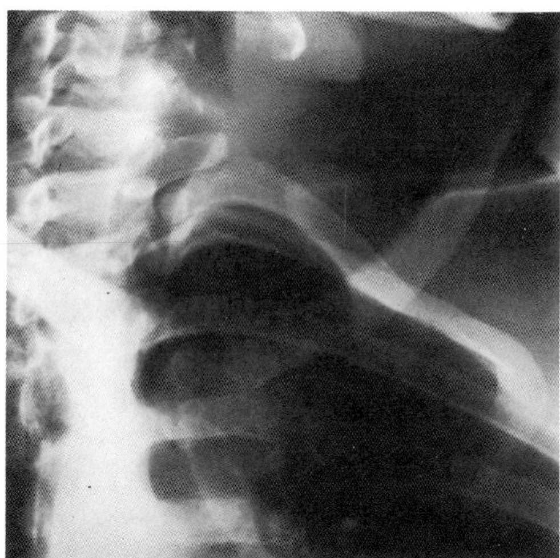

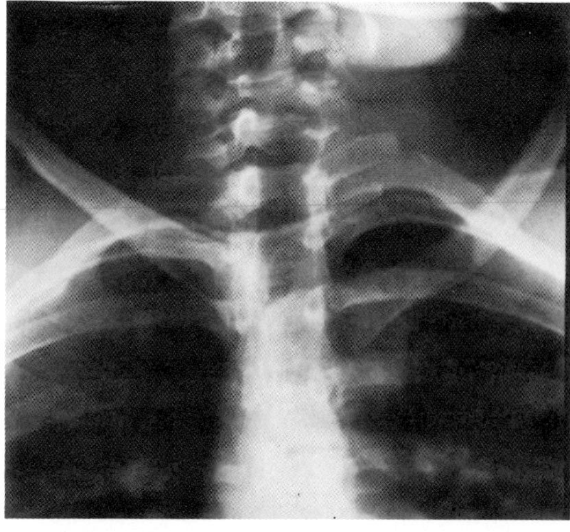

Fig. 11-161. Routine roentgenograms of the sternoclavicular joint are difficult to interpret, even though a posterior dislocation of the left sternoclavicular joint is clinically evident.

a view that comes close to being a 90-degree cephalocaudal lateral view of the sternoclavicular joints. In the Hobbs view, the patient is seated at the x-ray table, high enough to lean forward over the table. The cassette is on the table top, and the lower anterior rib cage is against the cassette (Fig. 11-162). The patient leans forward so that the nape of his flexed neck is almost parallel to the table top. The flexed elbows straddle the cassette and support the head and neck. The x-ray source is above the nape of the neck, and the beam passes through the cervical spine to project the sternoclavicular joints onto the cassette on the table top.

Laminagrams and stereos are helpful but difficult to obtain and interpret in the emergency department.

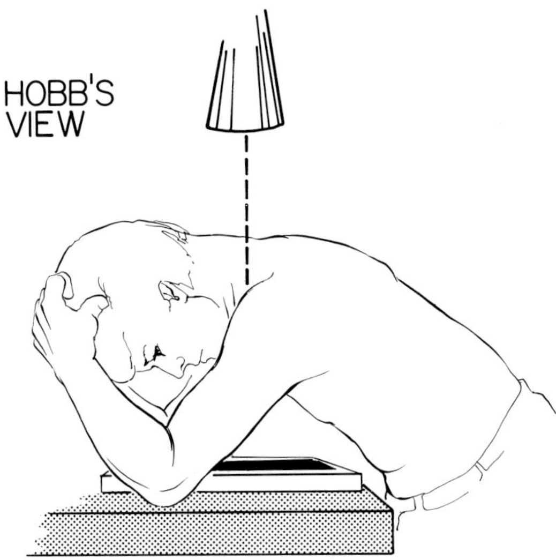

Fig. 11-162. Positioning of the patient for roentgenography of the sternoclavicular joint as recommended by Hobbs. (Redrawn from Hobbs, D. W.: Radiology, *90*:801, 1968)

Suggested Roentgenographic Technique

This should rightfully be called the serendipity technique, because that's the way it was developed. I found, accidentally, that the next best thing to having a true cephalocaudal lateral view of the sternoclavicular joint is a 40-degree cephalic tilt view.

The patient is positioned on his back squarely and in the center of the x-ray table. The tube is tilted at a 40-degree angle off of the vertical and is centered directly at the manubrium (Fig. 11-163). A **non-grid** 11 × 14-inch cassette is placed

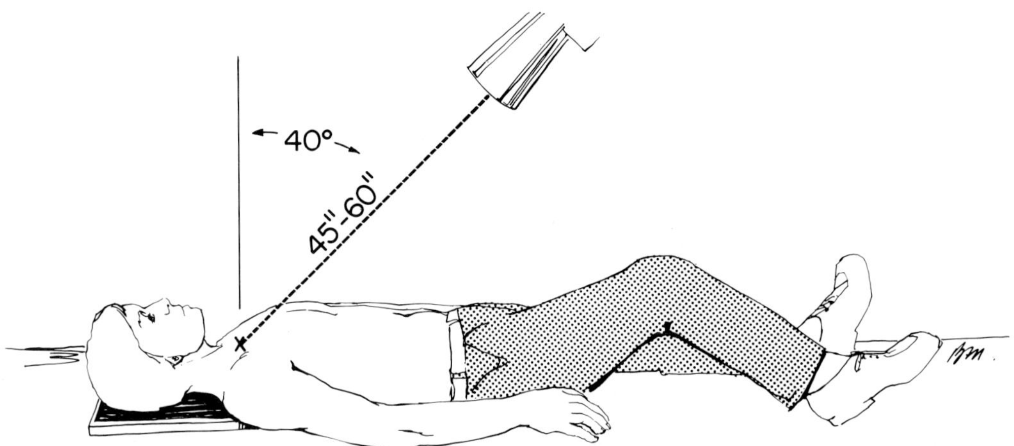

Fig. 11-163. Positioning of the patient to take the cephalic tilt roentgenogram of the sternoclavicular joint. The x-ray tube is tilted 40 degrees from the vertical position and is aimed directly at the manubrium. The cassette should be large enough to receive the projected images of the medial halves of both clavicles. In children, the tube distance should be approximately 45 inches; with thicker-chested adults, the distance should be 60 inches.

squarely on the table top and under the patient's upper shoulders and neck, so that the beam aimed at the manubrium will project the clavicles onto the middle of the film. The cone is adjusted so that the medial one-half to two-thirds of both clavicles will be seen on the film. It is important to note that the cassette should be placed squarely on the x-ray table top (i.e., not angulated or rotated) and that the patient should be positioned squarely on top of the cassette.

For children, the distance from the tube to the cassette is 45 inches, but in adults whose anteroposterior chest diameter is greater, the distance should be 60 inches. The technical setting of the machine is essentially the same as for a posteroanterior view of the chest.

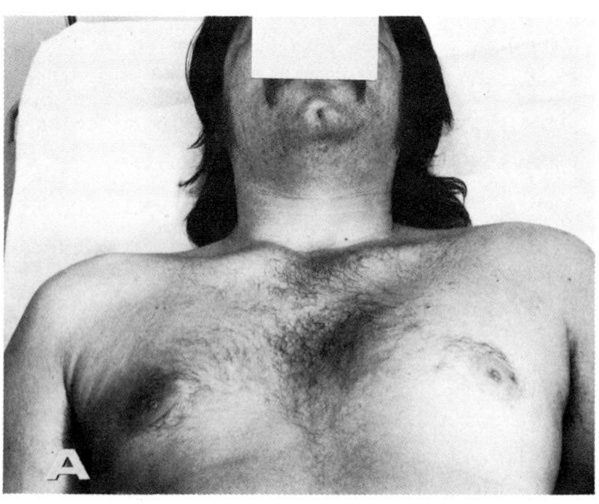

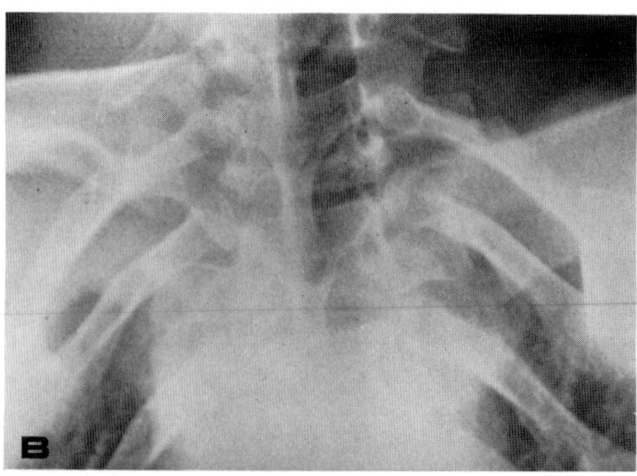

Fig. 11-164. (*A*) When the medial clavicles are viewed from the level of the patient's knees, it is apparent that the right medial clavicle is anteriorly dislocated. (*B*) In the 40-degree cephalic tilt roentgenogram, the right medial clavicle is superiorly displaced from the level of the left (normal) medial clavicle, indicating an anterior dislocation.

For example, imagine that your eyes are at the level of the patient's knees and you are looking up toward his clavicles at a 40-degree angle. If the right sternoclavicular joint were dislocated anteriorly, the right clavicle would appear to be displaced more anteriorly or riding higher on an imaginary horizontal line when compared to the normal left clavicle (Fig. 11-164). The reverse is true when the right sternoclavicular joint is dislocated posteriorly (i.e., the right clavicle would be displaced posteriorly or riding lower on an imaginary horizontal plane than the normal left clavicle). The idea, then, is to take a 40-degree cephalic tilt roentgenogram of both medial clavicles and compare the relation to an imaginary line of the injured clavicle and the uninjured one (Fig. 11-165).

TREATMENT OF DISLOCATION TO THE STERNOCLAVICULAR JOINT AND CARE AFTER REDUCTION

Traumatic Injuries

Type I. The joint is stable but painful. Ice for the first 12 to 24 hours followed by heat is helpful. The upper extremity should be immobilized in a sling for 3 to 4 days, and then, gradually, the patient can regain use of his arm in everyday activities.

Type II. For subluxation of sternoclavicular joint ice is recommended for the first 12 hours, followed by heat for the next 24 to 48 hours. The joint may be in anterior or posterior subluxation, which can be reduced by drawing the shoulders backward as if reducing and holding a fracture of the clavicle. A clavicle strap can be used to hold the reduction. A sling and swathe should also be used to hold up the shoulder and to prevent motion of the arm. The patient should be protected from further possible injury for 4 to 6 weeks. DePalma[874] sug-

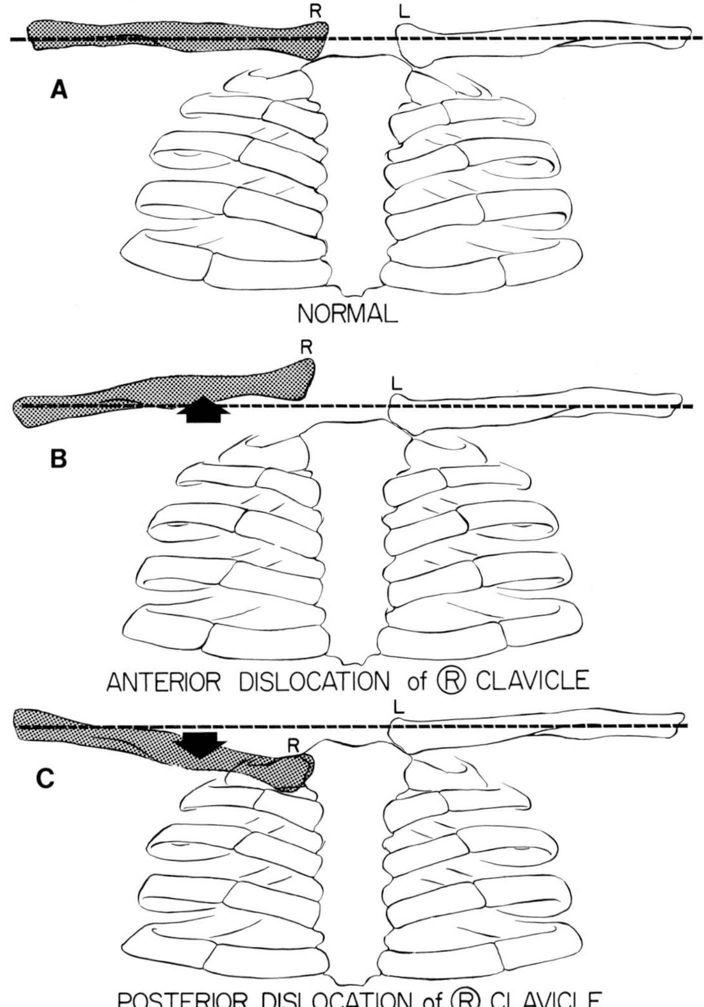

Fig. 11-165. Interpretation of the cephalic tilt roentgenogram of the sternoclavicular joints. (*A*) In the normal individual, both clavicles appear on the same imaginary line drawn horizontally across the film. (*B*) In a patient with anterior dislocation of the right sternoclavicular joint, the medial half of the right clavicle is projected above the imaginary line drawn through the level of the normal left clavicle. (*C*) If the patient has a posterior dislocation of the right sternoclavicular joint, the medial half of the right clavicle is displaced below the imaginary line drawn through the normal left clavicle.

gests a plaster figure-of-eight dressing, and McLaughlin[914] recommended the same type of treatment that would be used for fracture of the clavicle, with the addition of a sling to support the arm. Allman[845] prefers the use of a soft figure-of-eight bandage with a sling, and occasionally uses adhesive strapping over the medial end of the clavicle. When in certain circumstances the subluxation cannot be reduced, some authors[851,874] recommend repair of the ligaments and temporary internal fixation of the sternoclavicular joint with pins drilled from the clavicle into the sternum. Postoperatively DePalma[874] applies a plaster figure-of-eight cast and, in addition, supports with a sling and swathe; the pins and the cast are removed after 6 weeks.

Occasionally, following conservative treatment of a Type II injury, the pain lingers on and the symptoms of popping and grating persist. This may require joint exploration. Bateman[851] has commented on the possibility of finding a tear of the intraarticular disc, which should be excised. Duggan[875] reported a case in which, several weeks after an injury to the sternoclavicular joint, the patient still had popping in the joint. Through a small incision, Duggan exposed the capsule, and out through the capsule popped the intraarticular disc, which looked like "an avulsed fingernail." Following repair of the capsule, the patient had no more problems. If degenerative changes become severe in the sternoclavicular joint, excision of the medial clavicle over to the attachment of the costoclavicular ligament may be required.

Type III. Dislocation of the sternoclavicular joint may be anterior or posterior.

Treatment of Anterior Dislocation of the Sternoclavicular Joint

Technique of Closed Reduction. Closed reduction of the sternoclavicular joint may be accomplished with general anesthesia. Some authors recommend the use of narcotics or muscle relaxants. The patient is placed on his back on the edge of the table with a sandbag between the shoulders. With the upper extremity in 90 degrees of abduction and extension, traction is applied in line with the clavicle (Fig. 11-166A). If reduction is not accomplished, the gentle pressure directed posteriorly can be applied to the anteriorly displaced clavicle. In some instances, the reduction is quite stable, whereas, in others, it is unstable when the traction is released. An alternative technique of reduction is to put your knee between the scapulae of the seated patient and pull both shoulders back. Usually, if both shoulders are held back, the reduction can be maintained.

Care After Reduction. The shoulder can be held back with a soft figure-of-eight dressing, a commercial clavicle strap harness, or a plaster figure-of-eight cast. Some authors recommend a bulky pressure pad over the anterior medial clavicle, held in place with elastic tape. A sling and swathe should be worn in addition to the figure-of-eight bandage, because it holds up the shoulder and prevents motion of the arm. Immobilization should be maintained at least 6 weeks, and then the arm should be protected for another 2 weeks before strenuous activities are undertaken.

Many anterior closed reductions of the sternoclavicular joint are unstable (i.e., even with the shoulders held back, the joint is in subluxation). You then must decide whether to accept the subluxation or to perform open reduction of the joint.

Operative Repairs and Care After Reduction. DePalma[874] recommends the use of two 5⁄64-inch pins drilled from the clavicle into the manubrium with repair of the ligaments. Postoperatively, he holds the patient in a plaster figure-of-eight cast and in a sling and swathe for 6 weeks. At that time the immobilization is discontinued, and the pins are removed.

Brown[860] recommends open reduction and internal fixation of all acute or chronic dislocations of the sternoclavicular joint. He uses one pin inserted obliquely from the clavicle into the manubrium. The pin is inserted into the clavicle 2 to 3 inches lateral to the joint so that there is an oblique positioning of the pin. In addition, he divides the medial 2 to 3 inches of the clavicular head of the sternocleidomastoideus muscle to prevent upper displacement of the proximal clavicle.

Lunseth and Frankel[911] have used a modified Burroughs[862] technique wherein the subclavius tendon is used to strengthen the costoclavicular ligaments, and a pin is placed across the sternoclavicular joint for 6 weeks.

Omer[922] has described a technique in which, along with the sternoclavicular capsular ligament and the costoclavicular ligament repair, he performs a step-cut osteotomy of the medial clavicle. In addition, he detaches the origin of the sternocleidomastoid from the medial segment of the clavicle, to prevent upward displacement of the medial segment and tension on the ligament repairs. Motion of the upper extremity then occurs in the osteotomy site, which heals later.

Treatment of Posterior Dislocation of the Sternoclavicular Joint

Careful Examination of the Patient. Complications are common with posterior dislocation of the sternoclavicular joint, and the patient should receive prompt atten-

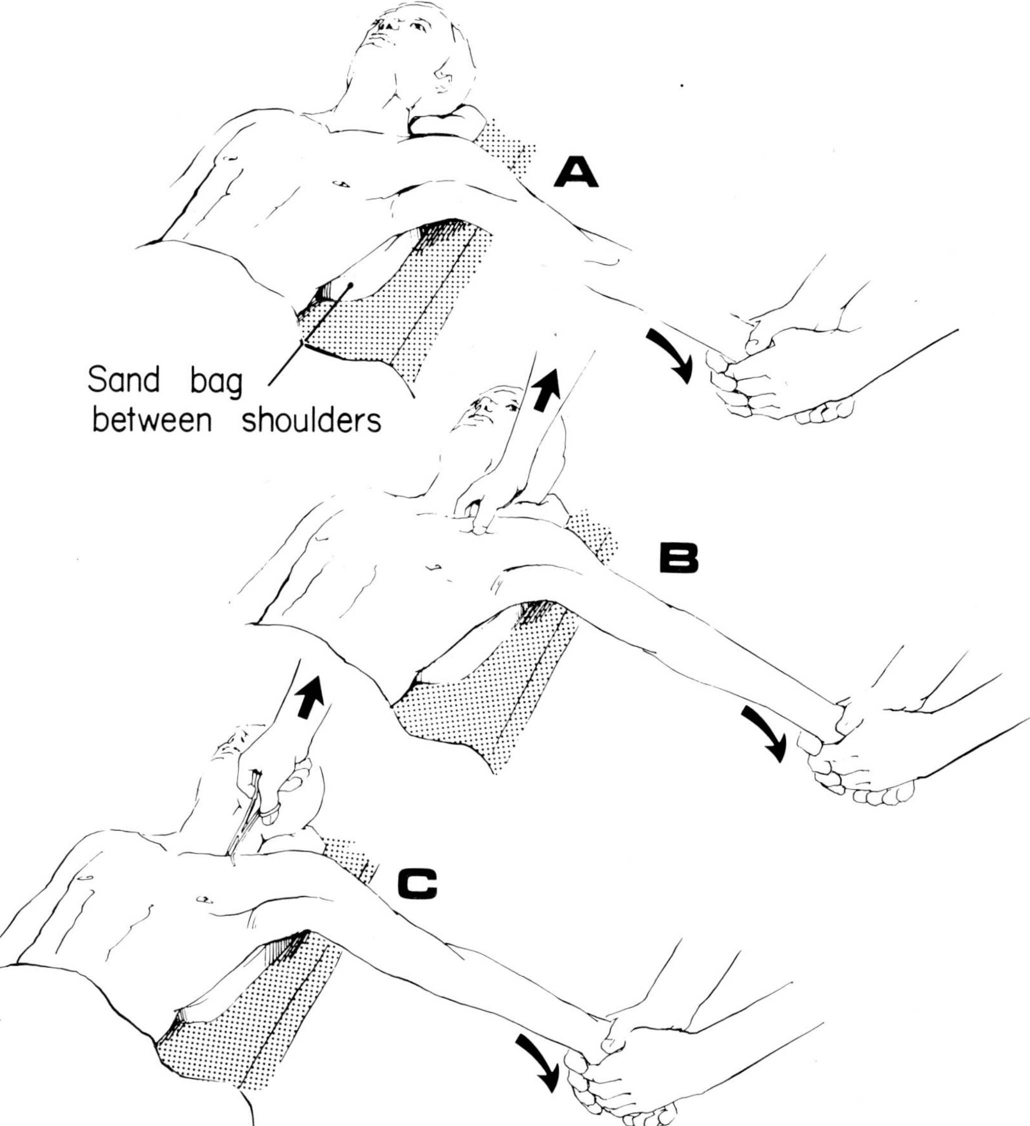

Fig. 11-166. Technique of closed reduction of the sternoclavicular joint. (*A*) In positioning the patient for closed reduction of the sternoclavicular joint, a sandbag should be placed between the shoulders. Traction is then applied to the arm in abduction and in slight extension. In anterior dislocations, direct anterior pressure may be required to replace the medial end of the clavicle. (*B*) In posterior dislocations of the sternoclavicular joint, in addition to the traction, it may be necessary to lift with the fingers to dislodge the clavicle from behind the manubrium. (*C*) In stubborn cases of posterior dislocations of the sternoclavicular joint, a sterile towel clip may be used to grasp the medial end of the clavicle to lift it laterally and anteriorly.

tion. A careful physical examination should be done to rule out damage to the pulmonary and vascular systems. General anesthesia is used ordinarily, because of the severe pain and muscle spasm. However, some authors recommend the use of intravenous narcotics and muscle relaxants. Heinig[890] has successfully used local anesthesia to reduce the dislocation. If specific complications are noted, then the appropriate consultant should be advised. Worman and Leagus[945] reported a posterior dislocation of the sternoclavicular joint in which it was noted, at surgery, that the displaced clavicle had put a hole into the right pulmonary artery. The clavicle had prevented exsanguination, because the vessel was impaled on it; had he performed a closed reduction, the result could have been disastrous.

From a review of the earlier literature, it would appear that the treatment of choice for posterior sternoclavicular dislocation was by operative procedures. However, since the 1950's, the treatment of choice of posterior sternoclavicular dislocation is closed reduction.[863,868,877,887,890,913,914,917,925,933,939] Some authors,[925,939] who opened the first retrosternal dislocation, were amazed at how easily the dislocation reduced under direct vision, and thereafter they used closed reductions with complete success.

Technique of Closed Reduction. The patient is placed on his back with the dislocated shoulder near the edge of the table. A sandbag is placed between the shoulders (Fig. 11-166A). Lateral traction is applied to the abducted arm, which is then gradually brought back into extension. This may be all that is necessary to accomplish the reduction. Too much extension can bind the anterior surface of the dislocated medial clavicle on the back of the manubrium. Occasionally, it may be necessary to grasp the medial clavicle with your fingers, to dislodge it from behind the manubrium (Fig. 11-166B). If this fails, the skin can be prepped and a sterile towel clip used to grasp the medial clavicle to apply lateral and then anterior traction (Fig. 11-166C). The clavicle usually reduces with an audible snap or pop, and it is practically always stable. In fact, all of the cases that have been treated closed have been stable.

Some authors[876] have reported that they have accomplished reduction simply by having the patient lie on his back on folded towels or by putting a knee between the scapulae of the seated patient and pulling the shoulders back. Stein[939] has utilized skin traction on the abducted and extended arm to accomplish the reduction gradually.

Should closed maneuvers fail, operative intervention must be performed, as the patient cannot tolerate the clavicle posteriorly displaced into his mediastinum. The procedure should be performed in such a manner as to disturb as few of the ligamentous structures as possible. Ordinarily, at the time of surgical reduction, the joint is stable and internal fixation is unnecessary.

After reduction, the shoulders should be held back for 4 to 6 weeks with a figure-of-eight dressing or one of the commercially available figure-of-eight straps used to treat fractures of the clavicle (Fig. 11-167).

Technique of Operative Reduction and Postoperative Care. Essentially the techniques that are used for open reduction of the anterior dislocation can be utilized for the posterior dislocations. Elting,[876] reporting on four cases of posterior sternoclavicular dislocation, used Kirschner wires from the clavicle into the sternum and then supported the repair of the sternoclavicular joint with a short toe extensor tendon. Denham and Dingley[871] recommend the use of Kirschner wires from the clavicle into the sternum in the management of posterior displacement of the medial clavicle from the epiphysis. Greenlee[885] reported an interesting case, in which the posterior sternoclavicular dislocation could not be reduced at surgery until an assistant pulled the arm out from under the drapes. The reduction was then dramatic and stable. In one case, Stein[939] used braided wire from the clavicle to the first rib to stabilize the sternoclavicular joint, and Kennedy[902] advocated wire fixation supplemented with a fascial repair of the ligaments. Brooks and Henning[859] have recommended the use of a 1.9-mm. smooth Kirschner wire following open reduction of posterior displaced epiphyseal injury. The wire is inserted retrograde as follows: The wire is first drilled into the epiphysis of the clavicle, across the sternoclavicular joint, into the manubrium, and out through the skin below

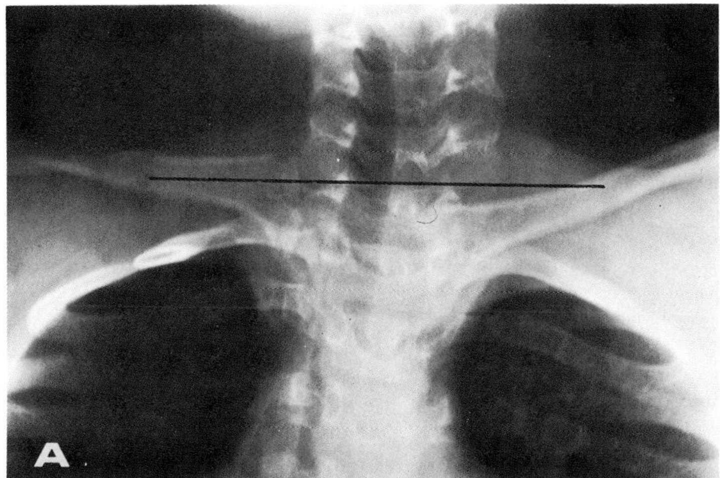

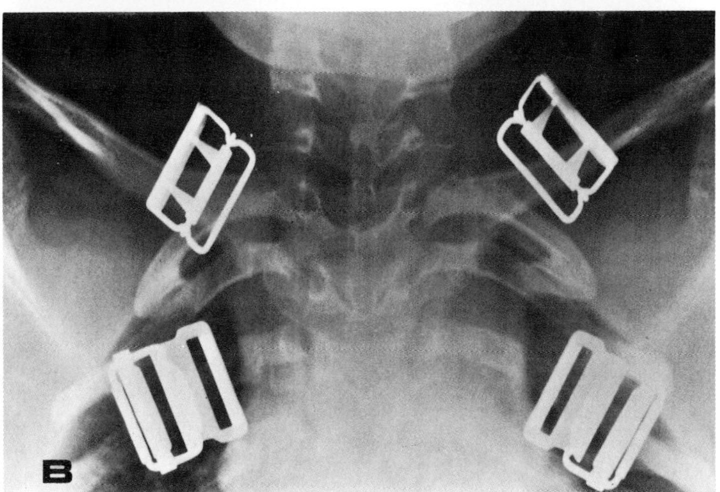

Fig. 11-167. (*A*) Posterior dislocation of the left sternoclavicular joint as seen on the 40-degree cephalic tilt roentgenogram in a 12-year-old boy. Note that the left medial clavicle is displaced inferiorly to the normal right medial clavicle. (*B*) Following the closed reduction the medial ends of both clavicles are on the same horizontal plane. Note the buckles of the figure-of-eight clavicular harness, which is used to hold the shoulder back after reduction.

the opposite clavicle. Following reduction of the epiphyseal fracture, the pin is drilled retrograde back into the clavicle. The pin is left projecting out of the skin and bent into a hook. The postoperative care is essentially the same as that described under operative procedures for reduction of anterior dislocation of the sternoclavicular joint (i.e., no motion and firm immobilization of the shoulder for 6 weeks, when the ligaments have healed and/or when the pins are removed).

Recurring and Old Unreduced Dislocations of the Sternoclavicular Joint

Conservative Approach. It has been stressed by the majority of authors that most patients who have cases of recurrent or long-standing sternoclavicular joint dislocation are asymptomatic and require no treatment. Essentially all of the cases reported have been anterior, except for the case reported by Holmdahl,[893] which could have been a recurrent posterior dislocation.

There are several basic approaches to replacing and maintaining the medial end of the clavicle in its normal articulation with the manubrium. Fascia lata, suture, internal fixation across the joint, subclavius tendons, arthrodesis, osteotomy of the medial clavicle, and resection of the medial end of the clavicle have been advocated.

Surgical Reconstructions. *Replacement of the Sternoclavicular Ligament with*

Strips of Fascia Lata. Bankart[850] and Milch[916] used fascia between the clavicle and the manubrium. Lowman[908] used a loop of fascia in and through the sterno-clavicular joint, so that it acts like a ligamentum teres in the hip. Speed[937] and Key and Conwell[903] have reported on the use of a fascial loop between the clavicle and the first rib. Allen[844] recommended the use of a fascial strip from the medial clavicle to the second rib. Bateman[851] utilizes fascia latae to reconstruct a new sternoclavicular ligament.

Rigid Internal Fixation Across the Sterno-clavicular Joint. Speed[937] inserted an ivory peg from the clavicle into the manubrium. Another technique uses pins across the sternoclavicular joint.

Use of Subclavius Tendon. Burrows[862] recommends the use of the subclavius tendon as a substitute for the costoclavicular ligament. The origin of the subclavius muscle is from the first rib just 6 mm. lateral and 1.3 cm. anterior to the attachment of the costoclavicular ligament.[882,883] The insertion of the tendon is to the inferior surface of the junction of the middle third, with the outer third of the clavicle and the muscle fibers arising from the tendon to be inserted into the inferior surface mid-third of the clavicle (Fig. 11-154). The muscle fibers coming off the tendon look like feathers on a bird's wing. Burrows detaches the muscle fiber from the tendon, does not disturb the origin of the tendon, and then passes the tendon through drill holes in the anterior proximal clavicle.

In comparing his operation with the use of free strips of fascia, Burrows said that it is "safer and easier to pick up a mooring than to drop anchor; the obvious mooring is the tendon of the subclavius separated from its muscle fiber and suitably re-aligned." Lunseth and Frankel[911] have reported a modified Burrows procedure with a threaded Steinmann pin across the joint.

Osteotomy of the Medial Clavicle. Omer,[922] following repair or reconstruction of the ligaments, creates a step-cut osteotomy lateral to the joint and detaches the clavicular head of the sternocleidomastoid muscle from the proximal fragment (see p. 772).

Resection of the Medial End of the Clavicle. McLaughlin,[914] Pridie,[928] Bateman,[851] and Milch[916] all have recommended excision of the medial clavicle when degenerative changes are noted in the joint (Fig.

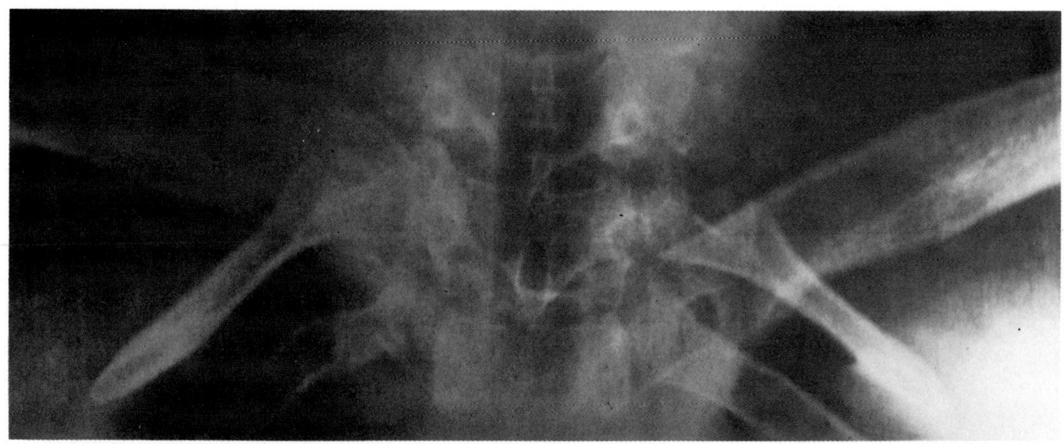

Fig. 11-168. This patient had an open reduction and pin fixation 4 years prior to this roentgenogram. Note that on the 40-degree cephalic tilt view, the right medial clavicle is still dislocated upward. Because of persistent pain and popping in the joint, the proximal end of the right clavicle medial to costoclavicular ligament was excised and symptoms were relieved.

11-168). Care should be taken not to remove the medial clavicle beyond the attachments of the costoclavicular ligament.

Rice[930] performed a bilateral arthrodesis of the sternoclavicular joints and reinforced the operation with kangaroo tendons in a patient with habitual dislocations. He did not report adequate follow-up results. This technique is reported only for historical interest. It should **not** be performed, because the clavicle must elevate and rotate to allow elevation of the arm.

TREATMENT OF EPIPHYSEAL FRACTURES

The management of epiphyseal injuries in the shoulder of an adult is applicable only to the medial end of the clavicle. As has been described, the clavicle is the first long bone to ossify, and it is the last major bone in the body to close its epiphyses. The epiphysis on the medial end of the clavicle does not appear on roentgenograms until about the 18th year and unites with the medial clavicle around the 25th year[882,883] (Fig. 11-169).

In 1966, when I first recognized and treated a case of fracture through the epiphysis of the medial clavicle, I thought that it might be an original observation as I could not find any references on the subject. Denham and Dingley,[871] in 1967, reported three cases of medial epiphysis injury, in patients aged 14 to 16, in which they demonstrated at surgery that the pathology was indeed an epiphyseal slip of the medial clavicle. In 1972, Brooks and Henning[859] presented a paper in which they concluded from nine cases that many sternoclavicular dislocations and fractures of the medial clavicle were indeed separations through the medial clavicle epiphysis.

As it turns out with most "new ideas" in orthopaedics, John Poland[927] wrote a text in 1898 entitled *Traumatic Separation of the Epiphysis.* In this beautifully illustrated and written text, Poland reviewed several French articles that evaluated over 60 cases of separation of the medial epiphysis of the clavicle simulating sternoclavicular dislocations. He discussed the anatomy of the joint and the classifications of the injury and described methods of treatment.

He described in detail an article by Verchere written in 1886, which probably represents the first published report of a death caused by posterior dislocation of the sternoclavicular joint:

A 20-year-old man, following a severe crushing injury, died on the seventh day, of subcutaneous emphysema. Autopsy revealed that the inner third of the right clavicle was detached of its periosteum, and its smooth rounded end was displaced posteriorly and had produced a perforation of the pleural sac about the size of

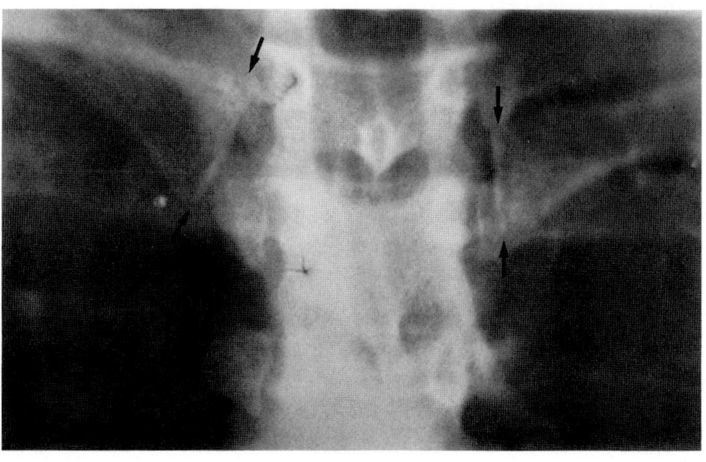

Fig. 11-169. An anteroposterior view of the medial ends of both clavicles demonstrates the thin, wafer-like appearance of the epiphysis of the medial clavicle (*arrows*).

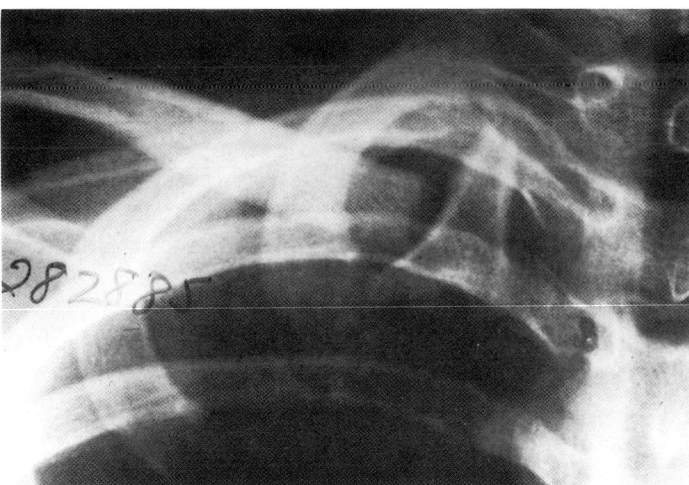

Fig. 11-170. Type I epiphyseal separation of the medial clavicle associated with the fracture of the shaft of the clavicle with 90 degrees rotation of the segment.

a 2-franc piece. The hole was in the left lung, whereas the ipsilateral lung escaped injury. The report very clearly described that the sternoclavicular joint was not injured and that the 5-mm.-wide epiphyseal plate was held firmly in place by the ligaments about the joint. The specimen of the separated epiphysis was placed in the Dupuytren Museum.

Poland went on to describe that the capsular ligament is primarily attached to the epiphysis of the medial clavicle, and that with injury, the epiphysis is held by the capsular ligament and stays with its articulation with the manubrium.

I first recognized this entity in 1966 when I was trying to replace a fracture dislocation of the medial clavicle in a 16-year-old boy. The fragment was 3.7 cm. long and had rotated 90 degrees from the long axis of the clavicle (Fig. 11-170). In my eagerness to explore the anatomy, the fragment of clavicle, which had been completely stripped of its periosteum, fell onto the floor! However, the sternal end of the fragment did not have a smooth cartilaginous articular surface. It was rough, like the end of a chicken bone when the epiphysis has been pulled off. The costoclavicular ligaments were intact to the

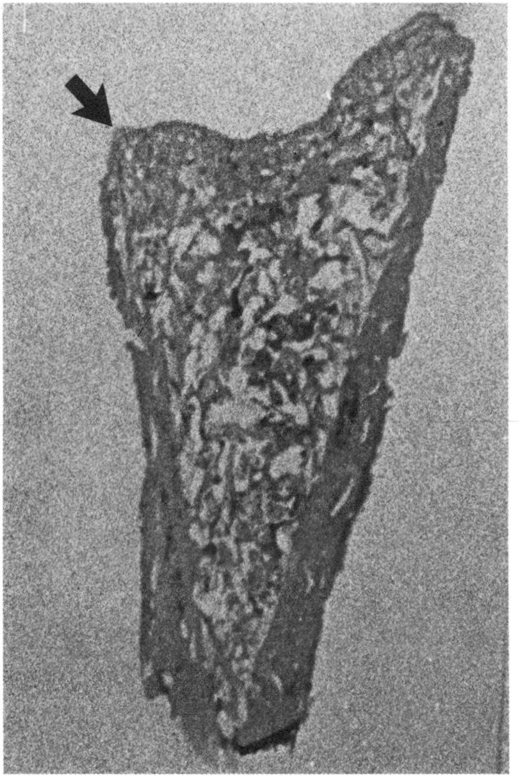

Fig. 11-171. Microscopic examination of the medial end of the fragment of the clavicle shown in Fig. 11-170 (*arrow*) which was "removed" revealed the provisional zone of calcification of the metaphysis. This indicates that the epiphysis of the medial clavicle was still in its normal position, adjacent to the manubrium held by the sternoclavicular ligaments. The epiphyseal injury characteristically has occurred through the zone of hypertrophy.

periosteum inferiorly, and in the most medial corner of the periosteal tube was a dense structure that could be taken for the intraarticular disc ligament—*or* it could have been the unossified epiphysis. Treatment consisted of closing the periosteal tube. Later, microscopic studies of the most medial end of the fragment revealed the provisional zone of calcification of the metaphysis, indicating that indeed there had been a separation through the epiphyseal plate and that it had occurred through the zone of hypertrophy (Fig. 11-171). Serial roentgenograms revealed a gradual replacement of the medial clavicle, and after 18 months, the entire defect had been replaced with bone (Figs. 11-172; 11-173). The patient was and still is a manual laborer; he has a full range of motion and essentially no pain (Fig. 11-174).

Since 1966 in other cases of "dislocation of the sternoclavicular joint," I have been able to document with the 40-degree cephalic-tilt roentgenogram that the injury really was an epiphyseal fracture, because the thin wafer-like disc has remained in its normal articulation with the manubrium, while the metaphysis and shaft were displaced. Some of the epiphyseal fractures have been Type II injuries with a small fragment of the metaphysis remaining with the epiphysis. Obviously, before the epiphysis ossifies at the age of 18, you can't be sure whether a displacement about the sternoclavicular joint is a dislocation of the sternoclavicular joint or a fracture through the epiphyseal plate.

Despite the fact that there is significant displacement of the shaft with either a Type I or a Type II epiphyseal fracture the periosteal tube remains in its anatomical position, and the attaching ligaments are intact to the periosteum (i.e., the costoclavicular ligaments inferiorly and the capsular and interarticular disc ligaments medially; Fig. 11-172).

Anterior Displacement of the Medial Clavicle. If the epiphyseal injury is recognized, or if the patient is under the age of 25, closed reduction as has been described for anterior dislocation of the sternoclavicular joint should be performed, and the shoulders should be held back in a clavicular strap or figure-of-eight dressing for 3 to 4 weeks. Healing is prompt in epiphyseal fractures, and remodelling will occur at the site of the deformity.

Posterior Displacement of the Medial Clavicle. Closed reduction of this injury should be performed in the manner de-

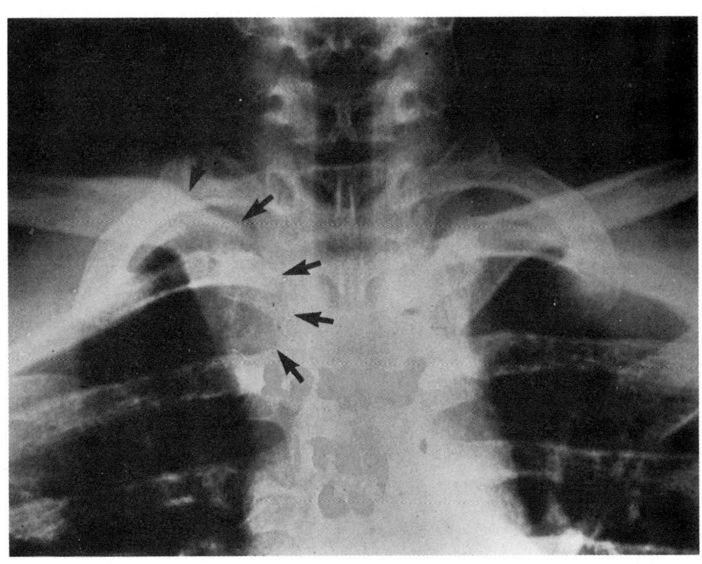

Fig. 11-172. An anteroposterior roentgenogram of the sternoclavicular joints taken 18 months after the medial 3.8 cm. of the proximal clavicle was "removed" reveals that total regeneration of the clavicle has been accomplished by the intact periosteal tube and the epiphysis (*arrows*).

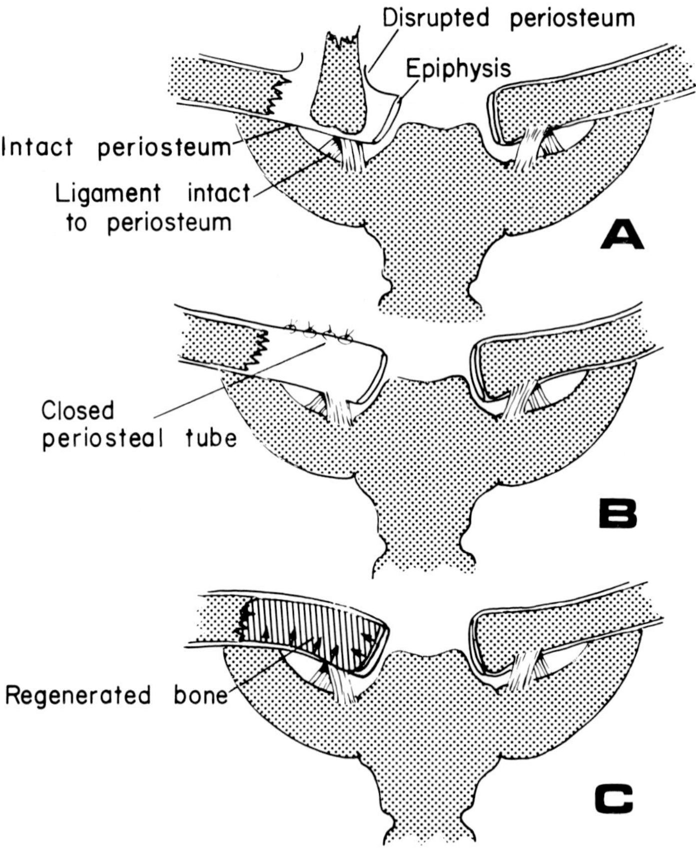

Fig. 11-173. Schematic drawing of the fracture and an epiphyseal injury of the medial 3.8 cm. of the clavicle of the patient shown in Fig. 11-170. (*A*) The fragment with its metaphysis has been separated from the epiphyseal plate and is partially displaced out of the periosteal tube. (*B*) The defect in the periosteal tube has been closed. Note that the coracoclavicular ligaments are intact and are attached inferiorly to the periosteal tube. The epiphysis has remained and its anatomical position has been maintained against the manubrium by the sternoclavicular capsular ligaments. (*C*) At 18 months the medial 3.8 cm. of the clavicle has been replaced by new bone formation from the epiphysis and periosteum.

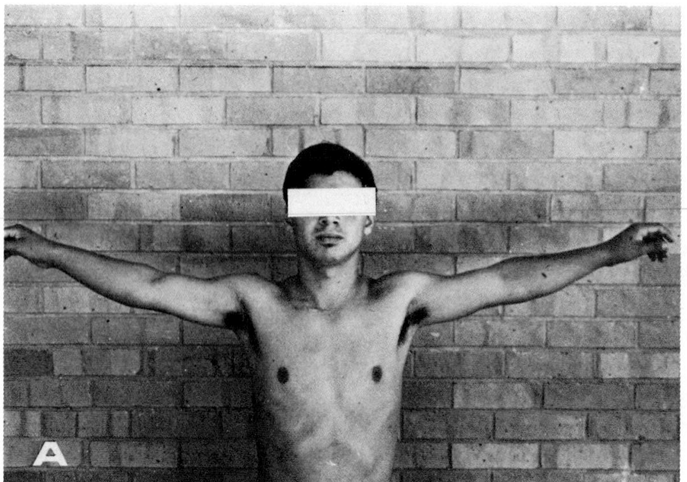

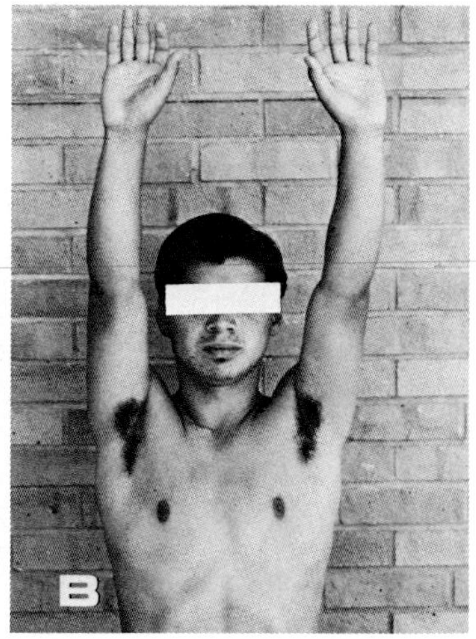

Fig. 11-174. (*A, B*) Eighteen months after the regrowth of the medial segment of the clavicle, the patient shown in Figs. 11-170 to 11-173 was asymptomatic, had a full range of motion, and was performing manual labor.

scribed for posterior dislocation of the sternoclavicular joint. Unlike anterior displacements of the medial clavicle, the reduction will be stable with shoulders held back in a figure-of-eight dressing or strap. Immobilization should continue for 3 to 4 weeks.

Atraumatic Injuries

Voluntary or Habitual Dislocation

This rarely occurs and can be confused with the recurring anterior subluxation or dislocation. The condition is usually not painful, and treatment should consist of explaining the problem to the patient and urging that the joint not be dislocated deliberately because of the danger of developing traumatic arthritis.

Congenital or Developmental Dislocation

This also is a very rare problem, and the treatment depends upon the exact anatomical part that is missing or abnormally developed.

Spontaneous Dislocation

The subluxation that is associated with aging is rarely painful.[856,858] If the symptoms become intolerable to the patient, the medial end of the clavicle can be excised as has been described. Spontaneous dislocation that is associated with an infection[880] may well be quite painful, and the treatment of choice is proper medication and possibly an excision of the medial end of the clavicle.

AUTHOR'S PREFERRED METHOD OF TREATMENT

Sprains

Type I Injury

Ice followed by heat, with the use of a sling, gives relief of pain. Ordinarily, after 3 to 5 days, the patient can use the arm for everyday activities.

Type II Injury

In addition to the ice and heat that have been described, a soft well-padded figure-of-eight clavicle strap is used. If this does not give enough relief of pain, the arm should be held in a sling. If the medial end of the clavicle is prominent anteriorly and the patient gets relief by gently displacing it backward, I suggest, in addition, the use of three or four compresses folded and held in place over the medial clavicle with elastic tape.

Type III Injury

In general, I manage all dislocations of the sternoclavicular joint by closed reduction. Essentially all of the posterior dislocations, when reduced, are stable when the shoulders are held back in a figure-of-eight strap. Many of the anterior dislocations are unstable, but I accept the deformity, as I believe it is less of a problem than the potential problems of operative repair and internal fixation.

Anterior Dislocation

Method of Reduction and Care After Reduction

The reduction is accomplished with the patient in the seated position; both shoulders are pulled back, occasionally over my knee, and held in a well-padded figure-of-eight strap and a sling. Ordinarily, pain is controlled with narcotics, and muscle relaxants may be used intravenously. The patients are kept in the clavicular strap and sling for approximately 4 to 6 weeks, at which time they gradually regain range of motion and begin strengthening exercises.

Most of the injuries of the sternoclavicular joint I have taken care of have been in young adults, under the age of 25, and I believe that a significant number, if not the majority, are *not* dislocations but Type I and II epiphyseal fractures which heal promptly with conservative treatment.

Some of the patients with anterior dislocations of the sternoclavicular joint treated by conservative means have persistent deformity which can become symptomatic.

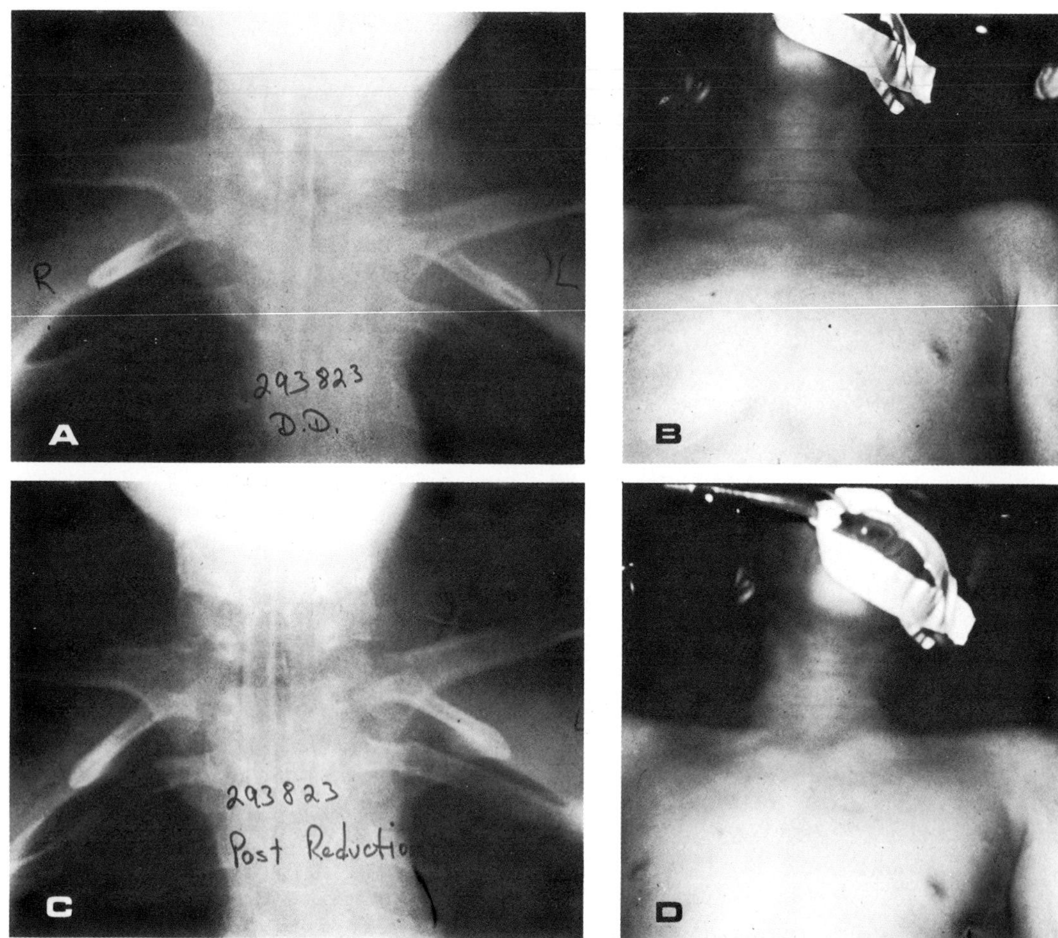

Fig. 11-175. Posterior dislocation, or Type I epiphyseal separation, of the left sternoclavicular joint in a 12-year-old boy. (*A*) A 40-degree cephalic tilt roentgenogram reveals that the left clavicle is significantly lower on the horizontal plane, than the normal right clavicle. (*B*) Before reduction, the left clavicle is essentially invisible, and only the remaining prominence of the superior corner of the manubrium is present. (*C*) In the post-reduction 40-degree cephalic tilt roentgenogam, the left clavicle has been restored to the same horizontal level as the normal right clavicle. (*D*) Clinically both clavicles are now evident. Note the swelling in the vicinity of the left sternoclavicular joint.

In my experience, however, this rarely occurs.

Posterior Dislocation

It is very important to take a very careful history and to perform a very careful physical examination to document whether there was or is any compression of the great vessels in the neck, the esophagus, or the trachea. If there are symptoms of pressure on the mediastinum, the appropriate specialist should be contacted. I do not believe that operative techniques are required to reduce the acute posterior sternoclavicular joint dislocation. Further, once reduced closed, the joint is stable (Fig. 11-175).

Method of Reduction and Care After Reduction

The patient is placed on his back with a sandbag between the scapulae to extend the shoulders. The dislocated shoulder should be at the edge of the table, so that extension of the shoulder can be obtained. If the patient is having *extreme* pain and muscle spasm and is quite anxious, general anesthesia is required; otherwise narcotics, muscle relaxants, or tranquilizers are given through an established intravenous infusion. First gentle traction is applied on the abducted arm in line with the clavicle while countertraction is supplied by an assistant who steadies the patient on the table. The traction on the abducted arm is increased gradually while the arm is brought into extension. Reduction usually occurs with an audible pop or snap. If the traction in abduction and extension is not successful, then an assistant grasps the clavicle in an effort to dislodge it and lift it anteriorly from behind the manubrium. Occasionally, in a stubborn case, it is impossible to obtain a secure grasp on the clavicle. The skin should then be surgically prepped and a sterile towel clip used to gain purchase on the medial clavicle percutaneously. Then the combined traction, through the arm and the towel clip, plus the lifting force of the towel clip, reduce the dislocation.

If the posterior dislocation cannot be reduced under general anesthesia with complete muscle relaxation and using a towel clip to grasp the medial clavicle, open reduction should be performed. Following the reduction, the sternoclavicular joint is stable even with the arm at the patient's side. However, I always hold the shoulders back in a well padded figure-of-eight clavicle strap for 3 to 4 weeks.

The complications of unreduced posterior dislocation are numerous. Therefore dislocation should be managed—by closed or open reduction, or, in a long-standing case, by resection of the inner end of the clavicle.

Epiphyseal Fracture of the Medial Clavicle

I am of the opinion that many, if not most, of the anterior and posterior injuries of the sternoclavicular joint in patients under 25, which are and have been interpreted as "dislocations of the sternoclavicular joint," are fractures through the medial epiphysis of the clavicle. Many authors have observed at the time of surgery that the intraarticular disc ligament stays with the manubrium, and I agree with them. However, in addition, I submit that the unossified or ossified epiphyseal disc also stays with the manubrium; anatomically it is lateral to the articular disc ligament, is held in place by the capsular ligament, and

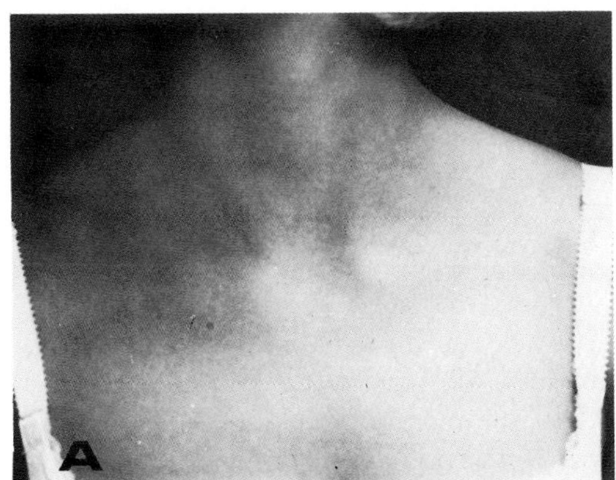

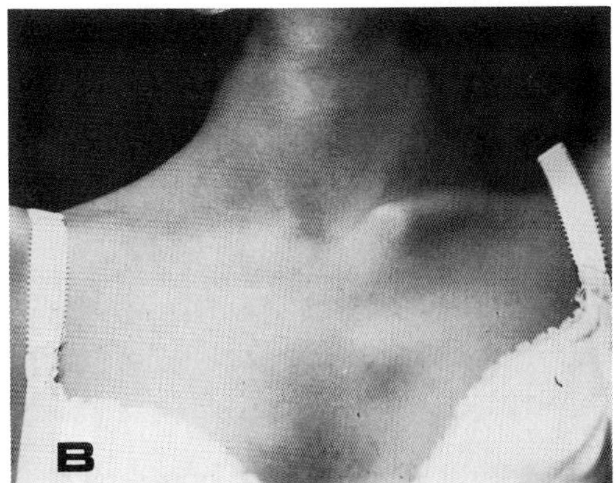

Fig. 11-176. Voluntary or habitual dislocation of the sternoclavicular joint. (*A*) Normal appearance of the sternoclavicular joints in a 23-year-old woman. (*B*) Subluxation of the left sternoclavicular joint with certain overhead movements of the upper extremity. This type of subluxation or dislocation is usually completely asymptomatic.

could be mistaken for the intraarticular disc. Therefore, because of the rapid healing capabilities of epiphyseal fractures and the potential remodelling of deformities, anterior and posterior displacement of the medial end of the clavicle are managed by closed reduction. Open reduction of the epiphyseal injury is seldom indicated (perhaps in the case of an irreducible posterior displacement). After reduction, the shoulders are held back with a figure-of-eight strap or dressing for 3 to 4 weeks.

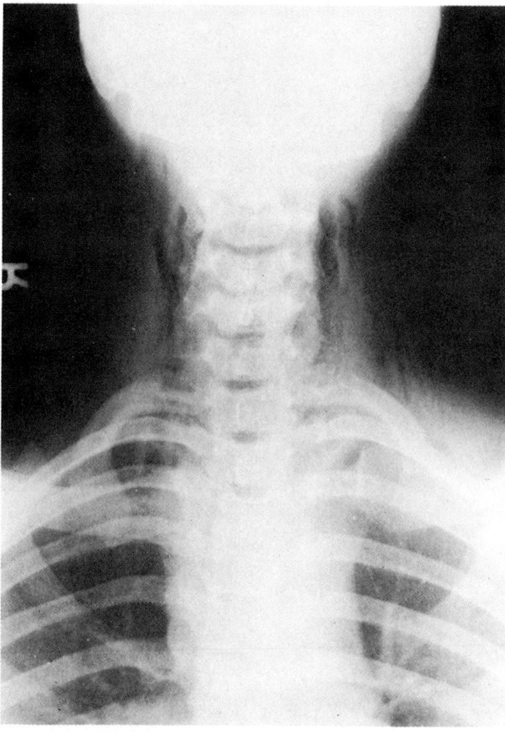

Fig. 11-177. Complication of posterior dislocation of the left sternoclavicular joint. The roentgenogram demonstrates massive subcutaneous emphysema about the soft tissues of the neck. The next day the patient was unable to swallow and noted a change in the quality of his voice. His condition became worse, and laryngoscopy revealed a small laceration of the esophagus. The patient developed a large abscess in the neck and superior mediastinum and and later developed osteomyelitis of the left medial clavicle. (Borowiecki, B., *et al.*: Joint. Arch. Otolaryngol., 95:185-187, 1972)

Recurrent Dislocation of the Sternoclavicular Joint

Many, if not most, patients with recurrent dislocation are asymptomatic, and treatment is unnecessary. Should the recurring dislocations become painful and should arthritic changes be noted, I recommend excision of the medial end of the clavicle.

Unreduced Dislocation of the Sternoclavicular Joint

The symptomatic anterior dislocation of the sternoclavicular joint is treated best by resecting the proximal portion of the clavicle medial to the costoclavicular ligaments. If the costoclavicular ligaments are disrupted and the medial clavicle is displaced upward or anteriorly, I recommend the use of the subclavius tendon as a living ligament to reconstruct the coracoclavicular ligament, to hold the remaining medial clavicle down to the first rib. In addition, to prevent the medial clavicle from being pulled upward while the subclavius tendon is healing, I would detach the medial 3.8 cm. of the clavicular head of the sternocleidomastoid. The posteriorly displaced clavicle can produce many complications, and therefore the symptomatic or asymptomatic posteriorly dislocated sternoclavicular joint must be reduced, or the inner end of the joint must be excised.

Voluntary or Habitual Dislocation of the Sternoclavicular Joint

I have seen three patients with this problem, and all have been young ladies between 16 and 24. All have been totally asymptomatic. They were referred because of the lump that appeared at the sternoclavicular joint when the arms were raised overhead (Fig. 11-176). I explained to them that this condition might become symptomatic and require excision of the medial end of the clavicle and urged that they refrain from deliberately performing the subluxation. Should the joint become symptomatic with degenerative changes, I would recommend excision of the medial end of the clavicle.

COMPLICATIONS OF DISLOCATION OF THE STERNOCLAVICULAR JOINT

The complications that occur at the time of dislocation of the sternoclavicular joint are primarily limited to the posterior dislocations. About the only complication that occurs with the anterior dislocation of the sternoclavicular joint is a "cosmetic bump" from incomplete reduction or late degenerative changes. The following complications have been reported secondary to the retrosternal dislocation: pneumothorax and laceration of the superior vena cava;[945] pressure or rupture of the trachea;[924] venous congestion in the neck; rupture of the esophagus with abscess and osteomyelitis of the clavicle[857] (Fig. 11-177); pressure on the subclavian artery in an untreated patient;[895,938] occlusion of the subclavian artery late in a patient who was not treated;[938] compression of the right common carotid artery by a fracture dislocation of the sternoclavicular joint;[895] brachial plexus compression;[913] hoarseness of voice, onset of snoring, voice changes from normal to falsetto with movement of the arm;[857,902,920] difficulty in swallowing;[870,924,938] and dyspnea.[885,902,917,933,941]

Worman and Leagus,[945] in an excellent review of the complications associated with posterior dislocations of the sternoclavicular joint, reported that 16 of 60 patients reviewed from the literature had suffered complications of the trachea, esophagus, or great vessels. I should point out that even though the incidence of complications was 25 per cent, only three deaths have been reported as a result of the injury.[884,902,927]

However, four deaths have been reported from the complications of performing surgery on the sternoclavicular joint,[866,907,920,933] and three near-deaths.[860,923,945] All of the deaths and near deaths have resulted from migration of Steinmann pins or Kirschner wires, used to stabilize the sternoclavicular joint at the time of surgery, into the heart, pulmonary artery, innominate artery, or aorta. In some cases, the entire pin migrated and, in others, a broken pin did (Fig. 11-178). Tremendous leverage force is applied to pins across the sternoclavicular joint, and fatigue breakage of the pins is common. Pins placed across the sternoclavicular joint always must be removed, and should fracture of the pin occur, the distal pin in the manubrium *must* be removed (Fig. 11-178). I wish to emphasize that I *do not* recommend open reduction of the joint, and I do not recommend transfixing pins across the sternoclavicular joint.

Brown[860] has reported an incidence of three complications in ten operative cases, two from broken pins and one, a near death, in which the pin penetrated the back of the manubrium and entered into the right pulmonary artery.

Omer,[922] in a review of 14 military hospitals, reported on 15 patients who had elective surgery for reduction and reconstruction of the sternoclavicular joint. Eight patients were followed by the same house staff longer than 6 months with the following complications: Of the five patients who had internal fixation with metal, two developed osteomyelitis, two had fracture of the pin with recurrent dislocation, and one had migration of the pin into the mediastinum with recurrent dislocation. Of the three patients who had soft-tissue reconstructions, one developed recurrent dislocation with drainage, one developed recur-

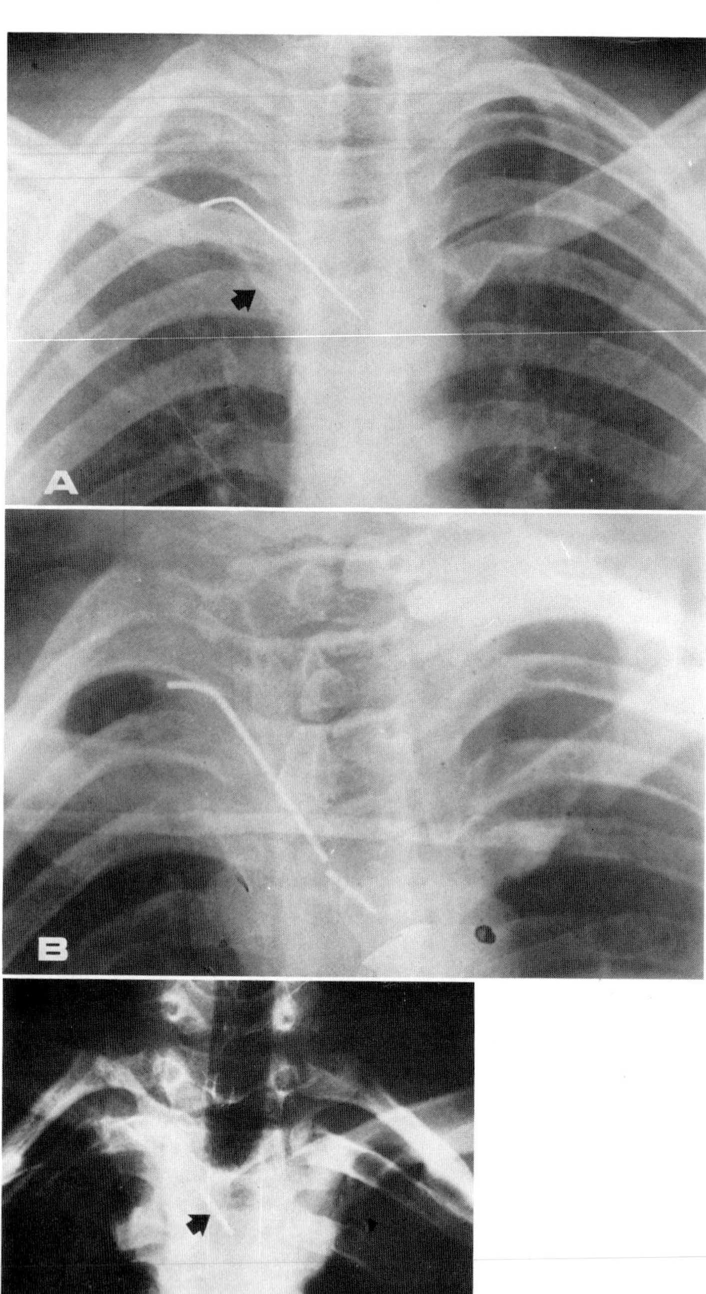

Fig. 11-178. Complications with pins across the sternoclavicular joint. (*A*) Postoperative anteroposterior roentgenogram with small size Steinmann pins across the sternoclavicular joint. This dislocation occurred in a 13-year-old boy and probably was a Type II epiphyseal injury. Note the fragment of the medial inferior clavicle in its normal relationship, and note that the joint has not been reduced (*arrow*). (*B*) At 4 weeks, at the time of pin removal, a fracture of the pin was noted. (*C*) Broken pins cannot be left in the manubrium, because they may migrate into the mediastinum with serious consequences. Moral of the story: Do not use pins across the sternoclavicular joint.

rent dislocation, and the third developed arthritis and extremity weakness and was discharged from the Service. Omer commented on this series of complications: "It would seem that complications are common in this rare surgical problem." To Omer's comment I can only add amen!

TOTAL DISLOCATION OF THE CLAVICLE

According to Beckman,[853] who described the 16th case in the literature, a report of a total dislocation was first published by Porral in 1831. Only three of the 16 were in children, ages 13 to 14. Severe trauma is the usual cause (e.g., compression of both shoulders when the patient is crushed between two vehicles; falls from great heights; a house falling in on the patient). In all of the reported cases, the medial end of the clavicle was anterior and the lateral end of the clavicle was up and posterior. In some instances, the posterior displacement is so severe that the lateral head of the clavicle is lying at the level of the spine of the scapula. Beckman states that the end results of the conservative management in previously presented patients were ideal in only 40 per cent, and a good functional result was noted in 66 per cent. In the case that he presented, that of a 13-year-old boy who was compressed and crushed under a car, it was decided that surgery would give better results. The medial clavicle was dislocated anterior to the sternum; the lateral end of the clavicle was superiorly dislocated and displaced beneath the trapezius muscle; the clavicle was not fractured, but had been completely stripped free of its periosteum.

Treatment consisted of replacing the bone in its periosteal and soft-tissue sleeve, which was repaired with sutures. Beckman called the operation "a bloody reposition of the clavicle." He reports that the end result was quite satisfying, both from a functional and from an anatomical point of view.

DISLOCATION OF THE SCAPULA

Dislocation of the scapula is a rare entity. The entire scapula is displaced forward and externally rotated, and the inferior tip of the scapula is caught and locked between the posterolateral ribs. The condition is quite painful, and any motion of the upper extremity increases the pain.

Treatment consists of traction on the hyperabducted arm as the scapula is externally rotated by pushing on its vertebral border. After reduction, the arm should be immobilized in a sling and swathe for 2 weeks.

My personal thanks to the following physicians who, knowing of my special interest in the shoulder, have sent me x-rays of interesting cases which I have used in this chapter: Roberto Barja, Major, USA (MC); Charles D. Hummer, Jr., M.D.; Charles S. Neer, II, M.D.; William B. Reinbold, M.D.; John H. Smith, Jr., M.D.; John E. Stewart, M.D.; Hilario Trevino, M.D.; James D. Wimpee, M.D.; and Carter R. Rowe, M.D.

REFERENCES

FRACTURES ABOUT THE SHOULDER

Fractures of the Proximal Humerus

1. Albee, F. H.: Restoration of shoulder function in cases of loss of head and upper portion of the humerus. Surgery, *32*:1-19, 1921.
2. Baker, D., M., and Leach, R. E.: Fracture-dislocation of the shoulder. Report of three unusual cases with rotator cuff avulsion. J. Trauma, *5*:659-664, 1965.
3. Bateman, J. E.: The shoulder and neck. ed. 1. Philadelphia, W. B. Saunders, 1972.
4. Böhler, L.: Die Behandlung von Verrenkungsbrüchen der Schulter. Deutsche Zschr. Chir., *219*:238-245, 1929.
5. Brostrom, F.: Early mobilization of fractures of the upper end of the humerus. Arch. Surg., *46*:614, 1943.
6. Caldwell, J. A.: Treatment of fractures in the Cincinnati General Hospital. Ann. Surg., *97*:174-177, 1933.
7. Caldwell, J. A., and Smith, J.: Treatment of unimpacted fractures of the surgical neck of the humerus. Amer. J. Surg., *31*: 141-144, 1936.
8. Codman, E. A.: The Shoulder. Boston, Thomas Todd, 1934.
9. Dehne, E.: Fractures of the upper end of the humerus. A classification based on the etiology of trauma. Surg. Clin. N. Amer., *25*:28-47, 1945.
10. DePalma, A. F.: Surgery of the Shoulder. ed. 2. Philadelphia, J. B. Lippincott, 1973.
11. DePalma, A. F., and Cantilli, R. A.: Fractures of the upper end of the humerus. Clin. Orthop., *20*:73-93, 1961.
12. Dingley, A., and Denham, R.: Fracture-dislocation of the humeral head. A method of reduction. J. Bone Joint Surg., *55A*: 1299-1300, 1973.
13. Edelman, G.: Immediate therapy of complex fractures of the upper end of the humerus by means of acrylic prosthesis. Presse Med., *59*:1777-1778, 1951.
14. Einarsson, F.: Fractures of the upper end of the humerus. Discussion based on follow-up of 302 cases. Acta Orthop. Scand., *32* [Suppl.]:10-209, 1958.
15. Fairbank, T. J.: Fracture subluxations of the shoulder. J. Bone Joint Surg., *30B*: 454-460, 1948.
16. Frankau, C.: A manipulative method for the reduction of fractures of the surgical neck of the humerus. Lancet, *2*:755, 1933.
17. Funsten, R. V., and Kinser, P.: Fractures and dislocations about the shoulder. J. Bone Joint Surg., *18*:191-198, 1936.
18. Garceau, G. J., and Coglang, S.: Early physical therapy in the treatment of fractures of the surgical neck of the humerus. J. Indiana Med. Ass., *34*:293-295, 1941.
19. Gardner, E., and Gray, D. J.: Prenatal development of the human shoulder and acromioclavicular joints. Am. J. Anat. *92*: 219-276, 1953.
20. Griswold, R. A., Hucherson, D. C., and Strode, E. C.: Fractures of the humerus treated with hanging cast. South. Med. J., *34*:777-778, 1941.
21. Gold, A. M.: Fractured neck of the humerus with separation and dislocation of the humeral head. Bull. Hosp. Joint Dis., *32*:87-99, 1971.
22. Gurd, F. B.: A simple effective method for the treatment of fractures of the upper two-thirds of the humerus. Amer. J. Surg., *47*:443-453, 1940.
23. Hall, R. H., Isaac, F., and Booth, C. R.: Dislocations of the shoulder with special reference to accompanying small fractures. J. Bone Joint Surg., *41A*:489-494, 1959.
24. Henderson, R. S.: Fracture dislocation of the shoulder with interposition of long head of the biceps. J. Bone Joint Surg., *34B*:240-241, 1952.
25. Henson, G. F.: Vascular complications of shoulder injuries, a report of two cases. J. Bone Joint Surg., *38B*:528-531, 1956.
26. Hermann, O. J.: Fractures of the shoulder joint with special reference to the correction of defects. American Academy of Orthopaedic Surgeons Instructional Course Lectures, *2*:359-370, 1944.
27. Howard, N. J., and Eloesser, L.: Treatment of fractures of the upper end of the humerus, an experimental and clinical study. J. Bone Joint Surg., *16*:1-29, 1934.
28. Hudson, R. T.: The use of the hanging cast in treatment of fractures of the humerus. Southern Surgeon, *10*:132-134, 1941.
29. Hundley, J. M., and Stewart, M. J.: Fractures of the humerus: a comparative study in methods of treatment. J. Bone Joint Surg., *37A*:681-692, 1955.
30. Jones, L.: Reconstructive operation for non-reducible fractures of the head of the humerus. Ann. Surg., *97*:217-225, 1933.
31. ———: The shoulder joint—observations

on the anatomy and physiology with analysis of reconstructive operation following extensive injury. Surg. Gynecol. Obstet., *75*:433-444, 1942.

32. Jones, R.: On certain fractures about the shoulder. Irish J. Med. Sci., *78*:282-291, 1932.
33. Kelly, J. P.: Fractures complicating electroconvulsive therapy and chronic epilepsy. J. Bone Joint Surg., *36B*:70-79, 1954.
34. Key, J. A., and Conwell, H. E.: Fractures, Dislocations, and Sprains. ed. 5. St. Louis, C. V. Mosby, 1951.
35. Knight, R. A., and Mayne, J. A.: Comminuted fractures and fracture-dislocations involving the articular surface of the humeral head. J. Bone Joint Surg., *39A*: 1343-1355, 1957.
36. Kocher, T.: Beitrage zur Kenntniss einiger praktisch wichtiger Fracture-neformen. Basel, Carl Sollman, 1896.
37. Krueger, F. T.: Vitallium replica arthroplasty of shoulder: care of aseptic necrosis of proximal end of humerus. Surgery, *30*:1005-1011, 1951.
38. LaFerti, A. D., and Nutter, P. D.: The treatment of fractures of the humerus by means of hanging plaster cast—"hanging cast." Ann. Surg., *114*:919-930, 1955.
39. MacDonald, F. R.: Intra-articular fractures in recurrent dislocations of the shoulder. Surg. Clin. N. Amer., *43*:1635-1645, 1963.
40. Machmull, G., and Weeder, S. D.: Bilateral fracture of the humeral heads; cases with bilateral fracture of the anatomical and surgical necks of the humeri due to convulsion. Radiology, *55*:736-739, 1950.
41. McLaughlin, H.: Trauma. Philadelphia, W. B. Saunders, 1959.
42. ———: Dislocations of the shoulder with tuberosity fracture. Surg. Clin. N. Amer., *43*:1615-1620, 1963.
43. Meyerding, H. W.: Fracture-dislocation of the shoulder. Minnesota Med., *20*:717-726, 1937.
44. Michaelis, L. S.: Comminuted fracture-dislocation of the shoulder. J. Bone Joint Surg., *26*:363-365, 1944.
45. Milch, H.: The treatment of recent dislocations and fracture-dislocations of the shoulder. J. Bone Joint Surg., *31A*:173-180, 1949.
46. Moseley, H. F.: Shoulder Lesions. ed. 3. Edinburgh, E. & S. Livingstone, 1969.
47. Neer, C. S., II: Articular replacement for the humeral head. J. Bone Joint Surg., *37A*:215-228, 1955.
48. ———: Indications for replacement of the proximal humeral articulations. Amer. J. Surg., *89*:901-907, 1955.
49. ———: Degenerative lesions of the proximal humeral articular surface. Clin. Orthop., *20*:116-124, 1961.
50. ———: Prosthetic replacement of the humeral head—indications and operative technique. Surg. Clin. N. Amer., *43*: 1581-1597, 1963.
51. ———: Displaced proximal humeral fractures. Part 1. Classification and evaluation. J. Bone Joint Surg., *52A*:1077-1089, 1970.
52. ———: Displaced proximal humeral fractures. Part II. Treatment of three-part and four-part displacement. J. Bone Joint Surg., *52A*:1090-1103, 1970.
53. ———: Replacement arthroplasty for glenohumeral osteoarthritis. J. Bone Joint Surg., *56A*:1-13, 1974.
54. Neer, C. S., II, Brown, T. H., and McLaughlin, H.: Fracture of the neck of the humerus with dislocation of the head fragment. Amer. J. Surg., *85*:252-258, 1953.
55. Neer, C. S., II, and Horwitz, B. S.: Fractures of the proximal humeral epiphyseal plate. Clin. Orthop., *41*:24-31, 1965.
56. Neviaser, J. S.: Complicated fractures and dislocations about the shoulder joint. American Academy of Orthopaedic Surgeons Instructional Course Lectures. *44A*:984-998, 1962.
57. Prillaman, H. A., and Thompson, R. C.: Bilateral posterior fracture dislocation of the shoulder. J. Bone Joint Surg., *51A*: 1627-1630, 1969.
58. Richard, A., Judet, R., and Rene, L.: Acrylic prosthetic construction of the upper end of the humerus for fracture-luxations. J. Chir., *68*:537-547, 1952.
59. Roberts, S. M.: Fractures of the upper end of the humerus. An end result study which shows the advantage of early active motion. J.A.M.A., *98*:367-373, 1932.
60. Rowe, C. R., and Marble, H.: Shoulder girdle injuries. *In* Cave, E. F. (ed.): Fractures and Other Injuries. Chicago, Year Book Medical Publishers, 1958.
61. Sante, H. E.: Fractures about the upper end of the humerus. Ann. Surg., *80*:103-114, 1924.

62. Sever, J. W.: Fracture of the head of the humerus. Treatment and results. New Eng. J. Med., *216*:1100-1107, 1937.
63. Stimson, B. B.: A manual of fractures and dislocations. ed. 2. Philadelphia, Lea & Febiger, 1947.
64. Thompson, F. R., and Winant, E. M.: Unusual fracture subluxations of the shoulder joint. J. Bone Joint Surg., *32*: 575-582, 1950.
65. ———: Comminuted fracture of the humeral head with subluxation. Clin. Orthop., *20*:94-96, 1961.
66. Valls, J.: Acrylic prosthesis in a case with fracture of the head of the humerus. Bal. Soc. Orthop. Trauma, (Argentina), *17*: 61, 1952.
67. Vander Ghirst, M., and Houssa, R.: Acrylic prosthesis in fractures of the head of the humerus. Acta Chir. Belg., *50*:31, 1951.
68. Watson-Jones, R.: Fractures and Joint Injuries. ed. 5. vol. 2. Baltimore, Williams & Wilkins, 1955.
69. Whitson, T. B.: Fractures of the surgical neck of the humerus—a study in reduction. J. Bone Joint Surg., *36B*:423-427, 1954.
70. Winfield, J. M., Miller, H., and LaFerte, A. D.: Evaluation of the hanging cast as a method of treating fractures of the humerus. Amer. J. Surg., *55*:228-249, 1942.

Fractures of the Clavicle

71. Abbott, L. C., and Lucas, D. B.: The function of the clavicle. Ann. Surg., *140*: 583-599, 1954.
72. Adams, F.: The Genuine Works of Hippocrates. vol. 2. New York, William Wood & Co., 1891.
73. Allman, F. L.: Fractures and ligamentous injuries of the clavicle and its articulation. J. Bone Joint Surg., *49A*:774-784, 1967.
74. Badgley, C. E.: Sports injuries of the shoulder girdle. J.A.M.A., *172*:444-448, 1960.
75. Barrett, J.: The clavicular joints. Physiotherapy, *57*:268-269, 1971.
76. Berkheiser, E. J.: Old ununited clavicular fractures in the adult. Surg. Gynecol. Obstet., *64*:1064-1072, 1937.
77. Billington, R. W.: A new (plaster yoke) dressing for fracture of the clavicle. South. Med. J., *24*:667, 1931.
78. Conwell, H. E.: Fractures of the clavicle. J.A.M.A., *90*:838-839, 1928.
79. Conwell, H. E., and Reynolds, F. C.: Key and Conwell's Management of Fractures, Dislocations, and Sprains. ed. 7. St. Louis, C. V. Mosby, 1961.
80. Cooper, A.: A treatise on dislocations and fractures of the joints. Lilly & Wait and Carter & Hendee, 2nd American Edition from the 6th London Edition, Boston, 1832, p. 375-377.
81. Cayford, E. H., and Tees, F. J.: Traumatic aneurysm of the subclavicular artery as a late complication of fractured clavicle. Can. Med. Ass. J., *25*:450-452, 1931.
82. Coyner, W. W., and Tompkins, S. F.: Open reduction of the clavicle; a review of forty cases. Presented at Clinical Conference, University of Oklahoma Medical Center, November, 1968.
83. Das, A. K., and Deb, H. K.: Synovioma of the clavicle. Report of a case. J. Internat. Coll. Surg., *35*:776-780, 1961.
84. Elting, J. J.: Retrosternal dislocation of the clavicle. Arch. Surg., *104*:35-37, 1972.
85. Fetterman, L. E.: Automobile head restraint injury. J.A.M.A., *214*:1328, 1970.
86. Gardner, E.: The embryology of the clavicle. Clin. Orthop., *58*:9-16, 1968.
87. Ghormley, R. K., Black, J. R., and Cherry, J. H.: Ununited fractures of the clavicle. Amer. J. Surg., *51*:343-349, 1941.
88. Guilfoil, P. H., and Christiansen, T.: An unusual vascular complication of fractured clavicle. J.A.M.A., *200*:72-73, 1967.
89. Howard, F. M., and Shafer, S. J.: Injuries to the clavicle with neurovascular complications. J. Bone Joint Surg., *47A*:1335-1346, 1965.
90. Inman, V. T., and Saunders, J. B. deC M.: Observations on the function of the clavicle. Calif. Med., *65*:158-166, 1946.
91. Jarman, J. B.: Treatment of fractures of the middle third of the clavicle in adults. Presented at Clinical Conference, University of Oklahoma Medical Center, March, 1963.
92. Kini, M. G.: A simple method of ambulatory treatment of fractures of the clavicle. J. Bone Joint Surg., *23*:795-798, 1941.
93. Kite, J. H.: Congenital pseudarthrosis of the clavicle. South. Med. J., *61*:703-710, 1968.
94. Kreisinger, V.: Sur le traitement des fractures de la clavicle. Rev. Chir., *16*:376, 1927.
95. Kremens, V., and Glauser, F.: Unusual sequela following pinning of medial clavicular fracture. Amer. J. Roentgenol., *74*:1066-1069, 1956.
96. Lee, H. G.: Treatment of fracture of the

clavicle by internal nail fixation. New Eng. J. Med., *234*:222-224, 1946.
97. Lester, C. W.: The treatment of fractures of the clavicle. Ann. Surg., *89*:600, 1929.
98. Lucas, D. B.: Function and surgery of the clavicle. Summary of Paper Presented at the 21st Annual Meeting of the Western Orthopaedic Association, Santa Barbara, California, October, 1957.
99. ———: Biomechanics of the shoulder joint. Arch. Surg., *107*:425-432, 1973.
100. Malgaigne, J. F.: Treatise on fractures. Philadelphia, J. B. Lippincott, 1859.
101. Marie, P., and Sainton, P.: On hereditary cleidocranial dysostosis. Clin. Orthop., *58*:5-7, 1968.
102. Mayer, J. H.: Non-union of fractured clavicle. Proc. Roy. Soc. Med., *58*:182, 1965.
103. Mazet, R.: Migration of a Kirschner wire from the shoulder region into the lung. Report of two cases. J. Bone Joint Surg., *25*:477-483, 1943.
104. Moore, T. O.: Internal pin fixation for fracture of the clavicle. Amer. Surg., *17*: 580-583, 1951.
105. Moseley, H. F.: The clavicle: its anatomy and function. Clin. Orthop., *58*:17-27, 1968.
106. Müller, M. E., Allgower, M., and Willenegger, H.: Manual of Internal Fixation. New York, Springer-Verlag, 1970.
107. Murray, G.: A method of fixation for fracture of the clavicle. J. Bone Joint Surg., *22*:616-620, 1940.
108. Neer, C. S., II: Nonunion of the clavicle. J.A.M.A., *172*:1006-1011, 1960.
109. ———: Fracture of the distal clavicle with detachment of the coracoclavicular ligaments in adults. J. Trauma, *3*:99-110, 1963.
110. ———: Fractures of the distal third of the clavicle. Clin. Orthop., *58*:43-50, 1968.
111. Neviaser, J. S.: Injuries in and about the shoulder joint. American Academy of Orthopaedic Surgeons Instructional Course Lectures, *13*:187-216, 1956.
112. ———: The treatment of fractures of the clavicle. Surg. Clin. N. Amer., *43*:1555-1563, 1963.
113. Packer, B. D.: Conservative treatment of fracture of the clavicle. J. Bone Joint Surg., *26*:770-774, 1944.
114. Patel, C. V., and Adenwalla, H. S.: Treatment of fractured clavicle by immediate partial subperiosteal resection. J. Postgrad. Med., *18*:32-34, 1972.
115. Penn, I.: The vascular complications of fractures of the clavicle. J. Trauma, *4*: 819-831, 1964.
116. Quesana, F.: Technique of roentgen diagnosis of fractures of the clavicle. Surg. Gynecol. Obstet., *42*:4261-4281, 1926.
117. Quigley, T. B.: Management of simple fractures of clavicle in adults. New Eng. J. Med., *243*:286-290, 1950.
118. Rowe, C. R.: An atlas of anatomy and treatment of midclavicular fractures. Clin. Orthop., *58*:29-42, 1968.
119. Rush, L. V., and Rush, H. L.: Technique of longitudinal pin fixation in fractures of clavicle and jaw. Miss. Doctor, *27*:332, 1949.
120. Sakellarides, H.: Pseudarthrosis of the clavicle. J. Bone Joint Surg., *43A*:130-138, 1961.
121. Sayre, L. A.: A simple dressing for fracture of the clavicle. Amer. Pract., *4*:1, 1871.
122. Shauffer, I. A., and Collins, W. V.: The deep clavicular rhomboid fossa. J.A.M.A., *195*:778-779, 1966.
123. Stone, P. W., and Lord, J. W.: The clavicle and its relation to trauma to the subclavian artery and vein. Amer. J. Surg., *89*:834, 1955.
124. Trynin, A. H.: The Böhler clavicular splint in the treatment of clavicular injuries. J. Bone Joint Surg., *19*:417-424, 1937.
125. Urist, M. R.: Complete dislocation of the acromioclavicular joint. J. Bone Joint Surg., *28*:813-837, 1946.
126. Watson-Jones, R.: Fractures and Joint Injuries. vol. 2. Baltimore, Williams & Wilkins, 1955.
127. Worcester, J. N., and Green, D. P.: Osteoarthritis of the acromioclavicular joint. Clin. Orthop., *58*:69-73, 1968.
128. Young, C. S.: The mechanisms of ambulatory treatment of fractures of the clavicle. J. Bone Joint Surg., *13*:299-310, 1931.

Fractures of the Scapula

129. Anderson, L. D.: Fractures. *In* Crenshaw, A. H. (ed.): Campbell's Operative Orthopaedics. ed. 5. St. Louis, C. V. Mosby, 1971.
130. Aston, J. W., and Gregory, C. F.: Dislocation of the shoulder with significant fracture of the glenoid. J. Bone Joint Surg., *55A*:1531-1533, 1973.
131. Bateman, J. E.: The shoulder and neck. ed. 1. Philadelphia, W. B. Saunders, 1972.
132. Benton, J., and Nelson, C.: Avulsion of the coracoid process in an athlete. J. Bone Joint Surg., *53A*:356-358, 1971.

133. Charlton, M. R.: Fractures of the neck of the scapula. Northwest. Med., *37*:18-20, 1938.
134. Comolli, A.: Ober ein deutliches Zeichen bei gewissen Schulter-Blattbruchen. Zentralbl f. Chir., Leipz, *59*:937-944, 1923.
135. Cooper, A.: Lectures on Principles and Practice of Surgery. ed. 3. Boston, Lilly & Walt., 1831.
136. Cotton, F. J., and Brickley, W. J.: Treatment of fracture of neck of scapula. Boston Med. Surg. J., *185*:326-329, 1921.
137. Coves, W. P.: Fracture of coracoid process. New Eng. J. Med., *212*:727-728, 1935.
138. DePalma, A. F.: Surgery of the Shoulder. ed. 2. Philadelphia, J. B. Lippincott, 1973.
139. Findlay, R. T.: Fractures of the scapula. Ann. Surg., *93*:1001-1008, 1931.
140. ———: Fractures of the scapula and ribs. Amer. J. Surg., *38*:489-494, 1937.
141. Fischer, W. R.: Fracture of the scapula requiring open reduction. Report of a case. J. Bone Joint Surg., *21*:459-461, 1939.
142. Golding, C.: Radiology and orthopaedic surgery. J. Bone Joint Surg., *48B*:320-332, 1966.
143. Harmon, P. H., and Baker, D. R.: Fracture of scapula with displacement. J. Bone Joint Surg., *25*:834-838, 1943.
144. Heatly, M. D., Breck, L. W., and Higinbotham, N. L.: Bilateral fracture of scapula. Amer. J. Surg., *71*:256-259, 1946.
145. Hitzrot, T. M., and Bolling, R. W.: Arch. Prov. Chir., *18*:574, 1909.
146. ———: Fracture of the neck of the scapula. Ann. Surg., *63*:215-234, 1916.
147. Key, J. A., and Conwell, H. E.: Fractures, Dislocations and Sprains. ed. 5. St. Louis, C. V. Mosby, 1951.
148. Köhler, A., and Zimmer, E. A.: Borderlines of the Normal and Early Pathologic in Skeletal Roentgenology. Amer. ed. 3. New York, Grune and Stratton, 1968.
149. Kummel, B. M.: Fractures of the glenoid causing chronic dislocation of the shoulder. Clin. Orthop., *69*:189-191, 1970.
150. Landoff, B. A.: Hitherto undescribed injury of the coracoid process. Acta Clin. Scand., *89*:401-406, 1943.
151. Liberson, F.: Os acromiale—contested anomaly. J. Bone Joint Surg., *19*:683-689, 1937.
152. Longabourh, R. I.: Fracture simple, right scapula. *In* Notes on cases of surgical interest. U. S. Naval Med. Bull., *27*:341, 1924.
153. McCally, W. C., and Celly, D. A.: Treatment of fractures of the clavicle, ribs, and scapula. Amer. J. Surg., *50*:558-562, 1940.
154. McLaughlin, H. L.: Trauma. Philadelphia, W. B. Saunders, 1959.
155. Madsen, E.: Bandage for fractured scapula. Chirurg., *12*:531-532, 1940.
156. Nettrour, L. F., Krufky, E. L., Mueller, R. E., and Raycroft, J. F.: Locked scapula: intrathoracic dislocation of the inferior angle. A case report. J. Bone Joint Surg., *54A*:413-416, 1972.
157. Neviaser, J.: Traumatic lesions. Injuries in and about the shoulder joint. American Academy of Orthopaedic Surgeons Instructional Course Lectures, *13*:187-216, 1956.
158. Newell, E. D.: Review of over 2000 fractures in past 7 years. South. Med. J., *20*:644-648, 1927.
159. Nunley, R. C., and Bedini, S. J.: Paralysis of the shoulder subsequent to a comminuted fracture of the scapula: rationale and treatment methods. Phys. Ther. Rev., *40*:442-447, 1960.
160. Ramin, J. E., and Viet, H.: Fractures during electroshock therapy. Amer. J. Psychiat., *110*:153-154, 1953.
161. Rounds, R. C.: Isolated fracture of the coracoid process. J. Bone Joint Surg., *31A*:662-663, 1949.
162. Rowe, C. R.: Fractures of the scapula. Surg. Clin. N. Amer., *43*:1565-1571, 1963.
163. Rowe, C. R., and Marble, H.: Shoulder girdle injuries. *In* Cave, E. F. (ed.): Fractures and Other Injuries. Chicago, Year Book Medical Publishers, 1958.
164. Rush, L. V.: Fracture of coracoid process. Ann. Surg., *90*:1113-1114, 1929.
165. Stein, R. E., Bone, J., Korn, J., and Wolff, W. I.: Axillary artery injury in closed fracture of the neck of the scapula: A case report. J. Trauma, *11*:528-531, 1971.
166. Steindler, A.: The Traumatic Deformities and Disabilities of the Upper Extremities. Springfield, Ill., Charles C Thomas, 1946.
167. Tachdijan, M. O.: Pediatric Orthopaedics. Philadelphia, W. B. Saunders, 1972.
168. Wilson, P. D.: Experience in the Management of Fractures and Dislocations (Based on Analysis of 4390 Cases) by the Staff of the Fracture Service, Mass. General Hospital, Boston. Philadelphia, J. B. Lippincott, 1938.

DISLOCATIONS ABOUT THE SHOULDER

Anterior Dislocations of the Shoulder

169. Adams, F. L.: The Genuine Works of

Hippocrates. vols. 1, 2. New York, William Wood & Co., 1886.
170. Adams, J. C.: Recurrent dislocations of the shoulder. J. Bone Joint Surg., *30B*: 26-38, 1948.
171. ———: The humeral head defect in recurrent anterior dislocations of the shoulder. Brit. J. Radiol., *23*:151-156, 1950.
172. Albert, E.: Arthodese bei einer habituellen luxation der schultergelenkes. Klin. Rundschau, *2*:281-283, 1898.
173. Alldred, A.: Subscapularis transplant for recurrent dislocation of the shoulder. J. Bone Joint Surg., *40B*:354, 1958.
174. Amorth, G., and Lazzari, E.: Voluntary dislocations of the shoulder. Riv. Deg. Infort. Mall. Prof., *49*:494-500, 1962.
175. Antoine, H. A.: De l'allongement des membres luxes apres la reduction de la luxation. Gaz. Med. Paris, *3*:621-622, 1836.
176. Artz, T., and Huffer, J. M.: A major complication of the modified Bristow procedure for recurrent dislocation of the shoulder. J. Bone Joint Surg., *54A*:1293-1296, 1972.
177. Asplund, G.: Ein operierter Fall von Willkurlicher (Habituelwillkurlicher) hinterer Schultergelenkluxation. Acta Chir. Scand., *87*:103-112, 1942.
178. Aston, J. W., Jr., and Gregory, C. F.: Dislocation of the shoulder with significant fracture of the glenoid. J. Bone Joint Surg., *55A*:1531-1533, 1973.
179. Augustine, R. W.: Repair of dislocation of the shoulder using modern Magnuson technique. Amer. J. Surg., *91*:736-741, 1956.
180. Aupecle, P., Briet, S., and Butin, J.: Luxation anterointerne de l'Epaule droit. Lyon Chir., *60*:101-103, 1964.
181. Babbitt, D., and Cassidy, R.: Obstetrical paralysis and dislocation of the shoulder in infancy. J. Bone Joint Surg., *50A*:1447-1452, 1968.
182. Badgley, C. E., and O'Connor, G. A.: Combined procedure for the repair of recurrent anterior dislocation of the shoulder. J. Bone Joint Surg., *47A*:1283, 1965.
183. Bailey, R. W.: Acute and recurrent dislocation of the shoulder. J. Bone Joint Surg., *49A*:767-773, 1967.
184. ———: Acute and Recurrent Dislocation of the Shoulder. Instructional Course Lectures 18, J1, p. 70-74, 1962-69.
185. Bankart, A. S. B.: Recurrent or habitual dislocation of the shoulder joint. Brit. Med. J., *2*:1132-1133, 1923.
186. ———: Dislocation of the shoulder-joints: *In* Robert Jones' Birthday Volume. A Collection of Surgical Essays. London, Oxford University Press, 1928.
187. ———: The pathology and treatment of recurrent dislocation of the shoulder joint. Brit. J. Surg., *26*:23-29, 1939.
188. Bardenheuer: Die Verletzungen der oberen extremitaten. Deutsche Chir., *63*: 268-418, 1886.
189. Bateman, J. E.: The shoulder and environs. ed. 1. St. Louis, C. V. Mosby, 1955.
190. ———: Gallie technique for repair of recurrent dislocation of the shoulder. Surg. Clin. North Amer., *43*:1655-1662, 1963.
191. ———: The Shoulder and Neck. Philadelphia, W. B. Saunders, 1972.
192. Bennett, G. E.: Old dislocations of the shoulder. J. Bone Joint Surg., *18*:594-606, 1936.
193. Blazina, M. E., and Satzman, J. S.: Recurrent anterior subluxation of the shoulder in athletes—a distinct entity. J. Bone Joint Surg., *51A*:1037-1038, 1969.
194. Blom, S., and Dahback, L. O.: Nerve injuries in dislocations of the shoulder joint and fractures of the neck of the humerus. Acta Chir. Scand., *136*:461-466, 1970.
195. Boicev, B.: Sulla lussazione abituale della spalla. Chir. Organi Mov., *23*:354-370, 1930.
196. Bonnin, J. G.: Transplantation of the Tip of the Coracoid Process for Recurrent Anterior Dislocation of the Shoulder. J. Bone Joint Surg., *51B*:579, 1969.
197. ———: Transplantation of the coracoid tip. A definitive operation for recurrent anterior dislocation of the shoulder. R. Soc. Med., *66*:755-758, 1973.
198. Bost, F., and Inman, V. T.: The pathologic changes in recurrent dislocation of the shoulder. A report of Bankart's operative procedure. J. Bone Joint Surg., *24*: 595-613, 1942.
199. Boyd, H. B., and Hunt, H.: Recurrent dislocation of the shoulder. J. Bone Joint Surg., *47A*:1514-1520, 1965.
200. Brav, E. A.: An evaluation of Putti-Platt reconstruction procedure for recurrent dislocation of the shoulder. J. Bone Joint Surg., *37A*:731-741, 1955.
201. ———: Ten years experience with Putti-Platt reconstruction procedure. Amer. J. Surg., *100*:423-430, 1960.
202. Brav, E. A., and Jefferess, V. H.: Simplified Putti-Platt reconstruction for recurrent shoulder dislocation. A preliminary report. Western J. Surg. Obstet. Gynecol., *60*:93-97, 1952.

203. Broca, A., and Hartmann, H.: Contribution a l'etude des luxations de l'epaule. Bull. Soc. Anat. Paris, *4*:312-336, 1890.
204. ———: Contribution a l'etude des luxations de l'epaule. Bull. Soc. Anat. Paris, *4*:416-423, 1890.
205. Brockbank, W., and Griffiths, D. L.: Orthopaedic surgery in the 16th and 17th centuries. J. Bone Joint Surg., *30B*:365-375, 1948.
206. Brown, F. W., and Navigato, W. J.: Rupture of the axillary artery and brachial plexus palsy associated with anterior dislocation of the shoulder—report of a case with successful vascular repair. Clin. Orthop., *60*:195-199, 1968.
207. Bryan, R. S., DiMichele, J. D., Ford, G. L., and Cary, G. R.: Anterior recurrent dislocation of the shoulder. Clin. Orthop., *63*:177-180, 1969.
208. Caird, F. M.: The shoulder joint in relation to certain dislocations and fractures. Edinb. Med. J., *32*:708-714, 1887.
209. Calandriello, B.: Revisione critica della cura chirugica della lussazione abituale di spalla. Arch. "Putti" Chir. Org. Movimento, *1*:359-387, 1951.
210. ———: The pathology of recurrent dislocation of the shoulder. Clin. Orthop., *20*:33-39, 1961.
211. Calvet, J., LeRoy, M., and Lacroix, L.: Luxations de l'epaule et lesions vasculaires. J. Chir., *58*:337-346, 1942.
212. Cave, E. F. (ed.): Fractures and Other Injuries. Chicago, Year Book Publishers, 1958.
213. Clairmont, P., and Ehrlich, H.: Ein neues Operations-verfahren zur Behandlung der habituellen Schulterluxation mittels Muskelplastik. Verhandl. Deutschen Ges. Chir., *38*:79-103, 1909.
214. Clark, K. C.: Positioning in Radiography. ed. 2. London, William Heinemann, Ltd., 1941.
215. Codman, E. A.: The Shoulder. G. Miller and Co., Medical Pub. Inc., Brooklyn, New York, 1934.
216. Collins, H. R., and Wilde, A. H.: Shoulder instability in athletes. Orthop. Clin. North Amer., *4*:759-773, 1973.
217. Conforty, B.: Boytchev's procedure for recurrent dislocation of the shoulder [Abstr.] J. Bone Joint Surg., *56*:386, 1974.
218. Connolly, J.: X-ray defects in recurrent shoulder dislocations. J. Bone Joint Surg., *51A*:1235-1236, 1969.
219. Conwell, H. E., and Reynolds, F. C.: Key and Conwell's Management of Fractures, Dislocations, and Sprains. ed. 7. St. Louis, C. V. Mosby, 1961.
220. Cooper, A.: A Treatise on Dislocations and Fractures of the Joints. (2nd American edition from the 6th London edition) Boston, Lilly, Wait, Carter, and Hendee, 1832.
221. Cozen, L.: Congenital dislocation of the shoulder and other abnormalities. Arch. Surg., *35*:956-966, 1935.
222. Cramer, F.: Resection des Oberarmkopfes wegen habitueller Luxation (Nach einem im arztlichen Verein zu Wiesbaden gehaltenen Vortrage). Berliner Klin. Wochenschr., *19*:21-25, 1882.
223. Crenshaw, A. H. (ed.): Campbell's Operative Orthopaedics. ed. 5. vols. 1, 2. St. Louis, C. V. Mosby, 1971.
224. Cubbins, W., Callahan, H., and Scuderi, C.: The reduction of old or irreducible shoulder dislocation. Surg. Gynecol. Obstet., *58*:129-135, 1934.
225. Curr, J. F.: Rupture of the axillary artery complicating dislocation of the shoulder. Report of a case. J. Bone Joint Surg., *52B*:313-317, 1970.
226. D'Angelo, D.: Lussazione volontaria della spalla (presentazione di quattro casi). Arch. "Putti", *17*:142-147, 1962.
227. Das, S. P., Saha, A. K., and Roy, G. S.: Observations on the tilt of the glenoid cavity of scapula. J. Anat. Soc. India, *15*:114, 1966.
228. Davis, A. G.: A conservative treatment for habitual dislocation of the shoulder. J.A.M.A., *107*:1012-1015, 1936.
229. Day, A. J., MacDonell, J. A., and Pedersen, H. E.: Recurrent dislocation of the shoulder. Clin. Orthop. *45*:123-126, 1966.
230. De Anquin, C. E.: A reliable operative procedure for recurrent dislocation of the shoulder. J. Bone Joint Surg., *43A*:26, 1961. Scientific Exhibit, AAOS Meeting, Miami Beach, Florida, Jan. 8-13, 1961.
231. ———: Recurrent dislocation of the shoulder—roentgenographic study. J. Bone Joint Surg., *47A*:1085, 1965.
232. Debevoise, N. T., Hyatt, G. W., and Townsend, G. B.: Humeral torsion in recurrent shoulder dislocations. Clin. Orthop., *76*:87-93, 1971.
233. Delitala, F.: Contributo al tratt amento della lussazione abituale della spalla. *In* Moseley, H. F. (ed): Recurrent Dislocation of the Shoulder. Montreal, McGill Univ. Press, 1961.
234. Delorme, D.: Die Hemmungsbander des

Schultergelenks und ihre Bedeutung fur die Schulterluxationen. Arch. Klin. Chir., *92*:79-101, 1910.
235. DePalma, A. F.: Recurring dislocation of the shoulder. A symposium. J. Bone Joint Surg., *39B*:9-58, 1948.
236. ———: Recurrent dislocation of the shoulder joint. Ann. Surg., *132*:1052-1065, 1950.
237. ———: Surgery of the Shoulder. ed. 1. Philadelphia, J. B. Lippincott, 1950.
238. ———: Factors influencing the choice of a modified Magnuson procedure for recurrent anterior dislocation of the shoulder—with a note on technique. Surg. Clin. North Amer., *43*:1647, 1963.
239. ———: Surgery of the Shoulder. ed. 2. Philadelphia, J. B. Lippincott, 1973.
240. DePalma, A. F., and Silberstein, C. E.: Results following a modified Magnuson procedure in recurrent dislocation of the shoulder. Surg. Clin. North Amer., *43*: 1651-1653, 1963.
241. DePalma, A. F., Cooke, A. J., and Prabhakar, M.: The role of the subscapularis in recurrent anterior dislocations of the shoulder. Clin. Orthop., *54*:35-49, 1967.
242. Dickson, J. A., and O'Dell, H. W.: Phylogenetic study of recurrent anterior dislocation of the shoulder joint. Surg. Gynecol. Obstet., *95*:357-365, 1952.
243. Dickson, J. A., Humphries, A. W., and O'Dell, H. W.: Recurrent Dislocations of the Shoulder. Edinburgh, E. & S. Livingstone, 1953.
244. Dickson, J. W., and Devas, M. B.: Bankart's operation for recurrent dislocation of the shoulder. J. Bone Joint Surg., *39B*: 114-119, 1957.
245. Didiee, J.: Le radiodiagnostic dans la luxation recidivante de l'epaule. J. Radiol. Electrol., *14*:209-218, 1930.
246. Downing, F. H.: The operative treatment for anterior dislocation of the shoulder. J. Bone Joint Surg., *51A*:811-812, 1969.
247. Du Toit, G. T., and Roux, D.: Recurrent dislocation of the shoulder. A 24-year study of the Johannesburg stapling operation. J. Bone Joint Surg., *38A*:1-12, 1956.
248. Du Toit, J. G.: Recurrent dislocation of the shoulder. Orthopaedic Correspondence Club Letter, August, 1969.
249. Ebel, R.: The cause of axillary nerve paresis in shoulder luxations. Monatsschr. Unfallheilkd, *76*:445-449, 1973.
250. Edeland, H. G., and Stefansson, T.: Block of suprascapular nerve in reduction of acute anterior shoulder dislocation. Acta Anesth. Scand., *17*:46-49, 1973.
251. Eden, R.: Zur Operation der habituellen Schulterluxation unter Mitteilung eines neuen Verfahrens bei Abriss am inneren Pfannenrande. Deutsch. Ztschr. Chir., *144*:269-280, 1918.
252. Eden-Hybbinette, R.: Technique of Palmer and Widen. *In* Crenshaw, A. H. (ed.): Campbell's Operative Orthopaedics. ed. 5. vol. I. St. Louis, C. V. Mosby, 1971.
253. Editorial. Voluntary dislocation of the shoulder. Brit. Med. J., *4*:505, 1973.
254. Eve, F. S.: A case of subcoracoid dislocation of the humerus with the formation of an indentation on the posterior surface of the head. Medico-Chirug. Trans. Soc. London, *63*:317-321, 1880.
255. Eyre-Brook, A. L.: The morbid anatomy of a case of recurrent dislocation of the shoulder. Brit. J. Surg., *29*:32-37, 1943.
256. ———: Recurrent dislocation of the shoulder. Lesions Discovered in Seventeen Cases. Surgery Employed, and Intermediate Report on Results. J. Bone Joint Surg., *30B*:39-48, 1948.
257. ———: Recurrent dislocation of the shoulder. Physiotherapy, *57*:7-13, 1971.
258. Fahey, J.: Anatomy of the shoulder. American Academy of Orthopaedic Surgeons Instructional Course Lectures, *4*: 186-190, 1947.
259. Finsterer, H.: Die operative Behandlung der habituellen Schulterluxation. Deutsch. Ztschr. Chir., *141*:354-497, 1917.
260. Flower, W. H.: On pathologic changes produced in the shoulder joint by traumatic dislocation. Trans. Path. Soc. London, *12*:179-200, 1861.
261. Froimson, A., and Alfred, K. S.: Sesamoid bone of the subscapularis tendon. J. Bone Joint Surg., *43A*:881-884, 1961.
262. Gallie, W. E., and LeMesurier, A. B.: An operation for the relief of recurring dislocations of the shoulder. Trans. Amer. Surg. Ass., *45*:392-398, 1927.
263. ———: Recurring dislocation of the shoulder. J. Bone Joint Surg., *30B*:9-18, 1948.
264. Gandin, J., and Gandin, R.: Oudards operation and its variants in recurrent dislocation of shoulder—statistical study of 139 late results. Chirurgie, *99*:779-786, 1973.
265. Gardner, E.: The prenatal development of the human shoulder joint. Surg. Clin. North Amer., *43*:1465-1470, 1963.

266. Gardner, E., and Gray, D. J.: Prenatal development of the human shoulder and acromioclavicular joints. Amer. J. Anat., *92*:219-276, 1953.
267. Gartland, J. J., and Dowling, J. J.: Recurrent anterior dislocation of the shoulder joint. Clin. Orthop., *3*:86-91, 1954.
268. Genovesi, A.: Contributo alla conoscenza della lussazione volontaria della spalla. Arch. Putti, *17*:268-275, 1962.
269. Giannestras, N. J.: Magnuson-Stack procedure for recurrent dislocation of the shoulder. Surgery, *23*:794-798, 1948.
270. Gibson, A.: Recurrent dislocation of the shoulder joint. Can. Med. Ass. J., *11*:194-199, 1921.
271. Gjores, J. E., and Nilsonne, U.: Prognosis in primary dislocation of the shoulder. Acta Chir. Scand., *129*:468-470, 1965.
272. Glessner, J. R.: Intrathoracic dislocation of the humeral head. J. Bone Joint Surg., *43A*:428-430, 1961.
273. Golding, C.: Radiology and orthopaedic surgery. J. Bone Joint Surg., *48B*:320-332, 1966.
274. Grant, J. C. B.: Method of Anatomy. ed. 7. Baltimore, Williams & Wilkins, 1965.
275. Grieg, D.: On true congenital dislocation of the shoulder. Edinb. Med. J., *4*:157-175, 1923.
276. Griffiths, D. L.: Reducing dislocated shoulder. J. Bone Joint Surg., *32B*:678-679, 1950.
277. Guney, F.: Methods in surgery of habitual shoulder dislocation and its results, with special reference to the Eden-Brun method. Helv. Chir. Acta, *40*:329-338, 1973.
278. Hall, R. H., Isaac, F., and Booth, C. R.: Dislocation of the shoulder with special reference to accompanying small fractures. J. Bone Joint Surg., *41A*:489-494, 1959.
279. Hark, F. W.: Habitual dislocation of the shoulder joint. Arch. Surg., *56*:522-527, 1948.
280. Hays, M. B.: Glenoid osteotomy for treatment of recurrent dislocations of the shoulder. J. Bone Joint Surg., *51A*:811, 1969.
281. Hejna, W. F., Fossier, C. H., Goldstein, T. B., and Ray, R. D.: Ancient anterior dislocation of the shoulder. J. Bone Joint Surg., *51A*:1030-1031, 1969.
282. Helfet, A. J.: Coracoid transplantation for recurring dislocation of the shoulder. J. Bone Joint Surg., *40B*:198-202, 1958.
283. Henderson, M. S.: Habitual or recurrent dislocation of the shoulder. Surg. Gynecol. Obstet., *33*:1-7, 1921.
284. ———: Tenosuspension operation for recurrent or habitual dislocation of the shoulder. Surg. Clin. North Amer., *5*:997-1007, 1949.
285. Hermodsson, I.: Rontgenologische Studien uber die traumatischen und habituellen Schultergelenk-Verrenkungen nach vorn und nach unten. Acta Radiol., [Suppl. 20]:1-173, 1934.
286. Heymanowitsch. Z: Ein Beitrag zur operativen Behandlung der habituellen Schulterluxationen. Zbl. Chir., *54*:648-651, 1927.
287. Hildebrand: Zur operativen Behandlung der habituellen Schuterluxation. Arch. Klin. Chir., *66*:360-364, 1902.
288. Hill, H. A., and Sachs, M. D.: The grooved defect of the humeral head. A frequently unrecognized complication of dislocations of the shoulder joint. Radiology, *35*:690-700, 1940.
289. Hippocrates: Works of Hippocrates with an English Translation by W. H. S. Jones and E. T. Withington. London, William Heinemann, 1927.
290. Hoover, R. D.: Dislocation of the shoulder: a method of reduction. Clin. Orthop., *58*:296, 1968.
291. Howell, A. B.: Speed in Animals. Chicago, University Press, 1944.
292. Hussein, M. K.: Kocher's method is 3,000 years old. J. Bone Joint Surg., *50B*:669-671, 1968.
293. Hybbinette, S.: De la transplantation d'un fragment osseux pour remedier aux luxations recidivantes de l'epaule; constatations et resultats operatoires. Acta Chir. Scand., *71*:411-445, 1932.
294. Ilfeld, F. W., and Holder, H. G.: Recurrent dislocation of the shoulder joint. J. Bone Joint Surg., *25*:651-658, 1943.
295. Inman, V. T., Saunders, J. B. de C. M., and Abbott, L. C.: Observations on the function of the shoulder joint. J. Bone Joint Surg., *26*:1-30, 1944.
296. Jeffery, C. C.: Recurrent dislocation of the shoulder. J. Bone Joint Surg., *41B*:623, 1959.
297. Jekic, M.: Rare case of bilateral shoulder dislocation. Langenbeck Arch. Chir., *334*:931, 1973.
298. Jens, J.: The role of the subscapularis muscle in recurring dislocation of the shoulder. J. Bone Joint Surg., *34B*:780-781, 1964.
299. Joessel, D.: Ueber die Recidine der Humerus-Luxationen. Deutsch. Ztschr. Chir., *13*:167-184, 1880.
300. Jones, F. W.: Attainment of upright positions of man. Nature, *146*:26-27, 1940.

301. Kazar, B., and Relovszky, E.: Prognosis of primary dislocation of the shoulder. Acta Orthop. Scand., *40*:216-224, 1969.
302. Keiser, R. P., and Wilson, C. L.: Bilateral recurrent dislocation of the shoulder (atraumatic) in a 13-year-old girl. Report of an unusual case. J. Bone Joint Surg., *43A*:553-554, 1961.
303. King, Thomas: Recurrent dislocation of the shoulder. Med. J. Austral., *1*:697-700, 1947.
304. Kingsley, J. S.: Comparative Anatomy of the Vertebrates. Philadelphia, Blakiston, 1917.
305. Kocher, T.: Eine neue Reductionsmethode fur Schulterverrenkung. Berlin. Klin., *7*: 101-105, 1870.
306. Kuhns, L. R., Sherman, M. P., Poznanski, A. K., and Holt, J. F.: Humeral-head and coracoid ossification in the newborn. Radiology, *107*:145-149, 1973.
307. Kummel, B. M.: Fractures of the glenoid causing chronic dislocation of the shoulder. Clin. Orthop., *69*:189-191, 1970.
308. ———: The syndrome of anterior-capsular derangement of the shoulder. Orthop. Rev., *1*:7-12, 1972.
309. Kuster, E.: Ueber habituelle schulter Luxation. Verh. Deutsch. Ges. Chir., *11*: 112-114, 1882.
310. Lacey, T., II: Reduction of anterior dislocation of the shoulder by means of the Milch abduction technique. J. Bone Joint Surg., *34A*:108-109, 1952.
311. Laing, P. G.: The arterial blood supply of the adult humerus. J. Bone Joint Surg., *38A*:1105-1116, 1956.
312. Lam, S. J. S.: Irreducible anterior dislocation of the shoulder. J. Bone Joint Surg., *48B*:132, 1966.
313. Lambdin, C. S., Young, S. B., and Unsicker, C. L.: A modified Bankart Putti-Platt shoulder capsulorrhaphy. J. Bone Joint Surg., *53A*:1237, 1971.
314. LeClerk, J.: Chronic subluxation of the shoulder. J. Bone Joint Surg., *51B*:778, 1969.
315. Leffert, R. D., and Seddon, H.: Infraclavicular brachial plexus injuries. J. Bone Joint Surg., *47B*:9-22, 1965.
316. Leguit, P.: Recurrent dislocations of the shoulder. J. Int. Coll. Surg., *20*:741-749, 1953.
317. Leslie, J. T., and Ryan, T. J.: The anterior axillary incision to approach the shoulder joint. J. Bone Joint Surg., *44A*: 1193-1196, 1962.
318. Levy, L. J.: Anterior axillary incision in the repair of recurrent dislocation of the shoulder. J. Bone Joint Surg., *49A*:204, 1967.
319. Lewis, W. H.: The development of the arm in man. Amer. J. Anat., *1*:145-184, 1902.
320. Liebolt, F. L., and Furey, J. G.: Obstetrical paralysis with dislocation of the shoulder. J. Bone Joint Surg., *35A*:227-230, 1953.
321. Little, M. G. A.: Dislocation of the shoulder (reduction). J. Bone Joint Surg., *47B*: 809, 1965.
322. Lucas, D. B.: Biomechanics of the shoulder joint. Arch. Surg., *107*:425-432, 1973.
323. Luckey, L. A.: Recurrent dislocation of the shoulder. Amer. J. Surg., *77*:220-222, 1949.
324. MacAusland, W. R.: Recurrent anterior dislocation of the shoulder. Amer. J. Surg., *91*:323-331, 1956.
325. MacDonald, F. R.: Intra-articular fractures in recurrent dislocation of the shoulder. Surg. Clin. North Amer., *43*:1635-1645, 1963.
326. Mackenzie, A. B.: Recurrent dislocation of the shoulder. J. Bone Joint Surg., *38B*: 601, 1956.
327. McLaughlin, H. L.: Discussion of acute anterior dislocation of the shoulder by Toufick Nicola. J. Bone Joint Surg., *31A*: 172, 1949.
328. ———: Trauma. Philadelphia, W. B. Saunders, 1959.
329. ———: Recurrent anterior dislocation of the shoulder. Amer. J. Surg., *99*:628-632, 1960.
330. McLaughlin, H. L., and Cavallaro, W. U.: Primary anterior dislocation of the shoulder. Amer. J. Surg., *80*:615-621, 1950.
331. McLaughlin, H. L., and MacLellan, D. I.: Recurrent anterior dislocation of the shoulder II. A comparative study. J. Trauma, *7*:191-201, 1967.
332. McMurray, T. B.: Recurrent dislocation of the shoulder. J. Bone Joint Surg., *43B*: 402, 1961.
333. Magnuson, P. B.: Treatment of recurrent dislocation of the shoulder. Surg. Clin. North Amer., *25*:14-20, 1945.
334. Magnuson, P. B., and Stack, J. K.: Bilateral habitual dislocation of the shoulders in twins, a familial tendency, J.A.M.A., *144*:2103, 1940.
335. ———: Recurrent dislocation of the shoulder. J.A.M.A., *123*:898-892, 1943.
336. Malgaigne, J. F.: Traite des fractures et des luxations J. B. Bailliere, Paris, 1855, J. B. Lippincott, 1859.
337. Maxwell, J. S.: Staple introducer for re-

current dislocation. Brit. Med. J. *1*:588, 1946.
338. ———: Recurrent shoulder dislocation. Lancet, *1*:467, 1947.
339. May, V. R., Jr.: A modified Bristow operation for anterior recurrent dislocation of the shoulder. J. Bone Joint Surg., *52A*: 1010-1016, 1970.
340. Mead, N. C., and Sweeney, H. J.: Bristow procedure. Spectator Letter, July 9, 1964.
341. Metcalfe, J. W.: The Bankart operation for recurrent dislocation of the shoulder. U. S. Navy Med. Bull., *47*:672-675, 1947.
342. Middeldorpf, M., and Sharm, B.: De nova humeri luxationis specie. Clinique Europenne, vol. II. 1859, Dissert. Inag. Breslav, 1859.
343. Milch, H.: Treatment of dislocation of the shoulder. Surgery, *3*:732-740, 1938.
344. Milgram, J. E.: Shoulder anatomy (the shoulder symposium). American Academy of Orthopaedic Surgeons Instructional Course Lectures, *3*:55-68, 1946.
345. Montagu, A.: An Introduction to Physical Anthropology. Springfield, Ill., Charles C Thomas, 1947.
346. Moseley, H. F.: Shoulder Lesions. ed. 1. Springfield, Ill., Charles C Thomas, 1945.
347. ———: The use of a metallic glenoid rim in recurrent dislocation of the shoulder. Can. Med. Ass. J., *56*:320-321, 1947.
348. ———: The use of a metallic glenoid rim in recurrent dislocation of the shoulder. Amer. J. Surg., *80*:615, 1950.
349. ———: Experiences with recurrent dislocations of the shoulder. Can. Orthop. Ass., June 25, 1955. J. Bone Joint Surg., *38B*:780, 1956.
350. ———: Recurrent Dislocation of the Shoulder. Montreal, McGill University Press, 1961.
351. ———: The Basic Lesions of Recurrent Anterior Dislocation. Surg. Clin. North Am., *43*:1631-1634, 1963.
352. Moseley, H. F., and Overgaard, B.: The anterior capsular mechanism in recurrent anterior dislocation of the shoulder. J. Bone Joint Surg., *44B*:913-927, 1962.
353. Murphy, I. D.: Sliding bone graft for connection of recurrent anterior dislocation of the shoulder. J. Bone Joint Surg., *50A*: 1270, 1968.
354. Nelson, C. L.: The use of arthrography in athletic injuries to the shoulder. Orthop. Clin. North Amer., *4*:775-785, 1973.
355. Nelson, W. E., and Skagerberg, D.: Recurrent shoulder dislocations—modified Magnuson repair. J. Bone Joint Surg., *49A*:202-203, 1967.
356. Neviaser, J. S.: An operation for old dislocation of the shoulder. J. Bone Joint Surg., *30A*:997-1000, 1948.
357. ———: The treatment of old unreduced dislocations of the shoulder. Surg. Clin. North Amer., *43*:1671-1678, 1963.
358. Neviaser, J. S., and Tobin, W. J.: Humeral torsion in relation to recurrent dislocations of the shoulder, Read at Meeting of the Interurban Club, Washington, D.C., 1959.
359. Nicholson, J. T.: Recurrent dislocation of the shoulder. J. Bone Joint Surg., *32B*: 510-511, 1950.
360. Nicola, T.: Recurrent anterior dislocation of the shoulder. J. Bone Joint Surg., *11*: 128-132, 1929.
361. ———: Recurrent dislocation of the shoulder—its treatment by transplantation of the long head of the biceps. Amer. J. Surg., *6*:815, 1929.
362. ———: Anterior dislocation of the shoulder. The role of the articular capsule. J. Bone Joint Surg., *24*:614-616, 1942.
363. ———: Acute anterior dislocation of the shoulder. J. Bone Joint Surg., *31A*:153-159, 1949.
364. ———: Recurrent dislocation of the shoulder. Amer. J. Surg., *86*:85-91, 1953.
365. Noordenbos, W.: Beenplastiek bij habitueele schouderluxatie. Ned. T. Geneesk, *82*:1784, 1938.
366. Odgers, S. L., and Hark, F. W.: Habitual dislocation of the shoulder joint. Surg. Gynecol. Obstet., *75*:229-234, 1942.
367. O'Donoghue, D. H.: Treatment of Injuries to Athletes. ed. 2. W. B. Saunders, Philadelphia, 1970.
368. Ogilvie, H.: Recurrent dislocation of the shoulder. The Johannesburg staple driver. Brit. Med. J., *1*:362, 1946.
369. Olsson, O.: Degenerative changes of the shoulder joint and their connection with shoulder pain. Acta Chir. Scand., [Suppl. 181]:1-130, 1953.
370. Osmond-Clarke, H.: Habitual dislocation of the shoulder. The Putti-Platt operation. J. Bone Joint Surg., *30B*:19-25, 1948.
371. ———: Recurrent dislocation of the shoulder. J. Bone Joint Surg., *47B*:194, 1965.
372. Oster, A.: Recurrent anterior dislocation of the shoulder treated by the Eden-Hybbinette operation. Follow-up on 76 cases. Acta Orthop. Scand., *40*:43-52, 1969.
373. Oudard, P.: La luxation recidivante de l'epaule (variete antero-interne) procede operatoire. J. Chir., *23*:13, 1924.
374. ———: Le traitment de la luxation re-

cidivante de l'epaule (variete antero-interne par la butee osseuse). Rev. Med., *1*:305, 1946.
375. Palmar, I., and Widen, A.: The bone-block method for recurrent dislocation of the shoulder joint. J. Bone Joint Surg., *30B*:53-58, 1948.
376. Palumbo, L. T., and Quirin, L. D.: Recurrent dislocation of the shoulder repaired by Magnuson stack operation. Arch. Surg., *60*:1140-1150, 1950.
377. Palumbo, L. T., Sharpe, W. S., and Nejdl, R. J.: Recurrent dislocation of the shoulder repaired by the Magnuson-Stack operation. Arch. Surg., *81*:834-837, 1960.
378. Patel, M. R., Pardee, M. L., and Singerman, R. C.: Intrathoracic dislocation of the head of the humerus. J. Bone Joint Surg., *45A*:1712-1714, 1963.
379. Perkins, G.: Rest and movement. J. Bone Joint Surg., *35B*:521-539, 1953.
380. Perthes, G.: Uber Operationen bei habitueller Schulterluxation. Deutsch. Ztschr. Chir., *85*:199-227, 1906.
381. Pettersson, G.: Rupture of the tendon aponeurosis of the shoulder joint in anterior inferior dislocation. Acta Chir. Scand., [Suppl.] *77*:1-187, 1942.
382. Pilz, W.: Zur Rontgenuntersschung der habituellen Schulterverrenkung. Arch. Klin. Chir., *135*:1-22, 1925.
383. Plummer, W. W., and Pott, F. N.: Two cases of recurrent anterior dislocation of the shoulder. J. Bone Joint Surg., *7*:190-198, 1925.
384. Ponseti, I. V., and Shepard, R. S.: Lesions of the skeleton and of other mesodermal tissues in rats fed sweet pea seeds. J. Bone Joint Surg., *36A*:1031-1058, 1954.
385. Popke, L. O. A.: Zur Kasuistik und Therapie der inverterirten und habituellen Schulterluxation. Inaug. Dissert., Halle, 1882. H. F. Moseley: Recurrent Dislocation of the Shoulder, McGill Un. Press, Montreal, 1961.
386. Pridie, K. H.: Bankart's operation for recurrent dislocation of shoulder. J. Bone Joint Surg., *38B*:589-590, 1956.
387. Raney, R. B.: Andry and the orthopaedia. J. Bone Joint Surg., *31A*:675-682, 1949.
388. Raney, R. B., and Miller, O. L.: The Nicola operation of recurrent dislocation of the shoulder—a review of 26 cases. South. Med. J., *35*:529-532, 1942.
389. Reeves, B.: Arthrography of the shoulder. J. Bone Joint Surg., *48B*:424-435, 1966.
390. ———: Experiments on the tensile strength of the anterior capsular structures of the shoulder region. J. Bone Joint Surg., *50B*:858, 1968.
391. Rice, E.: Experience with the Putti-Platt shoulder reconstruction. Paper presented to Clinical Conference, University of Oklahoma School of Medicine, Oklahoma City, Oklahoma, November 1967.
392. Robertson, R., and Stack, W. J.: Diagnosis and treatment of recurrent dislocation of the shoulder. J. Bone Joint Surg., *29*:797-800, 1947.
393. Rokous, J. R., Feagin, J. A., and Abbott, H. G.: Modified axillary roentgenogram. A useful adjunct in the diagnosis of recurrent instability of the shoulder. Clin. Orthop., *82*:84-86, 1972.
394. Rowe, C. R.: Prognosis in dislocations of the shoulder. J. Bone Joint Surg., *38A*:957-977, 1956.
395. ———: Acute and recurrent dislocations of the shoulder. J. Bone Joint Surg., *44A*:998-1008, 1962.
396. ———: Symposium on Surgical Lesions of the Shoulder. J. Bone Joint Surg., *38A*:977-1012, 1956.
397. ———: Anterior dislocation of the shoulder. Surg. Clin. N. Amer., *43*:1609-1614, 1963.
398. ———: The surgical management of recurrent anterior dislocations of the shoulder using a modified Bankart procedure. Surg. Clin. N. Amer., *43*:1663-1666, 1963.
399. ———: The results of operative treatment of recurrent dislocation of the shoulder. Surg. Clin. N. Amer., *43*:1667-1670, 1963.
400. Rowe, C. R., and Sakellarides, H. T.: Factors related to recurrences of anterior dislocations of the shoulder. Clin. Orthop., *20*:40-47, 1961.
401. Rowe, C. R., and Pierce, D.: The enigma of voluntary recurrent dislocation of the shoulder. J. Bone Joint Surg., *47A*:1670, 1965.
402. Rowe, C. R., Pierce, D. S., and Clark, J. G.: Voluntary dislocation of the shoulder. A preliminary report on a clinical, electromyographic, and psychiatric study of 26 patients. J. Bone Joint Surg., *55*:445-460, 1973.
403. Rubin, S. A., Gray, R. L., and Green, W. R.: Scapular **Y** diagnostic aid in shoulder trauma. Radiology, *110*:725-726, 1974.
404. Rupp, F.: Ueber ein vereinfachtes Operationsverfahren bei habitueller Schulterluxation. Deutsch. Z., Chir., *198*:70-75, 1926.

405. Ryan, A. J.: Recurrent dislocation of shoulder. J.A.M.A., *195*:173, 1966.
406. Saha, A. K.: Theory of Shoulder Mechanism. Springfield, Ill., Charles C Thomas, 1961.
407. ———: Anterior recurrent dislocation of the shoulder. Treatment by latissimus dorsi transfer with follow-up in 22 cases. J. Int. Coll. Surg., *39*:361-373, 1963.
408. ———: Anterior recurrent dislocation of the shoulder. Acta Orthop. Scand., *39*: 479-493, 1967.
409. ———: Dynamic stability of the glenohumeral joint. Acta Orthop. Scand., *42*: 491-505, 1971.
410. ———: Mechanics of elevation of glenohumeral joint. Its application in rehabilitation of flail shoulder in upper brachial plexus injuries and poliomyelitis and in replacement of the upper humerus by prosthesis. Acta Orthop. Scand., *44*:668-678, 1973.
411. Saha, A. K., Das, N. N., and Chakravarty, B. G.: Treatment of recurrent dislocation of shoulder: past, present, and future. Studies on electromyographic changes of muscles acting on the shoulder joint complex. Calcutta Med. J., *53*:409-413, 1956.
412. Said, G. Z., and Medro, I.: Glenoidplasty as a treatment for recurrent anterior dislocation of the shoulder. Acta Orthop. Scand., *40*:777-787, 1970.
413. Schlemm, F.: Ueber die Verstarkungsbander am Schultergelenk Arch. Anat., Physiol. Wissenschaft. Med., p. 45, 1853.
414. Schulz, T. J., Jacobs, B., and Patterson, R. L.: Unrecognized dislocations of the shoulder. J. Trauma, *9*:1009-1023, 1969.
415. Schwartz, D. I.: Bankart shoulder repair made easier. J. Bone Joint Surg., *45A*: 1334, 1963.
416. ———: Bankart shoulder repair made easier. Clin. Orthop., *56*:69-72, 1968.
417. Sever, J. W.: Recurrent dislocation of the shoulder joint. J.A.M.A., *76*:925-927, 1921.
418. Skogland, L. B., and Sundt, P.: Recurrent anterior dislocation of the shoulder. The Eden-Hybbinette operation. Acta Orthop. Scand., *44*:739-747, 1973.
419. Smith, W. S., and Klug, T. J.: Anterior dislocation of the shoulder—a simple and effective method of reduction. J.A.M.A., *163*:182-183, 1957.
420. Speed, K.: Recurrent anterior dislocation at the shoulder; operative cure by bone graft. Surg. Gynecol. Obstet., *44*:468-477, 1927.
421. Spence, A. J.: European travelling scholarship, 1959. J. Bone Joint Surg., *43B*: 176-179, 1961.
422. Stimson, L. A.: An easy method of reducing dislocations of the shoulder and hip. Med. Record, *57*:356-357, 1900.
423. Strauss, M. B.: The shoulder—roentgenological evaluation of recurrent anterior instability. [Unpublished paper].
424. Strauss, M. B., Wrobel, L. J., Cady, G. W., and Neff, R. S.: Radiological confirmation of anterior shoulder and instability. Department of Orthopaedics, Naval Regional Med. Center, San Diego, California, 1974. [Unpublished paper].
425. Sudaron, F.: The results of the modified Nosske-Oudard-Bazy-Savic operation for recurrent dislocation of the shoulder. J. Bone Joint Surg., *48B*:855, 1966.
426. Sverdlov, I. M., Arenberg, A. A., and Ahitnitsky, R. E.: Voluntary Subluxation of the Shoulder. Central Institute of Traumatology and Orthopaedics, 1962.
427. Symeonides, P. P.: The significance of the subscapularis muscle in the pathogenesis of recurrent anterior dislocation of the shoulder. J. Bone Joint Surg., *54B*:476-483, 1972.
428. Tavernier, L.: The recurrent luxation of the shoulder. J. Bone Joint Surg., *12*:458-461, 1930.
429. Thomas, T. T.: Habitual or recurrent anterior dislocation of the shoulder. Amer. J. Med. Sci., *137*:229-246, 1909.
430. ———: Habitual or recurrent dislocation of the shoulder. Forty-four shoulder operations in 42 patients. Surg. Gynecol. Obstet., *32*:291-299, 1921.
431. Thompson, F. R., and Moga, J. J.: The combined operative repair of anterior and posterior shoulder subluxation. Audiovisual Program, American Academy of Orthopaedic Surgeons, Jan. 10, 1965.
432. Townley, C. O.: The capsular mechanism in recurrent dislocation of the shoulder. J. Bonc Joint Surg., *32A*:370-380, 1950.
433. ———: The dislocating shoulder: anatomy, pathology, pathogenesis. J. Bone Joint Surg., *45A*:1335, 1963.
434. ———: Intrinsic glenohumeral anatomy and its relation to recurrent shoulder dislocation. J. Bone Joint Surg., *47A*:1276, 1965.
435. ———: Recurrent shoulder dislocations: pathogenesis and pathology. Clin. Orthop., *44*:280, 1966.
436. Tronzo, R. G.: Reduction of dislocated shoulders using methocarbamol. J.A.M.A., *184*:110-112, 1044-1046, 1963.

437. Truchly, G.: Modified Putti procedure for the recurrent dislocation of the shoulder. Scientific Exhibit, American Academy of Orthopaedic Surgeons, Jan. 20-25, 1968.
438. Truchly, G., and Thompson, W. A. L.: Simplified Putti-Platt procedure. J.A.M.A., *179*:859-862, 1962.
439. Tullos, H. S., and King, J. W.: Throwing mechanism in sports. Orthop. Clin. N. Amer., *4*:709-720, 1973.
440. Turek, S. L.: Orthopaedics—Principles and Their Application. ed. 2. Philadelphia, J. B. Lippincott, 1967.
441. Vare, V. B., Jr.: The Treatment of Recurrent Dislocation of the Shoulder. Surg. Clin. North Am., *33*:1703-1710, 1953.
442. Viek, P., and Bell, B. T.: The Bankart shoulder reconstruction. J. Bone Joint Surg., *41A*:236-242, 1959.
443. Warwick, R., and Williams, P. L.: Gray's Anatomy. ed. 35. Philadelphia, W. B. Saunders, 1973.
444. Watson, D. M. S.: The evolution of the tetrapod shoulder girdle and forelimb. J. Anat., *52*:1-63, 1918.
445. Watson-Jones, R.: Dislocation of the shoulder joint. Proc. R. Soc. Med., *29*: 1060-1062, 1936.
446. ———: Note on recurrent dislocation of the shoulder joint. Superior approach causing the only failure in 52 operations for repair of the labrum and capsule. J. Bone Joint Surg., *30B*:49-52, 1948.
447. ———: Recurrent dislocation of the shoulder. [Editorial.] J. Bone Joint Surg., *30B*:6-8, 1948.
448. ———: Fractures and Joint Injuries. 2 vols. ed. 4. Baltimore, Williams & Wilkins, 1957.
449. Weber, B. G.: Operative treatment for recurrent dislocation of the shoulder. Injury, *1*:107-109, 1969.
450. West, E. F.: Intrathoracic dislocation of the humerus. J. Bone Joint Surg., *31B*:61-62, 1949.
451. White, M.: Some late results of dislocation of the shoulder. Trans. Roy. Med. Chir. Soc. Glasgow, *22*:243-248, 1929.
452. Willard, D. P.: The Nicola operation for recurrent dislocation of the shoulder. Ann. Surg., *103*:438-443, 1936.
453. Wolff, E. F.: Transposition of the biceps brachii tendon to repair-luxation of the canine shoulder joint. Vet. Med/Sac, *69*: 51-53, 1974.
454. Zanoli, R.: Appraisal of the geriatric patient. Clin. Orthop., *11*:12, 1958.
455. Zimmerman, L. M., and Veith, I.: Great Ideas in the History of Surgery. Clavicle, Shoulder, Shoulder Amputations. Baltimore, Williams & Wilkins, 1961.

Complications of Anterior Dislocation of the Shoulder

456. Antal, C. S., Conforty, B., Engelberg, M., and Reiss, R.: Injuries to the axillary nerve due to anterior dislocation of the shoulder. J. Trauma, *13*:564-566, 1973.
457. Archambault, R., Archambault, H. A., and Mizeres, N. J.: Rupture of the thoracoacromial artery in anterior dislocations of the shoulder. Amer. J. Surg., *97*:782-783, 1959.
458. Babcock, J. L., and Wray, J. B.: Analysis of abduction in a shoulder with deltoid paralysis due to axillary nerve injury. Clin. Orthop., *68*:116-120, 1970.
459. Barnes, R.: Traction injuries of the brachial plexus in adults. J. Bone Joint Surg., *31B*:10-16, 1949.
460. Bateman, J. E.: Neurovascular syndromes about the shoulder. American Academy of Orthopaedic Surgeons Instructional Course Lectures, *18*:247-257, 1961.
461. ———: Nerve injuries about the shoulder in sports (treatment of injuries to the shoulder girdle symp.) J. Bone Joint Surg., *49A*:785-792, 1967.
462. ———: Nerve injuries about the shoulder in sports. Instructional Course Lecture 18. J. Bone Joint Surg., *49A*:785-792, 1967.
463. Blom, S., and Dahlback, L. O.: Nerve injuries in dislocations of the shoulder joint and fractures of the neck of the humerus. Acta Chir. Scand., *136*:461-466, 1970.
464. Bonney, G.: Prognosis in traction injuries of the brachial plexus. J. Bone Joint Surg., *41B*:4-35, 1959.
465. Brown, F. W., and Navigato, W. J.: Rupture of the axillary artery and brachial plexus palsy associated with anterior dislocation of the shoulder. Clin. Orthop., *60*:195-199, 1968.
466. Brown, J. T.: Nerve injuries complicating dislocation of the shoulder. J. Bone Joint Surg., *34B*:526, 1952.
467. Bunts, F. E.: Nerve injuries about the shoulder joint. Trans. Amer. Surg. Ass., *21*:520-526, 1903.
468. Calvet, J., Leroy, M., and Lacroix, L.: Luxations de l'epaule et lesions vasculaires. J. Chir., *58*:337-348, 1941-42.
469. Chauvenet, A., and Daraignez, J.: Sur deux cas de rupture traumatique de lar-

tere axillaire. Mem. Acad. Chir., *68*:132-136, 1942.

470. Cranley, J. J., and Krause, R. J.: Injury to the axillary artery following anterior dislocation of the shoulder. Amer. J. Surg., *95*:524-526, 1958.
471. Cubbins, W. R., Callahan, J. J., and Scuderi, C. S.: The reduction of old or irreducible dislocations of the shoulder joint. Surg. Gynecol., Obstet., *58*:129-135, 1934.
472. Curr, J. F.: Rupture of the axillary artery complicating dislocation of the shoulder. J. Bone Joint Surg., *52B*:313-317, 1970.
473. d'Aubigne, R. M.: Nerve injuries in fractures and dislocations of the shoulder. Surg. Clin. N. Amer., *43*:1685-1689, 1963.
474. Dehne, E., and Hall, R. M.: Active shoulder motion in complete deltoid paralysis. J. Bone Joint Surg., *41A*:745-748, 1959.
475. Duchenne, G. B.: Physiology of Motion. Philadelphia, J. B. Lippincott, 1949.
476. Ebel, R.: The cause of axillary nerve paresis in shoulder luxations. Monatsschr. Unfallheilkd., *76*:445-449, 1973.
477. Gariepy, R., Derome, A., and Laurin, C. A.: Brachial plexus paralysis following shoulder dislocation. Can. J. Surg., *5*:418-421, 1962.
478. Gibson, J. M. C.: Rupture of the axillary artery following anterior dislocation of the shoulder. J. Bone Joint Surg., *44B*:114-115, 1962.
479. Gryska, P. F.: Major vascular injuries—principles of management in selected cases of arterial and venous injury. New Eng. J. Med., *266*:381-385, 1962.
480. Guibe, M.: Des lesions des vaisseaux de l'aiselle qui compliquent les luxation de l'epaule. Rev. Chir., *44*:580-583, 1911.
481. Henson, G. F.: Vascular complications of shoulder injuries. J. Bone Joint Surg., *38B*:528-531, 1956.
482. Jardon, O. M., Hood, L. T., and Lynch, R. D.: Complete avulsion of the axillary artery as a complication of shoulder dislocation. J. Bone Joint Surg., *55*:189-192, 1973.
483. Johnston, G. W., and Lowry, J. H.: Rupture of the axillary artery complicating anterior dislocation of the shoulder. J. Bone Joint Surg., *44B*:116-118, 1962.
484. Kirker, J. R.: Dislocation of the shoulder complicated by rupture of the axillary vessels. J. Bone Joint Surg., *34B*:72-73, 1952.
485. Leborgne, J., LeNeel, J. C., Mitard, D., Monfort, J., Roy, J., Visset, J.: Lesions of the axillary artery and its branches following to closed injury of the shoulder. Apropos of 10 cases. Ann. Chir., *27*:587-594, 1973.
486. Lusskin, R., Campbell, J. B., and Thompson, W. A.: Post-traumatic lesions of the brachial plexus: Treatment by transclavicular exploration and neurolysis or autograft reconstruction. J. Bone Joint Surg., *55A*:1159-1176, 1973.
487. McKenzie, A. D., and Sinclair, A. M.: Axillary artery occlusion complicating shoulder dislocation. Amer. Surg., *148*: 139-141, 1958.
488. Milton, G. W.: The circumflex nerve and dislocation of the shoulder. Brit. J. Phys. Med., *17*:136-138, 1954.
489. ———: The mechanism of circumflex and other nerve injuries in dislocation of the shoulder and the possible mechanism of nerve injuries during reduction of dislocation. Austral. New Zealand J. Surg., *23*:24-30, 1953-55.
490. Mumenthaler, M., and Schliack, H.: Lasionen Peripherer Nerven. Stuttgart, Georg Thieme Verlag, 1965.
491. Pollock, L. J.: Accessory muscle movements in deltoid paralysis. J.A.M.A., *79*: 526-528, 1922.
492. Ray, B. S.: Injuries to the nerves about the shoulder. (Reconstruction of the shoulder joint symp.), Instructional Course Lecture, *2*:371-376, 1944.
493. Rob, C. G., and Standeven, A.: Closed traumatic lesions of the axillary and brachial arteries. Lancet, *1*:597-599, 1956.
494. St. John, F. B., Scudder, J., and Stevens, D. L.: Spontaneous rupture of axillary artery. Ann. Surg., *121*:882-890, 1945.
495. Seddon, H. J.: Nerve lesions complicating certain closed bone injuries. J.A.M.A., *135*:691-694, 1947.
496. ———: Peripheral nerve injuries. Nerve Injuries Committee of Medical Research Council. Special Report ser. 282. London, Her Majesty's Stationery Office, 1954.
497. Steenburg, R. W., and Ravitch, M. M.: Cervicothoracic approach for subclavian vessel injury from compound fracture of the clavicle: considerations of subclavian-axillary exposures. Ann. Surg., *157*:839-846, 1963.
498. Stener, B.: Dislocation of the shoulder complicated by complete rupture of the axillary artery. J. Bone Joint Surg., *39B*: 714-717, 1957.
499. Stevens, J. H.: Brachial Plexus Paralysis. *In* Codman, E. A.: The Shoulder, Brooklyn, New York, G. Miller & Co., 1934.
500. Van der Spek: Rupture of the axillary ar-

tery as a complication of dislocation of the shoulder. Arch. Chir. Neerl., *16*:113-118, 1964.
501. Watson-Jones, R.: Fractures and Joint Injuries, ed. 4. vol. 2. Edinburgh, E. & S. Livingstone, 1960.
502. White, J. C., and Hawelin, J.: Myelographic sign of brachial plexus avulsion. J. Bone Joint Surg., *36A*:113-118, 1954.

Posterior Dislocation of the Shoulder

503. Abbott, L. C., Saunders, J. B., Hagey, H., and Jones, E. W.: Surgical approaches to the shoulder joint. J. Bone Joint Surg., *31A*:235-255, 1949.
504. Adams, J. C.: Recurrent dislocation of the shoulder. J. Bone Joint Surg., *30B*:26-38, 1948.
505. Andrze, J. R., Lipski, W., and Maliszewski, A.: Unusual case of shoulder dislocation. Chir. Narz. Ruchu Orthop. Pol., *38*: 545-548, 1973.
506. Arden, G. P.: Posterior dislocation of both shoulders, report of a case. J. Bone Joint Surg., *38B*:558-563, 1956.
507. Arndt, J. H., and Sears, A. D.: Posterior dislocation of the shoulder. Amer. J. Roentgenol., *94*:639-645, 1965.
508. Asplund, G.: Ein operierter Fall von willkurlicher Hinterer Schultergel-enkluxation. Acta Chir. Scand., *87*:103-112, 1942.
509. Bankart, A. S. B.: The pathology and treatment of recurrent dislocation of the shoulder joint. Brit. J. Surg., *26*:23-29, 1938.
510. Bell, H. M.: Posterior fracture dislocation of the shoulder. A method of closed reduction—a case report. J. Bone Joint Surg., *47A*:1521-1524, 1965.
511. Bennett, G. E.: Shoulder and elbow lesions of the professional baseball pitcher. J.A.M.A., *117*:510-514, 1941.
512. Bermann, M. M.: Dislocation of shoulder: x-ray signs. [Letter to the editor.] New Eng. J. Med., *283*:600, 1970.
513. Bibley, D. L.: Posterior dislocation of the shoulder joint. Brit. Med. J., *1*:1345-1346, 1957.
514. Blackett, C. W., and Healy, T. R.: Roentgen studies of the shoulder. Amer., J. Roentgenol., *37*:760-766, 1937.
515. Bloom, M. H., and Obata, W. G.: Diagnosis of posterior dislocation of the shoulder with use of Velpeau axillary and angle-up roentgenographic views. J. Bone Joint Surg., *49A*:943-949, 1967.
516. Blumensaat, C.: Die Lageabweichungen und Verrenkungen der Kniescheibe. Ergebn. Chir. Orth., *31*:149-223, 1938.
517. Bohler, L.: Treatment of Fractures. ed. 4. Bristol, John Wright & Sons, 1935.
518. Bost, F. C., and Inman, V. T.: The pathological changes in recurrent dislocation of the shoulder. A report on Bankart's operative procedure. J. Bone Joint Surg., *24*: 595-613, 1942.
519. Boyd, H. B.: Recurrent posterior dislocation of the shoulder. J. Bone Joint Surg., *54B*:379, 1972.
520. Boyd, H. B., and Hunt, H. L.: Recurrent dislocation of the shoulder. The staple capsulorrhaphy. J. Bone Joint Surg., *47A*: 1514-1520, 1965.
521. Boyd, H. B., and Sisk, T. D.: Recurrent posterior dislocation of the shoulder. J. Bone Joint Surg., *54A*:779-786, 1972.
522. Brown, W. H., Dennis, J. M., Davidson, C. N., Rubin, P. S., and Fulton H.: Posterior dislocation of shoulder. Radiology, *69*:815-822, 1957.
523. Budd, F. W.: Voluntary bilateral posterior dislocation of the shoulder joint. Clin. Orthop., *63*:181, 1969.
524. Cameron, B. M.: Recurrent posterior dislocation of the shoulder. Texas J. Med., *51*:33-35, 1955.
525. Carter, C., and Sweetman, R.: Recurrent dislocation of the patella and of the shoulder. Their association with familial joint laxity. J. Bone Joint Surg., *42B*:721-727, 1960.
526. Cave, E. F.: Fractures and Other Injuries. Chicago, Year Book Publishers, 1961.
527. Chattopadhyaya, P. K.: Posterior fracture-dislocation of the shoulder. J. Bone Joint Surg., *52B*:521-527, 1970.
528. Codman, E. A.: The Shoulder. Boston, Thomas Todd & Co., 1934.
529. Cohen, H. H.: Acute posterior bilateral dislocation of the shoulder. Bull. Hosp. Joint Dis., *26*:175-180, 1965.
530. Cooper, A.: A treatise on dislocations and fractures of the joints. [2nd Amer. ed. from the 6th London Ed.] Boston, Lilly & Wait & Carter & Hendee, 1832.
531. ———: On the dislocation of the os humeri upon the dorsum scapula, and upon fractures near the shoulder joint. Guy's Hosp. Rep., *4*:265-284, 1839.
532. ———: A treatise on dislocations and fractures of the joints. B. B. Cooper, Editor, London, John Churchill, p. 391, 1842.
533. ———: A Treatise on Dislocations and Fractures of the Joints. New Edition, Edited by B. B. Cooper, Philadelphia, Lea, and Blanchard, p. 341, 1844.

534. Coover, C.: Double posterior luxation of the shoulder. Penn. Med. J., *35*:566-567, 1932.
535. DePalma, A. F.: The Management of Fractures and Dislocations. ed. 2. Philadelphia, J. B. Lippincott, 1973.
536. Detenbeck, L. C.: Posterior dislocations of the shoulder. J. Trauma, *12*:183-192, 1972.
537. Dimon, J. H., III: Posterior dislocations and posterior fracture-dislocation of the shoulder. A report of 25 cases. South. Med. J., *60*:661-666, 1967.
538. ———: Posterior dislocation and posterior fracture-dislocation of the shoulder. Clin. Orthop., *58*:297, 1968.
539. ———: Posterior dislocations and posterior fracture-dislocations of the shoulder. Clin. Orthop., *65*:262, 1969.
540. Dorgan, J. A.: Posterior dislocation of the shoulder. Amer. J. Surg., *89*:890-900, 1955.
541. Eden, R.: Zur Operation der habituellen Schulterluxation. Dtsch. Ztschr. Chir., *144*:269-280, 1918.
542. Ellerbroek, N.: Beobachtungen uber Schulterluxationen nach hinten nebst einer Ubersicht uber alle vom 1. Januar 1890 bis 1. januar 1907 in der Gottinger chirurigschen Poliklinik beobachteten Luxationen. Dtsch. Ztschr. Chir., *92*:453, 1908.
543. English, E., and Macnab, I.: Recurrent posterior dislocation of the shoulder. Can. J. Surg., *17*:147-151, 1974.
544. Eyre-Brook, A. L.: Recurrent dislocation of the shoulder. Lesions discovered in 17 cases, surgery employed, and intermediate report on results. J. Bone Joint Surg., *30B*:39-46, 1948.
545. ———: Posterior dislocation of the shoulder. J. Bone Joint Surg., *54B*:760, 1972.
546. ———: Posterior dislocation of the shoulder. South African Med. J., *47*:2139, 1973.
547. Fairbank, H. A. T.: Birth palsy: subluxation of the shoulder joint in infants and young children. Lancet, *1*:1217-1223, 1913.
548. Figiel, S. J., Figiel, L. S., Bardenstein, M. B., and Blodgett, W. H.: Posterior dislocation of the shoulder. Radiology, *87*: 737-740, 1966.
549. Fipp, G. J.: Simultaneous posterior dislocation of both shoulders. Clin. Orthop., *44*:191-195, 1966.
550. Fried, A.: Habitual posterior dislocation of the shoulder joint. A report of 5 operated cases. Acta Orthop. Scand., *18*:329-345, 1949.
551. Giannestras, N. J.: Discussion of traumatic posterior (retroglenoid) dislocation of the humerus. *In* J. C. Wilson, and F. M. McKeever. J. Bone and Joint Surg., *31A*: 172, 1949.
552. Gilula, L. A.: Roentgen rounds #1. Orthop. Rev., *2*:53-55, 1973.
553. Goodfellow, J. W., and Boldero, J. L.: Bilateral synchronous posterior dislocation of the shoulder. Brit. J. Surg., *46*:413-415, 1959.
554. Greenhill, B. J.: Persistent posterior shoulder dislocation: its diagnosis and treatment by Putti-Platt repair. J. Bone Joint Surg., *54B*:763, 1972.
555. Gregorie, R.: Luxation recidivante de l'epaule. Anatomie pathologique et pathogenie. Rev. Orthop., *24*:15-36, 1913.
556. Harmon, P. H.: The posterior approach for arthrodesis and other operations on the shoulder. Surg. Gynecol. Obstet., *81*:266-268, 1945.
557. Henderson, M. S.: Habitual or recurrent dislocation of the shoulder. Surg. Gynecol. Obstet., *33*:1-7, 1921.
558. Henry, A. K.: Exposure of long bones and other surgical methods. New York, William Wood and Company, 1927.
559. Hill, H. A., and Sachs, M. D.: The grooved defect of the humeral head. A frequently unrecognized complication of dislocations of the shoulder joint. Radiology, *35*:690-700, 1940.
560. Hill, N. A., and McLaughlin, H. L.: Locked posterior dislocation simulating a "frozen shoulder". J. Trauma, *3*:225-234, 1963.
561. Hindenach, J. C. R.: Recurrent posterior dislocation of the shoulder. J. Bone Joint Surg., *29*:582-586, 1947.
562. Honner, R.: Bilateral posterior dislocation of the shoulders. Austral. New Zealand J. Surg., *38*:269-272, 1969.
563. Hoyt, W. A., Jr.: Etiology of shoulder injuries in athletes. J. Bone Joint Surg., *49A*:755-766, 1967.
564. Hybbinette, S.: De la transplantation d'un fragment osseux pour remedier aux luxations recidivantes de l'epaule. Acta Chir. Scand., *71*:411-443, 1932.
565. ———: Traite Des Fractures et des luxations. J. B. Bailliere, 2, 433-434, Paris, 1855.
566. Inman, V. T., Saunder, J. B., and Abbott, L. C.: Observations on the function of the shoulder joint. J. Bone Joint Surg., *26*: 1-30, 1944.

567. Jacobs, B. W., Patterson, R. L., and Schultz, T. J.: Shoulder dislocations associated with seizure disorders. J. Bone Joint Surg., *52A*:824, 1970.
568. Jones, R.: Injuries to Joints. London, Oxford University Press, 1926.
569. Jones, V.: Recurrent posterior dislocation of the shoulder. J. Bone Joint Surg., *40B*: 203-207, 1958.
570. Jordan, H.: New technique for the roentgen examination of the shoulder joint. Radiology, *25*:480-484, 1935.
571. Key, J. A., and Conwell, H. E.: The Management of Fractures, Dislocations and Sprains. ed. 5. St. Louis, C. V. Mosby, 1951.
572. King, T.: Recurrent dislocation of the shoulder. Med. J. Austral., *1*:697-700, 1947.
573. Kretzler, H. H.: Paper presented to the American Academy of Orthopaedic Surgeons Meeting, January, 1974.
574. Kretzler, H. H., and Blue, A. R.: Recurrent posterior dislocation of the shoulder in cerebral palsy. J. Bone Joint Surg., *48A*: 1221, 1966.
575. Langford, O., and Rockwood, C. A.: Posterior dislocations of the shoulder. Exhibit at American Academy of Orthopaedic Surgeons, New York, 1965.
576. l'Episcopo, J. B.: Restoration of muscle balance in the treatment of obstetrical paralysis. New York J. Med., *39*:357-363, 1939.
577. Lindholm, T. S.: Recurrent posterior dislocation of the shoulder. Acta Chir. Scand., *140*:101-106, 1974.
578. McLaughlin, H. L.: Discussion of acute anterior dislocation of the shoulder. Nicola, T.: J. Bone Joint Surg., *31A*:172, 1949.
579. ———: Posterior dislocation of the shoulder. J. Bone Joint Surg., *34A*:584-590, 1952.
580. ———: Posterior dislocation of the shoulder. J. Bone Joint Surg., *44A*:1477, 1962.
581. ———: Locked posterior subluxation of the shoulder—diagnosis and treatment. Surg. Clin. N. Amer., *43*:1621-1622, 1963.
582. McLaughlin, H. L., and Cavallaro, W. U.: Primary anterior dislocation of the shoulder. Amer. J. Surg., *80*:615-621, 1950.
583. Malgaigne, J. F.: Traite des fractures et des luxations. Paris, J. B. Bailliere, 1855.
584. Mauck, R. H., and Clements, E. L.: Bilateral posterior shoulder dislocation. An orthopaedic case. Va. Med. Mth., *93*:452-454, 1966.
585. May, H.: The regeneration of joint transplants and intracapsular fragments. Ann. Surg., *116*:297-310, 1942.
586. ———: Nicola operation for posterior subacromial dislocation of the humerus. J. Bone Joint Surg., *25*:78-84, 1943.
587. Messner, D. G.: Posterior dislocation of the shoulder: with or without associated fractures. J. Bone Joint Surg., *48A*:1220-1221, 1966.
588. Michaelis, L. S.: Internal rotation of the shoulder. Report of a case. J. Bone Joint Surg., *32B*:223-224, 1950.
589. Miller, E. R., and Lusted, L. B.: Progress in indirect cineroentgenography. Amer. J. Roentgenol., *75*:56-62, 1956.
590. Mollerud, A.: A case of bilateral habitual luxation in the posterior part of the shoulder joint. Acta Chir. Scand., *94*:181-186, 1946.
591. Moore, B. H.: A new operative procedure for brachial birth palsy (Erb's paralysis). Surg. Gynecol. Obstet., *61*:832-835, 1935.
592. Moseley, H. F.: Athletic injuries to the shoulder region. Amer. J. Surg., *98*:401-422, 1959.
593. Moullin, C. W. M., and Keith, A.: Notes on a case. Backward dislocation of the head of the humerus caused by muscular action. Lancet, *1*:496, 1904.
594. Mynter, H.: Subacromial dislocation from muscular spasm. Ann. Surg., *36*:117-119, 1902.
595. Neer, C. S., II: Fractures of the distal third of the clavicle. Clin. Orthop., *58*:43-50, 1968.
596. Neviaser, J. S.: Posterior dislocations of the shoulder: diagnosis and treatment. Surg. Clin. N. Amer., *43*:1623-1630, 1963.
597. ———: The treatment of old unreduced dislocations of the shoulder. Surg. Clin. N. Amer., *43*:1671-1678, 1963.
598. Nicola, T.: Recurrent dislocation of the shoulder. Amer. J. Surg., *86*:85-91, 1953.
599. Nobel, W.: Posterior traumatic dislocation of the shoulder. J. Bone Joint Surg., *44A*:523-538, 1962.
600. O'Conner, S. J., and Jacknow, A. S.: Posterior dislocation of the shoulder. J. Bone Joint Surg., *37A*:1122, 1955.
601. ———: Posterior dislocation of the shoulder. Arch. Surg., *72*:479-491, 1956.
602. Palmer, I., and Widen, A.: The bone block method for recurrent dislocation of the shoulder joint. J. Bone Joint Surg., *30B*:53-58, 1948.
603. Pear, B. L.: Dislocation of the shoulder. X-ray signs. [Correspondence] New Eng. J. Med., *283*:1113, 1970.

604. Percy, L. R.: Recurrent posterior dislocation of the shoulder. J. Bone Joint Surg., *42B*:863, 1960.
605. Perkins, G.: Rest and movement. J. Bone Joint Surg., *35B*:521-539, 1953.
606. Preston, M. F.: Fractures and Dislocations, Diagnosis and Treatment. St. Louis, C. V. Mosby, 1915.
607. Prillaman, H. A., and Thompson, R. C.: Bilateral posterior fracture dislocation of the shoulder. A case report. J. Bone Joint Surg., *51A*:1627-1630, 1969.
608. Reeves, B.: Recurrent posterior dislocation of the shoulder. Proc. Roy. Soc. Med., *56*:897-898, 1963.
609. Rendich, R. A., and Poppel, M. H.: Roentgen diagnosis of posterior dislocation of the shoulder. Radiology, *36*:42-45, 1941.
610. Robert, A., and Wickstrom, J.: Prognosis of posterior dislocation of the shoulder. Acta Orthop. Scandinav., *42*:328-337, 1971.
611. Rockwood, C. A., Jr.: The diagnosis of acute posterior dislocation of the shoulder. J. Bone Joint Surg., *48A*:1220, 1966.
612. Rowe, C. R.: Prognosis in dislocation of the shoulder. J. Bone Joint Surg., *38A*: 957-977, 1956.
613. Rowe, C. R., and Ye, L. K.: A posterior approach to the shoulder joint. J. Bone Joint Surg., *26*:580-584, 1944.
614. Rowe, C. R., Pierce, D. S., and Clark, J. G.: Voluntary dislocation of the shoulder. A preliminary report on a clinical, electromyographic, and psychiatric study of 26 patients. J. Bone Joint Surg., *55*:445-460, 1973.
615. Rubin, S. A., Gray, R. L., and Green, W. R.: Scapular Y-diagnostic aid in shoulder trauma. Radiology, *110*:725-726, 1974.
616. Samilson, R. L., and Miller, E.: Posterior dislocations of the shoulder. Clin. Orthop., *32*:69-86, 1964.
617. Scaglietti, O.: The obstetrical shoulder trauma. Surg. Gynecol. Obstet., *66*:868-877, 1938.
618. Scott, D. J., Jr.: Treatment of recurrent posterior dislocation of the shoulder by glenoplasty. Report of 3 cases. J. Bone Joint Surg., *49A*:471-476, 1967.
619. Scougall, S.: Posterior dislocation of the shoulder. J. Bone Joint Surg., *37B*:355, 1955.
620. ———: Posterior dislocation of the shoulder. J. Bone Joint Surg., *39B*:726-732, 1957.
621. Sever, J. W.: Obstetrical paralysis. Surg. Gynecol. Obstet., *44*:547-549, 1927.
622. Shaw, J. T.: Bilateral posterior fracture-dislocation of the shoulder and other trauma caused by convulsive seizures. J. Bone Joint Surg., *53A*:1437-1440, 1971.
623. Shepherd, E.: Simultaneous posterior dislocation of both shoulders. J. Bone Joint Surg., *42B*:728-729, 1960.
624. Sillar, P.: Surgical treatment of habitual posterior dislocation of the shoulder joint. Magy Traumatol. Orthop., *15*:146-150, 1972.
625. Sjovall, H.: A case of spontaneous backward subluxation of the shoulder treated by the Clairmont-Ehrlich operation. Nord. Med. (Hygeia), *21*:474-476, 1944.
626. Speed, K.: A Textbook of Fractures and Dislocations. ed. 2. Philadelphia, Lea & Febiger, 1928.
627. Stimson, L. A.: Fractures and Dislocations. ed. 3. Philadelphia, Lea Brothers, 1900.
628. Taylor, R. G., and Wright, P. R.: Posterior dislocation of the shoulder. Report of six cases. J. Bone Joint Surg., *34B*:624-629, 1952.
629. Thomas, M. A.: Posterior subacromial dislocation of the head of the humerus. Amer. J. Roentgenol., *37*:767-773, 1937.
630. Thompson, J. E.: Anatomical methods of approach in operations on the long bones of the extremities. Ann. Surg., *68*:309-329, 1918.
631. Toumey, J. W.: Posterior recurrent dislocation of the shoulder treated by capsulorrhaphy and iliac bone block. Lahey Clin. Bull., *5*:197-201, 1946-1948.
632. Warrick, C. K.: Posterior dislocation of the shoulder joint. J. Bone Joint Surg., *30B*:651-655, 1948.
633. ———: Posterior dislocation of the shoulder joint. Brit. J. Radiol., *38*:758-761, 1965.
634. Watson-Jones, R.: Recurrent dislocation of the shoulder. J. Bone Joint Surg., *30B*: 6-8, 1948.
635. ———: Fractures and Other Joint Injuries. ed. 4. vol. 2. Baltimore, Williams & Wilkins, 1956.
636. Weber, B. G.: Operative treatment for recurrent dislocation of the shoulder. Injury, *1*:107-109, 1969.
637. Weissman, S. L., and Torok, G.: Bilateral recurrent posterior dislocation of the shoulder. Report of a case. J. Bone Joint Surg., *40A*:479-482, 1958.
638. Wickstrom, J.: Birth injuries of the brachial plexus; treatment of defects in the shoulder. Clin. Orthop., *23*:187-196, 1962.

639. Willard, D. P.: The Nicola operation for recurrent dislocation of the shoulder. Ann. Surg., *103*:438-443, 1936.
640. Wilson, J. C., and McKeever, F. M.: Traumatic posterior (retroglenoid) dislocation of the humerus. J. Bone Joint Surg., *31A*:160-172, 1949.
641. Wood, J. P.: Posterior dislocation of the head of the humerus and the diagnostic value of lateral and vertical views. U.S. Navy Med. Bull., *39*:532-535, 1941.
642. Zachary, R. B.: Transplantation of teres major and latissimus dorsi for loss of external rotation at the shoulder. Lancet, *2*:757-761, 1947.

Inferior Dislocation of the Glenohumeral Joint

643. Conwell, H., and Reynolds, F.: Key and Conwell's Management of Fractures, Dislocations and Sprains. ed. 7. St. Louis, C. V. Mosby, 1961.
644. Cozen, L.: Congenital dislocations of the shoulder and other abnormalities. Arch. Surg., *35*:956-966, 1935.
645. DePalma, A. F.: Surgery of the Shoulder. Philadelphia, J. B. Lippincott, 1973.
646. Falkner, E. A.: Luxatio erecta of the shoulder joint. Med. J. Austral., *1*:227-228, 1916.
647. Hermodsson, I.: Rontgenologische Studien uber die traumatischen und habituellen Schultergelenkverrenkungen nach unten. Translated by H. Moseley and B. Overgaard, Montreal, McGill University Press, 1963.
648. Laskin, R. S., and Sedlin, E. D.: Luxatio erecta in infancy. Clin. Orthop., *80*:126-129, 1971.
649. Lynn, F. S.: Erect dislocation of the shoulder. Surg. Gynecol. Obstet., *39*:51-55, 1921.
650. McLaughlin, H. L.: Trauma. Philadelphia, W. B. Saunders, 1959.
651. Middeldorpf, M., and Scharm, B.: De nova humeri luxationis specie. Clinique Europenne. Vol. II. Dissert Inag. Breslau, 1859.

Superior Dislocation of the Glenohumeral Joint

652. Speed, K.: Fractures and Dislocations. ed. 4. Philadelphia, Lea & Febiger, 1942.
653. Stimson, L. A.: A Practical Treatise on Fractures and Dislocations. ed. 7. Philadelphia, Lea & Febiger, 1912.

Acromioclavicular Dislocation

654. Abbott, L. C., Saunders, J. B., Hagey, H., and Jones, E. W.: Surgical approaches to the shoulder joint. J. Bone Joint Surg., *31A*:235-255, 1949.
655. Adams, F. L.: The Genuine Works of Hippocrates. vols. 1, 2. New York, William Wood, 1886.
656. Ahstrom, J. P., Jr.: Surgical repair of complete acromioclavicular separation. J.A.M.A., *217*:785-789, 1971.
657. Alexander, O. M.: Dislocation of the acromioclavicular joint. Radiography, *15*:260, 1949.
658. Alldredge, R. H.: Surgical treatment of acromioclavicular dislocations. J. Bone Joint Surg., *47A*:1278, 1965.
659. Allman, F. L., Jr.: Fractures and ligamentous injuries of the clavicle and its articulation. J. Bone Joint Surg., *49A*:774-784, 1967.
660. Anderson, M. E.: Treatment of dislocations of the acromioclavicular and sternoclavicular joints. J. Bone Joint Surg., *45A*:657-658, 1963.
661. Anderson, R., and Burgess, E.: Acromioclavicular dislocation — a conservative method of treatment. Northwest. Med., *38*:40, 1939.
662. Arner, O., Sandahl, U., and Ohrling, H.: Dislocation of the acromioclavicular joint —review of the literature and report of 56 cases. Acta Chir. Scand., *113*:140-152, 1957.
663. Aufranc, O. E., Jones, S. N., and Harris, W. H.: Complete acromioclavicular dislocation. J.A.M.A., *180*:681-682, 1962.
664. Badgley, C. E.: Sports injuries of the shoulder girdle. J.A.M.A., *172*:444-448, 1960.
665. Bailey, R. W.: A dynamic repair for complete acromioclavicular joint dislocation. J. Bone Joint Surg., *47A*:858, 1965.
666. Bailey, R. W., O'Connor, G. A., Tilus, P. D., and Baril, J. D.: A dynamic repair for acute and chronic injuries of the acromioclavicular area. J. Bone Joint Surg., *54A*:1802, 1972.
667. Baker, D. M., and Stryker, W. F.: Acute complete acromioclavicular separations. J.A.M.A., *192*:689-692, 1965.
668. Barnhart, J. M., Fain, R. H., Dewar, F. P., and Stein, A. H.: Acromioclavicular joint injuries. Clin. Orthop., *81*:199, 1970.
669. Barr, J. S.: Dislocations of the clavicle. *In* Wilson, P. D. (ed.): Experience in the Management of Fractures and Dislocations. Philadelphia, J. B. Lippincott, 1938.

670. Batchelor, J. S.: Splint for fractured clavicle and acromioclavicular dislocation. Lancet, *2*:690, 1947.
671. Bateman, J. E.: Athletic injuries about the shoulder in throwing and body-contact sports. Clin. Orthop., *23*:75-83, 1962.
672. ———: The Shoulder and Neck. Philadelphia, W. B. Saunders, 1972.
673. Bearden, J. M., Hughston, J. C., and Whatley, G. S.: Acromioclavicular dislocation: method of treatment. J. Sports Med., *1*:5-17, 1973.
674. Beckman, T.: A case of simultaneous luxation of both ends of the clavicle. Acta Chir. Scand., *56*:156-163, 1923.
675. Behling, F.: Treatment of acromioclavicular separations. Orthop. Clin. N. Amer., *4*:747-757, 1973.
676. Benson, R. A.: Acromioclavicular dislocation. U. S. Naval Med. Bull., *34*:341-342, 1936.
677. Bertwistle, A. P.: Acromioclavicular dislocation and sprain. Clin. J., *66*:76-77, 1937.
678. Birkett, A. N.: The result of operative repair of severe acromioclavicular dislocation. Brit. J. Surg., *32*:103-105, 1944-45.
679. Bloom, F. A.: Wire fixation in acromioclavicular dislocation. J. Bone Joint Surg., *27*:273-276, 1945.
680. Bohler, L.: Treatment of Fractures. ed. 4. Baltimore, William Wood, New York, 1935.
681. Bonnin, J. G.: Complete Outline of Fractures. London, William Heinemann, 1941.
682. Bosworth, B. M.: Acromioclavicular separation. New method of repair. Surg. Gynecol. Obstet., *73*:866-871, 1941.
683. ———: Calcium deposits in the shoulder and subacromial bursitis. Motion of acromioclavicular joint. J.A.M.A., *116*:2477-2482, 1941.
684. ———: Acromioclavicular dislocation: end results of screw suspension treatment. Ann. Surg., *127*:98-111, 1948.
685. ———: Complete acromioclavicular dislocation. New Eng. J. Med., *241*:221-225, 1949.
686. Bowers, R. F.: Complete acromioclavicular separation. Diagnosis and operative treatment. J. Bone Joint Surg., *17*:1005-1010, 1935.
687. Brandt, G.: Die behandlung der verrenkung im acromiolen Schlusselbeingelenk. Klin. Med., *51*:526-528, 1956.
688. Brosgol, M.: Traumatic acromioclavicular sprains and subluxations. Clin. Orthop., *20*:98-107, 1961.
689. Bundens, W. D., and Cook, J. I.: Repair of acromioclavicular separations by deltoid-trapezius imbrication. Clin. Orthop., *20*:109-114, 1961.
690. Bunnell, S.: Fascial graft for dislocation of the acromioclavicular joint. Surg. Gynecol. Obstet., *46*:563-564, 1928.
691. Cadenat, F. M.: The treatment of dislocations and fractures of the outer end of the clavicle. Internat. Clin., *1*:145-169, 1917.
692. Caldwell, G. D.: Treatment of Fractures. New York, Paul Hoeber, 1943.
693. ———: Treatment of complete permanent acromioclavicular dislocation by surgical arthrodesis. J. Bone Joint Surg., *25*:368-374, 1943.
694. Campbell, W. C.: Operative Orthopaedics. St. Louis, C. V. Mosby, 1971.
695. Campos, O. P.: Acromioclavicular dislocation. Amer., J. Surg., *43*:287-291, 1939.
696. Carrell, W. B.: Dislocation at the outer end of clavicle. J. Bone Joint Surg., *10*:314-315, 1928.
697. Codman, E. A.: The Shoulder. ed. 1. Boston, Thomas Todd & Co., 1934.
698. Colson, J. H. C., and Armour, W. J.: Sports Injuries and Their Treatment. Philadelphia, J. B. Lippincott, 1961.
699. Cooper, A.: A Treatise on Dislocations and Fractures of the Joints. 2nd American ed. from 6th London ed. Boston, Lilly & Wait and Carter & Hendee, 1832.
700. Cooper, E. S.: New method of treating long-standing dislocations of the scapuloclavicular articulation. Amer. J. Med. Sci., *41*:389-392, 1861.
701. Copher, G. H.: A method of treatment of upward dislocation of the acromial end of the clavicle. Amer. J. Surg., *22*:507-508, 1933.
702. Currie, D. I.: An apparatus for dislocation of the acromial end of the clavicle. Brit. Med. J., *1*:570, 1924.
703. DePalma, A. F.: The role of the disks of the sternoclavicular and acromioclavicular joints. Clin. Orthop., *13*:7-12, 1959.
704. ———: Surgical anatomy of the acromioclavicular and sternoclavicular joints. Surg. Clin. N. Amer., *43*:1540-1550, 1963.
705. ———: Surgery of the Shoulder. ed. 2. Philadelphia, J. B. Lippincott, 1973.
706. DePalma, A. F., Callery, G., and Bennett, G. A.: Variational anatomy and degenerative lesions of the shoulder joint. American Academy of Orthopaedic Surgeons Instructional Course Lectures, *6*:255-281, 1949.
707. Dewar, F. P., and Barrington, T. W.: The

treatment of chronic acromioclavicular dislocation. J. Bone Joint Surg., *47B*:32-35, 1965.

708. Dillehunt, R. B.: Luxation of the acromioclavicular joint. Surg. Clin. N. Amer., *7*: 1307-1313, 1927.
709. Dohn, K.: Luxatio acromioclavicularis supraspinata. Acta Orthop. Scand., *25*:183-189, 1956.
710. Dunlop, J.: Dislocations of the outer end of the clavicle. Calif. West. Med., *26*:38-40, 1927.
711. Eikenbary, C. F., and LeCocq, J. F.: The operative treatment of acromioclavicular dislocations. Surg. Clin. N. Amer., *13*: 1305-1314, 1933.
712. Elkin, D. C., and Cooper, F. W., Jr.: Resection of the clavicle in vascular surgery. J. Bone Joint Surg., *28*:117-119, 1946.
713. Ferguson, A. B., Jr., and Bender, J.: The ABC's of Athletic Injuries and Conditioning. Baltimore, Williams & Wilkins, 1964.
714. Fulton, W. A.: A treatment for greenstick fractures and for dislocations of the clavicle. Lancet, *43*:383-385, 1923.
715. Gallie, W. E.: Dislocations. New Eng. J. Med., *213*:91-98, 1935.
716. Gardner, E., and Gray, D. J.: Prenatal development of the human shoulder and acromioclavicular joints. Amer. J. Anat., *92*:219-276, 1953.
717. Gatewood, L. C.: Dislocation of the outer end of the clavicle. Surg. Clin. N. Amer., *3*:1193-1197, 1919.
718. Giannestras, N. J.: A method of immobilization of acute acromioclavicular separation. J. Bone Joint Surg., *26*:597-599, 1944.
719. Gibbens, M. E.: An appliance for the conservative treatment of acromioclavicular dislocation. J. Bone Joint Surg., *28*:164-165, 1946.
720. Girard, P. M.: Acute acromioclavicular dislocation. Bull. U.S. Army Med. Dept., *82*:5, 1944.
721. Glick, J.: Acromioclavicular dislocation in athletes. Orthop. Rev., *1*:31-34, 1972.
722. Goldberg, D.: Acromioclavicular joint injuries: modified conservative form of treatment. Amer. J. Surg., *71*:529-531, 1946.
723. Gradoyevitch, B.: Coracoclavicular joint. J. Bone Joint Surg., *21*:918-920, 1939.
724. Gurd, F. B.: The treatment of complete dislocation of the outer end of the clavicle. An hitherto undescribed operation. Ann. Surg., *113*:1094-1098, 1941.
725. Haggart, G. E.: The treatment of acromioclavicular joint dislocation. Surg. Clin. N. Amer., *13*:683-688, 1933.
726. Hamill, R. C.: Acromioclavicular dislocation. Internat. Clin., *3*:130-132, 1920.
727. Hart, V. L.: Treatment of acute acromioclavicular dislocation. J. Bone Joint Surg., *23*:175-176, 1941.
728. Henry, M. D.: Acromioclavicular dislocations. Minnesota Med., *12*:431-433, 1929.
729. Holestein, A., Lewis, G. B., and Sturtz, H.: Experience in the treatment of acromioclavicular dislocation. J. Bone Joint Surg., *48A*:1224, 1966.
730. Horn, J. S.: The traumatic anatomy and treatment of acute acromioclavicular dislocation. J. Bone Joint Surg., *36*:194-201, 1954.
731. Howard, N. J.: Acromioclavicular and sternoclavicular joint injuries. Amer. J. Surg., *46*:284-291, 1939.
732. Hoyt, W. A., Jr.: Etiology of shoulder injuries in athletes. J. Bone Joint Surg., *49A*: 755-766, 1967.
733. Inman, V. T., Saunders, J. B., and Abbott, L. C.: Observations on the function of the shoulder joint. J. Bone Joint Surg., *26*: 1-30, 1944.
734. Inman, V. T., McLaughlin, H. D., Neviaser, J., and Rowe, C.: Treatment of Complete Acromioclavicular Dislocation. J. Bone Joint Surg., *44A*:1008-1011, 1962.
735. Jacobs, B., and Wade, P. A.: Acromioclavicular joint injury. End result study. J. Bone Joint Surg., *48A*:475-486, 1966.
736. Jay, G. R., and Monnet, J. C.: The Bosworth screw in acute dislocations of the acromioclavicular joint. Presented at Clinical Conference, University of Oklahoma Medical Center, April, 1969.
737. Johnston, T. B., Davies, D. V., and Davies, F. (eds.): Gray's Anatomy. ed. 32. London, Longmans, Green, and Co., 1958.
738. Kennedy, J. C.: Complete dislocation of the acromioclavicular joint. J. Trauma, *8*:311-318, 1968.
739. Kennedy, J. C., and Cameron, H.: Complete dislocation of the acromioclavicular joint. J. Bone Joint Surg., *36B*:202-208, 1954.
740. Key, J. A., and Conwell, H. E.: The Management of Fractures, Dislocations, and Sprains. ed. 3. St. Louis, C. V. Mosby, 1942.
741. Laing, P. G.: Transplantation of the long head of the biceps in complete acromioclavicular separations. J. Bone Joint Surg., *51A*:1677-1678, 1969.
742. Lazcano, M. A., Anzel, S. H., and Kelly, P. J.: Complete dislocation and subluxation of the acromioclavicular joint. End

results in 73 cases. J. Bone Joint Surg., *43A*:379-391, 1961.
743. Liberson, F.: The role of the coracoclavicular ligaments in affections of the shoulder girdle. Amer. J. Surg., *44*:145-157, 1939.
744. Litton, L. O., and Peltier, L. R.: Athletic Injuries. Boston, Little, Brown, 1963.
745. Lucas, D. B.: Biomechanics of the shoulder joint. Arch. Surg., *107*:425-432, 1973.
746. McCurrich, H. J.: Calcification of the bursa of the coracoclavicular ligament. Brit. J. Surg., *26*:329-332, 1938.
747. Macey, H. B.: Separation of acromioclavicular joint. Report of a case. Proc. Staff Meeting, Mayo Clin., *11*:683-684, 1936.
748. McLaughlin, H. L.: On the "frozen" shoulder. Bull. Hosp. Joint Dis., *12*:383-393, 1951.
749. ———: Trauma. Philadelphia, W. B. Saunders, 1959.
750. ———: Rupture of the rotator cuff. J. Bone Joint Surg., *44A*:979-983, 1962.
751. McLaughlin, H. L., and Cavallaro, W. U.: Primary anterior dislocation of the shoulder. Amer. J. Surg., *80*:615-621, 1950.
752. McMurray, T. P.: A Practice of Orthopaedic Surgery. Baltimore, William Wood, 1937.
753. McNealy, R. W.: Dislocations and fracture-dislocations occurring at the acromioclavicular articulation. Illinois Med. J., *41*:202-205, 1922.
754. Madsen, B.: Osteolysis of the acromial end of the clavicle following trauma. Brit. J. Radiol., *36*:822, 1963.
755. Mazet, R. J.: Migration of a Kirschner wire from the shoulder region into the lung. Report of two cases. J. Bone Joint Surg., *25A*:477-483, 1943.
756. Meyerding, H. W.: The treatment of acromioclavicular dislocations. Surg. Clin. N. Amer., *17*:1199-1205, 1937.
757. Michele, A. A.: New Treatment of Acromioclavicular Dislocation. Clin. Orthop., *63*:245, 1969.
758. Millbourn, E.: On injuries to the acromioclavicular joint. Treatment and results. Acta Orthop. Scand., *19*:349-382, 1950.
759. Mitchell, A. B.: Dislocation of outer end of clavicle. Brit. Med. J., *2*:1097, 1926.
760. Moffat, B. M.: Separation of the acromioclavicular joint. Surg. Gynecol. Obstet., *41*:73-74, 1925.
761. Morisi, M., and Ferrabosch, P.: Treatment of acromioclavicular dislocation with percutaneous synthesis of the axis. Arch. Orthop., *68*:1148-1156, 1955.
762. Morrison, G. M.: Cast of acromioclavicular dislocation. J. Bone Joint Surg., *39A*:238-239, 1948.
763. Moseley, H. F.: Shoulder Lesions. ed. 2. New York, Paul Hoeber, 1953.
764. ———: Athletic injuries to the shoulder region. Amer. J. Surg., *98*:401-422, 1959.
765. Moseley, H. F., and Templeton, J.: Dislocation of acromioclavicular joint. J. Bone Joint Surg., *51B*:196, 1969.
766. Moshein, J., and Elconin, K. B.: Repair of acute acromioclavicular dislocation, utilizing the coracoacromial ligament. J. Bone Joint Surg., *51A*:812, 1969.
767. Mumford, E. B.: Acromioclavicular dislocation. J. Bone Joint Surg., *23*:799-802, 1941.
768. Murray, G.: Fixation of dislocations of the acromioclavicular joint and rupture of the coracoclavicular ligament. Can. Med. Ass. J., *43*:270-273, 1940.
769. ———: The use of longitudinal wires in the treatment of fractures and dislocations. Amer. J. Surg., *67*:156-167, 1945.
770. Neviaser, J. S.: Acromioclavicular dislocation treated by transference of the coracoacromial ligament. Bull. Hosp. Joint Dis., *12*:46-54, 1951.
771. ———: Acromioclavicular dislocation treated by transference of the coracoacromial ligament. Arch. Surg., *64*:292-297, 1952.
772. ———: Complicated fractures and dislocations about the shoulder joint. J. Bone Joint Surg., *44A*:984-998, 1962.
773. ———: Acromioclavicular dislocation treated by transference of the coracoacromial ligament. Clin. Orthop., *58*:57-68, 1968.
774. Nicol, E. E.: Miners and mannequins. J. Bone Joint. Surg., *36B*:171-172, 1954.
775. Nielsen, W. B.: Injury to the acromioclavicular joint. J. Bone Joint Surg., *45B*:207, 1963.
776. Norrell, H., and Llewellyn, R. C.: Migration of a threaded Steinmann pin from an acromioclavicular joint into the spinal canal. A case report. J. Bone Joint Surg., *47A*:1024-1026, 1965.
777. Nutter, P. D.: Coracoclavicular articulations. J. Bone Joint Surg., *23*:177-179, 1941.
778. Odelberg, A.: Operative method for dislocation of the acromioclavicular joint. Acta Chir. Scand., *98*:507-510, 1949.
779. O'Donoghue, D. H.: Treatment of injuries to athletes. Philadelphia, W. B. Saunders, 1970.
780. ———: Treatment of injuries to athletes. ed. 2. W. B. Saunders, 1970.

781. Olsson, D.: Degenerative changes of the shoulder joint and their connection with shoulder pain. Acta Chir. Scand. [Suppl.]: *181*:1-130, 1953.
782. Orofinio, C. S., and Stein, A. H., Jr.: Operative treatment for recent and complete tears of the acromioclavicular ligaments. Amer. J. Surg., *85*:760-763, 1953.
783. Patterson, W. R.: Inferior dislocation of the distal end of the clavicle. J. Bone Joint Surg., *49A*:1184-1186, 1967.
784. Pearson, G. R.: Radiographic technic for acromioclavicular dislocation. Radiology, *27*:239, 1936.
785. Phemister, D. B.: The treatment of dislocation of the acromioclavicular joint by open reduction and threaded-wire fixation. J. Bone Joint Surg., *24*:166-168, 1942.
786. Pilcher: Dislocation of the acromial end of the clavicle. New York Med. J., *43*: 419-420, 1886.
787. Pillay, V. K.: Significance of the coracoclavicular joint. J. Bone Joint Surg., *49B*: 390, 1967.
788. Poirier, P., and Rieffel, H.: Mechanisme des luxations sur acromiales de la clavicule. Arch. Gen. Med., *1*:396-422, 1891.
789. Powers, J. A., and Bach, P. J.: Acromioclavicular separations—closed or open treatment. Clin. Orthop., *104*:213-223, 1974.
790. Pridie, K.: Dislocation of acromioclavicular and sternoclavicular joints. J. Bone Joint Surg., *41B*:429, 1959.
791. Quesada, F.: Technique for the roentgen diagnosis of fractures of the clavicle. Surg. Gynecol. Obstet., *42*:424-428, 1926.
792. Quigley, T. B.: [Correspondence.] New Eng. J. Med., *241*:431, 1949.
793. ———: Injuries to the acromioclavicular and sternoclavicular joints sustained in athletics. Surg. Clin. N. Amer., *43*:1551-1554, 1963.
794. Quigley, T. B., and Banks, H.: Progress in the Treatment of Fractures and Dislocations. Philadelphia, W. B. Saunders, 1960.
795. Rawlings, G.: Acromioclavicular dislocations and fractures of the clavicle. A simple method of support. Lancet, *2*:789, 1939.
796. Riddel, J.: Dislocation of the acromioclavicular joint. Brit. Med. J., *1*:697, 1926.
797. Roberts, S. M.: Acromioclavicular dislocation. Anatomical exposure of the outer end of the clavicle and the coracoid process. Amer. J. Surg., *23*:322-324, 1934.
798. Rowe, C. R.: Symposium on surgical lesions of the shoulder. Acute and recurrent dislocation of the shoulder. J. Bone Joint Surg., *44A*:977-1012, 1962.
799. Rowe, M. J.: Nylon bone suture. Surgery, *18*:764-768, 1945.
800. Ryan, A. J.: Medical Care of the Athlete. New York, McGraw-Hill, 1962.
801. Sage, F. P., and Salvatore, J. E.: Injuries of acromioclavicular joint. Study of results in 96 patients. South. Med. J., *56*: 486-495, 1963.
802. Schneider, C. C.: Acromioclavicular dislocation. Autoplastic reconstruction. J. Bone Joint Surg., *15*:957-962, 1933.
803. Scott, J. C., and Orr, M. M.: Injuries to the acromioclavicular joint. Injury, *5*:13-18, 1973.
804. Shaar, C. M.: Upward dislocation of acromial end of clavicle. Treatment by elastic traction splint. J.A.M.A., *92*:2083-2085, 1929.
805. Shands, A. R., Jr.: Handbook of Orthopaedic Surgery. ed. 2. St. Louis, C. V. Mosby, 1940.
806. ———: An analysis of the more important orthopaedic information. Surgery, *16*:569-616, 1944.
807. Soule, A. B., Jr.: Ossification of the coracoclavicular ligament following dislocation of the acromioclavicular articulation. Amer. J. Roentgenol., *56*:607-615, 1946.
808. de Sousa, A., and Veiga, A.: Calcification of the coracoclavicular ligaments after acromioclavicular dislocation. J. Bone Joint Surg., *33B*:646, 1951.
809. Speed, K.: A Textbook of Fractures and Dislocations. ed. 4. Philadelphia, Lea & Febiger, 1942.
810. Spigelman, L.: A harness for acromioclavicular separation. J. Bone Joint Surg., *51A*:585-586, 1969.
811. Stephens, H. E. G.: Stuck nail fixation for acute dislocation of the acromioclavicular joint. J. Bone Joint Surg., *51B*:197, 1969.
812. Stewart, R.: Acute acromioclavicular joint dislocation. Minnesota Med., *29*:357-360, 1946.
813. Stubbins, S. G., and McGaw, W. H.: Suspension cast for acromioclavicular separation and clavicle fractures. J.A.M.A., *169*:672-675, 1959.
814. Thiemeyer, J. S.: A method of repair of symptomatic chronic acromioclavicular dislocation. Ann. Surg., *140*:75-85, 1954.
815. Thorndike, A.: Athletic Injuries. Philadelphia, Lea & Febiger, 1956.
816. Thorndike, A., Jr., and Quigley, T. B.: Injuries to the acromioclavicular joint. A

plea for conservative treatment. Amer. J. Surg., *55*:250-261, 1942.

817. Tossy, J. D., Mead, N. C., and Sigmond, H. M.: Acromioclavicular separations: useful and practical classification for treatment. Clin. Orthop., *28*:111-119, 1963.
818. Tourney, J. W.: Surgery of the acromioclavicular joint. Surg. Clin. N. Amer., *29*: 905-912, 1949.
819. Tristan, T. A., and Daughteridge, T. G.: Migration of a metallic pin from the humerus into the lung. New Eng. J. Med., *270*:987-989, 1964.
820. Trynin, A. H.: Conservative treatment for complete dislocation of the acromioclavicular joint. J. Bone Joint Surg., *16*:713-715, 1934.
821. Tucker, W. E., and Armstrong, J. R.: Injury in Sport. Springfield, Ill., Charles C Thomas, 1964.
822. Tyler, G. T.: Acromioclavicular dislocation fixed by a Vitallium screw through the joint. Amer. J. Surg., *58*:245-247, 1942.
823. Urist, M. R.: Complete dislocation of the acromioclavicular joint. The nature of the traumatic lesion and effective methods of treatment with an analysis of 41 cases. J. Bone Joint Surg., *28*:813-837, 1946.
824. ———: The treatment of dislocation of of the acromioclavicular joint. Amer. J. Surg., *98*:423-431, 1959.
825. ———: Complete dislocation of the acromioclavicular joint. J. Bone Joint Surg., *45A*:1750-1753, 1963.
826. Usadel, G.: Zur Behandlung der Luxatio claviculae supraacromialis. Arch. Klin. Chir., *200*:621-626, 1940.
827. Vargas, L.: Repair of complete acromioclavicular dislocation, utilizing the short head of the biceps. J. Bone Joint Surg., *24*:772-773, 1942.
828. Varney, J. H., Coker, J. K., and Cawley, J. J.: Treatment of acromioclavicular dislocation by means of a harness. J. Bone Joint Surg., *34A*:232-233, 1952.
829. Wagner, C.: Partial claviculectomy. Amer. J. Surg., *85*:259-265, 1953.
830. Wakeley, C. P. G.: Stabilization of the acromioclavicular joint. Lancet, *2*:708-710, 1935.
831. Warner, A. H.: A harness for use in the treatment of acromioclavicular separation. J. Bone Joint Surg., *19*:1132-1133, 1937.
832. Watkins, J. T.: An operation for the relief of acromioclavicular luxations. J. Bone Joint Surg., *7*:790-792, 1925.
833. Watson-Jones, R.: Fractures and Joint Injuries. ed. 4. vol. II. Baltimore, Williams & Wilkins, 1956.
834. Weaver, J. K., and Dunn, H. K.: Treatment of acromioclavicular injuries, especially complete acromioclavicular separation. J. Bone Joint Surg., *54A*:1187-1197, 1972.
835. Weitzman, G.: Treatment of acute acromioclavicular joint dislocation by a modified Bosworth method. J. Bone Joint Surg., *49A*:1167-1178, 1967.
836. Wertheimer, L. G.: Coracoclavicular joint. J. Bone Joint Surg., *30A*:570-578, 1948.
837. Wilson, P. D., and Cochrane, W. A.: Fractures and dislocations. Immediate management, after care, and convalescent treatment, with special reference to the conservation and restoration of function. Philadelphia, J. B. Lippincott, 1925.
838. Wolin, I.: Acute acromioclavicular dislocation. J. Bone Joint Surg., *26*:589-592, 1944.
839. Worchester, J. N., and Green, D. P.: Osteoarthritis of the acromioclavicular joint. Clin. Orthop., *58*:69-73, 1968.
840. Zanca, P.: Shoulder pain: involvement of the acromioclavicular joint. Analysis of 1,000 cases. Amer. J. Roentgenol., *112*: 493-506, 1971.
841. Zaricznyj, B.: Late reconstruction of the ligaments following acromioclavicular separation. [Unpublished paper].
842. Zimmerman, L. M., and Veith, I.: Great Ideas in the History of Surgery. Baltimore, Williams & Wilkins, 1961.

Dislocation of the Sternoclavicular Joint

843. Abbott, L. C., and Lucas, D. B.: The function of the clavicle; its surgical significance. Ann. Surg., *140*:583-599, 1954.
844. Allen, A. W.: Living suture grafts in the repair of fractures and dislocations. Arch. Surg., *16*:1007-1020, 1928.
845. Allman, F. L.: Fracture and ligamentous injuries of clavicle and its articulations. J. Bone Joint Surg., *49A*:774-784, 1967.
846. Anderson, M. E.: Treatment of dislocations of the acromioclavicular and sternoclavicular joints. J. Bone Joint Surg., *45A*: 657-658, 1963.
847. Bachmann, M.: Swelling of the sternoclavicular joint. Israel Med. J., *17*:65-72, 1958.
848. Baker, E. C.: Tomography of the sternoclavicular joint. Ohio State Med. J., *55*: 60, 1959.

849. Bancroft, F. W., and Murray, D. B.: Function of the clavicle. Ann. Surg., *140*:583-599, 1954.
850. Bankart, A. S.: An operation for recurrent dislocation (subluxation) of the sternoclavicular joint. Brit. J. Surg., *26*:320-323, 1938.
851. Bateman, J. E.: The Shoulder and Neck. Philadelphia, W. B. Saunders, 1972.
852. Bearn, J. G.: Direct observation on the function of the capsule of the sternoclavicular joint in clavicular support. J. Anat., *101*:159-170, 1967.
853. Beckman, T.: A case of simultaneous luxation of both ends of the clavicle. Acta Chir. Scand., *56*:156-163, 1923.
854. Berkhina, F. O.: Traumatic dislocations of clavicle, Orthop. Traumatol., *9*:11-26, 1935.
855. Bloom, F. A.: Wire fixation in acromioclavicular dislocation. J. Bone Joint Surg., *27*:273-276, 1945.
856. Bonnin, J. G.: Spontaneous subluxation of the sternoclavicular joint. Brit. Med. J., *2*:274-275, 1960.
857. Borowiecki, B., Charow, A., Cook, W., Rozycki, D., and Thaler, S.: An unusual football injury, posterior dislocation of the sternoclavicular joint. Arch. Otolaryngol., *95*:185-187, 1972.
858. Bremner, R. A.: Nonarticular, noninfective subacute arthritis of the sternoclavicular joint. J. Bone Joint Surg., *41B*:749-753, 1959.
859. Brooks, A. L., and Henning, G. D.: Injury to the proximal clavicular epiphysis. J. Bone Joint Surg., *54A*:1347-1348, 1972.
860. Brown, J. E.: Anterior sternoclavicular dislocation—a method of repair. Amer. J. Orthop., *31*:184-189, 1961.
861. Brown, R.: Backward and inward dislocation of the sternal end of the clavicle. Surg. Clin. N. Amer., *7*:1263, 1927.
862. Burrows, H. J.: Tenodesis of subclavius in the treatment of recurrent dislocation of the sternoclavicular joint. J. Bone Joint Surg., *33B*:240-243, 1951.
863. Butterworth, R. D., and Kirk, A. A.: Fracture dislocation of the sternoclavicular joint—case report. Virginia Med. Monthly, *79*:98-100, 1952.
864. Cave, A. J. E.: The nature and morphology of the costoclavicular ligament. J. Anat., *95*:170-179, 1961.
865. Cave, E. F.: Fractures and Other Injuries. Chicago Year Book Medical Publishers, 1958.
866. Clark, R. L., Milgram, J. W., and Yawn, D. H.: Fatal aortic perforation and cardiac tamponade due to a Kirschner wire migrating from the right sternoclavicular joint. South. Med. J., *67*:316-318, 1974.
867. Codman, E. A.: The Shoulder. Boston, T. Todd, 1934.
868. Collins, J. J.: Retrosternal dislocation of the clavicle. J. Bone Joint Surg., *54B*:203, 1972.
869. Conway, A. M.: Movements at the sternoclavicular and acromioclavicular joints. Phys. Ther. Rev., *41*:421-432, 1961.
870. Cooper, A.: A Treatise on Dislocations and Fractures of the Joints. 2nd Amer. ed. from the 6th London ed. Boston, Lilly & Wait and Carter & Hendee, 1832.
871. Denham, R. H., Jr., and Dingley, A. F., Jr.: Epiphyseal separation of the medial end of the clavicle. J. Bone Joint Surg., *49A*:1179-1183, 1967.
872. DePalma, A. F.: The role of the disks of the sternoclavicular and acromioclavicular joints. Clin. Orthop., *13*:222-233, 1959.
873. ———: Surgical anatomy of acromioclavicular and sternoclavicular joints. Surg. Clin. N. Amer., *43*:1541-1550, 1963.
874. ———: Surgery of the Shoulder. ed. 2. Philadelphia, J. B. Lippincott, 1973.
875. Duggan, N.: Recurrent dislocation of sternoclavicular cartilage. J. Bone Joint Surg., *13*:365, 1931.
876. Elting, J. J.: Retrosternal dislocation of the clavicle. Arch. Surg., *104*:35-37, 1972.
877. Ferry, A., Rook, F. W., and Masterson, J. H.: Retrosternal dislocation of the clavicle. J. Bone Joint Surg., *39A*:905-910, 1957.
878. Fisk, G. H.: Motion at the shoulder joint. Can. Med. Ass. J., *50*:213-216, 1944.
879. Fitchet, S. M.: Cleidocranial dysostosis; hereditary and familial. J. Bone Joint Surg., *11*:838-866, 1929.
880. Glickman, L. G., and Minsky, A. A.: "Case reports"—enlargement of one sternoclavicular articulation: a sign of congenital syphilis. Radiology, *28*:85-86, 1937.
881. Gorman, J. B., Stone, R. T., and Keats, T. E.: Changes in the sternoclavicular joint following radical neck dissection. Amer. J. Roentgenol., *111*:584-587, 1971.
882. Grant, J. C. B.: Method of Anatomy. ed. 7. Baltimore, Williams & Wilkins, 1965.
883. Gray's Anatomy: ed. 35. (British) Edited by Warwick, R. & Williams, P. L. Philadelphia, W. B. Saunders, 1973.
884. Greenlee, D. P.: Posterior dislocation of

the sternal end of the clavicle. J. Bone Joint Surg., *39A*:905, 1944.

885. ———: Posterior dislocation of the sternal end of the clavicle. J.A.M.A., *125*:426-428, 1944.

886. Gunson, E. F.: Radiography of sterno-clavicular articulation. Radiog. & Clin. Photog., *19*:20-24, 1943.

887. Gunther, W. A.: Posterior dislocation of the sternoclavicular joint. J. Bone Joint Surg., *31A*:878-879, 1949.

888. Gurd, F. B.: Surplus parts of skeleton; recommendation for excision of certain portions as means of shortening period of disability following trauma. Amer. J. Surg., *74*:705-720, 1947.

889. Haas, S. L.: The experimental transplantation of the epiphysis. J.A.M.A., *65*: 1965-1971, 1915.

890. Heinig, C. F.: Retrosternal dislocation of the clavicle: early recognition, x-ray diagnosis, and management. J. Bone Joint Surg., *50A*:830, 1968.

891. Hobbs, D. W.: Sternoclavicular joint: a new axial radiographic view. Radiology, *90*:801-802, 1968.

892. Hollinshead, W. H.: Pectoral region, axilla, and shoulder. Anat. for Surgeons, *3*:265-268, 1958.

893. Holmdahl, H. C.: A case of posterior sternoclavicular dislocation. Acta Orthop. Scand., *23*:218-222, 1953-54.

894. Hotchkiss, L. W.: Double dislocation of the sternal end of the clavicle. Ann. Surg., *23*:600, 1896.

895. Howard, F. M., and Shafer, S. J.: Injuries to the clavicle with neurovascular complications. J. Bone Joint Surg., *47A*:1335-1346, 1965.

896. Howard, N. J.: Acromioclavicular and sternoclavicular joint injuries. Amer. J. Surg., *46*:284-291, 1939.

897. Hoyt, W. A.: Etiology of shoulder injuries in athletes. J. Bone Joint Surg., *49A*:755-766, 1967.

898. Inman, V. T., Saunders, J. B., and Abbott, L. C.: Observations on shoulder joint. J. Bone Joint Surg., *26*:1-30, 1944.

899. Jones, R.: Injuries of Joints. ed. 2. London, Oxford University Press, 1917.

900. Kallimoaki, J. L., Vitanen, S. M., and Virtama, P.: Radiological findings of sternoclavicular joints in rheumatoid arthritis. Acta Rheum. Scand., *14*:233-240, 1969.

901. Kattan, K. R.: Modified view for use in roentgen examination of the sternoclavicular joints. Radiology, *108*:8, 1973.

902. Kennedy, J. C.: Retrosternal dislocation of the clavicle. J. Bone Joint Surg., *31A*: 74-75, 1949.

903. Key, J. A., and Conwell, H. E.: The Management of Fractures, Dislocations and Sprains. ed. 5. St. Louis, C. V. Mosby, 1951.

904. King, J. M., Jr., and Holmes, G. W.: Review of 450 roentgen ray examination of shoulder. Amer. J. Roentgenol., *17*:214-218, 1927.

905. Kurzbauer, R.: The lateral projection in roentgenography of the sternoclavicular articulation. Amer. J. Roentgenol., *56*: 104-105, 1946.

906. Lee, H. M.: Sternoclavicular dislocations. Trans. Minneapolis Surg. Soc., *20*:480-482, 1937.

907. Leonard, J. W., and Gifford, R. W.: Migration of a Kirschner wire from the clavicle into pulmonary artery. Amer. J. Cardiol., *16*:598-600, 1965.

908. Lowman, C. L.: Operative correction of old sternoclavicular dislocation. J. Bone Joint Surg., *10*:740-741, 1928.

909. Lucas, D. B.: Biomechanics of the shoulder joint. Arch. Surg., *107*:425-432, 1973.

910. Lucas, G. L.: Retrosternal dislocation of the clavicle. J.A.M.A., *193*:850-853, 1965.

911. Lunseth, P., Chapman, K., and Frankel, V.: Surgical treatment for chronic dislocation of the sternoclavicular joint. [Unpublished paper].

912. McCaughan, J. S., and Miller, P. R.: Migration of Steinmann pin from shoulder to lung. J.A.M.A., *207*:1917, 1969.

913. McKenzie, J. M. M.: Retrosternal dislocation of the clavicle. A report of two cases. J. Bone Joint Surg., *45B*:138-141, 1963.

914. McLaughlin, H.: Trauma. Philadelphia, W. B. Saunders, 1959.

915. Mehta, J. C., Sachdev, A., and Collins, J. J.: Retrosternal dislocation of the clavicle. Injury, *5*:79-83, 1973.

916. Milch, H.: The rhomboid ligament in surgery of the sternoclavicular joint. J. Internat. Coll. Surg., *17*:41-51, 1952.

917. Mitchell, W. J., and Cobey, M. C.: Retrosternal dislocation of clavicle. Med. Ann. D. C., *29*:546-549, 1960.

918. Moseley, H. F.: Athletic injuries to the shoulder region. Amer. J. Surg., *98*:401-422, 1959.

919. Mouchet, A.: Luxation sternoclavicular avant; reduction sanglante. Rev. Orthop., *28*:99-100, 1942.

920. Nettles, J. L., and Linscheid, R.: Sterno-

clavicular dislocations. J. Trauma, *8*:158-164, 1968.

921. O'Donoghue, D. H.: Treatment of Injuries to Athletes. ed. 2. Philadelphia, W. B. Saunders, 1970.

922. Omer, G. E.: Osteotomy of the clavicle in surgical reduction of anterior sternoclavicular dislocation. J. Trauma, *7*:584-590, 1967.

923. Pate, J. W., and Wilhite, J.: Migration of a foreign body from the sternoclavicular joint to the heart—a case report. Amer. Surg., *35*:448-449, 1969.

924. Paterson, D. C.: Retrosternal dislocation of the clavicle. J. Bone Joint Surg., *43B*: 90-92, 1961.

925. Peacock, H. K., Brandon, J. R., and Jones, O. L.: Retrosternal dislocation of the clavicle. South. Med. J., *63*:1324-1328, 1970.

926. Pendergrass, E. P., and Hodes, P. J.: Rhomboid fossa of the clavicle. Amer. J. Roentgenol., *38*:152-155, 1937.

927. Poland, J.: Separation of the epiphyses of the clavicle. *In* Traumatic Separation of Epiphyses of the Upper Extremity. London, Smith, Elder, and Co., 1898.

928. Pridie, K.: Dislocation of acromioclavicular and sternoclavicular joints. J. Bone Joint Surg., *41B*:429, 1959.

929. Quigley, T. B.: Injuries to the acromioclavicular and sternoclavicular joints sustained in athletics. Surg. Clin. N. Amer., *43*:1551-1554, 1963.

930. Rice, E. E.: Habitual dislocation of the sternoclavicular articulation—a case report. Oklahoma State Med. J., *25*:34-35, 1932.

931. Ritvo, M., and Ritvo, M.: Roentgen study of the sternoclavicular region. Amer. J. Roentgen. Ther., *53*:644-650, 1947.

932. Rodrigues, H.: Case of dislocation inwards of the internal extremity of the clavicle. Lancet, *1*:309-310, 1843.

933. Salvatore, J.: Sternoclavicular joint dislocation. Clin. Orthop., *58*:51-55, 1968.

934. Silberberg, M., Frank, E. L., Jarrett, S. R., and Silberberg, R.: Aging and osteoarthritis of the human sternoclavicular joint. Amer. J. Pathol., *35*:851-865, 1959.

935. Simurda, M. A.: Retrosternal dislocation of the clavicle. A report of 4 cases and a method of repair. Can. J. Surg., *11*:487-490, 1968.

936. Snyder, C. C., Levine, G. A., and Dingman, D. L.: Trial of a sternoclavicular whole joint graft as a substitute for the temporomandibular joint. Plast. Reconstr. Surg., *48*:447-452, 1971.

937. Speed, K.: A Textbook of Fractures and Dislocations. ed. 4. Philadelphia, Lea & Febiger, 1942.

938. Stankler, L.: Posterior dislocation of clavicle. Brit. J. Surg., *50*:164-168, 1962.

939. Stein, A. H.: Retrosternal dislocation of the clavicle. J. Bone Joint Surg., *39A*:656-660, 1957.

940. Turek, S. L.: Orthopaedics. ed. 2. Philadelphia, J. B. Lippincott, 1967.

941. Tyler, H. D. D., Sturrock, W. D. S., and Callow, F. M.: Retrosternal dislocation of the clavicle. J. Bone Joint Surg., *45B*:132-137, 1963.

942. Waskowitz, W. J.: Disruption of the sternoclavicular joint an analysis and review. Amer. J. Orthop., June:176-179, 1961.

943. Watson-Jones, R.: Fractures and Joint Injuries. ed. 4. vol. 2. Baltimore, Williams & Wilkins, 1956.

944. Williams, H. H.: Oblique views of the clavicle. Radiog. and Clin. Photog., *5*:191-194, 1929.

945. Worman, L. W., and Leagus, C.: Intrathoracic injury following retrosternal dislocation of the clavicle. J. Trauma, *7*:416-423, 1967.

Author Index

Vol. 1: pp. 1-816; vol. 2: pp. 817-1495.

Numbers in *italics* indicate mention in a reference. Numbers in Roman type indicate mention in the text.

B

D

E

F

I

J

M

N

S

U

Y

Z

Subject Index

Vol. 1: pp. 1-816; Vol. 2: pp. 817-1495.

Numerals in italics indicate a figure, "t" following a page number indicates a table.

A

B

C

D

I

J

K

O

Q

R

S

T